Pediatric Primary Care

A Problem-Oriented Approach

THIRD EDITION

Editor-in-Chief
M. William Schwartz, MD
Associate Dean Primary Care Education
Professor of Pediatrics, University of Pennsylvania School
of Medicine, The Children's Hospital of Philadelphia,
Philadelphia, Pennsylvania

Associate Editors
Thomas A. Curry, MD
Associate in General Pediatrics, Geisinger Medical Group—Pottsville,
Pottsville, Pennsylvania

A. John Sargent, MD
Associate Professor of Psychiatry and Pediatrics, University of
Pennsylvania School of Medicine, Director, General, Child, and
Adolescent Psychiatry, Philadelphia Child Guidance Center,
Philadelphia, Pennsylvania

Nathan J. Blum, MD
Assistant Professor of Pediatrics, University of Pennsylvania School
of Medicine, Children's Seashore House, Philadelphia, Pennsylvania

Joel A. Fein, MD
Assistant Professor of Pediatrics, University of Pennsylvania School
of Medicine, The Children's Hospital of Philadelphia, Philadelphia,
Pennsylvania

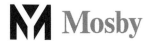

St. Louis Baltimore Boston Carlsbad Chicago Naples New York Philadelphia Portland
London Madrid Mexico City Singapore Sydney Tokyo Toronto Wiesbaden

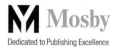

Mosby

Dedicated to Publishing Excellence

**A Times Mirror
Company**

Vice President and Publisher, Medicine: Anne S. Patterson
Editor: Laura De Young
Associate Developmental Editor: Jennifer Byington Geistler
Project Manager: Chris Baumle
Production Editor: Michelle R. Fitzgerald & Anthony Trioli
Design Manager: Nancy J. McDonald
Manufacturing Supervisor: William A. Winneberger, Jr.

Third Edition
Copyright © 1997 by Mosby–Year Book, Inc.

Previous editions copyrighted 1987, 1990

Printed in the United States of America
Composition by Graphic World
Printing/binding by Maple Vail Book Manufacturing Group

Mosby–Year Book, Inc.
11830 Westline Industrial Drive
St. Louis, Missouri 63146

Library of Congress Cataloging-in-Publication Data

Pediatric primary care : a problem-oriented approach / editor-in
  -chief, M. William Schwartz ; associate editors, Thomas A. Curry . . .
  [et al.]. — 3rd ed.
        p.   cm.
    Includes bibliographical references and index.
    ISBN 0-8151-8054-3
    1. Pediatrics.   2. Primary care (Medicine)   I. Schwartz, M.
  William, 1935-
    [DNLM: 1. Pediatrics.   2. Primary Health Care—methods.   WS
  100P957   1996]
  RJ47.P39   1996
  618.92—dc21
  DNLM/DLC
    for Library of Congress   96-53905
  98 99 00 01 / 9 8 7 6 5 4 3 2   CIP

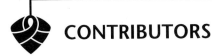

CONTRIBUTORS

James L. Ackerman, DDS
Senior Dentist, The Children's Hospital of
Philadelphia, Philadelphia, Pennsylvania

Evaline A. Alessandrini, MD
Assistant Professor of Pediatrics, University of
Pennsylvania School of Medicine, The Children's
Hospital of Philadelphia, Philadelphia, Pennsylvania

Herbert B. Allen, MD
Clinical Associate Professor, Department of
Dermatology, University Affiliate

Steven M. Altschuler, MD
Associate Professor and Acting Chairman,
Department of Pediatrics, Division Chief, Division
of Gastroenterology and Nutrition, University of
Pennsylvania School of Medicine, Philadelphia,
Pennsylvania

Robert Anolik, MD
President, Allergy and Asthma Specialists, PC
Clinical Assistant Professor, University of
Pennsylvania School of Medicine, Clinical Affiliate,
The Children's Hospital of Philadelphia,
Philadelphia, Pennsylvania

Laurie Robbins Appelbaum, MD
Medical Director, Community Programs Division,
Child Guidance Center, The Children's Hospital of
Philadelphia, Philadelphia, Pennsylvania

Linda Arnold
Fellow in Gastroenterology, The Children's Hospital
of Philadelphia, Philadelphia, Pennsylvania

Balu H. Athreya, MD
Professor of Pediatrics, Director, Pediatric
Rheumatology Center, A. I. DuPont Children's
Hospital, Wilmington, Delaware

Jeffrey R. Avner, MD
Associate Professor of Pediatrics, Albert Einstein
College of Medicine, Associate Director, Pediatric
Emergency Service, Jacobi Medical Center Bronx,
New York

Robert N. Baldassano, MD
Assistant Professor of Pediatrics, University
of Pennsylvania School of Medicine, Pediatric
Gastroenterologist, The Children's Hospital of
Philadelphia, Philadelphia, Pennsylvania

Marleen Ann Baron, MA, CCC/SLP
Acting Director, Department of Speech-Language,
Pathology, Children's Seashore House, Philadelphia,
Pennsylvania

Louis M. Bell, MD
Associate Professor of Pediatrics, University of
Pennsylvania School of Medicine, Attending

Physician, Sections of Emergency Medicine and
Infectious Diseases, The Children's Hospital of
Philadelphia, Philadelphia, Pennsylvania

Henry G. Berger, PhD
Clinical Associate Professor, University of
Pennsylvania School of Medicine, Staff,
Pennsylvania Hospital, Philadelphia, Pennsylvania

Judy C. Bernbaum, MD
Associate Professor of Pediatrics, University of
Pennsylvania School of Medicine, Director, Neonatal
Follow-Up Program, The Children's Hospital of
Philadelphia, Philadelphia, Pennsylvania

Nathan J. Blum
Assistant Professor of Pediatrics, University of
Pennsylvania School of Medicine, Children's
Seashore House, Philadelphia, Pennsylvania

John T. Boyle, MD
Professor of Pediatrics, Case Western Reserve School
of Medicine, Cleveland, Ohio

Lawrence W. Brown
Assistant Professor of Pediatrics, University of
Pennsylvania School of Medicine, Division of
Neurology, The Children's Hospital of Philadelphia,
Philadelphia, Pennsylvania

Deborah Calvert
Social Worker, Neonatal Follow-up Program, The
Children's Hospital of Philadelphia, Philadelphia,
Pennsylvania

William B. Carey, MD
Clinical Professor of Pediatrics, University of
Pennsylvania School of Medicine, Director, Section
on Behavioral Pediatrics, The Children's Hospital of
Philadelphia, Philadelphia, Pennsylvania

Carol Carraccio, MD
Associate Professor of Pediatrics, Director, Resident
Education, University of Maryland, Baltimore,
Maryland

Rosemary Casey, MD
Assistant Professor of Pediatrics, University of
Pennsylvania School of Medicine, General Pediatric
Faculty Practice, The Children's Hospital of
Philadelphia, Philadelphia, Pennsylvania

Anthony C. Chang, MD
Fellow, Pediatric Cardiology, The Children's Hospital
of Philadelphia, Philadelphia, Pennsylvania

Edward B. Charney, MD (deceased)
Professor of Pediatrics, University of Pennsylvania
School of Medicine, The Children's Hospital of
Philadelphia, Philadelphia, Pennsylvania

Kwaku Chene-Frempong
Professor of Pediatrics, Associate Director, Sickle Cell Center, University of Pennsylvania School of Medicine, The Children's Hospital of Philadelphia, Philadelphia, Pennsylvania

Cindy W. Christian, MD
Assistant Professor of Pediatrics, University of Pennsylvania School of Medicine, The Children's Hospital of Philadelphia, Medical Director, Child Abuse Program, The Children's Hospital of Philadelphia, Philadelphia, Pennsylvania

Robert Ryan Clancy, MD
Professor of Neurology and Pediatrics, University of Pennsylvania School of Medicine, Senior Neurologist, The Children's Hospital of Philadelphia, Philadelphia, Pennsylvania

Bernard J. Clark III, MD
Associate Professor of Pediatrics, University of Pennsylvania School of Medicine, Senior Cardiologist, The Children's Hospital of Philadelphia, Philadelphia, Pennsylvania

Liana R. Clark, MD
Clinical Assistant Professor of Pediatrics, The Children's Hospital of Philadelphia, Philadelphia, Pennsylvania

Paulo Ferrez Collett-Solberg, MD
Department of Endocrinology and Diabetes, Pediatric Endocrinology Fellow, The Children's Hospital of Philadelphia, Philadelphia, Pennsylvania

Mary Ellen Conley, MD
Professor of Pediatrics, Department of Immunology, St. Jude Children's Research Hospital, Memphis, Tennessee

Joseph A. Cox, MD
Assistant Professor of Surgery, University of Cincinnati School of Medicine, Cincinnati Children's Hospital, Cincinnati, Ohio

James E. Crawford, MD
Fellow, Child Abuse and Neglect/General Pediatrics, Department of General Pediatrics, The Children's Hospital of Philadelphia, Philadelphia, Pennsylvania

Robert S. Cummings, MD
Resident, Orthopedic Surgery, Allegheny University Health Systems, Philadelphia, Pennsylvania

Thomas A. Curry, MD
Associate in General Pediatrics, Geisinger Medical Group—Pottsville, Pottsville, Pennsylvania

JoAnn D'Agostino, RN
Nurse Coordinator, Neonatal Follow-up Program, The Children's Hospital of Philadelphia, Philadelphia, Pennsylvania

Anna-Maria DaCosta, MD
Clinical Assistant Professor, University of Pennsylvania School of Medicine, Children's Seashore House, Philadelphia, Pennsylvania

Gary R. Diamond, MD
Associate Professor of Ophthalmology, Allegheny University Health Systems, Philadelphia, Pennsylvania

Janet Etzi, MD
Associate Professor, Immaculata University, Bryn Mawr, Pennsylvania

Deborah L. Eunpu, MS, CGC
Director, Genetic Counseling Training Program, Beaver College, Glenside, Pennsylvania, Therapist, Penn Council for Relationships, Philadelphia, Pennsylvania

Maureen A. Fee, MD
Associate Professor of Pediatrics, Developmental and Behavioral Pediatrics, St. Christopher's Hospital, Philadelphia, Pennsylvania

Joel A. Fein, MD
Assistant Professor of Pediatrics, University of Pennsylvania School of Medicine, The Children's Hospital of Philadelphia, Philadelphia, Pennsylvania

John W. Foreman, MD
Professor of Pediatrics, Chief, Division of Pediatric Nephrology, Department of Pediatrics, Duke University Medical Center, Durham, North Carolina

Sidney Friedman, AB, MD
Professor of Pediatrics Emeritus, University of Pennsylvania School of Medicine, Senior Cardiologist, Division of Cardiology, The Children's Hospital of Philadelphia, Philadelphia, Pennsylvania

Susan Friedman, MD
Clinical Assistant Professor of Pediatrics, University of Pennsylvania School of Medicine, The Children's Hospital of Philadelphia, Philadelphia, Pennsylvania

Marsha Gerdes
Developmental Psychologist, Neonatal Follow-up Program, The Children's Hospital of Philadelphia, Philadelphia, Pennsylvania

William Gianfagna, MD
General Pediatrics, Geisenger Medical Center, Danville, Pennsylvania

Gail L. Ginder, MA, MSPH
Consultant to Health Profession, Healdsburg, California

Kenneth R. Ginsburg, MD, MSEd
Assistant Professor of Pediatrics, University of Pennsylvania School of Medicine, Assistant Professor of Pediatrics, The Children's Hospital of Philadelphia, Philadelphia, Pennsylvania

Marie M. Gleason, MD
Clinical Associate Professor of Pediatrics, University of Pennsylvania School of Medicine, Director, Outpatient and Community Cardiology, The Children's Hospital of Philadelphia, Philadelphia, Pennsylvania

Marc Gorelick, MD
Assistant Professor of Pediatrics, Emergency
Medicine, University of Pennsylvania School of
Medicine, The Children's Hospital of Philadelphia,
Philadelphia, Pennsylvania

Ernest M. Graham, MD
Assistant Professor, Obstetrics-Gynecology,
University of Pennsylvania School of Medicine,
Philadelphia, Pennsylvania

Lawrence D. Hammer, MD
Associate Professor, General Pediatrics, Stanford
University, Stanford, California

Mark L. Helpin, DMD
Associate Professor of Dentistry, University of
Pennsylvania School of Dental Medicine, Director,
Pediatric Dental Medicine, The Children's Hospital
of Philadelphia, Philadelphia, Pennsylvania

Richard W. Hertle, MD
Assistant Professor of Ophthalmology, University of
Pennsylvania School of Medicine, Attending Staff,
The Children's Hospital of Philadelphia, Director,
Adult Ocular Motility Service, The Scheie Eye
Institute, Philadelphia, Pennsylvania

Bradley R. Hoch, MD
Private Practice, Gettysburg, Pennsylvania

Gordon R. Hodas, MD
Clinical Associate Professor of Psychiatry, University
of Pennsylvania School of Medicine, Consultant
Psychiatrist, Child Guidance Center, Children's
Hospital of Philadelphia, Philadelphia, Pennsylvania

Dee Hodge III, MD
Assistant Clinical Professor of Pediatrics, University
of California School of Medicine, San Francisco,
California, Director, Emergency Department,
Children's Hospital, Oakland, Oakland, California

Paul J. Honig, MD
Professor of Pediatrics, Director, Pediatric
Dermatology, University of Pennsylvania School of
Medicine, The Children's Hospital of Philadelphia,
Philadelphia, Pennsylvania

Kelly A. Kane, DO
Department of Pediatrics, Doctor's Hospital,
Columbus, Ohio

Bernadette Kappen
Director, Overbrook School for the Blind,
Philadelphia, Pennsylvania

Gregory F. Keenan, MD
Assistant Professor of Medicine and Pediatrics,
Department of Rheumatology, University of
Pennsylvania School of Medicine, Philadelphia,
Pennsylvania

Thomas L. Kennedy III, MD
Clinical Professor of Pediatrics, Yale School of
Medicine, Department of Pediatrics, Bridgeport
Hospital, Bridgeport, Connecticut

Janice Key
Associate Professor of Pediatrics, Medical University
of South Carolina, Director of Adolescent
Development, Charleston, South Carolina

Brent R. King, MD
Assistant Professor of Emergency Medicine and
Pediatrics, Director, Division of Pediatric Emergency
Medicine, The Medical College of Pennsylvania,
Philadelphia, Pennsylvania

Richard M. Kravitz, MD
Assistant Professor, Department of Pediatrics,
University of Pennsylvania School of Medicine,
Director, Asthma Care Program, Attending
Pulmonologist, The Children's Hospital of
Philadelphia, Philadelphia, Pennsylvania

Stephen D. Kronwith, MD, PhD
Assistant Clinical Professor, Department of
Ophthalmology and Visual Sciences, Albert Einstein
College of Medicine, Bronx, New York

Beverly Lange, MD
Professor of Pediatrics, Department of Pediatrics,
University of Pennsylvania School of Medicine,
Philadelphia, Pennsylvania

Craig D. Lapin, MD
Assistant Professor of Pediatrics, Pediatric Pulmonary
Division, Connecticut Children's Medical Center,
University of Connecticut School of Medicine,
Hartford, Connecticut

Don LaRossa, MD, FAAP, FACS
Professor of Surgery (Plastic), University of
Pennsylvania School of Medicine, Director, Cleft Lip
and Palate Program, The Children's Hospital of
Philadelphia, Philadelphia, Pennsylvania

Mary Min-chin Lee, MD
Assistant Professor of Pediatrics, Pediatric Endocrine
Unit, Department of Pediatrics, Massachusetts
General Hospital, Harvard Medical School, Boston,
Massachusetts

Mary B. Leonard, MD
Instructor of Pediatrics, University of Pennsylvania
School of Medicine, The Children's Hospital of
Philadelphia, Philadelphia, Pennsylvania

Lorraine E. Levitt Katz, MD
Assistant Professor of Pediatrics, University of
Pennsylvania School of Medicine, The Children's
Hospital of Philadelphia, Philadelphia, Pennsylvania

Susan E. Levy, MD
Clinical Associate Professor of Pediatrics, University
of Pennsylvania School of Medicine, Clinical
Attending, Children's Seashore House, Philadelphia,
Pennsylvania

John Loiselle, MD
Assistant Professor of Pediatric Emergency Medicine,
The Medical College of Pennsylvania, St.
Christopher's Hospital for Children, Philadelphia,
Pennsylvania

William J. Malone, MD
Associate, Department of Pediatrics, Geisinger
Medical Center, Danville, Pennsylvania

Catherine Manno, MD
Associate Professor of Pediatrics, University of
Pennsylvania School of Medicine, The Children's
Hospital of Philadelphia, Philadelphia, Pennsylvania

Maria R. Mascarenhas, MBBS
Assistant Professor of Pediatrics, University of
Pennsylvania School of Medicine, Director, Nutrition
Support Service, The Children's Hospital of
Philadelphia, Philadelphia, Pennsylvania

Joyce Elizabeth Mauk, MD
Assistant Professor of Pediatrics, University of
Pennsylvania School of Medicine, Co-Director,
Biobehavioral Program, Children's Seashore House,
Philadelphia, Pennsylvania

Beth Leonberg McCoy, MS, MA, RD, CS, CNSD
Director, Department of Clinical Nutrition, The
Children's Hospital of Philadelphia, Philadelphia,
Pennsylvania

Steven E. McKenzie, MD, PhD
Associate Professor of Pediatrics, Thomas Jefferson
University, Philadelphia, Pennsylvania, A. I. DuPont
Children's Hospital, Wilmington, Delaware

Marianne Mercugliano, MD
Assistant Professor of Pediatrics, University of
Pennsylvania School of Medicine, Co-Director,
Attention Deficit Hyperactivity Disorder Evaluation
and Treatment Program, Children's Seashore House,
Philadelphia, Pennsylvania

Linda J. Michaud, MD
Associate Professor of Clinical Surgical Medicine and
Rehabilitation and Clinical Pediatrics, University of
Cincinnati Medical Center, Director, Division of
Pediatric Rehabilitation, Children's Hospital Medical
Center, Cincinnati, Ohio

Karen Miller, MD
Clinical Instructor in Pediatrics, University of
Maryland, Baltimore, Maryland

Thomas Moshang, Jr., MD
Professor of Pediatrics, University of Pennsylvania
School of Medicine, Division Chief, Division of
Pediatric Endocrinology/Diabetes, The Children's
Hospital of Philadelphia, Philadelphia, Pennsylvania

Michael N. Needle, MD
Assistant Professor of Pediatrics, The University
of Pennsylvania School of Medicine, Attending
Physician, The Children's Hospital of Philadelphia,
Philadelphia, Pennsylvania

Michael E. Norman, MD
Clinical Professor, Department of Pediatrics,
University of North Carolina School of Medicine,
Chairman of Pediatrics, Carolinas Medical Center,
Charlotte, North Carolina

Jerrold S. Olshan, MD
Senior Fellow, Division of Pediatric Endocrinology,
University of Pennsylvania School of Medicine,
Senior Endocrinology Fellow, The Children's
Hospital of Philadelphia, Philadelphia, Pennsylvania

Lee M. Pachter, DO
Associate Professor of Pediatrics and Anthropology,
University of Connecticut School of Medicine, St.
Francis Hospital and Medical Center, Hartford,
Connecticut

Roger J. Packer, MD
Chairman of Neurology, Children's National Medical
Center, Professor of Neurology and Pediatrics, The
George Washington University, Clinical Professor of
Neurology, Georgetown University, Washington, DC

Louis Pellegrino, MD
Assistant Professor of Pediatrics, University of
Pennsylvania School of Medicine, Attending
Physician, The Children's Hospital of Philadelphia,
Children's Seashore House, Philadelphia,
Pennsylvania

David A. Piccoli, MD
Associate Professor of Pediatrics, University
of Pennsylvania School of Medicine, Director,
Gastroenterology Division, The Children's Hospital
of Philadelphia, Philadelphia, Pennsylvania

Richard Polin, MD
Professor of Pediatrics, University of Pennsylvania
School of Medicine, The Children's Hospital of
Philadelphia, Philadelphia, Pennsylvania

Mortimer Poncz, MD
Professor of Pediatrics, Division of Hematology, The
Children's Hospital of Philadelphia, Philadelphia,
Pennsylvania

William P. Potsic, MD
Professor, Department of Otorhinolaryngology: Head
and Neck Surgery, University of Pennsylvania School
of Medicine, Director, Pediatric Otolaryngology and
Human Communication, The Children's Hospital of
Philadelphia, Philadelphia, Pennsylvania

Graham E. Quinn, MD
Associate Professor of Ophthalmology, The
Children's Hospital of Philadelphia, University
of Pennsylvania School of Medicine, Scheie Eye
Institute, Philadelphia, Pennsylvania

R. Beverly Raney, Jr., MD
Professor of Pediatrics, University of Texas Health
Sciences Center at Houston, Chief, Non-Neural Solid
Tumor Section, Department of Pediatrics UTMD,
Anderson Cancer Center, Houston, Texas

Anthony L. Rostain, MD
Associate Professor of Psychiatry and Pediatrics,
University of Pennsylvania School of Medicine,
Philadelphia Child Guidance Center, Philadelphia,
Pennsylvania

Richard M. Rutstein, MD
Assistant Professor of Pediatrics, University of
Pennsylvania School of Medicine, Medical Director,
Special Immunology Service, The Children's Hospital
of Philadelphia, Philadelphia, Pennsylvania

Michael E. Ryan, DO
Geisinger Medical Center, Danville, Pennsylvania

Joseph W. St. Geme, III, MD
Assistant Professor of Pediatrics and Molecular
Microbiology, Washington University School of
Medicine, Attending in Pediatrics and Pediatric
Infectious Diseases, St. Louis Children's Hospital,
St. Louis, Missouri

A. John Sargent, MD
Associate Professor of Psychiatry and Pediatrics,
University of Pennsylvania School of Medicine,
Director, General, Child, and Adolescent Psychiatry,
Philadelphia Child Guidance Center, Philadelphia,
Pennsylvania

Marta Satin-Smith, MD
Assistant Professor of Pediatrics, East Virginia School
of Medicine, Kings Daughter Hospital, Norfolk,
Virginia

Thomas F. Scanlin, MD
Professor of Pediatrics, University of Pennsylvania
School of Medicine, Director, Cystic Fibrosis Center,
The Children's Hospital of Philadelphia,
Philadelphia, Pennsylvania

David B. Schaffer, MD
Professor, Department of Ophthalmology, University
of Pennsylvania School of Medicine, Chairman,
Division of Ophthalmology, The Children's Hospital
of Philadelphia, Philadelphia, Pennsylvania

Craig M. Schramm, MD
Associate Professor of Pediatrics, Pediatric
Pulmonary Division, Connecticut Children's
Medical Center, University of Connecticut
School of Medicine, Hartford, Connecticut

M. William Schwartz, MD
Professor of Pediatrics, University of Pennsylvania
School of Medicine, The Children's Hospital of
Philadelphia, Philadelphia, Pennsylvania

Donald F. Schwarz, MD, MPH
Associate Professor of Pediatrics, University
of Pennsylvania School of Medicine, Director,
Adolescent Clinic, Acting Director of General
Pediatrics, Philadelphia, Pennsylvania

Steven M. Schwarz, MD
Professor of Pediatrics, State University of New York
Health Science Center, Chairman, Department of
Pediatrics, Long Island College Hospital, Brooklyn,
New York

Toni Seidl, RN, ACSW, LSW
Clinical Associate, University of Pennsylvania School
of Medicine, Social Work Supervisor, The Children's
Hospital of Philadelphia, Philadelphia, Pennsylvania

Steven M. Selbst, MD
Associate Professor of Pediatrics, University of
Pennsylvania School of Medicine, Emergency
Department, The Children's Hospital of Philadelphia,
Philadelphia, Pennsylvania

Kathryn Sexton, MD
Private Practice, Pediatrics, Greenbrae, California

Kathy N. Shaw, MD, MS
Assistant Professor of Pediatrics, University of
Pennsylvania School of Medicine, Attending
Physician, Emergency Department, The Children's
Hospital of Philadelphia, Philadelphia, Pennsylvania

Henry H. Sherk, MD
Professor of Orthopedic Surgery, Allegheny
University Health Systems, Philadelphia,
Pennsylvania

Gail B. Slap, MD, MSc
Director, Adolescent Medicine, Associate Professor of
Medicine and Pediatrics, University of Pennsylvania
School of Medicine, The Children's Hospital of
Philadelphia, Philadelphia, Pennsylvania

Kim Smith-Whitley, MD
Assistant Professor of Pediatrics, University of
Pennsylvania School of Medicine, Sickle Cell Center,
The Children's Hospital of Philadelphia,
Philadelphia, Pennsylvania

Howard M. Snyder III, MD
Professor of Urology in Surgery, University of
Pennsylvania School of Medicine, Associate Director,
Division of Pediatric Urology, The Children's
Hospital of Philadelphia, Philadelphia, Pennsylvania

Philip R. Spandorfer
Pediatric Resident, The Children's Hospital
of Philadelphia, Philadelphia, Pennsylvania

Steven D. Spandorfer, MD
Fellow in Obstetrics, Cornell Medical Center,
New York

Charles A. Stanley, MD
Professor of Pediatrics, University of Pennsylvania
School of Medicine, Senior Endocrinologist,
Assistant Director, CRC, The Children's Hospital
of Philadelphia, Philadelphia, Pennsylvania

Annie G. Steinberg, MD
Assistant Professor, Department of Psychiatry,
University of Pennsylvania School of Medicine,
Director of Psychiatry, Children's Seashore House,
Director, Deafness and Family Communication
Center, Philadelphia, Pennsylvania

William Tarry, MD
Associate Professor, Urology and Pediatrics, West
Virginia University Health Sciences Center,
Morgantown, West Virginia

Bruce Taubman, MD
Clinical Associate Professor, Department of Pediatrics
Division of Gastroenterology, University of
Pennsylvania School of Medicine, Philadelphia,
Pennsylvania

Fred W. Tecklenburg, MD
Associate Professor of Pediatrics, Medical University
of South Carolina, Director, Division of Critical Care,
Department of Pediatrics, Medical University of
South Carolina, Charleston, South Carolina

Jonathan E. Teitelbaum, MD
Division of Pediatric Gastroenterology, New England
Medical Center, Boston, Massachusetts

John M. Templeton Jr., MD
Professor of Pediatric Surgery, The Children's
Hospital of Philadelphia, University of Pennsylvania
School of Medicine, Associate Surgeon, The
Children's Hospital of Philadelphia, Philadelphia,
Pennsylvania

Andrew M. Tershakovec, MD
Assistant Professor, Department of Pediatrics,
University of Pennsylvania School of Medicine,
Assistant Physician, The Children's Hospital of
Philadelphia, Philadelphia, Pennsylvania

Symme W. Trachtenberg, MSW, ACSW, LSW
Clinical Associate, Social Work in Pediatrics,
University of Pennsylvania School of Medicine,
Director of Social Work, Children's Seashore House,
Philadelphia, Pennsylvania

William R. Treem, MD
Professor of Pediatrics, Chief, Division of Pediatric
Gastroenterology and Nutrition, Duke University
Medical Center, Durham, North Carolina

Nicholas Tsarouhas, MD
Assistant Director of Pediatrics, R.W. Johnson School
of Medicine, Director of Pediatric Emergency
Department, Cooper Medical Center, Camden, New
Jersey

David Turkewitz, MD
Director of Pediatrics, York Hospital, York,
Pennsylvania

Stuart Alan Weinzimer, MD
Fellow, Division of Endocrinology and Diabetes, The
Children's Hospital of Philadelphia, Philadelphia,
Pennsylvania

Jeffrey C. Weiss, MD
Professor of Clinical Pediatrics, University of
Arizona, Head, Section of General and Community
Pediatrics, Phoenix Children's Hospital, Phoenix,
Arizona

William J. Wenner, Jr., MD
Assistant Professor, University of Pennsylvania
School of Medicine, Division of Gastroenterology and
Nutrition, The Children's Hospital of Philadelphia,
Philadelphia, Pennsylvania

Ralph F. Wetmore, MD
Associate Professor, Otolaryngology: Head and Neck
Surgery, University of Pennsylvania School of
Medicine, Associate Surgeon, The Children's
Hospital of Philadelphia, Philadelphia, Pennsylvania

James F. Wiley II, MD
Associate Professor of Pediatrics, University of
Connecticut Health Center, Director, Pediatric
Emergency Department, Connecticut Children's
Medical Center, Hartford, Connecticut

English D. Willis, MD
Director, Pediatric Service, Mercy Health Medical
Center, Philadelphia, Pennsylvania

Robert W. Wilmott, MD
Associate Professor of Pediatrics, University of
Cincinnati College of Medicine, Director, Pulmonary
Medicine, Children's Hospital Medical Center,
Cincinnati, Ohio

Flaura Koplin Winston, MD, PhD
Clinical Assistant Professor of Pediatrics, University
of Pennsylvania School of Medicine, The Children's
Hospital of Philadelphia, Philadelphia, Pennsylvania

George A. Woodward, MD
Assistant Professor of Pediatrics, University of
Pennsylvania School of Medicine, Director of
Transport Services, The Children's Hospital of
Philadelphia, Philadelphia, Pennsylvania

Elaine H. Zackai, MD
Associate Director, Pediatrics and Genetics Director,
Clinical Genetics Center, The Children's Hospital of
Philadelphia, Philadelphia, Pennsylvania

Moritz M. Ziegler, MD
Professor of Pediatric Surgery, University of
Cincinnati School of Medicine, Chief, Pediatric
Surgery, Cincinnati Children's Hospital, Cincinnati,
Ohio

Kathleen Zsolway, DO
Assistant Professor of Pediatrics, University of
Pennsylvania School of Medicine, The Children's
Hospital of Philadelphia, Philadelphia, Pennsylvania

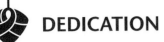 DEDICATION

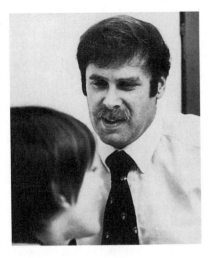

Ed Charney, a model clinical educator, loved both teaching and clinical duties. I marveled at his enthusiasm for his patients; he treated each person as a special individual. He offered time and patience to listen to his patients' needs and problems, and he offered hope to many. Charney loved to teach, and he won many awards for his special efforts. Prior to his death, Ed Charney was promoted to Professor of Pediatrics and received the Dean's award for clinical teaching.

Letters from his patients always included thanks for his care. In the last months of his life, Ed's patients offered to help him cope with his illness. The people's warmth and sincerity were special tributes to his kindness. He is a role model for many young pediatricians.

Ed came to Children's Hospital of Philadelphia for an internship and returned as a junior faculty after his service in the Navy. Always a generalist, he focused on the care of children with chronic illness, especially those with myelomeningocele. He was a leader in his field, in both practice and publication of his observations.

Special memories of Ed include his devotion to his wife Linda, and his daughters Laura and Rebecca; his neat office and appearance; his love of desserts, indiscriminate if chocolate chips were not available; his noncomplaining ways— even when he had much to complain about, he worked harder to help others. From him, we learned many lessons: 1) Redefine what is important; 2) Treasure the present; 3) Complain less and help others more; 4) Use your skills to help someone who needs you; and 5) Reach out to your family and friends.

With this legacy, we echo the words of James Whitcomb Riley: "I cannot say and I will not say, that he is gone, he is just away."

M.W.S.

To Susan, David, Charles, Burte, and Sloan

To Vicky and Ethan

To Barbara and Daniel

To Anne, Thomas, Bridgid, and Helen

To Meredith, Erin, Jonathan, and Patrick

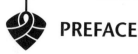

PREFACE

Revising this textbook for the third edition offered an opportunity to update the material, to determine what new concepts and directions were occurring, and to open up an opportunity for a new group of talented authors to publish their ideas. Additionally, it is a chance to reflect on the past 10 years when the first edition was initiated and to consider the changes that have occurred. Ten years ago, HIV infections were mentioned briefly. Lyme disease was a rare diagnosis; there were few if any clinics devoted to Lyme disease diagnosis and misdiagnosis. Managed care was something that occurred elsewhere. Strep infections were easily treated with penicillin. A 10-year review documents the rapid changes in medicine.

This edition was a pleasant opportunity to update the changes in diagnosis and treatment of many common problems. New chapters were added, expanding the scope of primary care pediatric issues. Contributions of new authors provided different perspectives and new energy to the content. The enthusiasm and promptness of these authors are appreciated. Once again, the "38 rule" seemed to hold true here. For example, in the first edition, I noticed prospective authors either responded eagerly or with great hesitation. In most cases, the positive responses came from those authors who were less than 38 years of age—another triumph for youth.

Special thanks to the people who helped to complete this project. Wendy Buckwalter started the project at Mosby. Her enthusiasm and hard work kept the project focused. She turned the job over to Jennifer Byington Geistler and Laura De Young at Mosby who helped with the final stages. The production was masterfully managed by Michelle Fitzgerald and Anthony Trioli. The associate editors, Nate Blum, Tom Curry, Joel Fein, and John Sargent, helped with the planning and editing of the chapters. Their cooperation and skills contributed to the quality of the project. I enjoyed working with them.

Sadly, two special friends are no longer with us. David Cornfeld, a friend and mentor, died in 1993. His companionship and advice are still missed. He was a kind ear, a validator of feelings, and a competitor for arcane vocabulary. Ed Charney, a former associate editor, died in 1994. We worked together on the first two editions of this book, as well as many other projects. His work with children with chronic illness set a standard for pediatricians. Both gentleman are irreplaceable and are constantly missed.

Ten years have gone by. We look to the future with enthusiasm and hope that the transformation of medicine will be good for children and their caretakers. Looking at the new medical students and residents, I think the future will be full of optimistic, talented people. The right ingredients for an optimistic start.

M. William Schwartz, MD
Philadelphia, Pennsylvania

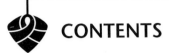

CONTENTS

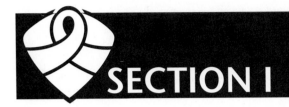

SECTION I

Well-Child Care

Well-child care (health supervision) is an integral part of the practice of medicine for those involved in the care of children and adolescents. The concept of care rendered in anticipation of problems to prevent disease serves as the foundation of primary care.

This section focuses on the content of the well-child visit. The first three chapters examine the purpose of the office visit, offer suggestions regarding the conduct of the interview, and develop a framework for examining what is to be accomplished by the visit.

Chapters 6 through 19 offer points peculiar to the physical examination of the various age groups and present topics that are frequently encountered during the evaluation of the patient and in discussion with the family.

The last seven chapters address a variety of issues that touch on the daily practice of well-child care. These include immunization practice, screening programs, obesity, accident prevention, television, day care, acquired immune deficiency syndrome (AIDS) education, the sports evaluation, and divorce.

CHAPTER 1

Expanded Office Visit

Gordon R. Hodas

Primary care physicians exert an important influence in helping children and parents to function competently. An ongoing primary care relationship becomes most significant by providing continuity that decreases parental anxiety while promoting parental competence and caretaking. The family gains a sympathetic, knowledgeable, and reliable professional who can serve as both an expert and a catalyst for the parents and child during the child-rearing years.

To promote family competence over time, the physician must learn who the child's family actually is. With two-parent biologic families, the physician should try to form a relationship with each parent. With single-parent families, the physician should get to know an involved grandmother or a boyfriend, whenever possible. When biologic parents have remarried and both parents remain actively involved with the child, the physician should try to develop positive relationships with both households.

Although medical expertise is indispensable to the physician, the development of a trusting doctor-family relationship depends more on certain personal qualities of the physician that, although intangible, are also unmistakable. This skill development starts with expressing respect toward the child and family and accepting them in a nonjudgmental manner. There should be empathy, whereby the physician acknowledges an appreciation of the family's goals and frustrations. The physician should display energy and enthusiasm in relating to the child and family, as well as patience in response to questions and doubts. The physician should be able to rely on a sense of humor at appropriate moments, while at other times stimulating motivation in a firm yet supportive manner. Finally, the physician should maintain and convey a sense of hopefulness and a belief in family competence.

The physician who believes that parenting, despite its frustrations and uncertainties, should be an essentially happy experience can convey this belief to the family, thereby promoting a positive family orientation from the beginning. During times of major disappointment, the physician can help the family call on its strengths to meet the immediate crisis and eventually move ahead in an adaptive way.

This commitment to work with the family's competence and strength in all clinical situations has been called the *health focus,* because the ultimate task of the physician is to promote healthy functioning and effective coping in dealing with well-child care, acute minor illness, medical and psychosocial emergencies, and chronic illness.

In the following discussion, the implementation of some of the above goals will be illustrated with respect to a routine pediatric visit of a well or sick child. The same principles would also apply in acute and emergency situations.

THE ROUTINE PEDIATRIC VISIT

As shown in Table 1-1, the routine pediatric visit has three components: the interview, the physical examination, and the wrap-up. Each of these parts of the visit has medical tasks and associated interpersonal tasks; the latter are intended to promote the competence of the child and parents and to strengthen the doctor-patient relationship. We will frequently refer to child and "parents." Although we realize that often only the mother in a two-parent family attends routine visits for a well or sick child, it is strongly recommended that the primary care physician try to involve the other parent as often as possible, so that information and decision making regarding the child can

TABLE 1-1
Components of a Routine Pediatric Visit

	MEDICAL TASK	INTERPERSONAL TASK
Interview	Chief complaint; history-taking	Connecting; establishing leadership; developing an agenda
Physical examination	Screening for illness	Creating a therapeutic experience; involving child and parents; communicating information
Wrap-up	Summarizing medical findings	Addressing the agenda; encouraging questions; formulating future goals

be more fully shared. When the physician suggests to mothers that they invite their husbands, a surprising number of fathers do come in. Even more fathers attend when invited directly by the physician, for example, during hospital contact following the birth of a newborn. The presence of both parents at least some of the time enables the physician to better understand the child's family and builds a solid foundation for future interventions during medical or psychosocial crises. With single-parent mothers, frequently another adult (mother's own mother, sister, or boyfriend) shares caretaking responsibilities; the mother should be encouraged to bring this person at least some of the time.

The Interview

With both initial and follow-up visits, the objectives of the pediatric interview are essentially the same. Medically, the goal is to determine the nature of any chief complaints and then to obtain data about them through history-taking. The physician has additional interpersonal psychosocial tasks; the overall goals are to promote family competence, to expand and broaden the data base, and to ensure that each office visit is goal directed and of value to the child and parents. For example, if the parents come in with recent problems, the physician also should inquire about recent successes. With parents focused on the child's ailing body, the physician also should address the child's overall physical, social, and emotional development and his/her family context. In this way, the physician defines his/her area of interest as encompassing not just the child's sick body, but the child as a whole and as part of the family.

The physician has two major psychosocial tasks during the pediatric interview: "connecting" with the family and establishing leadership.

Listed below are the important aspects of *connecting* that involve the physician's establishing himself/herself with the child and family as a concerned, approachable helper:

1. Putting the family at ease
2. Setting the tone
3. Relating to all adults
4. Relating to the child

The physician puts the family at ease in concrete ways such as introducing himself/herself, greeting each family member warmly by preferred name, showing fondness for the child, providing chairs, and encouraging everyone to take off coats and relax. In effect, the physician connects by setting the desired tone for the visit, which is one of respect, collaboration, and hopefulness. This tone is achieved both verbally through direct comments to the child and parents and nonverbally through the physician's manner in relating to the group. The need to relate to all adults as well as to the child constitutes the final element of successful physician connecting. In this way, everyone has a chance to contribute, more information is obtained, and the physician demonstrates that the verbal child is a person whose ideas should be respected. In addition, the physician who develops a relationship with the child at the beginning of the visit will encounter a less anxious, more cooperative child during the physical examination.

The contacting of various family members is a continuous process occurring throughout the interview, examination, and wrap-up. The physician will need to develop a comfortable style that enables him/her to shift attention from one person to another in a smooth, relatively inconspicuous way. One danger is overfocusing on the mother, who is often most eager to talk, to the relative exclusion of the father and child. If the father is to continue to attend visits and to perceive the physician as helpful, it is essential that the physician address him regularly. Similarly, by encouraging the child to contribute, the physician paves the way for a positive relationship for many years, hopefully through adolescence. Initial contact with each family member should occur within the first several minutes of the interview, as the physician engages each person briefly in "small talk." Each person again should be sought out as data are gathered about the child and any presenting problem.

Establishing leadership occurs almost simultaneously with connecting.

1. Relating with confidence
2. Organizing data-gathering
3. Broadening the focus
4. Developing an agenda for the visit
5. Promoting competence

The physician can establish leadership by relating confidently to the child and parents. Confidence is conveyed through firm handshakes, consistent eye contact, and a resonating voice that invites comments without being tentative. The physician's energy and enthusiasm in approaching the family also instill confidence. He/she further establishes leadership by providing the structure for organized data-gathering and helping parents to focus their concerns from the outset so that limited time can be utilized in a clearly defined manner.

Another important aspect of physician leadership involves broadening the focus. The family, especially early in the doctor-patient relationship, typically comes in with narrow expectations of their physician, as someone to give shots and treat the child when ill. Although these activities are essential aspects of the physician's responsibilities, they do not incorporate other interests of a physician providing "primary care." The physician can convey his/her broader interests—including developmental, social, and family concerns; the importance of medical continuity; and the promotion of family competence—indirectly through questions and directly by defining his/her role as the primary care physician.

During a particular visit, the broadening of the focus can take many forms. We recommend that the physician write down at the end of each visit the pertinent issues to be reviewed at the next visit. At that visit, the physician listens carefully to the parents' expressed concerns, then inquires about issues that the parents have not raised. On this basis, the physician can develop with the parents an agenda of specific goals for the immediate visit, which may include medical, developmental, behavioral, and family issues.

The promotion of child and family competence can occur as part of a continuing process as the physician successfully connects and establishes leadership during the office visit. Over time, the family comes to view the physician as a committed ally who also educates and challenges whenever indicated.

Physical Examination

The pediatric physical examination has a therapeutic potential that has not been fully exploited. Presenting medical concerns can be addressed by the physician in a way that promotes competence and reassurance, orienting the parents and child toward health and coping. Table 1-2 shows the role of the physical examination in promoting certain developmental psychosocial tasks of children and their parents. As these tasks are met, the likelihood of potential problems for each period is reduced. The four developmental periods considered are: 1) infancy through the second year of life; 2) the preschool period, ages 2 to 5 years; 3) the school-aged period, ages 5 to 12 years; and 4) adolescence, ages 12 to 18 years. Three major goals of the physician during the physical examination extend through each developmental period and are therefore not listed each time. These goals are the following: 1) promoting positive relationships with each parent; 2) promoting a focus on health whereby competence is highlighted under adverse as well as routine conditions; and 3) creating a therapeutic experience for the child and parents while conducting the examination.

Infancy (Table 1-2) is a particularly vulnerable time for parents, yet the outcome of this period may set the tone for subsequent development. Newborns, especially first-born infants, often precipitate a crisis of anxiety and uncertainty for parents, unprepared for the demands of their new role. The infant may be seen as fragile and "not a real person." If the child should be temperamentally difficult or develop colic, the crisis intensifies.

It is in this context that the physical examination can be quite therapeutic, promoting the parents' attachment by revealing the healthy

TABLE 1-2
Role of the Physical Examination in Promoting Psychosocial Tasks

	DEVELOPMENTAL TASKS*	POTENTIAL PROBLEMS	ROLE OF THE PHYSICAL EXAMINATION
Infancy (to second year of life)	Understanding infant's needs* Promoting infant's security and trust* Developing parental attachment* Developing mutual parental support*	Lack of infant-parent attachments Child as source of stress Impaired physical or emotional development Parental anxiety or depression; marital crisis Child abuse or neglect	Educating parents, relieving anxiety "Humanizing" the infant Demonstrating gentle, consistent approach to infant Promoting parental competence with infant Creating a sense of adventure Promoting joint involvement in parenting Encouraging private time
Preschool period (ages 2–5 yrs)	Gaining sense of initiative and separateness Developing sociability Pursuing eagerness to learn Promoting child's curiosity and separateness while remaining vigilant*	Separation anxiety Withdrawal and restrictive play Somatic symptoms Parental overinvolvement or parental neglect	Developing physician's separate relationship with child Promoting spontaneity and curiosity Promoting use of play Educating parents Promoting appropriate level of parental involvement Containing impact of acute minor illness
School-aged period (5–12 yrs)	Developing sense of accomplishment Strengthening sense of autonomy Developing positive self-esteem Encouraging exploration and responsibility*	Somatic complaints School refusal Depression Conduct disorders	Promoting child's relationship with physician Giving child more information and responsibility Respecting modesty Reinforcing child's cooperation Helping child begin to develop reasonable sense of control over body Promoting parents' view of child as competent Containing impact of acute minor illness
Adolescence (12–18 yrs)	Strengthening sense of independence and responsibility Developing stable body image and sense of control over body Dealing with sexuality Negotiating issues of independence and closeness Encouraging expression of adolescent's own ideas and concerns*	Somatic complaints Substance abuse Conduct disorders Depression and suicide attempts Pregnancy Eating disorders Promiscuity Pregnancy Eating disorders Overdependency Runaway behavior Psychosis Depression Conduct disorders	Examining adolescent alone, keeping parent informed Relating to adolescent as competent and responsible Explaining body changes Encouraging pride in body Respecting modesty Explaining body changes Encouraging pride in body Relating to adolescent as competent and responsible Allotting time for special concerns (sexuality, drugs, alcohol, dieting, exercise, peers, family) Allotting time for special concerns

*Denotes parental task; otherwise, psychosocial task of child.

newborn to be strong, capable, and very much a person. The physician uses the examination to illustrate the child's capabilities and vulnerabilities and to show how to approach the infant, demonstrating gentleness, consistency, eye contact, expressions of affection, and an absence of punitiveness. These efforts help "humanize" the infant for the parents. The infant is further transformed to a source of pleasure when the physician talks to him/her, uses humor, and points out the infant's smiling and other reflexes. Because the physician's demonstration is for both parents, joint parental involvement as well as parental competence with the infant are promoted, and the potential dangers of failed attachments are rendered less likely. The physician can try to create a sense of adventure for the parents, as they both watch and help the child grow.

The preschool child (Table 1-2) is a verbal being, separate from parents and desiring to establish areas of competence. There is great interest in using speech, being sociable, and learning. The physician therefore now maintains an active relationship with the child as well as the parents and promotes the child's spontaneity, curiosity, and play. Participation is encouraged. The physician also utilizes the examination to assess parent-child relationships and to promote appropriate levels of parental involvement.

The tasks of the school-aged child (Table 1-2) include developing a sense of accomplishment, strengthening the sense of autonomy, and elevating self-esteem in the process. Therefore, while continuing to relate to the parents as the primary caretakers, the physician devotes further efforts toward building a relationship with the child. The child is addressed frequently, given more information and responsibility, and helped to begin to develop a reasonable sense of control over his/her body. The child's physical modesty is always respected through use of gowns. The parents are encouraged to see the child as competent.

During adolescence (Table 1-2), important developmental tasks include the continued development of a sense of independence and a sense of responsibility, the development of a stable body image and a sense of control over one's body, and coming to terms with one's sexuality. The physician sees the adolescent alone, keeping parents informed of major health issues. Relating to the adolescent as competent and responsible, the physician can utilize the examination to discuss

such topics as physical growth, exercise, diet, weight control, acne, and menstruation.

With the adolescent the doctor encourages questions and tries to promote a positive body image and a sense of control over one's body. By offering confidentiality except in cases of attempted or threatened suicide, the physician can encourage discussion of other highly personal areas such as sexuality, birth control, drugs and alcohol, peers, and family relationships.

Summarized below are interpersonal goals and techniques, as developed by Honig and associates, that promote participation and competence during a single physical examination of a verbal child:

- Promoting relationship with child
  Providing transition from history to physical examination
  Engaging child in conversation
  Using humor
  Explaining procedures
  Allaying fears
  Encouraging curiosity
  Encouraging cooperation
  Communicating information
- Promoting relationship with parents
  Offering compliment(s) about child
  Promoting eye contact with child
  Promoting direct parental participation
  Communicating information

These techniques are meaningful to a physician who has a genuine commitment to develop a doctor-family relationship based on collaboration and respect. The two major goals are promoting the relationship with the child and promoting the relationship with the parents.

With the child, the physician should strive to diminish anxiety and encourage participation as much as possible. Toward this end, the physician should announce the physical examination and allow a brief transition from history-taking to the examination so that the child is not startled. The child can be given a chance to finish undressing or to climb onto the examining table. To initiate the examination itself, the physician should explain at the child's level what will be taking place, attempting to allay fears, promote understanding, and encourage cooperation. The doctor should reassure the child that the parents are there and should ask the child to cooperate. As the examination unfolds, the physician should try to maintain an ongoing dialogue with the child, at times turning to address the parents.

Some of the conversation can be related to topics of interest to the child, and some should involve the physician's explaining each aspect of the examination and reassuring the child about his/her body. The physician can engage the child's curiosity through "tricks of examination," asking the child questions, and offering a stethoscope or hammer for the child to try out.

Although the physical examination is often a special time between physician and child, it is nevertheless important that the parents participate in the process. Compliments about the child serve to orient the parents positively. Promoting eye contact between parents and child is important not only for the child but for the parents as well. With younger children, a mother may participate directly when the child is examined on her lap. Parents also may participate by providing information and by helping the child to cooperate during the examination. The role of parents is especially important when shots must be given. The physician has several ways to prepare the child: simple explanations, recalling an earlier shot, using humor, and offering a toy or a familiar object. After the shot, the physician can "make peace" in several ways such as offering a kind word or a plastic strip bandage. Nevertheless, it is the parents' reassurance and comforting that matter most to the child during and after the procedure.

Finally, the physician should provide information to parents during the physical examination; this relieves anxiety and adds further legitimacy to the physician's conclusions during the wrap-up.

Wrap-Up of the Pediatric Visit

The wrap-up, or summary, of the pediatric visit affords the physician the opportunity to tie together disparate questions and findings so that the visit becomes therapeutic and important themes are reinforced. This goal is achieved in a variety of ways:

- Addressing agenda of visit
- Highlighting themes
- Decreasing family anxiety
- Encouraging questions
- Formulating future goals
    Medical
    Developmental
    Behavioral or psychiatric
- Assigning tasks

First, the physician addresses the agenda agreed on earlier in the visit. Typically, this includes one or more medical concerns plus a behavioral or parenting question. If the physician has properly focused the interview and has utilized the physical examination strategically to promote his/her objectives, the wrap-up becomes the final step in a process already underway.

Thephysician should direct comments to both par- ents and to the child, allowing frequent opportunities for questions and clarification. The physi- cian's summary should be relatively brief so that it can be easily understood. In beginning a discussion, the physician should try to use the family's own words and phrases. Physician clarity will help decrease anxieties of the parents and child.

Once the presenting concerns have been addressed, the physician can encourage the family to formulate future goals. These goals fall into three categories: medical, developmental, and behavioral or psychiatric. Medical goals may pertain to a current illness, a past illness, or the ongoing management of a chronic illness. Developmental goals may apply to the child, the parents, or both. Issues for the child include safety and anticipatory guidance, sibling and peer relationships, and development of interests and other aspects of independent functioning. Issues for the parents include the need for shared parenting and mutual support and the need for some privacy for the couple. Parents also must deal with additional planned and unplanned events that impact on the child or family, such as a job change, an illness, or the birth of a new baby. Behavioral and psychiatric issues that involve the child or adolescent vary in severity and may include anxiety, withdrawal, disobedience, depression, suicide attempts, substance abuse, and psychosis. Issues that may involve the parents include severe marital conflict or divorce, parental depression, and substance abuse.

When confronted with significant developmental, behavioral, or psychiatric issues, the primary care physician must decide whether to manage them himself/herself or initiate psychiatric referral. The task of referral is easier when parents themselves identify a problem and request help. However, the physician who has serious concerns about a child or the family must be prepared to express this concern directly and to recommend psychiatric consultation if indicated. In such instances, it is important for the physician to propose psychiatric consultation constructively and to reaffirm his/her own continuing primary care involvement.

A special challenge of the pediatric visit is for the physician to create a balance between direct problem solving and problem solving on the part of the family. Toward that goal, the physician may at times conclude many routine pediatric visits by assigning tasks to the family. These tasks may involve a change in behavior on the part of the parents, the child, or both. The value of tasks is that they promote independent problem solving by the family while also maintaining the physician's presence as a catalyst for change during the interval between visits.

BIBLIOGRAPHY

Brazelton TB: *Doctor and patient,* New York, 1970, Dell Publishing.

Carey WB, Sibinga MS: Avoiding pediatric pathogenesis in the management of acute minor illness, *Pediatrics* 49:553, 1972.

Diller LH: On giving good advice successfully, *Fam Syst Med* 4:78, 1986.

Glenn ML: *On diagnosis: A systemic approach,* New York, 1984, Brunner/Mazel.

Glenn ML: Toward collaborative family-oriented health care, *Fam Syst Med* 3:466, 1985.

Hodas GR, Honig PJ: An approach to psychiatric referrals in pediatric patients: Psychosomatic complaints, *Clin Pediatrics* 22:167, 1983.

Hodas GR, Honig PJH, Montalvo B: *Interpersonal aspects of the pediatric physical examination,* William Penn Funded Grant, 1979–1982.

Honig PJ, Lieberman R, Malone C, et al: Pediatric-psychiatric liaison as a model for teaching pediatric residents, *J Med Ed* 51:929, 1976.

Klaus MH, Kennell JH: *Maternal infant bonding,* St. Louis, 1976, CV Mosby.

McDaniel S, Campbell TL: Physicians and family therapists: The risk of collaboration, *Fam Syst Med* 4:4, 1986.

Rinaldi RC: Positive effects of psychosocial interventions on total health care: A review of the literature, *Fam Syst Med* 3:417, 1985.

PART ONE

Communication Skills

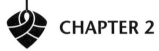

CHAPTER 2

Patient-Physician Communication

M. William Schwartz

WHY COMMUNICATION IS IMPORTANT

Good patient care requires good communication skills. If the patient is satisfied and follows the treatment plan, we efficiently use our time and funds. Poor communication between the physician and patient leads to low compliance and dissatisfaction resulting in less successful outcomes.

One purpose of the patient visit is to make the right diagnosis and plan the appropriate treatment. Another goal is to set the tone for maximizing patient compliance, establishing continuity of care, and building relationships that will foster better health and disease prevention. If the goal of the visit were only to make a diagnosis, we could handle most encounters with a computer to obtain information.

Computers, however, have trouble applying weights to the facts. They do not react to facial expressions and body language or make judgments about pain that is evident with a patient's change in voice or position. They do not minimize a complaint of pain in one history and expand the history for more detail in another. They do not see the anxiety of the family members or ask about their concerns. We should not fear being replaced by a computer in the data

gathering segment of the patient visit but accept the unstated challenge to expand the interaction beyond collecting facts to make a diagnosis.

This chapter offers insights that can improve your communication skills so that your patients will view their meetings with you positively. It also will help to decrease the number of difficult encounters with patients. In this discussion, the interview is divided into three main segments: beginning, middle, and end. Each section offers advice about the technical and the psychosocial considerations. As with any other technique or tool, the same approach or style should not be used with all patients. These skills should be applied at the appropriate time and adjusted to the patient's needs and problems.

THE INTERVIEW

The office should be comfortable for the patients and the doctor. Having both parties sit sends a signal that the visit will not be rushed and that the patient has the doctor's full attention. When possible, barriers such as desks should be removed.

Before asking the who, what, and where questions about the problem, take a few minutes to set the tone of the visit. This can help facilitate the flow of information and improve the quality of

TABLE 2-1
Opening Statements and Comments

OPENERS	COMMENTS
What can I do for you today?	Focuses on "I, the Doctor," rather than "you, the patient."
What seems to be the problem?	"Seems" implies that the patient is making up the problem.
How long have you had your sore throat?	Forces the patient into short answers—may not allow patient to tell the story.
What brought you here today?	Too broad—you can get an answer ranging from "the bus" to the symptom.
What did you expect to accomplish with this visit?	Slightly awkward but should be addressed sometime in the visit.
How are things?	Allows the patient to discuss what is important and to begin to tell the story.
Tell me about your . . .	Open ended—gives the control of the interview to the patient to start with the communication.

the communication. Good eye contact, identification of those present, and handshakes, when appropriate, help build the impression of an unhurried person who wants to help the patient and is ready to listen to the patient describe the problem. A brief period of socialization will help establish you as a concerned person. This phase, called *joining*, consists of comments about some article of clothes or jewelry, a vacation or family event, or concern about transportation. These comments, admittedly awkward at first, give the signal that you care about the person as an individual, not a disease. In pediatric practice, this is easier because children often get dressed up to see the doctor and may be wearing a new shirt or piece of jewelry or carrying a special toy. Just think how positive you feel when others notice something about you. In some cases, if the patient seems unresponsive to these gestures or appears eager to get to the problem, the attention should be quickly directed toward the medical problem.

We struggle with the opening statements and change them as our experience increases. Whatever words you use will work well with some patients and not as well with others. Open-ended questions work best. Table 2-1 includes some opening statements with comments about how patients perceive them.

Middle Segment

In the middle of the interview, the patient has the opportunity to tell the "whole story" with some direction and focus by the physician. This is the time to hear the patient's agenda and accomplish what the computer would do in collecting the facts that lead you to a diagnosis. At this time we

also work with the patient to establish relationships, clarify hazy concepts, and develop the treatment plan (Table 2-2).

Ending

We use many methods, both physical and oral, to indicate the end of the visit (Table 2-3). A transition statement such as "before we leave, let me summarize what I gained from this meeting and see how that fits with what you feel" prepares the patient for the visit end and allows the patient to respond. Other comments such as "I am interested in hearing what you are going to tell your (wife, mother, friend) about the problem" offers the patient the opportunity to repeat what you have told him/her without making patients feel as if they are being tested. It also gives you a chance to hear how the patient has understood the disease, cause, or prognosis. A question such as "anything else I should know" again signals the visit end is near while giving the patient a chance to discuss concerns not yet mentioned.

Handing the patient a prescription or instruction sheet will indicate the session is over. Standing up from your chair clearly indicates that you are finished with the interview. Glancing at your watch is the least effective indicator. This indicates that you have other things to do and may make the patient feel that you lost interest.

STRATEGIES FOR COMMUNICATION

A variety of techniques should be part of your communication toolbox. Like tools, they are not used every time with every patient but should be

TABLE 2-2
Technical Skills That Improve Communication

	GOOD QUESTIONS	POOR QUESTIONS (WHEN FOLLOWING AS A RESPONSE TO THE PATIENT'S REPLY)	COMMENTS
Open-ended questions	Tell me about your pain.	Do you have chest pain? Or, you don't have any chest pain, do you?	Closed questions do not allow the patient to tell the story of the problem.
Establishing connections (listening)	Let me stop here to summarize what I have heard.	I'd like to change the subject now.	Summarizing gives the patient evidence that you heard what was said. Moving on to a new topic may be premature because the patient may want to tell you more information.
Clarify	Can you tell me what you mean by constipation?	You mentioned constipation, how long have you had it?	Lack of definition may be confusing later. Assumes you know what the patient means by constipation—hard stool? straining? infrequent stooling?
Identify mood and act appropriately	You seem a little down today. What's happened?	I know how you feel.	The patient is the only one who knows how he/she feels.
Setting agenda	Did you bring in a list of topics you want to cover today? What did you want to accomplish today? I heard a list of concerns you have. Which ones have the highest priority for this visit?	I heard you mention fatigue, shortness of breath, and headaches. Where does your head hurt?	You, rather than the patient, have decided on the priority of the problem list.

readily available for the appropriate situation. Similar to a lumbar puncture or insertion of an arterial line, the practitioner needs these skills but does not use them on every patient.

Open-Ended Questions

We gain important information and form interpretations about the problem by allowing the patient time to tell the story of the disease. Open-ended questions guide the thrust of the dialogue while encouraging the patient to answer the questions with descriptions rather than with brief "yes/no" responses. Some inquiries have to be less open, especially in the beginning of a system review. These questions can be followed by more exploration, such as "tell me about it." You should monitor your style, making sure that only a minimum of questions allow the patient to answer with a one- or two-word response. You may have a tendency to see a healthy looking patient and "tell" a question by stating "you don't

have any pain or do you?" rather than "do you have any chest pain?" You may miss important information if telling questions becomes your interview style.

Establishing Connections (Listening)

Patients state the reason for poor compliance centers on the feeling that the doctor did not understand the problem or did not hear what they were trying to say. We must indicate to the patient that he/she is getting our full attention, which means attentive listening, eye contact, nods, and comments that indicate you understand the patient. Establishing connections is like an indicator light signaling that the patient's words were heard and you are processing this information. Because we do not have such an electronic signal to tell the patient about our listening status, we must do this orally, repeating the major statement—"the pain starts in the morning and does not wake you up at night . . . ";

TABLE 2-3
Ways to End the Visit

ORAL	PHYSICAL
Transition statement—"As we come to the end of the visit . . ."	Giving a prescription or instruction sheet
Summarize—"This is what I heard . . ."	Written summary of visit in brief outline form
Summarize—"What will you tell your _____ about the diagnosis?"	
"Anything else I should know?"	
Discussion of tasks to be accomplished before the next visit	Written instructions
Approval—"You have done an excellent job of managing the fever."	Writing an "A" on the instruction sheet

making a periodic summary—"let me stop here to summarize. The pain occurs in the morning and is not relieved with meals . . . "; making a transition summary—"before we move on to the next section, let me summarize what I have heard and what information I am using to make the diagnosis, start the treatment, etc."

When you speak to someone for whom English is a second language, you often wonder if they understood what you said when they respond "yes." Did they mean "yes" or is this a polite comment that does not reflect comprehension. Instead of guessing, it is better to solicit comments that qualify the "yes." Ask them "why" they said "yes" or to elaborate. Think of the patient as one who has medicine as a new second language. Request some kind of acknowledgment that the connections are being maintained by asking questions that require more than a "yes or no" answer. Likewise, keep sending out signals that you have made connections that are active and responding to the patient's message.

Interruptions impede the listening process and create another conflict—the patient wants to tell a story about the illness as he/she experienced it; you want to get the facts and determine the treatment. One study of internists by Beckam and Frankel showed that the average time allowed for the patient's opening statement was 18 seconds before the doctor broke in with a question. Try to discipline yourself to allow the patient to continue for a few minutes before you begin the questions. This strategy may actually save time as you work with the patient.

Identify the Patient's Mood and Anxiety Level and Act Appropriately

How does one react to a patient with a different affect? If you are the serious type and your patient is comical, do you act more solemn in order to get the patient to tone down the humor? If the patient is sad, do you speak more cheerfully? Sometimes this approach works; other times it causes the patient to accentuate the differences, thinking that by strengthening that affect, they will have you notice their state. This dilemma is called the "electric blanket syndrome" and is described by Karofsky and Keith. This analogy uses the image of an electric blanket with a temperature regulator on each side of the bed but with a crossed-wire connection. In other words, the control box on side A affects the person on side B and vice versa. When the temperature was too cool on side A, the person on side A turned up the regulator to send more heat. Side B received the extra heat, which prompted the person on side B to turn down the thermostat. This further cooled side A, which prompted the person on side A to turn up the heat again. You can see the similarities between this syndrome and differences in style in communication. In general, it is better to adjust to the patient's mood initially and then discuss the mood—"You seem a little down today" or "It is nice that you are in such a good mood. What happened?"

Patient's Agenda

The patient should be considered an expert in his/her own right and as such has unique perspectives and valuable insights into his/her physical state, functional state and quality of life (Roter and Hall 1992).

There are times when the interview does not go well despite good technical style, gathering important information, and making a diagnosis that agrees with the facts. The patient seems unhappy with the encounter or does not follow the treatment plan. Why? Many reasons can apply, but sometimes patients have another agenda. For example, you may want to find out the cause of the abdominal pain and the patient may want to change schools. Few teenagers will list possible pregnancy or obesity as the presenting problem, but they may use a common problem such as exhaustion or abdominal pain as the ticket of admission to see you. A mother may say, "I came to you for my child's cough," when she really means, "I am concerned about his lack of friends." It is as if you were working in two different areas of concern. These separate circles may be so far apart that they prevent effective communication; other times the spheres overlap enough that further questioning clarifies the purposes of the two parties, thereby improving communication. Periodically consider these possible differences in your agendas to assess communication quality with the patient.

If at the end of the visit when your hand is on the doorknob, the family begins to tell you a concern that was not mentioned in the visit, you have failed to determine the patient's agenda. Realizing that the opportunity to tell you the rest of the story is being lost, the last-minute disclosure is the patient's or family's final chance to interject the new problem list into the meeting. How much better it would be if the concerns were mentioned during the visit when time could be managed better. This awkward situation can be prevented by exploring the agenda earlier.

How do you avoid this problem? First, move beyond your personal concerns and recognize that the patient does have an agenda. At the appropriate time, bring the agenda into the discussion. Assess the degree of commonality of the agendas and explore the differences and possible explanations for them. Try to find a common area of interest. Work on the common items and look for successful resolution to the problems. With further time and stronger rapport, some agenda items may become common concerns for both you and the patient (Table 2-4).

Sequencing of Information Gathering

Your conduct of the physical examination can result in a patient misunderstanding your actions and becoming fearful that there is a serious problem that you are not disclosing. This fear can be heightened when you listen carefully to the heart for what may be longer than usual. After listening to the heart intently, a statement such as "you have a very healthy heart" may relieve the patient's fears, whereas saying nothing or "hmm" creates tension. Sometimes, for efficiency, you may perform the review of systems and the physical examination concurrently. In these situations, you should ask the review of systems questions before you do that segment of the physical examination. If you do the reverse and listen to the chest before asking about family

TABLE 2-4
Uncovering the Patient's Agenda at Various Points in the Interview

INTERVIEW	AGENDA
Beginning	Tell me about your concerns.
Middle	Right now I see there are two issues you have. Are there any others?
	From my examination, I find a healthy boy, but you have a list of problems about your son and a sad look on your face as I am telling you about my findings of a normal boy. Help me understand your concerns.
	You keep bringing up the unfair teacher. What are your ideas about how that relates to the cough?
	Is there anything else I should know?
End	I think your problem will decrease when you exercise more.
	You seem to feel that a chest x-ray is needed. Can we come up with a plan?
	To me, the pain is related to the diet. How does that fit with your thoughts?

history of chest disease, for example, you suggest that you heard something that prompted the suspicion of tuberculosis or other chest disease.

Silence

In the early stages of medical training, silence is an enemy to be fought with any type of speech, either meaningful or empty. With more experience, you can use the silence as an effective aid, signaling patients that you are still listening and they should continue to speak. Silence can prompt patients to speak about something that is significant on their agenda. Silence also may serve as a time-out period, which allows you to regroup when you feel some strong emotions or negative feelings. Without the silence, you may react or say something regrettable.

Note Taking

We often have the dilemma of trying to keep eye contact and to listen attentively while making sure to record adequately the information. Some people can remember the facts and record them accurately at a future time. Most, however, will either forget details and make sketchy notes or make errors in note writing when relying on memory. The tension of listening versus note writing is lessened when the interviewer acknowledges that there is a need to make a few notes, asks permission to write some notes, and quickly returns to listening.

SPECIAL TECHNIQUES

When a physician finishes a standard interview with a patient who has presented a vague story, he/she may have an uneasy feeling that there is more important missing information. There may be difficulty in summarizing what has been heard. The "who, what, where, and when" line of questioning may not always be sufficient to remove the vagueness. This may be the time to ask the five questions listed below.

- Why did you come? What is wrong?
- Why did you come today?
- What would you like me to do?
- What do you think is wrong?
- What do others think is wrong?

In a classic paper about six children with a cough, Yudkin discusses the second diagnosis. Describing six children with a cough, he points out the fallacy of trying to make one diagnosis per patient. He suggests that the following questions be included in the interview: "Why did you come to see me?" and "Why did you come today?" These questions may uncover the patient's second agenda and bring into the discussion concerns that are not easily articulated but need to be.

The five-question approach, an extension of Yudkin's concept, attempts to explore the patient's agenda. "Why did you come?" is answered in the chief complaint. "Why did you come today?" may present some difficulty if not phrased in a friendly, open manner. The importance of this question is to learn what caused the patient to feel that this was the time to seek care. Obviously we need to avoid making patients feel uncomfortable and having them interpret this as a pejorative, condescending question meaning "why didn't you come in sooner?" or "why didn't you wait a little longer?"

A young couple visited a pediatrician with a baby 6 months of age who had a fever. As commonly occurs, there was no source of fever and the infant looked well. The diagnosis of virus was made with instructions for fever control and a return visit if any change occurred. Late Friday night, 5 days later, the parents placed a frantic call that the baby was worse. The pediatrician feared that the child had meningitis and worried about a lawsuit. Much to his surprise, he examined a happy baby with no fever. After the relief passed, the doctor inquired about the reason for the return visit. The parents stated that this was their first baby and the next day the grandparents were making their initial visit. They knew that the baby was sick so the parents wanted another check-up on Friday to allow them to say that the baby was examined the night before and declared healthy—a far cry from meningitis and legal problems.

"What do you want me to do?" again explores the patient's agenda. This is not an offering of an open menu to the laboratory tests. If the patient wants another x-ray or blood test, you do not have to feel obligated to order the test. This question does, however, serve as another place for discussion and resolution of differences, if they exist. Doctors who need to have strong control over visit proceedings will feel threatened by this question; those who feel the visit is more of a partnership toward solving the problem will welcome the exchange.

"What do you think is wrong?" helps the patient participate in the discussion. The tendency to hear the various problems, set priorities, and investigate what you think is important leaves the patient out of the process. "What do you think is wrong?" also can clarify the patient's agenda and initiate a dialogue, allowing the patient to voice concerns and tell the story. Many parents, for example, may tell you the main problem but may also be concerned about leukemia. They have heard stories of leukemia starting with a fever, rash, bruise, fatigue, or lumps—signs and symptoms that cover a large percentage of the reasons that prompt a visit to the doctor. Even if it is clear to you that the bruise is from trauma or the fever is from otitis media, you need to be sensitive to the parent's concern. If there is a high level of anxiety, you may want to pause and find out what the parents are thinking. Stating that you are curious about the parents' explanation of the problem or diagnosis, however silly, can express concerns you have not considered but should address. Maybe even opening up this discussion with, "Many people come here worrying about diseases that they have recently heard about, such as Lyme disease, cancer, or leukemia. Have you ever had those

fears?" This question may evoke a response of denial or a pause and acknowledgment. Probing about a sensitive topic should not be utilized in every situation but may be productive when there is more anxiety than one would expect from the primary problem.

"What do others think is wrong?" is a look at the unofficial health advisor network that may be in play. A patient may seem unsure why he/she is in the office. These patients lack emotion about the problem and may not show concern appropriate to the chief complaint. Someone else may be concerned or may be advising the parent to seek attention for a problem that the parent did not recognize. Comments from a family member or friend such as "the child looks pale—have you had her checked for worms?" often influence parents who had not seen a problem.

Talk-show host Larry King said, "I never learned anything when I was talking." When dealing with a difficult situation, check on the amount of talking by the two parties. Create a chart with two columns, "doctor talking" and "patient talking," and make a note every minute of the interview (Table 2-5). If the majority of check marks are in the "doctor talking" column, this indicates that you talked too much and did not give the patient a chance to relate his/her story.

Assume the Diagnosis and Get the Details

Depending on the patients and our experiences, cultures, and backgrounds, we have different levels of comfort when discussing some issues with patients. Sexual activity, drug use, birth control, medication compliance, and family relationships are only a few of the topics that are either often avoided or glossed over in the interview. When asked in a nonjudgmental way, closed questions, such as "do you use drugs?," may elicit an truthful response. Other questioning styles may be more effective, such as "what kind of drugs do you use?" or "what happened to you when you experimented with drugs?" and may yield an honest answer (Table 2-6). The approach is not judgmental but shows an expression of curiosity and concern.

Approval

Most of us like to hear that we are doing a good job, especially when we are either proud of our accomplishments or unsure if we made the right decisions. We should take advantage of our role and offer encouraging words about performance, judgments, decisions, or family events. "That was nice," "You are doing so well for a new parent," "Great!," "Wasn't that thoughtful?" all signal approval for these activities. These words affect even the most secure and confident listener. A sophisticated parent appreciates a few words such as "Nice job—A+" written on the instruction sheet at the conclusion of a visit.

The Day History

Finding out the day's activities gives you insight into the patient's life, child-rearing style, ability to cope with multiple stimuli, and support systems. Asking a patient to describe a typical day will start the discussion. Most people are happy to tell you about their lives and welcome your questions. Far from being a diary of concise terms about feeding and activities, the historian should be encouraged to name the activity and to interpret the decisions that led to the action. For example, when the parent states that the baby woke at 7 A.M., you should ask, "How did you know the baby was awake?" You may learn that the baby was asleep down in its own room, in the parent's bedroom, or in the parent's bed. You may find out that the father made noise when he woke up to go to work at 6 A.M., the other kids were too noisy, or the mother woke up the baby to feed it so that task would be completed before preparing breakfast for the other children. You gather the pulse of the family as well as the time pressures and organization skills. The descriptions about activities at supper time provide many insights because this is the time of day

---

TABLE 2-5
Who's Doing the Talking?

MINUTE	DOCTOR TALKING	PATIENT TALKING
1		X
2	X	
3		X
4		X
5		X
6	X	
7		X
8		X
9	X	

Note: This diagram shows the patient did most of the talking during the visit. This can indicate that the patient has had the chance to relate the history and the doctor was listening.

TABLE 2-6
Questions That Uncover Details of an Assumed Diagnosis

DIRECT QUESTIONS	INDIRECT DETAIL QUESTION
Do you and your wife have fights?	What do the kids do when you fight?
Do you drink alcohol?	What kind of beer do you like?
	How much beer do you drink?
Do you use condoms?	What kind of condom do you use?
	How often do you use them?
Do you and your mother disagree?	How do you resolve the disagreements with your mother?
What is the dose of medicine you are taking?	Describe the color and size of your seizure medicine.

when the parents have most demands on their time. Meals need preparation, children have needs, and stress may be high from the employment situation. Adults are called on to be parents, spouses, first-aid providers, tutors, chefs, cleaners, and many other roles. Asking who helps to cope with these demands, what contribution each spouse, if present, makes, and what support systems exist give you insights that are not forthcoming if you ask, "How are things at home?"

The information gained from the day history helps you to assess the child's personality and temperament, the parenting skills, the support systems, and level of stress. This information will be useful when working on a treatment plan such as trying to fit in a medication schedule or explanation.

The Patient-Centered Interview

The concepts and tactics to improve communication allow the patient to communicate better about the problem and move the focus of the interaction from the physician data gatherer and diagnosis-maker to the patient who has the problem. The patient-centered interview has been articulated by Smith and Hoppe as an integration of the patient's and physician's roles and interests in discussing the problem. To accomplish this level of communication, the physician has to yield some control of the meeting and the patient must be comfortable in talking about the issues.

During the past decade, many articles have been published about the patient-centered interview, some of which are listed in the bibliography. The patient-centered interview allows patients to tell the story of the illness and how it affects him/her and the support systems. Derived from Gestalt, in an article by Koffka, the theory proposes that people are continuously developing a story that portrays what is most important in their lives. Our task in the interview is to make a diagnosis and to allow the patients to tell their stories, symptoms, fears, and the meaning of the illness. Finding and fixing the illness is only a part of the goal of the meeting. To successfully participate, the doctor has to transfer some control of the communication to allow the patient to tell the story and also retake control to guide the conversation and to obtain appropriate information to make the diagnosis and plan the treatment. Patient-centered communication presents the psychosocial content of the patient's life. Physician-centered communication only details the organic illness. The benefits of patient-centered communication are illustrated in Table 2-7. The patient comes to the doctor with an idea of what is wrong, what he/she expects from the visit, and fears about what the problem may be. Our task is to let the patient express these ideas and concerns.

Commonly, the preoperative visit consists of a succession of students, residents, nurses, and fellows who enter the room, acknowledge the impending surgery, ask about the doses of the present medications, obtain informed consent, and leave with the information needed to complete the record. Often no one has asked the patient about the fears of the impending major procedure or the change in the lifestyle that this illness may produce. The patient needs a chance to express these feelings, and the physician may learn important information by addressing these concerns.

TABLE 2-7
The Patient-Centered Interview

PATIENT	DOCTOR-CENTERED RESPONSE	PATIENT-CENTERED RESPONSE
Is there anything wrong with the baby?	The baby is fine—everything is normal.	What were you concerned about?
This was my first pregnancy.	Did you have any illness or take any medicine?	Tell me about it.
I found out I had a positive tuberculosis test.	What test did they use to diagnose it?	How did you feel when you found out?
This was the second asthma attack.	Did the medication control it?	How did it affect you?

Adapted from Smith RC, Hoppe RB: The patient's story: Integrating the patient- and physician-centered approaches to interviewing. *Ann Intern Med,* 1991, 115:470–477.

SUMMARY

This chapter has offered some interviewing hints and discussed the benefits of moving away from the "medical model" interview and the find it/fix it approach toward a broader focus with an inclusion of the patient. This approach offers better compliance, relationships, and trust.

The skillful communicator will meld the pairs of activities, considering the doctor's agenda and the patient's agenda as well as working with both the doctor-centered and the patient-centered interview. This means yielding some control, establishing a humanistic approach, and developing a partnership with the patient.

BIBLIOGRAPHY

Baron RJ: An introduction to medical phenomenology: I can't hear you when I'm listening, *Ann Intern Med* 103:606–611, 1985.

Beckam HB, Frankel RM: The effect of physician behavior on the collection of data, *Ann Intern Med* 101:692–696, 1984.

Conversation failure: Case studies in doctor-patient communication, Frederic Platt Tacoma: Life Sciences Press, 1992.

Del Banco T: Enriching the doctor-patient relationship by inviting the patient's perspective, *Ann Intern Med* 116:414, 1992.

Helfer R: An objective comparison of the pediatric interviewing skills of freshman and senior medical students, *Pediatrics* 45:623–627, 1970.

Karofsky P, Keith: Electric blanket syndrome, *Clin Ped* 20:279, 1981.

Koffka D: *Principles of gestalt psychology,* New York, 1935, Harcourt Brace and World.

Korsch B, Gozzi EK, Francis V: Gaps in doctor patient communication I. Doctor-patient interaction and patient satisfaction, *Pediatrics* 42:855–871, 1968.

Levenstein JH, Brown JB, Weston WW, et al: Patient centered interviewing. In Stewart M, Roter D, editors: *Communicating with medical patients,* ed 2, Newbury Park, 1990, Sage Publications.

Lipkin M, Putnam SM, Lazarre A: *The medical interview,* New York, 1995, Springer-Verlag.

Platt F, Keller VF: Empathetic communication: A teachable and learnable skill, *J Gen Intern Med,* 9:222–226, 1994.

Roter DL, Hall JA: *Doctors talking with patients—patients talking with doctors,* Westport, 1992, Auburn House.

Smith RC, Hoppe RB: The patient's story: Integrating the patient- and physician-centered approaches to interviewing, *Ann Intern Med* 115:470–477, 1991.

Spiro H: What is empathy and can it be taught?, *Ann Intern Med* 116:843–846, 1992.

Yukid S: Six children with coughs, *Lancet* 561–563, 1961.

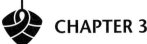

CHAPTER 3

The Problematic Physician-Patient Relationship

Henry G. Berger

Janet Etzi

This chapter will take up the multifaceted issue of approaching difficult situations in the context of medical care. It will attempt to construct a mind-set for minimizing problems and working them through as they arise. By analyzing difficult situations according to a few simple principles, the clinician will be able to maximize the chances of working them out to successful completion.

RELOCATING THE DIFFICULTY

The issue of managing the difficult patient has long been discussed in terms of locating the difficulty within the patient. Personality types have been listed and delineated to enlighten the clinician, and advice has been given on how to manage one's own feelings, which inevitably arise when dealing with difficult patients. These are useful measures, but they fail to address the ways in which even the most pleasant, compliant patient can trigger problems in the consultation room. Locating the difficulty within the dyad, which is the interaction between physician and patient, will shed light on the processes of 1) avoiding the exacerbation of conflicts, and 2) constructing a working alliance. The usefulness of this approach is found in its generalizability to any problem situation arising between patient and physician. Expanding the notion of the dyad to include the physician-family interaction leads to new ways of thinking about the communication. The benefit of changing the frame of reference from the difficult patient to the problematic interaction lies in its applicability to many types of problems that may arise between the physician and patient.

The Patient

In focusing on the interaction between the physician and patient we see both parties contributing in their own way to the development of the dyad. The combination of any particular patient with any particular physician results in a unique dyad. Recognizing the attributes of each side and how these attributes blend for desired effects or conflict with each other to prevent desired effects increases the physician's capacity to anticipate potential problems and to utilize all available methods at his/her command so that an optimal alliance may be established.

As one part of the dyad, the patient or the parent of the patient brings a great deal into the interaction. Focusing exclusively on the patient runs the risk that the problems will be automatically perceived as arising in and from the patient. In our reframing of this issue we find that what the patient contributes to the interaction, problematic or not, only has an effect in conjunction with what the physician contributes. It is the combination that is of interest here; therefore, the process of resolving conflicts will be applied to the interaction, not to the patient unilaterally, nor to the physician unilaterally.

In this context then we want to know what the patient brings to the dyad. Before entering the consultation room, the patient has his/her own expectations of the doctor and what the doctor will do. There may be a preconception that the doctor has all the answers. The patient may assume that he/she will be very active in the evaluation treatment process or may assume the opposite, that he/she will take on a passive onlooker role, taking orders as they come, never bothering to consider personal reactions. The patient may be someone who sees no need for giving a history or other important information, content to allow the doctor to do all the work.

Patients bring fears and anxieties into the consultation room. However, every patient has an idiosyncratic way of responding and behaving under the influence of those fears. It is helpful to keep in mind that fears about medical conditions, justified or not, touch on deeply ingrained beliefs about the physical body and its hidden mechanisms. In addition, every individual has unconscious beliefs and expectations regarding issues of being taken care of and protected from harm, as well as related feelings of helplessness. Because these feelings and expectations are usually far from conscious awareness, their influence will be felt in a particularly elusive and sometimes unruly way. They can invade the physician-patient interaction surreptitiously, leaving the physician upset or irritated before realizing why.

Patients have their own interpretations of symptoms, which can range from the realistic to the bizarre. This issue is of particular importance when treating a child and communicating with the family of that child. Common powerful feelings of shame, anger, and guilt will make the physician work to contain them or manage them in some other fashion.

There are special issues to consider when dealing with a family. For example, it is not always clear who is making the decisions concerning the patient; consequently it may not be obvious that any one family member is the primary source of information or the one with whom the doctor should be communicating. It may be important to consider what role an illness plays in ongoing family dynamics. Have there been other illnesses that the family now connects to the current illness, interpreting it as more or less serious than it really is, reading into it meanings and perhaps dangers that have no relevance? Is there a feeling of guilt and responsibility in a parent of a sick child, or implicit anger and blaming of another family member for the current illness. These and other issues will emerge in the family's communication patterns and style of handling crises, and will inevitably affect their decision-making abilities as well as their interactions with the physician.

Additional matters to consider when grappling with difficult interactions with patients is that of the patient's or family's relationship with the physician. Is the primary bond with the doctor, or is the family only connected to a clinic? Is the doctor their primary physician, looking forward to a long-standing relationship? What is the impact of economic and accessibility changes in medicine on this family? What is the family's history with other physicians, which may color their current expectations? These factors and others frame the patient-physician dyad. The extent that the physician is aware of their potential influence on the communication and interactions with patients and their families will improve the way any related problems or obstacles to treatment are handled.

The Physician

Every physician has a set of expectations about what the role should be. Some take on an authoritarian stance, expecting compliance from patients unconditionally. Others expect to adopt a linear problem-solving approach to patients with a clear-cut goal in mind. Physicians may expect a friendly relationship with patients, or to be appreciated by them. It is not unusual to hope for gratification from solving the problem presented by the illness and from the work of curing.

Past experiences that physicians have had with a certain kind of patient, perhaps with a particular illness, will have an impact on interactions with current patients. Presuppositions about this person or illness to the present situation may not apply. Included in this category of physician-related factors are reactions to various ethnic/racial groups that touch on the doctor's capacity for stereotyping others.

A factor that is perhaps of particular importance has to do with what is going on in the physician's life at the time. Conflicts, events, or difficulties involving family and children may be acting as current stressors and bringing extra burdens into the dyad. The physician may be anxious about a particular illness leading to self doubt and questioning of skills in relation to that illness. Some physicians may overidentify with certain patients and respond idiosyncratically; for example, a physician may become overly solicitous or, at the other extreme, may become remote and distant as a way of managing overidentification. The level of experience of the physician indirectly influences the approach to the difficulties. The physician may rely on a rigid problem solving style, whereas other less experienced physicians may feel anxious in facing a new problem.

A few mundane issues that also color the doctor-patient interaction include time constraints, what happened with the previous patient, or what is known about the following patient. There can be any number of matters going through the physician's mind on a given day.

MISMATCHES

The following three examples will serve to illustrate how physicians and patients contribute to the nature of the interactions between them and provide some solutions to the problems that arise. The first example shows the kind of conflict that can emerge when a particularly demanding patient meets a defensive physician.

Case 1

Dr. B was a senior resident completing her training. She had always been intolerant of her own shortcomings, self-critical, and hypersensitive to the criticism of others. During the time that Dr. B met Family A, her own father was suffering from a recurrent illness. Family A had a family member being treated for a similar illness. They often reacted to their anxiety by taking a demanding, critical, and adversarial position in relation to the treatment and guidance offered by Dr. B. This combination would lead one to expect a problematic encounter, which, in fact, was the case. When Dr. B was no longer able to contain herself, she responded to threats by the patient with angry outbursts of her own. The focus of much of the conflict revolved around whether some tests were necessary or if Dr. B was acting overcautiously.

Matters were resolved when a senior physician intervened. The intervention consisted of a review of the treatment plan with the family, which presented a recommendation but allowed the family choices. The senior physician neither felt nor behaved as if his authority was being questioned. Instead he presented himself as a source of information and experience.

Case 2

The next example illustrates what can happen when the doctor focuses on the individual patient, unaware of how the powerful family interactions are affecting the patient and the treatment. This kind of scenario might be characterized as "tunnel vision doctor meets cinemascope family." Problems arise when the doctor gets caught up in the family system not recognizing the impact it has on the interaction.

Dr. D, a competent and concerned pediatrician, was known for being particularly respectful of the rights of older patients in managing their care. He himself had a somewhat rebellious past and character that allowed him to work comfortably in his chosen field. His particular inclinations, however, proved problematic in working with T, an older adolescent, diagnosed with a severe gastrointestinal disorder. In the course of her illness, T's mother also had undergone a serious illness requiring surgery. The two illnesses had the effect of magnifying conflicts within the family concerning T's autonomy and struggle for independence.

T's treatment, an issue surrounding her illness, became a focal point of this conflict. Dr. D overtly and covertly sided with T, the adolescent, exacerbating conflict with the family. The mother then responded to Dr. D as a representative of her daughter and her daughter's unacceptable behaviors. Because T did realistically require family guidance and support and was not yet able to manage important decisions completely independently, this complicated her care. By overtly siding with T, Dr. D alienated the parents who then were unable to comply with the appropriate recommendations concerning T.

This problem was resolved when matters reached a crisis. Emergency surgery became necessary and all members of this drama were able to reorganize themselves into a team. Refocusing on the family allowed Dr. D to create an effective treatment and team. Dr. D was correct in respecting and encouraging adolescent autonomy. It is necessary, however, to understand how this family is dealing with that particular issue.

Case 3

The third discussion involves Dr. E, a much admired oncologist devoted to the welfare of her patients. Dr. E also was noted for maintaining an optimistic and positive attitude in the face of serious life-threatening illnesses with which she dealt.

L was an appealing, intelligent child aged 9 years who had been diagnosed with a serious but treatable malignancy. L's family, devastated by their son's illness, were understandably even more prone to indulge L, a tendency that they had prior to his diagnosis. Part of L's treatment included regular, particularly painful, traumatic procedures that L was unable to tolerate. It was determined that L could be anesthetized safely during these procedures, a solution readily accepted by the family. Dr. E, however, initially was strongly opposed to this option, citing possible complications from the anesthesia despite reassurances to the contrary from experts in anesthesiology. In the course of discussing this problem, Dr. E admitted that she was also determined that L would not begin to take "the easy way out," a policy that she feared would handicap L's future abilities to handle crises. One can only speculate that this particular issue was significant to Dr. E for more personal reasons, based on personal experiences of her own. Nonetheless, Dr. E was finally persuaded to allow L to undergo general anesthesia with the promise by a consultant that this indulgence would be managed in later counseling.

The above examples are given to demonstrate how problems can be potentiated by a mismatch of physician and patient or family. These examples also point to more specific problems in establishing a working relationship between physician and patient as well as specific physician characteristics that contribute to the development of conflict with the patient. These factors will now be discussed more fully in the next section.

GENERAL PRINCIPLES FOR APPROACHING PATIENT-PHYSICIAN INTERACTIONS

This section will outline and discuss several general principles to be used in approaching interactions with patients that have the potential for conflict and miscommunication. Each of the principles addresses what can be done to maintain a healthy, productive alliance with the patient and to minimize any difficulties arising with the patient. It is important here to recognize that none of these principles can necessarily avoid difficulties or eliminate conflicts and trouble altogether in the doctor-patient relationship.

First, it is important for the physician to reflect as much as possible on those factors mentioned above that might influence judgment and performance. In other words, self-awareness of one's own biases, limitations, and vulnerabilities will prevent further magnification of problems that require balanced management. On a day-to-day basis, recognition of particularly strong stressors or demands is essential for maintaining such a balance. For example, to the extent possible the physician should avoid those patients experienced as most difficult when he/she is especially rushed, exhausted, or otherwise distracted. It is *good* practice to seek help, obtain a consultation or a second opinion, or even refer those patients and families who are most overwhelmingly difficult. Some warning signals include a sense of great anxiety or despair when anticipating an appointment or undue preoccupation with a particular case. The willingness of the physician to examine his/her own reactions is probably the single most effective antidote to troubled therapeutic relationships.

The second powerful tool available to the physician in avoiding problems is the effort to establish a relationship early in treatment. Naturally this means that time be taken not only to acquaint oneself personally with the patient and family but to try and uncover those problems that may interfere with treatment. The physician who takes the time to do this has a better chance of building trust and a good rapport with the patient. Approaching patients with this goal in mind may assist in reassuring frightened or suspicious patients or disarming hostile patients. It also will help to uncover early on future problems that are likely to arise, allowing the physician to anticipate possible strategies.

In addition to establishing a relationship with the patient, the physician must take time to set appropriate goals and limitations. This will have the effect of minimizing problems that arise with patients who feel entitled to the doctor's time and efforts. Dependent patients who look to the physician for an excessive degree of reassurance will benefit from early clarification of goals in as much as this is possible. There are patients who are prone to idealize the doctor and his/her efforts and who would become profoundly disappointed at the slightest hint of "failure" or uncertainty. Outlining treatment aims clearly can minimize patients' tendencies to distort interactions, and setting limits early may prevent unrealistic expectations and future disappointments.

Finally, if one observes experienced physicians, one is struck by their ability to fit their approach to the demands of their patients while at the same time maintaining their own identity. They demonstrate how it is possible to adapt to the needs of their patients and have their responses flow naturally according to their own style and personality. One physician may use humor to support a frightened family, whereas another may find it more comfortable to reveal some of his/her own history and experience. When dealing with a particularly hostile family, for example, the experienced physician is able to convey firmness and sympathy in his/her own individual manner. Experience allows the physician to remain calm, to avoid becoming engaged in unnecessary argument, or to unwittingly signal abandonment. In a sense, the recognition of a patient's needs and the use of appropriate responses is a definition of professionalism.

Referring to the examples given above, one can see the problems resulting by ignoring these principles. In all cases, time spent in establishing an initial relationship and working out a realistic treatment plan and goals would have been beneficial.

SUMMARY

In summary, when the focus of attention broadens from the patient to the interaction between the patient and family and physician, it is easier to comprehend problems and potential solutions. A clear understanding of factors affecting both sides of the relationship, self-awareness on the part of the physician, and sufficient early efforts given to the establishment of a relationship with the patient and family are all ways of avoiding or minimizing difficulties. Finally, a willingness to seek advice and a recognition of one's own limitations are also crucial in working with difficult or demanding patients.

BIBLIOGRAPHY

Fritz GK, Mattison RE, Nurcombe B, Spirito A: *Child and adolescent mental health consultation in hospitals, schools, and courts,* Washington, DC, 1993, American Psychiatric Press.

Groves JE: Taking care of the hateful patient, *N Engl J Med* 298(16):883–887, 1978.

Kanaha RJ, Bibring GL: Personality types in medical management. In Zinberg NE, editor: *Psychiatry and medical practice in a general hospital,* New York, 1964, The International University Press.

Lewis M, King RA, editors: *Child and adolescent psychiatric clinics of North America,* Philadelphia, 1994, WB Saunders.

Oken D: Difficult and obnoxious patients. In Oken D, Lakovics M, editors: *A clinical manual of psychiatry,* New York, 1981, Elsevier.

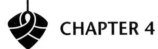

CHAPTER 4

The Patient-Physician Relationship: What Parents Want from Their Doctor

Gail L. Ginder
Kathryn Sexton

The relationship between parents and their child's doctor is like no other. The mother and father are placing their trust in another human being to take care of their cherished child.

The parents' expectations are enormous. The doctor must be accurate, warm, loving, responsive, respectful, and compassionate. But the factor that determines whether parents consider their child's doctor to be a "good doctor" is the quality of the relationship between the physician and the family.

Fostering trust and confidence among patients and their parents benefits the physician, too.

- When the relationship with the patient is strong and trust is developed over time, the patient is more likely to do what the doctor recommends and adhere to therapeutic regimen. If the patient follows through with what the physician recommends it is far more likely that the patient will have a positive health outcome.
- There is growing evidence that shows that one major way to avoid lawsuits is to have positive communication with patients. Relationship problems (not financial incentives) are consistently cited as the major reason behind a patient's decision to sue.
- When patients have a positive trusting relationship with their child's doctor, they will be generally happier and will complain less. When patients are happy, the physician's practice will be more satisfying.

There has been a great deal of research on what makes this relationship effective. In general, the research has shown that what patients want from their doctor is technical competence, adequate information about their medical problems, and a warm, cooperative atmosphere.

This chapter focuses on six major elements that contribute to an effective parent-physician relationship: competence, compassionate treatment, information and agendas, respect, involvement in decisions about care, and responsiveness.

Each of these elements will be treated in a section of this chapter with specific suggestions about what the physician can do to foster their development.

COMPETENCE

The patient needs to know that the physician possesses a high level of competence and technical expertise. Because the parent does not have the background to judge clinical competence, he/she uses measures that are familiar to draw conclusions about a physician's technical ability.

One mother described it simply, "I don't know what the doctor looks for when he examines my son when he is not feeling well, I just look for results from the treatment." Because many childhood health problems are easily treatable, the results are often positive.

In addition to positive results, the most common way parents will evaluate the competence of the physician is through the quality of the personal interaction: Was the doctor warm and gentle with my child? Did I understand what the doctor was saying to me? Was the office staff friendly? Did the doctor listen to my opinions about my child's health? Did the doctor make my child feel comfortable? Did we feel like our concerns were important? Did the doctor return my calls quickly?

What Parents Want To Tell Their Child's Doctor

Be Thorough

Show us that you are doing a thorough examination and tell us what you are doing when you are doing it. If you are discovering something during the examination, tell us: "It looks to me like her ears are clear, and there is no infection."

When There Is a Problem Tell Us What You Know—and Do It Quickly

We are always fearing the worst, so when you hesitate, it makes us imagine the unthinkable. When you are still unsure, tell us you are unsure. Tell us how you will go about finding an answer and how and when you will communicate that answer to us.

Anticipate Problems My Child Might Face or Questions I Might Have

Tell me about potential complications associated with my child's illness, possible side effects of a particular medication, or even predictable developmental problems that my child might face. Draw on your experience with other parents to anticipate questions I might have but haven't thought of yet (eg, "you might be wondering about the implications of another round of antibiotics for your daughter").

COMPASSIONATE TREATMENT

Parents want their children to develop a foundation for a lifetime of positive health care. They want their child to look forward to going to the doctor as a friendly guide. Like parents, the child will judge the physician on the basis of the personal interaction: Was the doctor nice to me? Did the doctor hurt me? Did the doctor make me laugh? Did I feel special? Did the doctor care about me?

If the child leaves with the feeling that the doctor cares about him/her, then the foundation for positive health care is being established.

What Parents Want To Tell Their Child's Doctor

Begin Slowly

Take a few minutes at the beginning of our visit to let us know you care about us. Talk to me and talk to my child. Ask me how things are going in general with my child's health. Ask my child how school is going. Even in a short visit, take time to connect.

Get Down To My Child's Level

Imagine how it would be for you if you were only 30 inches tall and were constantly asked to deal with someone two times your size. Bend down when you are talking or let the child sit on the examination table so that you can look each other in the eye.

Speak Directly To My Child

As soon as my child begins to understand—certainly by age 4 years—ask my child how she is feeling or where it hurts. Then ask me if I have observed anything or have anything else to add. When you're examining my child, tell her what you are doing and why you're doing it.

Treat Me Like an Individual

I know that you have a very busy schedule and that you can't remember the details about every one of your patients. I also know that you've probably heard the problem I am about to describe to you 5000 times before. The most powerful thing you can do is make me feel like our problems are unique (they are to us), that our concerns are important, and that you care about us. Maybe you could make a note in the chart about something I told you last time I came in.

Be Kind, Warm, and Gentle

Go beyond the words. Let my child know that you hope she feels better soon. Tell my child that you know her broken arm hurts a great deal and that you will work as quickly as you can to make it better.

Listen

When you ask a question, wait for the answer before you move on to the next question. Sometimes it takes a while for me to remember the examples that you've asked for. Sometimes it takes time for my child to get up the nerve to describe how he is feeling. Listen to what my child is communicating. If he is saying that everything is all right, but he is saying it with droopy shoulders and no eye contact, take some time to find out what is really going on.

INFORMATION AND AGENDAS

In one important study in the literature about physician-patient communication, physicians were asked to estimate how much time they spend educating a patient. Their estimates were compared with actual audio tapes of visits. The physicians' estimates ranged from 5 to 7 minutes, but the audio tapes showed that the physicians were spending about 1 minute educating the patient (Waitzkin and Stoeckle 1976).

No matter how much time is actually spent educating the patient about health matters, it will never be enough if the specific questions brought by the parent are not directly answered. Whereas the doctor will have many office visits in one day, the parent has only one. The parent has hours, maybe days or even a week, to think about what he/she wants from this visit.

For an annual check-up for her 3-year-old child, it isn't unusual for a parent to come with a written list of discussion items that might include her child's limp, how much milk she should be drinking, whether or not it is OK to sleep on a foam mattress, and how to tell if the daycare center is all right for her child. The doctor, too, has his/her own priorities for discussion.

If the two agendas include the same issues, both the parent and the physician leave satisfied. If the parent only makes it halfway through her list, she can leave quite dissatisfied. However, if the doctor works only with the parent's agenda, too much time may be given to unimportant problems and not enough to critical developmental issues.

Agendas: What Parents Want To Tell Their Child's Doctor

Listen To My Concerns, Then Prioritize (With Me) How We Will Spend Our Time Together

After you've given me an opportunity to list all of the concerns, say something like, "After I take time to do a thorough examination, let's first discuss Johnnie's eating and sleeping hab-

its and his adjustment to school. Then we'll take the time that is left to address your other concerns."

Remember That You Don't Have To "Fix" Everything That I Might Be Concerned About

Often I just need a little reassurance. Sometimes I need a name of someone else who can help with a particular problem. Sometimes I need to get something off my chest.

Questions

When a parent brings a child to the doctor for an urgent problem, the parent's need for information will be immediate and will supersede any other form of discussion. In this situation, the physician can assume that the parent has the following questions and wants all of them answered as quickly as possible:

- **What is wrong with my child?**
  Unspoken: How serious is it? How do you know that is the problem?
- **What are you going to do or recommend for my child?**
  Unspoken: Are you going to do anything that will hurt my child?
- **Why are you suggesting this rather than that?**
  Unspoken: Are you giving this problem the serious consideration it deserves? How do you know it's not something more serious?
- **What will happen next?**
  Unspoken: When will my child be well? How will I know there is improvement?
- **When should I call you back?**
  Unspoken: Will you call me? When should I bring my child in for a follow-up visit?
- **What are the long-term implications?**
  Unspoken: Will my child play basketball again? Will we be able to go on our family vacation this year?

Even when every effort is made to be responsive to the parents' agenda and to address their concerns, any attempts to communicate information will be incomplete without attention to the way the information is delivered.

Information: What Parents Want To Tell Their Child's Doctor

Give Clear Explanations

When you are delivering news about my child's condition, be clear and precise. We want to be told exactly what the situation is. If you leave anything out, we will start imagining the worst. If you are unsure of a diagnosis, tell us you are unsure, tell us what you will do to find out what is wrong, and tell us what possibilities you have eliminated.

Go Beyond the Words

One parent tells the story of her 7-day-old infant, hospitalized for jaundice. At 2 A.M., the worried and sleepless mother called the doctor. The doctor was surprised at the depth of the parent's concern and was tempted to simply reassure her that the treatment for jaundice was fairly straightforward. Instead, he asked her to tell him more about her concerns. The mother burst into tears and revealed, "Before my son was born, I had a daughter who died before I could bring her home from the hospital. I'm afraid that the same thing will happen with my son." The doctor began to understand and offered her as much reassurance as he could and explained (again) the treatment her son was receiving. He suggested that she try and get some rest because her son would be coming home soon and she would need all of her strength to take care of her newborn baby. She felt enormously relieved because the conversation helped her to understand what she was really worried about. She was very appreciative of the doctor's willingness to go beyond her initial concerns.

Avoid Using Medical Terms

While you are conducting an examination or determining the extent of a fracture, remember that the technical terms for what is going on mean very little to me. Explain everything simply. Anticipate the questions I might have. "What questions do you have?" is a far more useful question than "Do you have any questions?"

Tell Me What All This Means

If my child is injured or seriously ill, the only thing that matters at all to me is whether he will recover and to what extent his functioning will return to normal. My son will also want to know what the illness means, but in a more practical way. To him the big question is whether or not he will play football again and when. *While you are busy developing*

a diagnosis, we are more concerned with outcome.

Be Very Clear About Follow-Up

Let me know the conditions under which I should bring my child in again. Tell me what I should look for to know he's getting better. Let me know when I can relax again.

RESPECT

Parents want to hear that they are capable, that the physician has confidence they can handle the situation, and that they are doing the right things. Reassurance from their child's doctor goes a long way toward giving the parents the necessary tools to care for their child's health.

One parent described why she was so committed to her child's doctor. "She listens to me and validates my intuition as a mom. She takes the time to answer any questions we might have without making them seem foolish or insignificant."

What Parents Want To Tell Their Child's Doctor

Trust Me

Let me know you have faith in my abilities to do the best for my child. Tell me it's OK to rely on mother's intuition. Let me know that my perceptions of the problem are very important.

One mom described how her child's doctor assessed a problem: "I was worried about my son's high fever so I immediately called his doctor. She asked several questions about his symptoms, then said, 'How does he seem to you? How is this different from other fevers he has had? Is he acting like he's very, very sick?' My views of his illness were very important to her."

Listen To Me and Try To Understand My Point of View

Even when my ideas about my child or about health care differ from yours, acknowledge my point of view and try to understand it. *What I believe will influence how I care for my child.*

It is important to me that you pay attention to these beliefs. If you think I am wrong about something, tell me and explain why.

Acknowledge My Positive Actions Toward My Child's Health

Let me know when I am doing something right. This has a very powerful effect and will encourage me to do more of the same. Acknowledgment is easy to do, takes very little time, and has a long-lasting effect.

Let Me Know That It's OK To Be Concerned About My Child

One mom described an interaction she had with her child's doctor when her child was 6 months old: "One morning when I realized I had been up twice in the night to make sure my daughter was still breathing, I decided to call the doctor and ask if all this worry was 'normal.' He made me laugh and also reassured me when he said, 'I'll tell you what's normal. You'll probably worry some every day for the rest of her life. Now, let's talk about last night's worries and see if we can put them in perspective.'"

Show Me That You Really Understand What I Am Going Through

Be genuine with me. It's all right to share your personal reactions occasionally. It's all right to give an example about your own children once in awhile (eg, "My child went through that at age 5, too."). When I hear that you've been through some of the same things I am going through, I feel more connected and am more likely to open up and tell you what is really going on.

INVOLVEMENT

One of the biggest differences in what parents want today versus what they wanted 20 years ago is the extent to which they want to be involved in their child's care. Most parents today expect to be involved in decisions that affect their child's health. The major benefit is obvious—when parents thoroughly understand the situation by being involved in decisions, they are far more likely to carry out the treatment for their child.

One parent described why she was so commit-ted to her child's doctor: "He always listens to what I have to say. Together, we make decisions about which direction to go. We all benefit."

What Parents Want To Tell Their Child's Doctor

Let Me Know When I Can Be Involved and When There's Only One Course of Action

For some problems, there is only one clear-cut course of treatment that is appropriate. For most problems, it is a judgment call and there is plenty of room to involve me in a decision. Even for something as simple as an ear infection, there is a decision to be made about when to prescribe antibiotics and when to try to let it heal without medication.

One parent described an interaction with her child's doctor: "I brought my child in because he was coughing and had a cold. The doctor said that my child's ear was slightly infected and described two options for treating the infection. He asked me if my child gets ear infections often. When I told him no, he explained he has probably had infections before and in all likelihood they've cleared up on their own. He said that we could give my son an antibiotic to treat the mild infection or we could give it a chance to clear up on its own. In the latter case I could call if a fever appears or if he started to have pain. He explained that the only down side to that approach is that I might have to deal with a crying child in the middle of the night. Because I am very reluctant to give my child medication, we chose the second course of treatment. I appreciated being included in the decision and was very appreciative of my doctor's approach."

Ask My Opinion

Don't be hesitant to ask, "What do you think the problem is?" This can be helpful in two ways. First, I just might be right. I bring a wealth of information about my child that you don't have, and I may have an idea that you haven't considered yet. If I am wrong, however, what I am thinking will influence my ability to hear your diagnosis and suggestions for treatment. It is important for you to know what I am thinking so that you can dispel any worries or misunderstandings I have about my child's condition.

RESPONSIVENESS

No discussion about what parents want to tell their child's doctor would be complete without addressing the topic of how available the child's doctor is. Ideally, parents want their child's doctor to be available 24 hours a day, to make house calls whenever there is a problem, and to return telephone calls promptly.

Obviously this is not possible, but there are changes that can be made to provide a greater sense of responsiveness in even the busiest practice.

What Parents Want To Tell Their Child's Doctor

Don't Rush When You Are With Me

Let me know that during the time you are with me, my child and I are the most important concern in the world. Unless there's a real emergency, don't let anyone interrupt. If you know in advance that our time will be limited, tell me as soon as you walk into the room. When we are not able to address all of my concerns, tell me how they will be addressed (eg, phone call, another follow-up appointment, or a conversation with the nurse).

Make Your Office Comfortable

Remember that your office reflects who you are. If your receptionist or nurse is rude, I will generalize this behavior to the whole visit and my experience with you will be negative.

Organize the Office So Waiting Is Minimal

Manage your office so that waiting is minimal. This is a very important factor to many parents and a factor on which we will base our decision of whether or not to change physicians. Although waiting for any doctor can be undesirable, problems associated with a wait with sick children are magnified intensely. Consistent long waits can indicate lack of organization and can even raise questions about a physician's competence.

Acknowledge a Long Wait When It Does Occur

Ask your office staff to let me know how long the wait is likely to be. This helps me change my expectations and will reduce anxiety that can be created with a long wait. Give me an opportunity to reschedule if the wait is really excessive. Finally, if you know that I've waited to see you, thank me for waiting or apologize for the conditions that created the wait. It makes a big difference when the acknowledgment comes directly from you.

Have a System So You Know When My Need Is Urgent. I Need a Way To Gain Access To You When It Is Urgent

If I know that such a system exists, I will be more willing to wait for responses to my everyday questions. Always let me know when I am likely to hear back from you.

Follow-Up When My Child Is Really Ill

The importance of a personal unsolicited call from my child's doctor asking how she is doing cannot be overstated. This one act goes a long way to demonstrate caring, warmth, and compassion.

SUMMARY

In their relationship with their child's physician, parents want to be listened to, respected, informed, and involved. Small daily acts from a follow-up telephone call to eye-level communication with the child, to consulting with parents in decisions on medication build a relationship of trust and caring that have far-reaching consequences for the health of the patient, the confidence of the parent, and the satisfaction the physician feels in his/her practice.

BIBLIOGRAPHY

Avery JK: How the medical "lawsuit pie" is cut: Lawyers tell what turns some patients litigious, *Med Malpract Prev* July/Aug:35–37, 1986.

Beckman HB, Markakis KM, et al: The doctor-patient relationships and malpractice: Lessons from plaintiff depositions, *Arch Intern Med* 154:1365–1370, 1994.

Keller V, Carroll JG: A new model for physician-patient communication, *Pat Edu Counsel* 23: 131–140, 1994.

Leebov W, Vergare M, Scott G: *Patient satisfaction: A guide to practice enhancement,* Oradell, 1990, Medical Economics Books.

Meichenbaum D, Turk DC: *Facilitating treatment adherence,* New York, 1987, Plenum Press.

Waitzkin H, Stoeckle JD: Information control and the micropolitics of health care, *Soc Sci Med* 10:263–276, 1976.

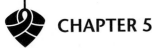

CHAPTER 5

Cultural Considerations in Pediatrics

Lee M. Pachter

Successful clinical practice of pediatrics requires bidirectional flow of information between the practitioner and the patient and family. The communication necessary for this flow may at times be hampered due to differing perspectives, experiences, and backgrounds of the physician and patient. These differences can occur between any physician and patient but may be most evident as the cultural distance between people increases. This is often the case when individuals come from different ethnocultural backgrounds. A person's approach to illness-related matters depends on his/her experiences with the health care system, personal and family beliefs and practices, as well as culturally normative beliefs and practices, which are passed on from individual to individual and generation to generation. In this chapter, the provision of culturally sensitive and competent health care is examined. *Culturally sensitive health care* can be defined as an approach to clinical practice in which the beliefs, attitudes, and lifestyles of the patient are respected; the clinician appreciates that ethnic values, cultural orientation, and linguistic issues are important inputs into the conceptualization of health and illness; and the practitioner is aware and sensitive to variations in

beliefs and practices within cultural groups and, in doing so, avoids labeling and stereotyping. An appreciation and understanding of how ethnocultural beliefs and practices shape a patient's approach to health-related matters will help the physician to communicate more effectively and create a clinical environment wherein the most optimal health outcomes may be accomplished.

EXPLANATORY MODELS

One way to assess the differences between the health beliefs and practices of patients and physicians is to understand the differences in explanatory models of sickness. An *explanatory model* is the way an individual conceptualizes a sickness episode. It includes beliefs and practices concerning what causes sickness, how sicknesses are categorized, what happens inside the body during sickness, what are the signs and symptoms of a particular sickness, how activities and roles change when one is sick, and ways of treating and healing sickness. One common difference in the explanatory models of doctors and patients is that, in general, doctors' models are often based on the concept of *disease* (a pathophysiologic state of impairment or dysfunction), whereas patients' models center on the experience of *illness* (the perception of dysfunction and how that perception affects an individual as a biological and social being). The "sick role," as well as decisions to seek health care, are based on illness concerns. Illness may not necessarily correlate with biomedical disease categories; it can be considered a more subjective experience. Patients may have a disease but not be ill, such as those with chronic diseases (*eg*, cancer, cystic fibrosis) in remission or those with subclinical prodromes. Conversely, individuals often assume the role of being ill without having a biomedical disease. It has been estimated that 70% to 90% of all visits to primary care practitioners are due to illness episodes without serious biomedically defined diseases.

An individual's illness beliefs and practices are influenced by one's familial and cultural background. The primary care provider who has contact with patients and families from diverse cultural backgrounds must be sensitive to differences in defining and expressing sickness and illness in different groups.

Although culturally defined health beliefs and behaviors are components of a patient's explanatory model, it is important to point out that individuals subscribe to the beliefs and values of a group in varying degrees. The concept of *intracultural diversity,* that is, the knowledge that there is often as much diversity of beliefs, values, and practices within groups as there is between groups, is a crucial concept if the practitioner is to steer clear of simplistic and stereotypic beliefs about members of different cultural groups. Culture can be thought of as providing an individual with a "menu" of choices regarding beliefs, values, and behaviors. It is up to the individual to pick and choose from this menu his/her personal style and approach to health and illness matters.

CULTURALLY DETERMINED CONCEPTS ABOUT THE BODY AND ITS FUNCTION

Many cultural groups have beliefs regarding the body and its function that may be at odds with standard biomedical knowledge. For example, blood and other body fluids are the focus of many health beliefs. Individuals from different ethnocultural groups may describe blood as high, low,

bad, thin, hot, cold, weak, or strong. The primary care practitioner must be aware that these terms have very specific cultural meanings in some groups. For example, the term *high blood* may, to a traditional African-American, refer to a condition characterized by an increase in the amount of blood in the body, possibly secondary to strong emotions or eating too much rich food, which, if untreated, may be thought to back up into the brain and cause a stroke. Traditional treatment may consist of ingesting astringent substances, such as vinegar, which are believed to thin out the blood. The health care practitioner must be aware of this alternative meaning, especially if he/she is trying to explain hypertension to a family. In this context, the use of the term *high blood* may create misunderstanding that could possibly lead to compliance problems (the treatment of hypertension requires chronic therapy, whereas the treatment for high blood is not prolonged, because medicine taken for a long time will make the blood too thin). The belief that medications taken in excessive amounts or over a long period of time may weaken the blood of an individual has been described in different cultural groups and may be one contributory factor toward poor compliance. The culturally sensitive physician should be specific in using medical terms and inquire about patient- or parent-held beliefs regarding how medications and therapies work inside the body, including beliefs and concerns about potentially negative effects of our therapies.

CULTURALLY INFLUENCED IDEAS ABOUT ILLNESS CAUSATION

Patients very often have theories regarding the causes of illness that may seem at odds with the biomedical paradigm. In the patient's perspective, these beliefs fit into an internally logical and consistent system. Traditional African-Americans may talk about natural and unnatural illnesses, Latinos may define illness as hot or cold, suburban white "New Agers" may discuss illness in terms of internal energy fields, and Southeast Asians may refer to wind as a causative agent of illness. These theories of illness causation are different from biomedical beliefs, but rarely does an individual exclusively use either the "folk" or "biomedical" system. Individuals usually approach illness in a pluralistic manner, picking and choosing from many different belief systems.

For example, an individual may go to a spiritual healer or folk healer to work on the cause of an illness, while at the same time go to a physician to alleviate the symptoms of illness.

FOLK ILLNESSES AND FOLK REMEDIES

Sometimes sickness episodes are defined and labeled differently by physicians and patients. Even when both the doctor and patient agree on the definition of an illness episode (*eg*, asthma, "cold," stomach virus), the explanatory models of two individuals are never totally concordant. These differences become greater when the patient defines the sickness episode in terms that are not similar to biomedical disease categories. When these illness beliefs are commonly known within a cultural group, they are referred to as *folk illnesses* (Box 5-1):

Evil eye beliefs include parental concerns that another individual is jealous of a baby or child and secretly covets the child. Because of this jealousy, a bad influence or spell may be put on the child, causing a variety of illness symptoms such as lack of appetite, crying, and decreased activity level. Parents may place amulets on their child to guard against the evil eye. The pediatrician should be aware that some bracelets or charms that are put on a child may be more than just decorative jewelry and should be respectful of the parent's desire to keep the object on the child. *Empacho* is a digestive illness thought to be caused by dietary indiscretion, resulting in food or other ingested materials getting "stuck" to the wall of the stomach. Treatment includes dietary changes, massage, and possibly going to a folk healer who is known to help treat this illness. Because parents may take a child to the physician even if they think the child may have empacho, the pediatrician who cares for Latino patients should become aware of the specific beliefs about empacho in

his/her community and have a knowledge of the additional treatments that a child may undergo for mild gastrointestinal complaints. Many of the folk treatments for empacho are harmless and could even be incorporated into the medical treatment plan for mild gastroenteritis (*eg*, massage, herbal teas, dietary restrictions).

Other ethnocultural remedies may be mistaken for signs of child abuse. Examples include coining, cupping, and moxibustion. These practices have been described in various cultural groups, including Southeast Asians, Latinos, and Eastern Europeans. *Coining* refers to briskly rubbing the edge of a coin over oiled skin, which creates patterns of ecchymosis (Fig. 5-1). *Cupping* consists of placing a heated glass or cup on the skin, which creates a bruise when the cup cools and a suction effect results. *Moxibustion* entails the placing of small amounts of burning herbs or incense on the skin. These practices produce skin lesions that may be misinterpreted

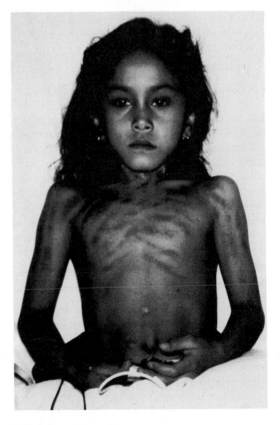

FIG 5-1
An 8-year-old girl with coining marks on chest.

BOX 5-1
Examples of Folk Illnesses That May Affect Children

Mal de ojo, malocchio, and other evil eye beliefs (Latino, Mediterranean, Middle Eastern cultures)
Empacho (Latino cultures)
Susto/fright (Latino cultures)
Caida de la mollera/fallen fontanelle (Mexican)

as signs of abuse, but they are not because abuse connotes a willful attempt to harm the child. These practices are done with the intent to help heal or cure a child's illness. The culturally sensitive physician should discuss his/her concerns about the practices in an open and respectful manner and work with the family in identifying alternative treatments that are culturally appropriate and less painful.

Nonbiomedical remedies are often used during many sickness episodes, not just during illnesses that are categorized as "folk." Again, different explanatory models that individuals use create limitless combinations of biomedical, personal, and cultural therapies. Complementary treatments include homeopathy, spiritual healing, megavitamin therapy, herbal remedies, energy techniques, and lifestyle changes. These alternative and complementary therapies are not only utilized by members of ethnocultural minority groups but are practiced by Anglo-Saxon patients as well. The sensitive practitioner should attempt to combine biomedical treatment plans with nonbiomedical practices that are not harmful. Doing this will place the medical treatment plan within a context that fits the patient's beliefs and lifestyle.

PHYSICIAN-PATIENT INTERACTION

All cultures have rules regarding roles and acceptable interaction between people. To many, physicians are regarded as authority figures. Some cultural groups treat authority figures with quiet respect and may not ask questions, because this would be considered inappropriate behavior. The physician must be supportive in this situation and should encourage questions in a nonintimidating way. Other cultures place greater emphasis on a more egalitarian exchange; the physician may mistake this form of interaction as being overly aggressive when this is in fact not the intent.

Nonverbal communication is also dependent on cultural norms. What is considered appropriate and comfortable with regard to personal space, physical contact, and eye contact differs from culture to culture. Some cultures have strict rules regarding what is appropriate physical and eye contact with members of the opposite sex. Traditionally oriented individuals from these groups may interpret direct eye contact (considered an indication of empathy and caring in the culture of medicine) as either intimidating or "staring down." The physician who works with patients from different cultural backgrounds must gain an appreciation of what is socially acceptable within that culture.

Language Barriers

The potential for miscommunication is greatest when the primary care provider and the patient or family do not speak the same language. In the best of all possible worlds, health care practitioners should become fluent in the languages of their patients. A realistic alternative is to have interpreters available when the need arises.

Certain rules should be followed when choosing and using an interpreter.

1. Whenever possible, children should not be used as interpreters for their parents; this may result in disruption of social roles and relations and puts the child in a stressful situation.
2. Do not ask a stranger from the waiting room to act as an interpreter; this would result in a breech of patient confidentiality and may strain the doctor-patient relationship.
3. It would be appropriate in most cases to use as a translator an adult that the patient or parent brings to the visit for this purpose, but be aware that the nonprofessional interpreter may have limited medical knowledge and may also editorialize.
4. Always ask the patient or parents if the designated interpreter is acceptable to them.
5. Maintain eye contact with the patient or parent who is receiving the information; you may pick up important nonverbal clues.
6. Ask the interpreter to translate as literally as possible; make sure he/she understands the medical terms that you use.

DIETARY HABITS

Diet and food preference are not only personal choices but also are culturally determined. In pediatric practice, food plays a very important role. Proper nutrition is essential to the growing child, many of our treatment plans involve food as a form of therapeutic intervention, and food is used as a palatable medium to facilitate medicine taking. It is important to know which foods are appropriate and available in the community, and also to know any general health beliefs and behaviors that may affect the diet.

Every ethnic group has specific food preferences that largely determine dietary intake. The practitioner needs to be aware of the staple foods in the cultural group when making nutritional recommendations. A simple but effective way of providing culturally appropriate nutritional counseling is to make up lists of foods rich in different nutrients (eg, protein, carbohydrates, and specific vitamins) that are commonly consumed by the particular ethnic group.

SUMMARY

Cultural affiliation and culturally normative beliefs and practices provide one of the inputs that an individual may use when deciding how to approach a health or illness-related matter. It is only one of many variables that account for an individual's health beliefs and practices. The culturally sensitive physician should be aware of how cultural values and beliefs may affect a person's definition of health and illness, the conceptualization of sickness, the acceptable behaviors that communicate distress, and the ways in which patients relate to the health care provider and the clinical setting. The culturally sensitive physician has the knowledge and appreciation of the normative beliefs, practices, and communicative styles that may be commonly seen in a cultural group, and uses this knowledge as subtext when working with a specific patient and family. A very important aspect of culturally sensitive health care is the appreciation that individuals act as individuals; we as health care practitioners should not base our perceptions of a patient solely on his/her ethnic or cultural heritage.

When the physician becomes aware of patient-held beliefs or practices that may be different than those we have learned in our medical education, he/she should try to find out the origins of these beliefs and practices. Often they are manifestations of a system of beliefs that are consistent and logical (but different from biomedicine). If the specific practices are harmful, the physician should attempt to replace them with culturally acceptable alternatives. If they are not harmful, we should try to find innovative ways to combine these practices with our biomedical plans. This does not require us to personally accept these alternative practices or theories of health and illness. It only requires us to be open and flexible, and to acknowledge and respect the diversity of beliefs and values that individuals may have.

BIBLIOGRAPHY

Eisenberg DM, Kessler RC, Foster C, et al: Unconventional medicine in the United States: Prevalence, costs, and patterns of use, *N Engl J Med* 328:246–252, 1993.

Guarnaccia PJ, Pelto PJ, Schensul SL: Family health culture, ethnicity, and asthma: Coping with illness, *Medical Anthropology* 9(3):203–224, 1985.

Harwood A: *Ethnicity and medical care,* Cambridge, 1981, Harvard University Press.

Harwood A: The hot-cold theory of disease: implications for treatment of Puerto Rican patients, *JAMA* 216(7):1153–1158, 1971.

Kleinman A, Eisenberg L, Good B: Culture, illness, and care: Clinical lessons from anthropologic and cross-cultural research, *Ann Intern Med* 88(2):251–258, 1978.

Pachter LM: Culture and clinical care: Folk illness beliefs and behaviors and their implications for health care delivery, *JAMA* 271(9): 690–694, 1994.

Pachter LM, Bernstein B, Osorio A: Clinical implications of a folk illness: *Empacho* in mainland Puerto Ricans, *Med Anthropol* 13: 285–299, 1992.

Pachter LM, Cloutier MM, Bernstein BA: Ethnomedical (folk) remedies for asthma in a mainland Puerto Rican community, *Arch Pediatr Adolesc Med* 149:982–988, 1995.

Putsch RW III: Cross-cultural communication: The special case of interpreters in health care, *JAMA* 254(20): 3344–3348, 1985.

Snow LF: Folk medical beliefs and their implications for care of patients. *Ann Intern Med* 81:82–96, 1974.

PART TWO

The Newborn Infant

CHAPTER 6

The Newborn Examination

David Turkewitz

The newborn examination and subsequent communication with the parents are challenging yet honored responsibilities for the physician. In the event of a healthy newborn, a physician's reassurance alleviates anxiety that might interfere with parenting. A discharge examination with the parents present is a wonderful way to assess parental bonding and assure all questions are answered. In the event of a problem, sensitive dialogue with the parents lays the foundation for the difficult decisions that need to be made.

Because the current length of stay for newborn care is between 1 to 2 days, the physician may have only one opportunity to see the newborn. The examination typically is accomplished within 5 minutes. To develop a high level of efficiency and competency, the practitioner should have a set routine with little room for deviation. The range of normal findings needs to be appreciated, and the physician should never feel uncomfortable asking a colleague for a second opinion. All major or minor malformation should be recorded because single or multiple findings may point to a genetic or environmentally acquired syndrome.

HISTORY

Printed, standardized check sheets are helpful in obtaining a complete prenatal and perinatal history. Key maternal data includes medical background, previous obstetrical history and current pregnancy details such as infections, drug use, vaginal bleeding, premature labor, gestational dates, glucose control, hypertension, cigarette or alcohol consumption, timing of membrane rupture, stages of labor, fetal heart rate and relationship to contractions, and type of delivery and presentation. Newborn details include status of the newborn, presence or absence of resuscitative efforts, and reviewing the Apgar score. The Apgar score is based on rating the newborn's color, cry, tone, reflex irritability, and heart rate at 1 and 5 minutes. Depressed Apgar scores are an indicator of perinatal asphyxia, prematurity, maternal drug or anesthetic exposure, or fetal conditions leading to cardiorespiratory compromise. Although the Apgar score can be used to guide the resuscitative efforts, the score does not have the prognostic weight previously assumed. Most children with cerebral palsy had normal Apgar scores, and most children with low Apgar scores do not develop cerebral palsy.

General Impression

A healthy baby should arouse easily when stimulated. At rest, the newborn maintains both arms and legs in a flexed position that reflects previous normal intrauterine positioning. After the first several minutes of life, the newborn's central color should be pink. Initial acrocyanosis is normal as is mottling of the extremities. Breathing should be effortless. Respiratory rates that are either too fast or too slow require urgent evaluation. The latter accompanied by cyanosis is indicative of impending cardiorespiratory failure.

Vital Signs

A normal heart rate range for newborns is 120 to 160 beats per minute, although lower heart rates in as low as the 80s can be seen in resting newborns, and heart rates of 180 to 200 can be seen when stimulated. Systolic blood pressures range from 60 to 90 mm of mercury. Respiratory rates are normally between 30 to 60 breaths per minute. Once stabilized, the newborn's temperature range is normally between 36.5 to 37.5° C. Any deviation of an infant's vital signs from normal should prompt the clinician to search for an explanation and initiate treatment once the etiology is determined. Although overbundling can cause temperature elevation over 38° C, this can be easily corrected by retaking the temperature after a short period of being unbundled.

GESTATIONAL AGE AND GROWTH ASSESSMENT

Gestational age is estimated by maternal date of conception and a review of specific examination parameters. By definition, a term infant is between 38 to 42 weeks gestational age. One of the initial gestational age assessment tools was the Dubowitz score. This system graded an array of physical and neurologic parameters and was divided into two parts: external signs (*eg*, edema, skin opacity, lanugo, ear firmness) and neurological signs (*eg*, posture, ankle dorsiflexion, arm recoil, scarf sign, ventral suspension). The new Ballard score both simplified and extended the utility of the previous scoring systems to include extremely premature infants. The physical as-

sessment portion of the Ballard score is based on skin (friable and transparent to leathery and wrinkled); lanugo (none to plentiful); plantar surface (no creases to creases over entire sole); breast bud (imperceptible to raised areola with stippling surrounding the nipple); eye/ear (lids fused to open eyes and soft to stiff earlobe cartilage); and genitalia (male—flat to pendulous scrotum with deep rugae, female—prominent clitoris and visible labia minora to labia majora covering much of the clitoris and all the labia minora). The neurologic portion assesses truncal and extremity neuromuscular tone.

Once the gestational age is determined, the examiner graphs the height, weight, and head circumference on standardized newborn growth tables. If a newborn is small for gestational age (SGA), the practitioner should search for causes of intrauterine compromise such as congenital infection, maternal illness, malnutrition, or cigarette or alcohol abuse. A large for gestational age (LGA) newborn is most commonly due to maternal hyperglycemia but could also be due simply to a familial large size predisposition or an uncommon endocrine condition such as neonatal hyperinsulinemia. Marked microcephaly suggests a central nervous system malformation or a congenital infection from cytomegalovirus. Macrocephaly with or without a bulging fontanelle usually suggests hydrocephalus.

The Skin

A newborn's skin should be pink and warm to the touch. Translucent skin is seen with prematurity, and thickened, peeling skin is a sign of postmaturity. Fine body hair noted on the shoulders, forehead, and lower back is called *lanugo*. The amount of lanugo peaks around 38 weeks gestation and by 1 month of age, most lanugo is gone. Bruising and petechiae may be seen on the newborn's presenting part or when the delivery is assisted by either forceps or vacuum extraction. Diffuse or localized unexplained purpura requires evaluation for infection or a bleeding disorder.

Birthmarks can be detected on nearly every newborn, and the overwhelming majority are benign. The nevus simplex, a flat capillary hemangioma, is the most common vascular nevus and can be located on the nape of the neck, scalp, forehead, eyelids, and nasal bridge. This should be distinguished from the nevus flammeus, which does not fade with aging and is

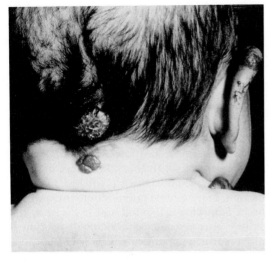

FIG 6-1
Capillary hemangioma.

associated with visceral and nervous system vascular malformations. Raised vascular hemangiomas are commonly referred to as *strawberry hemangiomas.* These present as flat, faint telangiectasias in the newborn period and do not become palpable until after a few weeks of age (Fig. 6-1). Mongolian spots are common in dark-skinned newborns and are usually located on the buttocks, lower back, and thighs. Despite similar blue coloration, these should not be confused with the cutaneous findings of child abuse. Congenital pigmented and sebaceous nevi are seen in approximately 0.5% to 2% of newborns. These should be carefully noted because factors such as appearance, size, and location determine whether diagnostic referral and excision may be needed.

There are several transient skin eruptions particular to the newborn. Erythema toxicum is an erythematous, macular, papular, and occasionally vesiculopustular eruption, which is a nearly universal finding in lightly pigmented children. The onset occurs within the first few days of life, and the rash is gone by a week. If vesicles or pustules predominate, evaluation may be indicated to rule out infectious etiologies such as candida or staphylococcus infection. Transient neonatal melanar pustulosis is rare in caucasians and is more common in dark-skinned newborns. The vesicles are very superficial and are typically unroofed with the first bathing, leaving a tran-

sient, fine scale and dark pigment at the site. Milia are small, white-tipped papules usually located on the nasal bridge, cheeks, or chin.

Jaundice is the cutaneous manifestation of hyperbilirubinemia. As the bilirubin concentration rises, jaundice progresses in a cephalad to caudal direction. Generally in light-skinned babies, bilirubin values of 5, 8, 12, 15, and above 20 mg/dL, respectively, correspond to jaundice involving the face, upper chest, lower chest and abdomen, proximal extremities, and distal extremities.

HEAD AND NECK

The head should be assessed for size and shape. The diamond-shaped anterior fontanelle should be open 1 to 4 cm on each side of the midline and depressed. The posterior fontanelle is smaller and may be closed at birth. A distinct ridge at the suture line indicates an overriding bone, which is usually caused by molding. This condition resolves promptly with postnatal head growth and must be distinguished from craniosynostosis, an early fusion of suture lines, which may require neurosurgical intervention. The degree and number of synostotic sutures can be predicted by the head shape. A demarcated swelling over the head scalp that does not cross suture lines usually represents a subperiosteal bleed called a *cephalhematoma.* A caput succedaneum is an area of soft-tissue edema of the scalp, which can be differentiated from cephalohematomas by the location across suture lines and the resolution within days.

The eyes should be examined for size, shape, and orientation. Epicanthal folds and a relatively flat nasal bridge can give the appearance of pseudostrabismus. An upward slant to the palpebral fissure is common in Down syndrome, whereas a downward slant may be seen with fetal alcohol syndrome. Conjunctival injection or discharge may be due to an infection or irritant reaction to topical agents such as silver nitrate. Small subconjunctival hemorrhages are common and not a concern. The ophthalmoscope should be used to determine the presence of the red reflex bilaterally to screen for congenital problems of the lens, cornea, and retina. Visual acuity of the newborn is approximately 20/600. The examiner should note the newborn's ability to transiently maintain eye fixation on close objects.

The size, shape, and orientation of the auricles should be noted. Malformations and malposition of the ear and periauricular skin tags are associated with renal anomalies and hearing deficits. An otoscopic examination adds little information and is not obligatory unless external abnormalities are evident.

Because newborns are preferentially obligate nose breathers, obstruction of the nares in the newborn period presents with respiratory distress. In particular, a newborn who is pink when crying and cyanotic when not suggests choanal stenosis or atresia. This condition can be evaluated by gently passing a lubricated 5- or 8-French catheter down each naris.

The oral cavity should be inspected and palpated for clefts and submucosal defects. At the junction of the soft and hard palates, there may be small inclusion cysts called *Epstein pearls*. Natal teeth are unusual and are either due to the presence of defective dental buds or premature eruption of otherwise normal primary dentition. Defective dentition has shallow roots and should be removed to eliminate the risk of aspiration.

The neck should be examined for masses and range of motion. Congenital torticollis represents a head tilt caused by shortening of the sternocleidomastoid muscle. This condition is commonly associated with deformational orthopedic problems such as tibial torsion and metatarsus adductus along with rare abnormalities of the cervical spine. Lymph nodes are not palpable in the newborn and if found suggest congenital infection. A cystic hygroma is a congenital lymphatic malformation found in the neck region. This lesion presents as a boggy swelling with poorly defined margins, and an infant with this condition requires specialty referral.

CHEST AND CARDIOVASCULAR EXAMINATION

The chest of the newborn should be inspected, palpated, and auscultated. The clavicles should be without bony irregularities. A paucity of movement of either arm is a clue to a possible clavicular fracture on the side. Engorgement of the breast bud is a transient, physiologic condition. Chest motion should be symmetric with each respiration. Asymmetric motion suggests an abnormality such as pneumothorax, cystic malformation of the lung, or diaphragmatic hernia. The latter condition may be associated with a scaphoid abdomen. No rales, wheezes, or rhonchi should be heard.

The examiner should be able to distinguish the first heart sound, splitting of the second heart sound, and the presence or absence of murmurs. Benign murmurs are usually located at the left lower sternal border and are rarely greater than 2/6 intensity. These murmurs do not radiate widely, and upper and lower extremity pulses should be easily palpable. Murmurs over the precordium should be distinguished from the murmur of peripheral pulmonic stenosis, which has a faint blowing sound and is heard in the axillas. Any murmur associated with cardiorespiratory distress, unexplained cyanosis, poor perfusion, weak pulses, feeding difficulties, auscultory findings different than the benign murmur, or ill appearance mandates prompt investigation and referral to a pediatric cardiologist. Unfortunately, the presence of a normal chest radiograph and electrocardiogram does not ensure the absence of life-threatening congenital heart disease.

ABDOMEN

The abdomen should be soft and protuberant. The umbilical stump is examined prior to or immediately after clamping the cord for the presence of two arteries and one vein. The arteries can be distinguished by the thicker muscular wall. Excessive fullness of the cord can be seen with an omphalocele, a midline defect in the abdominal wall. Umbilical hernias are common, and almost all resolve within the first years of life. The liver edge may be palpable 1 to 2 cm below the costal margin. The spleen tip usually cannot be felt. Any abdominal masses need to be evaluated, and approximately 50% of these masses are renal in origin. The rectum should be examined to ensure patency and normal placement.

GENITALIA

The female newborn has a predominately large clitoris. Hymenal tissue is always present and is usually redundant. Hymenal tags are normal. A white mucoid discharge is often noted, which resolves within the first 2 weeks of life. In the

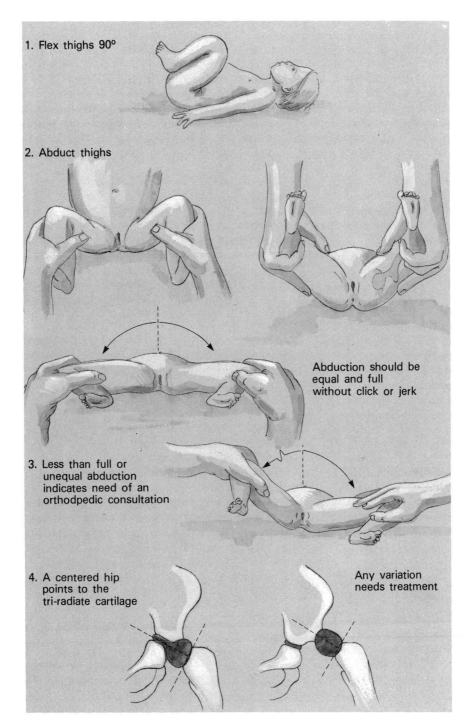

1. Flex thighs 90°

2. Abduct thighs

Abduction should be
equal and full
without click or jerk

3. Less than full or
unequal abduction
indicates need of an
orthodpedic consultation

4. A centered hip
points to the
tri-radiate cartilage

Any variation
needs treatment

FIG 6-2
Examination of an infant for a congenital dislocated hip.
Correct placement of the thumb and finger, overlying the
head of the femur during abduction, should be noted.

male newborn, both testes should be palpable within the scrotum. Scrotal fullness, either unilateral or bilateral, is usually due to a hydrocele, a persistent fluid collection caused by a patent processus vaginalis. If fullness is also found overlying the superficial ring in the lower inguinal area, an inguinal hernia should be suspected and an attempt should be made to reduce the scrotal sac. The scrotum should also be carefully examined to note the presence or absence of testicles of proper size and consistency. The penis should be examined for presence of hypospadias and a chordee on the ventral portion of the shaft. If present, consultation with a urologist or pediatric surgeon is mandatory prior to circumcision.

EXTREMITIES

All joints should have a full range of motion, and no fixed deformities should be noted. Bowing of the legs and flexible metatarsus varus of feet are both common findings and are due to intrauterine constraint. Neither condition requires referral. The hands and feet should be checked for supernumery digits and syndactyly. Due to the frequency of hip dysplasia and the deleterious consequences of delayed diagnosis, examination of the hips is critical. In the Ortalani maneuver, the infant's thighs are flexed to a right angle position and fully abducted. Each hip should be examined separately, while the other hand stabilizes the pelvis. If the hip is dislocated, the examiner will feel a clunk as the hip settles back into the acetabulum. This maneuver should be

followed by abducting each flexed thigh, while pressure is applied along the long axis of the femur in the direction of the posterior lip of the acetabulum. If a clunk is felt, the hip can be subluxed or dislocated (Fig. 6-2). If either maneuver is positive, orthopedic consultation is mandatory. Asymmetry of creases and shortening of the affected limb are not useful signs in the neonatal period to assess hip dislocation.

NEUROLOGIC SYSTEM

The newborn should arouse easily when stimulated. Stimulation typically produces extension of both the arms and legs. When held in ventral suspension, the newborn is capable of maintaining momentary head and leg extension before fatiguing. The newborn's muscular tone should provide some resistance to movement. Floppiness or hypotonia and excessive tightness or hypertonia are abnormal and may result from wide-ranging etiologies such as direct central nervous system injury, asphyxia, metabolic causes, and infectious disease. Persistent clonus often accompanies hypertonic conditions.

SUMMARY

The newborn examination requires a thorough yet time-efficient approach. Through attention to routine and examination details, the physician can accomplish this task and provide the parents with appropriate anticipatory guidance and the newborn with timely intervention if needed.

BIBLIOGRAPHY

Alper J, Holmes LB, Mihm MC: Birthmarks with serious medical significance: Nevocellular nevi, Sebaceous nevi, and multiple cafe au lait spots, *J Pediatr* 95:696, 1979.

Aronsson DD, Goldberg MJ, Kling TF, Roy DR: Developmental dysplasia of the hip, *Pediatrics* 94:201, 1994.

Ballard JL, Novak KZ, Driver M: A simplified score for assessment of fetal maturation of newly born infants, *Pediatrics* 95:769, 1979.

Constantine NA, Kraemer HC, Kendall-Tackett MA, et al: Use of physical and neurologic

observations in assessment of gestational age in low birth weight infants, *J Pediatr* 110:921, 1987.

Dubowitz LMS, Dubowitz V, Goldberg C: Clinical assessment of gestational age in the newborn infant, *Pediatrics* 77:1, 1970.

Hoyme HE: Minor malformations significant or insignificant? *Am J Dis Child* 141:947, 1987.

Jorgenson RJ, Shapiro SD, Salinas CF, Levin LS: Intraoral findings and anomalies in neonates, *Pediatrics* 69:577, 1982.

Lieberman A, Carmi R, Bar-Ziv Y, Karpus M: Congenital nasal stenosis in newborn infants, *J Pediatr* 120:124, 1992.

Nelson KB, Ellenberg JH: Antecedents of cerebral palsy: Multivariate analysis of risk, *N Engl J Med* 315:81, 1986.

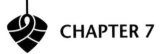

CHAPTER 7

Problems of Newborn Care

Thomas A. Curry

Health supervision of the infant less than 1 year of age requires the ability to separate specific disease entities from everyday occurrences that are variations or minor deviations from normal.

Many needless diagnostic studies and therapeutic trials have resulted from the physician's overreaction to the infant who regurgitates after feeding, has difficulty passing a bowel movement, or is awake all night crying. However, each symptom requires a thoughtful approach because it may be the harbinger of a significant medical problem. The communication of information to the family in a manner that lessens anxiety and improves parental confidence is a challenge.

The following is a discussion of problems (listed in alphabetical order) that are frequent topics of concern at the time of a health supervision visit.

CAROTENEMIA

A common concern in infant health care is a deep yellow coloration of the infant's skin. On occasion, a family member associates this development with neonatal jaundice, which can produce a great deal of anxiety for the family.

On physical examination, the skin has a distinct yellow appearance, without evidence of scleral icterus. The dietary history reveals inges-

tion of foods containing carotenoids over a prolonged period of time. These foods include carrots and squash.

The coloration of the skin is harmless and does not require treatment. The color lessens after a change in dietary intake is accomplished.

CRYING AND GAS

The crying, fussy, gassy infant is a frequent source of anxiety to parents, extended family, and consequently to the primary care physician.

Causes of Recurrent Pain

- Feeding problems
    Technique (too much air, nipple inappropriate)
    Volume of feeding
    Breast-feeding and technique
- Problems related to gastrointestinal (GI) tract
    Reflux
    Constipation
    Allergy to milk
- Head or neck
    Mental retardation
    Otitis media
    Eyes (glaucoma, abrasion)
    Ears (infection, deafness)
- Abdomen (hernia, intussusception, torsion testicles, fissure)

- Extremities (fracture, ingrown toenails, hair strangulation)
- Urinary tract
    Infection
    Obstruction

The fact that infants have fussy periods and that the symptom complex of colic develops in some has resulted in a number of folk and traditional remedies for the situation. The number of approaches in itself is testament to the inadequacy of the treatment methods.

Colic is an infant's episodic fussiness or crying (after the immediate newborn period) that is persistent over hours and days and that does not respond to simple comforting measures. During the episode, the infant will cry as if in pain and pull up the legs. Often the abdomen will be hard. Occasionally, relief is evident with passage of flatus. The attack may last for hours. Treatment of colic is discussed in Chapter 9.

A detailed history is valuable in conveying to the family the physician's earnestness in dealing with the problem. Important points include family history of colic, review of birth history, feeding history (including rate of flow from the nipple), formula changes, technique of burping, and stool pattern. Social history should focus on current family stress regarding the newborn, parents' relationship, financial problems, health problems, and expectations of the infant. This is an important time to find out if the mother is fatigued physically and emotionally, if she has free time, and how much help is available to her.

A complete physical examination should be performed. Points to be emphasized include: central nervous system (CNS), ears, eyes, mouth (dentition), abdomen (hernia, intussusception), extremities (fracture), and rectum. Announcing several times during the examination that the results of the physical examination are normal helps build the confidence of the parents.

If the history and physical examination, including review of growth to date, fail to point to any of the suggested causes of crying in infancy, little in the way of laboratory studies is required. Some physicians would insist that a urinalysis and a urine culture be obtained.

There are a number of infants who have periodic fussiness that does not fit the definition of colic. These infants do not meet the parental or extended family concept of the "good" baby. Familiarity with the literature in regard to infant temperament is very helpful in reassuring parents that the pattern of behavior with which they are dealing is not a sign of disease (see Chapter 10). Reassurance that the crying or gassy infant's symptoms are not beyond the expectation of normal variation can be helpful. The family must perceive that the physician is interested and willing to take action if there is a further development of symptoms. If the physician gives the family the impression of unwillingness or reluctance to discuss the problem because of its trivial nature, little resolution of their anxiety can be expected.

CONJUNCTIVITIS

Conjunctivitis is a frequent problem during the first year of life. Symptoms that appear in the nursery immediately after the instillation of chemical drops or antibiotic must be distinguished from infection that occurs during the first few days of life. Gonorrheal ophthalmia produces a profuse, purulent discharge with lid swelling. It occurs during the first week of life. Gonorrheal ophthalmia may be delayed by the use of silver nitrate or antibiotic ointments in the nursery.

Infections that occur after the infant is discharged from the nursery are frequently caused by bacteria or *Chlamydia.* The cause cannot be assumed on the basis of the time sequence alone. Patients with infection caused by *Chlamydia* may also have a cough. If the infant has had excessive tearing preceding the development of infections, evaluation for dacryostenosis may be necessary after treatment of the infection. In the older infant, conjunctivitis in the presence of an upper respiratory tract infection should suggest careful evaluation of the tympanic membranes for otitis media.

It is frequently stated that all episodes of conjunctivitis require Gram staining (for intracellular diplococci), Giemsa staining (for inclusion blennorrhea), and culture (for gonococci and chlamydia). It should be kept in mind that this laboratory approach can be extremely expensive and may not be necessary in every circumstance if the infant is older than 1 month. The development of monoclonal antibody testing to identify *Chlamydia* may ease the problem of documenting the cause of conjunctivitis, because culturing *Chlamydia* is a difficult procedure for most community hospital laboratories.

Treatment of conjunctivitis depends on the cause. Gonococcal ophthalmia requires intense, inpatient therapy. Treatment of chlamydial conjunctivitis includes the use of oral erythromycin rather than topical agents alone. Prolonged treatment may prove to be of value in preventing chlamydial pneumonitis.

Most cases of bacterial conjunctivitis can be treated with an ophthalmic solution of sodium sulfacetamide. Explaining to the parents the expected response time and making arrangements for a return call or visit are equally important to the institution of treatment. If the condition fails to improve after 48 hours of treatment, a culture should be obtained.

The parents of an infant with dacryostenosis should be informed of the probability of recurrence. Guidelines for appropriate surgical referral vary with geographic location. Many physicians think that surgical correction before the infant is 9 months of age is rarely necessary.

CONSTIPATION

Constipation and questions related to what is perceived by parents as constipation are among the most frequent inquiries made of a primary care physician. Underlying the problem is a common misunderstanding with regard to neonatal stool patterns. The difficulty in dealing with the symptom is compounded by the occurrence of life-threatening conditions that can present as constipation during this time period (eg, Hirschsprung disease, hypothyroidism, infant botulism).

The diagnosis and treatment of constipation must be grounded in a thorough history that includes description of stool consistency and frequency. Newborns, particularly breast-fed infants, may have a stool as infrequently as once per week. If the stool is soft, of appropriate volume, and produced with moderate effort, even though it may occur once every several days, constipation does not exist.

In reviewing family history, there can be a family predisposition to constipation or a family can be overly concerned regarding constipation. If there was delay in passage of the first stool and the infant always had difficulty with stool passage, the history can be suggestive of Hirschsprung disease. Hypothyroidism is suggested by the following signs and symptoms: jaundice as a newborn, large tongue, and umbilical hernia. A history that includes difficulty with feeding such as poor suck, decreasing volume of intake, respiratory symptoms, and poor muscle tone

indicates the need for further investigation to rule out infant botulism.

Physical examination includes evaluation of growth velocity and determination of the presence of the following: jaundice; large tongue; umbilical hernia; poor head control; testing of reflexes; sensory examination, particularly in lower extremities; and abnormalities of vertebral column. A rectal examination must be performed. A forward-placed anus has been associated with constipation. Partial rectal stenosis may be evident on examination. Failure to elicit an anal wink points to neurologic defect. Absence of stool in the ampulla can suggest Hirschsprung disease. If the stool is present in the rectum, a neurologic cause is less likely.

Hirschsprung disease can be confirmed with a barium enema study demonstrating a narrow segment of colon. Rectal manometry is occasionally used in diagnosis. Findings of neither test are definite, and biopsy for presence of ganglion cells is necessary.

If a physician is convinced that no underlying cause of constipation exists, a variety of approaches have been used. Dietary manipulations may include a decrease in the volume of formula or decrease in amount of cereal. Additional fruit or water may be helpful. Administration of a nonabsorbable carbohydrate (malt soy extract) provides an improved stool pattern after the second day of administration. Although dietary manipulation is helpful in most cases, a rare patient may require use of a stool softener (dioctyl sodium) or glycerin suppository.

A glycerin rectal suppository for infants will frequently provide prompt relief of constipation. Unfortunately, parents will often resort to this technique with great frequency despite admonitions to the contrary.

In infants, mineral oil is not usually needed because it may lead to pneumonary aspiration and poor absorption of fat-soluble vitamins.

CRADLE CAP

Cradle cap, a crusted scaling area on the scalp, is a frequent finding at the time of physical examination of the neonate. It is important to distinguish cradle cap as an isolated physical finding rather than a more generalized condition such as seborrhea, eczema, and psoriasis. Inquiry should be made regarding a family history of such conditions. Other points to cover in the history

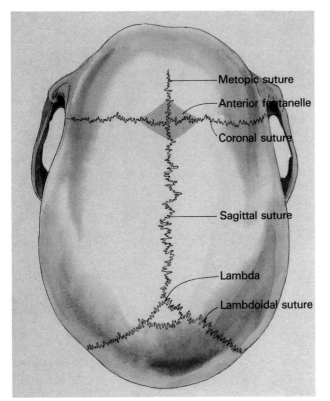

Metopic suture

Anterior fontanelle

Coronal suture

Sagittal suture

Lambda

Lambdoidal suture

FIG 7-1

Cranial sutures present in the newborn. The specific types of craniosynostosis are determined by the suture or sutures involved in the process.

include the treatment attempted by the family prior to the office visit. Some parents apply baby oil after the completion of shampooing. This practice temporarily improves the appearance of the scalp but after a period of time only leads to further increase in the amount of scaly material present.

On physical examination the oily scaling crust may be obvious or exposed by gentle abrasion with the fingernail. The presence of a rash behind the ears, on the neck, on the extensor surfaces, and in the diaper area should alert the physician that the condition may not solely be related to common cradle cap.

The major treatment of cradle cap is daily washing with a baby shampoo. The family should be instructed that vigorous shampooing is not precluded by the presence of a patent anterior fontanelle. Some families are hesitant regarding care of the scalp for fear of injuring the fontanelle. Frequently, this assurance is all that is needed to prevent a more extensive condition from developing.

When a diffuse process is present, the dry crusted material may be loosened with baby oil and gentle brushing. The oil treatment should be applied only prior to shampooing and only to aid in lifting the dried material from the scalp. Frequently, an antiseborrheic shampoo is necessary to complete the process. This should not be used routinely for shampooing but only in the initial stages of removal of cradle cap.

CRANIOSYNOSTOSIS

Craniosynostosis is the premature closing or fusion of one or more of the suture lines present in the skull of the neonate. Knowledge of the condition is important, because diagnosis when the infant is at an early age affords the best opportunity to avoid long-term medical complications related to increases in intracranial pressure and to prevent development of a configuration of the face and head that is esthetically unacceptable to some families.

Craniosynostosis can occur as part of a multisystem congenital condition such as Crouzon disease or Apert syndrome, or it may be an isolated finding. Diagnosis is suspected as a result of the specific configuration of the skull, palpation of a ridge along a given suture line, or

TABLE 7-1
Craniosynostosis

DIAGNOSIS	SUTURE	SHAPE
Plagiocephaly	Unilateral coronal synostosis	Facial asymmetry
Trigonocephaly	Metopic synostosis	Triangular configuration
Acrocephaly, oxycephaly	Coronal and lambdoidal	High, peaked, conical skull
Brachycephaly	Coronal and lambdoidal	Short, broad cranium
Scaphocephaly	Sagittal synostosis	Long, narrow cranium

abnormal head circumference. The diagnosis can be suspected at birth but may not be evident until an early well-child examination.

The myriad of terms used in describing craniosynostosis can be confusing to the practitioner who deals with the condition on an infrequent basis. The specific type of craniosynostosis is determined by the suture or suture line involved. An understanding of the condition is aided by reference to the common suture lines present in the newborn: sagittal, coronal, lambdoidal, and metopic (Fig. 7-1). Fusion of a specific suture results in growth in a direction parallel to the suture line that is fused. The resulting configuration of the skull is given a specific diagnosis: plagiocephaly, brachycephaly, scaphocephaly, acrocephaly, oxycephaly, and trigonocephaly (Table 7-1).

The urgency with which surgery must be performed depends on the involvement of multiple sutures. Some conditions mandate surgery when the infant is approximately 6 weeks of age. Other conditions (scaphocephaly) may not have implications other than cosmetic results, and occasionally parents will refuse to have surgery performed, particularly if a parent or close relative has a skull with a similar shape. Craniosynostosis in conjunction with other anomalies may require a clinical evaluation for genetic dysmorphology.

Diagnosis can frequently be confirmed with a radiograph of the skull, although a negative finding (absence of heaped-up suture margins) does not rule out the problem. Neurosurgical consultation at an early date is recommended.

DERMOID

A lump on the skull, often first palpated by a parent, needs immediate clarification to allay anxiety and begin treatment when indicated. The lesion is not always noticed at birth or as part of the newborn examination and may not be questioned until the infant is several months of age. A frequent location of palpable lesions is the occipital region; another common location is the supraorbital region, at the lateral margin of the eyebrow.

The primary differential diagnosis includes dermoid structure, lymph node, and sebaceous cyst. The location of the lesion helps to make the diagnosis. Dermoids occur at a suture line, because they are composed of embryologically derived tissue at the site where two cranial bones are joined. When a lesion is located in the occipital region, attempts should be made to define it in relation to the posterior auricular lymph nodes and the occipital nodes. A dermoid is usually midline between these anatomic markers. The dermoid has a fluid-filled consistency and is smooth surfaced; it is not fixed to the underlying structures if it is superficial to the bone. The intradeploic dermoid cannot be moved. A sebaceous cyst will frequently have a dimple present in the overlying skin.

Although many physicians will obtain radiographs of the skull to determine if there is an underlying bone defect, the absence of bone abnormalities is not conclusive evidence of the absence of an intracranial connection to the lesion. Midline lesions are particularly likely to be intradeploic.

Referral of a child with this lesion to an experienced surgical-anesthesia team is appropriate.

DIAPER RASH

Rash in the diaper area is a recurrent problem during the infant's first year of life. It is important to obtain a history of the rash and of the attempts made to care for it prior to instituting treatment.

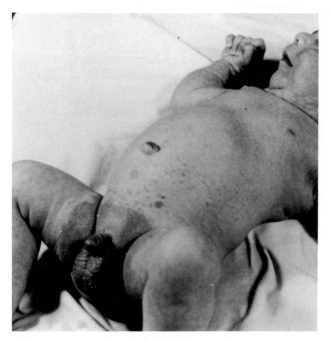

FIG 7-2
Monilial diaper rash demonstrating satellite lesions at the border of the rash.

The type of diaper used should be ascertained. Cloth diapers, washed at home and worn in conjunction with occlusive rubber pants, can frequently lead to maceration and inflammation of the skin. The use of antibiotics, particularly for the treatment of otitis media, can be associated with changes in bowel flora that permit overgrowth of fungus. Prior treatment with ointments and creams such as the use of neomycin-containing products may have exacerbated the underlying condition. Application of petroleum jelly can also lead to maceration and worsening of the condition.

Physical examination should not be restricted to the diaper area. The mouth should be examined for thrush. Evidence of coexisting rash behind the ears and on the scalp, intertriginous areas, face, extensor surfaces, and trunk may lead to a diagnosis of a more generalized skin condition that happens to be exacerbated in the diaper area. These conditions include seborrhea, eczema, and psoriasis.

Although the diaper area may have similar appearance for rashes of diverse cause, certain physical findings are helpful. A pustular eruption extending up to the umbilicus is consistent with a localized staphylococcal dermatitis. An intense red eruption with small satellite lesion or blister at the border of the rash is present with a monilial eruption (Fig. 7-2).

Treatment consists of removal of the offending agents. If diapers are washed at home, particular efforts should be made regarding rinsing the diaper of residual material. Occlusive diapering that prevents evaporation of moisture from the layers of material next to the skin must also be altered.

If there is extensive inflammation and weeping, treatment with a modified Burow solution applied with a soaking diaper and followed by air drying is an important first step. If a specific cause such as staphylococcal or monilial infection is evident, an antibacterial or antifungal agent is appropriate. Use of multiple-agent creams is discouraged by many dermatologists. Contact dermatitis may be treated with a 1% hydrocortisone preparation. Potent fluorinated creams should not be used because they cause skin atrophy.

Occasionally an area of extreme skin breakdown exists, particularly in the perianal region. This results in the infant crying at the time of stool passage and the contact of stool with the skin. It is appropriate to use an occlusive petrolatum only over the area of breakdown to prevent contact with stool. It must be stressed to the

parent that the petrolatum is only meant to protect the area and not as a primary treatment. A perianal streptococcal infection should be considered as part of the differential diagnosis if the rash is localized to this anatomic region.

DRUG ABUSE EFFECT ON NEONATE

The infant who was exposed to drugs in utero as a result of maternal drug abuse or addiction is an infant at risk. In addition to in-utero exposure, an infant may have continuous drug effect if the mother is breast feeding and abusing drugs. Attributing signs and symptoms in the newborn to exposure to a specific street drug is difficult. Careful clinical observation of infants born to mothers with a single drug addiction as opposed to polydrug addiction has permitted the development of defined clinical syndromes, such as fetal alcohol syndrome.

Obtaining a history of maternal drug abuse prior to delivery may be difficult. The physician need only be reminded of the pervasiveness of drug use and abuse in our society to realize the likelihood that at least some of the infants under his/her care have had drug exposure in utero. The assumption that this problem is restricted to portions of our population fails to take into account the extent to which cocaine and other drugs are viewed as recreational drugs by the age group in their reproductive years.

A physician needs to consider a diagnosis of neonatal drug withdrawal when there is a history of drug use during pregnancy and when a breast-fed infant has symptoms of drug withdrawal. The American Academy of Pediatrics Committee on Drugs has suggested the mnemonic "WITH-DRAWAL" to aid in evaluating such symptoms.

Symptoms of Neonatal Drug Withdrawal*

W = Wakefulness
 I = Irritability
 T = Tremulousness, temperature variation, tachypnea
H = Hyperactivity, high-pitched persistent cry, hyperacusia, hyperreflexia, hypertonusrhea

D = Diarrhea, diaphoresis, disorganized suck
R = Rub marks, respiratory distress, rhinor-rhea
A = Apneic attacks, autonomic dysfunction
W = Weight loss or failure to gain weight
A = Alkalosis (respiratory)
L = Lacrimation

Other symptoms of drug withdrawal include hiccups, vomiting, photophobia, and twitching.

With the widespread implementation of early discharge of newborns from the hospital, the physician needs to be mindful that although the symptoms may be present at birth or shortly afterward, definitive symptoms may not be evident until after the infant is discharged.

Treatment of a drug-addicted infant would normally take place in a hospital setting. Although pharmacologic therapy is not needed in a large percentage of infants, careful attention to caloric requirements, temperature regulation, and the changing clinical picture require initial inpatient assessment and treatment.

Hospitalization also permits the development of long-range plans for the infant at risk. Specific areas that need to be addressed include treatment of parental addiction, parental involvement in the care of the infant, and identification of social service support in the months after discharge. An infant who has been withdrawn from drugs can have subacute symptoms that last several months.

The parent who is already under stress may have trouble dealing with the irritable, difficult to console baby. The infant of the mother receiving methadone is at risk for developmental delay, neurologic abnormalities in development of muscle tone, and nystagmus. Long-term medical involvement is necessary in addition to support from experienced social service professionals.

HERNIA

Hernias in the newborn usually involve questions of the location of the hernia and the appropriate timing of surgery (Fig. 7-3). Any lump or bulge in the inguinal region deserves consideration of a surgical consultation. Indirect inguinal hernias are common in the neonatal period. Although surgery is occasionally delayed until the infant sustains an appropriate weight gain, establishing prompt surgical contact is impor-

---

*From American Academy of Pediatrics Committee on Drugs: Neonatal drug withdrawal. *Pediatrics* 72: 896, 1983. Used by permission.

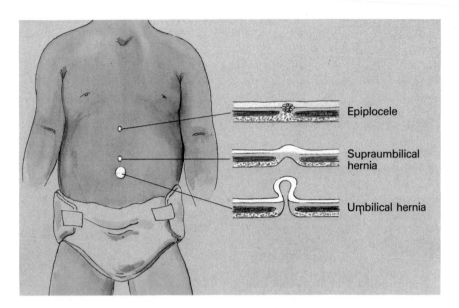

FIG 7-3
The anatomic location of midline defect in relation to umbilicus helps to determine the need for surgical cor- rection. A true umbilical hernia rarely requires early surgical intervention.

tant. Another factor indicating surgical consul- tation is the occasional occurrence of an ovary or fallopian tube at the site of the inguinal hernia in the female infant. At times parents will report the presence of an inguinal bulge that will be gone by the time the infant is examined. The parents' observation should not be dismissed, because the hernia may slip back through the abdominal wall defect. An experienced examiner can frequently palpate a thickened spermatic cord or the tunica vaginalis rubbing on itself (silk glove sign) on the side of the previously observed bulge.

Umbilical hernias are approached differently. An umbilical hernia does not need surgical clo- sure at an early age. Even large defects can close spontaneously, so observation and counseling are the best treatment. Many surgeons recom- mend waiting until the child is 4 or 5 years of age before closure is necessary. It is necessary to remind the parent that old-time therapies (such as an umbilical band or placing a coin over the hernia) are not useful and in rare cases can cause problems, particularly contact dermatitis.

Remnant umbilical structures such as a patent urachus or omphalomesenteric duct remnant may also be present. Any weeping lesion or structure with intermittent drainage or friable appearance should be considered a potential congenital rem- nant and appropriate consultation sought.

Hernias located in the midline but cephalad to the umbilicus do not close spontaneously. It is inappropriate to defer referral awaiting sponta- neous closure of these supraumbilical hernias. An epiplocele is a midline defect with herniation of fatty tissue.

JAUNDICE

Jaundice persisting or developing after the infant is discharged from the newborn nursery merits an organized approach. Many primary care physicians now perform an initial in-office evaluation of a newborn 2 days after discharge from the hospital or birthing center. The reasons for this practice are varied, but one reason in- volves the frequency with which jaundice is noted at the time of this initial evaluation.

Historical points to be reviewed include prior history of jaundice in the extended family, the ethnic backgrounds of parents, and the previous neonatal history of the child's older siblings. Details of the pregnancy including symptoms of infection should be ascertained. The perinatal history must be reviewed. If the infant was not under the care of the practitioner during the newborn period, discussion with the attending physician or a review of the nursery records is

TABLE 7-2
Comparison of Types of Hyperbilirubinemia

DIRECT HYPERBILIRUBINEMIA	INDIRECT HYPERBILIRUBINEMIA
Hepatitis (variety of causes)	High red blood cell destruction
Inborn error (galactosemia)	Hemolysis
Cystic fibrosis	Congenital defect of red blood cell
Sepsis	Resolved hematoma
α-Antitrypsin deficiency	Deficiency of glucose-6-phosphate dehydrogenase, pyruvate
Biliary atresia	kinase deficiency
Infection	Deficient β-glucuronyl transferase activity
	Type I (Crigler-Najjar disease)
	Type II
	Breast feeding
	Familial-transmitted neonatal hyperbilirubinemia
	Maternal diabetes
	Pyloric stenosis or other congenital obstruction
	Hypothyroidism

helpful. If the infant had jaundice in the nursery, a review of laboratory evaluation obtained at that time is important. If the infant is breast feeding, history should include the frequency of nursing, the use of water supplements, and the identification of the poorly feeding, excessive sleeping, dehydrated infant. Inquiry should be directed at the infant's activity level, including the level of alertness, eye contact, and response to a voice. The presence of vomiting, including the characteristics and color of emesis, should be documented. Stool and urinary patterns are also important historical points.

At the time of physical examination, documentation of weight and the change since discharge from the nursery should be noted. In addition to this documentation, the physician should note head circumference, presence of hematoma, and results of funduscopic examination (including evaluation for cataracts and chorioretinitis). The presence of rash (including petechiae), hepatosplenomegaly, umbilical hernia, large tongue, and dry skin are all points that should be covered.

The possible conditions on which the differential diagnosis is based are numerous. If the child is breast fed and if the findings of the historical and physical examination fail to point to a specific pathologic process, a less aggressive approach to diagnosis is warranted. A minimal laboratory diagnosis would include a bilirubin fractionation, and blood type and Rh typing should be done if not performed while the infant was in the newborn nursery.

The interruption of breast feeding when an infant is jaundiced and the use of phototherapy to treat hyperbilirubinemia are treatment options that have been reexamined in recent years. A full-term infant who is healthy and does not have hemolysis as a cause of jaundice may not merit extensive attempts at identification of the cause of the jaundice or vigorous treatment with phototherapy. Newman and Maisles have presented an argument for a kinder, gentler approach with interruption of nursing at bilirubin levels of 16 to 25 mg/dL and the use of phototherapy at levels of 17.5 to 22 mg/dL.

Findings of laboratory tests that aid diagnosis include results of bilirubin fractionation, hemoglobin level, leukocyte count, platelet count, reticulocyte count, blood type, results of Coombs test, and review of the peripheral smear. Liver function tests and urine tests for reducing substances should also be performed (Table 7-2).

NASAL STUFFINESS

Nasal stuffiness, usually a benign condition, is confused with an infection or allergy. Historical information helps to assess the significance of the problem. The physician should determine the extent to which the nasal congestion interferes with the infant's sleep. Does the infant wake frequently during the night? Is there a noticeable drainage at the time of waking? Does the nasal congestion interfere with feeding? Inquiry as to whether the stuffiness bothers the infant, parent, or grandparent can sometimes place the problem in perspective. Convincing a parent that a growing infant who sleeps through the night and feeds without difficulty does not need treatment of a stuffy nose takes time but may help avoid an endless round of medication and symptomatic trials.

Nasal stuffiness that occurs in the infant during fall and winter months may be related to the heating system and breathing warm air with the resultant drying of mucus in the nose. There is no drainage associated with this problem. Use of a humidifier is frequently helpful. However, if this maneuver prompts the development of mold in the bedroom or creates an increase in the dust mite population, further problems may ensue in an allergy-prone infant. On occasion, physical examination will reveal a dry mucus plug in the nares. Parental smoking, especially in a closed winter-time environment, may exacerbate the infant's nasal congestion.

If drainage has been present since birth, particularly unilaterally, consideration should be given to anatomic abnormalities such as choanal atresia. Passage of a feeding tube designed for infants will help to define the problem. Rarely is a foreign body a problem in this age group. Foreign bodies usually produce a foul-smelling discharge.

Occasionally, an infant will have persistent purulent drainage. It is appropriate to culture this material and consider antibiotic therapy for a documented bacterial rhinitis. If there is a recurrent problem, inquiry should be made regarding parental manipulation of the nares with a bulb syringe. Persistent purulent drainage should lead to consideration of an ethmoid sinus infection and radiographs of those structures.

Therapy for nasal stuffiness with decongestant or decongestant-antihistamine medication is discouraged because of frequent reactions, particularly to the antihistamine. Overuse of topical nasal decongestant results in rhinitis medicamentosus.

SEPARATION ANXIETY

As an infant approaches 6 months of age, he/she will frequently become fretful and distressed when the parent leaves. This situation is termed *separation anxiety*. Variations in separation anxiety can present in the toddler. A new or inexperienced parent will be informed by friends or family that separation anxiety is a result of "spoiling" the infant. If the parents have been warned prior to the occurrence of separation anxiety (most often as part of anticipatory guidance at the 4-month visit), feelings of poor parenting or guilt can be avoided. Separation anxiety should be discussed in terms of normal development such as sitting, crawling, and other milestones.

The following suggestions can be helpful to parents. The development of a routine is important, so that the mother and father have definite time periods away from the infant. Reassurance that they are not "bad" parents to have time away from the infant must be verbalized and occasionally emphasized. The parents of an infant who experienced medical problems in the newborn nursery must particularly be encouraged to take time out from parenting.

Frequently a routine can be set up to have a reliable high-school student stay with the infant for an hour several times a week after school or for mothers to share baby-sitting duties for infants of similar ages. This program should be followed despite the fact that the infant may cry when the parents leave.

Occasionally parents will develop routines that emphasize coming and going in excess. Overstatements that "mom is leaving now" or on her return "did you miss your mom?" only serve to underline the mother's and infant's anxiety.

Reassurance that in time the intensity of the separation anxiety will abate may be helpful. Most important, the parents should be told this is a normal developmental stage through which the child must pass. They should be encouraged to help the child work through this separation rather than to be in constant attendance and delay the child's development.

INGROWN TOENAILS

Ingrown toenails can occur during the first year of life. Some physicians believe they are seen more often when restrictive clothing (tight socks, sleeper pajamas) is worn by the infant. The condition usually resolves if the parent is instructed to avoid tight clothing for the infant and to care for the nail properly. Proper care includes cutting the nail straight across rather than on a diagonal at the outer edges and applying gentle pressure at the nail margin after bathing the infant to eventually lift the nail plate above the

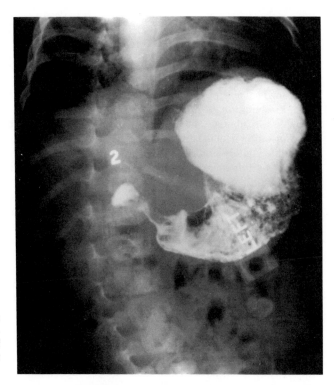

FIG 7-4
Pyloric stenosis demonstrated by a barium swallow study. The procedure must be performed with care to avoid consequences of aspiration. This study has been replaced by the ultrasound in many centers.

adjoining skin. Rarely is nail removal necessary when the infant is this age.

VOMITING, REGURGITATION

The difficulty for the primary care physician in assessing recurrent vomiting includes identifying those infants who have surgical causes (pyloric stenosis, intestinal obstruction), pinpointing those infants who require diagnostic evaluation for gastroesophageal reflux (GER), deciding what diagnostic tests should be performed and in what sequence, and avoiding unnecessary studies and consultation for the vast majority of infants who regurgitate small amounts after feeding without any underlying cause.

Causes of Recurrent Vomiting
- Feeding
  Excess air
  Overfeeding
- CNS disease
- Metabolic acidosis
- Infection
  Sepsis
  CNS infection
  Urinary tract infection
- Drugs
  Aspirin
  Antibiotics
- Esophageal reflux
- Surgical
  Obstruction (pyloric, intussusception)
  Appendicitis
- Spitting of newborn

Questions to be answered in the evaluation of vomiting include: Has the vomiting been present since the infant's birth or is it a new development? When does the vomiting occur in relation to feeding? After the infant vomits, does he/she want to be refed? What is the color and what is the volume of vomitus? Does the infant show other signs of illness?

Physical examination must include documentation of weight, change of weight, and a plot of weight on the percentile graph. CNS examination should include head circumference, status of fontanelle, extraocular movement, and presence of appropriate reflexes. Chest examination should include evaluation for evidence of aspiration such as wheezing. Abdominal examination includes evaluation for signs of obstruction and a mass lesion, and a rectal examination should be performed.

Most obstructive lesions of the gastrointestinal tract that are congenital are diagnosed prior to the infant's discharge from the nursery (eg, tracheoesophageal fistula, duodenal atresia). Pyloric stenosis can present in the infant from the first week until several months of age, although the usual presentation is at 3 to 6 weeks of age. With pyloric stenosis, the vomiting is forceful and projectile. The infant is frequently hungry immediately after vomiting. Despite traditional thinking, pyloric stenosis does not occur more frequently in first-born boys.

Experienced physicians can make a diagnosis of pyloric stenosis by palpation of the tumor located lateral to the midline in the right upper quadrant. Ultrasound is helpful in making a diagnosis. Care must be exercised when performing a barium swallow study to avoid aspiration pneumonia (Fig. 7-4).

Sepsis can present as vomiting, and the physician should think of CNS and renal infection as a possible cause.

Gastroesophageal reflux occurs commonly and has been associated with a number of conditions that include asthma, anemia, and failure to thrive. The infant vomits at any time, from immediately after feeding to several hours later. The volume varies with each episode. The emesis may be preceded by crying and irritability. A variety of studies are available, with no one study currently being used universally. The traditional barium swallow study will fail to identify reflux in many cases. Overreading and overmanipulation of the abdomen may result in false-positive findings. A milk scan with technetium is slightly more sensitive but the pH probe is presently the best diagnostic test.

Once diagnosis has been confirmed, therapy should start with small, frequent, thickened feedings and prone positioning. A mainstay of therapy for years had been upright feeding; however, Orenstein and others have demonstrated a lack of efficacy of the upright feeding. Although vomiting may persist, the patient may thrive. If growth velocity decreases, wheezing or other signs of pulmonary aspiration appear, or symptoms of esophagitis develop, treatment with metoclopramide or other prokinetic agents is attempted. Consideration of fundoplication is necessary for the infant in whom conservative medical treatment fails to control symptoms.

BIBLIOGRAPHY

Carey WB: The effectiveness of parent counseling in managing colic, *Pediatrics* 84:333–334, 1994.

Chasnoff IJ: Cocaine, pregnancy, and the growing child, *Curr Probl Pediatr* 22:302–321, 1992.

Fernbach SK, Feinstein KA: Radiologic evaluation of the child with craniosynostosis, *Neurosurg Clin North Am* 2:569–585, 1991.

Fuchs SF, Jaffe D: Vomiting, *Pediatr Emerg Care* 6:164–170, 1990.

Guarisco JL: Congenital head and neck masses in infants and children, *Ear Nose Throat J* 70:75–82, 1991.

LaVoo EJ, Paller AS: Common skin problems during the first year of life, *Pediatr Clin North Am* 41:1105–1119, 1994.

Loening-Baucke V: Management of chronic constipation in infants and toddlers, *Am Fam Physician* 49:397–406, 1994.

Newman TB, Maisels MJ: Evaluation and treatment of jaundice in the term newborn: A kinder, gentler approach, *Pediatrics* 89:809–818, 1992.

O'Hara MA: Ophthalmia neonatorum, *Pediatr Clin North Am* 40:715–725, 1993.

Orenstein SR, Whitington PF, Orenstein DM: The infant seat as treatment for gastroesophageal reflux, *N Engl J Med* 309:760–763, 1983.

Singalavanija S, Frieden IJ: Diaper dermatitis, *Pediatr Rev,* 16:142–147, 1995.

Singer L, Farkas K, Kliegman R: Childhood medical and behavioral consequences of maternal cocaine use, *J Pediatr Psychol* 17:389–406, 1992.

Skinner MA, Grosfeld JL: Inguinal and umbilical hernia repair in infants and children, *Surg Clin North Am* 73:430–449, 1993.

Sondheimer JM: Gastroesophageal reflux in children, *Gastrointest Endosc Clin North Am* 4:55–74, 1994.

CHAPTER 8

Infant Nutrition

David Turkewitz

Although recommendations on infant feeding in the not-too-distant past were predominately based on style rather than substance, current practices place a greater emphasis on a blending of art and science. This is a positive trend because the history of infant feeding practices contained periods in which the value of breast feeding was downplayed and nutrient deficiencies were common due to poorly conceived general advice, promotion of cow's milk, and inadequate proprietary formulas.

This chapter is organized into five sections: breast feeding, formula feeding, use of cow's milk in infancy, vitamin and mineral requirements, and a sampling of nutritional caveats.

BREAST FEEDING

There is a broad consensus shared by the Committees on Nutrition of both the American Academy of Pediatrics and the Canadian Pediatric Society that breast feeding is superior to all other forms of nutrition for the newborn and young infant.

Positive Features of Breast Feeding

1. Reduction in infant mortality and morbidity from sepsis, gastroenteritis, and respiratory tract infections
2. Reduction in the frequency of otitis media
3. Reduction in the frequency of food allergy
4. Promotion of positive psychosocial development through enhanced maternal infant bonding and resultant child-rearing behaviors
5. Less costly and more convenient
6. Less gastrointestinal intolerance and lower incidence of functional constipation
7. Possibly enhanced neurodevelopment

Contraindications for Breast Feeding

There are few true contraindications to breast feeding. Breast infections, if appropriately recognized and treated, are not contraindications, nor are urinary tract infections, group B streptococcal infections, or cytomegalovirus. Active tuberculosis does present an increased risk. While hepatitis B active infections pose a risk, use of hepatitis immune globulin immediately after birth, along with the hepatitis B vaccine series, greatly reduces the risk of HBV transmission. Acute varicella infection, active herpetic or syphilitic lesions around the breast, areola, or nipple are each contraindications to ongoing breast feeding.

Hints for Successful Breast Feeding

The successful promotion of breast-feeding practices requires more than a knowledge of the theoretic benefits of breast feeding. In addition, the health care provider needs the practical knowledge and counseling skills required to facilitate first the initiation and then the maintenance of breast feeding. If the physician lacks either the expertise or the time, these responsibilities can be shared with or delegated to a well-trained nursing staff and a lactation consultant.

In the prenatal period, the reasons why breast feeding is the best form of nutrition for the newborn should be discussed along with any specific family concerns and considerations. It is important to assess the availability of family and community resources such as breast-feeding support groups such as La Leche league.

Starting Breast Feeding

The newborn should be breast fed within minutes after delivery. Most babies are alert and nurse well in this period, and this single intervention has been shown to improve the likelihood of successful lactation. Use of maternal systemic analgesics and anxiolytics should be minimized.

Resolving Nipple Problems

Proper positioning of the maternal infant dyad is the single most important key to avoiding most nipple problems. If the infant's suck is painful to the mother, the infant is malpositioned or not properly latched on the areolar tissue. Use of prescreened educational breast-feeding videos can assist in avoiding initial problems by displaying proper positioning; latch-on techniques, and methods to remove the feeding newborn from the breast. The best treatment of nipple problems is prevention. Nipple shields have no role in the approach to sore nipples and, in fact, contribute to breast-feeding failure.

Patterns of Breast Feeding

By describing feeding styles to the mother, some anxiety can be avoided. Five patterns of feeding describe almost all newborns.

Barracudas vigorously, promptly, and energetically grasp the nipple. Everyone is happy.

Excited ineffectives grasp at the nipple, suck a few times, lose the nipple, and then start screaming. Quieting the baby and again offering the breast helps. Once milk letdown occurs, these babies adjust.

Procrastinators put off nursing until the milk letdown. These babies cannot be forced or prodded. These babies tend to lose up to 12% of their birth weight within the first week of life before regaining the weight and subsequently doing fine.

Gourmets insist on mouthing the nipple, tasting a bit of milk, and then losing suction on the nipple. These babies cannot be rushed, and only patience is needed.

Resters prefer short nursing periods alternating with rests. These babies also cannot be prodded to go faster.

Introducing Water

Neither routine water nor formula supplementation have any role at the beginning of breast feeding. Additional water offers none of the needed calories for the newborn. Because hypocaloric intake promotes exaggerated hyperbilirubinemia, water feedings may promote, rather than prevent, this condition.

Mixing Breast Feeding and Formulas

Formula supplementation in the first few days of life lessens the likelihood of successful breast feeding, possibly because of reinforced improper sucking techniques.

How Often To Breast Feed

Initial frequent breast feeding with the goal of eight or more times during each day facilitates maternal lactation and lessens the likelihood of jaundice.

How Babies Physically Respond To Breast Feeding

Parents also need to know that breast-fed babies initially lose more weight than their bottle-fed counterparts, urinate less, and are more likely to be jaundiced. None of this should elicit concern provided the newborn looks well otherwise, maternal letdown has occurred, and there are no feeding problems.

Hints For Breast Feeding When the Mother Goes Home

Once at home, the mother should be comfortable and well rested. If possible, household responsibilities should be delegated to others aside from the mother. Bottle feedings should not be routinely used for the first few weeks. Close support following hospital discharge (phone calls, visiting nurse, office check within a few days) is preferred. This provides early reinforcement for the parents and allows for earlier detection of problems such as dehydration, malnutrition, and severe hyperbilirubinemia.

The Difference Between Engorgement and Mastitis

Engorgement, a common sequela of milk stasis, must be distinguished from mastitis. Engorgement typically involves both breasts being warm, firm, and tender. There are no systemic symptoms. Engorgement is treated by alleviating potential nipple problems caused by poor positioning, increasing the frequency of feedings, utilizing warm local soaks to facilitate letdown, and prescribing rest for the mother. Mastitis is usually unilateral. A single portion of the breast is involved in a wedgelike distribution. That area is warm, red, and tender. Systemic symptoms such as fever and malaise may be present. Treatment includes recognizing and treating the causes of milk stasis as discussed previously and adding systemic antibiotics such as cephalexin that cover the most usual pathogen, staphylococcus.

Maternal Drug Use During Breast Feeding

The clinician should begin with the assumption that any medicine taken by the mother may possibly pass through the breast milk and be absorbed by the infant. Although most maternal drugs result in no measurable untoward effects, this does not assure an idiosyncratic or rare event will not occur.

Therefore, any maternal drug use should be closely scrutinized. The following list of drugs to avoid is not intended to be all-inclusive or absolute (in certain circumstances, the benefits may outweigh potential risks). If the clinician is uncertain, resources such as the American Academy of Pediatrics Committee on Drugs, a La Leche League representative, or local pharmacist can be contacted.

Drugs to Avoid During Breast Feeding

Drugs of abuse such as:

- Alcohol
- Stimulants
- Depressants
- Hallucinogens
- Nicotine
- Narcotics

Drugs with specific therapeutic uses such as:

- Anxiolytics
- Antidepressants
- Chemotherapeutic agents
- Antipsychotics
- Radioactive compounds used for nuclear medicine studies

Miscellaneous drugs such as:

- Aspirin
- Bromocriptine
- Chloramphenicol
- Clemastine
- Ergotamines
- Iodine-containing agents
- Isoniazid
- Lithium
- Metoclopramide
- Metronidazole
- Phenobarbital

- Primidone
- Sulfur-containing agents

Drugs That Have No Effect On Breast-Feeding Infants

- Ampicillin
- Cephalosprorins
- Erythromycin
- Furosemide
- Haloperidol
- Hydralizine

FORMULA FEEDING

When breast feeding is not chosen, formula feeding is an acceptable alternative to support an infant's nutritive needs. Bottle feedings allow others to share in the early feedings and may be more convenient for the mother working outside the home. Most commercial formulas are made from modified cow's milk with vegetable oil substituted for cow's milk fat. These breast-milk substitutes closely approximate the caloric concentration, 20 kcal/oz, and nutrient blend found in breast milk. Standards for infant formulas are set and periodically updated by the American Academy of Pediatrics Committee on Nutrition. The Food and Drug Administration utilizes these guidelines in establishing regulations that are further mandated by the Infant Formula Act. Infant formulas are available as a concentrate, powder, or ready-to-feed formula. Consumer choice is based on cost and convenience.

When To Use Formulas Made From Other Protein Sources

In addition to cow's milk–based formulas, there is a variety of formulas for infants with special needs such as cow's milk allergy, lactose intolerance, malabsorptive disorders, and metabolic diseases such as phenylketonuria. Although soy formulas are frequently chosen for presumptive milk allergy, the cross-reactivity between soy and milk protein limits the utility of this therapeutic change. Unfortunately, a wide variety of symptoms and signs such as colic, constipation, excessive gas, and skin rashes, to name a few, have been falsely attributed to formula allergy or intolerance. In particular, there is no indication in a full-term infant for utilizing low-iron formulas.

COW'S MILK FEEDING

Does Whole Milk Feeding Have a Place In the First Year of Life?

Previously, cow's milk feedings had been endorsed in the first year of life, but this practice can no longer be recommended as a reasonable substitute for formula or breast feeding. Ingestion of cow's milk in early infancy is associated with iron deficiency due to the small amount of iron in cow's milk and enteric blood loss induced by the antigenic cow's milk protein. The higher solute load of cow's milk compared with infant formula places young infants at risk for dehydration. Because cow's milk contains limited amounts of certain essential fatty acids, vitamin C, zinc, and other trace substances, nutritional deficiencies are possible. Similarly, skim milk and low-fat milks cannot be routinely endorsed. The reduced caloric concentration of defatted milk may promote overconsumption leading to excessive protein and solute intake.

Will a Baby Get Enough Nutrients From Milk Feedings?

Ad libitum intake of formula results in an average ingestion of 150 to 210 mL/kg/day. This amount supplies the caloric needs of 100 to 135 kcal/kg/day that are required to sustain the expected gains of 20 to 30 g/day in the first 6 months and 15 to 25 g/day from 7 to 12 months of age. When used as the sole form of intake, either breast milk or infant formula can meet all the nutritional needs of the infant in the first 6 months of life. In the next 6 months, continued breast feeding or infant formula is recommended along with the introduction of solid feedings.

WHEN TO INTRODUCE SOLID FOODS

Arguments for withholding beifost (solid or semisolid foods) during the first few months of life include the potential for gastrointestinal, allergic, pulmonary, and metabolic derangements. In fact, even young infants can effectively digest infant cereals—the risk of inducing food allergies is only relevant to a small group of infants predisposed to atopic disease, early solid feedings can be accomplished without aspiration, and foods can be selected with low-solute loads. This should not be misconstrued as an endorsement for the early introduction of solid feedings. On the contrary, because solid feeds offer no advantage over sole feeding with formula or breast milk in the first 6 months of life and the potential for the problems listed exists, early solid feedings should be firmly discouraged. Although anecdotes abound touting the benefits of early solid feedings to promote nighttime sleep, the literature does not support this contention.

Generally applicable recommendations for starting solids include infant older than 3 months of age; parents perceive the infant is not satisfied by liquid feedings; infant displaying clear behavioral preference for solid feedings; and formula consumption of more than 40 oz a day. Additional special circumstances include breast-fed infant with slow weight gain despite what appears to be adequate lactation and infants with gastroesophageal reflux on trials of thickened bottle feedings. Otherwise, solids can be withheld until approximately 6 months of age.

Strategy For Introducing Solid Foods

Once a decision has been made to introduce solids, a prudent approach suggests starting with small amounts, increasing the amount slowly, and adding no more than one food at a time. Infant cereals are easily digested, provide a good caloric source, and are iron supplemented. These characteristics promote infant cereals as the first solid baby food. Following this, either vegetables or fruits can be slowly introduced. Yellow and green vegetables should be added in balanced amounts to avoid caroteinemia, a benign skin discoloration due to excessive dietary carotene. Because methemoglobinemia can result from high nitrate intake, excessive feedings with beets, spinach, and collard greens should be avoided. Meats are expensive and add a relatively high protein load. Infant meats should be added after the infant is on an array of cereals, fruits, and vegetables. Yogurt is an excellent milk substitute and has an added advantage of easy digestibility due to the bacterial lactases in the yogurt. Because high sugar content may contribute to obesity and poor eating habits, dessert foods are unnecessary. There are no data to support the benefits of adding salts to infant feedings, and there is information that suggests the development of essential hypertension may be partially due to hormonal and renal adjustments to high salt ingestion in infancy. Due to the increased risk of aspiration, foods such as nuts, popcorn, raw carrots, meat, fruits with seeds, celery, fish with bones, hot dogs, cherries, and grapes should be avoided. Regardless of the type of food, infants should never be allowed to run while chewing food. The ability to handle textures varies considerably because some infants gag more easily than others and preferences vary. Most babies are ready for three feedings a day with planned snacks and finger foods by 6 to 9 months of age. The exact timing and schedule should be largely dictated by the family lifestyle.

Vitamins and Minerals

Vitamins and minerals, with the exception of fluoride, are incorporated into infant formulas in amounts designed to meet nutritional needs. In 1994, fluoride supplementation recommendations were reduced due to the increased incidence of dental fluorosis. Fluoride dosage is unnecessary in those municipalities with adequately fluoridated water supplies. Although previous controversies existed concerning the adequacy of breast milk to provide vitamin D needs, current information suggests no vitamin supplementation is routinely needed in breast-fed infants who have a typical exposure to sunlight. Because there is widespread vitamin and mineral fortification of common foods, routine vitamin and iron supplementation is probably unnecessary, but on the other hand is not harmful. The recommended dietary allowances (RDAs) are established and updated periodically by the Food and Nutrition Board of the National Academy of Sciences, National Research Council. The Food and Drug Administration utilizes these RDAs to establish the United States' RDAs, which are set to minimize the risk of specific deficiencies and excesses.

Fluoride

After 6 months of age 0.25 mg/day of fluoride is recommended for breast-fed infants and those who have ready-to-feed formulas or if the water supply does not have fluoride.

CAVEATS AND CLINICAL PEARLS

Providing proper nutritional counseling allows parents to promote healthy lifestyles for their children and to enjoy parenting. Unfortunately, entrenched rituals exist that serve little purpose aside from producing extra work with no benefit. This section outlines several commonly misunderstood caveats.

Water

Water used for formula preparation does not have to be boiled unless the water source is potentially contaminated. Likewise, utensils and bottles only need to be cleaned, not sterilized. Routine water supplementation is unnecessary for infants who are solely breast or formula fed even in the summertime.

Introducing Bottle Feeding

By introducing intermittent bottle feedings at 4 weeks of age to a previously completely breast-fed baby, breast feeding will not be compromised, and the infant usually will easily take the bottle. This allows the mother some guilt-free time away from the baby, allows the father to participate in feedings, and makes things easier for anyone else watching the baby. Although on-demand breast-fed babies are typically overweight by 2 to 4 months of age, this is not a problem. By 4 to 8 months, the rate of weight gain slows without any specific intervention.

Irregular Eating Patterns

Food jags, food dislikes, and occasional refusal to eat are common. Patience and struggle avoidance usually works best. A simple strategy that allows an infant to self-select small foods works best.

Use of Cups

The introduction of cup feedings should coincide with the infant's acquisition of good truncal control and the ability to purposefully and steadily grasp objects. These skills are usually acquired between 6 to 12 months of age. Bottle feedings are best eliminated between 9 to 18 months of age. The elimination of bottle feedings is easy provided the family is comfortable either putting or throwing the bottles away and not attempting a slow withdrawal of bottle feedings. The latter strategy often leads to prolonged confrontational infant crying. This is often the parents' first realization that rational explanations are ineffective when used as a parenting techniques in infancy and early childhood.

Nighttime Feedings

Nighttime feedings by 4 months of age are usually habitual. If the baby is gaining weight well, abrupt elimination of nighttime feedings or substituting water feedings works best.

Juices

Juices are primarily useful in softening bowel movements once solids are begun. Dietary constipation can be avoided by titrating the amount and type of juice in the infant's diet. Juices also facilitate iron absorption from sources such as infant cereals. Not surprisingly, excessive juice consumption due to its osmotic load is associated with chronic diarrhea of infancy.

SUMMARY

This chapter provides the clinician with a framework to provide nutritional advice and counseling. Through appropriate anticipatory guidance, sensitive collaborative discussions, and close regular periodic office visits, the clinician can both ensure the infant's proper nutrition and teach a parenting style that should meet the needs of each family.

BIBLIOGRAPHY

American Academy of Pediatrics Committee on Nutrition: *Pediatric nutrition handbook,* Illinois, 1993, American Academy of Pediatrics.

Beaton GH: Nutritional needs during the first year of life: Some concepts and perspectives, *Pediatr Clin North Am* 32(2):275, 1984.

Chandra RK, Shakuntla P, Hamed A: Influence of maternal diet during lactation and use of formula feeds on development of atopic eczema in high risk infants, *Br Med J* 299:228, 1989.

Cunningham AS, Jelliffe DB, Jelliffe EF: Breastfeeding and health in the 1980s: A global epidemiologic review, *J Pediatr* 118(5):659, 1991.

Dewey KG, Heinig MJ, Nommsen-Rivers LA: Differences in morbidity between breastfed and formula-fed infants, *J Pediatr* 126:696, 1995.

Freed GL, Clark SJ, Lohr JA, Sorenson JR: Pediatrician involvement in breast feeding promotion: A national study of residents and practitioners, *Pediatrics* 96:490, 1995.

Freed GL, Landers S, Schandler RJ: A practical guide to successful breast-feeding management, *Am J Dis Child* 145:917, 1991.

La Leche League: *The womanly art of breastfeeding,* Illinois, 1987, La Leche League International.

Lawrence RA: Breastfeeding: *A guide for the medical profession,* St. Louis, 1989, Mosby–Year Book.

Losch M, Dungy CI, Russell D, Dusdieker LB: Impact of attitudes on maternal decisions regarding infant feeding, *J Pediatr* 126:507, 1995.

Martinez JC, Maisels MJ, Otheguy L, et al: Hyperbilirubinemia in the breast-fed newborn: A controlled trial of four interventions, *Pediatrics* 91:470, 1993.

Myers MG, Fomon SJ, Koontz FP, et al: Respiratory and gastrointestinal illness in breast and formula fed infants. *Am J Dis Child* 138(7): 629, 1984.

Shulman RJ, Wong WW, Irving CS, et al: Utilization of dietary cereal by young infants, *J Pediatr* 103:23, 1983.

Tisacane A, DeVizia B, Valiante A, et al: Iron status in breast-fed infants, *J Pediatr* 127:429, 1995.

CHAPTER 9

Infant Colic Syndrome

Bruce Taubman

Infant colic is a syndrome in which healthy infants with normal growth and development, who are usually less than 3 months of age, have episodes of excessive, seemingly inconsolable crying for no apparent reason. The problem, which occurs in 10% to 20% of infants, can begin any time after birth but rarely before 1 week of age and in most cases improves significantly by 3 months of age. Behavior diaries show that these infants cry more than 2 hours a day, although parents almost always report that the crying lasts longer than 3 hours per day. The crying usually occurs at the same time of day, most often in the evening. During the crying episodes the infants are described as drawing their legs up, hardening the abdomen, turning red, and passing flatus. The infant often appears to the observer to be having abdominal pain.

The cause and treatment of the syndrome are controversial. Three major theories have been put forth. One theory assumes, because of their appearance, that these infants cry because of abdominal pain. Some believe the pain is secondary to increased abdominal gas and recommend frequent burping and simethicone for the treatment of colic. Others have looked to milk protein allergy as the cause of the abdominal pain. Jakobsson's group has published two reports showing improvement in a significant number of colicky infants given hydrolyzed casein formula and one report showing improvement in breast-fed infants when their mothers were placed on a milk-free diet. However, these reports included infants with vomiting or diarrhea, which would exclude infant colic syndrome as usually defined.

Those who assume that infant colic syndrome is caused by abdominal pain have suggested various medications for treating it. The only drug found to be effective in controlled studies is dicyclomine. The side effects of this medication include lethargy and sedation, and its effectiveness may be related more to its sedative action than to antispasmodic properties. There have been reports of apnea and death in infants given dicyclomine, and the manufacturer has warned against its use in infants.

Another popular theory of infant colic syndrome is that the immature nervous system in infants causes them to be extremely sensitive to external stimuli; thus the crying is nonspecific and unavoidable. Attempts to quell such crying result in further stimulation of the infant and more crying. Advocates of this theory recommend putting the crying, seemingly inconsolable infant down and letting him/her cry, thereby decreasing the stimulation to the infant. To date there is only one clinical study, by Taubman in 1984, of the effectiveness of such an approach. Six parents of colicky infants were introduced to this theory and counseled to let their babies cry when they become inconsolable. There was no decrease in crying among this small group of infants. The approach was successful in helping the parents, in that five of the six felt better after treatment.

The third major theory concerning infant colic syndrome states that the crying begins as an attempt by the infant to communicate wants and needs and continues, often to the point of extreme agitation and inconsolability when the parents misinterpret these cries and respond incorrectly.

Treatment involves counseling the parents to help them interpret infant signals more effectively by treating infant crying as a form of communication. The effectiveness of parental counseling in the management of the infant colic syndrome has been shown to be effective in several published studies.

COUNSELING TECHNIQUE

Parents of infants with infant colic syndrome present many different chief complaints, including "Our infant has a lot of gas or is gassy all the time"; "Our infant cries every evening no matter what we do"; "My baby is having episodes of severe abdominal pain." In taking the history from these parents, try to determine if these babies meet the criteria for having infant colic syndrome. It is important to be sure there are no other symptoms other than excessive crying and perhaps the association of the passage of flatus. Ask specifically about vomiting, diarrhea, or constipation. Look for any preconceived concepts of infant behavior held by the parents that may interfere with their responding appropriately to their infant's cries. Are they truly feeding on demand or are they reluctant to feed their baby freely because of concern about infant obesity? Do they have an aversion to the use of a pacifier? Are they afraid they will spoil their baby if they hold him/her too much? Do they believe infants should sleep a specific number of hours during certain times of the day?

After taking the history, a physical examination should be done carefully to discover any source of pain, such as otitis media, incarcerated inguinal hernia, testicular swelling, or a hair wrapped around a digit. A rectal examination should be done. A tight band in the anal canal can cause discomfort and crying with attempts at bowel movements. If found it can be easily dilated with the finger.

If after the history and physical examination you find the infant's symptoms meet the criteria for infant colic syndrome, the important concepts of infant crying and infant colic should be explained to the parents; for example, "It may appear to you that your infant is crying because of abdominal pain. This is because whenever babies cry, whether from hunger, sleepiness, or ear pain, they often look like they have abdominal pain. They draw their legs up, turn red, harden the abdomen, and pass gas. However, after taking a history and careful physical examination, I am sure your infant is not in pain. Normal infants, such as yours, rarely cry because of pain. They cry to communicate their wants and needs. You may think your infant's crying is inconsolable. This is because infant cries can be difficult to interpret. Some infants become so agitated after crying a good while that no response can calm them."

If the parents find these concepts difficult to accept, as many do, completion of a 72-hour behavior diary with precoded 12-hour diary sheets is helpful. They record the time each activity begins and ends, adding any relevant comments. The following list suggests codes to be used in recording the diary.

ACTIVITY CODE
    S = Sleeping alone (not held)
  SH = Sleeping held
   F = Feeding
AAH = Awake, alone, and happy (not held; in crib, infant seat, swing)
AAC = Awake, alone, and crying
AHH = Awake, held, and happy
AHC = Awake, held, and crying
   B = Bathing

The diary allows you to quantitate the amount of crying and can be used to monitor treatment. It is difficult to get accurate information about the circumstances of the infant crying and the parental response to it by talking to the parents. The diaries give you this information. You can determine whether the parents assume all crying is pain related and only respond by walking the baby. It can be determined how much time the parents allow the infant to cry before responding. The type of responses the parents try, in what order, and how logical these responses are can also be evaluated.

After reviewing the behavior diary it is necessary to meet again with the parents and go over the information with them. For example, "Your infant is really crying a lot. Most infants cry 1 to 1½ hours a day, and your infant is crying 3 hours a day. By responding differently to the baby, we can decrease the crying significantly." The parents are instructed to assume that crying is communication and try one of five responses: feeding, offering a pacifier, putting the baby to sleep, holding the baby, or stimulating him/her. If one response does not work quickly, they are to move on to another one, trying to find the correct response before the baby becomes agitated. Never just let the baby cry. The primary care provider should review the diary, pointing out specific episodes of crying and suggesting alternate responses. Finally, the parents are given an instruction sheet on how to respond to the infant's crying (Box 9-1).

The parents should continue the behavior diaries and have them reviewed every 2 to 3 days until improvement is observed.

BOX 9-1
INSTRUCTIONS FOR PARENTS ON INFANT COLIC SYNDROME

Your baby's cry is the way the infant signals you about needs. When the baby cries you respond immediately and try to determine what the infant wants. The baby's cry is a signal for one of the following:

1. **The baby is hungry.**
   Many babies do not feel hunger at regular intervals. There may be days when the baby wishes to feed frequently and other times when he/she wants to feed less often. Feed the baby whenever appropriate. You will not overfeed the infant.
2. **The baby is not hungry but wants to suck.**
   There will be times when the baby does not want the bottle or full breast but does want to suck. The baby will take a pacifier readily at these times.
3. **The baby wants to be held.**
   If an infant cries because he/she wants to be held, holding will quickly stop the crying. You will not spoil the infant or make it a habit. If the baby continues to cry while being held, try something different.
4. **The baby is bored and wants stimulation.**
   This can be achieved by playing with the baby or putting him/her in an infant seat in a room where there is a lot of activity, such as the kitchen while you are cooking.
5. **The baby is tired and wants to sleep.**
   Try putting the baby down in a dark quiet room. If fussing, you can leave the baby alone, but the infant should be picked up if crying loudly.

You decide in what order to try these suggestions.

NOTE
1. If after trying one of these suggestions the baby continues to cry, try another. Do not persist in any one item if the infant continues to cry.
2. Before you pick up a crying baby, be sure the baby is awake and not just crying in his/her sleep.
3. If you think the baby is tired, it is all right to leave the baby alone while crying, as long as the crying is off and on and does not last more than 5 minutes.

If at their first visit the parents seem receptive to a discussion of crying as communication, an attempt can be made to counsel without the use of the behavior diaries.

Good anticipatory guidance can often prevent the occurrence of the infant colic syndrome. When talking to new parents, the concept of crying as communication should be explained. The importance of responding to infant cries in the development of a healthy infant-parent attachment should be discussed. Parents should be advised to feed the infant on demand and not to be reluctant to hold their baby or use a pacifier. They should be discouraged from just letting their baby cry. When parents report that their infant is at times fussy, explain he/she is trying to communicate some desire that has not occurred to them. They should be encouraged to be flexible in their response at these times. They can try feeding more frequently, holding the baby more, or offering a pacifier. Such advice should go a long way in preventing infant colic syndrome.

BIBLIOGRAPHY

Adams LM, Davidson M: Present concepts of infant colic, *Pediatr Ann* 16:817–820, 1987.

Carey WB: The effectiveness of parent counseling in managing colic, *Pediatrics* 94:333–334, 1994.

Illingworth RS: Three months colic, *Arch Dis Child* 29:165–174, 1954.

Taubman B: Clinical trial of the treatment of colic by modification of parent-infant interaction, *Pediatrics* 74:995–1003, 1984.

Taubman B: Parental counseling compared with elimination of cow's milk or soy milk protein for treatment of infant colic syndrome: A randomized trial, *Pediatrics* 81:756–761, 1988.

Wessel MA, Cobb JC, Jackson EB, et al: Paroxysmal fussing in infancy, sometimes called "colic," *Pediatrics* 14:421–424, 1954.

CHAPTER 10

Children's Temperaments

William B. Carey

When parents complain to their pediatrician about their child's behavior, the doctor is often at a loss as to how to proceed from that point to a mutually satisfactory solution. The first step, after briefly defining the concern and determining what kind of help the family is seeking, is usually to sort the problem into one of three major groups: 1) a true adjustment problem, involving dysfunction in one of the main behavioral and emotional areas of social competence, school performance, self-relations, or thinking and feeling; 2) a temperamental variation, such as shyness or resistance to change, which is normal but may be annoying to the caretakers; or 3) truly normal, average behavior, such as decreased appetite or resistance to parental direction around 18 months, which is misperceived as abnormal by an uninformed or overstressed parent.

Pediatricians are likely to refer the patient with definite behavior problems to mental health specialists when they do not feel able to handle them without help; they attempt to manage the misperceptions through education, reassurance, and sometimes referral of the parent for indicated professional assistance. However, pediatricians may not deal with the temperament variations as skillfully because their education generally has not included instruction in identifying these problems and in helping parents understand and cope with them. At times normal temperament variations are erroneously interpreted as parental misperceptions or, on the other hand, are regarded as real but are due to parental mismanagement or abnormalities of brain function.

This chapter aims to help the reader improve his/her accuracy of clinical diagnosis and appropriateness of handling children's temperament variations.

CHILD'S CONTRIBUTION TO DEVELOPMENT AND BEHAVIOR

In the first half of this century the field of child development was dominated by environmentalism, the belief that all differences in behavior could be accounted for by the impact of the environment in prior experiences. By the 1950s it was becoming increasingly evident that the parent-child interaction is what really matters for behavioral outcome and that the child contributes as much to this result as does the environment. The child's participation could be either through interactions of normal variations in temperament with the environment or by the expression of deviations of the central nervous system, such as those presumed to underlie specific disabilities in learning.

The concept of aberrant nervous system function has caught on readily, as can be seen in the current surge in diagnosing attention deficit hyperactivity disorder. However, despite the extensive research performed and reported in the temperament field, child health and educational professionals of various disciplines have demonstrated little knowledge about temperament and apparently seldom make use of it in practical settings.

REALITY, NATURE, AND SIGNIFICANCE OF TEMPERAMENT

Definition

By *temperament* we mean the behavioral style of the individual, the "how" of behavior, or the characteristic way the person experiences and reacts to the environment, not his/her abilities (the what) or adjustment (the why or how much). Temperament is not simply a fabrication of parents, as some academic researchers have maintained. It can be observed and measured in the office, laboratory, or home. We rely heavily on parents' reports in clinical situations and research because mothers know their children better than anyone else, and because there is as yet no observational technique that is sufficiently comprehensive to match the rich data set provided by parents. The reports of parents may be distorted by a variety of influences, but all appropriately designed studies have, with suitable questioning, given us a picture of at least moderate validity, certainly accurate enough for clinical management. Temperament is indeed real and matters to children and their caretakers.

A useful image to demonstrate the nature of temperament is the child aged 5 years who has learned to tie his/her shoes. The achievement of this skill is a normal developmental milestone for that age. Whether the child exercises this skill or prefers to have a parent do it instead is a measure of adjustment or motivation. But the child's temperament will determine how it is done. Active, persistent, and negative Albert may do it rapidly with a frown on his face. Inactive, positive Barbara may perform it slowly, singing merrily all the while. Active, unadaptable, nonpersistent Charlie may delay doing it until he has run around the house for a while. Distractible Doris may tie her shoes part way, become diverted by the fascination of passing cars, but eventually return to the job. The same developmental level and motivation can be expressed in many different ways.

Dimensions

Children can be rated according to the following nine temperament characteristics originally described by Thomas and Chess (1977): activity, biological rhythmicity, initial approach or withdrawal in new situations, adaptability, intensity of reactions whether positive or negative, prevailing positive or negative mood, persistence/attention span, distractibility, and sensory threshold (Box 10-1). The other current conceptualizations of temperament were neither clinically derived nor clinically applied.

Clusters

According to Chess and Thomas, the nine characteristics tend to cluster in several clinically significant groups: the difficult child (irregular,

---

BOX 10-1
TEMPERAMENT CHARACTERISTICS

Activity: The amount of motion during sleep, eating, play, dressing, bathing, etc.

Rhythmicity: The regularity of physiologic functions such as hunger, sleep, and elimination.

Approach/withdrawal: The nature of initial responses to new stimuli, such as people, situations, places, foods, toys, and procedures.

Adaptability: The ease or difficulty with which reactions to stimuli can be modified in a desired way.

Intensity: The energy level of responses regardless of quality or direction.

Mood: Amount of pleasant and friendly or unpleasant and unfriendly behavior in various situations.

Persistence/attention span: The length of time particular activities are pursued by the child with or without obstacles.

Distractibility: The effectiveness of extraneous stimuli in interfering with ongoing behaviors.

Sensory threshold: The amount of stimulation, such as sounds or light, necessary to evoke discernible responses in the child.

Data from Thomas A, Chess S: *Temperament and Development.* New York, 1977, Brunner/Mazel.

---

withdrawing, low in adaptability, intense, and negative), the easy child (the opposite characteristics of the difficult child), and the slow-to-warm-up (shy) child (similar to the difficult child but less intense). Because the difficult cluster is found in 10% to 15% of the population, the pediatrician can count on dealing with two or three of these "spirited" children each day, the aversiveness being expressed and responded to in various ways. The shy children are a little less numerous (5%–15%) and less noticeable because of their lower intensity.

Some other characteristics such as impulsivity have been proposed but are not widely accepted. Several additional clusters such as task orientation, sociability, flexibility, and reactivity have been suggested by other researchers. A more general term, *temperament risk factors* has been recommended to describe any temperament characteristic or group of characteristics that can under certain circumstances predispose to excessive stress and conflict with the caretakers and to specific reactive or secondary problems in the child's physical health, development, or behavior.

Temperament traits are not the same as problems in behavior or other functions, nor do they necessarily lead to them. Chess and Thomas cite that the most important factor is "goodness of fit," or the degree of consonance or dissonance between the child's temperament and the values and expectations (or the understanding and tolerance) of the caretakers. The stress generated by the incompatibility leads to reactive problems in the child and the parents. Almost any temperament characteristic may be regarded as welcome or stressful depending on the preferences of the caretakers, but some traits such as negativity or low adaptability probably have the smallest chance of being considered desirable. For example, some parents may welcome an intense child, whereas others find the vigorous emotional expression intolerable and seek to repress it.

Origins

Approximately half of these behavioral style characteristics have been shown to be determined by genetic processes, the other half arising from various nongenetic physical factors such as health status and from the psychosocial environment.

Stability

Despite the strong genetic component, these behavioral traits have only a low consistency from one day to the next in the newborn period. After the transient pregnancy and perinatal effects have worn off, the genetic influences become increasingly evident. By 3 years of age, the traits have become much more consistent, achieving moderate stability by middle childhood. These traits are never completely fixed or changeable.

EFFECTS OF A CHILD'S TEMPERAMENT ON THE PARENTS

Some children are by nature harder to care for than others. Whether or not the child is sociable or vigorous makes a great difference in the quality of the interactions of caretaking. Parents find it hard to be affectionate with infants who are consistently negative. Setting limits is not easy when the child is slow to accept and adapt to changed parental requirements. Instruction is difficult with inattentive children. Different children require different rearing strategies.

In addition to the impact of the child's temperament on the interaction, the temperament also affects how caretakers think and feel about themselves. Easy children generally make their parents feel competent and happy. However, studies have documented how children with difficult temperament influence parental mood, self-esteem, satisfaction in parenting, and spousal relationships. One study showed that marital satisfaction decreased significantly between the pregnancy and 4 months postpartum with the birth of a difficult infant but remained about the same with other infants. Pediatricians can help parents recognize and deal with these feelings if they understand the nature of the problem.

MANAGING PARENTAL CONCERNS

As mentioned previously, when parents express concern to the pediatrician about a child's behavior, it is likely to fall into one of three major categories: 1) a normal element of behavior that is misperceived as aberrant, such as thumb sucking in infants and toddlers; 2) a normal temperamental variation, such as shyness or persistence, which may be annoying to the parents but is not a deviation; and 3) a true behavioral adjustment problem involving dysfunction in one or more areas.

If the problem is one of parental misperception, the solution lies either in supplying the necessary information or in assisting the parent to find help for the personal problems that are depriving them of their ability to appreciate the normality of the child.

On the other hand, a temperament risk factor such as the difficult child characteristics may be causing an excess of friction with the parents because they do not understand it or have not learned how to tolerate it. Some simple principles guide the general handling of bothersome temperament differences when there is no behavior problem and are described below.

Assessment

When parents are concerned about the child's behavior, it is helpful for the clinician to identify the child's temperament profile. Methods commonly used are parent interviews, questionnaires, clinical observations, or some combination of these methods. Full descriptions of the currently available methods are found in several specialized textbooks as listed in the bibliography. A list of the five questionnaires developed for different ages by Carey, McDevitt, and associates is found in Box 10-2. For routine clinical care the pediatrician usually can obtain sufficient temperament information by brief, informal interviewing, but, when there is substantial concern about behavior, a complete temperament profile, which can be obtained from a questionnaire, is needed. At present, however, clinicians who are well acquainted with these issues have not recommended a routine screening of all children's temperaments at any fixed time because of the work involved, the probable lack of usefulness if things are going well, and the danger of misuse by poorly informed professionals.

Difficult Temperament

Of the various temperament risk factors one might encounter, the difficult child cluster is the most likely to provoke parental concern, to call for identification, and to require professional assistance. Several steps can help the parents in this situation.

Recognition

Recognition of the pattern by the pediatrician or other primary care person is a necessary first phase.

Revision

Revision of the parents' understanding and handling of the problem can then follow. General counseling provides them with information, perspective, and confidence. Specific counseling gives them coping skills to handle the individual abrasive behaviors better. Four books listed in the bibliography are available for parents to supplement pediatric advice.

Relief

Relief for the parents from the stress of rearing a difficult child should be recommended. It consists of various environmental interventions: mobilizing assistance from friends and relations, putting the child in daycare, taking occasional evenings and weekends away from the child, and participating in well-run support groups with parents who have similar concerns.

Referral

Referral to a mental health specialist should seldom be necessary for normal temperament risk factors such as shyness, stubbornness, and

---

BOX 10-2
HOW TO OBTAIN TEMPERAMENT QUESTIONNAIRES

Listed below are the addresses for obtaining the five temperament questionnaires constructed by the team headed by Drs. Carey and McDevitt.*

1) **Early Infancy Temperament Questionnaire** (for infants aged 1 to 4 months): Barbara Medoff-Cooper, PhD, University of Pennsylvania School of Nursing, Philadelphia, PA 19104-6096.
2) **Infant Temperament Questionnaire-**Revised (for infants aged 4 to 8 months): William B. Carey, MD, Division of General Pediatrics, Children's Hospital of Philadelphia, Philadelphia, PA 19104-4399.
3) **Toddler Temperament Scale** (for children aged 1 to 3 years): William Fullard, PhD, Department of Educational Psychology, Temple University, Philadelphia, PA 19122.
4) **Behavioral Style Questionnaire** (for children aged 3 to 7 years): Sean C. McDevitt, PhD, 11225 North 28th Drive, Suite C103, Phoenix, AZ 85029.
5) **Middle Childhood Temperament Questionnaire** (for children aged 8 to 12 years): Robin L. Hegvik, PhD, Suite 210, Falcon Building, 1240 West Chester Pike, West Chester, PA 19382.

Information on internal consistencies and retest reliabilities is available in published papers.

---

*Please send a contribution of $15 for each scale to help cover expenses. You may make as many photocopies as you wish, but any changes in wording or format must be approved by the authors.

---

low adaptability. Such consultations should be reserved for the moderate or severe reactive behavior problems that the pediatrician feels unable to help, but rarely for the temperament itself. For example, the pediatrician should help the parents cope with low adaptability but may need to recommend a referral when the interactions with the low adaptability have led to a pattern of chronic oppositional behavior.

COUNSELING FOR BEHAVIOR PROBLEMS

Parental concern about the child's behavior may be due to a true behavior adjustment problem, which may involve the child's temperament, other factors, or both. When dissonance in the interaction between the child's temperament and the demands and expectations of the environment is leading to reactive symptoms in the child's physical health, development, or behavior, the intervention should try to reduce the conflict and excessive stress in that interaction so that the secondary problem diminishes and eventually is resolved. It is important to stress that these clinical problems usually arise in essentially normal children with variable environments that are generally more incompatible than pathologic. For example, an unadaptable child may be coerced into adjusting rapidly to a complex situation, such as the arrival of a younger sibling or placement with a rigid school teacher, resulting in rebellious and antisocial behavior. The main element of the therapeutic plan would be to suggest alternative methods of management to improve the fit and restore consonance, such as making introductions to changes more gradual and providing more emotional support during the process.

The child's temperament is not a "disorder" in itself and is not changed by the intervention, but it can be accommodated more comfortably by revised parental care. If the intervention includes giving the parents a thorough understanding of the child's behavioral style, they should be able to limit occurrences of similar conflicts in the future. As children get older, they can learn to modify the expression of their distressing temperaments, such as when the shy child discovers ways to push him/herself into novel situations to avoid the embarrassment of missing desired experiences.

TEMPERAMENT'S ROLE IN PHYSICAL HEALTH

Probably all pediatricians have witnessed the interactions of temperament and physical health but may not have fully understood their extent. There are two principal types of interactions: 1) those predisposing to some problems, such as accidents, child abuse, child neglect, bottle mouth caries, failure to thrive, excessive weight gain in infants, colic, sleep disturbances, and recurrent abdominal pains and headaches; and 2) those affecting the management and outcome of other conditions, such as over- or underresponse to illness and to diagnostic and therapeutic procedures, over- and underutilization of medical care, and similarly varied reactions to hospitalizations and surgery. For example, fussy infants are likely to be fed more and to gain weight faster,

and irritable children tend to get medical attention faster for illnesses involving pain, such as otitis media. Irritable children may be given too much attention, whereas easier children may not get enough. Pediatric care providers will improve the quality of their services if they keep such important influences in mind.

TEMPERAMENT'S IMPACT ON SCHOOL PERFORMANCE

In the past decade the importance of children's temperament in several aspects of their schooling has been established, especially by the work of Keogh and Martin: 1) Scholastic achievement is significantly related to several characteristics, particularly the task orientation cluster of high persistence/attention span, low distractibility, and low activity. This relationship holds true for the whole range of the student body, not just for a special category of individuals who are having educational difficulties. 2) Teacher attitudes toward students are influenced by the pupils' temperament traits. Teachers prefer children with high task orientation, greater flexibility (high approach and adaptability and positive mood), and low reactivity (low activity and intensity and high threshold). Teacher attitudes affect their handling of students and thus probably also the students' performance. 3) Behavior and health problems affect children at school in much the same way they do at home. 4) The relationship of temperament to attention deficit hyperactivity disorder (ADHD) has not yet been satisfactorily delineated, but it appears that much of the behavior now diagnosed as ADHD is probably due to normal variations of temperament fitting poorly with environmental values and expectations at school rather than to the supposed brain malfunction.

This issue of brain malfunction overdiagnosis has been dealt with elsewhere in detail (Carey and McDevitt, 1985). Some of the problems with the current ADHD construct include a lack of coherence as a syndrome, an unclear differentiation from normal behavior, the fact that many children with the behaviors supposedly defining the disorder are functioning satisfactorily or even well, and the observation that the commonest characteristic of children receiving this diagnosis today is probably not inattentiveness or activity but low adaptability.

Teachers could begin now to broaden their use

of the concept of temperament in their daily work. When problems in school performance occur, an appraisal of the child's temperament, along with the evaluations of cognition, motivation, and achievement, would greatly enrich the diagnostic process. Pediatricians would greatly increase their skill in management of school problems if they were to include normal temperamental variations in their differential diagnosis and avoid the overdiagnosis of brain malfunction.

TEMPERAMENT IN RESPONSE TO ENVIRONMENTAL STRESSORS

Children are challenged by a variety of environmental stressors and crises, including the birth of siblings, school entry, parental separation and divorce, hospitalization and death of family members, and various natural and civilian disasters.

Several factors affect children's responses to these events, some increasing vulnerability and others providing protection: 1) the trauma itself—its nature, intensity, duration, and the degree of exposure to it; 2) emotional support—the availability and supportiveness of the parents and other trusted adult figures; 3) age and gender of the child; and 4) the child's temperament. Although not well studied, the temperament of the child, or his/her reaction style, appears to be an important but generally unappreciated determinant of the nature and magnitude of the child's response.

Professional persons charged with helping children and their families through these crises should be aware of these varied factors in children's responses and keep them in mind during evaluations and management. The clinician should try to separate out the part of the observed behavior that is typical of the child's reaction style (eg, loud screaming or silence in the face of adversity) from that which is usually expected in the particular situation. The surface display may not be an accurate measure of the real impact.

CONCLUSION

Pediatricians deal with children's temperament and its interactions and consequences throughout every day's work, but often without recognizing it for what it is and how much it matters for the child and the caretakers. When a child's temperament is properly identified and managed with understanding and tolerance, pediatric and parental care are greatly improved. Parents and children then can live more happily together, and pediatricians can rightly feel that they are living up to their potential as front-line mental health counselors.

BIBLIOGRAPHY

*Budd L: *Living with the active alert child. Groundbreaking strategies for parents* (revised and enlarged), Seattle, 1993, Parenting Press.

Carey WB: The difficult child, *Ped Rev* 8:39–45, 1986.

Carey WB: Pediatric assessment of behavioral adjustment and behavioral style. In Levine MD, Carey WB, Crocker AC, editors: *Developmental-behavioral pediatrics,* ed 2, Philadelphia, 1992, WB Saunders.

Carey WB: What pediatricians need to know about temperament, Focus & Opinion: *Pediatrics* 1:268–274, 1995.

Carey WB, Jablow MM: Your child's temperament. What it is. What it does. How to work with it (tentative title). New York, Macmillan USA, Simon & Schuster, (in press).

Carey WB, McDevitt SC, editors: *Clinical and educational applications of temperament research,* Amsterdam/Lisse, 1989, Swets & Zeitlinger.

Carey WB, McDevitt SC, editors: *Prevention and early intervention. Individual differences as risk factors for the mental health of children. A festschrift for Stella Chess and Alexander Thomas,* New York, 1994, Brunner/Mazel.

Carey WB, McDevitt SC: *Coping with children's temperament. A guide for professionals,* New York, 1995, Basic Books.

Chess S, Thomas A: *Temperament in clinical practice,* New York, 1986, Guilford.

Kohnstamm GA, Bates JE, Rothbart MK, editors:

*Books for parents

Temperament in childhood, New York, 1989, Wiley.

*Kurcinka MS: *Raising your spirited child,* New York, 1991, HarperCollins.

Porter R, Collins GM, editors: *Temperamental differences in infants and young children,* London, 1982, Pitman.

Thomas A, Chess S: *Temperament and development,* New York, 1977, Brunner/Mazel.

*Turecki S, Tonner L: *The difficult child* (revised edition), New York, 1989, Bantam.

CHAPTER 11

Primary Care of the Preterm Infant

Judy C. Bernbaum
Susan Friedman
JoAnn D'Agostino
Marsha Gerdes
Deborah Calvert

The survival of infants with low birth weight has markedly improved with advances in neonatal care. The result is a significant decrease in the mortality rate among the extremely low birth weight infants—those weighing less than 1000 g or even less than 750 g. Of 3.75 million live births annually in the United States, the number of infants who are born weighing less than 1500 g is small (45,500), and the number weighing less than 1000 g at birth is even smaller (17,500; almost 5000 of these infants weighed less than 500 g). This population comprises a disproportionally high percentage of children at risk for medical, neurologic, and developmental problems. As more infants with low birth weight enter the pediatric population, physicians must become expert in managing their unique medical conditions, in addition to monitoring their developmental progress and recognizing early signs of neurologic disorders. Routine physical examinations are usually not sufficient for such children; more time is needed in their assessment and in discussions with their parents than in those of the typically well child. Physicians can play a major role in the identification of problems early in their evolution. Their efforts can have a major effect on the prevention or further progression of a child's disabilities.

This chapter includes a review of conditions frequently encountered by physicians caring for the preterm infant who has been discharged from the neonatal unit.

GROWTH

Some general statements may be made regarding growth patterns of preterm infants. During the initial period of acute illness, there is usually some growth delay, followed by improving growth and then rapid "catch-up" growth. Most catch-up growth occurs during the first 2 years of life, and it is important to optimize nutrition during this period to maximize growth potential.

Following this period, growth rates tend to parallel those in standard growth charts. A significant percentage of preterm infants will remain less than normal weight compared with full-term children.

Evaluation of growth patterns often provides valuable information regarding an infant's well-being. Conversely, inadequate nutrition can impede recovery from chronic illness such as bronchopulmonary dysplasia (BPD). Because preterm infants are at risk for growth problems, it is important to monitor growth closely.

When the physician is plotting anthropometric measurements to determine growth percentiles, corrected ages should be used to adjust for the infant's premature birth. Corrected ages can be determined by subtracting the number of weeks the infant was born prematurely from the chronologic age. Most assessments of growth are based on corrected ages until the infants are 2.5 years old (corrected age) after which time chronologic ages are used. Growth charts standardized on a large population of healthy preterm infants are available through Ross Products. If unavailable, standard growth charts may be used.

Head circumference in preterm infants is usually the first growth parameter to exhibit catch-up gain, often resulting in a head circumference percentile that is significantly higher than weight and height percentiles. In most cases, this situation can be attributed to catch-up growth after a period of adequate nutrition. However, rapid head growth also may be due to ventricular dilation (associated with intraventricular hemorrhage [IVH]) or a head that is growing while the rest of the body does not due to poor nutritional status.

Cranial ultrasonography is indicated in any infant who demonstrates signs of hydrocephalus, such as widely split sutures, tense fontanelle, irritability, alterations in normal behavior and activity level, vomiting, or "sun-setting" (an increased amount of sclera seen above the iris caused by the eyes deviating downward). Ultrasound also should be done for an infant with a history of IVH who is demonstrating unusually rapid head growth. Conversely, head circumference that is more than three standard deviations below the mean places the child at high risk for significant developmental disability in the future.

When the weight falls in percentiles significantly lower than length or when all growth velocity decreases, poor nutritional status or malnutrition is suggested. Special attention should be paid to growth measurements at birth and at discharge, nutritional status during hospitalization, results of cranial ultrasonography, and the status of ongoing illnesses such as BPD, congenital heart disease, malabsorption syndromes associated with necrotizing enterocolitis, and poor feeding due to oral motor dysfunction.

NUTRITION

At the time of discharge from the hospital, the healthy preterm infant's dietary needs are similar to those of full-term neonates. The milk source for preterm infants after reaching term gestation (or weight of approximately 2000 g) may be breast milk, a commercial 20- to 24-cal/oz infant formula, or other special formula (indicated because of milk intolerance, increased calcium requirements, or malabsorption resulting from bowel resection). Neocare (Ross Products), a transition formula specially suited to the preterm infant prior to discharge, is now available for those infants who need slightly higher caloric density and mineral content. Whole cow's milk is not suitable for preterm infants until 12 months of age.

Increased nutritional needs are frequently encountered in preterm infants with ongoing medical problems such as BPD, congenital heart disease, malabsorption, or feeding disorders. These infants often require a 24- to 30-kcal/oz formula to maintain growth, which can be accomplished by concentrating the formula alone (up to 27 kcal/oz) or by also adding caloric supplements such as vegetable oil (8.0 kcals/mL), medium-chain triglycerides (MCT oil, 7.6 kcals/mL), microlipids (4.5 kcals/mL), or glucose polymers (2 kcals/mL). Care should be taken to maintain the proper ratio of fat, carbohydrate, and protein.

Mothers of preterm infants who desire to breast feed should be strongly encouraged and supported throughout the hospitalization as well as at discharge. The breast milk of such mothers has been found to be well suited to the nutritional needs of the preterm infant during the first few weeks of life. For this reason, pooled breast milk should not be used for preterm infants.

After the first few weeks, breast milk matures and will no longer meet the caloric and mineral (particularly calcium) requirements of most preterm infants. Commercial fortifiers (such as Enfamil Human Milk Fortifier [Mead Johnson] and Similac Natural Care [Ross Products]) should then be added to the breast milk.

Breast feeding a small preterm infant often requires increased support and expert guidance. Such teaching should therefore be initiated well before discharge if possible. If there is particular concern about ensuring adequate caloric intake while breast feeding is being established, a supplemental nursing system (such as Lact-Aid) may be used initially, filled with either pumped breast milk (with additional fortifier if desired) or premature formula. The use of such a system allows for adequate stimulation of milk production by the breast, which is not true with supplemental bottles. By the time of discharge, mature breast milk is generally nutritionally adequate for the healthy preterm infant.

If necessary, a high-calorie liquid fortifier such as Similac Natural Care (Ross Products) can be used as a supplement in a supplemental nursing system.

Solid feedings should be initiated according to the guidelines of the American Academy of Pediatrics (AAP) for full-term infants. When counseling parents of preterm infants, however, dietary recommendations should be based on the infant's corrected age, not chronologic age. Solid foods should be initiated when any one of three criteria is met: the infant consistently consumes more than 32 oz of formula per day for 1 week; the infant weighs 6 to 7 kg; or the infant is 6 months old, corrected age.

Larger infants may not be satisfied with 32 oz of formula and may need to begin solid foods as early as 4 months, corrected age. Starting solid foods before 4 months is not recommended by the AAP. The premature introduction of solid foods may lead to gastrointestinal allergy, contribute to overeating, or lead to feeding problems as a result of lack of neuromuscular readiness for solid feedings. Refer to the section on infant feeding in Chapter 8 for additional dietary guidelines.

NUTRITIONAL SUPPLEMENTATION

Multivitamins
A number of factors place the preterm infant at risk for vitamin deficiencies during the first weeks of life. Low body stores of vitamins, possible defects in absorption (particularly of fat-soluble vita-

mins), and low intakes of formula may contribute to deficiency states. The AAP Committee on Nutrition recommends that a multivitamin supplement that provides the equivalent of the recommended dietary supplements for the full-term infant be supplied to preterm infants during the first weeks of life. After the infant is consuming more than 300 kcal/day or when body weight exceeds 2.5 kg, a multivitamin supplement is no longer needed, but it is a convenient method for providing the few nutrients such as vitamin D and iron that still may be required.

For infants who demonstrate poor growth because of recurrent or chronic illness or poor caloric intake, administration of multivitamin supplements should continue. These infants may benefit from special dietary counseling from a clinical nutritionist.

Iron
Low birth weight infants are especially susceptible to the development of iron deficiency anemias because their store of iron is much smaller than that of full-term infants and is insufficient to last over a prolonged period of rapid growth. Without supplemental iron, the preterm's body stores of iron will be depleted sometime after 2 months of age rather than after 4 to 6 months of age, as in normal full-term infants. The Committee on Nutrition recommends that low birth weight infants receive 2 mg of iron per kg per day starting at 2 months of age or earlier. Sufficient iron for the prevention of iron deficiency in preterm infants can be supplied through the use of iron-fortified formula or multivitamin preparations containing iron. Infants who have received multiple blood transfusions may have some protection against iron deficiency anemias because of the high iron content in packed red blood cells, 5 mg/10 mL, but because of rapid growth rates they should still receive supplementation according to the above recommendations. Preterm infants should receive iron supplements in either vitamins or formula until they have made the transition to solid foods and are consuming adequate amounts of iron-fortified cereals.

Vitamin E
Vitamin E deficiency in preterm infants during the first several weeks of life can be attributed to several factors, including limited tissue stores at birth, relative dietary deficiency, intestinal mal-

absorption, and rapid growth. After the development of mature digestive and absorptive capacity, tocopherol absorption improves and vitamin E levels rise.

Preterm formulas generally meet the vitamin E requirements for preterm infants. The addition of a daily multivitamin supplement that contains 5 IU of vitamin E may help correct vitamin E deficiency and achieve physiologic levels of 0.8 to 1.8 mg/dL. This supplementation may be particularly important when these infants are receiving iron-fortified formula, because iron may increase the susceptibility of infants to vitamin E deficiency. Infants receiving vitamin E supplementation should have periodic serum vitamin E levels checked. Supplemental vitamin E is generally not needed once full feedings are achievable.

Fluoride

The AAP Committee on Nutrition recommends initiating fluoride supplementation at 6 months of age in full-term breast-fed infants, in formula-fed infants whose community water supply is not optimally fluoridated, and in infants receiving ready-to-feed formula. These recommendations should be followed for preterm infants as well.

ISSUES IN THE CARE OF PRETERM INFANTS

Primary Immunizations

The AAP recommends that diphtheria and tetanus toxoids and pertussis vaccine (DTP), hemophilus influenza type B, hepatitis B vaccine, live oral poliomyelitis vaccine (OPV) be administered to prematurely born infants at the appropriate postnatal age. If the infant remains in the hospital, the OPV can be initiated at the time of discharge, or inactivated poliovirus vaccine (IPV) can be given at routine intervals instead.

Recent research supports these recommendations and demonstrates that preterm infants immunized with a full dose of these vaccines at routine intervals (8, 16, and 24 weeks after birth) are capable of producing a protective serologic response. There is no need to use a reduced dosage of these vaccines. Most important, a high percentage of preterm infants demonstrate *inadequate* protection (most commonly against pertussis) if given a reduced dosage of DTP at routine intervals.

Infants older than 6 months of age with chronic lung disease, such as BPD, and their primary caretakers should receive influenza virus vaccine in areas where this virus is known to be particularly virulent. Studies have just been completed that suggest that respiratory syncytial virus (RSV)-specific immunoglobulin can prevent the serious sequelae of RSV in highly susceptible infants and is expected to be used clinically during the winter months.

Each year the Center for Immunization Practices Advisory Committee publishes updated immunization recommendations that should be followed.

Hearing

Early identification of hearing loss is key to the promotion of normal language development. Being born prematurely places an infant at increased risk for hearing loss. The AAP Joint Committee on Infant Hearing in its 1994 Position Statement has recommended that all neonates at risk for hearing loss be screened prior to 3 months of age. Those neonates identified to be at risk for hearing loss include:

1. Family history of hereditary childhood sensorineural hearing loss.
2. In utero infections, such as cytomegalovirus, rubella, syphilis, herpes, and toxoplasmosis.
3. Craniofacial abnormalities, including those with morphologic abnormalities of the pinna and ear canal.
4. Birth weight less than 1500 g (3.3 lbs.)
5. Hyperbilirubinemia at a serum level requiring exchange transfusion.
6. Ototoxic medications, including but not limited to the aminoglycosides, used in multiple courses or in combination with loop diuretics.
7. Bacterial meningitis.
8. Apgar scores of 0 to 4 at 1 minute or 0 to 6 at 5 minutes.
9. Mechanical ventilation lasting 5 days or longer.
10. Stigmata or other findings associated with a syndrome known to include a sensorineural and/or conductive hearing loss.

There are several methods available for screening for hearing loss. Because a loss of 30 dB in the 500- to 4000-Hz frequency can interfere with normal language development, it is important that the screening method selected be able to detect a hearing loss in this range.

Regardless of the results of an initial hearing screening, language development and articulation in high-risk infants should be closely monitored and a repeat hearing evaluation should be considered if concerns arise.

Retinopathy of Prematurity

Preterm infants are at increased risk for retinopathy of prematurity (ROP). Multiple factors have been implicated in development of ROP; those most closely linked include low birth weight, short gestation, and prolonged oxygen therapy. ROP is a disease of overgrowth of the developing retinal vessels and may lead to significant scarring and distortion of the retina. ROP has been classified into five stages, with the fifth stage the most severe.

Most ROP is reversible and may regress completely; however, it is important that severe active disease be identified early to minimize sequelae. The AAP recommends that infants born at less than 35 weeks' gestation or who weighed less than 1800 g and required supplemental oxygen be screened for ROP prior to discharge or at 5 to 7 weeks of age if still hospitalized. Infants born at less than 30 weeks' gestation or who weigh less than 1300 g should be examined regardless of oxygen exposure. The schedule for further evaluation is generally determined by the ophthalmologist who examines the infant. Several methods for minimizing sequelae of severe ROP, such as cryotherapy and laser therapy, are available for use by the ophthalmologist if ROP is identified early.

Infants with ROP are at a greater risk for refractive errors as well as more severe sequelae depending on the severity of ROP. For this reason, the preterm infant with previously diagnosed ROP requires close ophthalmologic follow-up throughout life.

Rickets

Very low birth weight infants, those requiring long-term parenteral alimentation, those with prolonged treatment with furosemide, those with gastrointestinal malabsorption, those with cholestatic liver disease, and those with fat malabsorption are at increased risk for rickets. Rickets also has been reported in breast-fed preterm infants who did not receive vitamin and mineral supplementation.

Routine monitoring of serum calcium, phosphorous, and alkaline phosphatase levels, and if abnormal, periodic examination of bone radiographs, will allow early detection of this condition in infants with one or more of these risk factors. Screening should be done once the infant is on full enteral feedings (or earlier) and repeated before discharge.

Prevention of rickets consists of providing adequate dietary calcium and vitamin D through the use of premature infant formulas with the addition of 10% calcium gluconate and phosphorus as needed. Supplementation with 400 IU/day of vitamin D is also recommended. Treatment of rickets consists of first correcting any calcium and phosphorus deficiencies (and magnesium also, if low), followed by vitamin D at a dose of 1000 to 2000 IU/day for 6 to 8 weeks.

Nephrocalcinosis

Renal calcification is increasingly recognized as a complication in preterm infants, especially those with extremely low birth weight and those receiving diuretic therapy with furosemide, which increases calcium excretion through the immature kidneys. Screening for nephrocalcinosis includes evaluation for microscopic hematuria. If this screen is abnormal, abdominal ultrasonography to document the presence of calcifications is warranted. If confirmed, the need for diuretics should be reconsidered and altered if current therapy includes furosemide. If furosemide cannot be discontinued, chlorothiazide should be added to decrease calcium excretion in the urine. Follow-up ultrasound studies are suggested to document any progression or regression. Documentation of any renal stones should prompt screening for urinary tract infections as well as referral to a nephrologist if infection is found.

Periventricular Leukomalacia

Ischemic injury of the periventricular white matter can lead to the development of periventricular leukomalacia (PVL). The presence of a watershed area between the end zones of the cerebral arterial supply in the immature brain places the preterm infant at risk for PVL. Depending on the location of the PVL, whether or not cysts are present, and the size of any cysts still present, the child with PVL may be at a significantly increased risk for the development of cerebral palsy, developmental delay, and, in some instances, visual impairment.

Infants in whom PVL is suspected should have close neurodevelopmental follow-up. Serial ultrasonography is recommended in infants in

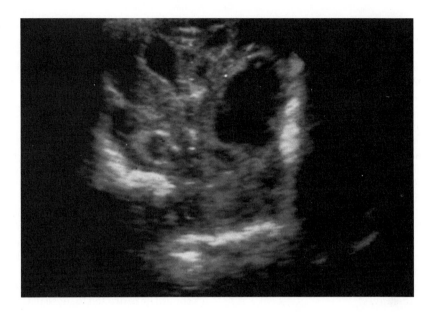

FIG 11-1
Ultrasound study of the head of an infant shows large residual cystic lesions resulting from periventricular leu- komalacia. These were not evident on initial ultrasono- grams obtained during the early neonatal period.

whom PVL is suspected, because cystic changes can develop several weeks to months after the initial insult (Fig. 11-1).

Feeding Problems

Although most feeding problems in the preterm infant population occur during the neonatal pe- riod, many infants exhibit long-term or recurrent problems in both sucking and swallowing. The cause of these feeding problems is often multi- factorial. Delayed onset of oral feedings may lead to immature oral motor skills. Abnormal oral motor reflexes and/or low oral muscle tone may cause feeding difficulties. Abnormal (aversive) behavioral responses to feeding may result from negative experiences (such as intubation and suctioning) during the neonatal period. Under- lying illness such as BPD or congenital heart disease may cause easy tiring or oxygen desatu- ration with feedings. Finally, refusal to continue a feeding may occur because of discomfort from gastroesophageal reflux.

All of these problems are amenable to therapy if they are properly identified and appropriate intervention is begun. Depending on their train- ing, either a pediatric speech pathologist or oc- cupational therapist can develop a feeding pro- gram that would be most appropriate once a particular feeding problem is identified. Man-

agement of any underlying lung disease or con- genital heart disease should be optimized, and evaluation for gastroesophageal reflux should be considered.

Gastroesophageal Reflux

Although not unique to preterm infants, gastro- esophageal reflux is more common in the prema- ture population; the presentation and therapy for preterm infants is similar to that described for full-term infants. However, it is important to remember that gastroesophageal reflux occasion- ally may be associated with apnea and should be considered in an apnea work-up. It also should be considered in the infant who exhibits poor oral feeding, aspiration pneumonia, worsening pul- monary status, and irritability with no apparent cause.

Apnea

Apnea in premature infants is most likely caused by the immature brain failing to trigger automatic breathing. Bradycardia often accompanies the apnea. Use of a pneumogram or thermistor, with a 12- to 24-hour recording of heart rate and respiratory rate variability, will often document the presence of apnea and bradycardia and help determine the appropriate therapeutic interven- tion.

Although apnea usually originates in the central nervous system, the acute onset or increase in frequency of apnea should warrant further investigation. Conditions such as infection, IVH, and anemia commonly have apnea as their initial sign. Apnea also may be associated with gastroesophageal reflux in some infants.

The mainstay of therapy for apnea of prematurity is theophylline or caffeine, pharmacologically similar agents that are both central stimulants. Some infants may require continued therapy even after initial hospital discharge. Preterm infants, as they mature neurologically, normally "outgrow" apnea and bradycardia. Theophylline or caffeine levels should be monitored, however, and maintained at therapeutic levels if central nervous system–induced apnea persists. Often an infant will require home cardiorespiratory monitoring in addition to or in lieu of drug therapy.

The need for monitoring or medication is usually determined prior to the infant's initial hospital discharge. It is the physician's task to decide when it is appropriate to withdraw either therapy. Some general principles should be followed. At least 1 month should elapse after the infant's discharge before theophylline or caffeine is withdrawn. If the infant is being monitored at home and no episodes of apnea or bradycardia occur, then the infant should be allowed to "outgrow" the medication by not increasing the dosage as the baby's weight increases. If episodes of apnea persist or increase in frequency, the theophylline or caffeine dosage can be increased after other possible causes have been evaluated.

Once medication has been discontinued in the infant who is being monitored, 1 to 2 months with no monitor alarms or episodes of apnea should elapse before obtaining a pneumogram. Most often the pneumogram can be performed at home. Interpretation of results should help to determine any further monitoring needs. The majority of infants have no medication or monitoring needs beyond 6 months, adjusted age.

Bronchopulmonary Dysplasia

Many preterm infants have BPD, a condition that develops as a sequel to respiratory distress syndrome. What role oxygen therapy, ventilatory support, or lung immaturity play in its cause is unclear. Infants with BPD often have prolonged oxygen needs or require a combination of fluid restriction, diuretic, or bronchodilator therapy even after discharge from the nursery. Depending on the clinical evaluation for signs of respiratory distress, these therapies can be altered and eventually withdrawn as the child matures.

Diuretics

Infants with BPD are often given diuretics in addition to fluid restriction to decrease the amount of excess lung and total body water. Drugs in common use include furosemide, chlorothiazide, and spironolactone.

When diuretics are given on an outpatient basis, the infant's oral intake, estimates of output, weight gain, and serum electrolytes should be closely monitored. Because of potential electrolyte abnormalities associated with diuretics, potassium chloride supplements are often used with all diuretics except spironolactone. Diuretics should be restricted to those patients in whom there is an apparent clinical response to the medication. Although uncommon, nephrocalcinosis has been reported in infants given furosemide. Most often these drugs do not need to be increased as the child gains weight if there are no clinical signs or symptoms of right ventricular failure or pulmonary edema.

The medication can be withdrawn when the child has grown to a weight that results in the drug being subtherapeutic on a milligram per kilogram basis, as long as respiratory stability is maintained. Weaning the child from a diuretic requires frequent evaluations of body weight, nutritional and fluid intake, vital signs, and auscultation of the chest.

Bronchospasm

Many infants with mild residual BPD develop evidence of bronchospasm with viral illnesses or environmental irritants. Their airways are quite hyperreactive. In many respects they have similar clinical symptoms as children with asthma. Unlike those with asthma, however, most infants "outgrow" BPD-related bronchospasm by 1 to 2 years of age. Because physicians are not accustomed to seeing bronchospasm in a child younger than 1 or 2 years, BPD-related bronchospasm in the infant is often incorrectly diagnosed as bronchitis or pneumonia, and antibiotics or cough medicine are often administered. Antibiotics are usually not warranted unless a bacterial process is suspected. Cough medicines, especially those containing antihistamines, should be used with

TABLE 11-1
Weaning a Patient from Supplemental Oxygen: Sample Schedule*

	AMOUNT OF OXYGEN (PER MIN)
At hospital discharge	0.5 L at all times
1 mo after discharge	0.5 L during feedings and sleep, 0.25 L when awake
2 mo	0.25 L at all times
3 mo	0.25 L during feedings and sleep, room air when awake
4 mo	Room air at all times

*Schedule assumes clinical stability, adequate weight gain, and documentation of adequate oxygen saturation. Intervals may vary depending on these criteria.

caution, because their use may lead to the development of inspissated secretions, leading in turn to worsening of pulmonary symptoms.

The use of bronchodilators, administered either orally or via an inhaled nebulized solution, is appropriate intervention for bronchospasm related to BPD. In contrast to previous beliefs, these infants do have bronchial smooth muscle that is responsive to such medication. Albuterol, terbutaline, and metaproterenol are all selective β_2 agonists and can be administered in the oral or nebulized form. Theophylline, a methylxanthine, is less tolerated but is used in dosages similar to those used in children with asthma. Infants receiving theophylline should be closely monitored for evidence of theophylline sensitivity or toxicity, such as tachycardia, vomiting, and irritability. These side effects are less often experienced when using the nebulized form of medication.

These medications can be used during acute episodes either for short periods (3 to 7 days) or for several weeks until symptoms resolve. If symptoms do not resolve, readjustment of medications may be warranted or further investigation of other possible causes for the bronchospasm may be indicated.

As with asthma, maintenance doses of one or more of these medications may be needed if the infant has recurrent episodes of bronchospasm.

During acute exacerbations, either adding a second bronchodilator (eg, theophylline or metaproterenol) or decreasing the interval between nebulized inhalation treatments can function to achieve the desired relief.

Another medication being used more commonly is cromolyn disodium. This drug acts as a mast cell membrane stabilizer and may be useful in the child with frequent episodes of bronchospasm. It is a medication given by inhalation (20 mg three times a day) and is most effective if given as routine prophylaxis.

Oxygen Requirements

Dependence on supplemental oxygen varies with the severity of BPD. If the infant is otherwise medically stable, the need for supplemental oxygen should not necessarily preclude consideration for discharge. The supplemental oxygen required should usually be no more than 2 L/min delivered via nasal cannula. Outpatients should be followed-up at frequent intervals and weaned slowly, depending on clinical stability (weight gain, good pulmonary reserve during periods of activity or feeding, and lack of significant intercurrent pulmonary illness). Ideally, if there is access to a device to measure oxygen saturation (pulse oximetry), weaning can be done with more accuracy. These measurements should be done when the infant is at rest, during periods of activity and feeding, and when crying to determine if any desaturation occurs relative to the resting state.

If the infant is medically stable based on the above criteria and not anemic, the weaning process can begin. The most important rule is to wean gradually. Studies have shown that infants with BPD who are receiving optimal oxygen demonstrate better weight gain, attain corrected age–appropriate milestones more readily, and have fewer intercurrent respiratory illnesses than do those with borderline oxygenation. A typical weaning schedule is shown in Table 11-1. Infants should be kept on their bronchodilator and only if necessary, their diuretic regimen, until completely weaned to room air.

Rehospitalization

Rehospitalization is common in infants with BPD, especially in the first year of life. Recurrent episodes of bronchospasm that are difficult to treat on an outpatient basis may be precipitated by exposure to environmental irritants such as cigarette or fireplace smoke, paint fumes, insecticides, or kerosene heaters and exposure to other people with respiratory viruses. In particular, infants with BPD are at higher risk for contracting debilitating respiratory symptoms secondary to RSV, adenovirus, and influenza viruses. The physician should recommend that every effort be made to avoid exposure to these potential irritants.

Studies have shown a much higher rate of rehospitalization in the preterm population during the first year of life. The need arises most often from pulmonary illnesses, but poor weight gain, minor surgical procedures, gastroesophageal reflux, or apnea and bradycardia are also frequent causes. Although most episodes warrant rehospitalization, the physician should be sensitive to the effects these repeated "disruptions" have on the family unit and attempt to treat the infant as much as possible as an outpatient.

NEUROLOGIC PROBLEMS

Abnormalities of muscle tone and posture are the most common neurologic abnormalities encountered in preterm infants. Several reports in the literature describe transient muscle tone abnormalities in premature infants during the first 12 to 18 months. In general these abnormalities are evident within the first 3 months after discharge and begin to resolve by the time the child is 12 months, corrected age. In a full-term infant, abnormal muscle tone during the first year of life is relatively rare and is associated with an increased risk for neurologic handicaps. In the preterm infant, however, it is more common and may not carry the same prognostic importance. Misinterpretation of the significance of muscle tone abnormalities during the infant's first year of life may result in *inaccurately* describing normal premature infants as neurologically handicapped. Therefore caution should be used when labeling a condition as cerebral palsy before the infant is 18 months, corrected age. If, however, there is evidence of hemiparesis of known cause (*eg*, porencephalic cyst or periventricular leukomalacia), especially with residual cyst formation, the diagnosis of cerebral palsy may be used earlier and with more certainty.

The most common abnormality of tone is increased extensor tone of the lower extremities.

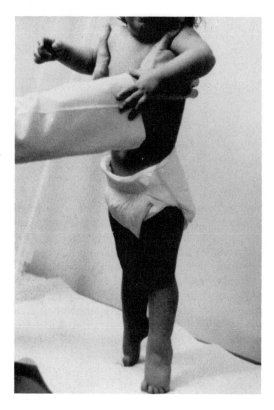

FIG 11-2
Demonstration of neurologic examination of infant with increased extension tone of lower extremities. Note stiff knees and pointed toes.

Figure 11-2 shows increased extensor tone seen in the lower extremities of an infant aged 6 months, corrected age. When placed in a position of support, this infant demonstrates marked knee stiffening and toe-pointing, as well as rigidity about the hip musculature. Residual hypertonicity persistent beyond 12 months is usually limited to a mild to moderate degree of toe-walking, which becomes evident when the child begins to walk unassisted. As expected, when lower extremity hypertonicity does not resolve by 1 year of age, these children can demonstrate a delay in walking because they are more unstable than if they were able to walk with their feet flat on the floor.

Preventive corrective measures in infancy include proper positioning so as not to reinforce and exacerbate this abnormally increased tone. It is therefore strongly recommended that these children not be placed in positions of support, such as in a walker or jumper or standing in a parent's lap. When significant lower extremity

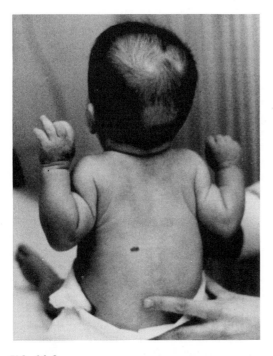

FIG 11-3

Demonstration of scapular retractions seen in hypertonicity of shoulder girdle, trapezius, and upper extremities.

hypertonicity persists that interferes with normal ambulatory skills, referral to an orthopedic surgeon may be appropriate for consideration of casting for tendon stretching or for possible release of the hamstring or Achilles tendon to ensure adequate ambulation.

Figure 11-3 shows hypertonicity of the shoulder girdle and trapezius musculature, as well as upper extremity increased flexor tone. This posture is commonly referred to as "scapular retractions." When this increased tone persists until 6 to 9 months of age the infant is unable to perform the lateral-propping protective reflex and parachute reflex, respectively, because the infant is unable to extend his/her arms to the side or to the front. This also markedly affects independent sitting, reaching, and midline activities and can be a cause of frustration for the infant. This type of muscle tone problem is amenable to treatment with specific positions that encourage the shoulders to be brought forward, in an attempt to break up the shoulder girdle muscle hypertonicity so that reaching can be more adaptive.

Compared with the incidence of hypertonicity, decreased muscle tone is encountered in preterm infants less frequently. Hypotonicity affecting

the trunk can be evidenced as a slumped posture when the infant aged 6 months is placed in a sitting position. Hypotonicity of the trunk musculature will delay the onset of sitting until the second half of the first year. Muscle hypotonicity can also be evident as the persistence of an exaggerated head lag on pull-to-sit or head bobbing with the infant in a sitting position at 6 months, corrected age. Less frequently one can see hypotonicity of either the upper or the lower extremities evidenced by an inability of the infant to bear weight on his/her legs in vertical suspension or on the arms in prone position; both abilities are expected in an adjusted age infant aged 3 to 4 months.

Some infants may demonstrate mixed tonal abnormalities. The most common is truncal hypotonicity coexisting with lower extremity hypertonicity.

Although it is an area of much controversy (because the natural history of these abnormalities suggests that they resolve some time within the second year of life), formal physical therapy intervention is recommended when the tone abnormality is sufficiently involved that it affects the infant's functional status or delays the acquisition of key developmental milestones. The physical therapist can assist the child to develop adaptive measures for overcoming a functional disability.

One last neurologic problem encountered in the preterm population is the persistence of primitive reflexes. Some premature infants have reflexes such as the asymmetric tonic neck, Moro, or grasp reflexes that persist beyond 4 months, of adjusted age, which are thought to be normal for full-term infants. Although this finding is commonly encountered in full-term children with neurologic abnormalities such as cerebral palsy, a mild persistence of primitive reflexes in the preterm infant is usually not such an ominous sign.

DEVELOPMENTAL OUTCOME

The primary care physician can play an important role in promoting the normal development of a preterm infant. The responsibilities are twofold: to screen for mental, motor, and behavioral dysfunctions for which this population is at risk and to provide emotional and educational support to parents whose task is made more difficult by the stressful neonatal period.

Screening for developmental disabilities is mandatory. Despite an improved outlook on the outcome of low birth weight infants, there remains a higher incidence of mental retardation, cerebral palsy, and learning problems in the preterm population. The majority of infants who weigh between 1000 and 1500 g at birth are intellectually normal after the first year of life; the remainder, approximately 10% to 13%, do have moderate or major delays in development. This percentage represents a major improvement over the 89% incidence of handicaps in low birth weight infants born in the 1950s. The outlook for infants weighing less than 1000 g at birth is less positive. Approximately 15% to 20% of these infants have moderate to major delays in development. Of those infants weighing less than 800 g at birth, approximately 25% are delayed developmentally.

In addition to the children who have moderate to major developmental delays, another large population of preterm children has been identified with learning problems. These are children of all birth weights who, despite normal intelligence as measured with IQ tests, have problems learning in school and often require special education. Deficits have been documented in perceptual-motor integration skills, impulse control, attention span, language skills, and integration of sensory stimuli. These learning disabilities are more difficult to identify before school age but can have a significant impact on the affected child and family.

Screening by the community physician can be accomplished with assessment tools. The Denver Developmental Screening Test or more informal developmental interviews will provide enough information to the physician that a decision for further evaluation can be made. Interpretation of the results of the developmental examination must be done in coordination with evaluation of vision and hearing abilities because any sensory impairment, even mild, can cause abnormalities in intellectual performance.

At this time, there are no separate norms for the development of preterm infants, so we must employ those norms standardized for a healthy term population. To correct for this difference, it is advisable to use the infant's age corrected for 40 weeks' gestation rather than the birth date. Because the developmental progress of low birth weight infants is more consistent with age from conception, using this adjusted age prevents the

evaluator from being overly concerned when the infant lags behind his/her chronologic age behavior. The use of adjusted age becomes unnecessary when the infant reaches a chronologic age of 2.5 years because the time span between birth and 40 weeks has become a smaller fraction of the total age. Even with correction for prematurity, these infants often demonstrate developmental lags in the first year of life. For example, most infants at the corrected age of 6 months are still not sitting upright and have only clumsy reaching skills. By the corrected age of 12 months, most infants have "caught up" to their corrected age.

Although the study of risk factors or causes of developmental handicaps has not yielded data definitive enough to predict later outcome, some factors have been identified that place a low birth weight infant at higher risk for problems: IVH (grade 3 or 4), need for transport to a tertiary care center, birth asphyxia, extended need for mechanical ventilation, BPD, and social factors.

IVH, as discussed previously, ranges from small bleeding to greater and more damaging bleeding. Developmental follow-up studies have reported that only grade 3 and 4 bleeding are associated with a risk for handicap. In particular, cerebral palsy is a frequent finding; often some children will have no accompanying delays in intellectual skills. Periventricular leukomalacia is a relatively rare brain injury that is frequently associated with mental retardation and visual impairment. Birth asphyxia, as defined by Apgar score of less than 3 at 1 and 5 minutes, is associated with poor developmental outcome. Children requiring extended mechanical ventilation, usually an indication of BPD, generally perform in the low-average range and often demonstrate more significant delays in the preschool years while the disease is still active. The impact of social class variables such as maternal education, family income, and knowledge of child development often emerge as stronger predictors of later outcome.

Referral for further assessment and therapeutic intervention should take place when there are concerns about a specific aspect of a child's development; when there is overall delay from the child's adjusted age; when uneven or abnormal development is present; or when parents seek more specific or extensive information than the physician has time or background to give.

Because problems seen in the first year of a

preterm infant's life are often transient, the decision to refer is often difficult; however, early referral is appropriate for this high-risk population. Each state will provide free education and therapeutic services for children from birth to 3 years who demonstrate delays.

Community physicians have the opportunity to affect the developmental progress of low birth weight infants by supporting the family. When these infants go home, they are quite different from full-term infants. Feeding and weight gain may still be a concern, sleeping and waking patterns are confused, their appearance is still disparate from that of a full-term infant, and most important, parents usually have concerns about their child's future development and may not think of the child as "normal." By showing parents the strengths and weaknesses and personality of their infant, informing them of developmental sequence, and even suggesting appropriate play and learning activities, physicians have been found to have a positive impact on parent-child relationships. Parents of low birth weight infants have experienced numerous stresses and may seek support from community physicians; by their sensitivity to the parents' concerns, physicians can help improve the family environment for the developing child.

IMPACT ON THE FAMILY

The stresses on families of preterm infants during the hospitalization are overt and dramatic. For families of preterm infants who require medically complicated home care the stresses continue to be significant after discharge. Because of these home care needs the family centers its attention on the child and normal activities become extremely difficult.

Siblings often feel neglected because not only has a new baby come home but one that demands extra attention. The impact on these families after discharge can be described in three phases: euphoria, despair, and acceptance. Euphoria occurs during the first few weeks after discharge. The parents experience the thrill of having their child home. They finally feel like parents. Despair sets in once the parents realize that there are ongoing issues related to their child's neonatal illness. Exhaustion may predominate. The parents may realize the child is much sicker and more developmentally delayed than they

thought. During the final phase, acceptance, the parents start to integrate the child with complex medical needs into their lives. By accepting their child and the attendant life style the family is able to resume a more normal life. However, physicians should be aware of issues of chronic grief, which is a continuous process for the families who do not have a "normal" child. Failure to meet significant developmental milestones can be very difficult for these families. For the families whose preterm infants are growing, developing, and have no significant ongoing medical needs the stresses are more subtle and possibly difficult to recognize.

Many of the stresses on the families of preterm infants after discharge are described in what Green and Solnit call the "vulnerable child syndrome." Despite the infant's recovery from illness, the parents continue to experience anxiety because they perceive their infant as fragile, vulnerable, and having special needs. The behavior of the parent and child is adversely affected by this continuing belief.

The parents' perception of an infant's vulnerability persists for several reasons. Questions of the infant's survival that preoccupied the parents' emotions during the hospitalization linger after discharge. Parents also appear to lack confidence in their parenting ability. This may be due to an interruption in the normal development of parenting skills as a result of a prolonged hospitalization, or it may be related to persistent feelings that the hospital staff is more competent at caretaking. Feeling that they should be constantly happy about the infant's arrival home, parents may have difficulty admitting and expressing normal frustrations of parenting and latent anger about separation. Concerns over problems with the child's future development often lead to parental feelings that the infant remains sick, different from other infants, and warrants special status in the family.

Several parent-infant behavior problems frequently result in:

1. Feeding problems, including overfeeding and underfeeding.
2. Difficulty in separation from the mother. Mother feels that only she can do the care and wants no one else involved.
3. Overindulgence and overpermissiveness. Families have difficulty setting disciplinary limits on the child, thus interfering with nor-

mal development. The child becomes dependent, demanding, and out of control; the child, not the parent, is running the household.

What can be done to prevent the vulnerable child syndrome? First, the parents of preterm infants need more time with their physician. All the concerns that parents of full-term infants have are exaggerated in parents of preterm infants. It is important to establish rapport with the family, be sensitive to their needs, and provide support. The family needs to feel comfortable in expressing their fears and concerns to their physician. Second, families should be encouraged to normalize the caretaking of their preterm infant and their daily activities. The promotion of the normalization process is critical in the development of a healthy parent-child relationship. Third, encourage the families to be firm. Assist the parents in setting disciplinary limits and schedules. Give them permission to set limits and be in control. Fourth, educate the parents about developmental delays in preterm infants that are common and in most cases temporary.

It is important that the infant with developmental delays be enrolled in an early intervention program as soon as possible. The intervention program not only promotes developmental progress but provides an opportunity for parental involvement. As a result of direct parental involvement, the parents have a more realistic view of their child's abilities and needs.

Finally, if the parent's worries are recognized, a careful explanation and continued clarification of the infant's true health status can alleviate unnecessary concerns and promote more effective use of the primary care physician.

BIBLIOGRAPHY

American Academy of Pediatrics: Joint Committee on Infant Hearing, 1994 Position Statement, *Pediatrics* 95(1), 1995.

Ballard RA: *Pediatric Care of the ICN Graduate,* Philadelphia, 1988, WB Saunders.

Bernbaum JB, Daft A, Anolik R, et al: Response of preterm infants to diphtheria-tetanus-pertussis immunizations, *J Pediatr* 107:184–188, 1985.

Bernbaum JC, Hoffman-Williamson M: *Primary care of the preterm infant,* St. Louis, 1991, Mosby–Year Book.

Feinberg E: Family stress in pediatric home care, *Caring* 38–41, 1985.

Forbes GB, Woodruff CW: *Pediatric nutrition handbook,* ed 2, Elk Grove Village, 1985, American Academy of Pediatrics.

Green M, Solnit AJ: Reactions to the threatened loss of a child: A vulnerable child syndrome, *Pediatrics* 34:58, 1964.

Groothuis JR, Rosenberg AA: Home oxygen promotes weight gain in infants with bronchopulmonary dysplasia, *Am J Dis Child* 141:992–995, 1987.

Guidelines for perinatal care, Elk Grove, IL, 1992, American Academy of Pediatrics.

Hack M, Taylor HG, Klein N, et al: School-age outcomes in children with birthweights under 750g, *N Engl J Med* 331(12):753–759, 1994.

Harrison H: *The premature baby book,* New York, 1983, St Martin's Press.

Hurt H: Symposium on continuing care of a high-risk infant, *Clin Perinatol* 11:1, 1984.

McCormick MC, Brooks-Gunn J, Workman-Daniels K, et al: The health and developmental status of very low birth weight children at school age, *JAMA* 267(16):2204–2208, 1992.

Ross G: Mortality and morbidity in very low birthweight infants, *Pediatr Ann* 12:1, 1983.

Saigal S, Szatmari P, Rosenbaum R, et al: Cognitive abilities and school performance of extremely low birth weight children and matched term control children at age 8 years: A regional study, *J Pediatr* 118(5):751–760, 1991.

Silverman WA, Flynn JT: Contemporary issues in fetal and neonatal medicine. Retinopathy of prematurity, Boston, 1985, Blackwell Scientific Publications.

Vohr B, Hack M: Developmental follow-up of low-birth-weight infants, *Pediatr Clin North Am* 29:1441, 1982.

PART THREE

The Toddler and Older Child

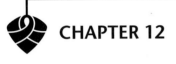

CHAPTER 12

Examination

Rosemary Casey

Watching and helping children grow gives the primary care physician special insight into human development. Variations in the physical and emotional growth of normal children make this aspect of practice both interesting and challenging. Parents who do not have the experience or knowledge of ranges of development look to the physician to determine if their child has a problem or is in the range of normal development. Therefore, the practitioner needs to keep in mind the common developmental issues that occur at various segments of the child's life and be prepared to help and advise the families.

These chapters focus on the physical and emotional issues of the toddler. The physical examination is highlighted, rather than covered completely, as it is assumed that the reader has experience in physical examinations. Next a range of normal developmental issues is discussed in a practical manner, describing a spectrum of expected concerns of parents.

APPROACH TO THE EXAMINATION

The examining room should be a warm, safe environment. Children who feel cold will shiver and cry. Begin by talking to the child: ask questions, tell a story, show an instrument, and help the child relax. As your examination proceeds, keep your hands and equipment warm, avoid quick, jerky movements, and continue to speak to the child in a calm, confident tone of voice. Use the power of suggestion to your advantage and do not ask the child's permission to perform the examination. It is usually better to say, "Show me how still you can be while I look in your ears" than to ask, "May I look in your ears?"

The order of the examination must be tailored to the child's age, degree of fear, and specific complaints. Generally, it is best to postpone the objectionable parts until the end. Much of the examination can be done with a young child sitting in the parent's lap.

Although sometimes impossible to avoid, restraint should be used as little as possible. It is surprising how frequently physicians hold children down unnecessarily. A child's natural reaction is to struggle to escape, thus making the examination much more difficult to perform. A moment used to calm a child is generally time well spent.

The physician should not rush into the physical examination with frightening instruments and poking fingers. Even while taking a history, much information can be learned by observing the child and parent. The child's posture and movements and overall comfort should be noted. Degree of illness, general development, and speech skills should be determined. Some assessment of growth, nutrition, and hydration should be made. This is a particularly good time to assess respiration, to get an initial view of the skin, and to note any specific abnormal odors. The parent-child interaction and the child's personality and fearfulness also can be noted at this time.

The following discussion includes common problems in physical diagnosis. For more detailed information consult the text by Barness.

BLOOD PRESSURE

Children 3 years of age and older should have their blood pressure (BP) measured annually. The rubber bladder in the cuff should cover approximately 75% of the upper arm length and should be long enough to completely encircle the arm. Cuff selection should always be based on arm size, not age. Cuffs that are too narrow will yield an artificially high BP.

The child should be relaxed and in a sitting position. Inflate the cuff to 20 to 30 mm Hg above the level at which the pulse can no longer be palpated. Next, release the pressure slowly, about 2 to 3 mm Hg per second, until a clear tapping sound is heard. This is the first Korotkoff sound and corresponds to the systolic pressure.

There is some disagreement about whether the fourth (muffling) or fifth (disappearance of all sounds) Korotkoff phase should be used as the measurement of diastolic pressure. The standard children's BP charts (Figs. 12-1 and 12-2) generally use the fourth sound, but the pressure at which sounds disappear should probably also be recorded. The most common causes of error in BP determination are incorrect cuff selection, poor measurement technique, and an upset or anxious child.

Measurement of BP above the 95th percentile for age should be repeated on at least three separate occasions. Only if the BP is persistently elevated should the child be considered hypertensive. These children should undergo a careful history and physical examination to determine the extent of the further diagnostic evaluation.

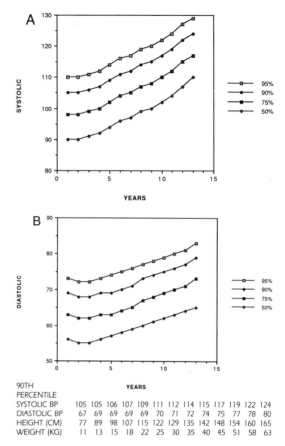

90TH PERCENTILE													
SYSTOLIC BP	105	105	106	107	109	111	112	114	115	117	119	122	124
DIASTOLIC BP	67	69	69	69	69	70	71	72	74	75	77	78	80
HEIGHT (CM)	77	89	98	107	115	122	129	135	142	148	154	160	165
WEIGHT (KG)	11	13	15	18	22	25	30	35	40	45	51	58	63

FIG 12-1

Age-specific percentiles for blood pressure measurements in boys 1 to 13 years of age; Korotkoff phase IV (K4) used for diastolic BP. [From Horan MJ, et al: Report of the Second Task Force on Blood Pressure Control in Children–1987. *Pediatrics* 79:1-25, 1987. With permission.]

HEIGHT, WEIGHT, HEAD CIRCUMFERENCE

The evaluation of a child's height, weight, and head circumference requires the proper use of appropriate growth charts. After the first year of life and until adolescence, a child's growth pattern is normally parallel to the percentile lines. Growth patterns that cross over percentile lines are often the first sign of some medical, emotional, or social problem. One note of caution: if a child's standing height is plotted on a chart standardized for supine length, the resultant percentiles will be falsely low.

For children whose measurements fall outside the normal ranges, tables and charts that make

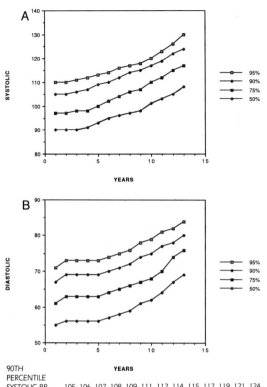

90TH PERCENTILE	YEARS											
SYSTOLIC BP	105	106	107	108	109	111	112	114	115	117	119	121	124
DIASTOLIC BP	69	68	68	69	69	70	71	73	74	75	76	77	79
HEIGHT (CM)	80	91	100	108	115	122	129	135	141	147	153	159	165
WEIGHT (KG)	11	14	16	18	22	25	29	34	39	44	50	55	62

FIG 12-2

Age-specific percentiles for blood pressure measurements in girls 1 to 13 years of age; Korotkoff phase IV (K4) used for diastolic BP. [From Horan MJ, et al: Report of the Second Task Force on Blood Pressure Control in Children–1987. *Pediatrics* 79:1-25, 1987. With permission.]

adjustments for parental size should be used. The method of Weaver to adjust for parental head circumference is especially helpful in the evaluation of children with large heads. With both height and head circumference, the finding of an abnormal rate of growth, known as the *growth velocity,* is usually more clinically important than is an abnormal measurement on a single occasion. (*See* also the chapter on growth problems, Chapter 42.)

SKIN

Bruises due to normal play activity are generally irregular in shape and are usually located on the distal extremities. In contrast, bruises from child abuse with an instrument are found on the trunk, buttocks, face, and proximal extremities and often reflect the shape of the instrument used to inflict the trauma. A bruise progresses through the following stages: 0 to 2 days, swollen, tender; 0 to 5 days, red, blue; 5 to 7 days, green; 7 to 10 days, yellow; 10 to 14 days, brown; and 2 to 4 weeks, clear.

Mongolian spots are gray or blue-black large macular lesions, usually located in the lumbosacral area and the buttocks. They are seen in 90% of black children, 80% of Asian children, and 10% of white children. This discoloration usually fades spontaneously by adulthood and should not be confused with bruising from child abuse.

Café-au-lait spots are present in 10% to 20% of normal individuals but can also be seen in persons with neurocutaneous disorders. Six or more lesions that are 1.5 cm in diameter are presumptive evidence of neurofibromatosis in adults. In children under 6 years of age, the criterion for this diagnosis is the presence of five lesions, each 0.5 cm or larger.

Acquired pigmented moles usually develop when a child is between 2 and 6 years of age or during adolescence; consequently, by adulthood the average person has approximately 30 lesions. Fears about malignancy are unfounded unless the lesion shows rapid growth, irregular borders or nodularity, irregular darkening or bluish discoloration, an erythematous halo, spontaneous bleeding or scarring, or unless it is associated with pain or pruritus. A hypopigmented halo should not cause concern if the central nevus has benign characteristics.

The management of congenital melanocytic nevi remains controversial and depends on estimates of melanoma risks, timing of surgery, and cosmetic issues. Giant congenital melanocytic nevi have a definite premalignant potential of 1.8% to 13% before the age of 5 years. Therefore total excision of a giant congenital melanocytic nevus is recommended, as soon after birth as possible. Smaller lesions may be excised later in life (but before puberty) as long as they have a benign appearance and stable growth.

When a normally hydrated child's skin and subcutaneous tissue are pinched and then released, there is a brisk snapping back to the original position. A delay in return, called *tenting,* indicates poor turgor and dehydration.

Hypernatremia may give the skin a "doughy" feel.

A common cause of hair loss is traction alopecia. Tight braiding can cause hair loss at the margins of the hairline or where the hair is parted.

LYMPH NODES

Lymphoid tissue grows steadily during childhood, then gets progressively smaller at puberty. Discrete, movable, nontender nodes up to 3 mm in diameter are normally found and can be as large as 1 cm in the cervical and inguinal regions without raising concern. Enlarged occipital and posterior scalp nodes are often seen in children with minor scalp problems such as seborrhea. Enlarged inguinal nodes are particularly common in the warm months when children run barefoot. Palpable supraclavicular nodes should never be considered normal; they are usually associated with systemic or intrathoracic disease.

TEETH

In addition to looking for obvious caries, the physician should determine the number, position, and color of the teeth. In early stages caries appear as dull, opaque, whitish discolorations. The examiner should make a special effort to view the posterior aspect of the upper incisors, a common site for "baby-bottle" caries.

Table 12-1 shows the schedule for normal tooth eruption. Early or delayed tooth eruption can be seen in normal children; however, it is also associated with many specific syndromes and systemic disorders.

The deciduous (baby) teeth are normally separated by spaces. They may erupt in an irregular alignment but can realign spontaneously. The primary care physician should have the older child "open and bite" to observe for malocclusion.

Tooth discoloration that is extrinsic (superficially located on enamel surface) may be caused by poor oral hygiene, diet, or oral medications

TABLE 12-1
Chronology of Human Dentition*

| | | | PRIMARY OR DECIDUOUS TEETH | | | |
| | CALCIFICATION | | ERUPTION | | SHEDDING | |
TEETH	BEGINS	COMPLETE	MAXILLARY	MANDIBULAR	MAXILLARY	MANDIBULAR
Central incisors	5th fetal mo	18–24 mo	6–8 mo	5–7 mo	7–8 yr	6–7 yr
Lateral incisors	5th fetal mo	18–24 mo	8–11 mo	7–10 mo	8–9 yr	7–8 yr
Cuspids (canines)	6th fetal mo	30–36 mo	16–20 mo	16–20 mo	11–12 yr	9–11 yr
First molars	5th fetal mo	24–30 mo	10–16 mo	10–16 mo	10–11 yr	10–12 yr
Second molars	6th fetal mo	36 mo	20–30 mo	20–30 mo	10–12 yr	11–13 yr

| | | | SECONDARY OR PERMANENT TEETH | | | |
| | | CALCIFICATION | | ERUPTION | | |
		BEGINS	COMPLETE	MAXILLARY	MANDIBULAR	
Central incisors		3–4 mo	9–10 yr	7–8 yr	6–7 yr	
Lateral incisors	Maxillary	10–12 mo	10–11 yr	8–9 yr	7–8 yr	
	Mandibular	3–4 mo				
Cuspids (canines)		4–5 mo	12–15 yr	11–12 yr	9–11 yr	
First premolars (bicuspids)		18–21 mo	12–13 yr	10–11 yr	10–12 yr	
Second premolars (bicuspids)		24–30 mo	12–14 yr	10–12 yr	11–13 yr	
First molars		Birth	9–10 yr	6–7 yr	6–7 yr	
Second molars		30–36 mo	14–16 yr	12–13 yr	12–13 yr	
Third molars	Maxillary	7–9 yr	18–25 yr	17–22 yr	17–22 yr	
	Mandibular	8–10 yr				

*Adapted from Losch PK: Harvard School of Dental Medicine.

(such as iron). Unlike intrinsic discoloration, these stains can be removed with a wet gauze pad or scraped off by the dentist.

GAIT AND STANCE

Most neonates are bowlegged, but by the age of 3 to 4 years children display a knock-kneed stance (valgus angulation of about 10°). By the time the child is 7 years of age the knock-kneed appearance has usually spontaneously resolved.

A young child learns to walk with a wide-based gait. Foot contact with the floor is not with the heel but rather with the toe or the foot flat. Tip-toe gait should disappear by the time the child is 2 years of age. The angle of toeing-out (that angle between the axis of the foot and the line of gait progression) is normally about 10°; an angle of toeing-out greater than 30° is considered abnormal.

In children, toeing-in is commonly due to metatarsus adductus, internal tibial torsion, or increased femoral anteversion. These conditions are evaluated by examining the sole of the foot, determining the thigh-foot angle, and measuring the limits of internal and external rotation of the hip (Fig. 12-3). The normal range of thigh-foot angle is between 0° and 30° of external rotation, but in children with tibial torsion some degree of internal rotation is seen (Fig. 12-4). Hip rotation is best measured with the knee flexed and the child in the supine position. Internal rotation greater than 70° is indicative of femoral anteversion.

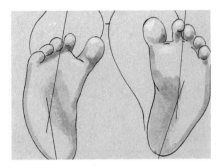

FIG 12-3
Metatarsus adductus examination demonstrates medial deviation of the forefoot.

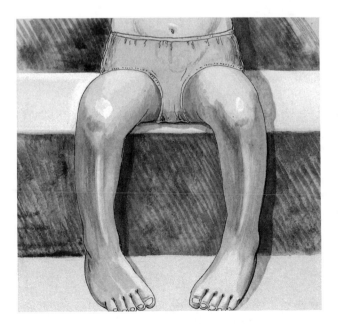

FIG 12-4
Tibial torsion with internal rotation of the foot.

BIBLIOGRAPHY

Barness LA: *Manual of pediatric physical diagnosis,* Chicago, 1981, Year Book Medical Publishers.

Gundy JH: *Assessment of the child in primary health care.* New York, 1981, McGraw-Hill.

Hoekelman R: Pediatric examination. In Bates BA, editor: *Guide to physical examination,* Philadelphia, 1979, JB Lippincott.

Horan MJ, et al: Report of the Second Task Force on blood pressure control in children—1987, *Pediatrics* 79:1–25, 1987.

Hurwitz S: *Clinical pediatric dermatology,* Philadelphia, 1981, WB Saunders.

Jacobs AH, Hurwitz S: The management of congenital nevocytic nevi, *Pediatr Dermatol* 2:143–156, 1984.

Lowrey GH: *Growth and development of children,* Chicago, 1973, Year Book Medical Publishers.

Staheli L: Torsional deformity, *Pediatr Clin North Am* 24:799–811, 1977.

Weaver DD, Christian JC: Familial variation of head size and adjustment for parental head circumference, *J Pediatr* 96:990–994, 1980.

CHAPTER 13

Care of the Toddler and Older Child

Rosemary Casey
Jeffrey C. Weiss

PROBLEMS

Rosemary Casey

BEHAVIORAL PROBLEMS

Although the developmental tasks are the same for all children, each child approaches the challenge with his/her own temperament, genetic and environmental influences, and parental expectations, which results in a broad range of normal development. Thomas and Chess have demonstrated that the child's individual characteristics play an important role in the developmental process. They describe three configurations of temperament, although some children do not fit neatly into a single category.

The "easy child" is characterized by regularity, positive-approach responses to stimuli, high adaptability to change, and mild or moderate intensity. The "difficult child" has irregularity, negative-withdrawal responses to new stimuli, nonadaptability to change, and intense mood expressions, which are frequently negative. The third group of children has a combination of negative responses of mild intensity to new stimuli, with slow adaptability after repeated contact; hence this group is called "slow to warm up." In discussing the clinical applications of temperament, Carey has pointed out that an awareness of a child's temperament is particularly helpful in diagnosing behavioral problems. For example, parents commonly ask for help because their child is "hyperactive." A physician who is aware of that child's behavioral style can direct the parent's attention toward the more relevant questions of attention or distractibility. Temperament alone does not predict a child's success or failure in achieving developmental goals. The same child who is considered withdrawn in one family may be praised as easygoing by another family. The physician, aware of the interaction between parental values and the child's behavioral style, can distinguish between behavioral problems that require treatment and normal behavioral differences.

There have been few studies on the incidence and prevalence of behavioral problems in preschool children. In an epidemiologic study of children aged 3 years in London, Richman, Stevenson, and Graham found that 7% had moderate to severe problems and 15% had mild behavioral problems. The percentage of mothers worried about their child's behavior was highest when the child was 3 years of age.

This section will focus on the more common behavioral problems of the toddler and older child, with particular emphasis on the normal limits and signs that intervention is necessary.

SEPARATION ANXIETY

Separation anxiety, a developmentally appropriate response for preschoolers, occurs after the child's removal from major attachment figures such as parents or from home. A child evolves from a toddler who is struggling with independence to a first-grader who is comfortable in the world of peers. Fraiberg and others have suggested that some anxiety may be crucial to the child's development of a mature ego structure. Parents who overprotect their children or quickly prevent the child from feeling anxious about an unpleasant experience place these children at risk for separation anxiety disorder. This diagnosis should not be made during the preschool years or the first months of school attendance. If an older child describes persistent morbid fears or phobias of kidnapping, accidents, or dying, there is cause for concern. These children frequently have nightmares and difficulty falling asleep, particularly if they are away from home. Their anxiety can present as a physical complaint such as headache or stomachache or can manifest itself as school avoidance. In children with a

separation anxiety disorder, further psychiatric evaluation and help are needed.

FEARS AND PHOBIAS

Young children have a variety of common fears, including fears of animals, darkness, and loud noises. Girls are more fearful, and the incidence peaks at 3 years of age. School-age children also fear ghosts, monsters, and certain animals, but they shift their fears to more abstract concepts such as dying. Fear can be a healthy emotion. It is often appropriate and helpful in preventing physical injury. Fear is unhealthy when it becomes excessive, spreads into other areas, and interferes with the child's normal activities. Young children who still think of their parents as endowed with special powers can usually overcome small anxieties with parental reassurance. Older children use many different approaches in overcoming their fears. Some children intellectualize their fears; others play through their terrors by acting macho or reading monster and horror stories. Most children succeed in handling their fears, and phobias are rare. Phobia is defined as persistent, excessive fear of a specific object that results in a desire to avoid that object or situation. The usual fear of insects or darkness would not be considered a phobia unless avoidance of the object was significantly stressful for the child and interfered with normal social functioning. Children with phobias know that they shouldn't be afraid, don't want to be afraid, and suffer the consequences of avoidance behaviors. The prognosis for these children is good, but treatment by experienced psychiatrists or psychologists is needed.

AGGRESSIVENESS, SHYNESS, PEER REJECTION

The child aged 2 years is still egocentric and engages mostly in parallel play with his/her peers. During the preschool years the child gradually learns to understand things from the perspective of others. By elementary-school age, the child must be ready for rule-governed competitive and cooperative play. Each child negotiates this transition in his/her own way. Some use objects, such as teddy bears and special blankets. Others are fascinated with "superheroes" as they cope with their own vulnerability. Certain children are shy and cling more to their parents; others are more aggressive and even defy adult authority. Parental concerns about their child being "withdrawn" or "aggressive" should be dealt with in the context of a broad normal range.

It is critical that a toddler develop a healthy self-esteem and that this sense of self-worth be sustained through the school years. Thomas and Chess note that the development of self-esteem must be a social process because the child has no a priori way of assessing his/her achievements. The judgments of parents and others provide the initial standards. Parents need to strike a balance between being highly critical and approving to excess everything a child does.

Youngsters use aggression as a defense against imagined danger or as a way of coping with conflicting emotions (eg, "hugging" the new baby strenuously enough to hurt). When kept in its place, aggression can be a healthy way of coping with fears, but the primary care physician must warn parents to set limits for their children. A child who loses control enough to strike a parent or be destructive is frightened and needs to have the parent step in and regain control. Extreme aggressiveness includes multiple episodes of disobedience, fighting, extreme competitiveness, and social egocentricity. This aggressiveness can lead to social isolation. Because this behavior usually will not be evident during the office visit, the physician should ask the parents or teachers to describe the duration of this behavior, the frequency of events, and specific consequences (such as injuries to other children). Unusual aggressiveness can begin during the preschool years and continue into early adulthood. The differential diagnosis of aggressive conduct disorder includes psychomotor seizures and brain damage secondary to severe trauma or infection. If these disorders are ruled out, the primary care physician can treat moderate forms of aggressiveness, but the more severe forms need to be referred for psychiatric intervention.

Children also experience shyness, daydreaming, peer rejection, and withdrawal in their socialization. The shy or isolated child tends to do well in the long run if the shyness is not accompanied by peer rejection. The daydreamer is defined by Gattman as one who is usually "off task" in the classroom, shy and anxious, neither accepted nor rejected but ignored by peers. Shyness and daydreaming must be distinguished from mental retardation, severe language delay, seizure disorders, hearing deficits, and childhood psychosis. The withdrawal seen in children with schizoid disorder is far more extreme than normal social reticence. These children are seclusive, generally unable to express strong feelings, and have few if any friends. When forced into social participation, they may become very irritable or even destructive. The primary care physician can thus distinguish these children from those with shy or sensitive temperaments.

TEMPER TANTRUMS

Temper tantrums occur commonly in children between the ages of 6 months and 6 years; they are most frequent between the ages of 1 and 3 years and should decrease over time. Tantrums reflect a child's struggle to become more autonomous. They can be caused by frustration at failing to master a developmental task but frequently are manipulative. If a parent allows a child to get his/her way through tantrums, the child will continue to use temper tantrums as a predominant way of interacting with adults and peers. This behavior will interfere with the child's learning appropriate social interactions such as sharing, taking turns, and making the correct verbal request. When parents ask about how to deal with temper tantrums, the physician should elicit an explicit history, looking for the frequency, specific circumstances of the tantrums, and the parents' feelings about or reactions to the child's behavior. It is normal for a parent to feel angry or frustrated, but parents who relate only negative comments (eg, "She's always been evil") are telling you there is a significant parent-child interaction problem. In general, the parental response should help the child regain self-control (this can be done by holding the younger child or calling a "cooling-off period" in a safe place for the older child). It is important that the parent follow through to be sure that the temper tantrum has not allowed the child to get his/her own way. For example, if the child was trying to avoid something like picking up toys, the parent should physically guide him/her to tidying up after the child has regained control. Discipline should include praise for the desired behavior and disapproval of the undesired behavior. Temper tantrums that control the household or are constant indicate that parent and child have lost control. Barkley provides an excellent resource for pediatricians in his book, *Defiant Children: A Clinician's Manual For Parent Training.* His program is helpful in counseling parents of children between 2 and 11 years of age who display noncompliant behavior alone or in conjunction with other oppositional disorders. Children with more severe developmental psychopathologic disorders may need further help.

THUMB SUCKING

Sucking is a normal infant behavior, and nonnutritive sucking is a self-regulatory, pleasurable, consoling activity for infants. Approximately one third of infants will persist in sucking their thumbs as toddlers. If parents ignore this behavior, most children will relinquish the habit between the ages of 4 and 5 years. Parents should not intervene before the ages of 4 to 6 years. Punitive measures, bitter-tasting substances, or embarrassing comments rarely work and may have a deleterious effect by depriving the child of a positive coping mechanism. Parents raise reasonable concerns about the dental implications of thumb sucking. The primary care physician should recommend a dental evaluation for children who persist in sucking their thumbs after 4 years of age.

SEXUALITY

The healthy development of sexuality occurs well before adolescence. In her book *The Magic Years,* Fraiberg stresses that giving a child facts about sex education is not sufficient. Parents, through their example and attitudes, teach children about identification with members of their own sex. This is a very important developmental task for the preschool period. It is inevitable that infants and toddlers discover the relationship between exploring their genitals and arousal and pleasure. Masturbation probably occurs in all children of both sexes. It is a normal part of development that only becomes a problem if the child persists in masturbating in public places where it is socially unacceptable. Parents must be taught not to overreact and to help the child learn that masturbation is not an evil act but something that should be done in privacy. The older child who persists in masturbating openly or in clinging to the genitals without apparent pleasure is manifesting anxiety that requires further attention.

TOILET TRAINING

A prerequisite for successful toilet training is bowel and bladder control, which is determined mainly by maturation and generally occurs between 1 and 3 years of age. However, toilet training is also a classic example of the toddler's struggle for autonomy. The outcome of this struggle is largely determined by the child's temperament, the parents' attitudes, and the parent-child interaction. It is usually successful when parents adopt a relaxed, nonthreatening approach once the child is ready. Brazelton refers to this as a "child-oriented approach to toilet training." In this method parents are taught to wait until the child is physically and psychologically ready (approximately at the age of 2 years). The "potty chair" is casually introduced, and gradually the child moves from sitting down on it with clothes on to changing his/her soiled diapers on it, and eventually to using the potty chair correctly by himself/herself. Whenever the child fails or resists going to the next step, parents are urged to wait and reassure the child. Some of the pressure is taken off the parents because the focus is on the child's achievement. Most children should have bowel and daytime urine control by 3 to 3.5 years of age. Nocturnal bladder control should be achieved by the age of 5 to 6 years.

In general, any child older than 2.5 years of age who is not toilet trained after several months of trying can be assumed to be resistant. An organic cause for toilet training resistance is rare. Urinary tract infection is probably the most common cause of daytime wetting; other causes include bubble bath urethritis, urgency incontinence, ectopic ureter, and neurogenic bladder. Children with dysuria, weak urine stream, constantly damp underwear, or wetting while running to the toilet require medical evaluation. However, most children who resist toilet training are involved in a power struggle. Schmitt has outlined a plan for treating toilet training refusal. He suggests that parents transfer all responsibility for using the toilet to the child, that major incentives be used, and that the child's progress be charted. Children should not be punished for accidents, and the babysitter or daycare center should use the same approach. Brazelton's no-pressure approach to toilet training was successful in 98% of children by the age of 36 months.

BREATH HOLDING

Breath-holding spells are frightening sudden episodes in which a child cries, appears to hold his/her breath, then becomes limp and occasionally develops tonic-clonic movements. These spells occur in 5% of children between age 6 months to 6 years and are commonly categorized as either cyanotic or pallid. The cyanotic type is usually precipitated by frustration or anger; the pallid type is triggered more by painful stimuli. The cry is more obvious in the cyanotic episodes in which the child proceeds to hold his/her breath in expiration, becomes cyanotic, unresponsive, and then sometimes twitches or develops opisthotonos. In the pallid type the breath holding or apnea is very brief before the child progresses to the same sequence of events.

The differential diagnosis must distinguish between a seizure disorder and breath holding, although cardiac disease and causes of tetany should be considered. Results of physical examination of the breath holder are normal, and a careful history should rule out seizures. A precipitating factor is always present in breath holding and rarely noticed before a seizure. Cyanosis or pallor usually occurs during or after a seizure, but it directly precedes the jerking movements in a breath-holding spell. The electroencephalogram (EEG), not necessary in most cases, is usually normal.

The physician should first reassure the family that the child does not have a seizure disorder and that there are no serious sequelae from breath-holding spells. All children outgrow these episodes by grade school age. Parents should be advised to treat these children normally and not spoil them in order to avoid temper tantrums. Anticonvulsants are not efficacious and should not be used for breath-holding spells.

SHOES FOR TODDLERS

Jeffrey Weiss

Concerns about foot abnormalities are expressed and questions about shoes and corrections are asked during most well-child visits. Most of the problems can be handled without referral if a few principles and concepts are appreciated.

Shoe Construction

Shoe construction is divided into two major parts, the sole and the upper. The upper should be pliable and porous enough to allow for moisture evaporation. Because the ankle requires no additional support from shoes, either high-top or low-cut shoes are acceptable. A young child is less likely to step out of a high shoe; however, the leather must be flexible enough so as not to restrict ankle movement. The counter is that part of the upper that surrounds the heel and helps to maintain the shape of the rear portion of the shoe.

The sole of a shoe may have several components: the insole, outsole, filler, and welt (Fig. 13-1). The upper can be stitched directly to an outsole or connected to the sole using an extra piece of leather called a *welt*. Welt construction is considered sturdiest and is used when wedges are applied to the shoes. In general, the sole should be flexible, bending easily at the ball of the foot.

The area of the shoe under the midportion of the arch of the foot is called the *shank*. Some specialists feel that a firm (steel) shank helps reinforce the arch and prevents the muscle strain that is caused by an elevated heel. Because heel elevation is really not a desirable feature for a young child's shoe, the shank is not necessary.

Shoes may have an inflare, outflare, or straight shape, depending on the angles formed by the axes of the front and rear portions of the last. The normal childhood foot is not straight but rather shows a mild forefoot inflare.

Little agreement exists among professionals concerning which shoe features are necessary for children with normal feet or helpful for children with foot deformities. Studies that compare the beliefs of pediatricians, podiatrists, orthopedic surgeons, and shoe fitters demonstrate wide differences in opinions about "proper" sole material

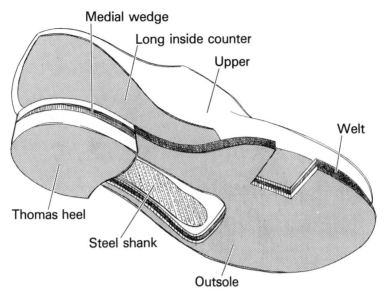

Medial wedge

Long inside counter

Upper

Welt

Thomas heel

Steel shank

Outsole

FIG 13-1
Diagrammatic representation of the components of a shoe.

and flexibility, shoe height, last shape, and shank stiffness. These disagreements among professionals, which confuse parents, result from a lack of objective data about the efficacy of various shoe features. Nowhere is this problem clearer than in the "great sneaker vs shoe debate."

Questionnaire studies show that about 77% of pediatricians and 65% of podiatrists believe that sneakers are adequate as regular footwear for children, yet only 37% of parents and 28% of shoe salespeople agree that sneakers are good for the feet. There is really no evidence that wearing sneakers results in flatfoot or any foot deformity, but other questions about shoes with rubber or crepe soles have been raised. Some authors believe that rubber is actually less flexible than leather and that rubber's high coefficient of friction results in heat and moisture buildup and an increased frequency of tripping on certain types of floor surfaces. Other experts claim that the nonskid rubber sole will prevent slipping. Some argue that because sneakers come in a limited number of widths, proper fit can be a problem that may result in blisters and foot irritation. These opinions are neither supported nor refuted by any data from well-designed clinical studies.

Problems Caused By Shoes

Wearing shoes can cause various irritations and inflammations of the skin of the foot. Pressures and friction due to poorly fitting shoes commonly affect the medial part of the large toe, the tips of the toes, the Achilles tendon area, the skin under the external malleolus, and the lateral aspect of the base of the fifth metatarsal. Irritation over the first metatarsophalangeal joint, known as "shoe bite," is due to leather rubbing the foot under the break (crease) of the shoe. Various substances used in the manufacture of shoes can cause shoe dermatitis, especially if excessive perspiration and moisture buildup are also present. Offending agents include rubber cements, chromates in chrome-tanned leather, nickel in lace eyelets, dyes, and antimildew preparations in shoe linings. Vesicles on the dorsum of the foot are most likely a contact dermatitis from one of these chemical agents. Patch-testing kits are available to determine the responsible agent.

Children do not develop athlete's foot, but another more serious shoe-related infection is *Pseudomonas* osteomyelitis, which can follow a puncture wound. A recent study has demonstrated that *Pseudomonas* can be cultured from the interior rubber layers of the sole in about 10% of those sneakers that have been worn.

SUMMARY

Certain points should be kept in mind by the primary care physician who counsels parents about children's shoes:

1. Shoes are worn for protection. There is no evidence to suggest that shoes are needed for support of any part of the normal foot.
2. Until a child is walking, a sock or other cloth covering is appropriate foot protection. Shoes do not help a child learn to walk better or sooner.
3. A child should be able to walk freely and naturally while in footgear. The sole must flex easily when the child walks, and ankle movement should be unrestricted.
4. The bottom of the shoe should be flat. A convex surface will cause side-to-side instability, and an elevated heel may stress the arch.
5. Skin irritations commonly result from new or poorly fitting shoes. In general, shoes that are a little large are better for a child than those that are too small. Parents can be advised that shoes should be replaced before their child's toes press against the front end of the upper.
6. The upper should be made of a porous material to allow for evaporation of moisture and perspiration.
7. Shoes will not correct structural foot deformities. Flexible flatfoot, bowleg, knock-knee, and toeing-out are all seen as part of normal development. These deformities (unless severe, asymmetric, or painful) generally require no special shoes. An orthopedist may be consulted for severe foot problems.

BIBLIOGRAPHY

Barkley RA: *Defiant children: A clinician's manual for parent training,* New York, 1987, Guilford Press.

Bleck EE: The shoeing of children: Sham or science? *Dev Med Child Neurol* 13:188–195, 1971.

Brazelton TB: A child-oriented approach to toilet training, *Pediatrics* 29:121–128, 1962.

Cowell HR: Shoes and shoe constructions, *Pediatr Clin North Am* 24:791–797, 1977.

Dyment PG, Bogan PM: Pediatrician's attitudes concerning infant's shoes, *Pediatrics* 50:655–657, 1972.

Fisher MC, Goldsmith JF, Gilligan PH, et al: Sneakers as a source of *Pseudomonas aeruginosa* in children with osteomyelitis complicating puncture wounds of the foot. Presented at Interscience Conference on Antimicrobial Agents and Chemotherapy (abstract 729), Las Vegas, Oct 1983.

Fraiberg S: *The magic years,* New York, 1959, Charles Scribner's Sons.

Gabel S: *Behavioral problems in childhood,* New York, 1981, Grune & Stratton.

Levine M, Carey W, Crocker A, et al: *Developmental behavioral pediatrics,* ed 2, Philadelphia, 1992, WB Saunders.

Lombroso CT, Lerman P: Breathholding spells (cyanotic and pallid infantile syncope), *Pediatrics* 39:563–581, 1967.

Richman N, Stevenson I, Graham P: Prevalence of behavior problems in 3-year-old children: An epidemiological study in a London borough, *J Child Psychol Psychiatry* 16:277–287, 1975.

Rincover A: *The parent-child connection.* New York, 1988, Random House.

Schmitt BD: Toilet training refusal: Avoid the battle and win the war, *Contemp Pediatr* 32–50, 1987.

Seder JI, Dyment PG: Infant's shoes: Attitudes of podiatrists and pediatricians, *J Podiatr Assoc* 70:244–246, 1980.

Staheili LT, Giffin L: Corrective shoes for children: A survey of current practice, *Pediatrics* 65:7–13, 1980.

Tax HR: *Podopediatrics,* Baltimore, 1980, Williams & Wilkins.

Thomas A, Chess S: *Temperament and development,* New York, 1977, Brunner Maizel.

Weiss JC, DeJong A, Packer E, et al: Purchasing infant shoes: Attitudes of parents, pediatricians and store managers, *Pediatrics* 67:718–720, 1981.

CHAPTER 14

Sleep Disorders

Anthony Rostain

Sleep disorders are common during childhood and vary according to the age of the child. In infancy, most problems are related to falling asleep and nightwaking. Toddlers and pre-schoolers have difficulties with falling and staying asleep, night terrors, nightmares, and enuresis. For older children, nightmares, insomnia, and sleepwalking are the most common complaints related to sleep. Although estimates vary widely, a majority of children will have some type of sleep disorder during childhood.

Although most sleep problems improve with minimal or no intervention, sleep disorders that are associated with organic or psychiatric illness are important to recognize and treat appropriately.

The duration of sleep changes with maturation (Table 14-1). The newborn sleeps for periods of 3 to 4 hours, with waking periods lasting 1 to 2 hours. At 1 month of age most infants sleep slightly longer at night, and by 5 months of age most sleep more than 7 hours at a time. There is a gradual decline in the length of time spent sleeping: during the second year it averages 12 to 13 hours, with one nap during the day; from the ages of 2 to 5 years, it decreases to about 11 hours without a nap; and by adolescence it reaches the adult average of 7 to 8 hours. It is important to keep in mind that sleep patterns vary among individuals and that they are related to temperament, maturation, activity level, habits, parent-child interactions, and family characteristics. All of these factors must be assessed when evaluating a sleep disorder.

GENERAL APPROACH TO PROBLEMS OF SLEEP

Problems with sleep will be noted either as a primary complaint by the parents or as an item in the review of the child's overall behavior and development. Parents may not be aware of a problem if there are separation issues between parent and child or if there are general parenting difficulties. Management will depend on the physician's relationship with the family, the parents' ability and willingness to change, and the duration and severity of the problem.

The strategy for evaluating sleep disorders centers on differentiating three general types of problems: mild behavioral problems stemming from either parenting difficulties or "lack of fit" between the child's temperament and the family environment; stress-related sleep disturbances that are part of a significant pattern of family dysfunction or psychiatric illness; and organically based sleep disorders, which may be primary or secondary to other physical illnesses.

Chief Complaint

The chief complaint is likely to vary according to the age of the child. Infants will have difficulty falling asleep, with waking in the middle of the night, with poorly established sleeping-waking cycles, and with fears associated with separation from parents. Toddlers tend to have problems described by parents as "can't sleep," "won't sleep," or "gets out of bed." Older children may complain of insomnia, nightmares, night terrors, sleepwalking, sleeptalking, or nocturnal enuresis. Adolescents tend to have difficulties with insomnia or hypersomnia.

Differential Diagnosis

Evaluation of a sleep disorder will depend on the age of the child and the nature of the complaint (Table 14-2).

History

The child's sleep milestones should be reviewed to find out at what time the child first slept through the night, stopped taking naps, and started having sleep disturbances. Current day-night sleep habits should be discussed, including naps, duration of night sleep, schedule and regularity of sleep, whether the child is a "light" or "heavy" sleeper, where the child sleeps (in relation to parents and siblings), and whether there are other people in the child's room. Prebedtime activities and bedtime rituals (*eg,* story time, snacks, goodnight kisses) should also be reviewed. Special consideration should be given to details in the bedtime routine that may aid in diagnosis (*eg,* scary bedtime stories or television programs, too much physical activity before bedtime, irregular habits, no fixed schedule). Some children have trouble sleeping because they are overtired.

It is important to inquire about parental responses to the sleep problem: Who is most worried? Why? How have they expressed this concern? If both parents seem to agree, what do they think is going on? If they disagree, are they communicating with each other? In this latter instance, it is very important to hear from *both* parents and to solicit their ideas in a nonjudgmental fashion. It is also helpful to inquire about the impact that the problem is having on the family. Are the parents losing sleep because of the child's problems? How are other siblings affected? What changes in family routines has the problem produced? Has it affected their parenting? Is it creating problems in the marriage? The answers to these questions will help determine the severity and complications of the problem and will aid in assessing the family's level of concern.

The presence of family stresses should be explored because sleep problems often begin in

TABLE 14-1
Typical Daily Sleep Time*

AGE	AVERAGE HOURS OF SLEEP (±1 HR)
Premature (29 wk gestation)	20
Newborn (full term)	18
Infant (3–9 mo)	14
1–2 yr	13
2–3 yr	12
3–4 yr	11
4–5 yr	10
6–12 yr	9.5
13–15 yr	8
16–19 yr	7.5

*From Ferber R, Rivinus M: *Med Times* 107:71, 1979. Used by permission.

TABLE 14-2
Common Sleep Problems by Age

AGE	PROBLEM	DIFFERENTIAL DIAGNOSIS
Infant	Nighttime waking	Normal variation
	Irregular sleep cycle	Immaturity
Toddler	Nighttime waking	Separation anxiety
	"Can't sleep"	Illness; parental disagreement (marital problems)
Preschool-aged	"Can't sleep"	Separation anxiety
	"Won't go to bed"	Fears of aggression
	"Gets out of bed"	Ineffective disciplining
	Nighttime waking	Parental anxiety; parental disagreement
School-aged	Nighttime waking	Nightmares; night terrors; sleepwalking/sleeptalking; enuresis; family stress; primary sleep disorder
School-aged and adolescent	Insomnia	Depression; anxiety; stress-related syndrome; attention deficit; delayed sleep phase syndrome
	Hypersomnia	Narcolepsy, idiopathic central nervous system hypersomnia, sleep-associated airway obstruction, chronic viral illness, Kleine-Levin syndrome

response to other family problems. Often it helps to preface such questions with a statement such as, "Kids can be sensitive to problems going on in the family, and these can cause the child to have problems sleeping. Is there anything that might be upsetting your child at home?" or "How are things at home?"

Finally, a family history of sleep disorders, neurologic diseases, or psychiatric illness must be ruled out. These must be explored carefully to ascertain any hereditary conditions or predispositions to sleep disturbances.

Evaluation

The most important aspects of the physical examination include a careful neurologic examination, a close inspection for evidence of central nervous system anomalies or brain damage, and a comprehensive developmental assessment. Most organic causes for sleep disorders can be ruled out after a thorough evaluation of this type.

The child's temperament should be assessed. Is the child somewhat overactive and demanding? Is he/she quiet and withdrawn? What kind of emotional issues is the child facing? The interaction between parents and child should be evaluated. Is there evidence of excessive manipulation? Does the child seem to obey the parents or is he/she generally disrespectful? Do the parents seem to have difficulty disciplining the child? Is the child perhaps being treated as older or younger than his/her age? Are the parents in agreement over issues of discipline? These questions are best answered by carefully observing the family in the office and by providing feedback to parents if other behavior problems are noted by the physician. Quite often sleep problems are a manifestation of behavioral rather than primary sleep disturbances.

On occasion the clinician may encounter a child with a sleep problem that is organic. If sleep apnea, narcolepsy, or seizures are strongly suspected, workup may necessitate an electroencephalogram, a tape cassette recording, or a videotape or time-lapse recording of the child's sleep. At this point most physicians would refer the patient to a sleep clinic or a psychiatrist.

TREATMENT

The treatment of sleep problems should be approached with several goals: to help the family break a repetitive cycle of interrupted sleep, reassure parents of the absence of organic disease, ameliorate symptoms, and help parents adopt an approach that they are likely to execute successfully. Although medications such as sedatives (antihistamines) or hypnotics (chloral hydrate) are not advocated for long-term use, they are helpful if given for a few nights to disrupt an acute pattern. The following is a brief outline of the most common sleep problems encountered in office practice, listed by chief complaint.

Most Common Sleep Problems

"Wakes Up"

Nighttime waking may be due to immature diurnal rhythms or to delay in the development of "settling" in infants and to fear of separation in toddlers. In such cases parents need to be reassured that this situation is normal. Parents should be counseled to let the child cry for as long as necessary, to initiate bedtime rituals and positive rewards, and to avoid using hypnotics or other medications.

"Can't Sleep"

Often a child tries to go to sleep but has trouble falling asleep. This situation usually becomes a problem for children who are 2 years of age, who grow frightened of the dark, start to hear voices, or are too excited to sleep. Treatment involves instructing parents to *reassure* the child, with a bedtime story (or similar ritual), a night-light, or letting the child take a favorite object to bed. Parents should be cautioned against getting into bed with the child, because this is a difficult habit to break. The physician should verify that parents agree with him/her and that they have developed a plan that suits them. If the child has a delayed sleep phase and normally falls asleep later than the parents would like, it is possible to advance the onset of sleep by waking up the child earlier in the morning and preventing the child from taking naps during the day. Eventually the child will fall asleep at an earlier time.

"Won't Go to Bed"

Some children resist going to sleep, either by refusing to get ready for bed or by fussing or crying excessively once in bed. This problem can be due to separation anxiety, to concurrent stress, or to manipulative behavior. Treatment involves teaching parents to be patient with the child. There should be adequate preparation for bedtime, including frequent reminders at 1 hour, at 30 minutes, and at 15 minutes prior to beginning the bedtime routine. The routine should be consistent and predictable, with little variation. After the parents say goodnight to the child, they must leave the room and *not* return no matter how long the child cries. Although this is initially quite anxiety provoking for parents, such patience is quickly rewarded. The child soon understands that the parents are serious and eventually goes to sleep without protesting.

"Gets Out of Bed"

This problem usually follows one of two patterns. Either the child gets out of bed shortly after bedtime and disrupts parents' evening activities or the child awakens late at night and climbs into the parents' bed. The causes of this problem are similar to those mentioned previously. The difference is that parents tacitly consent to this behavior if they do not return the child directly to bed. Parents usually report ineffective attempts to reason with the child or to gently coax him/her back to bed.

Treatment consists of helping parents maintain *discipline.* Both parents need to agree on a consistent plan of action that they will carry out regardless of the child's protests. The specifics of such a plan will vary from family to family. Careful preparation for bedtime and predictable routines are recommended. Once the parents say goodnight, they should leave the room. The child must be monitored closely. If he/she is caught getting out of bed, parents must convey the seriousness of their intentions by using whatever safe and controlled measure they prefer. This must be repeated each time the child gets up. The child who climbs into the parents' bed must be taken back to his/her own bed immediately. Parents must be firm and unemotional in carrying out discipline of this sort, otherwise the child will find a way to persist in this behavior. It is also recommended that the parents praise the child the following morning for being so good and listening to them. "Big boys and girls sleep in their own bed," is a helpful comment that can be used to appeal to the child's wish to be more grown up.

Nightmares

Nightmares are frightening dreams that can awaken a sleeping child and cause him/her to cry. These dreams can be remembered and recounted by the child; when comforted by the parents, the child usually returns to sleep without difficulty. Nightmares are normal occurrences. As children get older, they can learn to orient themselves in their room and return to sleep without involving their parents.

Night Terrors

Night terrors are distinctive episodes of nighttime waking seen primarily in preschool-aged children. The child suddenly sits up in bed and begins screaming. Parents find the child quite aroused and agitated, with sweating, rapid breathing, and "glassy-eyed" staring. In contrast to nightmares, the child is not consolable. After a few minutes the child returns to sleep, with no later recall of the event. Night terrors are most frightening for parents and other family members; they need to be reassured that these are not serious or pathologic episodes. The episodes resolve spontaneously as the child grows older and do not require treatment. Use of diazepam or imipramine hydrochloride should be reserved for those children whose episodes are causing excessive family disruption or alteration of the child's behavior during the day.

Sleepwalking and Sleeptalking

Approximately 15% to 30% of all school-aged children experience one episode of sleepwalking, and 2% to 3% experience repeated episodes.

The child suddenly sits up in bed and clumsily begins to move about, occasionally arising and walking with no purpose. It is common for the child to speak in a slurred, monosyllabic, often incomprehensible manner. Repetitive finger and hand movements also can be observed. The child walks with a blank stare and seems more asleep than awake. Although capable of stumbling or bumping into furniture, the child usually avoids walking into objects. To prevent injuries, parents must use precautions such as stair guards and window bars. The episodes are otherwise harmless and usually resolve by adolescence.

The major differential diagnosis is psychomotor epilepsy, which usually produces more fatigue and confusion on awakening and is not associated with a return to bed, as with sleepwalking. If the sleepwalking or sleeptalking is thought by parents to be purposeful, a psychologic disorder should be suspected.

Insomnia in Older Children and Adolescents

Sleep problems in older children and adolescents are usually stress related. Problems include trouble falling asleep, frequent awakening during the night, early morning awakening, daytime napping, or a chronic feeling of being tired. The physician must carefully review daily sleeping and waking habits and must sensitively inquire into issues that may be upsetting the individual. Emotional problems in children and teenagers often present with complaints of insomnia. Depression, suicidal impulses, anxiety, drug usage, and other psychiatric disturbances must be investigated before making the diagnosis of a chronic sleep disorder. Treatment depends on the diagnosis and may necessitate referral for psychiatric care or counseling. In any case, these complaints must be taken seriously by the physician and should be handled expeditiously.

Many adolescents enjoy staying up late at night, a habit that can easily result in delayed sleep phase syndrome (DSPS). The circadian rhythm becomes readjusted, so that the adolescent has trouble falling asleep before 2:00 or 3:00 A.M. and cannot wake up before 10:00 or 11:00 A.M. the next day. School problems resulting from tardiness and absenteeism are a typical complaint. Parents report that the teenager cannot be awakened in the morning, and the adolescent complains that he/she cannot fall asleep until late at night. The primary treatment for DSPS is chronotherapy, which involves systematic advancing of the sleep-wake cycle until it is normalized. The adolescent's bedtime should be advanced by 3 hours (eg, from 2:00 A.M. to 5:00 A.M. to 8:00 A.M. to 11:00 A.M.) over 6 days until it is normalized. Resistance to this simple technique should raise a suspicion of psychologic difficulties in the patient or family.

Hypersomnia in Older Children and Adolescents

Too much sleep or excessive daytime sleepiness is termed *hypersomnia,* and may be due to various disorders. Narcolepsy consists of excessive daytime sleepiness, cataplexy ("drop attacks"), hypnogogic hallucinations, and sleep paralysis. It is characterized by sleep-onset rapid eye movement (REM) episodes and dissociation of the components of REM sleep. Treatment involves increasing the nocturnal sleep period and scheduling daytime naps. Occasionally low-dose pemoline or methylphenidate hydrochloride is used to control sleepiness. In idiopathic central nervous system hypersomnia, there is constant daytime sleepiness that is not associated with other symptoms or with disturbed sleep patterns. Although hypersomnia is poorly understood, there is speculation that it is associated with chronic viral illnesses such as infectious mononucleosis. Treatment with stimulants appears to be of little long-term benefit. Sleep-associated airway obstruction may result from a variety of structural abnormalities, including enlarged tonsils and adenoids, choanal atresia or stenosis, nasal septal deviation, enlarged tongue, cleft palate, and temporomandibular joint dysfunction. Associated signs include loud snoring, mouth breathing, frequent arousal during sleep, nocturnal enuresis, and a host of behavioral problems such as hyperactivity and poor school performance. An evaluation of the ears, nose, and throat and treatment are necessary for these conditions. Finally, Kleine-Levin syndrome is a rare, poorly understood pattern of excessive sleep, hyperphagia, and abnormal behavior (eg, irritability, motor unrest, excitement), which lasts for days or weeks and recurs on a regular basis from once to 12 times a year. These symptoms should result in prompt referral for psychiatric care.

BIBLIOGRAPHY

Anders TF, Sadeh A, Appareddy V: Normal sleep in neonates and children. In Ferber R, Kryger M, editors: *Principles and practice of sleep medicine,* Philadelphia, 1995, WB Saunders.

Beltramini AU, Hertzig ME: Sleep and bedtime behavior in preschool-aged children, *Pediatrics* 71:153, 1983.

Carey WB: Night waking and temperament in infancy, *J Pediatr* 84:756, 1974.

Carskadon MA, Anders TF, Hole W: Sleep disorders in childhood and adolescence. In Fitzgerald HE, Lester BM, Yogman MW, editors: *Theory and research in behavioral pediatrics,* vol 4, New York, 1988, Plenum Press.

Christopherson ER: Incorporating behavioral pediatrics in primary care, *Pediatr Clin North Am* 29:281, 1982.

DiMario FJ, Emery ES: The natural history of night terrors, *Clin Pediatr* 26:505, 1987.

Ferber R, Kryger M, editors: *Principles and practice of sleep medicine in the child,* Philadelphia, 1995, WB Saunders.

Ferber R: Behavioral "insomnia" in the child, *Psychiatr Clin North Am* 10:641, 1987.

Guilleminault C: Mononucleosis and chronic daytime sleepiness: A long-term follow-up study, *Arch Intern Med* 146:1333, 1986.

Guilleminault C: *Sleep and its disorders in children,* New York, 1987, Raven Press.

Hawkins DR, Taub JM, Van de Castle RL: Extended sleep (hypersomnia) in young depressed patients, *Am J Psychiatry* 142:905, 1985.

Kataria S, Swanson MS, Trevathan GE: Persistence of sleep disturbances in preschool children, *J Pediatr* 110:642, 1987.

Mark JD, Brooks JG: Sleep-associated airway problems in children, *Pediatr Clin North Am* 31:907, 1984.

Parkes JD: The parasomnias, *Lancet* ii:1021, 1986.

Richman N: Sleep problems in young children, *Arch Dis Child* 56:491, 1981.

Sheldon SH, Spine J-P, Levy HB: *Pediatric sleep medicine,* Philadelphia, 1992, WB Saunders.

Thorpy MJ, Glovinsky PB: Parasomnias, *Psychiatr Clin North Am* 10:623, 1987.

Zuckerman B, Stevenson J, Bailey V: Sleep problems in early childhood: Continuities, predictive factors, and behavioral correlates, *Pediatrics* 80:664, 1987.

PART FOUR

The Adolescent

CHAPTER 15

Examination

Gail B. Slap

Primary care physicians who deal with adolescent patients must adapt their interviewing skills to address patient concerns about body image, sexuality, independence, and life roles. They must be comfortable with the developmental tasks of adolescence, family interaction, gynecology, and psychiatry. This chapter reviews the routine examination of the adolescent patient and includes topics in the areas of development, gynecology, and contraceptive counseling. Other chapters relevant to adolescent care are found in Section V (delinquency, eating disorders, suicide, drug abuse, and family dynamics), Chapter 22 (Obesity), and Chapter 95 (Sexually Transmitted Disease).

Examination of the adolescent patient requires an understanding of the physical, cognitive, and social changes that occur with puberty. The interview and physical examination provide a natural opportunity to discuss developmental changes with the adolescent as well as to monitor growth and screen for disease. The successful interview requires balancing the adolescent's concern about confidentiality with the parents' request for information.

HISTORY

Legal Issues

Most states permit physicians to treat emancipated minors and patients older than 18 years of age without parental consent. The definition of emancipated minor, however, differs among the states. It usually implies 1) abdication of parental responsibilities, 2) adolescent financial independence, and 3) residence outside the parental home. In many states the age for provision of general medical care without parental consent is higher than for contraceptive care or treatment of substance abuse, pregnancy, and sexually transmitted disease. Important legal considerations in the treatment of nonemergent medical problems include maturity of the minor and assessment of the adolescent's best interests. Statutes and court precedents related to abortion change frequently and should be reviewed before proceeding in an individual case.

Health care providers should attempt to notify parents of an adolescent's medical care whenever possible. An adolescent who initially is reluctant to inform the parent frequently agrees to do so when the reasons for parental involvement are explained. Management usually is facilitated when the adolescent is supported by his/her parents.

Approach to the Adolescent Patient

The Department of Adolescent Health of the American Medical Association has compiled a concise set of Guidelines for Adolescent Preventive Services (GAPS). The guidelines are a series of preventive health measures to be delivered annually for patients aged 11 to 21 years. The content and frequency of the GAPS recommendations are shown in Figure 15-1. The interaction with the adolescent is most effective when the visit is well structured and conducted in a relaxed, sensitive manner.

Many adolescents talk more openly when interviewed without their parents. The health provider should meet the patient and parent together but conduct part of the interview with the adolescent alone. If the adolescent agrees, the physical examination should be completed while the parent remains in the waiting room. The parent then should be invited to join the adolescent in the office. This gives the provider an opportunity to review the history and physical examination with both the patient and parent, to obtain additional information from the parent, and to discuss the management plan.

Questions addressed to the adolescent should be open-ended. This encourages discussion rather than simple yes or no answers. Poor communication, downcast eyes, and withdrawal usually are not attributable to adolescent shyness alone. Depression is a common and often unrecognized problem in teenagers. A history of behavioral problems, poor school performance, psychosomatic complaints, or frequent medical visits points to the need for a thorough psychosocial history. This history often should include direct questioning about suicidal ideation or gestures.

Psychosomatic symptoms such as abdominal pain, headache, and chest pain are common during adolescence. If a psychosomatic disorder is suspected, several meetings with the patient and parents may help identify family dynamics that are contributing to the problem. Characteristics of the psychosomatic family include excessive parental anxiety about the adolescent's symptoms, rigidity, overprotectiveness, and lack of conflict resolution. For example, parents in the midst of marital conflict may focus their attention on the teenager's functional abdominal pain rather than on their own relationship. The adolescent's symptom draws the family together around a common issue but prevents resolution of the primary problem. An integrated, multidisciplinary approach often is needed in such situations to dispel anxiety about an organic cause and to focus attention on the psychodynamics involved.

Regardless of the presenting complaint, it may be difficult to obtain a full history until the adolescent is comfortable with the health provider. Information that is not essential for management, therefore, may be obtained more readily at a subsequent visit. The patient and parent should each leave the office with a card indicating the provider's name and telephone number. The adolescent should be encouraged to discuss all visits with the parent but also should feel free to call or schedule appointments as he/she thinks necessary.

Patient Profile, Development, and Present Illness

The interviewer should begin by asking why the adolescent decided to come in for the visit. The first visit should include a discussion of the adolescent's living arrangement, family members, grade and performance in school, sports or hobbies, and social milieu. Changes in the adolescent's family life (death, divorce, remarriage, new baby, change in residence or school) should be elicited. A clear notation of cigarette, alcohol, and drug use is essential.

A developmental history should be obtained from the patient and parents. This should include complications of the mother's pregnancy, labor, or delivery. The provider should note the child's length of gestation, birth weight, developmental milestones, and school history (special classes, grade repetition, peer relationships, absenteeism).

A summary of the pediatric medical record should be included in either the history of present illness or the past medical history.

Infectious Disease

Adolescents must be fully immunized against diphtheria, tetanus, poliomyelitis, measles, mumps, rubella, and hepatitis B (see Chapter 20). After the primary immunization series, diphthe-

Recommended frequency of GAPS preventive services.

Key and Notations:

● : Once per time period

■ : Yearly

◗ : Optional

HR: High Risk Category

1. Recommendation developed by the National Heart, Lung, and Blood Institute Second Task Force on Blood Pressure in Children.

2. Recommendation developed by the National Cholesterol Education Program: Report of the Expert Panel on Blood Cholesterol Levels in Children and Adolescents, 1991.

3. Recommendation developed by the Advisory Committee for Immunization Practices.

* Screening should be performed if the adolescent is currently sexually active.

** Screening should be performed if the adolescent female is sexually active or 18 years of age or older.

HR-1: Test should be performed if there is a family history of cardiovascular disease prior to age 55 or parental history of high cholesterol. Physician may choose to perform test if family history is unknown or if adolescent has multiple risk factors for future cardiovascular disease.

HR-2: Syphilis test should be performed on and HIV test offered to adolescents who are at high risk for infection. This includes having had more than one sexual partner in last six months, having exchanged sex for drugs, being a male who has engaged in sex with other males, having used intravenous drugs (HIV), having had other STDs, having lived in an area endemic for infection, and having had a sexual partner who is at risk for infection.

HR-3: Test should be performed on adolescents who have been exposed to active TB, have lived in a homeless shelter, have been incarcerated, have lived in an area endemic for TB, or currently work in a health care setting.

HR-4: Vaccination should be provided to adolescents who have had only one previous MMR.

HR-5: Vaccination should be given 10 years following previous dT booster.

HR-6: Hepatitis B virus vaccination (HBV) should be given to susceptible adolescents at high risk for infection (see HR-2).

	Early (11-14 yrs.)	Middle (15-17 yrs.)	Late (18-21 yrs)
Health Guidance			
Parenting	●	●	◗
Adolescent Development	■	■	■
Safety Practices	■	■	■
Diet and Fitness	■	■	■
Healthy Lifestyles (sexual behavior, smoking, alcohol and drug use)	■	■	■
Screening			
Hypertension[1]	■	■	■
Hyperlipidemia[2]	HR-1		●
Eating Disorders	■	■	■
Obesity	■	■	■
Tobacco Use	■	■	■
Alcohol & Drug Use	■	■	■
Sexual Behavior	■	■	■
Sexually Transmissible Diseases (STDs)			
Gonorrhea	■ *	■ *	■ *
Chlamydia	■ *	■ *	■ *
Genital Warts	■ *	■ *	■ *
Syphilis	HR-2	HR-2	HR-2
HIV Infection	HR-2	HR-2	HR-2
Cervical Cancer	■ *	■ *	■ **
Depression/Suicide Risk	■	■	■
Physical, Sexual or Emotional Abuse	■	■	■
Learning Problems	■	■	■
Tuberculosis	HR-3	HR-3	HR-3
Immunizations[3]			
Measles, Mumps, & Rubella	HR-4	HR-4	HR-4
Diphtheria & Tetanus		HR-5	
Hepatitis B	HR-6	HR-6	HR-6

FIG 15-1

Recommended frequency of Guidelines for Adolescent Preventative Services (GAPS).

ria and tetanus require boosters every 10 years throughout adulthood, with the vaccine for diphtheria reduced to one tenth the pediatric dose. All adolescents should have received a booster immunization for measles-mumps-rubella during late childhood. In addition, all adolescents should be immunized against hepatitis B.

There is no need to routinely screen all adolescents with chest radiography. Tuberculin skin testing is indicated for adolescents who are exposed to index cases and for screening of high-risk populations.

Sexual History

During adolescence, 60% of boys and 50% of girls have intercourse. Only 30% of sexually active teenagers, however, report that they consistently use contraception. Consequently, 40% of girls become pregnant by age 19 years. One quarter of all cases of sexually transmitted infections reported annually in the United States occur in teenagers who have not yet finished high school. It is imperative that the health care provider discuss sexual activity and contraceptive options with the adolescent. The sexually active girl must understand that gynecologic care is an integral part of her routine medical care. When the parents are out of the room, the adolescent should be asked if he/she is sexually active. A tactful approach is to ask what kind of contraception the patient uses.

An adolescent who is considering the onset of sexual activity should receive anticipatory guidance regarding contraception and the prevention of sexually transmitted illness. All adolescents, regardless of the preferred method of contraception, should be urged to use condoms to decrease the risk of infection. The health provider should serve as a counselor and educator and should be prepared to discuss the implications of sexual activity with the adolescent. Although the number of reported cases of AIDS among adolescents in the United States remains small, this population is clearly at risk for infection. An understanding of HIV transmission and prevention therefore is essential.

Substance Abuse

The most comprehensive data on drug and alcohol use among adolescents in the United States come from a 22-year study called "Monitoring the Future." Self-administered questionnaires were completed by 50,000 eighth through 12th graders in 1995. The results indicate a rise in illicit drug use, particularly marijuana, since 1991. More than 28% of eighth graders, 41% of 10th graders, and 48% of 12th graders have used at least one illicit drug. The most commonly used drugs among eighth graders are inhalants (22%) and marijuana (20%).

This increase in drug and alcohol use is associated with a decline in both the students' perceived risk of use and peer disapproval of use. Past trend analyses indicate that use rates will continue to increase until the attitudes about use reverse.

In addition to the disturbing trends in illicit drug use, alcohol binge drinking (five or more drinks at one time) has increased since 1992. Within the 2 weeks preceding the 1995 survey, one in seven 8th graders and one in four 10th and 12th graders reported binge drinking.

More than one fifth of students are daily cigarette smokers when they leave high school, and most begin smoking by the age of 13 years.

Adolescent drug abuse usually comes to medical attention only when behavioral problems, injuries, or overdose forces the patient and family to seek help. The adolescent may admit to drug use prior to these problems if assured that the parents will not be told. It is important, however, to involve the parents in their child's problem with drugs as soon as possible. Unexplained depression, difficulty in school, behavioral change, weight loss, tachycardia, or hypertension should lead the physician to consider drug abuse. The teenager should be questioned about drug use and suicidal ideation, should understand the ramifications of drug use and driving, and should be informed of the potential for accidental overdose. Parents who abuse alcohol themselves should be informed that there is little chance that their son or daughter will stop drinking until they stop their own drinking.

Nutritional History

The growth spurt that occurs during adolescence represents one of the most rapid developmental rates experienced during the human life cycle. Most adolescent girls require at least 2350 calories at the age of 11 years and 2500 calories at the age of 15 years. Adolescent boys require 200 to 600 calories more than girls of the same age. The increasing popularity of fast-food chains, macrobiotic diets, and rapid-weight-loss regimens place the adolescent at high risk for inadequate nutritional intake. The health care provider should determine if caloric intake is appropriate and should educate the patient and parent of nutritional requirements. It should be remembered that adolescent girls require 18 mg of iron daily, three times the amount in the average American diet.

Eating disorders are common in the adolescent population. The obese adolescent requires close supervision and support to maximize weight reduction and nutritional adequacy. The adolescent who has signs of weight loss, secretive eating habits, distorted body image, amenorrhea, delayed menarche, and other manifestations of anorexia nervosa or bulimia should be asked directly about restrictive eating, binge eating, self-induced vomiting, and use of laxatives or diuretics.

Menstrual History

The age of menarche, the interval and duration of menses, and the presence of dysmenorrhea should always be recorded in the adolescent girl's history. The average age of menarche in the United States is 12.8 years, and 95% of girls reach menarche by the age of 14.8 years. Worldwide, the mean age of menarche is 13.5 years, and 95% of girls reach menarche by the age of 15.5 years. Menses may be irregular due to anovulation for up to 2 years following menarche. The development of dysmenorrhea during middle or late adolescence often is associated with ovulation and increasing regularity of the menstrual cycle.

Menarche can occur at any time during puberty, but is most common at Tanner stage IV. Delayed puberty in girls is defined as no breast development by the age of 13 years or the absence of menses by age 15 years. Patients who meet these criteria should undergo a complete medical evaluation. It is important to document eating and exercise habits in young women with primary or secondary amenorrhea. There is some evidence that a critical body fat percentage is necessary to begin and maintain menstruation.

Family and Social History

The clinician has had an opportunity by this point in the history to discuss family and social issues with the adolescent on a one-to-one basis. Time should be set aside after the physical examination to discuss family medical history, intrafamily relationships, school performance, growth and development, and social maturation with the adolescent and parent together. Parents often are concerned that the adolescent's symptoms are an early manifestation of a disease that is present in another family member. It is especially important to inquire about a family history of hypertension, diabetes mellitus, and coronary artery disease. For example, hereditary hyperlipidemia is found in 30% of teenagers whose parent(s) had myocardial infarctions before the age of 50 years. These adolescents require education about risk factors for heart disease and close surveillance of their serum lipid levels.

This part of the history taking allows the provider both to obtain information from the parent and to observe the dynamics between the patient and parent. Some conflict or disagreement is to be anticipated as the adolescent strives to achieve independence. The manner in which the parent handles these conflicts is important. Parents who repeatedly preempt authority without allowing the adolescent to discuss his/her feelings often face prolonged or exaggerated rebellion. Conversely, parents who abdicate all authority may experience less conflict but often are faced with adolescents who are unable to set limits and who have difficulty achieving a smooth transition to adulthood. Both adolescent and parent may benefit from tactful suggestions for limit setting and conflict resolution.

PHYSICAL EXAMINATION

General Approach

The physical examination should be conducted without the parents present whenever the adolescent permits. This gives the health care provider and patient a chance to discuss normal adolescent development and sensitive issues such as sexual activity or substance abuse. Most adolescents are anxious to know if their height, weight, and sexual maturation are normal. The examiner should routinely discuss these observations both to reassure the patient and to clarify the expected changes of adolescence.

Each visit should include measurements of height, weight, blood pressure, and heart rate. Sexual development according to the method of Tanner, breast examination, genital examination in boys, pelvic examination in sexually active girls, scoliosis screening, skin examination, and visual-acuity testing should be done annually.

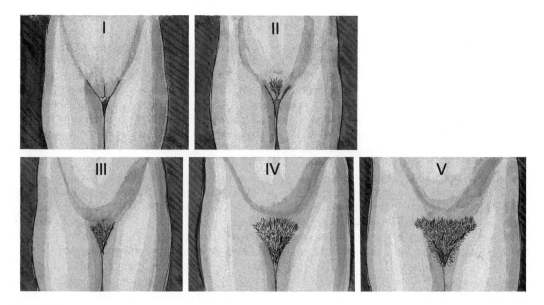

FIG 15-2

Stages of pubic hair growth in girls according to Marshall and Tanner: Stage I: no pubic hair; Stage II: long, pigmented hair over mons veneris or labia majora; Stage III: dark, coarse, curled hair spread sparsely over the mons veneris; Stage IV: abundant, adult-type sexual hair limited to the mons veneris; Stage V: sexual hair is adult-type in quantity and distribution, with spread to the medial aspect of the thighs. [Adapted from Marshall WA, Tanner JM: *Arch Dis Child,* 44:291–303, 1969.]

Growth and Development

Height and weight should be plotted on grids to indicate the percentiles for age. However, because chronologic age correlates poorly with adolescent development, Tanner stage also should be noted. Pubic hair growth (Fig. 15-2) and breast development (Fig. 15-3) in girls and pubic hair growth and genital development in boys (Fig. 15-4) are used to classify the sexual maturation of adolescents into one of five stages. If there are no signs of puberty by 15.2 years in a boy or 13.4 years in a girl, sexual development is considered delayed (Fig. 15-5). Furthermore, if more than 5 years elapse between thelarche and menarche in the girl or between initiation and completion of genital growth in the boy, the progression of puberty is considered abnormal. Full medical and endocrine evaluation are indicated for delayed initiation or progression of puberty.

Blood Pressure

Distribution norms for childhood and adolescent blood pressure (BP) were established in 1977 (*see* Figs. 15-1 and 15-2). Hypertension was defined as three BP readings greater than the 95th percentile obtained over 3 months. For most adolescents, a BP reading above the 95th percentile on the initial examination will fall within the normal range on subsequent visits. A single reading above the 90th percentile probably should be repeated in 6 months and yearly thereafter.

Scoliosis Screening

Idiopathic scoliosis affects 5% of adolescents. It usually becomes evident during the rapid growth phase (Tanner stage II to III in girls, Tanner stage III to IV in boys) and may progress very quickly during this time. Appropriate intervention requires early detection and close follow-up throughout puberty.

The physician first should observe the patient's back for asymmetry of the shoulders, scapulae, or pelvis (Fig. 15-6). The anterior chest should be examined for breast asymmetry. Next, the patient should be asked to bend forward to a 90° angle (Fig. 15-7). This accentuates the curvature and causes protrusion of the rib cage on the convex side of the curve (Fig. 15-8). The primary curve usually is to the right in idiopathic

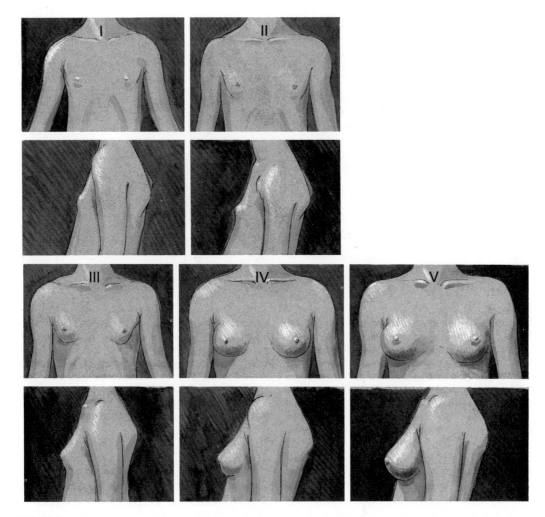

FIG 15-3
Stages of breast development in girls according to Marshall and Tanner: Stage I: no breast development; Stage II: breast budding, widening of areola and elevation on mound of subareolar tissue, erect papilla; Stage III: continued enlargement of breast and widening of areola without separation of their contours; Stage IV: areola and papilla project above the plane of the enlarging breast; Stage V: the mature breast, areola and breast in same plane, erect papilla. [Adapted from Marshall WA, Tanner JM: *Arch Dis Child,* 44:291–303, 1969.]

scoliosis and comprises the first part of the descriptive term (*eg,* thoracolumbar). The degree of scoliosis is then determined: mild scoliosis, less than 20° curvature; moderate, 20° to 40°; severe, more than 55°. A typical description might read, "Scoliosis, right thoracolumbar, moderate degree." If scoliosis is detected, leg lengths should be measured, a radiograph of the spine should be obtained, and the adolescent should be referred for orthopedic examination.

Breast Examination
Breast examination is important in both adolescent boys and girls. Gynecomastia occurs in 40% of adolescent boys and is most common at the age of 14 to 15 years. In 75% of the cases, it is bilateral and resolves within 2 years. Many boys with gynecomastia are too embarrassed to discuss their concerns with the health care provider; the physician should not wait until the patient asks about the gynecomastia but should reassure him

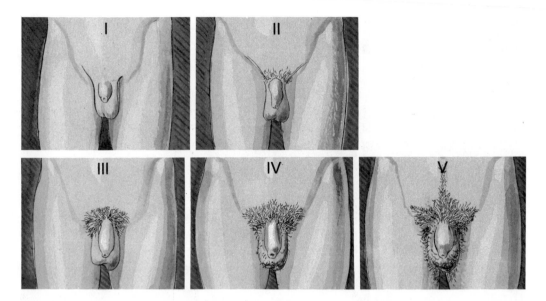

FIG 15-4

Stages of pubic hair growth and development of the external genitalia according to Marshall and Tanner. Description of stages of pubic hair: Stage I: no pubic hair; Stage II: long, downy, pigmented hair at and lateral to the base of the penis; Stage III: dark, coarse, curled hair at and lateral to the base of the penis; Stage IV: abundant, adult-type sexual hair limited to the pubic region, with no extension to the thighs; Stage V: sexual hair is adult-type in quantity and distribution, with spread to the medial aspect of the thighs. Description of genitalia stages: Stage I: prepubertal; Stage II: enlargement of the testes and scrotum; Stage III: lengthening of the penis, further enlargement of the testes and scrotum; Stage IV: increase in width and length of penis, further enlargement of testes and scrotum, increased pigmentation of scrotum; Stage V: adult size and shape of genitals. [Adapted from Marshall WA, Tanner JM: *Arch Dis Child,* 44:291–303, 1969.]

that it is a normal part of development that usually resolves spontaneously. Gynecomastia that persists for more than 2 years requires medical evaluation. If no cause is found and the adolescent is troubled by the breast enlargement, surgical repair can be considered.

Breast masses are a common finding in adolescent girls and usually represent benign fibroadenomas. These lesions are persistent, freely mobile, and usually do not require surgery. Cystic lesions are less common and usually resolve with needle aspiration. Carcinoma of the breast is extremely rare in the adolescent population.

Pelvic Examination

Every sexually active adolescent girl should have a pelvic examination performed as part of the routine physical examination. It should include speculum inspection of the vagina and cervix, Papanicolaou smear, endocervical swabs for gonorrhea and chlamydia, bimanual examination, and rectovaginal examination.

The first pelvic examination of the virginal adolescent should be done at age 18 years. It should always be done, regardless of age, in the adolescent with in utero exposure to diethylstilbestrol, unexplained abdominal or pelvic pain, menstrual abnormality, or vaginal discharge.

The examination should be explained thoroughly, with the aid of a pelvic model. If the adolescent refuses examination, it is best to delay it whenever possible rather than assume an aggressive approach that will interfere with subsequent follow-up and compliance. If the patient resists speculum or bimanual examination, a rectovaginal examination should be done and any discharge from the vagina should be examined microscopically and cultured.

Laboratory Evaluation

The laboratory tests for all adolescent patients include urinalysis, and hematocrit. All sexually active girls should have a Papanicolaou smear, endocervical culture for gonorrhea, endocervical

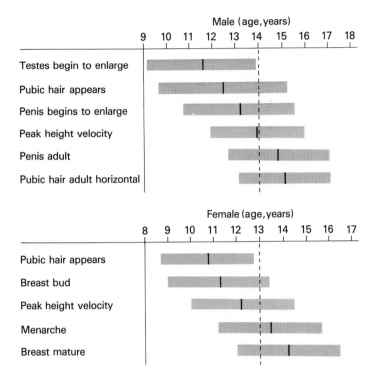

Male (age, years)

| | 9 | 10 | 11 | 12 | 13 | 14 | 15 | 16 | 17 | 18 |

Testes begin to enlarge

Pubic hair appears

Penis begins to enlarge

Peak height velocity

Penis adult

Pubic hair adult horizontal

Female (age, years)

| | 8 | 9 | 10 | 11 | 12 | 13 | 14 | 15 | 16 | 17 |

Pubic hair appears

Breast bud

Peak height velocity

Menarche

Breast mature

FIG 15-5

Normal timing of puberty in boys and in girls. Horizontal bars represent plus/minus 2 SD; vertical marks represent mean age of stage. [Adapted from Prader A, Constitutional delay of growth and puberty. In Chiunello G, Laron Z (ed): Proceedings of the Serono Symposia: Recent Progress in Pediatric Endocrinology, Orlando, 1977, Academic Press.]

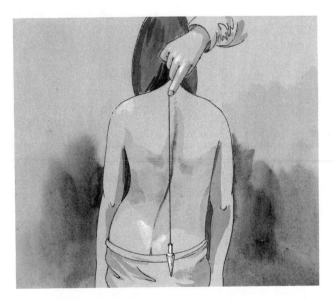

FIG 15-6

Observation of patient's back demonstrating asymmetry of the shoulders, scapula, and pelvis.

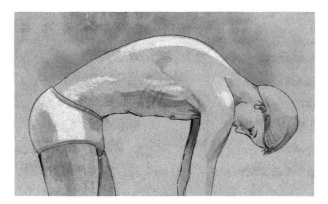

FIG 15-7
Correct forward bending position to accentuate curvature.

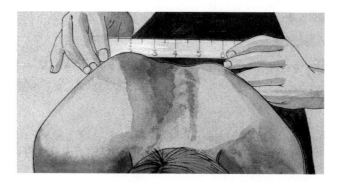

FIG 15-8
Protrusion of the rib cage evident on assuming forward bending position. Protrusion occurs on the convex side of the curve.

culture or antigen detection screen for *Chlamydia trachomatis,* and serologic testing for syphilis. All sexually active boys should have annual testing for urinary leukocyte esterase, urethral cultures for gonorrhea and chlamydia if positive, and serologic testing for syphilis.

The decision to screen adolescents for antibody to HIV should be based on the patient's risk for infection. The number of reported cases of AIDS among American adolescents aged 13 to 19 years remains small relative to the total number of reported cases. However, because of the future risk confronting a young person who is newly sexually active, the physician must be prepared to answer questions pertaining to HIV infection and to counsel adolescents about protection against infection.

SUMMARY

1. Most of the history should be obtained with the adolescent alone in the office. Time should be allowed after the physical examination to interview the adolescent and parents together and to discuss the physician's impressions.
2. The physical examination should be conducted without the parents in the room. Height, weight, BP, heart rate, Tanner stage, and examination for scoliosis should be included in each visit.
3. Pelvic examination should always be performed for the sexually active girl or for the girl with in utero exposure to diethylstilbestrol, abdominal or pelvic pain, menstrual abnormality, or vaginal discharge.

4. All adolescents should have a urinalysis, hematocrit, and cholesterol and triglyceride levels. Sexually active girls should have a Papanicolaou smear, endocervical cultures for gonorrhea and *C. trachomatis,* and RPR test. Sexually active boys should have urinary leukocyte esterase or urethral cultures for gonorrhea and *C. trachomatis* and a RPR test.

BIBLIOGRAPHY

American Medical Association: *AMA Guidelines for Adolescent Preventive Services (GAPS): Recommendations and rationale,* Baltimore, 1994, Williams & Wilkins.

Centers for Disease Control and Prevention: 1993 Sexually transmitted diseases treatment guidelines, *MMWR* 42(No. RR-14):1–102, 1993.

Congress of the U.S. Office of Technology Assessment: *Adolescent Health, Vol I. Summary and Policy Options,* OTA-H-468, Washington, U.S. Government Printing Office, April 1991.

Council on Scientific Affairs, American Medical Association: Confidential health services for adolescents, *JAMA* 269:1404–1407, 1993.

Horan MJ, et al: Report of the Second Task Force on blood pressure control in children—1987, *Pediatrics* 79:1–25, 1987.

Johnston LD, Bachman JG, O'Malley PM: *Summary of 1995 drug study results. University of Michigan News and Information Services.* Ann Arbor, 1995, University of Michigan.

Johnston LD, O'Malley PM, Bachman JG: *National Survey Results on Drug Use from the Monitoring the Future study, 1975-1993, Vol. I, Secondary School Students.* Rockville, National Institute on Drug Abuse, NIH Publication No. 94-3809.

Kulin HE, Reiter EO: Delayed pubertal development. In McAnarney ER, Kreipe RE, Orr DP, Comerci GD, editors: *Textbook of adolescent medicine,* Philadelphia, 1992, WB Saunders.

Slap GB, Jablow MM: *Teenage health care.* New York, 1994, Pocket Books.

Society for Adolescent Medicine: HIV infection and AIDS in adolescents. *J Adol Health* 15:427–434, 1994.

Sollom T: State actions on reproductive health issues in 1994, *Fam Plan Perspec* 27:83–87, 1995.

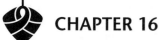

CHAPTER 16

Psychosocial Concerns of the Adolescent

English D. Willis

The psychosocial development that occurs during adolescence involves the accomplishment of several developmental tasks, the most important of which are establishing independence from parents, achieving a satisfying and realistic body image, establishing a meaningful and satisfying sexual relationship, and choosing a career and achieving economic stability. Progression through each of these developmental tasks is necessary if the adolescent is to establish a sense of identity and become a healthy adult.

The psychosocial development of adolescence may be classified into three phases: early (ages 10 to 14 years), middle (ages 15 to 17 years), and late (ages 17 years through early twenties). The adolescent's behavior is influenced by his/her phase of development. During each phase, adolescents concentrate on accomplishing a particular aspect of each developmental task. However, their psychosocial development both influences and is influenced by their ability to master each developmental task.

The assigned age range for each phase is arbitrary and varies among individuals and with different social and cultural backgrounds. Psychosocial development will also vary with differences in physical maturation. Because the range of normal pubertal development is so wide, adolescents of the same chronologic age who are at different levels of pubertal development will vary in their ability to accomplish each developmental task. In addition, adolescents at either end of the maturation spectrum, early vs late, will behave differently from the majority.

In the care of adolescents, knowledge of normal adolescent psychosocial and cognitive development is essential. The physician is able to monitor the maturational process of the adoles-

cent toward adulthood and counsel the parents about recent and anticipated changes in the behavior of their adolescent.

PHASES OF ADOLESCENCE

Early Adolescence

This phase of development usually occurs between the ages of 10 and 14 years. It is during this phase that young adolescents begin to establish independence. In their effort to develop a separate identity from their parents, they are often viewed as rebellious and difficult. Young adolescents may be quick to disagree with parents and take the opposite view on an issue to test parental values. They will often cast away hobbies or objects that link them to their childhood or demonstrate their dependence. The role of the primary care physician is to recognize these changes and to reassure the parents that this is normal separation behavior.

Emotionally, the adolescent will move away from the family toward peers of the same sex or other adults. These friends are often idolized and appear to be the center of the adolescent's "world." Adolescents within the same peer group develop similar patterns of dress, hairstyles, and speaking. It is important to the young adolescent to fit in and not appear different from his/her peers.

Coincident with psychosocial growth is pubertal development. Young adolescents must adjust to the physical changes that are occurring in their bodies. Enormous amounts of time are spent on grooming and on becoming acquainted with their new bodies. Young adolescents focus attention not only on their development but also on that of their friends, to see if their developmental changes are comparable. For the late or early maturing adolescent, this time can be particularly stressful. It is often beneficial to acknowledge the level of development and counsel the adolescent on the maturation process.

Early adolescence is the time of sexual curiosity. Masturbation and sexual play with same-sex friends is common. Two of three boys experience their first ejaculation through masturbation. Heterosexual intercourse is also occurring at an earlier age for many; thus the discussion of sexual activity and contraceptive counseling at an earlier age is appropriate.

Cognitive maturation, the transition from concrete to abstract conceptualization, begins during adolescence. Young adolescents think concretely and are unable to relate aspects of one experience to another or relate their present actions to future consequences. They frequently respond to questions literally, not figuratively. Knowledge of the young adolescent's thinking process is important for the physician trying to obtain an accurate history or provide counseling.

Middle Adolescence

During middle adolescence, ages 15 to 17 years, body awareness is heightened. Adolescents are concerned with their physical appearance and believe that others are also concerned. In an effort to become comfortable with their new bodies, greater time is invested in grooming, exercising, and experimenting with new images such as makeup and clothing styles. This is done with the purpose of developing a satisfying and realistic body image. However, their focused attention on themselves is a contributing factor to the self-centeredness of this age group.

Middle adolescents experience sexual drives and aggression and must learn to control and be comfortable with their sexuality. During this phase peer groups expand to include friends of the opposite sex. Taking risks and experimenting with sex, drugs, alcohol, and cigarettes is common. The increase in sexual activity among adolescents makes it imperative to obtain a sexual history and provide contraceptive counseling.

Experiences of adolescents are broadened by their relationships with adults outside the family. They are exposed to new and unfamiliar situations and lifestyles. Situations in the struggle for independence are often frightening and create an ambivalence in adolescents' separation process. This ambivalence may result in increased tension with parents and other family members.

Middle adolescents have a greater ability to think abstractly. Conceptualization expands beyond past and present experiences, and they are able to theorize. Their ability to understand spatial relationships and to utilize symbols improves. These new abilities are impressive to many adolescents and contribute to their already self-centered behavior.

Late Adolescence

Late adolescence is the period from age 17 through the early twenties. During this phase one of the primary developmental tasks facing the adolescent is selecting a career and achieving economic stability. With the completion of high school, future career decisions must be made. The array of available options and the concern for economic independence contribute to the stress of this period. Those adolescents electing to continue their education prolong this growth task because of their financial dependence on family or others.

The value system of older adolescents is changing. They are often idealistic, with rigid concepts of right and wrong. Causes are embraced with conviction. Peer-group relationships are replaced by individual friendships. Older adolescents are capable of developing close, caring, and intimate relationships with a member of the opposite sex. Most have obtained a secure and realistic physical image of themselves and are capable of committing themselves to relationships with others. Relationships with parents improve because the adolescents have established a sense of identity and are no longer threatened by seeking their parents' advice or counseling. Late adolescence therefore marks the period of integration of the various developmental tasks in an effort to become an adult.

THE EFFECT OF EARLY VS LATE PHYSICAL MATURATION

The stage of pubertal development in an adolescent appears to be a better correlate of psychosocial development than of chronologic age. Because the age range for normal pubertal development is so wide, there are great variations in behavior within any age group.

Differences in the behavioral characteristics of early- vs late-maturing adolescents have been shown. In a previous study, early-maturing boys were judged to be more popular, self-assured, poised, and athletic; the late-maturing boys were seen as less physically attractive, less poised, more attention-seeking, and more talkative. For girls, however, there were no clear advantages in being an early maturer. Early-maturing girls, compared with late-maturing girls, exhibited less prestige, popularity, and leadership qualities. The level of self-esteem was higher in the late-maturing girls than in those who had matured early.

A correlation also exists between academic performance and timing of physical maturation. Compared with early- and mid-maturing boys, late-maturing boys had less desire to complete college, were characterized less often as above average in intellectual abilities, and were less often in the upper third of their class for academic achievements. However, for girls a similar correlation between educational and intellectual achievements in early vs late maturation did not exist. This information may be important to the health care provider when discussing behavior and school performance with the adolescent boy and his parents.

BIBLIOGRAPHY

Conger JJ: *Adolescence and youth,* New York, 1973, Harper & Row.

Duke PM, Carlsmith JM, Jennings D, et al: Educational correlates of early and late sexual maturation in adolescence. *J Pediatr* 100:633–637, 1982.

Felice ME: Adolescence: General considerations. In Levine MD, Carey WB, Crocker AC, et al, editors: *Developmental-behavioral pediatrics,* Philadelphia, 1983, WB Saunders.

Felice ME, Friedman SB: Behavioral considerations in the health care of adolescents, *Pediatr Clin North Am* 29:399–413, 1982.

Gross RT, Duke PM: Adolescence: Effects of early versus late physical maturation on adolescent behavior. In Levine MD, Carey WB, Crocker AC, et al, editors: *Developmental-behavioral pediatrics,* Philadelphia, 1983, WB Saunders.

Hayes CD: *Risking the future: Adolescent sexuality, pregnancy and child bearing,* vol 1, Washington, 1987, National Academy Press.

Irwin CE Jr, Millstein SG: Biopsychosocial correlates of risk-taking behaviors in adolescence: Can the physician intervene? *J Adolesc Health Care* 7:825–965, 1986.

Marks A, Fisher M: Health assessment and screening during adolescence, *Pediatrics* 80 (suppl):135–158, 1987.

Neinstein LS: *Adolescent health care: A practical guide,* Baltimore, 1984, Urban and Schwarzenberg.

Slap GB: Normal physiological and psychosocial growth in the adolescent, *J Adolesc Health Care* 7:13s–23s, 1986.

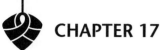

CHAPTER 17

Delayed Menarche (Primary Amenorrhea)

Janice Key

Menarche usually occurs during the second half of puberty in Tanner stages III and IV and after the growth rate has begun to decrease. Thelarche is the first sign of normal puberty and occurs between ages 8 and 12 years (mean, 11 years) with menarche following the onset of thelarche by 1 to 3 years. Therefore, delayed menarche (primary amenorrhea) is no menses by age 16 years or by 3 years after thelarche.

DIFFERENTIAL DIAGNOSIS OF PRIMARY AMENORRHEA

I. NORMAL PUBERTY
- Pregnancy
- Hypothalamic dysfunction
  Weight loss
  Obesity
  Stress
  Excessive exercise
  Chronic illness
  Medications
  Anorexia nervosa
- Abnormal structure
  Imperforate hymen
  Transverse vaginal septum
  Uterine adhesions (Asherman syndrome)
  Uterine agenesis (Mayer-Rokitansky sequence)
- Ovarian failure
  Galactosemia
  Ataxia-telangectasia
  Postinfectious
  Irradiation
  Chemotherapy
  Autoimmune
  Ovarian cyst/tumor
- Excessive androgens
  Polycystic ovary syndrome (Stein-Leventhal syndrome)
  Ovarian androgen syndrome
  Partial congenital adrenal hypertrophy
- Endocrinopathies
  Hypothyroidism
  Hyperprolactinemia

II. ABNORMAL PUBERTY
- Androgen insensitivity syndrome (testicular feminization)
- Ovarian failure
  Turner syndrome
  (*see* differential as above)
- Hypothalamic-pituitary dysfunction
  Adenoma/carcinoma
  Irradiation
  Chemotherapy
  Postinfectious
  Trauma
- Endocrinopathies
  17-α-hydroxylase deficiency
  Hypothyroidism

NORMAL PUBERTY

Although the differential diagnosis for primary amenorrhea is extensive, the initial approach should be to determine if puberty has occurred normally. The history should include a complete adolescent history (Home, Education, Activities, Depression, Sexual activity, and Substance use [HEADSS]), any recent weight change, exercise, medications, past medical history (especially chronic illnesses), review of systems, and a family history, as well as an exact determination of the timing and sequence of thelarche and adrenarche. The physical examination should include a general physical examination including height, weight, and vital signs, as well as a genital examination for Tanner staging, internal and external structure, and evaluation of estrogen effect. Estrogenization can be determined by examination of the vaginal epithelium. Once exposed to estrogen, the vaginal epithelium becomes a thicker squamous epithelium and therefore should not have visible vessels as are seen in the prepubertal vaginal epithelium.

Further evaluation and testing should be based on the history and physical examination. Patients with a history of normal puberty and a normal physical examination should have a pregnancy test followed by a progesterone challenge if the pregnancy test is negative. If estrogen is present to stimulate a proliferative endometrium, then progesterone (10 mg twice a day for 5 days) will convert the endometrium to a secretory phase and result in withdrawal vaginal bleeding within 2 weeks. A positive progesterone challenge usually indicates that the hypothelamic-pituitary-ovarian axis and uterine function are normal. Lack of withdrawal bleeding following progesterone may indicate an abnormality in one of these areas. Additional testing may include luteinizing hormone (LH) and follicle-stimulating hormone (FSH), prolactin, thyroid function tests and thyroid-stimulating hormone (TSH), and pelvic ultrasound (with vaginal probe).

ABNORMAL PUBERTY

Evaluation of a patient who has not had a normal puberty can be approached by determining if thelarche has occurred. Thelarche indicates the presence of estrogen and therefore also implies hypothalamic and pituitary stimulation. Patients who have had normal thelarche and adrenarche should be carefully examined for obstructions to vaginal flow, such as an imperforate hymen or transverse vaginal septum. If an abnormality cannot be found on examination, pelvic ultrasound (with vaginal probe) is indicated and may be followed by hysterosalpingogram. Patients also may be found to have an absent cervix and uterus by examination or by ultrasound. These patients should have a karyotype to differentiate androgen insensitivity (testicular feminization syndrome) (46,XY) from congenital absence of the Mullerian structures (Rokitansky sequence) (46,XX). Androgen insensitivity also can be suspected clinically if the patient has no pubic or axillary hair.

Patients who have not had thelarche also have a lack of estrogen due to ovarian failure or hypothalamic-pituitary dysfunction. These two categories can be differentiated by measuring LH and FSH. An elevated FSH indicates ovarian failure. These patients should have a karyotype to diagnose Turner syndrome (45,X; 46,XX/45,X; 46,XisoX; 45,X/46,XY). If the karyotype is normal, the patient should be evaluated further for ovarian failure, including ovarian autoantibodies for autoimmune premature ovarian failure, and also should be referred for an evaluation for 17-α-hydroxylase deficiency. Certain conditions are associated with premature ovarian failure including galactosemia, ataxia-telangiectasia, irradiation, chemotherapy, and postinfectious ovarian failure.

Patients who have not had thelarche and who have a low FSH have some form of hypothalamic-pituitary dysfunction. Further laboratory testing should be determined by the history and the physical examination of the patient. Initial tests may include thyroid function tests and TSH (hypothyroidism), prolactin (pituitary adenoma), and computed tomography or magnetic resonance imaging (pituitary or hypothalamic lesion).

BIBLIOGRAPHY

Blythe MB: Amenorrhea/Oligomenorrhea. *Adolescent Health Update* 4(1):1–7, 1992.
Polaneczky MM, Slap GB: Menstrual Disorders in the Adolescent: Amenorrhea. *Pediatr Rev* 13(2):43–48, 1992.

CHAPTER 18

Dysfunctional Uterine Bleeding

Ernest M. Graham

DEFINITIONS

Dysfunctional uterine bleeding (DUB) is bleeding from the uterine endometrium that is unrelated to organic, systemic, or iatrogenic causes. Most patients with DUB have anovulatory cycles; however, ovulatory cycles also can occur. Uterine bleeding secondary to such pathologic entities as blood dyscrasias, submucous myomas, endometrial polyps, uterine carcinoma, and accidents of pregnancy should not be considered dysfunctional.

Menorrhagia is prolonged (more than 7 days) or excessive (more than 80 mL) uterine bleeding occurring at regular intervals.

Metrorrhagia is a variable amount of uterine bleeding occurring at irregular but frequent intervals.

DIFFERENTIAL DIAGNOSIS

Pregnancy is the most common cause of abnormal bleeding in any woman of reproductive age. Initial attempts to diagnose DUB should be directed toward eliminating anatomic lesions of the reproductive tract and coagulation disorders as possible etiologic factors. Coagulation disorders are found in as many as 20% of adolescent girls who require hospitalization for abnormal uterine bleeding.

Disorders that may resemble DUB include:

- Intrauterine benign neoplasia (polyps, myomas)
- Reproductive tract malignancy (carcinoma of the cervix, corpus)
- Bleeding associated with early pregnancy (threatened abortion, ectopic pregnancy, hydatidiform mole) or the puerperium (subinvolu-

tion of the uterus placental polyp, retained products of conception)
- Blood dyscrasias (thrombocytopenic purpura, von Willebrand disease, platelet abnormalities)
- Cervical polyps or erosion
- Chronic endometritis
- Intrauterine synechiae
- Vaginal lesions
- Intrauterine device (IUD)

Other causes of abnormal uterine bleeding include:

- *Hypothalamus.* Dysfunction at the hypothalamic level is the most common abnormality responsible for anovulation. Emotional stress can cause disruption of hypothalamic function and lead to anovulation and DUB.
- *Pituitary.* Disruption of the normal menstrual cycle may be the earliest sign of pituitary neoplasia, which precedes amenorrhea. The finding of an elevated serum prolactin level may lead to the diagnosis of a prolactin-secreting pituitary adenoma.
- *Adrenal.* Adrenal hyperfunction, such as congenital adrenal hyperplasia, can lead to anovulatory cycles.
- *Thyroid.* Both hypothyroidism and hyperthyroidism may lead to anovulatory bleeding.
- *Drugs.* Many drugs, such as gonadal steroids, psychopharmacologic agents, and autonomic drugs, also have well-established inhibitory effects on the ovulatory process.

LABORATORY AIDS

1. Serum human chorionic gonadotropin (HCG) is used to rule out pregnancy.
2. Hemoglobin, serum iron, and serum ferritin

levels should be obtained because patients with DUB are at high risk for iron deficiency anemia. Iron replacement therapy should be started, if indicated.

3. Thyroid-stimulating hormone is used to rule out hypo- and hyperthyroidism.
4. Serum prolactin is used to rule out pituitary adenoma.
5. Prothrombin time/activated partial prothromboplastin time, platelets, and bleeding time are used to rule out coagulopathy, if suggested by history and physical examination.

PHYSICAL FINDINGS

Obesity is frequently associated with anovulation and DUB, probably because of the sequestration of estrogens in the body fat, which prevents the surge of luteinizing hormone required for ovulation to occur. Adipocytes also can convert androgens to estrogens, which becomes significant in the obese patient and can cause cycle disruption.

Undernutrition also can lead to DUB and eventually amenorrhea. Anorexia nervosa and vigorous exercise with or without significant weight loss have been associated with amenorrhea and anovulatory cycles.

PATHOPHYSIOLOGY

The predominant cause of DUB in the postmenstrual and premenopausal years is anovulation; during the rest of the reproductive years, most DUB is associated with ovulation.

Patients with anovulatory DUB have continuous estradiol production without corpus luteum formation and progesterone production. The steady state of estrogen stimulation leads to a continuously proliferating endometrium, which may outgrow its blood supply or lose nutrients with varying degrees of necrosis. In contrast to normal menstruation, uniform slough to the basalis layer does not occur, which produces excessive uterine blood flow.

Low levels of estrogen yield intermittent spotting, which may be prolonged but is generally light in quantity of flow.

Estrogen breakthrough bleeding is caused by high levels of estrogen. These high levels of estrogen and sustained availability lead to prolonged periods of amenorrhea followed by acute, often profuse, bleeds with excessive loss of blood.

Progesterone breakthrough bleeding occurs only in the presence of an unfavorably high ratio of progesterone to estrogen. In the absence of sufficient estrogen, continuous progesterone therapy, such as occurs with long-acting progestin contraceptives, will yield intermittent bleeding of variable duration, similar to low-dose estrogen breakthrough bleeding.

MANAGEMENT

No single approach is appropriate in the management of all patients with DUB. The treatment will depend on the amount of bleeding that has occurred and the patient's age, medical status, and desire to become pregnant.

Progestin Therapy

The ultimate treatment of choice for the majority of patients with anovulatory DUB is progestin therapy. For anovulatory bleeding, progestin therapy can be used to maintain a cyclic menstrual pattern and to prevent endometrial hyperplasia.

Orderly limited withdrawal bleeding can be accomplished by administration of medroxyprogesterone acetate, 10 mg daily for 10 days every month. A heavy period will occur at the end of the 10 days of progestin therapy, which is referred to as *medical curettage*. Medroxyprogesterone acetate may not interfere with spontaneous ovulation; therefore, a barrier method of contraception should be used if the patient is sexually active.

Combination Oral Contraceptives

Contraceptive pills are given for 21 days with a 7-day period between cycles to allow for withdrawal bleeding. An advantage of oral contraceptives over sequential estrogen and progestin administration is that the withdrawal bleeding is lighter. Birth control pills reduce menstrual flow by at least 60% in normal uteri.

Any of the oral combination tablets may be given as one pill four times a day for 5 to 7 days. This therapy is maintained despite cessation of flow within 12 to 24 hours. If flow does not abate, other diagnostic possibilities (polyps, incomplete abortion, and neoplasia) should be reevaluated.

Combination hormonal therapy produces structural rigidity in the endometrium. Continued random breakdown of formerly fragile tissue is avoided and blood loss is stopped.

The patient must be warned to expect heavy bleeding after cessation of hormonal therapy so that she will not view the withdrawal bleed as recurrent disease or failure of therapy.

After the withdrawal bleed, the patient is started on a low-dose cyclic combination pill (one pill a day).

High-Dose Estrogen Therapy

Use as much as 25 mg of premarin intravenously every 4 hours until bleeding stops (up to three doses can be given). In these cases progestin treatment will have no effect because there is insufficient tissue on which the progestin can exert action. Intravenous premarin is very effective in controlling the bleeding over a 12- to 24-hour period.

The intravenous estrogen must be followed by oral estrogen in a dose equivalent to 2.5 to 3.75 mg of conjugated estrogens daily.

After 3 weeks of estrogen therapy, a progestational agent should be given orally for 7 to 10 days together with estrogen to allow a more controlled withdrawal flow during that cycle.

In cases in which bleeding is less, lower oral doses of estrogen (1.25 mg of conjugated estrogens daily for 7 to 10 days) can be prescribed initially. All estrogen therapy must be followed by progestin coverage.

Danazol

Androgenic steroid has been shown to be useful in the treatment of DUB. Doses of 200 to 400 mg daily have been given over 12 weeks after careful pretreatment observation and evaluation.

Danazol causes a significant decrease in menstrual blood loss as well as an increased interval between bleeding episodes.

Some patients may ovulate when receiving this dose of danazol.

The most common side effects of danazol treatment are weight gain and skin disorders such as acne.

BIBLIOGRAPHY

American College of Obstetrics and Gynecology Technical Bulletin: Dysfunctional uterine bleeding. Number 134, Oct 1989.

Mishell DR: Abnormal uterine bleeding. In Herbst AL, Mishell DR, Stenchever MA, Droegemueller W, editors: *Comprehensive gynecology,* St. Louis, 1992, Mosby–Year Book.

Nelson L, Rybo G: Treatment of menorrhagia, *Am J Obstet Gynecol* 110:713, 1971.

Speroff L, Glass RH, Kase NG: Dysfunctional uterine bleeding. In *Clinical gynecologic endocrinology and infertility,* ed 4, Baltimore, 1989, Williams & Wilkins.

CHAPTER 19

Contraception

Philip R. Spandorfer
Steven D. Spandorfer

COUNSELING

During the transition from childhood to adulthood, adolescents develop physically, psychologically, and socially. It is during this time when adolescents attempt to assume responsibility and independence. Often adolescents will act contrary to the advice of their parents in an effort to exert their autonomy. Primary care physicians are fortunate to be able to offer counseling and guidance to the adolescent patient, particularly if a good rapport has been established. It is of the utmost importance for the physician to stress the confidentiality of the visit. Parents or guardians should only receive information at the adolescents' request or as required by law.

The physician should offer advice in an unbiased and nonjudgmental manner. Because sexuality can be a sensitive subject, the physician should determine the patient's attitudes about sexuality. An acceptable approach would involve first inquiring about the patient's feelings about teenagers engaging in sexual activity. The subject then could be directed more toward the individual patient's feelings about sexual activity, including whether or not the patient is sexually active. The worst offense a physician could commit is to assume the patient is not sexually active. Knowing a patient's views about sexual intercourse and other sexual activities better allows the physician to guide the patient in selecting a contraceptive agent.

Discussions about contraception also should include information about sexually transmitted diseases (STDs). Adolescents should be informed of the increasing incidence of cervical and pelvic infections as well as that of HIV infection and syphilis. Patients should understand which type of contraceptive agent protects against both pregnancy and STDs.

While discussing contraception with the adolescent, it is important to have the actual methods present for the teenager to see and touch. This demonstration will lead to better compliance with the chosen method. Actual failure rates of contraceptive methods often are much higher than theoretic failure rates, and this failure is very often secondary to patient noncompliance with a particular method. Compliance also will be higher if the adolescent feels that the method he/she will be using was his/her choice.

Other important factors to consider include pattern of sexual activity, cost, access to care, partner cooperation, and medical contraindications.

Adolescents participating in sexual intercourse infrequently may consider barrier methods preferable to hormonal methods, but a patient who engages in regular intercourse might prefer a noncoitus-related method such as the oral contraceptive pill. However, this patient should be reminded about the need for protection against STDs.

Cost is always an important consideration in choosing contraception. If a patient cannot afford a type of contraceptive agent, that method is obviously useless.

Access to care is an important consideration as well. A patient who is unable to attend regular clinic follow-up visits would be best served by using an agent that requires little to no follow-up such as the condom.

Patients who state that their partner refuses to participate in contraceptive matters should use a

TABLE 19-1
Women Experiencing Pregnancy in the First Year of Continuous Use

METHOD	LOWEST EXPECTED	TYPICAL
Norplant	0.3%	0.3%
Depo-Provera	0.3%	0.3%
Oral contraceptive pill	0.1%	—
Condom	2%	12%
Diaphragm	6%	18%
Cervical cap	6%	18%
Withdrawal	4%	18%
Spermicide	3%	21%
Vaginal sponge	6%	18%
No method	85%	85%

BOX 19-1
Contraindications to Use of Oral Contraceptive Pills

ABSOLUTE

Thromboembolic disease
Active liver disease
Coronary artery disease
Cerebrovascular disease
Hepatic adenoma
Breast cancer
Gynecologic cancer
Pregnancy
Undiagnosed abnormal vaginal bleeding

RELATIVE

Severe headaches
Hypertension
Diabetes
Gallbladder disease
Immobilization
Lactation
Depression
Seizure disorder
Recent surgery

method that can offer both contraception and protection from STDs (*eg*, the female patient whose partner refuses to wear condoms might achieve better protection using a diaphragm).

Medical contraindications should be considered for any patient receiving a particular method of contraception. These contraindications will be further discussed in the section on each of the various types of agents.

After selecting a type of contraception, the patient should receive thorough instructions on the proper techniques involved with using that method. The patient should be asked to demonstrate to the physician or nurse the correct use of the method. Written instructions should be given. A follow-up visit should be scheduled for all patients in a timely manner.

Table 19-1 refers to the percentage of women experiencing an accidental pregnancy in the first year of continuous use of a particular contraceptive.

CONTRACEPTIVE METHODS

Oral Contraceptives

The oral contraceptive continues to be one of the most common forms of adolescent birth control. The low-dose combined oral contraceptive has a 99% method effectiveness and a 98% use effectiveness. However, these failure rates are much higher in the teenage patient. Almost 60% of teenagers discontinue the oral contraceptive pill (OCP) within the first year of use.

The OCP prevents pregnancy through four major mechanisms: 1) the OPC prevents ovula-

tion; 2) the OCP causes the cervical mucus to thicken, which decreases the chance of penetration by sperm into the uterine cavity and also decreases the risk of upper tract infection; 3) the OCP decreases the overall receptivity of the endometrium for pregnancy; and 4) the OCP alters tubal motility and decreases the chance of conception in a particular cycle.

Physicians providing OCPs to women should understand the absolute and relative contraindications to them (Box 19-1). The OCPs most often used today contain less than 50 µg of estrogen and are considered low-dose estrogen OCPs.

The original data on side effects from OCPs were from studies using high-dose OCPs with greater than 50 µg of estrogen. Pulmonary emboli, stroke, and myocardial infarction are much less common in the lower-dose OCPs than in the original data from women using the higher-dose OCPs. These major cardiovascular side effects are seen more often in women who are aged more than 35 years and who smoke. More importantly, the mortality from using the low-dose OCPs is much less than that seen with pregnancy.

Commonly seen side effects of OCPs include breakthrough bleeding, weight gain, breast tenderness, nausea, acne, and possibly depression or mood changes. Typically, these side effects resolve after three to four cycles and all that is required is reassurance. However, these common minor side effects often concern the adolescent the most and may lead to discontinuation of the OCPs or missed medications, which may result in an unintended failure.

Mild elevation in the patient's blood pressure is noted in less than 5% of all patients. An elevation in blood pressure, although slight, is one of the important reasons to have a patient return for an examination within the first 3 months of beginning this method of contraception. In most patients discontinuation of the OCP is all that is necessary for the blood pressure to return to normal. Hepatobiliary side effects include a slight increase in hepatic adenoma and gallbladder disease.

Advantages of the OCP are many, including a decreased amount of menstrual blood loss, and thus, an overall decrease in iron-deficient anemia. Furthermore, decreased risks of ovarian cancer, endometrial cancer, benign breast disease, menorrhagia, dysmenorrhea, functional ovarian cysts, and pelvic inflammatory disease are demonstrated in patients that have used OCPs. It is important to stress to the adolescent interested in OCPs as a contraceptive method that although they decrease the incidence of pelvic inflammatory disease, they are not as good as barrier method forms of contraception in preventing the spread of STDs.

The combination OCPs contain both estrogen and progesterone components. The two estrogens used currently in the United States are ethinyl estradiol and mestranol, which is converted in the liver to the pharmacologically active ethinyl estradiol. Multiple progestins also are being used, all of which vary in their androgenic, estrogenic, and progesterone effects. OCPs are available in monophasic, biphasic, and triphasic strengths. The estrogen component remains constant, and the progesterone component is increased once or twice depending on if the compound is bi- or triphasic. The advantages of these triphasic OCPs is that they decrease the total amount of progesterone given.

The OCPs contain 21 days of hormonally active pills. The 28-day preparations also contain 7 days of inert ingredients in addition to the previously described 21 days of hormonally active pills. Menstruation occurs secondary to progesterone withdrawal during the inert pill days.

It is recommended that adolescents use the 28-day pack to decrease the confusion that can occur with the 21-day packs, which require the patient to remember to start a new pack 7 days after completing the previous pack.

The patient should be instructed to take the OCP once a day, preferably the same time each day. The OCP is most effective when taken this way. The most important pills are those in the very beginning of the cycle, and if a patient has been noncompliant with these pills it is best if she uses a back-up form of contraception for the remainder of that month.

If the patient forgets to take a pill, she should take two the next day and continue her regular schedule. If two pills are forgotten, she should take two pills as soon as she remembers and two the next day. If more than three pills are missed, she should be told to stop taking the pills for at least 7 days, ensure that she is not pregnant, allow a withdrawal bleed, and then restart a new pack of OCPs. It is important to emphasize the need for back-up contraception if any pills are missed, particularly those at the very beginning of the cycle.

A progestin-only pill is also available, which is often referred to as the *mini-pill*. It is less effective than the combination OCPs in the adolescent and is associated with a greater incidence of menstrual irregularities.

Depo-Provera

Depo-medroxyprogesterone acetate (Depo-Provera) is a long-acting, injectable progestin contraceptive. It is given as 150 mg as a deep muscular injection every 3 months. It recently has been approved by the Food and Drug Administration.

Depo-Provera's mechanism of action is to block the luteinizing hormone surge and prevent ovulation. Depo-Provera also thickens the cervical mucus to decrease the likelihood of sperm penetration as well as decreasing the endometrial receptivity for implantation.

Nearly 50% of all patients using Depo-Provera are amenorrheic after the first year. However, the most difficult side effect is the high rate of menstrual irregularities that occur. Other important side effects include mood changes, depression, nervousness, abdominal bloating, acne, hair loss (rare), headaches, and weight gain. Many women report that these side effects decrease over time.

When given as a regularly scheduled contraceptive agent every 3 months, Depo-Provera has a failure rate of less than one per 100 women. As with OCPs, the patient should be counseled that this method does not prevent STDs.

Contraindications include pregnancy, undiagnosed vaginal bleeding, breast cancer, stroke, phlebitis, and active liver disease.

Fertility returns over time—66% of patients attempting pregnancy after discontinuing Depo-Provera will achieve pregnancy in less than 18 months, and after 18 months this rate will increase to 93%.

Norplant

Norplant is a subdermal implant that contains levonorgestrel, a progestin. It is a long-acting contraceptive agent that is implanted into the woman's arm. It is composed of six matchstick-size capsules containing 36 mg of levonorgestrel. Once steady state is achieved, approximately 30 µg of levonorgestrel are released each day. The contraceptive agent will work for 5 years. The failure rate is 0.04%, and, if inserted within the first few days after menses, it is effective within hours.

Initially a higher failure rate occurred in women weighing more than 50 kg, but after revising the silastic capsule, the effectiveness is equivalent for the full 5-year period for all women.

Norplant's mechanism of action is based on the ability of progesterone to thicken the cervical mucus and decrease the endometrium's receptivity for implantation.

The primary side effect is irregular bleeding, which can vary from occasional spotting to heavy, prolonged bleeding. Some patients will, in fact, achieve amenorrhea. Others will continue to note monthly bleeding. It is important to counsel the patient about the irregular bleeding because the capsules must be removed to discontinue the contraceptive. Other side effects include headaches, acne, weight changes, and bloating.

Contraindications are similar to those of Depo-Provera.

After removal of the capsules, fertility returns quickly and is comparable to fertility experienced after discontinuation of barrier methods.

Once again, the adolescent should be cautioned that although Norplant is highly effective in preventing unintended pregnancies, it is not as effective as barrier methods in preventing STDs.

Condom

The importance of condom use should be stressed to all sexually active adolescents. The high rates of STDs among teenagers and the emergence of AIDS has made condom use extremely important as a prevention of STDs. No matter what form of contraception a patient uses, condom use should be encouraged. The latex condom has been shown to prevent the transmission of gonorrhea, chlamydia, herpes, trichomonas, and HIV. It should be emphasized that only the latex condom offers such protection.

The theoretic effectiveness of the condom (98%) is much higher than the actual effectiveness (90%). This difference is probably a result of the fact that the condom's effectiveness is so dependent on coitus-related activities. Spermicide use with the condom can increase its effectiveness.

Adolescents should be instructed on the proper application of a condom. It should be placed on an erect penis prior to penetration. A reservoir should be left at the tip to collect the sperm after ejaculation. The condom should be removed after ejaculation and should only be used once. The condom should be held in place during withdrawal.

Advantages to condoms are that they are cheap, are readily available, and can prevent STDs. Further advantages include safety and an almost zero rate of medical complications. Occasional patients will report allergies to latex condoms.

Disadvantages center around the fact that condoms are coitus dependent. The condoms are thought to decrease the pleasure derived from intercourse, which prevents many adolescent boys from using them.

Lubricants such as KY Jelly and saliva will not interfere with the condom's effectiveness; however, petroleum jelly should not be used because it may compromise the latex material.

A female condom also is now on the market. It is more expensive than the male condom but works in a very similar fashion.

Vaginal Spermicides

Vaginal spermicides contain nonoxynol-9 or octoxynol as a spermicide. The medicine's efficacy is a result of the surfactant's action on sperm, immobilizing or killing sperm on contact. Furthermore, these spermicidal agents are bactericidal and inactivate viruses.

These agents are often used in conjunction with other barrier methods including the condom, diaphragm, or cervical cap.

The theoretic failure rate of spermicidal agents is approximately 3%. However, because it is a coitus-related agent, it has an actual failure rate in the first year of almost 20%. Therefore, it should not be offered as a single contraceptive agent to the adolescent but rather used in conjunction with another form of barrier contraception.

The disadvantages also include occasional allergies to either the inert material or the spermicide itself.

Contraceptive Sponge

The contraceptive sponge is a recently introduced variety of barrier protection. It is a flattened disk of polyurethane that is impregnated with a spermicide and preservatives. The sponge should be moistened prior to insertion and should be inserted no more than 12 hours before intercourse. The sponge also should be left in the vagina at least 6 hours after intercourse. Furthermore, it should not be left in the vagina for more than 24 hours.

The sponge can be used for multiple episodes of intercourse within a 1-hour period. Other advantages of the sponge are that it does not require a fitting as does the diaphragm and that it is easy to use.

Data suggest that the failure rate is 13.3 pregnancies per 100-woman years of use. This failure rate is higher than that observed with hormonal methods but comparable to that of other barrier methods.

Diaphragm

Diaphragms are flexible pieces of rubber that are made to be placed in the vagina and cover the cervix. The diaphragm is available in three shapes: arcing spring, coil spring, and flat spring. Adolescent patients do best with the arcing spring because it is the easiest to insert. The arcing spring diaphragm forms an arc when compressed, which allows easy insertion and removal.

The diaphragm is available in sizes from 50 to 105 mm. The diaphragm should be properly fitted by the experienced clinician. The most common error in fitting a patient with a diaphragm is using a diaphragm that is too small. When properly fitted, the diaphragm should cover the cervix. The posterior part should be in the posterior fornix, and the anterior part should fit snugly against the pubic bone. The patient should feel comfortable with the diaphragm in place and also should be able to easily remove the diaphragm. The patient should return to the office in 1 to 2 weeks to ensure proper fitting. After childbirth, a patient should be refitted for a proper-fitting diaphragm.

The patient should be informed that a spermicide also should be used and that the diaphragm should be left in place at least 6 hours after intercourse (spermicide also must be reinserted between acts of intercourse). The diaphragm should be cleaned with soap and water and should be replaced yearly. If holes are detected, it should be discarded. Furthermore, the patient should be instructed to never leave the diaphragm in place longer than 24 hours to avoid possible toxic shock syndrome.

The failure rate, especially in the first year, is close to 20%. This is mostly due to lack of proper use. In the highly motivated couple its use-effectiveness is close to 98%.

Cervical Cap

The cervical cap, which functions as a barrier method, has been recently approved for use as a contraceptive agent. The cervical cap is a thimble-shaped dome of rubber that is used with a spermicide and is applied over the cervix. The cervical cap must be properly fitted. It is available in four sizes ranging from 22 to 31 mm inside diameter. Its theoretic and actual effectiveness are similar to that of the diaphragm (94% and 83%, respectively).

The insertion of the cervical cap tends to be more difficult than the diaphragm, although it is considered less messy. It is not necessary to use additional spermicide between acts of intercourse that occur within the initial 6-hour period. The cervical cap can be left in place up to 48 hours. Cleaning is similar to that of the diaphragm. Cervical cap users are more likely to complain of vaginal odor.

The cervical cap is not recommended for adolescents due to its difficulties with placement and removal.

Intrauterine Device

The intrauterine device (IUD) is recommended for use in patients who have had two or more pregnancies and who are in a stable, monogamous relationship. Adolescents generally do not meet these requirements and are not candidates for the IUD.

Sterilization

Sterilization is the most common form of birth control in the United States but is not suitable for the adolescent.

Natural Family Planning (The Rhythm Method)

Natural family planning methods use a woman's ability to predict her menstrual cycle. A woman predicts times when she is unlikely to be fertile based on the characteristics of factors such as her body basal temperature and cervical mucus. The adolescent will typically have very irregular cycles and will not know her body and her menstrual cycle well enough to effectively use natural family planning as a reliable method.

Therefore, this method is not recommended for the adolescent.

"Morning After Pill"

The "morning after pill" can be prescribed for up to 72 hours after unprotected intercourse in patients who are not pregnant. The risk of pregnancy when using the "morning after pill" is decreased by approximately tenfold or more. The total pregnancy rate is approximately 1.8%. The most common regimen is Ovral (50 μg of ethinyl estradiol; 0.5 mg of norgestrel) taken as two tablets as soon as possible and two more tablets 12 hours later. Nausea is very common. No side effects on the fetus have been noted in the case of a pregnancy. If a period does not occur within 2 to 3 weeks, a pregnancy test should be checked. Finally, the patient should be counseled concerning STDs and contraceptive agents.

BIBLIOGRAPHY

Center for Population Options: The facts: Teenage sexuality, pregnancy and parenthood, Washington, April 1987.

Connell EB: Barrier contraceptives, *Clin Obstet Gynecol* 32:377, 1989.

Dickey RP: *Managing contraceptive pill patients,* ed 5, Durant, 1987, Creative Informatics.

Fasoli M, Parazzinin F, Cecchetti G, et al: Postcoital contraception: An overview of published studies, *Contraception* 39:459, 1989.

Foster DC: Low dose monophasic and multiphasic oral contraception: A review of potency, efficacy and side effects, *Semin Reprod Endocrinol* 7:205, 1989.

Goldman JA, Dicker D, Feldberg D, et al: Barrier contraception in the teenager: A comparison of four methods in adolescent girls, *Pediatr Adolesc Gynecol* 3:59, 1985.

Greydanus DE, McAnarney R: Contraception in the adolescent: Current concepts for the pediatrician, *Pediatrics* 65:1, 1980.

Hatcher R, Guest F, Stewart F, et al: Contraceptive technology, 1986-87, ed 13, New York, 1986, Irvington Publishers.

Jones EF, Forrest JD, Goldman D, et al: Teenage pregnancy in developed countries: Determinants and policy implications, *Fam Plann Perspect* 17:53, 1985.

Kulig JW: Adolescent contraception: Non-hormonal methods, *Adolesc Gynecol* 36:717, 1989.

Lana ME, Arceo R, Sobero AJ: Successful use of the diaphragm and jelly by a young population: Report of a clinical study, *Fam Plann Perspect* 8:81, 1976.

Liskin L, Blackburn R, Ghani R: *Hormonal contraception: New long acting methods,* Population Information Program, The Johns Hopkins University Population Reports. Series K. No. 3 Mar–Apr 1987.

Oral contraception, *ACOG Technical Bulletin* 106:1–5, 1987.

Rosenfield A: Injectable contraception. In Carson SL, Derman RJ, Tyrer LB, editors: *Fertility control,* ed 1, Boston, 1985, Little, Brown, and Co.

Stone KM, Grimes DA, Magder LS: Personal protection against sexually transmitted diseases, *Am J Obstet Gynecol* 155:180, 1986.

Trussel J, Hatcher RA, Cates W, et al: Contraceptive failure in the U.S.: An update, *Stud Fam Plann* 21:51, 1990.

PART FIVE

Other Issues

CHAPTER 20

Immunizations

Michael E. Ryan
Kelly A. Kane

It is important to understand that the recommendations for vaccine use and schedules are constantly changing. New technologies not available today may be readily used tomorrow. Many new vaccines are in the development phase; therefore, this chapter serves as a general guide to immunizations and not a final update. The vaccines will be discussed in the order that they are routinely given.

HEPATITIS B

Recombinant vaccines for hepatitis B are now produced by two manufacturers using yeast, genetically modified to synthesize hepatitis B surface antigen (HBsAg). The vaccine is universally recommended, especially for infants and adolescents. Infants are at increased risk for developing chronic hepatitis B, and they have a better immunologic response to the vaccine. Adolescents are more likely to participate in risk-taking behaviors and therefore should be immunized. People who should not receive the vaccine include those who have had anaphylactic reactions to previous hepatitis B vaccination or yeast products. The vaccine schedule includes three intramuscular injections. Infants may receive the first dose in the newborn nursery.

Physicians normally administer the second dose 1 month after the first and the third dose 6 months after the first. Some latitude does exist in the schedule, but there should be at least 2 months between the second and third doses. The three-shot series may be completed using appropriate doses of the same vaccine or a combination of both vaccine brands for separate doses (see Table 20-1). The vaccine is 95% effective in infants, children, and adolescents. The most common adverse reactions include local reactions, fever, headache, and dizziness.

In patients who have been recently exposed to hepatitis B and are not vaccinated, hepatitis B immune globulin (HBIG) should be given concomitantly at a separate injection site, with the first dose of the vaccine. The vaccine series should then be completed as scheduled. Patients who have begun immunization but have not completed the three-dose series should resume it as scheduled and not repeat any doses. Immunocompromised patients and patients on dialysis need to receive the vaccine in higher doses but on the same schedule. Serologic screening for hepatitis B surface-antibody (Anti-HBs) is not necessary in normal children but should be performed for patients older than 49 years, patients who have received the vaccination in the gluteal region, patients with HIV infection, babies born to HBg-Ag–positive mothers, patients with high risk for exposure, and twice yearly for patients on dialysis. Pregnant women may receive the vaccine or HBIG, if necessary. The hepatitis B vaccine cannot be administered with the yellow fever vaccine, but it can be given with other routine childhood vaccines.

DIPHTHERIA

The diphtheria vaccine is made with a diphtheria toxoid and is available only in combination with other vaccine preparations. It is universally recommended for children from 2 months to 7 years of age in full dose or 6.7 to 12.5 flocculation units (Lf). In patients older than 7 years of age, a partial dose of diphtheria toxoid is used (less than 2 Lf). Patients who should not receive the vaccine include those who have suffered anaphylactic reactions to previous diphtheria-combination vaccines. The vaccine schedule begins in infancy with full-strength doses at the age of 2 months, 4 months, 6 months, 12 to 18 months, and 4 to 6 years. The partial-strength vaccine, combined with tetanus, is given in booster doses every 10 years thereafter. The vaccine's efficacy is best when those booster doses are given. The most common adverse reactions include localized tenderness, fever, drowsiness, fretfulness, and anorexia.

Anyone recently infected with diphtheria should be treated with antibiotics and antitoxin. Afterwards, such patients need to be given the vaccine, because endotoxin exposure does not always confer immunity. Patients who delay starting or have interrupted their vaccine series should complete their doses at the recommended intervals, with tetanus vaccine given after 7 years of age. Immunocompromised patients should receive the vaccine, and if at all possible, immunosuppressive therapy should be discontinued 1 month before vaccination. Pregnant women should receive the vaccine only if it is necessary. Physicians may administer the vaccine concurrently with other vaccines.

TETANUS

The tetanus vaccine contains tetanus toxoid and usually is given in combinations such as with other vaccines (see Table 20-1). Tetanus vaccina-

tion is universally recommended throughout life, unless the patient has had anaphylactic reactions to previous tetanus vaccinations. Case-by-case decisions should be made about administration to patients who have moderate to severe acute illness and those who have underlying neurologic diseases. The dose schedule is the same as for the diphtheria toxoid. Most studies show that the vaccine is 95% effective with the current vaccine schedule. Adverse reactions are usually minor local reactions but may also include fever.

If possible exposure to tetanus has occurred in an unimmunized patient, the wound should be thoroughly cleaned and debrided and tetanus immune globulin (TIG) should be administered, followed by appropriate immunization. Tetanus infection usually does not confer immunity. If the patient already has received three or more doses of tetanus vaccine and the wound is a clean minor wound no further immunization is necessary. If the patient has received fewer than three doses or if the wound is not a clean, minor wound, then tetanus and TIG may be required. When TIG is unavailable alternative treatments include antitoxin, intravenous immune globulin, and penicillin G for 10 to 14 days. Patients who have delayed starting immunizations or have interrupted their immunization schedules should complete their doses at recommended intervals, without repeating any doses. Immunize the immunocompromised patient, but for improved efficacy, consider discontinuing immunosuppressive therapy for 1 month before the vaccination. Pregnant women should be vaccinated only if necessary. Do not freeze the vaccine.

PERTUSSIS

Physicians use two different pertussis vaccines to immunize against pertussis. The first type is whole cell, made of whole, inactivated pertussis organisms. The second type is an acellular vaccine made of between two and four antigens thought to be important in developing immunity against pertussis. Adverse reactions are less common with the acellular vaccine. The vaccine is recommended universally in children less than 7 years of age. Patients may be vaccinated at 4 weeks of age in an outbreak situation. Patients who are not recommended to receive the vaccine include those who have experienced anaphylactic reactions to previous pertussis vaccines, those who have had new-onset central nervous system dysfunctions within 7 days of vaccine administration, and those who have an unstable seizure disorder. Those patients for whom the administration of the vaccine should be questioned include patients who are moderately to severely ill; have had previous vaccine reactions, such as 3 or more hours of inconsolable crying; have a fever of greater than 40.5° C within 48 hours of a pertussis vaccination; have had a convulsion, with or without fever, within 3 days of vaccine administration; and have shocklike symptoms. Whole-cell pertussis vaccine is currently recommended to be given at 2, 4, and 6 months of age. Acellular pertussis vaccine may be used in patients older than 1 year, specifically at 15 to 18 months and 4 to 6 years. Recent studies have established the efficacy of the acellular vaccine in patients less than 1 year of age, hoping to replace the whole-cell vaccine entirely. Vaccinations should be given intramuscularly in the deltoid or anterolateral thigh. With three vaccinations, 80% of patients are immune to pertussis.

Patients infected by recent exposure to pertussis should receive antibiotics and supportive care. Prophylaxis should be given to all household contacts and other close contacts irrespective of vaccination status. Patients who have documented pertussis infections have no need for pertussis immunization. Patients with delayed or interrupted immunization schedules should complete their doses at recommended intervals with the appropriate vaccine. Immunocompromised patients should receive the vaccine, but to improve immunogenicity, patients on immunosuppressive therapy should be taken off therapy for 1 month before the vaccination, if at all possible. The vaccine is usually administered in combination with other routine childhood vaccines.

A casual relationship between the diphtheria-tetanus-pertussis (DTP) vaccine and brain damage has not been demonstrated; if it does occur, it is extremely rare. Several large studies have found no association between the DTP vaccine and sudden infant death syndrome.

HAEMOPHILUS INFLUENZAE B

The *Haemophilus influenzae* B (HIB) vaccine is a conjugate vaccine made of capsular polysaccharides or oligosaccharides covalently linked to a carrier protein. It is produced as an individual vaccine and in combination with DTP (DTP-HIB). It is universally recommended in children, especially those 2 months to 1 year of age. Physicians should consider not giving the vaccine to patients who have moderate to severe acute illnesses. The vaccine is given at 2, 4, 6, and 15 months of age by intramuscular injection at sites separate from other vaccination injections. The vaccine's efficacy is very high, between 97.6% and 100%. Adverse reactions to HIB vaccine alone include local reactions, fever, and irritability.

Patients who have infections secondary to recent exposure to HIB should receive antibiotics and supportive therapy. Even if a child has a documented infection, vaccinations should continue until the child is older than 24 months of age. Three doses of HIB vaccine should be given to patients less than 6 months of age, in 1- to 2-month intervals, to properly develop immunity. Children older than 6 months of age but less than 5 years of age receive one to two doses at 2-month intervals. Children older than 5 years of age should receive only one dose of the HIB vaccine. Immunocompromised patients should receive the vaccination. Patients infected with HIB after vaccination should be evaluated for immunodeficiency, especially IgG_2 deficiency. As with other vaccines, premature infants should receive this immunization according to their chronologic age.

POLIOMYELITIS

There are two types of trivalent poliomyelitis vaccines available: an oral form that contains live, attenuated viruses (oral polio vaccine [OPV]) and an alternative vaccine containing inactivated, killed viruses (inactivated poliovirus vaccine [IPV]) that is administered as an intramuscular injection. Universal vaccination is recommended except for patients who have experienced anaphylactic reactions to previous poliomyelitis vaccines. Diarrhea and breast feeding are not considered contraindications to OPV or IPV. IPV should not be given to patients who have experienced anaphylactic reactions to streptomycin, neomycin, or polymyxin. OPV, as is true of all live-virus vaccines, should not be given to immunocompromised patients. In addition, OPV is not recommended for patients living in a household with an immunocompromised person; in those instances, IPV is recommended. The poliomyelitis vaccine schedule is 2, 4, and 6 to 18 months, and 4 to 6 years of age. The vaccines' efficacy is 95%. Many experts are now advising IVP at 2 and 4 months. Because OPV is a live, attenuated form of vaccine, rare cases of poliomyelitis infection have occurred secondary to the exposure of the vaccine virus in immunocompromised patients.

Patients who have had poliomyelitis infection should still be vaccinated because there are three virus types. If a patient is unimmunized at 18 years of age or older and is at risk for exposure through contacts or travel, IPV should be given in three doses, with a 2-month interval between the first and second dose and a third dose given 6 to 12 months after the second dose. If the patient is at high risk for exposure to wild poliomyelitis virus, OPV may be used. Children older than 1 year of age who are underimmunized should receive two doses of OPV with 2-month intervals or only the last dose of the three if two have already been given. A booster dose of OPV should then be given at 4 to 6 years of age. IPV and OPV are approved for pregnant women. The vaccine should not be delayed because unimmunized adults may live in the same household as infants receiving OPV. Every attempt should be made to immunize those adults with IPV, as previously recommended.

MEASLES

The measles vaccine contains live, attenuated virus. It is available alone and in combination with rubella, or mumps and rubella (MMR). MMR is the vaccine of choice in most situations. The MMR vaccine is universally recommended except for pregnant women, immunocompromised patients (except those with HIV) and patients who have experienced anaphylactic reactions to neomycin or previous measles vaccination. Patients born before 1957 and those who have positive serologies, documenting infection, should be considered immune and therefore do not require the vaccine. Patients who have received immune globulin preparations in the past 3 months should not receive the measles vaccine. Case-by-case consideration should be given for patients who have a history of seizures or anaphylactic reactions to egg ingestion. Re-

cent evidence suggests it is acceptable to give MMR vaccine even to those infants with a history of anaphylaxis to eggs. Careful observation after the MMR is necessary. MMR vaccine can be given with or after purified protein derivative (PPD) and varicella vaccine but should not be given less than 1 month before the PPD. The MMR vaccine should be given by subcutaneous injection in two doses at 12 to 15 months (not before 6 months of age) and either 4 to 6 years or 11 to 12 years of age. The vaccine's efficacy is 95%. Adverse reactions to the vaccine include rash and fever of greater than 39.4° C 1 week after vaccination, with increased risk of febrile seizures at that time. The vaccine is approved for lactating women, but only if it is necessary. Measles vaccination should be current in those traveling to measles-endemic areas. In questionable cases screening may be done to determine a patient's susceptibility. The MMR vaccine should be kept frozen or cold and is good for only 8 hours after reconstitution.

MUMPS

The mumps vaccine contains live, attenuated viruses. It is universally recommended for infants and children in combination with the measles and rubella vaccines. Contraindications to that vaccine have been mentioned previously. Special consideration should be given to revaccinating patients with MMR because mumps can occur even in highly vaccinated populations. Those born before 1957 who have had documented cases of mumps, or who are serologically positive for mumps should be considered immune and therefore do not require vaccinations. To be most effective, vaccination should be given at least 3 months after the last immunoglobulin infusion. Standard doses are given by subcutaneous injection at 12 to 15 months of age and either 4 to 6 or 11 to 12 years of age. Mumps vaccine seems to be less protective than either measles or rubella vaccine. Revaccination with mumps vaccine given as MMR does not appear to be harmful. Adverse reactions are generally rare, but they include fever, febrile seizures, parotitis, meningitis, encephalitis, rash, pruritus, purpura, and orchitis. Patients who have had recent exposure to mumps require supportive treatment, but not vaccination. For the underimmunized, one dose of mumps vaccine may be given up to adolescence. The mumps vaccine is most likely given to travelers as prophylaxis (given as MMR). Screening for susceptibility is optional. Vaccinated persons with MMR do not transit measles, mumps, or the rubella vaccine virus.

RUBELLA

The rubella vaccine contains live, attenuated virus (RA 27/3 strain) and is recommended for children over 12 months of age. Contraindications to the vaccine have been mentioned previously. The rubella vaccine should be given as MMR by subcutaneous injection at approximately 15 months of age. The vaccine is 98% effective. Adverse reactions include rash, fever, lymphadenopathy, and occasional arthritis/arthralgia, especially in postpubescent women.

In patients who delay starting immunizations, one dose of MMR should be administered up until adolescence. College students and travelers going to rubella-endemic areas should be up to date with their MMR vaccinations. All pregnant women should be screened for rubella immunity to prevent congenital rubella syndrome. Breast feeding is not a contraindication to postpartum immunization. Careful attention should be paid to documenting rubella immunity among those patients coming in contact with pregnant patients or susceptible infants.

VARICELLA

A vaccine is now available for universal use to protect patients from varicella infection. The vaccine, which contains a live, attenuated virus, is approved for patients who live with immunocompromised people and also for breast-feeding mothers; however, it is not approved for immunocompromised patients. This group would include patients with acute lymphocytic leukemia in remission for less than 1 year, patients who have received immune globulin products within the last 5 months, patients on steroid therapy not discontinued for 1 to 3 months for doses more than 2 mg/kg or 1 month for doses less than 2 mg/kg, pregnant women, patients who have had anaphylactic reactions to neomycin, and patients younger than 12 months of age. The vaccine should be given by subcutaneous injection in one dose to children older than 12 months (usually 15 months of age) and less than 13 years of age. In patients older than 13 years of age, two doses must be given 4 to 8 weeks apart. The varicella vaccine should be kept frozen and used within 30 minutes of reconstitution.

The vaccine is 95% effective, and it appears to reduce the incidence of herpes zoster. Adverse reactions include an attenuated form of chickenpox with a few lesions, fever, and an abbreviated course. Upper respiratory tract symptoms, headache, and fatigue are rarely reported. Some vaccinated people can be infectious to others, but the infection transmitted also produces the attenuated disease.

Screening for varicella immunity is optional for patients more than 18 years of age. It is not known how long the immunity secondary to the varicella vaccine lasts or whether booster doses may be needed. Salicylates should not be given to the patient within 6 weeks of the vaccine because of the risk of developing Reye syndrome. Research is being done on a vaccine combining varicella with the MMR vaccine.

PNEUMOCOCCUS

The pneumococcal vaccine, given by intramuscular injection, is not used for healthy children but only in patients older than 2 years of age with sickle cell disease, asplenia, or renal dysfunction (eg, nephrotic syndrome or chronic renal failure); immunosuppressed patients; and patients with cerebrospinal fluid leaks. Adverse reactions include local reactions, fever, rash, arthralgia, and idiopathic thrombocytopenia purpura exacerbation. Ongoing research holds promise for a conjugate vaccine that may be effective in infants.

INFLUENZA

The influenza vaccine recommended in certain children younger than 13 years of age is a split virus vaccine, which contains purified surface antigens from two types of influenza virus. Because there are yearly antigenic drifts in the influenza virus, a decision is made annually about which viral components will be used in the vaccine to protect against any changes that the virus would undergo. It is not usually recom-

TABLE 20-1

Recommended Ages for Administration of Currently Licensed Childhood Vaccines—July through December 1996

Vaccines are listed under the routinely recommended ages. *Bars* indicate range of acceptable ages for vaccination. *Shaded bars* indicate catch-up vaccination: at 11 to 12 years of age, hepatitis B vaccine should be administered to children not previously vaccinated, and varicella zoster virus vaccine should be administered to children not previously vaccinated, who lack a reliable history of chickenpox.

AGE ▶ VACCINE ▼	BIRTH	2 MOS	4 MOS	6 MOS	12[1] MOS	15 MOS	18 MOS	4–6 YRS	11–12 YRS	14–16 YRS
Hepatitis B[1,2] (Hep B)	Hep B-1	Hep B-2		Hep B-3					Hep B[2]	
Diphtheria, tetanus, pertussis[3] (DTP)		DTP	DTP	DTP	DTP[3] DTaP at 15+ m			DTP or DtaP	Td	
Haemophilus influenzae type B[4] (HIB)		HIB	HIB	HIB[4]	HIB[4]					
Poliomyelitis (OPV)[5]		OPV[5]	OPV	OPV				OPV		
Measles, mumps, rubella[6] (MMR)					MMR			MMR[6] or MMR[6]		
Varicella zoster[7] (VZV)					VZV				VZV[7]	

Approved by the Advisory Committee on Immunization Practices (ACIP), the American Academy of Pediatrics (AAP), and the American Academy of Family Physicians (AAFP).

[1] *Infants born to HbsAg-negative mothers* should receive 2.5 μg of Merck vaccine (Recombivax HB) or 10 μg of SmithKline Beecham (SB) vaccine (Energix-B). The second dose should be administered ≥ 1 month after the first dose.
Infants born to HbsAg-positive mothers should receive 0.5 mL hepatitis B Immune globulin (HBIG) within 12 hours of birth, and either 5 μg of Merck vaccine (Recombivax HB) or 10 μg of SB Vaccine (Energix-B) at a separate site. The second dose is recommended at 1 to 2 months of age and the third dose at 6 months of age.
Infants born to mothers whose HbsAg status is unknown should receive either 0.5 μg of Merck vaccine (Recombivax HB) or 10 μg of SB Vaccine (Energix-B) within 12 hours of birth. The second dose of vaccine is recommended at 1 month of age and the third dose at 6 months of age.

[2] Adolescents who have not previously received three doses of hepatitis B vaccine should initiate or complete the series at the 11- to 12-year-old visit. The second dose should be administered at least 1 month after the first dose, and the third dose should be administered at least 4 months after the first dose and at least 2 months after the second dose.

[3] DTP4 may be administered at 12 months of age, if at least 6 months have elapsed since DTP3. DtaP (diphtheria and tetanus toxoids and acellular pertussis vaccine) is licensed for the fourth and/or fifth vaccine dose(s) for children aged ≥15 months and may be preferred for these doses in this age group. Td (tetanus and diphtheria toxoids, absorbed, for adult use) is recommended at 11 to 12 years of age if at least 5 years have elapsed since the last dose of DTP, DTaP, or DT.

[4] Three H. influenzae type B (Hib) conjugate vaccines are licensed for infant use. If PRP-OMP (PedvaxHIB [Merck]) is administered at 2 and 4 months of age, a dose at 6 months is not required. After completing the primary series, any Hib conjugate vaccine may be used as a booster.

[5] Oral poliovirus vaccine (OPV) is recommended for routine infant vaccination. Inactivated poliovirus vaccine (IPV) is recommended for persons with a congenital or acquired immune deficiency disease or an altered immune status as a result of disease or immunosuppressive therapy, as well as their household contacts, and is an acceptable alternative for other persons. The primary three-dose series for IPV should be given with a minimum interval of 4 weeks between the first and second doses and 6 months between the second and third doses.

[6] The second dose of MMR is routinely recommended at 4 to 6 years of age or at 11 to 12 years of age, but may be administered at any visit, provided at least 1 month has elapsed since receipt of the first dose.

[7] Varicella zoster virus vaccine (Var) can be administered to susceptible children any time after 12 months of age. Unvaccinated children who lack a reliable history of chickenpox should be vaccinated at the 11- to 12-year-old visit.

mended that healthy children receive the influenza vaccine, but immunosuppressed patients and children with chronic lung disease, significant cardiac disease, sickle cell disease, and other hemoglobinopathies should be vaccinated. Others who should be considered for the influenza vaccine are children who have HIV infection, diabetes, chronic renal failure, chronic metabolic diseases and those on long-term salicylate therapy, as well as those who are in contact with these high-risk patients. The vaccine is administered by intramuscular injection and should be given in two doses with a 1-month interval for first-time vaccines. One dose of vaccine may be used in those patients who have had previous influenza vaccinations. Vaccine efficacy is variable according to age and health status, but it should create an attenuated influenza infection, which will make influenza less of a life-threatening illness for high-risk patients. Adverse reactions to the vaccine are minor and occur infrequently. Children who have anaphylactic reactions to egg ingestion should have skin tests and possibly should be desensitized before being considered for this vaccine. More appropriately, physicians should weigh the results of anaphylaxis versus the risk of influenza.

RABIES

Rabies immune globulin (RIG) is used for postexposure protection against the rabies virus, an RNA rhabdovirus. Local care should be given first to the open wound, followed by RIG and the first dose of the human diploid cell rabies vaccine (HDCV). With first exposure, and without previous vaccination, five doses of HDCV are required, with the last four being given on postexposure days 3, 7, 14, and 28. Where there has been a previous vaccination, two doses of HDCV are required, with the final dose given on the 3rd day after exposure. Reasons to administer rabies vaccine need to be individualized, and help from Public Health Departments may be required. Physicians should keep in mind that rabies is preventable but, if acquired, is almost always

fatal. Adverse reactions include local reactions, dizziness, abdominal pain, myalgia, headache, and, rarely, Guillain-Barré–like symptoms, that are self-resolving. Postvaccination syndrome occurs 21 days after vaccination in 6% of patients. The symptoms that occur include urticaria, arthritis and arthralgia, angioedema, nausea, vomiting, fever, and general malaise. This syndrome is self-resolving and rarely has any sequelae.

VACCINE ADVERSE EVENTS REPORTING SYSTEM

Vaccination information pamphlets with benefits and risks listed must be given to each parent or guardian before vaccination can be administered to their child.

Those who give vaccinations are required to report serious adverse events that occur, as well as the time of their occurrence. Vaccine Adverse Events Reporting System (VAERS) was established to provide a single system to collect and analyze all data from adverse events. Although vaccines must be tested for safety and immunogenicity, benefits and risks still must be evaluated.

VAERS forms are mailed yearly to physicians who are likely to give vaccinations. The VAERS form asks for information about the patient, the adverse event, and the vaccine type, manufacturer, and lot number. Additional forms, assistance in filling out forms, and other answers can be obtained by calling 1-800-822-7967.

The use of vaccines is evaluated by weighing the benefits and risks of the vaccine. Those benefits and risks change as use of each vaccine changes. As vaccine use evolves, the diseases that vaccines are designed to prevent also evolve, and vaccine recommendations must be reevaluated. Vaccination is an area of medicine that is in constant flux because of new technologies and the refinement of information about diseases and immunization. Therefore, it is important to keep updated and practice current recommendations. Current recommendations for vaccination are listed in Table 20-1.

BIBLIOGRAPHY

American Academy of Pediatrics Committee on Infectious Diseases: Recommendations for the use of live attenuated varicella vaccine, *Pediatrics* 95(5):791–795, 1995.

American Medical Association: *Prevention, diagnosis, and management of viral hepatitis: A Guide for primary care physicians,* 1995.

Chen RT: The Vaccine Adverse Event Reporting System (VAERS), *Vaccine* 12(6):542–550, 1994.

Peter G, editor: *1994 Red Book: Report of the Committee on Infectious Diseases,* ed 23, Elk Grove Village, 1994, American Academy of Pediatrics.

Recommended Childhood Immunization Schedule—United States 1995, *MMWR* 34(No. PR5): 1–9, 1995.

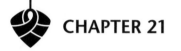

CHAPTER 21

Screening

Bradley R. Hoch

Screening is the evaluation of an asymptomatic population for the presence of a defined condition. Every facet of the evaluation of a "well child" is a screen. During the health supervision visit the health care provider is screening for the presence of multiple conditions that may place the child's health at risk.

Many physicians believe screening only involves laboratory evaluation. This narrow interpretation is not especially beneficial nor is it productive. If we as health care providers and parents care about the lives of our children, we must face reality. In the United States, accidents and homicides destroy the lives of more of our children then does anemia or renal disease. We must screen for the risk factors that affect the lives of our children, and we must find ways to alter these risks.

For what should we screen? Perhaps the most illuminating way to restate the question is, "What kills our children?" The Centers for Disease Control and Prevention (CDC) report that, "In the United States, 72% of all deaths among school-aged youth and young adults 5 to 24 years of age are from only four causes: motor vehicle crashes (30% of all deaths in this age group), other unintentional injuries (12%), homicide (19%), and suicide (11%)."

Obviously the risk of death is not the only criterion to be used when formulating the primary care screen. Other behaviors and environmental factors create significant morbidity.

Mass population screening programs are undertaken only after careful evaluation of cost effectiveness and potential benefit to the individual and to society. The condition being sought should be significant in frequency and severity. It should be treatable and should have a reasonable likelihood that early treatment will decrease morbidity and mortality. Therefore, the primary care physician, in an effort to maximize time and effectiveness, should plan screening in the office after a consideration of the same factors. This chapter presents the concept of screening as a necessary process during the health supervision visit.

SCREENING IN THE OFFICE

Screening by Interview

The provision of anticipatory guidance in the practitioner's office must begin with a screen. Anticipatory guidance is the sharing with the child's caregiver, and at a later age with the patient, information that will reduce the risk of morbidity and mortality. It is the crucial component of preventive medicine.

The delivery of anticipatory guidance should begin with a thorough screening of the parent's and the child's knowledge. This investigation will reveal which topics need to be discussed and in what depth. Thus, there is no need to waste the time of the physician or the parent by covering all topics of anticipatory guidance.

Perhaps the most efficient use of time in screening knowledge is through the use of a self-administered written or computerized test (Box 21-1). The screen should be age specific, may be kept with the patient's chart (thus allowing each physician to know what the other has covered), and should identify those areas of concern that warrant attention by the physician. This attention may then be given by the physician for greater emphasis, by auxiliary staff, by teaching tape, or by written material.

Topics for screening that can be derived from parental or patient knowledge include:

Nonintentional Injury

Any screening program must screen for those conditions that place the lives of our children at greatest risk. Accidental deaths are clearly the single greatest threat. Motor vehicular deaths are the largest subgroup. In the primary care setting the family's awareness of accident prevention should be assessed by screening. Areas needing improvement may then be discussed. One commercially available questionnaire for screening accident risk is The Injury Prevention Program (TIPP) from the American Academy of Pediatrics. The creation of a safe environment and the prudent education of the child and his/her caregiver are paramount.

Homicide and Suicide

Homicide is the second leading cause of death in the age group 15 to 24 years and the third leading cause of death in the age group 5 to 14 years. In certain subgroups homicide is the leading cause of death. In a 1993 CDC survey of high

---

BOX 21-1
Sample of Screening Questionnaire

BIRTH TO 1 YEAR OF AGE
Adapted from information contained in *Bright Futures*. The publication of *Bright Futures* was supported by the Maternal and Child Health Bureau and the Medicaid Bureau.
Respond to the following statements by writing "TRUE," "NOT TRUE," "DON'T KNOW."

1. We own and use a car seat.
2. Our crib is safe (slats not more than 2⅜ inches apart and firm mattress that fits snugly).
3. I do not plan to use a walker.
4. Smoke detectors are in our house and working.
5. The hot water heater thermostat is set at less than 120° F.
6. We never leave our baby in the bath tub alone or with a young child.
7. Our child may not ride with a driver who has been drinking.
8. I know infant CPR.
9. There are plug protectors on our electric sockets.
10. There are safety locks on our cabinets.
11. All poisonous substances are locked and out of reach.
12. We have syrup of ipecac in the house.
13. We have the Poison Control phone number on our phone.
14. I do not smoke.
15. No one may smoke in the house or car.
16. My child qualifies for Women, Infants, and Children (WIC).
17. I did not give my child whole cow's milk prior to 6 months of age.
18. I did not use low-iron formula.
19. My child does not live in or regularly visit a home built prior to 1960.
20. We are not remodeling a house built prior to 1960.

This questionnaire is presented as an example only and is not intended to be complete. Questionnaires appropriate to other age groups should be used at later visits.

---

school-aged students, 22.1% of students reported that they carried a gun, knife, or club at some time during the 30 days preceding the survey. Risk factors for violent behavior include poor parenting, untreated conduct disorder, social stress, poverty, and school failure. In an excellent review article concerning the role of the pediatrician in the prevention of violence, Rivara and Farrington state, "Screening for parenting problems should be an essential element of child health maintenance, beginning with the prenatal visit," and "Screening for behavior problems should become a routine part of health maintenance examinations."

The most common method of suicide is by firearms, the second by hanging, and the third by poisoning. Risk factors for suicide include verbal, physical, or sexual abuse; family history of depression or suicide; frequent separation from or loss of loved ones; incarceration; pregnancy; alcohol or drug use; and availability of firearms in the home.

Malignant Neoplasms
Cancer is the most common cause of death by disease in the age group 1 to 24 years. The American Cancer Society estimated that in 1996, 8300 new cases of cancer would be diagnosed in children, of which 2800 would be leukemia. They estimated that 1700 children would die in 1996 as a result of cancer. Childhood symptoms that may warrant special attention include unusual mass or swelling; unexplained paleness and loss of energy; sudden tendency to bruise; a persistent, localized pain or limping; prolonged unexplained fever or illness; frequent headaches, often with vomiting; sudden eye or vision changes; and excessive rapid weight loss. Risk factors for the development of cancer in childhood and also later in life should be sought. These risk factors include genetic factors (*eg*, trisomy 21, familial history of retinoblastoma), tobacco use, alcohol use, nutrition, and sunlight exposure.

Alcohol and Drug Use
The Youth Risk Behavior Surveillance of 1993 reports that 80.9% of high school students have had at least one drink during their lifetime, and 30% of students had had five or more drinks of alcohol on at least one occasion during the 30 days preceding the survey. More than 35% of high school students had, during the 30 days preceding the survey, ridden with a driver who had been drinking alcohol. Thirty-two percent of students have tried marijuana, and 4.9% have tried cocaine. Current usage of marijuana was reportedly 17.7% and of cocaine 1.9% during the 30 days preceding the 1993 survey.

Sexual Behavior
The tragedies of ill-considered sexual activity, such as teenage pregnancy with its resultant economic and personal disasters and sexually transmitted diseases including HIV infection, are major problems for our children and teenagers. The CDC reports that 53% of high school students have experienced sexual intercourse. Nationwide 1 million pregnancies occur each year in adolescents, and 10 million cases of sexually transmitted diseases occur annually in persons 15 to 29 years of age.

Smoking
The 1984 Surgeon General's Report states that smoking is the chief, single, avoidable cause of death in our society and the most important public health issue of our time. Sixty-nine percent of high school students report that they have tried cigarette smoking with 24.7% reporting "regular" use. The primary health care provider is in a unique position to alter the course of events. The physician comes in contact with children and adolescents who are the victims of passive smoking and is one of the few health professionals to come in contact with young adults. Perry and Silvis have reviewed the health consequences of tobacco smoke at each age level. They elucidate a prevention program for use in the primary care office and list the concepts behind that program. Screening the attitudes and usage of tobacco of each generation is crucial to the program.

Child Abuse
Child abuse is one of the paradoxes of human behavior. Of all substantiated cases of child abuse, 80% of the abusers are the mother or father. Ten percent of abusers are other relatives. In the nonrelative group of perpetrators (the remaining 10%), the most common perpetrator is the babysitter. The majority of child abuse cases involve neglect, and slightly more than half of the substantiated cases involve sexual abuse. In the babysitter subgroup more than 85% of cases involve sexual abuse. Common signs to trigger suspicion of child abuse include failure to thrive, malnutrition, unexplained bruises or fractures, sexual injuries, and sexually transmitted diseases. In their 1994 report, the Department of Public Welfare of Pennsylvania found that approximately 40% of reported cases of child abuse were eventually declared substantiated. Approximately 15% of substantiated reports are repeat reports on the same child. There were 2.2 fatalities per 100,000 children in the United States in 1991. Burns, suffocation, brain injuries,

and shaken baby syndrome were common causes of death.

School Problems

Neurodevelopmental variation, as influenced by a host of pathologic and nonpathologic factors, results in school problems for as many as 20% of children. Some problems are severe. Some are not. School problems include attention deficit disorder, language learning deficits, processing deficits, and dyslexia. The most common misdiagnoses for these children are lack of intelligence or lack of motivation. Several screening tools for use in the primary care physician's office now exist. Examples include: *The Pediatric Symptom Checklist* by Jellinek, et al, of the Child Psychiatry Service of Massachusetts General Hospital; *The Answer System* by Levine, Educators Publishing Service, Inc.; and *The Child Behavior Checklist* by Achenbach, of the Department of Psychiatry, University of Vermont.

Development

Developmental screening by the physician is an integral part of the assessment of the child. Developmental skills are often divided into the areas of gross motor, language, fine motor (adaptive skills) and personal, or social, skills. A delay in acquisition of these skills may indicate various physical or environmental problems. The screening process itself may be by self-administered questionnaire (Denver Prescreening Developmental Questionnaire [PDQ]), by staff or physician interview, and/or by physician examination. The "gold standard" for the primary care physician's office is the Denver Developmental Screening Test II. (*See* Chapter 120.)

Nutrition

Heart disease, cerebrovascular accidents, diabetes, hypertension, and obesity are diseases that have been shown to be directly linked to diet. The patient's current nutrition habits should be screened. Parents and children should be provided with nutrition information on subjects such as breast feeding, iron, calcium, sodium, fat content, fluoride, sugar, calorie content, folic acid, infant botulism, and dieting. Availability of nutritional counseling programs in the community, such as Women, Infants, and Children (WIC), should be made known.

Immunizations

The immunization rate in the United States needs improvement. The immunization status of each child should be reviewed at each visit—both health supervision visits and sick visits—and updated following the Academy of Pediatrics or CDC recommendations.

Screening By Physical Examination

Each time the physician places a stethoscope to the chest of a "well child" and performs a health supervision examination, a screening takes place. A representative sample of the topics commonly viewed as screens in the physical examination include:

Growth

The assessment of growth is a major responsibility of every physician who cares for children. Height and weight should be measured at each health supervision visit. Head circumference should be measured at each visit from birth until at least age 2 years. These values should be plotted on the child's growth chart, and the progression of growth should be analyzed. Normal variations in growth velocity, usually familial, may be noted. The growth pattern should also be analyzed for indications of pathology, such as malnutrition, hormone deficiency, systemic disease, hydrocephalus, and microcephaly. Various growth charts are available for the population at large, for premature children, and for children with trisomy 21.

Hearing

Every child should be screened for adequacy of hearing at each health supervision visit from birth. Premature infants are often screened by the tertiary care center prior to discharge with a brainstem auditory evoked response (BAER). Screening the hearing of the very youngest of patients is important. Many younger children with hearing loss can be fitted with hearing aids. In practical terms performing an adequate hearing screening on a young child is incredibly difficult. Most often the hearing of a child under 1 year of age is assessed by looking for the presence of eye blink, startle, or other movement of the child in response to a sudden loud sound. Parental observation can be extremely important. Questionnaires that check for the development of behaviors thought to be dependent on adequate hearing may be very useful. Other aids to gain

TABLE 21-1
Methods for Screening and Their Indications

AGE	SCREENING METHOD	INDICATIONS FOR REFERRAL
Newborn to 3 months	Red reflex	Abnormal or asymmetric
	Corneal light reflex	Asymmetric
	Inspection	Structural abnormality
6 months to 1 year	Red reflex	Abnormal or asymmetric
	Corneal light reflex	Asymmetric
	Differential occlusion	Failure to object equally to covering each eye
	Fix and follow with each eye	Failure to fix and follow
	Inspection	Structural abnormality
3 years (approximately)	Visual acuity*	20/50 or worse or 2 lines of difference between the eyes
	Red reflex	Abnormal or asymmetric
	Corneal light reflex/cover-uncover	Asymmetric/ocular refixation movements
	Stereoacuity**	Failure to appreciate random dot or Titmus Stereogram
	Inspection	Structural abnormality
5 years (approximately)	Visual acuity*	20/30 or worse
	Red reflex	Abnormal or asymmetric
	Corneal light reflex/cover-uncover	Asymmetric/ocular refixation movements
	Stereoacuity**	Failure to appreciate random cot or Titmus Stereogram
	Inspection	Structural abnormality

*Allen figures, HOTV, Tumbling E, or Snellen.
**Optional, sometimes advocated in lieu of visual acuity; Random Dot E Game, (RDE), Titmus Stereogram, Randot Stereograms.
(From The American Academy of Ophthalmology: *Comprehensive Pediatric Eye Evaluation, Preferred Practice Pattern®*, San Francisco, 1992, American Academy of Ophthalmology. With permission.)

more information about hearing relate to the determination of fluid behind the tympanic membrane. Pneumatic otoscopy and tympanometry are the methods utilized. After the age of 3 years, routine audiometry is possible. Screening is recommended at ages 4 to 5, 12, and 18 years.

Vision

The visual system should be assessed at each health supervision visit beginning at birth. The American Academy of Ophthalmology recommends the schedule listed in Table 21-1.

Blood Pressure

Blood pressure should be screened yearly beginning at 3 years of age according to the National Heart, Lung, and Blood Institute Task Force on Blood Pressure Control in Children. Mass screening programs for hypertension are not recommended. (*See* Chapter 48.)

Screening By Laboratory Evaluation

Anemia

Acceptable hemoglobin values are age related. The arbitrary cut-off usually chosen as the point for intervention or investigation is two standard deviations below the mean for age. Recommended screening for anemia is at 9 to 12 months of life. Some physicians also recommend screening at ages 2, 8, and 18 years. Other physicians recommend screening high risk groups only: 1) low socioeconomic status, 2) birth weight under 1500 g, 3) cow's milk given before age 6 months (not recommended), or 4) low-iron formula used (not recommended).

Urinalysis

There is wide disagreement among authorities as to the inclusion, frequency, and timing of urinalysis as a screen. Recommendations range from "do not include at all" to as frequently as "yearly in the sexually active male patient." Possible reasons for inclusion of a screening urinalysis include: 1) evaluation of renal function (red blood cells, protein); 2) detection of asymptomatic bacteriuria in the preschool population (white blood cells, bacteriuria); and 3) detection of gonorrhea or *Chlamydia trachomatis* infections in the asymptomatic sexually active male patient (positive leukocyte esterase dipstick). The prevalence of these problems is not especially great (but does approach 10% of sexually active male patients for *Chlamydia*). The sensitivity and specificity of the screening urinalysis is not high. Collection problems in children under 3 years of age may make the results of up to 30% of tests suspect. The test is, however, relatively inexpensive and continues to be recommended by the American Academy of Pediatrics at 6 months and 2, 8, and 18 years of life. The first morning void has the greatest reliability for screening.

Tuberculosis

The only acceptable tuberculosis screening device is now the purified protein derivative (PPD). PPD should be employed annually if the child is in a low socioeconomic group, resides in areas where tuberculosis is present, has exposure to tuberculosis, or has immigrant status. For individuals *not* at high risk, the American Academy of Pediatrics recommends screening at 1, 4, and 14 years of age.

Lead

Lead screening via a serum lead level should be performed at 6 months of age for children with significant risk factors and at 12 months of age for children with no significant risk factors. Screening thereafter is dependent on the data obtained and the risk level of the child. Significant risk factors include living in or regularly visiting (child care) a home with peeling or chipping paint built before 1960; living in or regularly visiting a house built before 1960 with ongoing renovation; living with an adult exposed to lead (*eg*, plumber, glass factory worker, automobile mechanic, highway construction worker, furniture refinisher, pottery or stained glass maker), or living near an active lead smelter or battery recycling plant.

Cardiac Risk

The American Academy of Pediatrics Committee on Nutrition has endorsed selective screening of cholesterol in children who are more than 2 years of age, have a parent or grandparent with early cardiovascular disease (onset at 55 years of age or younger), or have a parent or grandparent with a cholesterol of 240 mg/dL or higher. It is expected that nearly 25% of American children will meet the criteria for "selective" screening. Some experts, however, consider this recommendation controversial. Newman and colleagues argue that cholesterol-lowering diets are not very effective; that cholesterol-lowering drugs are not especially palatable or cheap, nor are they cost-benefit-risk proven for younger patients; and that data exist to show significant reduction in excess risk caused by hypercholesterolemia when treatment is begun in middle age. More research is needed before markedly restrictive diets and cholesterol-lowering drugs become widespread in the pediatric population.

Sickle Cell Anemia

Sickle cell status may be screened if the child has an African-American background—especially if there is a relative with sickle cell disease or trait. Many states include this in the newborn screening program.

Others

Screening of adoptees and recent immigrants may be indicated. These patients are screened for HIV, serology, hepatitis surface antigen, tuberculosis, and, in individuals from tropical areas, stools for ova and parasites.

SCREENING MASS POPULATIONS

The mass population screens most familiar to the primary care practitioner are those funded by governmental agency and consist of newborn screens, preschool-age screens, and various screens provided by the public schools.

Newborn screening in the first week of life is designed to detect various diseases at an early stage. Damage to the child may be ameliorated or prevented by this early screening. Most practitioners are aware that all 50 states screen for phenylketonuria (PKU) and for hypothyroidism. Surprisingly there is little consensus among the

TABLE 21-2
Newborn Screening by Incidence and Number of States*

DISEASE	INCIDENCE	NUMBER OF STATES PERFORMING
PKU	1:12,000	50
Hypothyroidism	1:4000	50
Sickle cell anemia (African-Americans)	1:400	40
Galactosemia	1:60,000	37
Maple syrup urine disease	1:250,000	23
Homocystinuria	1:250,000	22
Galactokinase deficiency	1:250,000	17
Biotinidase deficiency	1:250,000	13
Tyrosinemia	1:150,000	6
Congenital adrenal hyperplasia	1:12,000	6
Cystic fibrosis (Caucasians)	1:2500	3

*Figures valid as of 1992 [4].

states thereafter as to which additional screens are desirable (Table 21-2).

Newborn screening may give the practitioner a false sense of security. The practitioner must be careful not to assume that every case of PKU, hypothyroidism, and so forth has been detected by the newborn screen. If the presentation warrants, a second determination must be performed.

The role of the primary care practitioner in newborn screening has been summarized by Buist and Tuerck. The practitioner must be responsible for parental education regarding newborn screening including the concepts of false positives and negatives, must be responsible for supervising the collection and handling of screening samples, and must be responsible for adequate follow-up of abnormal results. It is failure to ensure that the laboratory results have returned and inadequate follow-up of abnormal results that account for the largest percentage of system failures.

Preschool mass screening programs are those mandated by the states or the federal government through Head Start, WIC, or The Early Periodic Screening and Diagnostic Testing Program.

Screens include vision, hearing, hemoglobin determination, lead levels, and growth assessment. Screens in the school-aged population include vision, hearing, oral health, growth, scoliosis, and physical examinations.

Other nations also fund mass population screenings. Japan, for example, provides the opportunity to screen for neuroblastoma in the first year of life. Some developing countries screen for low birth weight infants in an effort to target malnutrition. Some nations screen for developmental delays.

SUMMARY

The crux of the matter is clear: how does the primary care physician do a good job in a short period of time? For the health supervision visit the answer is also clear—one must employ screening to direct efforts and resources. The process finally employed must be carefully tailored to the needs of the patient and to the strengths of the physician. Screening must be well planned, and relevant.

BIBLIOGRAPHY

American Academy of Pediatrics: *Clinician's handbook of preventive services: Put prevention into practice,* Elk Grove Village, 1994, The American Academy of Pediatrics. Reprinted from *Clinician's handbook of preventive services,* United States Department of Health and Human Services, Public Health Service, 1994.

American Cancer Society: *Cancer facts and figures—1995,* Atlanta, 1995, American Cancer Society.

Bergman AB, Rivara FP: Sweden's experience in reducing childhood injuries, *Pediatrics* 88(1): 69–74, 1991.

Buist NRM, Tuerck JM: The practitioner's role in screening, *Pediatr Clin North Am* 2:199–211, 1992.

Centers for Disease Control and Prevention: Suicide among children, adolescents, and young adults—United States, 1980–1992, *MMWR* 44(15):289–291, 1995.

Centers for Disease Control and Prevention: Youth risk behavior surveillance—United States, 1993, *MMWR* 44(SS-1), 1995.

Department of Public Welfare of Pennsylvania: *7th annual child abuse report,* Harrisburg, 1994, Department of Public Welfare.

Frankenburg WK, Dodds J, Archer P, et al: The Denver II: A major revision and restandardization of the denver developmental screening test, *Pediatrics* 89(1):91–97, 1992.

Green M, editor: *Bright futures: Guidelines for health supervision of infants, children, and adolescents,* Arlington, VA, 1994, National Center for Education in Maternal and Child Health.

Levine MD: *Developmental variation and learning disorders,* Cambridge, 1987, Educators Publishing Service.

Marks A, Fisher M: Health assessment and screening during adolescence, *Pediatrics* 80(suppl 1), 1987.

Newman TB, Garber AM, Holtzman NA, et al: Problems with the report of the expert panel on blood cholesterol levels in children and adolescents, *Arch Pediatr Adolesc Med* 149:241–247, 1995.

Perry CL, Silvis GL: Smoking prevention: Behavioral prescriptions for the pediatrician, *Pediatrics* 79(5):790–798, 1987.

Rivara FP, Farrington DP: Prevention of violence, role of the pediatrician, *Arch Pediatr Adolesc Med* 149:421–429, 1995.

Schaffer SJ, Szilagyi PG, Weitzman M: Lead poisoning risk determination in urban population through the use of a standardized questionnaire, *Pediatrics* 93:159–163, 1994.

United States Bureau of the Census: *Statistical abstract of the United States—1994,* ed 114, Washington, 1994.

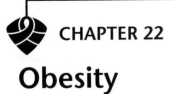

CHAPTER 22

Obesity

Lawrence D. Hammer

Obesity is one of the most common disorders of growth and nutrition affecting children and adolescents in the United States. The medical and psychological sequelae of obesity make its prevention, early recognition, and management important. Much is currently known about the development of body fatness during childhood and the risk factors and behavioral patterns that predispose to the development of obesity in children and adolescents. Because a specific organic cause of obesity is rarely present, the primary care physician must help the family implement a program of treatment based on modifying eating and activity patterns. This chapter includes definitions of obesity, the development of adipose tissue in children and adolescents, factors that contribute to excessive body fatness, and the diagnosis and treatment of obesity.

BACKGROUND

Definition and Prevalence of Obesity

Obesity is most simply defined as excessive body fatness. A number of definitions are used for clinical and research purposes. The most accurate methods of measuring body fatness used in research are not clinically practical because they involve the use of radioisotopes or underwater weighing to estimate body fatness.

One commonly accepted definition of obesity is weight greater than 120% of ideal body weight. Ideal body weight is derived from charts giving average weight for age, sex, and height. Another popular clinical method requires growth charts that plot weight as a function of height. Although helpful when confronted with a tall, heavy child, these charts are inadequate because they assume that weight for height is constant irrespective of age. These graphs and tables tend to overestimate body fatness in adolescents and underestimate it in younger age groups.

A good indicator of body fatness is the body mass index (weight divided by height squared). Body mass index, also known as *Quetelet's index,* can be compared with normative data based on age, sex, and race. The body mass index does not overestimate body fatness in short individuals or underestimate it in tall individuals to the same degree as weight for height. Body mass index greater than the 95th percentile for age and sex is an acceptable definition of obesity (Table 22-1).

A clinical estimation of body fatness is obtained by measurement of skinfold thickness with standard calipers. Skinfold thickness correlates highly with other measures of body fat and is more accurate than visual assessment or weight for height in diagnosing obesity. An accepted definition of obesity uses triceps skinfold thickness greater than the 85th percentile for age, race, and sex. Normative data are available for comparison with the patient's skinfold thick-

TABLE 22-1
Body Mass Index (Reference Values)*†

	MEN		WOMEN	
AGE (YR)	50%ILE	95%ILE	50%ILE	95%ILE
2	16.3	18.4	16.0	18.5
3	15.8	17.8	15.4	17.7
4	15.6	18.1	15.3	18.0
5	15.4	18.0	15.3	19.6
6	15.3	21.1	15.3	19.3
7	15.7	19.8	15.7	19.9
8	16.2	20.8	15.9	20.3
9	16.4	21.8	16.5	25.2
10	17.3	24.4	17.0	24.1
11	17.5	26.4	18.1	26.2
12	18.0	25.0	18.8	26.3
13	18.9	24.8	19.3	28.5
14	19.6	25.1	20.4	28.8
15	20.5	26.6	19.9	26.6
16	21.6	28.0	21.0	29.1
17	21.3	28.3	21.4	31.3
18	22.1	29.9	21.6	30.7

*Adapted from Najjar MF, Rowland M: Anthropometric reference data and prevalence of overweight. United States. 1976-1980. *Vital Health Stat [11]* 1987, 238. Rockville, Md. US Department of Health and Human Services, DHHS Publication No (PHS) 87-1688.
†Calculated as weight/height^2 (kg/m^2).

ness measurement (Table 22-2). The accuracy of skinfold thickness is increased by measuring multiple sites and summing or averaging these measurements; however, the single skinfold thickness measure is adequate for clinical purposes.

Obesity is seen in all parts of the world and in all ethnic groups. It is more prevalent with increasing age and is more common in women than in men. In childhood, prevalence correlates inversely with social class for boys and girls, whereas in adulthood obesity is most common in lower social class women and in upper class men. Data from national health surveys indicate that the prevalence of obesity in the United States has increased 54% among children aged 6 to 11 years and 39% among children aged 12 to 17 years, to 27% and 22%, respectively, in the decade preceding the National Health and Nutrition Examination Survey (NHANES) II conducted in 1976 to 1980.

Development of Adipose Tissue

The earliest stage of adipose tissue development occurs in utero. At birth the infant's body mass is 10% to 15% fat. Almost half the weight gained by

TABLE 22-2
Triceps Skinfold Thickness (Reference Values)*†

	MEN			WOMEN		
AGE (YR)	50%	85%	95%	50%	85%	95%
1	10	13.0	15.5	10.5	13.5	16.5
2	10	13.0	15.0	10.5	13.5	16.0
3	9.5	12.5	15.0	10.0	12.5	16.5
4	9.0	12.0	15.0	10.0	13.0	15.5
5	8.0	11.5	14.5	10.5	14.0	16.0
6	8.0	12.0	17.5	10.0	14.5	18.5
7	8.5	12.0	17.5	10.5	15.0	20.0
8	9.0	16.5	22.0	11.0	16.0	21.0
9	9.0	16.0	23.0	13.0	20.0	27.0
10	11.0	20.0	26.0	13.5	21.0	24.5
11	10.5	22.0	30.0	14.0	21.5	29.5
12	11.0	18.0	26.5	13.5	21.5	27.0
13	9.0	16.5	22.5	15.0	22.0	30.0
14	9.0	15.0	23.0	17.0	25.0	32.0
15	7.5	14.5	22.0	16.5	24.5	32.1
16	8.0	18.5	28.5	18.0	27.0	33.1
17	7.0	12.5	18.0	20.0	26.5	34.5
18	9.5	17.5	22.5	18.0	27.0	35.0

*Adapted from Najjar MF, Rowland M: Anthropometric reference data and prevalence of overweight. United States. 1976-1980. *Vital Health Stat [11]* 1987, 238. Rockville, Md. US Department of Health and Human Services, DHHS Publication No (PHS) 87-1688.
†Measured in millimeters.

the infant in the first 4 months of life is fat. By 1 year of age the child's body mass is 25% to 30% adipose tissue. The child's body fat decreases to 20% to 25% of its body mass by the age of 2 years and begins to increase again after the adipose rebound occurs. Girls have a greater increase of body fat during adolescence than boys, so that by early adulthood, a woman's body composition includes 15% to 30% adipose tissue, whereas in men body fat remains 15% to 20% of body mass.

These changes in body composition correlate with adipocyte development. Adipose tissue development involves cellular proliferation and hypertrophy. Proliferation leads to the formation of new adipocytes by cell division and is most important in infancy and childhood. In utero, adipocyte proliferation and limited lipid filling occur. Cellular studies have demonstrated that adipocyte number remains fairly constant during the first 12 months of life, whereas filling of adipocytes with lipid continues. Adipocyte size increases during the first year of life, reaching normal adult values when the child is 9 to 12 months of age. Adipocyte number then increases steadily from the age of 1 year through puberty. A second burst of adipocyte proliferation occurs

in puberty. In children who are obese, cell size and number are often increased. A proportionally greater increase in cell size than cell number characterizes individuals with adult-onset obesity. Whether development of an excessive number of fat cells during infancy and childhood contributes to the likelihood of obesity persisting into adulthood remains controversial. Factors that control adipocyte hyperplasia and hypertrophy are still incompletely understood.

Natural History of Obesity

There is a growing body of evidence that obesity in infancy or childhood strongly predicts later obesity. Correlation between birth weight and weight later in life is poor; however, at each successive stage of growth the presence of obesity increases the risk for later obesity when compared with nonobese infants or children. Approximately 25% of infants who are obese remain obese after childhood. The older and fatter the obese child the more likely obesity is to persist into adulthood. Thus approximately 50% of obese adolescent girls remain obese as adults. Children with an earlier adipose rebound are at an increased risk for persistent obesity.

Complicating the natural history of obesity in

childhood and adolescence is the effect of pubertal maturation on body fatness. Data from the Ten-State Nutrition Survey demonstrate that while boys undergo a decrease in percent body fat during early adolescence and a gradual increase later in adolescence and adulthood, girls begin to increase body fat prepubertally and continue to increase their body fat into adulthood.

Medical and Psychological Sequelae of Obesity

Obesity influences a variety of physiological and metabolic processes. During childhood, obesity leads to accelerated bone growth and skeletal maturation. Accelerated physical maturation with early menarche and decreased final height is often seen in obese girls. Metabolically, obesity leads to hyperinsulinemia, which increases with age in proportion to body fatness. This hyperinsulinemic state is accompanied by elevated levels of free fatty acids and glycerol. Growth hormone levels are decreased, despite accelerated growth. Decreased prolactin levels have also been reported. Levels of testosterone are decreased in some extremely obese boys. Although ovarian function is intact, obese girls suffer increased rates of amenorrhea and dysfunctional uterine bleeding. In such cases polycystic ovaries should be ruled out.

There is much interest in the effect of obesity in childhood on cardiovascular risk factors such as hyperlipidemia and hypertension. Hyperlipidemia is more common among obese children and adolescents. Cholesterol and triglyceride levels increase with increased weight, and obese children have been noted to have a higher prevalence of hypercholesterolemia and hypertriglyceridemia. Hypertension is also more common among obese children and adolescents. More than 25% of hypertensive adolescents are obese. Systolic and diastolic blood pressures correlate with skinfold thickness.

Other organ systems may be affected as well. Increased cholesterol turnover leads to an increased risk of cholelithiasis in obese children and adolescents. Orthopedic complications include slipped capital femoral epiphyses, Legg-Calvé-Perthes disease, and genu valgum. Intertriginous dermatitis is common. An increase in respiratory tract illness has been associated with obesity in toddlers under 2 years of age. Some patients with obesity have increased daytime sleepiness and hypoventilation (pickwickian syndrome). These patients are also at risk for obstructive sleep apnea and right ventricular failure.

Perhaps the greatest consequence of obesity in childhood or adolescence is its likelihood to persist into adulthood, when obesity is associated with increased morbidity and mortality from hypertension, diabetes, cardiovascular disease, and cerebrovascular accident (CVA). It is estimated that men who are twice their ideal body weight have 12 times the expected mortality for age, and those who are only 50% above ideal body weight have 1.3 to 2.0 times the expected mortality.

Significant psychosocial sequelae have been described in obese children and adolescents. The obese child is teased, ridiculed, and rejected. Many obese adolescents have poor self-esteem, abnormal body image, and difficulty developing peer relations, leading to withdrawal and social isolation. These psychological sequelae help perpetuate the disorder, because obese individuals often shy away from outdoor exercise and physical activity because of embarrassment over their appearance.

Pathogenesis and Differential Diagnosis

Obesity results from an excess of caloric intake over energy expenditure. Factors that influence caloric intake include feeding patterns, composition of the diet, availability of food, and preference for certain types of food. Factors that influence energy expenditure include basal and active metabolic rate and degree of day-to-day activity. At least 95% of obesity in childhood and adolescence may be considered exogenous, or due to an imbalance of these factors. The remaining 5% of children with obesity have either a syndrome associated with obesity or an underlying endocrinologic abnormality.

Most patients with obesity have an imbalance in energy intake and expenditure. Although it is commonly believed that obese individuals have lower basal metabolism than other individuals, obese adolescents have increased basal metabolic activity, probably secondary to increased lean mass. Although basal metabolism is not decreased, active energy utilization may be less in obese than nonobese individuals. The obese have a decreased thermogenic response to activity and carbohydrate intake, which may be a predisposing factor to the development or perpetuation of obesity. Energy utilization also decreases when obese patients are placed on hypocaloric diets. Because the obese individual does not necessarily consume more calories than the nonobese individual, this energy-conserving capability helps perpetuate the obese state.

Although overfeeding may lead to obesity, it does not appear necessary to maintain the obese state. Epidemiologic studies have not demonstrated significant differences in caloric intake or distribution of calories with respect to fat or carbohydrate in obese and nonobese children. In infancy, obesity may develop as a result of overfeeding by parents who mistake the infant's cry as an indication of hunger or who feed the infant beyond the point of satiety. Because infants less than 3 to 4 months of age do not regulate their intake as finely as older infants do, overfeeding can occur, thereby leading to excessive body fatness. Bottle feeding and earlier introduction of solid foods have been associated with more rapid doubling of birth weight; however, the efficacy of breast feeding in protecting against obesity has not been clearly demonstrated. Factors that influence intake during infancy, such as taste preference, appetite, and satiety, are still poorly understood.

Much evidence exists for a significant role of activity and exercise in moderating the effects of caloric intake on the development of obesity. Studies of infants have shown significant correlations between body weight and activity level. Among older children and adolescents, the obese appear to be less active than the nonobese. In addition, caloric energy expenditure per unit of activity is less in the obese adolescent than in the nonobese. It is not uncommon for obesity to develop after a serious illness requiring a period of bed rest and decreased physical activity. Once the obese state develops, decreased self-esteem and clumsiness often lead to further elimination of physical activity and exercise by the child or adolescent. Large periods of time spent watching television or engaged in other passive activity predispose to the development of obesity.

The relative importance of familial and genetic factors cannot be underestimated. Genetic factors exert a strong influence on the development of obesity. Approximately 40% of the offspring of one obese parent are obese, and 70% of the offspring of two obese parents are likely to be obese. Environmental modeling of dietary behavior and physical activity certainly influence

the child of obese parents, yet even adopted children raised from infancy resemble their biologic parents in fatness and not their adoptive parents. There may be genetic influences on metabolic rate and energy expenditure that underly this familial tendency.

Although many diagnostic entities are associated with obesity, the presence of normal or increased stature, normal gonadal development, and normal intelligence rules out most of these disorders. Inherited disorders and congenital syndromes account for only 2% to 3% of cases of obesity. Prader-Willi syndrome is characterized by obesity, hypogonadism, mental retardation, short stature, small hands and feet, and dysmorphic facies (down-turned triangular mouth, almond-shaped eyes, decreased bifrontal diameter). Infants with Prader-Willi syndrome are often hypotonic and have slow weight gain in infancy secondary to feeding problems; however, late in childhood hyperphagia and obesity develop. These children have severe behavioral problems in addition to mental retardation. Prader-Willi syndrome is the most common genetic obesity syndrome, occurring in one in 5000 to 10,000 births. It is usually sporadic, but 70% of cases are associated with deletions involving chromosome 15. DNA probe analysis is diagnostic in 95% of cases. The defect in Prader-Willi syndrome is probably hypothalamic. Lawrence-Moon-Biedl syndrome is characterized by obesity, mental retardation, short stature, polydactyly, retinitis pigmentosa, deafness, and hypogonadism. Vasquez syndrome is an X-linked disorder characterized by obesity, mental retardation, hypogonadism, and gynecomastia. Alstrom syndrome is characterized by obesity, deafness, diabetes mellitus, retinitis pigmentosa, short stature, and hypogonadism. Cohen syndrome is an autosomal recessive syndrome with obesity, hypotonia, and mental retardation, but without hypogonadism or short stature.

Several endocrine disorders, such as Cushing disease and hypothyroidism, also may be associated with obesity; however, their diagnosis is usually apparent from other clinical signs. In both Cushing disease and hypothyroidism the bone age is delayed, whereas most obese children have normal or advanced bone age. Patients with pseudohypoparathyroidism have short stature, hypocalcemia, and short fourth metacarpals in addition to obesity.

Children with central nervous system disease

also may be at risk for obesity due to hyperphagia or hypoactivity. Meningitis, brain tumors, CVA, and head trauma have all been associated with the onset of obesity.

DATA GATHERING

Evaluation of obesity in the child or adolescent should begin with a complete history and physical examination. Because the syndromes described previously account for only a small portion of childhood obesity and generally can be excluded with a good history and physical examination, few laboratory tests are needed in this evaluation. The history should include parental weight, the child's birth weight, early feeding history, age of onset of obesity, and information regarding the family's perception of the child's body habitus. It is important to obtain information regarding the feeding patterns of the household and the use of food within the family as reward or part of social functions. With older children it is important to inquire about school performance, peer relationships, relationships with members of the family, and the child's perception of his/her own body. A family history of obesity, hypertension, cardiovascular disease, diabetes, and CVA should be elicited. Any history of antecedent illness, hospitalizations, or surgery is pertinent.

A dietary history for weekday and weekend is useful, as are using a food diary and an interview with questions regarding food preferences, eating habits, snacks, where meals are eaten, and with whom. By inquiring into the family and child's eating habits, people, places, and moods commonly associated with foods are better understood. Some children binge eat, have compulsive patterns of eating, or respond to changes in emotional state with eating. Some obese children are particularly responsive to external stimuli such as the appearance, taste, or smell of food, while being unresponsive to internal cues such as a feeling of satiety. Information regarding physical activity also should be obtained, including information about daily habits such as reading and television watching. A weekday and weekend activity record is useful for this purpose.

The physical examination should include particular attention to the child's overall appearance, vital signs (especially blood pressure), dis-tribution of fat, the presence of striae and skin irritation, the child's stage of sexual maturation, and the presence of any orthopedic abnormalities, including scoliosis, genu valgum, and slipped capital femoral epiphyses. Accurate measurement of weight and height are mandatory and the measurement of skinfold thicknesses with calipers is recommended. To rule out a congenital syndrome, observe for hypogonadism, short stature, mental retardation, dysmorphic faces, and small extremities. Signs of hypoventilation would suggest "pickwickian" syndrome. A psychological evaluation of the child and family also may be helpful, and consultation with a mental health professional can provide useful diagnostic information.

The laboratory evaluation of the obese child is not routine but directed to ruling out any disease suggested by the history and physical examination. Because less than 5% of cases have an organic basis, the testing can be very limited. If the child is short for his/her age, a thyroid function test is needed. High-resolution chromosome analysis or DNA probe analysis can be ordered if the child has clinical signs of Prader-Willi syndrome. Urinalysis is useful as an initial screening for diabetes mellitus. A lipid profile is indicated to rule out hypercholesterolemia or hypertriglyceridemia, particularly in adolescents. If the child has a history of daytime sleepiness or apnea, obstructive sleep apnea syndrome should be evaluated in a sleep laboratory with an arterial blood gas determination, pulmonary function tests, electrocardiography, and otolaryngologic consultation. Obese adolescents with amenorrhea or dysfunctional bleeding should have a pelvic ultrasound examination to look for polycystic ovaries and gonadotropin levels to evaluate hypothalamic-pituitary function.

MANAGEMENT

Obesity is a lifelong disorder. Its treatment requires patience and motivation. The importance of intervention during childhood and adolescence arises from its immediate psychological and medical effects and the tendency for obesity to persist into adulthood, when the cardiovascular effects of excess weight become more apparent. Many adolescents are concerned about their weight and body image. Many feel they are fatter than they really are. During puberty the normal increase in adipose tissue comes at a time when youth are particularly sensitive to changes in their appearance. Adolescence should therefore be an ideal time to initiate a weight-loss program, yet the combination of increasing adipose tissue and a desire to be like others with respect to diet and recreational activities leave the adolescent highly resistant to treatment. Earlier the nutritional needs of the young child for growth and development make restriction of caloric intake potentially hazardous.

The guiding principle of treatment is to change behavior so that more energy is utilized by the child for activity, growth, and metabolic processes than is consumed. Treatment can be initiated at any age as long as the nutritional needs of the child are met. The younger the child the more direct involvement parents will have to have, but family cooperation is needed for treating children and adolescents of all ages.

Management of the school-aged child should be done with consideration of the nutritional requirements for growth and development. Caloric intake should be modified to provide a balanced diet without excess calories remaining for storage as fat. Reduction of caloric intake by 250 to 500 kcal/day can provide enough energy for growth without additional weight gain, particularly if restriction is focused on fatty and sweet foods. The usual goal of treatment at this age is limited reduction in weight or maintenance of weight over time while growth continues and the child's body composition normalizes. This process may take quite a while; each 20% over ideal body weight requires about a year of "catch-up" time without weight gain. If the child is severely obese, periods of caloric restriction may be needed to yield actual weight loss, but this should always be done cautiously so as to allow growth to proceed.

Modifying caloric intake during childhood requires change in the eating behavior of the parent as well as the eating habits of the child. Simple dietary counseling is not adequate. Knowledge of the family's own dietary habits, with use of food for reward, pleasure, or social interaction, is important. If the family eats together, are the children given the same foods as the parents and in the same quantities? Insisting on a clean plate contributes to unnecessary caloric intake. Many children learn at an early age that their eating gives their parents a sense of pleasure and feeling

of successful parenting. These children eat to please their parents rather than to satisfy their own nutritional needs or to enjoy the taste of food. The whole family may have an eating pattern that encourages excessive intake; treatment necessitates involvement of the whole family. The child should not be the target of treatment or the scapegoat in an obese family.

Treatment of obese children has generally focused on dietary modification, without sufficient emphasis on the role of exercise and increased activity in the reduction of adipose tissue and maintenance of weight. When used alone exercise programs are often inadequate for treating obesity, but when combined with dietary change, they can be a powerful tool for initiating and maintaining weight reduction. Exercise may be particularly important in the maintenance of reduced weight. Exercise facilitates the dietary approach and decreases the inactive time during the day, when excess caloric intake occurs. Activities that encourage family participation and reduction in television viewing are especially useful in treating the whole family. Exercises, sports, and games should be selected that are appropriate for the child's age and level of fitness. As treatment proceeds, exercises that are more vigorous and demanding may be recommended. It is most important to make exercise a regular habit. Walking to school or to other activities is a good beginning. Bicycling, swimming, skating, jogging, and cross-country skiing are suitable activities for the school-aged child. The obese child is usually self-conscious about appearance and is reluctant to participate in outdoor activities, be they individual or organized group sports. It is usually best to begin with activities after school two to three times per week and increase the frequency and vigor of the activity gradually as the child begins to lose some fatness and begins to feel proud of his/her progress.

Although there are no definitive rules about who should participate in the treatment of the obese child and how often the child should be seen, a team approach with frequent visits appears to work best. The physician may coordinate visits to the office for the initial and subsequent history, examination, and follow-up. A dietitian can be called on to obtain more extensive dietary information from the child and parents and give guidance for choosing foods. Specific diets may be useful initially in treatment, but ultimately the child and parent must learn to make appropriate choices for themselves. A counselor (eg, psychologist, psychiatrist, social worker) can be particularly helpful in establishing and maintaining the behavioral aspects of treatment, including reducing cues that stimulate eating, encouraging exercise, and reinforcing success. All of these components of treatment can be provided by the physician if desired; however, treatment may demand more time than is generally available in many practices. Visits for measurement of weight should be encouraged weekly, with positive reinforcement in the way of gold stars on a calendar or chart or other rewards (treats, privileges, money) given for achievement of reasonable goals, preferably not based on weight but rather on dietary modification and increased activity. Parents also should be rewarded for their achievements. Strong consideration should be given to the benefits of treating children and their parents in groups (see below).

Treating the Adolescent

The principles that apply to treatment of the younger child also apply to the adolescent. Energy expenditure must exceed energy intake if treatment is to succeed. The components of treatment are also the same: dietary modification and increasing exercise, with emphasis on changing eating behavior and daily activity patterns. The most successful treatment programs include a combination of these components reinforced with behavior modification.

The principles of dietary modification in adolescence again require provision of adequate calories for growth and development without excessive calories for fat storage. Adolescents interested in losing weight may be eager to try the latest fad diet. This should be discouraged because these diets, although usually successful in initiating weight loss, are generally unbalanced nutritionally for the growing teen. The physician or dietitian should work with the adolescent to develop a well-balanced diet that reduces daily caloric intake by approximately 500 calories and provides less than 20% of calories as fat, while maintaining a level of protein intake of at least 30% to 40% of daily intake. Reliance on dietary education and counseling is rarely successful in the long run, however, unless coupled with a program designed to modify eating behavior. Teens with severe obe-

sity (ie, greater than 100 lbs overweight) may benefit from a protein-sparing modified fast coupled with behavior modification and group support. Such patients should be carefully monitored by a physician experienced with this approach.

Exercise should be strongly encouraged in the adolescent as part of the treatment of obesity. In addition to utilizing excess calories, exercise leads to reduction in hyperinsulinemia and hypertension independent of its weight-reducing effect. After exercise, metabolic rate remains elevated for a time, appetite is temporarily reduced, and a sense of greater well-being is induced, which further enhances self-esteem and increases motivation for the achievement of weight loss. The greatest barrier that the obese adolescent must overcome is the initial hesitancy to exercise due to embarrassment and self-consciousness. Activities with other family members or alone rather than with peers may be more acceptable to the embarrassed teenager. Parents should be encouraged to join the adolescent in exercises such as walking, jogging, swimming, and bicycling. It is important to develop realistic goals for exercise. Periods of walking each day can be slowly increased before proceeding to jogging or bicycling. Over time the duration and strenuousness of the exercise program should be increased. Much positive reinforcement should be given for the achievement of even modest exercise goals, and a daily log of the adolescent's exercising will provide a proud reminder of progress over weeks and months.

It should be recalled that the obese adolescent often has a variety of psychological sequelae, such as anxiety, anger, and depression. The obese adolescent is at a disadvantage in developing important peer relations, particularly with members of the other sex. This is an important time for the development of confidence in dealing with social situations. These sequelae coupled with the frustration often experienced by the obese adolescent during treatment make the use of group meetings with other obese adolescents and an experienced therapist valuable. At these meetings adolescents share their frustrations, constructively discuss their eating behavior, and with the help of the therapist and support of the group, successfully begin to modify their behavior. Treatment programs in which parents attend a group separate from their obese children have been shown to be more effective than programs in which parents and children attend the same group together. Groups should meet at least once a week, particularly early in the treatment program, with an organized curriculum concerning behavior change and factors influencing behavior change. This group approach, with children and parents treated in separate groups, has been found to offer long-term benefits, when used with children or adolescents.

Behavior Modification in Treatment of Obesity

Techniques of behavior modification should be employed by the physician, counselor, or dietitian as a powerful adjunct to dietary restriction and exercise in the treatment of obesity. The use of behavior modification is helpful in this setting because exogenous obesity is often maintained by excessive eating occurring as a result of endogenous and environmental cues. Each individual's eating behavior should be carefully analyzed by the therapist guiding the treatment and its immediate antecedents and consequences discovered. Treatment involves altering and limiting exposure to the antecedent stimuli (called *stimulus control*) and reducing the reinforcing nature of the eating behavior. A child who overeats whenever an upsetting event occurs can be given alternative suggestions for responding to discomfort. A child who eats while doing homework in the kitchen might be encouraged to do his work in another part of the house where food will not be readily available. Reducing the amount of high-calorie food available in the house also helps (environmental control). Substitution of high-calorie food with snack items such as celery and carrots should be recommended. Rewarding the child with a dessert for finishing the rest of dinner should be avoided. The child who is not hungry should not be encouraged to clean his/her plate. Reducing time spent watching television and encouraging activity or exercise in the evening serves the dual purposes of reducing intake and increasing energy expenditure.

Positive reinforcement can be provided in a number of ways, such as with gold stars, special outings with the family, an extra visit to a favorite place, even a rare visit to the ice cream store. Most important is that reinforcement be given for change in behavior, such as change in eating patterns and exercise, using very modest and achievable goals, rather than rewarding weight loss per se. The obese adolescent easily begins losing weight with dietary restriction, but continued loss of weight is difficult. Reinforcement for behavior change is most important to ensure continued success with treatment.

A very powerful tool for achieving behavior change is self-monitoring. Self-monitoring involves recording as accurately as possible the behavior such as eating and its immediate surrounding behaviors, with attention to timing and location. Such a record provides the therapist with a highly accurate picture of where eating occurs, in what context, with whom the adolescent usually eats, and the events that precede and follow eating that may reinforce it. Knowledge of these cues for eating and the patterns of reinforcement help the therapist and the individual in treatment understand and limit exposure to the cues and change the pattern of behavior. Self-monitoring also increases the individual's insight into his/her own behavior and independently acts to help alter that behavior. Finally, self-monitoring provides a record of achievement and success for the adolescent as treatment proceeds and weight loss continues. Combining self-monitoring with a behavior contract provides a practical approach to the problem of realistic goal setting and reinforcement. A behavior change contract might specify a daily dietary goal (*eg*, the number of "red light" foods, as in Epstein's traffic light diet), a daily exercise goal, and a behavior such as keeping a daily food record. The child "contracts" with the parent for an agreed reward for fulfillment of the contract. The reward should be age appropriate and available soon after it is earned. Young children should be able to receive a reward twice weekly; a weekly reward is appropriate for the older child. Rewards need not be expensive; an extra outing alone with the parent or to a special event may be more meaningful than material gifts.

Maintenance of Weight Loss

Many programs for treating obesity report average losses of 1 to 2 kg/wk during treatment. Most programs also report gradual regaining of weight after treatment ends. The challenge of maintaining weight loss may be greater than the challenge of initial weight loss. Most treatments, from behavioral to controlled fasting, ultimately fail unless a maintenance program is included. Maintenance requires the continuation of moderation in dietary intake coupled with a regular program of exercise. Limited self-monitoring of intake, exercise, and weight are helpful. Continuation of stimulus reduction by keeping the environment free of high-calorie foods and avoiding situations in which dietary indiscretion occurs also helps. Monthly group meetings provide further impetus and reinforcement for behavior change. During the maintenance phase, periodic intensification of treatment with further dietary restriction for several months may encourage the obese youngster to stick with the program. Any soundly conceived weight loss program for the adolescent can only succeed if he/she continues in treatment. Maintaining adherence to a program is the greatest challenge for the therapist and patient. Weight loss is difficult, requiring long periods of dedication during which success and frustration often intermingle. The treatment program should reinforce adherence, even if other goals of behavior change and weight loss are not always met. Various contingency systems using payback regimens have been very successful as adjuncts to weight loss programs. Physicians should investigate group programs available in their communities that might be suitable for children or adolescents, particularly if coupled with regular follow-up and involvement by the physician.

Prevention
Because the treatment of obesity requires long periods of dedication and difficult changes in eating behavior and activity, the disorder is best prevented. Knowledge of risk factors can help target efforts at prevention. Families with parental obesity have an increased risk of obesity in the children. Particular attention to overfeeding and avoidance of excessive weight gain in the first few years of life is important. Restriction of caloric intake early in childhood should be done only with careful medical supervision. The use of food as reward should be discouraged. It is wise to discourage eating in front of the television or excessive snacking between meals. Feeding should not be forced or overly encouraged if the child is not hungry. Children should not be required to clean their plates and should be encouraged to avoid junk food and high-calorie snacks. Adolescents, in particular, are prone to irregularity in their diet. It is helpful if adolescents understand that it is normal to gain weight during puberty, especially for girls, but that excessive weight gain can be avoided by regular exercise and limitation of excessive intake. The whole family should be encouraged to exercise in moderation on a regular basis. Early emphasis on healthy diet and regular exercise should be the cornerstone of the physician's approach to healthy weight management.

BIBLIOGRAPHY

Agras WS, Kraemer HC, Berkowitz RI, et al: Does a vigorous feeding style influence early development of adiposity? *J Pediatr* 110:799–804, 1987.

Brown MR, Klish WJ, Hollander J, et al: A high protein, low calorie liquid diet in the treatment of very obese adolescents: long-term effect on lean body mass, *Am J Clin Nutr* 38:20–31, 1983.

Dietz WH, Gortmaker SL: Do we fatten our children at the TV set? Television viewing and obesity in children and adolescents, *Pediatrics* 75:807–812, 1988.

Dietz WH, Robinson TN: Assessment and treatment of childhood obesity, *Pediatr Rev* 14:337–343, 1993.

Epstein LH, Valoski A, Wing RR, McCurley J: Ten-year follow-up of behavioral, family-based treatment for obese children. *JAMA* 264:2519–2523, 1990.

Epstein LH, Wing RR: Behavioral treatment of childhood obesity, *Psych Bull* 101:331–342, 1987.

Freedman DS, Burke GL, Harsha DW, et al: Relationship of changes in obesity to serum lipid and lipoprotein changes in childhood and adolescence, *JAMA* 254:515–520, 1985.

Garn SM: Continuities and changes in fatness from infancy through adulthood, *Curr Probl Pediatr* 15:1–47.

Gortmaker SL, Dietz WH, Sobol AM, et al:

Increasing pediatric obesity in the United States, *Am J Dis Child* 141:535–540, 1987.

Poissonnet CM, LaVelle M, Burdi AR: Growth and development of adipose tissue, *J Pediatr* 113:1–9, 1988.

Roberts SB, Savage J, Coward WA, et al: Energy expenditure and intake in infants born to lean and overweight mothers, *N Engl J Med* 318:461–466, 1988.

Rolland-Cachera MF, Deheeger M, Bellisle F, et al: Adiposity rebound in children: A simple indicator for predicting obesity, *Am J Clin Nutr* 39:129–135, 1984.

Rosenbaum M, Leibel RL: Obesity in childhood, *Pediatr Rev* 11:43–55, 1989.

Stunkard AJ, Sorensen TI, Hanis C, et al: An adoption study of human obesity, *N Engl J Med* 314:193–198, 1986.

CHAPTER 23

Injury Prevention

Flaura Koplin Winston

Effective health counseling requires a knowledge of the epidemiology, pathophysiology, therapy, and prognosis of disease so that the practitioner can answer questions the patient and the family may have. Too many practitioners and parents have the misconception that injuries result from accidents—much like how, 200 years ago, infectious diseases were viewed as random, unpreventable events. Many people believe that children, especially boys, are destined to get hurt and that injuries in children are mild. Injuries are not inevitable and are often not mild; they surpass all other causes of childhood mortality combined.

Each year 10,000 children under the age of 15 years die of injuries. Many die instantaneously, before medical care can be administered. Death is only a part of the problem. For every child between the ages of 1 and 15 years who dies from injury, another 34 children are admitted to hospitals, many to be discharged with lifelong disabilities. Each year in the United States injuries lead to more than 10 million emergency room visits and, despite the best emergency medical care, permanently disable 50,000 children ages 14 years and under.

The key to minimizing this health crisis is injury prevention. Pediatricians can be effective in injury prevention with well-informed, well-timed anticipatory guidance. In this chapter, a practical overview of the epidemiology and biomechanics of unintentional injuries will be presented for children under the age of 15 years with a focus on the role of the pediatric primary care practitioner in injury prevention.

THE PRIMARY CARE PROVIDER ROLE IN INJURY PREVENTION

Injury prevention strategies exist in three phases: before, during, and after the injury-producing event occurs. The primary care practitioner has a role in each phase. In the following discussion and Table 23-1, the role of the practitioner in the prevention of firearm-related injuries is presented to illustrate this approach and then the generalized approach will be presented.

During the first phase of injury prevention, the pre-event phase, the practitioner should educate the family about characteristics of the child and his/her environment that increase the likelihood

TABLE 23-1

Example of the Role of the Pediatric Primary Care Practitioner in Injury Prevention: Counseling in the Prevention of Firearm Injuries

	CHARACTERISTICS TO ADDRESS AS PART OF HEALTH MAINTENANCE		
PHASE	CHARACTERISTICS OF THE CHILD	CHARACTERISTICS OF THE GUN	CHARACTERISTICS OF THE ENVIRONMENT
Pre-event	Young child 1. Curious 2. Interested in guns Older child 1. Depressed 2. Violent personality traits 3. Conflict resolution skills lacking	1. Firearms in the home 2. BB guns or realistic-looking toy guns in the home 3. Unlocked gun cabinet	1. Supervision 2. Access to a gun 3. Family, community, and peer attitudes toward guns 4. Knowledge of risk of accidental shootings
Event	1. Ease with which even a young child can pull a trigger 2. Suicidal ideation 3. Involvement in conflict 4. Gang-related activities	1. Type of gun (BB guns cause eye injuries) 2. Availability of ammunition 3. Absence of a trigger lock	1. Availability of crisis intervention services 2. Parental supervision 3. Metal detectors at schools
Post-event	1. Physical rehabilitative needs 2. Need for psychosocial services and counseling	1. Have guns been removed from the home? 2. Have remaining guns been unloaded and locked?	1. Availability of social support for child or family 2. Attitudes of family, peers, and community

of occurrence of an injury-producing event. With regard to firearm injuries, the event would be gaining access to a gun. Curious young children and depressed or violent older children are at risk for gaining access to a firearm when in a house with firearms and in an environment that condones the use of guns.

The next phase of injury prevention, the event phase, involves preventing the injury once the event has occurred. In this phase, the practitioner should be knowledgeable about injury mechanisms and be able to counsel regarding the effective use of safety devices. Triggers are easy to pull for even a very young child. For families that insist on keeping a gun in the house, the practitioner should inform them of several designs that exist to make guns more difficult to fire unintentionally, including trigger locks and loaded gun indicators. The presence of an unlocked handgun loaded with ammunition greatly increases the risk of injury once a young child or adolescent has access to the weapon.

During the final stage, the postevent stage, the emergency medical system has the primary role in the initial treatment of the injury once it has occurred. The primary care practitioner has the responsibility to understand the long-term complications of the injury in order to provide effective health maintenance to ensure optimal growth and development of the injured child and

to prevent future injuries. Physical rehabilitative services will be needed for the victim as well as additional services to address psychosocial issues that led to and resulted from the gun-related injuries.

PRE-EVENT PHASE OF INJURY PREVENTION: PREVENTION OF THE EVENT THAT WOULD LEAD TO INJURY

Injuries are common throughout childhood but the rate and type of injuries vary with the age and developmental level of the child (Table 23-2). Recognition of hazards, curiosity, level of skill mastery (eg, riding bicycles), and need for supervision all contribute to risk of injury. According to Baker and colleagues, boys, children with behavior problems, children with a history of injury, and children living in stressful situations, in particular, children living in poverty, are more prone to injuries. A strong knowledge of the epidemiology of injuries will provide the practitioner with the information necessary to guide the parents in assessing those aspects of the child and the environment that put the child at risk for injury.

Throughout childhood, motor vehicle collisions, fires, and drownings are potential causes of

TABLE 23-2
Most Common Causes of Unintentional Injury Deaths

AGE	CAUSES OF UNINTENTIONAL INJURY DEATH				
<1 yr	Motor vehicle collision	Aspiration	Fire	Drowning	Falls
1 to <2 yrs	Motor vehicle collision	Drowning	Fire	Pedestrian (nontraffic-related)	Aspiration and poisonings
2 to <5 yrs	Drowning	Fire	Motor vehicle collision	Pedestrian (traffic-related)	Aspiration and falls
5 to <10 yrs	Pedestrian (traffic)	Motor vehicle collision	Drowning	Fire	Bicycle collision
10 to 15 yrs	Motor vehicle collision	Drowning	Firearms	Fire	Bicycle collision

Adapted from Wilson MH, *et al:* Saving children: A guide to injury prevention, Oxford, 1991, Oxford University Press and Baker SP, *et al:* Head injuries incurred by children and young adults during informal recreation, *Am J Public Health* 84:649–652, 1994.

death. Prevention of injuries from these events should be emphasized with children of all ages. The importance of other injury mechanisms varies with age and should be emphasized for children at special risk for those injuries. For example, the importance of aspiration, suffocation, and falls as causes of injury death decreases after the first year of life, at which time nontraffic-related pedestrian injuries (*eg,* children struck by vehicles while playing in driveways) and poisonings gain importance. During the toddler years, curiosity and physical development surpass the child's ability to recognize hazardous situations, and the injury patterns reflect this change.

Pedestrian injury deaths become a leading cause of death in children ages 4 to 8 years and peak at age 6. Again, this pattern reflects the inability of young children to assess hazardous situations properly. Therefore, children should not be allowed to cross busy streets by themselves until the age of 9 years.

Bicycle-related deaths gain importance in school-aged children, and the head is the primary site of fatal bicycle-related injuries. Bicycles still remain hazardous for the preadolescent, but unintentional firearm deaths emerge as the third leading cause of unintentional injury death in this age group.

Most studies regarding injury rates are based on mortality data; however, deaths represent only a small fraction of the injured children. Although burns, playground- and sports-related injuries, and falls are important causes of injury morbidity, these events are rare in the injury

mortality data. Each year 100,000 children from birth to age 4 years require emergency medical treatment for scalds.

Incorporating Injury Epidemiology into Anticipatory Guidance

A logical time to provide anticipatory guidance is during the developmental evaluation at a well-child examination, but reinforcement should occur at all encounters, especially when a child is seen for an injury. After first assessing the child developmentally, the practitioner should share with the parents both the current capabilities of the child and the skills expected to be mastered in the near future that will put the child at risk for injury.

For example, when examining a child aged 4 months, the practitioner might note that the child has just begun to roll over. After reassuring the parents that the child is progressing well developmentally, the practitioner might discourage the use of baby walkers and warn the parents not to leave the child unattended while on a changing table, bed, or chair to prevent falls. The practitioner also should inform the parents that the child will soon be crawling and putting everything into his/her mouth, and it is at this time that the parents should begin "baby-proofing" their house.

The parents should be instructed to get down on their hands and knees in rooms in which the child will be crawling and look for hazards, such as uncovered outlets, hot objects that could be pulled to the floor, small objects (buttons, raisins, nuts) that could be aspirated, and stairs without baby gates. Finally, the practitioner might guide parents in strategies for prevention of injuries not attributable to characteristics of the child. These strategies include installing smoke detectors and automatic sprinkler systems to reduce the risk of injury from house fires, not leaving the child unattended in the bath to reduce the risk of drowning, lowering the hot water heater thermostat to reduce the risk of scalds, and using child safety seats to reduce the risk of injury in motor vehicle crashes.

This age-specific approach to anticipatory guidance for the preadolescent child is presented in the American Academy of Pediatric's TIPP program.

EVENT PHASE OF INJURY PREVENTION: PREVENTION OF THE INJURY ONCE THE EVENT HAS OCCURRED

With the best of intentions on the part of the parents and the practitioner, events will occur that put the child at risk for injury. If the child is properly protected, injury need not result. Effective use of safety devices is enhanced by instruction from a practitioner on their proper use before the event occurs. The key to understanding the use of specific safety devices is in understanding the pathophysiology and mechanisms of the specific injuries.

Injury results when a body is exposed to energy that surpasses the body's ability to absorb or dissipate the energy without structural or functional damage.

Much as viruses and bacteria are among the agents of infectious disease, energy is the agent of injury. Infectious diseases are prevented by minimizing the burden of viruses and bacteria on the body; injury is prevented by minimizing exposure to energy. It is second nature for a parent to make sure that the bath water is not too hot before putting the baby in the tub. This parent is minimizing thermal energy exposure to the child to prevent scalding. Thermal energy, or heat, is the agent that causes burns.

It is helpful to understand the relationship between water temperature and scalds in the effective minimization of thermal energy exposure. For adult skin, water at 119° F may cause pain but will not burn the skin. At 130° F, water

causes first- and second-degree burns within 29 seconds. At 140° F, an exposure of only 3 seconds is all that is required to cause serious injuries. Children's skin is thinner and is more susceptible to burn injuries than adult skin. Therefore, many childhood scald injuries could be prevented by setting the hot water heater thermostat to 120° to 125° F.

The energy involved in motor vehicle crashes and other forms of mechanical trauma is known as *mechanical energy.* Many safety technologies are aimed at the prevention of mechanical trauma and involve minimizing exposure to mechanical energy.

Mechanical energy is the agent that breaks bones and causes head injuries when tissues are stopped suddenly. Mechanical trauma can occur without impact, such as whiplash after rapid flexion-extension of the neck or avulsion fracture after twisting an ankle, but most commonly occurs with impact. One of the most lethal and disabling forms of mechanical injury is head trauma. Head trauma can occur with or without impact but the most severe forms of head trauma occur with impact.

What Happens During Head Impact?

The small portion of the skull that makes contact during head impact stops moving immediately. The adjacent skull continues to move and bends. If the energy of impact is high enough, a skull fracture results. The brain and blood vessels inside the skull continue to rotate relative to the skull after the impact, and, if the energy of impact is high enough, this motion causes the blood vessels to break and the nerves to stop transmitting impulses.

The mechanical energy involved in head impact increases the more sudden the impact. Hitting the head on concrete is a sudden, violent, short-duration impact and results in worse head injuries than the gentle, long-duration impact of hitting the head on foam. Many injury prevention strategies are aimed at preventing head injuries by lengthening the duration of impact and therefore reducing the impact energy transmitted to the head, often with the use of foam padding.

Prevention of Head Injuries During a Motor Vehicle Collision

During an impact, the vehicle decelerates suddenly and comes to an ultimate stop over a distance related to the amount the vehicle is crushed. For a frontal impact with a rigid barrier at a speed of 30 miles per hour, deceleration to a stop occurs over 2 feet. As the collision occurs, the vehicle begins to stop but the unrestrained passenger continues to move at the original speed of the vehicle. Because the knees contact the instrument panel early during the crash phase, before the vehicle has come to a complete stop, the knees experience a relatively low impact energy and then decelerate, or "ride down" the collision, relatively gently with the vehicle. The chest will impact next and then the head. For most passengers sitting against the seat back, the head is 2 feet from the windshield. In many crashes, the head will impact after the vehicle has come to a complete stop and will not benefit from any vehicle ride-down. Therefore, the head of an unrestrained occupant will be exposed to a sudden, violent, short-duration stop.

Unrestrained infants are at particular risk during motor vehicle collisions, especially if a passenger holds the infant in his/her lap. During the collision, the infant not only will experience a violent impact when thrown against the vehicle interior but also will be crushed by the passenger holding the infant.

Prevention strategies are aimed at increasing the occupant ride-down time during a collision by restraining the movement of the occupant in the vehicle. The restrained occupant stops with the vehicle, thereby coming to a more gentle stop than the unrestrained occupant.

Restraints must be used properly to achieve maximal benefit and to prevent injuries induced by the restraint system itself. Proper fit is the first consideration and should be based on size rather than age of the child. Infants who weigh less than 20 lbs should sit in rear-facing infant seats. Children between 20 and 40 lbs should sit in a forward-facing child safety seat.

Although many state laws stipulate that children who weigh 40 lbs can be restrained by a lap or lap-shoulder belt, neither is ideal for the 40-lb child. Lap-shoulder belts work by restraining the wearer at the shoulder, across the ribs, and over the anterior iliac spines. The force of impact is distributed over strong bony structures. However, belt systems as well as the size of the vehicle seat are designed for an average-sized adult man.

Because a child's thigh is shorter than the length of the car seat, the child will have to slide forward in the vehicle so that his/her knees can bend comfortably at the end of the seat. This shift changes the positioning of the lap portion of the seat belt so that it rides high over the delicate soft tissues of the abdomen, and seat belt–induced abdominal injuries can result. The shoulder portion of the belt system serves to restrain the motion of the upper torso and head and prevent head impact. However, the shoulder belt rides high over the child's neck rather than over the shoulder, and spinal cord injuries can occur. To alleviate this problem, belt-positioning booster seats are available for the older child. In addition to safety benefits, the child may find these boosters more comfortable because the knees bend at a natural spot and the belt system fits appropriately.

After choosing the appropriate restraint for the size of the child, the child must be placed appropriately in the restraint. It is important for parents to read the instruction manual for the restraint before using it. Safety seats must be adjusted to fit the child, the straps must be kept tight to the child, and the seat must be attached firmly to the vehicle. Unfortunately, safety seats are very complicated to use and are often used incorrectly. Remember, airbags today are not designed for use with children. Children should be placed in the back seat.

Prevention of Bicycle-Related Head Injuries

During a bicycle crash, the head is often the first body part to impact. The mechanical energy involved in the impact is transmitted directly to the skull and then to the brain and blood vessels as described previously. Helmets are designed to decrease energy transmitted to the head during impact in order to decrease the chance of significant head injury.

During a crash, the head crushes the foam liner in the helmet. As the foam liner is crushed, it applies sufficient force to slow the head to a relatively gentle stop, which protects the head from the potentially lethal levels of energy the head would sustain without a helmet. Helmets are designed to protect the head by absorbing and dissipating the impact energy. In addition, helmets are designed to spread a concentrated load over the entire head, protect against penetration, and remain on the wearer's head during an impact.

Until very recently, all helmets protected

TABLE 23-3
Examples of Effective Injury Prevention Strategies

PROBLEM	STRATEGIES
Motor vehicle crashes	Restraint systems appropriate for size; children should be placed in back seat (especially in vehicles with airbags)
Bicycle-related injuries	Helmets; clothing that increases visibility
Pedestrian injuries	Education, training, and supervision
House fires	Smoke detectors; automatic sprinkler systems; escape plans including easy egress from house
Near drownings	Life vests; child-proof pool fencing; supervision in pools and bathtubs; parental knowledge of CPR
Aspiration	No access to small objects and foods; parental knowledge of the Heimlich maneuver
Poisonings	Child-resistant caps; dispensing nonlethal amounts of medication per prescription; child-proof storage
Firearms	*See* Table 23-1
Falls	Discouraging use of baby walkers; carpet at the foot of stairs; multi-impact helmets for all sports

against a single impact. Once the foam crushed during impact, the helmet was no longer protective for future impacts and needed to be replaced. Therefore, a new generation of helmets is emerging, the multi-impact helmets. These helmets are made of new foams that crush during impact, thereby protecting the head even during bicycle-related impacts, but then recover after crushing. The foam is able to crush multiple times making these helmets ideal for sports involving many falls, such as rollerblading.

For helmets to have their maximal protective effect, they must be worn properly. Four key points should be considered when purchasing and fitting a helmet: Snell, Size, Straight, and Straps. A sticker from The Snell Memorial Foundation on the inside of the helmet assures the buyer that the helmet has passed the most rigorous pre- and postmarket testing currently available for helmets. The helmet should fit the child comfortably when placed on the head straight across the midforehead. Foam pads should be added to ensure a tight fit. Finally, the retention straps should be adjusted according to the manufacturer's instructions so that the helmet will not come off during an impact. Like safety seats, helmets are complicated to use and often are used incorrectly. Once a helmet is on, it should not be easily moved from side-to-side or front-to-back.

POSTEVENT PHASE INJURY PREVENTION: PREVENTION OF THE COMPLICATIONS OF AN INJURY

Injury prevention does not end once the child is injured. The effect the injury has on the child's life will depend upon the postinjury care the child receives. It is the responsibility of the primary care practitioner to ensure optimal recovery of the injured child. Health maintenance of the injured child involves close supervision for expected sequelae of injury and arranging the necessary ancillary services for the child.

Disability, as it pertains to head injury, in particular, is common and lifelong. It includes psychiatric, physical, and neurological consequences. In one 23-year follow-up study of children with head injury (90% of which were classified as mild), one third of the children reported physical, intellectual, and emotional problems resulting from the head injury. Personality changes, irritability, school learning difficulties, and memory and attention problems are common even after minor head injuries. In children, there are additional developmental considerations. Some effects of a head injury in a child aged 4 years with an excellent recovery may not be apparent until the child is required to perform complex thought processes used in, for example, science and computer programming.

The course to maximal recovery is long, often lasting from 6 months to 1 year. The burden of the rehabilitation is on the family, economically, emotionally, and socially. The enormous demands placed on the families of patients with head injuries often result in social isolation and divorce.

OVERALL STRATEGY FOR EFFECTIVE ANTICIPATORY GUIDANCE

Parents have a strong motivation to protect their children from hazards, but, at the same time, parents are busy and prefer strategies that are easy to use, inexpensive, and require no action (*eg,* automatic water temperature regulators built in to faucets) or one action (*eg,* lowering hot water heater thermostats). Strategies that require the constant vigilance of parents are destined to fail. *See* Table 23-3 for effective injury prevention strategies.

Well-timed counseling from a primary care practitioner, both during well-child examinations and during acute care visits for injuries, can quell the belief of the inevitability of childhood injury. Parents can be informed of effective ways to reduce the chance of injury by safeguarding their child in his/her environment. In addition, the frustration of the use of complicated safety devices can be lessened by careful instruction from the practitioner. Above all, the practitioner can serve as the patient's information resource for injury prevention strategies in the same way the practitioner educates about disease.

ADDITIONAL RESOURCES

The Insurance Institute for Highway Safety's Status Report
IIHS
1005 North Glebe Road
Arlington, VA 22201
(Free subscription)
Electronic mail notification of consumer product recalls by the Consumer Product Safety Commission.
Send your E-mail address to: cpscinfo-1@cpsc.gov to receive notification of recalls (free service)
Safe Ride News Publications
117 East Louisa Street
Suite 290
Seattle, WA 98102
(Paid subscription)
Bicycle Helmet Safety Institute's newsletter
BHSI
4611 Seventh Street South
Arlington, VA 22204
(Free subscription)
Firearms Safety Counseling Materials
The Center to Prevent Handgun Violence
PO Box 425
Bladensburg, MD 20710-9974
(Free information)
Consumer Reports
Consumers Union of the United States, Inc.
101 Truman Avenue
Yonkers, NY 10703-1057
(Paid subscription)
AAP Traffic Injury Prevention Program
1-800-CAR-BELT
(advice/resources for parents and professionals)

BIBLIOGRAPHY

Baker SP, Fowler C, Li G, et al: Head injuries incurred by children and young adults during informal recreation, *Am J Public Health* 84(4):649–652, 1994.

Baker SP, O'Neill B, Ginsburg MJ, et al: *The injury fact book,* ed 2, Oxford, 1992, Oxford University Press.

Bass JL, Christoffel KK, Widome M, et al: Childhood injury prevention counseling in primary care settings: A critical review of the literature, *Pediatrics* 4:544–550, 1993.

Consumer Reports Staff: Bicycle helmets, *Consumer Reports* 518–522, 1994.

Greenspan AI, MacKenzie EJ: Functional outcome after pediatric head injury, *Pediatrics* 94(4):424–243, 1994.

The Insurance Institute for Highway Safety: *Protecting child passengers: Crash tests by the IIHS,* Arlington, 1990, Insurance Institute for Highway Safety.

Lane JC: The seat belt syndrome in children. In Petrucelli E, editor: *Child occupant protection,* Warrendale, 1993, Society of Automotive Engineers.

McCormick MC: Accidental injury in primary care pediatrics. In Schwartz MW, editor: *Pediatric primary care: A problem oriented approach,* Chicago, 1990, Year Book Medical Publishers.

Rivara F, Farrington D: Prevention of violence: Role of the pediatrician, *Arch Pediatr Adolesc Med* 149:421–429, 1995.

The Snell Memorial Foundation: *The N-94 standard for protective headgear for use in nonmotorized sports,* St. James, New York, 1994, The Snell Memorial Foundation.

Stalnaker RL: Spinal cord injuries to children in real world accidents. In Petrucelli E, editor: *Child occupant protection,* Warrendale, 1993, Society of Automotive Engineers.

TIPP Revision Subcommittee: *A guide to safety counseling in office practice,* Elk Grove Village, 1994, American Academy of Pediatrics.

Wilson MH, Baker SP, Teret SP, et al: *Saving children: A guide to injury prevention,* Oxford, 1991, Oxford University Press.

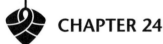

CHAPTER 24

Contemporary Issues: Day Care, Television, and AIDS Education

William Gianfagna

DAY CARE

Most children receive care in a home setting—the caregiver comes to the child's home or the child goes to the caregiver's home. The large majority of these caregivers are relatives. These small, home-based arrangements account for 60% of the children in day care. The remaining 40% of the children are involved in such diverse settings as preschool, nursery school, large group day care centers, and parent cooperative programs.

According to Pizzo, parents choose specific child care arrangements based on the reliability of the caregiver and caregiver's responsiveness and trustworthiness. The second most important factor is cost. Larger group care of younger children is much more costly than family care. Middle- and upper-income families have wider options for child care and can benefit from child care tax deductions, whereas low-income families have fewer options and tend to seek government-subsidized group care when family care is not available.

Despite the best efforts by working parents to provide for good alternative care for their child, most working mothers are ambivalent about child care. It is important for the practicing physician to acknowledge the feelings of working parents and to be supportive of these families.

Illness In Day Care

Parents often remark that their child seems to have more frequent illnesses after entering day care. Several studies comment on the incidence of respiratory tract illnesses in children in the general population. These studies indicate that there is an increased incidence of respiratory tract illnesses in children in varied day care settings in comparison with the incidence of respiratory tract illnesses in children in the general population. The incidence of minor respiratory tract illnesses is increased in the first 1 to 2 years of life for children in day care compared with children remaining at home, but there is no difference in illness frequency between the two groups after 2 years of age. Sample households in the Atlanta metropolitan area found a higher incidence of upper respiratory tract infections and ear infections in children younger than 5 years of age who attended day care. The increased incidence of ear infections, however, was only statistically significant in full-time enrollees. This study's figures estimate between 9% and 14% of upper respiratory tract infections and ear infections in children younger than 5 years of age occur as a result of attending day care. Because most upper respiratory tract illnesses are contagious both before clinical symptoms appear and after recovery, isolation of these children is ineffective in preventing spread.

The number of acute infectious gastrointestinal illnesses also is higher in children attending day care. This finding is particularly true in children younger than 3 years of age who are not yet toilet trained and have an increased propensity to oral-fecal contamination because of their personal health habits. Hand washing by both staff and children and separation of diaper changing areas and food preparation areas has been shown to dramatically decrease the incidence of diarrhea. Rotavirus, *Shigella, Campylobacter,* and *Yersinia* outbreaks have been described in day care. Weisman and colleagues investigated *Shigellosis* infection in day care attendees and its spread to other family members. They found that children attending day care are more likely to be a significant cause of intrafamiliar spread of the disease than those children who commonly are cared for at home.

Health care professionals also must consider certain parasitic infections in children in the day care setting. *Giardia lamblia* is a common enteric pathogen in day care attendees, and although most of the children with positive specimens are asymptomatic, treatment may be necessary if there is a community outbreak. Heijbel and colleagues recently reported chronic diarrhea in day care attendance due to the protozoon *Cryptosporidium.* The most frequent symptoms were vomiting associated with cough and watery stools that lasted for approximately 8 days. Oocysts can be diagnosed with special acid-fast staining of the stool.

Makintubee and colleagues demonstrated an increased incidence of primary serious *Hemophilus influenza* type B infection among children cared for outside the home. Although not all studies agree as to the magnitude of secondary cases, prophylaxis with rifampin is presently recommended for all day care contacts of an index case of *H. influenza* type B. This specific infection can now be considered largely preventable with the widespread availability of a conjugated hemophilus vaccine. This vaccine should be given to children starting at 2 months of age.

Other infections are recognized because of clinical illness transmitted to the parents of children in day care and to the caregivers of these children. Hepatitis A in infants and children is generally associated with a mild or asymptomatic illness and nearly always with complete recovery. In adults, however, recovery can be prolonged and may require hospitalization. Infection with and excretion of cytomegalovirus (CMV) is moderately increased in children raised at home. CMV infection is generally associated with mild symptoms, but infection in a pregnant woman poses potential serious risk to the developing fetus. Exposure to parvovirus B-19 infection (Fifth disease) can affect caretakers in the first half of pregnancy.

In recent years concern has escalated as to whether children with AIDS should attend day care. Ample evidence now exists to show that HIV, the infectious agent of AIDS, is transmitted only by sexual contact or by inoculation with blood products. Even in intimate family settings, there continues to be no evidence that HIV is transmitted by casual contact such as hand holding, sharing utensils, or kissing. The American Academy of Pediatrics Task Force on Pediatric AIDS has published guidelines for HIV-infected children in day care. Decisions should be made on an individual basis. Consideration should be given to the potential for other children to expose the child with AIDS to infections, the ability of the caregivers to deliver the kind of care needed to deal with such a physically and emotionally devastating illness, and whether the child could theoretically transfer the illness via open skin lesions. Even the child who bites does not represent significant risk because of the lack of evidence for transmission of HIV through saliva, which contains low concentrations of the virus. Clearly the common day care interactions of hugging, holding hands, kissing, diaper changing, and feeding do not represent high-risk activities for the transmission of HIV.

All children enrolled in day care should have a complete set of age-appropriate immunizations as recommended by the American Academy of Pediatrics.

With the release of the varicella vaccine, it is recommended that all children at 12 months of age receive the vaccine unless they are immuno-compromised or are receiving medications that induce immunodeficiency.

The ill child has become an additional source of stress for the working mother and her family. Should the sick child be cared for at day care or at home? Increasingly there is pressure to have the mildly ill child remain in day care. During illness children need familiar settings and may have increased demands for comforting. Families need to take these needs into consideration when deciding where the mildly ill child should stay while recuperating. The provisions of the particular day care center for extra space for isolation and for rest, as well as for the necessary staff to care adequately for sick children, must be considered. Day care centers for sick children are now being established to care for the mildly ill child. Clearly the needs of the child and others in the group must be balanced against the stress of increased maternal absenteeism. The need for having a prearranged strategy for the care of the child with a minor illness is an important topic that should be stressed by the primary care physician when discussing child care with the parent.

Child Development and the Family

The psychological and emotional effects of day care on children have always been major concerns of primary care physicians and parents alike. To date there is no evidence that well-supervised and attentive day care has any detrimental effects on child development. Strong parent-child attachment is maintained despite prolonged care away from the home. Infants at the ages of 12 to 15 months who have spent as much as 12 hours each day with day care providers will choose the parent over the day care provider when approached by a stranger. Firm conclusions as to the effects of childcare on infant attachment on infants less than 6 months of age are not yet available.

Howell reviewed the effects of day care and maternal employment on families. She concluded that when mothers are employed, both parents report that their marriages are as happy as other marriages. When both parents are pleased about the wife's employment, their marriages may even be reported to be happier than those marriages in which the spouse is not employed. Employed mothers often spend as much or more time on a one-to-one basis with their children and report more enjoyment in the care of the child than do nonemployed mothers. Firm conclusions as to the effects of child care on infant attachment are not yet available. According to the American Psychiatric Association Task Force on Day Care for Preschool Children, parents can be advised that under some circumstances, infant day care can increase the statistical likelihood of insecure attachment but that "good" infant day care can be a compensating factor.

Counseling Parents

There are many opportunities during health supervision visits for the primary care physician to offer advice and answer a family's questions on day care. One such entry point may arise in the initial newborn office visit by questioning the mother about her plans to return to work and asking about child care arrangements. The physician should be supportive of the parent and avoid casual comments that may increase the common feelings of guilt that plague working mothers. The physician can anticipate the health care needs of the child by asking if the caregiver will be able to keep the child with minor illness or bring the child to the physician's office if the illness required medical care. Box 24-1 summarizes some of the medical questions parents may wish to ask when evaluating day care. Individual family needs including cost and convenience also must be considered when the physician is

---

BOX 24-1
How to Evaluate Day Care

- Is the day care licensed and inspected regularly?
- What is the ratio of children to caregiver?
- Are changing areas and food preparation areas separate?
- How are minor illnesses handled?
- What provisions have been made to maintain safety and prevent injury in the day care center?
- Are children offered a variety of experiences to enhance development and learning?

---

questioned about which day care arrangements are most suitable.

Young children may benefit most by consideration of a setting with a low child-to-caregiver ratio (less than 8:1), as recommended by the American Academy of Pediatrics. Higher ratios are more acceptable for the child older than 4 years, especially if the duration of stay is short. Parents also should be encouraged to find the time before leaving the child to tell the caregiver any early signs of illness or other special needs of the child that day so that caregivers can be optimally responsive and prepared.

Hopefully, an acknowledgement of the needs of the family and child regarding day care as well as an appreciation of the importance of this issue to the community will ultimately help physicians provide improved health care for all children. Further research is needed to more fully elucidate the effects of child care on infants and children.

TELEVISION

Childhood television viewing is only second to sleeping as the most time-consuming activity. Various studies trace the average weekly viewing time of television from 23 hours of television per week for our preschoolers to an incredible 54 hours per week for children during ages 4 to 5 years. By the time of high school graduation, a typical child will have viewed 15,000 hours of television, as compared with having received 11,000 hours of classroom instruction. Children will see 200,000 violent acts on television by age 18 years and view over 14,000 sexual situations and innuendoes per year. It is hard to imagine that this quantity of television viewing would not

have a powerful emotional and social impact on our children.

The primary care physician possesses a unique opportunity for anticipatory guidance regarding television viewing and its effects as well as for challenging parents to optimize their child's enormous time investment in television. The expertise of health care providers on developmental and psychological issues of child health is being increasingly demanded by parents. This expertise should include information about television.

Many articles point to the negative aspects of television viewing on children. There are, however, potential positive effects of this medium on the growth and development of children. Television provides children with a stimulus for learning, and studies indicate that children do learn from television. Television can increase the child's contact with new vocabulary, expand the knowledge of the world around the child, and expose the child to different cultures and ways of thinking. Notable positive programming for children can be found by careful parental selection. "Sesame Street" and "Mr. Rogers' Neighborhood" have been extensively studied and are examples of format and pace that are specifically geared to the developmental and cognitive level of children. Public broadcasting stations present such worthwhile programs as the "National Geographic" specials and "Nova", which expose children to other cultures or ways of life and encourage interest in science and nature.

Violence

Few health care providers for children must be reminded that our children face an increasingly violent society. Television viewing also contributes to this barrage of violence. As Rothenberg states, "The average child will witness some 18,000 murders, countless bombings, beatings, robberies, torture—an average of approximately one per minute in the standard television cartoon for children under the age of 10." Although it is true that television shares the preponderant theme of violence with other media such as movies, magazines, and books, television is the most accessible and influential medium for most children. Wharton and Mandell present case reports of imitative child abuse by parents after viewing a made-for-television film.

Charren and colleagues suggest that pediatricians advocate for improved television quality and choices for family viewing rather than for legislative efforts to regulate exact program content. Action for Children's Television (ACT) exemplifies such an advocacy group.

Commercials

Repetitive exposure to commercials serves as another of television's potential influence on children. It is estimated that the average American child will receive nearly 350,000 commercial messages by his/her late teens. Most advertisers are quick to point out just how persuasive television commercials have become with young viewers and will spend millions of dollars to influence target age groups to buy (or coerce their parents to buy) certain products. Each Christmas season successful marketing and selling on television create "hot items" that soon cannot be found on the toy shelves to satisfy demand. Of all Saturday morning commercial messages, 60% to 80% are for sugared breakfast cereals or snacks, many of which will be incorporated into the child's diet. Children under 5 years of age have little ability to understand the selling intent of commercials, and children under 12 years of age are consistently unable to distinguish program content from commercial messages.

Commercials for drug use and health products also influence young audiences. In their study, Lewis and Lewis found that 70% of fifth and sixth graders believed all health messages and commercials they identified. The products advertised are trusted if a parent or the child uses the product. Heavy exposure to drug advertising leads children to believe that people are frequently sick and often need medication to make a quick recovery from illness.

Television viewing has other ill effects on child health. Dietz and Gortmaker in the National Health Examination survey demonstrate a unidirectional causal relationship of the number of hours of television viewing with obesity in adolescents. Controlling for other variables known to be associated with obesity, each additional hour of viewing was associated with a 2% increase in the prevalence of obesity in the age group 12 to 17 years. Only a history of prior obesity was more strongly linked than television viewing hours to later obesity in a prospective study of adolescents.

New Technology

Cable television, electronic television games, and the videocassette recorder (VCR) exemplify double-edged technologies that have expanded traditional network television. An increased variety of positive educational and entertainment programs and films are now available to children, because 65% of households own at least one VCR. These advances also allow for increased control by children and parents over the content and duration of viewing. However, a vast repertoire of sexually explicit and violent films can now enter the home by bypassing conventional censorship. Health care providers should remind parents of the ever pressing need to supervise and direct their child's exposure to these media. Overuse of electronic television games promotes physical inactivity at a time when American youth possess the lowest levels of physical fitness in years.

The American Academy of Pediatrics Committee on Communication specifically opposes the use of television-activated toys. These toys are energized by inaudible television broadcast signals. Many of these devices engage aggressive television figures in gun battles. The Committee expresses concern about the effects of these toys on the child's own creativity and imagination in play, particularly when television not only tells the child with what to play but now actually plays with the toy for the child as well.

Counseling Parents

What can health care providers do to improve the effects of television on their patients? The guidelines of San Francisco's Committee on Children's Television can offer some practical criteria to help parents evaluate television programming. The American Academy of Pediatrics also publishes patient educational material for parents regarding television. The Academy challenges parents to limit the time children spend in front of the television and to plan their viewing schedule in advance. Parents are encouraged to watch television along with their children so that they can act as interpreters of the program information and reinforce the positive experiences with a family discussion.

Physicians should be confident in informing parents, during the health supervision visits, of the effects of repeated television violence on the behavior and psyche of their children. Physicians can emphasize the importance of parental interpretation of the value systems and commercialism exposed by modern programming. Parents should be fully informed of the content of videotapes, computer games, and tapes brought into the home by children.

Physicians and health care providers for children interested in affecting public policy regarding television should contact local parent-teacher associations and regional television action groups. These coordinated action groups are working with parents and physicians toward the healthy and effective use of this most formidable teacher of our children—television.

AIDS EDUCATION

Since the discovery of HIV as the cause of AIDS, public health officials and others concerned with child health have been developing strategies to prevent the spread of AIDS. Because there is no cure for AIDS, one preventative strategy is the education of school-aged children and adolescents to reduce the chances that they will become infected. The school-aged pediatric and adolescent populations represent target groups likely to respond to educational efforts. The pediatric health care professional is in a position to be a positive force for appropriate AIDS education. A background in child development enables him/her to make recommendations on what is appropriate material to present on AIDS. Because of other health-related issues, the preexisting relationships with school nurses, administrators, and parents may be used to influence and guide decisions and policy on an AIDS curriculum. It is during general health education in the schools that most of the formal dissemination of information will take place. In addition, the primary care physician has the opportunity to directly discuss and answer questions about AIDS with both the child and family at the time of health supervision visits.

Early Elementary School
The primary purpose of AIDS education in the young school-aged child is to relieve anxiety about the AIDS epidemic. Because transmission occurs via sexual activity and from contact with infected blood, such as in sharing needles for intravenous drug abuse, young school-aged children are not commonly at high risk. Elementary school children should be told that AIDS is very hard to catch. Early school-aged children will, in the future, be in contact with children who have acquired AIDS in the perinatal period. It is important for them to know that touching someone or being in the same classroom with a child with AIDS will not cause them to get the disease. This scenario presents an additional opportunity to discuss and develop compassionate and accepting attitudes toward children with other handicaps in the classroom. Young children should be taught that medical scientists and physicians all over the world are working to find a cure for AIDS.

Middle School
The educational objectives in middle school consist of further discussion of the basic principles of transmission of HIV and presentation of the high-risk behaviors to be avoided. Children in this age group can begin to understand some of the basic principles of infectious disease and become acquainted with the concept of HIV as a microorganism, a living thing too small to be seen with the unaided eye. Middle school children should be taught that the infection can be spread by the use of a needle contaminated with the blood of an AIDS patient, from an infected mother to her baby during pregnancy, or from sexual contact either between a man and a woman or between two men. Most sources do not define the term *sexual contact* in their recommendations, but teachers and parents will need to be comfortable with some direct discussion of what the term means based on the age and experience of the group and the prevailing standards of the community. Such a discussion should give an awareness that people of all races and in all parts of the United States can become infected, and although most patients are adults, infants and teenagers can acquire the disease as well. Those who are infected can be without symptoms for a long time and still pass the disease to another person. The children should be told that they will not be able to look at a person and see anything that will tell them that he/she has AIDS. Reinforcement must be given to the idea that casual contact, such as sitting next to someone or being in the same classroom with a person with AIDS, is not dangerous. Children should be told that the way to avoid AIDS is to not

have sexual contact with another person and to not use intravenous drugs.

Junior and Senior High School

The adolescent and young adult not only need explicit information regarding the facts about AIDS, but the material must be presented in such a way that the adolescent believes that he/she should and can change personal behavior to prevent being infected with HIV. Adolescence not only represents a high-risk pediatric group, but they are the population segment with a dramatically increasing incidence of AIDS. Belying this statement is the tendency for adolescents to possess a sense of invulnerability and immortality and to engage in multiple behaviors that may place them at high risk of contracting HIV. These behaviors are well known to health professionals working with adolescents. By the age of 16 years, depending on the racial and ethnic groups examined, 30% to 50% of girls and 45% to 60% of boys report having had sexual intercourse. Fewer than 20% of all sexually active teenagers use any type of contraception, and each year in the United States more than 1 million teenage girls become pregnant. Sexually transmitted diseases infect more than 2 million adolescents each year. Illegal drug use is prevalent among adolescents and young adults, although the percentage of intravenous drug users remains small. AIDS is but one crisis area among many calling for a comprehensive approach to adolescent health education.

Adolescents should be taught that HIV is the cause of AIDS and that the initial illness may be a flulike syndrome, which will then disappear. The patient can remain asymptomatic for months or years; however, the disease still can be transmitted during this period. Additional information should be given about secondary infections, including pneumonia and meningitis. The children should be taught that the lymph glands throughout the body can become enlarged and that a rare type of cancer known as Kaposi sarcoma may develop. Specific details of how the virus can be transmitted should be stressed, including all types of vaginal, anal, and oral intercourse, both homosexual and heterosexual. AIDS can be transmitted by use of infected drug injecting equipment and by an infected mother to her unborn baby. It is important to discuss the theoretic possibility of transmission from deep mouth kissing if there is direct mucous membrane exposure to infected blood or saliva.

BOX 24-2
Basics of AIDS Education

Elementary School
- AIDS is a disease that is hard to catch.
- You cannot catch AIDS by being in the same room with a child with AIDS.
- All children with handicaps need your friendship and help.

Middle School
- Understand the basic principles of infectious disease and the micro-organism causing AIDS.
- Avoid high-risk behavior such as intravenous drug use and sexual intercourse.
- A mother with AIDS could infect her baby.
- Ordinary contact in classroom with a person with AIDS is not dangerous.
- Children and adults with chronic conditions need respect and support.

High School
- Discuss AIDS and common sexually transmitted diseases.
- Discuss cause of AIDS and emphasize that it is a fatal illness.
- Explore the necessary decision-making skills needed to avoid high-risk behaviors.
- Specify the high-risk behaviors to be avoided. Help students to locate sources of medical care.

Increased risk comes from unprotected intercourse between men and with multiple partners of either gender, such as men or women who are prostitutes. Adolescents should be informed that once infection occurs and symptoms appear, there is no cure and the patient will eventually die. Children and adolescents should feel optimistic, however, that worldwide research for a future vaccine offers the hope of protecting those not yet infected by the virus. Perhaps the most important message for adolescents is that the most effective way to eliminate the chance of infection with HIV and other sexually transmitted diseases is by not engaging in sexual contact and by not using illegal intravenous drugs. Parents, educators, and professionals should not be fearful of supporting sexual abstinence or letting the teenagers under their care know why they make this recommendation. Abstinence offers the teenager freedom from worry about pregnancy and other sexually transmitted diseases, freedom from overcommitment to one relationship, and the ability to maximize future plans and options. Educators can discuss the healthy ways to have romantic relationships during adolescence without sex. It is unrealistic, however, to believe that all adolescents will adopt this behavior strategy. Therefore, those adolescents who continue to be sexually active should be instructed to use latex condoms, carefully applied, during every act of sexual intercourse. The use of spermicides offers additional protection, although no method provides 100% protection.

Adolescents should be told where to obtain necessary medical services if they believe they may be already infected with HIV or any other sexually transmitted disease. It is important to encourage patients to be tested so that further spread can be eliminated and to inform the patients that although there is no cure, drugs can be used and appropriate medical care given.

Education and Behavior

Is there any evidence that education has any real impact in altering behavior in high-risk groups or in adolescents at risk for AIDS? Brown and Fritz have reviewed the medical literature and give mixed results. There is evidence that educational efforts are successful in changing behavior in homosexual and bisexual men and in intravenous drug abusers in San Francisco. However, the review of the success of sex education programs reveals that sex education does increase knowledge and dispel myths but that this knowledge does not necessarily lead to a change in behavior, such as the use of birth control or condoms with each sexual contact. Some AIDS prevention programs did lead to delay in initiation of intercourse and reduction in the number of sexual partners according to Kirby and Short. Which approaches will optimize AIDS education in adolescents and children? Behavior modification appears to be most successful if the program gives the adolescents decision-making skills and enables participants to practice coping with the pressures of how to say no to drugs or sexual intercourse. Children and adolescents conform to peer pressure as peers help move the adolescent away from the family toward independence. Programs with peers, or individuals whose opinion the peer group values, as role models may lead to successful transfer of information about AIDS into alteration of high-risk behaviors. Additional research is needed to assess the effectiveness of health decision making for adolescents and young adults.

BIBLIOGRAPHY

Action for Children's Television, Newtonville, MA.

American Academy of Pediatrics: *Health in day care: A manual for health professionals,* Elk Grove Village, 1987, American Academy of Pediatrics.

American Academy of Pediatrics, Committee on Communications: The commercialization of children's television and its effects on imaginative play. *Pediatrics* 81:900–901, 1988.

American Academy of Pediatrics, Committee on School Health Policy Statement: *Acquired immunodeficiency syndrome education in schools.* 82:278–280, 1988.

American Psychiatric Association, Task Force on Day Care for Preschool Children: Day care for early preschool children: Implications for the child and family. *Am J Psych* 150(8):1281–1287, 1992.

American Academy of Pediatrics, Task Force on Pediatric AIDS: *Pediatric guidelines for infection control of HIV (AIDS) in hospitals, medical offices, schools, and other settings,* Elk Grove Village, 1988, American Academy of Pediatrics.

Aronsen S, Gilsdorg J: Prevention and management of infectious disease in daycare. *Pediatr Rev* 7:259–267, 1986.

Asch-Goodkin J: AIDS: What do we teach the children? *Contemp Pediatr* 5:50–84, 1988.

Asch-Goodkin J: AIDS on the homefront: Schooling and foster care. *Contemp Pediatr* 5:76–90, 1988.

Barbour SD: Acquired immunodeficiency syndrome of childhood. *Pediatr Clin North Am* 34:247–268, 1988.

Brown LK, Fritz GK: AIDS education in the schools: A literature review as a guide to curriculum planning. *Clin Pediatr* 27:311–316, 1988.

Centers for Disease Control and Prevention: Guidelines for effective school health education to protect the spread of AIDS. *MMWR* 37(suppl S2): 1–9, 1988.

Centers for Disease Control and Prevention: Human immunodeficiency virus infection in the

United States: A review of current knowledge. *MMWR* 36(suppl S6):1–48, 1987.

Charren P, Gelber A, Arnold M: Media, children, and violence: A public prospective. *Pediatrics* 63:1–7, 1994.

Dersken DJ, Strasburger VC: Children and the influence of the media. *Prim Care* 21(4):747–758, 1994.

Dietz WH Jr, Gortmaker SL: Do we father our children at the television set? Obesity and television viewing in children and adolescents. *Pediatrics* 75:807–812, 1985.

Dietz WH Jr, Strasburger VC: *Curr Prob Pediatr* 21(1):8–31, 1991.

Fleming DW, et al: Childhood upper respiratory tract infections: To what degree is incidence affected by daycare attendance? *Pediatrics* 79:55–60, 1987.

Haskins R, Kotch J: Daycare and illness: Evidence, costs and public policy. *Pediatrics* 77(suppl):951–982, 1986.

Heijbel H, et al: Outbreak of diarrhea in a daycare center with spread to household members: The role of Cryptosporidium. *Pediatr Infect Dis J* 6:532–535, 1987.

Howell MC: Effects of maternal employment with child care. *Pediatrics* 52:327–343, 1973.

Janai H, Stutman HR, et al: Invasive Haemophilus influenzae type B infection: A continuing challenge. *Am J Infect Control* 18(3):160–166, 1990.

Kirby DJ, Short L: School based programs to reduce sexual risk behaviors: A review of effectiveness. *Pub Health Rep* 109(3):339–360, 1994.

Larger LM, Wachert GJ: the pre-adult health decisions making model: making directness/orientation to adolescent health related attitudes and behaviors. *Adolescence* 27(108):919–940, 1992.

Lewis CE, Lewis MA: The impact of television commercials on health related beliefs and behavior in children. *Pediatrics* 53:431–434, 1974.

Loda FA: Day care. *Pediatr Rev* 1:277–281, 1980.

Makintubee S, Istre GR, Wand JI: Transmission of invasive Hemophilus influenzae type B disease in daycare settings. *J Pediatr* 111:180–186, 1987.

Pizzo PD: Counselling parents about day care. *Pediatr Ann* 6:593–603, 1977.

Roberts CR, et al: Working mothers and infant care: A review of the literature. *AAOHN-J* 41(11):541–546, 1993.

Wharton R, Mandell F: Violence on television and imitative behavior impact on parenting practices. *Pediatrics* 75:1120–1123, 1985.

Wesiman JB, et al: The role of preschool children and daycare centers in the spread of Shigellosis in urban communities. *J Pediatr* 84:797–802, 1974.

Zuckerman DM, Zuckerman BS: Television's impact on children. *Pediatrics* 75:233–239, 1985.

ADDITIONAL INFORMATION

AIDS, sex, and you; facts about AIDS and drug abuse.

AIDS
1555 Wilson Boulevard, Suite 700
Rosslyn, VA 22209

National AIDS Information Line
1-800-342-AIDS

Understanding AIDS
Publication #HHS-88-8404
United States Department of Health and Human Services

Public Health Service, Centers for Disease Control and Prevention
PO Box 6003
Rockville, MD 20850

PARENT RESOURCES

Child Care Action Campaign
330 7th Avenue, 17th Floor
New York, NY 10001-5010
The Child Primer for Parents

National Association for the Education of Young Children
1509 16th Street, NW
Washington, DC 20036
Childcare Brochure #580

CHAPTER 25

Divorce

Anthony L. Rostain

Divorce is not a single event, but a long and complicated process involving a series of transitions, or stages, including predivorce, separation, adjustment, reorganization, and remarriage. These stages present different challenges to family members and occur over variable lengths of time.

STAGES OF DIVORCE

Predivorce

The predivorce stage is filled with emotional tension and marital conflict. As the marital crisis intensifies, children are often brought into the marital conflict and may develop behavioral changes or "moodiness."

Separation

The separation stage begins on the day that one spouse departs from the home. Profound disruption of daily routines takes place as negotiations begin over the terms of the divorce. Irrational and immature behavior is often demonstrated by both spouses. Financial problems, dependence on grandparents, and disruption of well-established social support networks all contribute to the regressive behavior commonly observed in the children.

The uncertainty, disorder, and confusion contribute to the children's sense of insecurity, and they may show signs of profound sadness, marked hostility, or apparent withdrawal. Emotional outbursts at home or at school and poor academic performance are common. Doctor visits for minor problems may suddenly increase, as if both parents and children are looking for reassurance from the trusted physician.

Adjustment

After a time, the family's changed circumstances require new coping mechanisms. Schedules are rearranged and living habits altered. The formerly unemployed housewife may take an outside job. New social supports for parents *and* children are enlisted with greater ease and frequency. After a fair amount of experimentation with different rules and routines in both the custodial and noncustodial households, the turmoil of earlier phases begins to subside. If antagonisms and resentments between parents develop into a recurrent pattern of challenges over parenting, mutual disrespect, and constant conflict, children will continue to be dragged into the parents' fights.

Reorganization

After new equilibrium is reached and life seems to be reorganized, the divorce appears to be an accepted fact of life. Routine parent-child issues reemerge with both custodial and noncustodial parents. Children's views and expectations of parents grow more balanced and secure. The child's sense of self, although altered, is more integrated.

Remarriage

Most divorced parents remarry. Initially this may precipitate strong emotional reactions from the children: stepparents can be challenged, angry or acting-out behavior may be directed at biological parents, and a new "readjustment" phase is initiated. In most cases, once it becomes clear to the children that they have not lost the remarried parent, family relationships eventually restabilize.

CHILD'S RESPONSE TO DIVORCE

The child's response to divorce varies according to a number of factors. Individual temperament, developmental level, predivorce adjustment, previous emotional difficulties, the role of the child in the parents' antagonisms prior to the split, the immediate circumstances of the divorce, and parental behavior in its aftermath all interact to determine the child's responses to the situation. For the most part, divorce is an extremely painful experience that initiates a grieving process in children. The characteristic features of this grief and mourning are similar to those of reactive depression. John Bowlby has identified four stages of grief following the death of a loved person: numbness or shock; yearning, searching for the lost figure; disorganization and despair; and reorganization. Children seem to go through a similar process after divorce. Unlike death, however, the more "voluntary" loss of one parent, who goes away but is not gone forever, can add confusion to the grieving process. Children ask, "How can I belong to two people who don't love each other?"

Many children remain torn between two warring parents who use the children to fight their battles. Love expressed to one parent is interpreted as rejection by the other one. The child may be made to feel guilty for his/her anger at the parents for divorcing. This guilt is complicated by an initial sense of helplessness that the child experiences when his/her efforts to help the parents stay together have failed.

The child's feelings of vulnerability and insecurity are intensified by the new life circumstances: fluctuating parental attention (due to parental grief and upset), unstable family routines, weakened family ties, high mobility, decreased economic resources, less available social support structures, and unpredictable parental behavior. The specific reactions will vary according to the child's age and level of cognitive and emotional functioning.

Infants may react with increased fretfulness, poor sleep, poor appetite, or decreased activity. Toddlers may react with regression in toilet habits, greater irritability, and more dependence on their mother. Preschoolers may become more aggressive, throw tantrums, have problems sleeping, become possessive of objects and people, and show signs of autoerotic activity. Older preschool children may become frightened, confused, and sad. Although their play, as well as their fantasies, may reflect denial of the divorce, children at this age tend to blame themselves for the breakup and often display a general bewilderment and helplessness.

Young school-aged children have a better cognitive understanding of the changes resulting from parental divorce. They can express sadness, longing, and the wish for reconciliation more directly, although they tend to become restless, whiny, moody, anxious, and aggressive. Many children can successfully deny some of these painful feelings and can find gratification outside the home. By contrast, grade-school children (ages 7 to 8 years) seem more affected by the divorce. They show pervasive sadness and grief, fear about the future, feelings of deprivation, and a strong sense of loss. They are often preoccupied with wishes for reconciliation and may experience conflicts in loyalty. Preadolescents react similarly but with more direct expressions of anger and shame. They appear more self-controlled and engage in a multitude of activities to cope with underlying feelings of loss and rejection. Some increase their participation in school-sponsored programs or attempt to master new skills. Others attempt to take on the role of the departed parent at home. A few may act out by lying or stealing in situations in which they are likely to get caught. The majority experience identity confusion, loneliness, powerlessness, and conflicts in loyalty. There may be somatic complaints (eg, headaches, cramps, abdominal pain) and a decline in both school performance and peer relationships. Occasionally these children may demonstrate precocious sexuality or assume the role of "parental child," both of which are responses marked by "pseudomaturity."

Adolescents are particularly vulnerable to parental divorce because of the primacy of their developmental task: separation and individuation. The teenager's "search for identity" can be disrupted and accelerated by divorce. Although they don't often feel responsible for the breakup, most express concerns about future personal and marital plans. They may become moralistic and self-righteous, especially in their attitudes toward the parent they believe to be "wrong." A majority will use distancing as a coping mechanism, such as general aloofness, self-involvement, increased social activity, rebelliousness, and staying away from home. Parents often complain that the adolescent does not seem to care about the family. This behavior may be an adaptive response insofar as it prevents the teenager from getting enmeshed with either parent, and it is consistent with the tasks of separation and individuation.

Most children survive their parents' divorce without major psychologic or emotional sequelae. With time and understanding from the primary adults responsible for their care, children eventually work through their grief and attain a stage of readjustment. Several risk factors for poor resolution of grief must be kept in mind, including continued parental conflict, depression or psychiatric illness in the custodial parent, continued family instability (nonresolution of divorce), overinvolvement of the custodial parent with the child, and previous emotional disorder in the child. Evidence of any of these conditions should alert the physician to the need for psychiatric referral.

Indications for Referral

- Child
  Depression
  Withdrawal from peer relationships
  Severe or persistent school problems
  Behavior problems
  Other signs of emotional maladjustment
- Family
  Parental conflict
  Parental depression
  Continued family instability
  Parental overinvolvement
  Other signs of family dysfunction

PEDIATRIC MANAGEMENT OF DIVORCE

The sensitive pediatrician or family physician can play an important child advocacy role for children when parents divorce. The physician is in a unique position to provide emotional support to the children, to help parents fulfill their responsibilities as parents, and to offer neutral, objective advice to parents who request it. The primary care physician's role is to offer immediate emotional first aid, to monitor the child's and the family's progress in coping with the divorce, to provide anticipatory guidance, and to offer referral to psychiatric or counseling services when these seem indicated. To do this, the physician must feel comfortable with his/her own feelings, must be familiar with the predictable responses of parents and children to the divorce process, and should know about the variety of community resources available to help families of divorce.

Although the practitioner usually hears of the divorce from one parent, it is important to speak with the other parent to be able to take a position of impartiality and respect for both spouses. The informant should be reassured that the physician is interested in providing support to the family during this difficult process. A subsequent appointment should be made to discuss issues related to the children's reactions to the divorce. It is preferable to meet with both parents together to emphasize that despite their divorce both will remain parents to the children. If the antagonism between them is too great, it will be necessary to meet separately. In either case, the physician should establish his/her expertise as a child advocate, primarily interested in preventing emotional problems in the children.

Immediate Steps

In the early stages of the divorce the physician should focus the counseling on communication and other issues that may be upsetting the children. When possible, both parents should inform the children of the divorce and explain the changes that the children can anticipate. Children will worry more if they are not informed in advance of the plans that will affect them. Stress the importance of extended family ties, of continuity of place and routine, and of parental acceptance of children's questions and expressions of sadness and anger. In these early stages children fear the loss of emotional support from *both* parents, who may be preoccupied with their own reactions to the breakup. It will be necessary for the physician to emphasize repeatedly the children's need to maintain contact with both parents.

The predictable responses of children of different ages also should be explained in a calm and objective manner. Because parents are filled with guilt about the emotional trauma their children are experiencing, they need to be reassured that although their children will undergo strong emotional reactions in the ensuing months, most children adjust to divorce without severe psychological disturbances. Parental guilt is itself an obstacle to the children's coping with divorce.

The physician should maintain contact with the noncustodial parent, which is usually the father. The father should understand his importance to the child, his current and future role in raising the child, and the need to maintain an open line of communication. By meeting with the father, the primary care physician is practicing preventive psychiatry and helping to promote an easier adjustment process for the children. By knowing the concerns, feelings, and attitudes of the noncustodial parent, the physician is better able to monitor the divorce process in an objective manner. Both sides of the story will become available, and a fuller picture will emerge.

Plan of Action

As a first step of the plan of action, the resources of each parent and of each child should be assessed. On the basis of their strengths and abilities, parents can be advised about rational allocations of responsibility in situations they must negotiate between themselves, such as visitation schedules, special events, discipline, school performance, purchase of clothing and other necessities, and transportation. Their obligations as parents must be clarified and met, or their children will suffer the consequences.

Potential problem areas should also be assessed. Over what issues are the parents in conflict? Are the parents responding appropriately to the children? Are they emotionally available to them? Are the children having a particularly hard time, and if so, why? Based on these concerns, the physician may decide to schedule several meetings to discuss problems that seem to be developing or to refer the family for counseling. The children should meet with the physician without the parents to assess their coping abilities and to provide reassurance and emotional support.

The physician's plan must include methods for maintaining open communication among members of the family as well as between family and physician. Children should be encouraged to express their feelings directly to their parents. Parents should be counseled about the evolution of feelings over time and about the process by which children and parents eventually achieve a new balance. The need for parents to talk to each other about child-rearing issues should be emphasized. All family members should be reassured that their physician is interested.

Custody

Custody battles are painful, ugly, and costly for everyone. If it appears that a custody fight is imminent, every effort should be made to refer the parents to a divorce counselor or mediator, a professional who specializes in helping parents to resolve custody disputes *outside* the courtroom. Because neither parent forfeits his/her right to pursue a legal judgment should this step fail to produce a mutually acceptable outcome, this alternative should be seriously considered by both parents.

If the physician is called into the courtroom to offer expert testimony, a few guiding principles should be kept in mind: 1) Use reason and sensitivity, and above all be honest. 2) Comment only on direct observations from interviews with the children and parents. 3) Try to offer an opinion regarding the preference of the child, the capacities of each parent, the strength of the parent-child bond, and the best chances for providing continuity of place, routine, and parental contact for the child. 4) Avoid having the child choose the custodial parent unless he/she is willing and is capable (adolescent-aged). 5) Avoid commenting on criticisms or accusations raised by either parent unless they are established as being true and are potentially harmful to the child. As child advocate, the physician should emphasize the child's right to visitation with the noncustodial parent, to maintenance of current lifestyle if possible, and to representation by an attorney if it appears that neither parent has the child's best interests in mind.

The choice of joint custody should always be considered when the possibility exists for both parents to work out their disagreements. For certain families joint legal custody has proved to be the best solution. It avoids a "winner-takes-all" situation and provides each parent with a sense of continued involvement in raising the children. Studies have shown that in cases in which the parents make the effort to cooperate, children adjust well.

The Two-Family Child

The concept of the "two-family child" is helpful in that it emphasizes the importance of *both* parents in the life of the child and serves to remind parents that any rivalry between them only harms the child. The child lives in two families, and these families should be as consistent as possible. It is natural for some differences to exist; but parents must try to maintain similar approaches to discipline, homework, housework, and daily routine.

If they are unable to agree with each other, parents will soon notice their children beginning to manipulate them, using arguments such as "At Mommy's house we do this" or "Daddy lets us stay up later than you do." As with nondivorced families in which parents fail to be consistent, children will play each parent against the other, making the task of discipline extremely difficult and frustrating.

The custodial parent should be encouraged to resume a normal life pattern as quickly as possible. Frequent contact with the noncustodial parent may be necessary in the early stages to reassure the children that they are still effective together as parents. The custodial parent should avoid confiding in the children and involving them in the emotional, financial, and social concerns of an adult. Commonly, the oldest child assumes a "parental" role in the home, but that child must avoid becoming a substitute for the departed spouse.

The noncustodial parent must not play "camp counselor" but should establish a home environment for the children that includes a stable living area, assigned tasks around the house, and regular bedtime and other routines. These are important insofar as they provide the children with a sense of belonging in the new home of the noncustodial parent. Visitation time should not be shared with other adults except on special occasions. The parent should wait for several months before introducing new lovers or friends to the children, and this should be planned well in advance.

Single-Parent Families

When the noncustodial parent has departed from the family and lost regular contact with the children, a single-parent family evolves. These families require special consideration from the physician. The first step is providing support to the parent and the children, who likely feel abandoned. Available resources from the extended family and the community need to be assessed and utilized.

Single parents need reassurance that they can manage the tasks of child rearing, albeit under different circumstances. The goal is to help the parent achieve a sense of authority, confidence, and competence in parenting. This may mean that the parent will need help from the oldest child or a grandparent. The partnership that results must be under the parent's control; other-

wise his/her authority will be undermined and a sense of helplessness will result.

As the family adjusts to its new situation, the physician will need to monitor the emotional development of the children to identify problems requiring psychiatric referral. The physician can anticipate having to spend extra time with single parents during times of crisis, developmental transition points, and whenever the family undergoes structural change.

Infrequent and irregular contact with the noncustodial parent presents a problem for the children. If possible, this parent should be contacted directly by the physician and encouraged to make regular visits and phone calls to the children. Usually the custodial parent is resentful and finds it difficult to hide this from the child. A sensitive pediatrician can create an opportunity for the child to discuss feelings about the missing parent. The child must be reminded that there is a caring adult who can accept him/her nonjudgmentally.

Daily Crisis Areas

Predictable problems of daily living can become crisis areas for families of divorce. The practitioner who employs foresight, sensitivity, and common sense can help divorcing parents avoid crises. The adults should understand that they need to work together as parents when the need arises, while also maintaining their "separateness" as divorced individuals. Consistency between parents does not imply they do everything exactly the same way but that they respect each other's individuality and avoid undermining the other's parental authority.

School

In the early stages of divorce the child may have problems with school performance and peer relationships. Both parents should be encouraged to inform the child's teacher about the divorce and to request that each of them be notified of any difficulties with the child's behavior or performance in school. Each parent should maintain interest in and knowledge of the child's academic development. Instead of parents blaming each other for the child's difficulties, school problems must be approached calmly and rationally. Parents should try to meet together with teachers to learn directly about the nature of the child's problems. Parents who are incapable of working together may need to be referred for therapy.

In these cases the physician must make use of his/her own relationship with the parents to convince both to accept the referral. Therapy is for the divorced family, not just the distressed child.

Special Events

Birthdays, holidays, school plays, recitals, athletic events, and graduations all require special consideration from parents. Despite negative feelings that the parents may continue to harbor toward each other, each parent must make an effort to attend events that hold special significance for the child. This does not require that they attend *every* event, nor that they go to these events together. However, children have a right to expect that their parents will show an appreciation for the special activities in which they are involved. In addition, parents must learn to explain directly to their children their reasons for choosing not to attend a particular occasion. It is not acceptable for parents to use the excuse that they do not want to encounter each other there; this will only make the child feel guilty and ashamed.

Ideally, parents should negotiate holiday and birthday plans well ahead of time. Differences must be worked out without involving the child in the dispute; otherwise these special occasions will become unhappy events marred by conflict and turmoil. Each parent should be warned against becoming competitive and using these events to prove they love the child most. This competition forces the child into loyalty conflicts. Finally, parents can expect the child to express sadness or anger or to voice reconciliation wishes during these moments. Parents may need to be reassured that these are natural feelings for the child and that eventually the parents will learn to take these feelings in stride.

Discipline

Divorced parents often need help concerning issues of discipline. During the early stages of the divorce, children may exhibit regressive or challenging behavior. Parents should not be alarmed to find increased testing of limits or acting out. If the parents are overwhelmed with guilt or are too self-absorbed with their own emotional turmoil, they will find it difficult to enforce limits in the home. The physician can be of most value by listening to the parent's concerns, providing another perspective on the child's (or the parent's) behavior, and helping parents anticipate conflict situations or devise strategies for carrying out disciplinary measures. The physician should emphasize the competence and responsibility of both parents for enforcing discipline. Often these problems resolve as the family reorganizes itself. Most problems can best be handled when there is consistency of approach between the custodial and noncustodial parents.

On occasion these problems become chronic. This situation may signal continuing parental conflict despite the divorce or may reflect the child's efforts to manipulate the parents and play them against each other. By misbehaving, the child also may be seeking attention, trying to rescue a depressed parent, or attempting to reunite the parents. It is important that the physician make a careful assessment of the entire family before glibly offering advice about discipline. The physician should not perpetuate the problem by siding with either parent or by giving repeated suggestions to a "helpless" parent who has been wronged by the ex-spouse.

Illness

When children get sick there is a danger that illness episodes will be used by parents to accuse each other of neglect. Parental guilt, already high, is quickly intensified when children are ill. The physician can confront this directly by clarifying that the child's sickness is *not* a reflection of poor parenting, by gently cautioning against parental overreaction, and by making certain that the separated parent knows about the illness and that his/her concerns are addressed.

Physicians can expect an increase in office visits for minor illnesses and physical complaints during the early stages of divorce. The child or parents may be looking for emotional reassurance from the physician, who must handle such situations sensitively and use them as opportunities to monitor the divorce process. If these visits become chronic, it is important to look for a pattern of parent-child interaction whereby parental anxiety causes the child to express his/her emotions through physical symptoms, which in turn causes parental overprotectiveness and enmeshment with the child. Skillful intervention is required to break this cycle. The physician may suggest that although the child does not appear to be too ill, it would be a good idea to schedule a return visit to see how things are going. Gradually the focus of such visits can shift from the physical complaints to the emotional issues that are troubling the child and the parent.

Remarriage

The remarriage of one or both parents signals the beginning of a new phase of family development. Of special concern to the pediatrician is the restructuring of roles in the new family. The success of this new family arrangement depends on a number of factors. First, the child needs to know that he/she still has access to the parent who has remarried and that this change does not mean abandonment or rejection. Second, the child needs to understand that the stepparent is *not* a replacement for the biological parent and that he/she is not being asked to choose one parent over the other. Third, the child has the right to express feelings about the stepparent and to develop a relationship with him/her independent of the remarried parent. Fourth, the stepparent has the right to provide both nurturance and discipline to the child in collaboration with the biological parent. This must be done within a framework that is mutually acceptable to biological parent, stepparent, and child. Finally, the new marriage partners must create a satisfying relationship independent of the child. The creation of a new "distance" between parent and child can be a painful process if the divorce has created parent-child bonds that are either very tight or very loose. The remarriage also can increase anxiety and competition between the biological parent and the stepparent of the same sex. The astute physician will be aware of these different dimensions and will be able to help locate the problem should difficulties arise. Efforts should be made to meet the stepparent and to offer the family ongoing support.

SUMMARY

Divorce has become a common experience for millions of children. It is a painful and complicated process involving a fundamental restructuring of family relationships, patterns of daily living, and definitions of personal identity. Primary health care practitioners who work with children are in a unique position to provide support, continuity, and guidance to families and to play an advocacy role for children affected by divorce. To do this successfully the practitioner must feel comfortable with his/her own feelings; must demonstrate concern, sincerity, and patience; must be knowledgeable about children's reactions to the divorce process; and must have a good understanding of the particular child and family—their strengths, weaknesses, needs, and resources. Effective intervention can minimize the emotional complications, provide direct support to the individuals involved, and give the practitioner a tremendous sense of personal as well as professional satisfaction.

BIBLIOGRAPHY

Anthony EJ: Children at risk from divorce: A review. In Anthony EJ, Kovpernic C, editors: *The child and his family—children at psychiatric risk,* New York, 1974, John Wiley & Sons.

Bowlby J: *Attachment and Loss,* vol 3, *Sadness and depression.* New York, 1980, Basic Books.

Brun G: Conflicted parents: High and low vulnerability of children to divorce. In Anthony EJ, Kovpernic C, Chiland C, editors: *The child and his family—vulnerable children,* New York, 1978, John Wiley & Sons.

Caplan G: Preventing psychological disorders in children of divorce: General practitioner's role, *Br Med J* 292:1431, 1986.

Caplan G: Preventing psychological disorders in children of divorce: Guidelines for the general practitioner, *Br Med J* 292:1563, 1986.

Child custody consultation: Report of the task force on clinical assessment in child custody, Chicago, 1982, American Psychiatric Association.

Derdyn AP: Children in divorce: Intervention in the phase of separation, *Pediatrics* 60:20, 1977.

Despert JL: *Children of divorce,* Garden City, 1962, Dolphin Books.

Francke LB: *Growing up divorced,* New York, 1983, Simon & Schuster.

Galper M: *Co-parenting,* Philadelphia, 1978, Running Press Book Publishers.

Gardner R: *The boys and girls book about divorce,* New York, 1971, Bantam Books.

Goldstein S, Solnit A: *Divorce and your child: Practical suggestions for parents,* New Haven, 1984, Yale University Press.

Grollman E, editor: *Explaining divorce to children,* Boston, 1969, Beacon Press.

Guidubaldi J, Perry JD: Divorce and mental health sequelae for children: A two-year follow-up of a nationwide sample, *J Am Acad Child Psychiatry* 24:531, 1985.

Hancock E: The dimensions of meaning and belonging in the process of divorce, *Am J Orthopsychiatry* 50:18, 1980.

Hazen BS: *Two homes to live in: A child's eye view of divorce,* New York, 1983, Human Sciences Press.

Hetherington EM, Cox M, Cox R: Long-term effects of divorce and remarriage on the adjustment of children, *J Am Acad Child Psychiatry* 24:518, 1985.

Hodges WF: *Intervention for Children of Divorce,* ed 2, New York, 1991, John Wiley & Sons.

Jellinek MS, Slovik LS: Divorce: Impact on children, *N Engl J Med* 304:557, 1981.

Kalter N, Pickar J, Lesowitz M: School-based developmental facilitation groups for children of divorce: A preventive intervention, *Am J Orthopsychiatry* 54:613, 1984.

Kalter N: Long-term effects of divorce on children: A developmental vulnerability model, *Am J Orthopsychiatry* 57:587, 1987.

Kappelman MM, Black J: Children of divorce: The pediatrician's responsibility, *Pediatr Ann* 9:343, 1980.

Krementz J: *How it feels when parents divorce,* New York, 1988, Alfred A Knopf.

Luepnitz D: *Child custody,* Lexington, 1982, Lexington Books.

McDermott JF: Divorce and its psychiatric sequelae in children, *Arch Gen Psychiatry* 23:421, 1970.

Ricci I: *Mom's house, dad's house,* New York, 1980, Macmillan Publishing.

Rofes EE: *The kids' book of divorce: By, for and about kids,* Lexington, 1981, Lewis Publishing.

Roman H, Haddad W: *The disposable parent,* New York, 1978, Holt Rinehart & Winston.

Shamsie J: Family breakdown and its effects on emotional disorders in children, *Can J Psychiatry* 30:281, 1985.

Sinberg J: *Divorce is a grown up problem: A book about divorce for young children and their parents,* New York, 1978, Avon Books.

Visher E, Visher J: *How to win as a stepfamily,* New York, 1982, Dembner Books.

Wallerstein J, Kelly J: *Surviving the break-up,* New York, 1980, Basic Books.

Wallerstein JS: Children of divorce: The psychological tasks of the child, *Am J Orthopsychiatry* 53:230, 1983.

Wallerstein JS: Children of divorce: Preliminary report of a ten-year follow-up of older children and adolescents, *J Am Acad Child Psychiatry* 24:545, 1985.

Wallerstein JS: Children of divorce: Emerging trends, *Psychiatr Clin North Am* 8:837, 1985.

Weiss RS: *Marital separation,* New York, 1975, Basic Books.

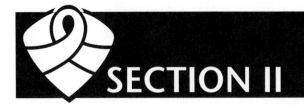

SECTION II

Assessing Signs and Symptoms

Assessing a patient's problems and organizing an evaluation challenges the primary care physician to be both complete and economical. This section highlights the major concerns for parents of sick children. After the common etiologies of the problem are listed, the major items are discussed in more detail. The discussion of the data-gathering process, history, physical examination, and laboratory testing includes hints and approaches for an office-based evaluation. Some problems that require the help of consultants are mentioned. The methods described should not be used as a prescription but should be modified in the light of the resources available in local practice.

Likewise, the flow sheets offer an approach to working through the problem. As in any such attempt to simplify the diagnostic process, there are other attractive options that work well so the approach suggested in the diagrams needs to be modified with common sense and practicality.

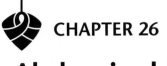

CHAPTER 26

Abdominal Masses

M. William Schwartz

Many abdominal masses are discovered by a parent while bathing or dressing the child or by the physician during routine physical examination. Rarely is the mass associated with other signs or symptoms such as pain or fever. The problem requires immediate attention, and the primary care physician should have an organized approach to expedite the evaluation and management of the abdominal mass.

DIFFERENTIAL DIAGNOSIS

Causes of Abdominal Masses

- **Trauma**
  Pseudocyst of the pancreas
- **Infection**
  Abscess
    Appendix
    Other
- **Allergic/immunologic**
  Large bladder
    Transverse myelitis
- **Endocrine–metabolic**
  Liver
    Glycogen storage disease
    Nutritional deficiency
    Kwashiorkor
    Hyperalimentation
- Spleen
    Gaucher disease
    Histiocytosis X
- Uterus
    Pregnancy
    Hematometria
- **Tumor**
  Liver
    Metastatic disease
    Neuroblastoma
    Wilms tumor

Gonadal tumor
Infiltrative disease
    Leukemia
    Histiocytosis
    Granuloma: tuberculosis, sarcoidosis
Spleen
    Leukemia
Kidney
    Wilms tumor
Adrenal gland
    Neuroblastoma
Lymphoid tissue
    Lymphoma
Connective tissue
    Rhabdomyosarcoma
- **Congenital**
Liver
    Cysts
    Congenital hepatic fibrosis
Spleen
    Congenital anemia
        Spherocytosis
Kidney
    Ureteropelvic obstruction
    Cystic disease: multicystic, polycystic
Dilated ureters
Bladder
    Urethral valves
Intestine
    Duplication
    Omental cysts
Ovary
    Dermoid
    Follicular cyst
- **Multiple etiologies**
    Ascites
    Constipation

Discussion

An effective organization of the differential diagnosis combines the age of onset with the location of the abdominal mass. Young children commonly have congenital causes, mainly genitourinary malformations or tumors such as Wilms tumor and neuroblastoma. Older children have infectious and oncologic masses. In adolescent girls, tumors, cysts, or teratomas may develop in the reproductive organs.

Newborns with abdominal masses may have either multicystic dysplasia or polycystic kidneys. Multicystic kidneys contain cysts of various sizes that may have surrounding islands of functional glomeruli that sustain life for a period of time, or they may have no functional tissue. This malformation may occur with urethral valves or pulmonary malformations, or it may be an isolated problem.

Polycystic kidneys may be "infantile" or "adult." These terms are somewhat misleading because both occur in infants and children. Infantile polycystic kidneys, an autosomal recessive disorder, consist of many dilated tubules that form sacules. Relatively few of the nephrons are functional, so the prognosis is poor. Some forms of polycystic kidneys are associated with liver cysts and fibrosis that typically cause portal hypertension in the third decade. The adult form has small cysts that remain functional and do not cause any clinical problems until adulthood when hypertension is the major problem. Within each group are many variations of anatomic changes and functional disability.

Ureteropelvic obstruction, the other frequent anomaly that presents as an abdominal mass in the newborn, is caused by narrowing at the juncture of the renal pelvis with the ureter. The stricture will cause hydronephrosis, which, if severe, will be discovered as an abdominal mass. In less severe cases, mild hydronephrosis may present as hematuria after mild trauma.

Patients with urethral valves may have lethargy or failure to thrive and an enlarged firm bladder. Often there are ureteral reflux and dilated tortuous ureters. A voiding cystourethrogram will outline the urethral valve and reflux, if present. Renal ultrasonography will demonstrate any associated hydronephrosis.

Wilms tumor and neuroblastoma are two main abdominal tumors of childhood. Few patients have any associated signs, although some have either hematuria or hypertension. Imaging of the mass with ultrasound or computed tomography (CT) will help differentiate the two masses. In the first year of life, a special form of neuro-

blastoma, stage IV, may regress without any specific treatment.

Dermoid cysts or cystic teratomas in adolescent girls are the most common ovarian tumor in children or adolescents. These tumors contain tissue from all three germ layers, including skin, hair, and sebaceous glands; 10% to 20% are bilateral. Usually detected on a rectal examination or coincidentally on an abdominal radiograph, the tumors may enlarge to present as an abdominal mass. The major complication of dermoid cysts are torsion and peritonitis, although most cause no symptoms.

Pseudocyst of the pancreas is seen in patients after trauma, usually in cases of child abuse. After it is damaged, the pancreas undergoes autodigestion and forms a pseudocyst. This mass, not easily palpable, is demonstrated with ultrasound studies. If the history does not reveal any major trauma, an investigation for child abuse should be undertaken.

A mass in the lower midabdomen frequently is shown to be an enlarged bladder, usually a neurogenic bladder. Neurologic problems, such as transverse myelitis or spinal trauma, may produce contraction of the bladder sphincter and urinary retention. Because the second to fourth sacral nerves innervate both the anal and bladder sphincters, stimulating the skin on the buttocks and looking for contraction of the anus serves as a test for the integrity of these spinal nerves.

DATA GATHERING

History

For most problems of abdominal masses, the history offers limited information. Age will help in some cases, because many congenital problems appear in infancy, such as infantile polycystic kidney and multicystic kidney. Most cases of Wilms tumor occur in children 3 to 5 years of age. Masses associated with reproductive organs usually appear during early adolescence.

Constipation is a common cause of masses in the left lower quadrant; therefore, a series of questions about constipation should be asked, including diet, frequency of bowel movements, medications, and left-sided pain. A history of blunt abdominal trauma should make one suspect a pseudocyst of the pancreas and child abuse. Growth charts should be completed to

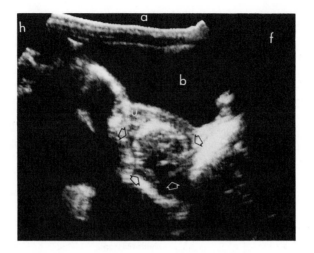

FIG 26-1

A 9-year-old child with chronic abdominal pain. Ultrasonography was helpful in outlining the mass with a calcification in the center (arrows). At surgery, the diagnosis of teratoma was confirmed. a = anterior; b = bladder; f = caudad; h = cephalad. [From Haffer JO, Slovis TL: Introduction to Radiology in Clinical Pediatrics, Chicago, 1984, Year Book Medical Publishers, p 110.]

determine if there is a growth problem that might suggest the possibility of urethral valves. Patients with urethral valves have a weak urinary stream.

Polycystic disease of the kidney is familial, so a family history may lead to the diagnosis.

Physical Examination

The physical examination will be more helpful in establishing the diagnosis. A description of an abdominal mass should include the location and degree of firmness, tenderness, and sharpness of the border. The location of the mass is usually related to the underlying structure. For example, a right upper quadrant mass is related to the liver: a left lower abdominal mass is associated with a feces-filled intestine or an ovary. Renal masses are in the flanks. Some masses, such as an omental cyst, are not in a fixed location but move as the patient's position changes.

The other characteristics of the mass (firmness, tenderness, and sharpness of the border) also aid in the focusing of the diagnostic possibilities. A hard liver should make one suspect a metastatic process, whereas a soft, full, and tender liver is congested, as seen in patients with heart failure or hypoalbuminemia. Likewise, the hard spleen may be infiltrated with cells from Gaucher disease, whereas the soft spleen is more likely from a hemolytic anemia. A large hard bladder is secondary to an obstruction, whereas a soft bladder is from a neurologic process such as a spinal cord injury or transverse myelitis. Most tumors are hard. Tenderness usually comes from a stretched capsule or impingement of the mass on other organs or nerves. Ill-defined borders may indicate a spreading tumor or a deep organ, in which case palpation is difficult because of overlying normal structures.

Common errors in physical diagnosis include not being able to recognize the spleen from the left kidney and not appreciating how far to the left of the midline the left lobe of the liver can appear. Often, this left lobe may be confused with the spleen.

Laboratory Evaluation

Ultrasonography has simplified the evaluation of abdominal masses (Fig. 26-1). Although it has taken some of the challenge from the bedside clinician who had impressive physical diagnostic skills, this test helps speed up the identification of the mass. In most cases, the organ can be identified, cysts located, and either a diagnosis can be made or direction can be given to the next step in the diagnostic process: biopsy, CT, or

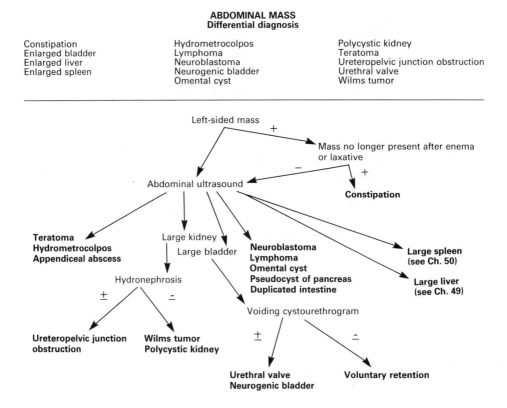

ABDOMINAL MASS
Differential diagnosis

Constipation
Enlarged bladder
Enlarged liver
Enlarged spleen

Hydrometrocolpos
Lymphoma
Neuroblastoma
Neurogenic bladder
Omental cyst

Polycystic kidney
Teratoma
Ureteropelvic junction obstruction
Urethral valve
Wilms tumor

FIG 26-2
Decision tree for differential diagnosis of abdominal masses.

magnetic resonance imaging. Ultrasonography has helped decrease the number of contrast radiologic studies, laparoscopies, and diagnostic biopsies. Cysts of any organ are easily outlined. Ureteropelvic obstruction, renal cysts, tumors, and thick-walled bladders are identified with ultrasonography. The origin of a large mass may be traced to the pelvis and calcifications identified that suggest the diagnosis of a pelvic teratoma.

Other helpful screening tests include the complete blood cell count, especially if anemia, malignancy, or infection is suspected. If there is anemia, further testing with reticulocyte counts and Coombs test will complete the screening (*see* Chapter 85 for anemia evaluation. Renal function tests, urine cultures, and serum chemical analyses are important when a mass from the genitourinary system is being considered.

Special testing is indicated by the specifics of the case. Tests such as abdominal CT may help the surgeon or oncologist better outline the mass.

Barium studies can better define a mass secondary to intestinal duplication. Screening for vanillylmandelic acid (VMA) or quantitative analysis of VMA will help confirm a neuroblastoma.

INDICATIONS FOR CONSULTATION OR REFERRAL

With the exception of the mass secondary to constipation, most patients with abdominal masses need consultation with appropriate specialists. If the left lower quadrant mass is thought to be secondary to constipation, an enema may relieve the primary problem, but further attention should be directed to the causes of this problem.

DISCUSSION OF ALGORITHM

Because many masses located on the left side are secondary to constipation, this possibility must be ruled out first. After that step, the masses must be evaluated expeditiously, because they may be malignant, infectious, or, if benign, cause pressure on other organs or torsion and progress to acute abdomen (Fig. 26-2). Other problems of pregnancy, trauma, and malnutrition should be considered, as well as anemia and hepatomegaly secondary to heart failure or liver disease.

Abdominal ultrasonography plays a pivotal role in the evaluation, because it demonstrates the characteristics of the mass and often suggests the correct diagnosis. The remainder of the evaluation will be determined from the results of ultrasonography.

BIBLIOGRAPHY

Bliss DP Jr, Coffin CM, Bower RJ, et al: Messenteric cysts in children, *Surgery* 115(5):57, 1994.

Bloom DA, Brosman J: Multicystic kidney, *J Urol* 120:211–215, 1978.

Caty MG, Shamburger RC: Abdominal tumors in infancy and childhood, *Pediatr Clin North Am* 40(6):1253–1271, 1993.

Ein SH, Darte JMM, Stevenson CT: Cystic and solid ovarian tumors in children—44 year review, *J Pediatr Surg* 5:148, 1970.

Goodman SN: Neuroblastoma screening data, *Am J Dis Child* 145:1415, 1991.

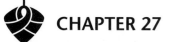

CHAPTER 27

Acute Abdominal Pain

Brent R. King

In the majority of children acute abdominal pain is caused by a self-limiting condition. The physician must distinguish these children from the few whose illness is more serious. In making this distinction, the clinician should be aware of the child's age and developmental level, because these factors influence the history, physical examination, and differential diagnosis. Whereas the older child and adolescent may be able to give a concise history of abdominal pain and to cooperate with the physical examination, the signs and symptoms in the younger child are more often nonspecific. Results of the physical examination can be misleading. Furthermore, many common childhood illnesses have features that may be confused with acute abdomen.

DIFFERENTIAL DIAGNOSIS

Common Causes of Acute Abdominal Pain

- **Trauma**
    Child abuse
- **Infection**
    Viral or bacterial gastroenteritis

Infections that may be confused with acute abdominal pain
> Pneumonia
> Urinary tract infection
> Otitis media
> Streptococcal pharyngitis
> Meningitis
> Mononucleosis
Mesenteric lymphadenitis
Sexually transmitted disease
- **Mechanical**
  Intussusception
  Volvulus
  Malrotation
  Testicular torsion
  Tortion of testicular appendage
  Ovarian torsion
- **Toxin**
  Food poisoning
  Accidental ingestion
- **Metabolic**
  Renal stone
  Diabetes
- **Inflammation**
  Anaphylactoid purpura (HSP)
  Inflammatory bowel disease
- **Other**
  Hemolytic uremic syndrome
  Dietary indiscretion
  Constipation
  Appendicitis
  Appendiceal abscess
  Functional abdominal pain
  Peptic ulcer
  Mittelschmerz
  Sickle cell anemia

Discussion

Trauma

Trauma is a rare cause of abdominal pain throughout childhood, and significant abdominal pain does not occur as a result of minor trauma. Any child with significant abdominal pain reported to result from incidental trauma such as a fall from bed should be considered an abused child until proved otherwise. Adolescents often participate in dangerous activities that may result in abdominal trauma, but because these activities may have been proscribed by their parents, they may be unwilling to explain the circumstances.

Trauma severe enough to cause significant intra-abdominal injury should be managed with the assistance of an experienced surgeon.

Gastroenteritis

Gastroenteritis is the most common cause of acute abdominal pain at any age. The infant usually has diarrhea, with or without vomiting, often preceded by symptoms of an upper respiratory tract infection. Fever also may be present. Stools will be passed more frequently and will be watery. The pain associated with gastroenteritis is colicky and diffuse. The examination may reveal hyperactive bowel sounds. Tenderness, if present, is most often diffuse. Viruses, especially rotavirus, commonly cause gastroenteritis in infants and young children. Bacterial pathogens include *Salmonella* and *Shigella,* and less commonly certain strains of *Escherichia coli* and *Campylobacter.* Diarrhea that is bloody or contains large numbers of white blood cells on microscopic examination is likely bacterial and should be sent for stool culture. Treatment is conservative and aimed at maintaining adequate hydration. Antibiotics should be withheld until stool culture results are available. Exhaustive evaluation is best reserved for those cases that do not resolve spontaneously.

Constipation

Constipation may cause abdominal pain, which is usually left-sided and colicky in nature. The stools are usually hard, and their volume may be either large or small. Abdominal distention is often present. The physician may be able to palpate doughy stools in the bowel. The possible causes of constipation are numerous, varying from functional to serious diseases such as Hirschsprung disease.

Intussusception

Intussusception, the process in which a segment of bowel telescopes into a more distal segment, is the leading cause of acute bowel obstruction in infants and is most common during the second 6 months of life. Most intussusception is ileocolic, although ileoileal intussusception does occur. The classic features of intussusception are colicky abdominal pain, vomiting, a sausage-shaped right upper quadrant mass, and bloody "currant jelly" stools. Patients frequently have periods of quietness or sleepiness. There may be a paucity of abdominal contents on palpation of the right lower quadrant (Dance sign). Some of these symptoms, including abdominal pain, may be absent, and therefore a high index of suspicion must be maintained. Diagnosis (and often reduction) may be accomplished with a barium enema study (air contrast enema has a lower success rate). In those cases in which the intussusception cannot be reduced or recurs, surgery is usually indicated, and a surgeon should be involved when the diagnosis is suspected. When intussusception is diagnosed in an older child, a search for an underlying disease is warranted.

Malrotation

Malrotation is a congenital condition in which the mesentery is abnormally attached to the bowel, allowing the bowel to twist. The patient usually has constant, severe abdominal pain and bile-stained vomitus. The onset may be acute or may be preceded by minor gastrointestinal symptoms, such as "feeding difficulty." Volvulus can cause extensive ischemic injury to the bowel in a short time, and emergency surgery is necessary. In the patient with suspected malrotation, plain flat and upright abdominal radiographs may demonstrate loops of small intestine overriding the liver. If volvulus has occurred, plain films often show air-fluid levels and dilated bowel loops proximal to the obstruction and a paucity of bowel gas distally. A barium esophagogram is usually diagnostic.

Colic

Colic syndrome occurs most frequently in infants younger than 3 months of age. The cause of colic is unknown, but the symptom complex consists of paroxysms of extreme irritability accompanied by apparent abdominal pain, with "drawing up" of the legs and a distended, tense abdomen. These episodes may persist for hours and tend to recur, usually in the late afternoon (see Chapter 9 for discussion of colic).

Appendicitis

Of all causes of acute abdominal pain in childhood, appendicitis causes the greatest concern. It can be difficult to diagnose, especially in children younger than 6 years of age. Appendicitis is most common during late childhood and early adolescence, with 12 years being the average age of occurrence. The pain begins as colicky, sometimes vague, periumbilical pain that increases in intensity and migrates to the right lower quadrant over 12 to 24 hours. However, only a third to half of affected children have these classic symptoms. In many children the pain begins in the right lower quadrant, and in others the pain does not migrate. Anorexia is present in the majority of children with appendicitis. Vomiting is also common, occurring after the onset of abdominal pain. The physical examination is often more helpful than the history. The patient usually appears ill and objects to any movement. Signs of peritoneal irritation are frequently present.

The diagnosis of appendicitis is made on clinical grounds. The laboratory data are often equivocal. Most patients have mild leukocytosis. Urinalysis is negative for white blood cells unless the inflamed appendix lies near the ureter, in which case a few leukocytes may be seen. Occasionally a fecalith will be seen on plain radiographs, but films are usually normal (Fig. 27-1).

The patient with suspected appendicitis should be seen by a surgeon without delay, because most appendixes rupture within 48 hours of the onset of symptoms. Those children in whom results of physical examination are equivocal but in whom the diagnosis is being considered should be admitted to the hospital for serial abdominal examinations.

A child with a history that includes symptoms of appendicitis, with sudden relief of pain followed by gradual return of pain and fever, probably has a ruptured appendix or an appendiceal abscess. Immediate surgical consultation is mandatory.

Mesenteric Lymphadenitis

Mesenteric lymphadenitis is a poorly understood disorder that can mimic appendicitis so closely that it may be difficult to differentiate the two. Mesenteric lymphadenitis sometimes occurs concurrent with or shortly after a viral infection. Adenovirus may play a role in this disease. Symptoms that help to differentiate mesenteric lymphadenitis include generalized lymphadenopathy, pain that is diffuse rather than localized, and lymphocytosis. In most cases the diagnosis is made either when a normal appen-

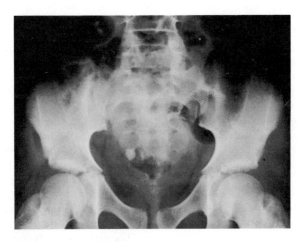

FIG 27-1

A 9-year-old child with abdominal pain. Calcification in the right lower quadrant was part of a teratoma. [From Haller JO, Slovis TL: Introduction to Radiology in Clinical Pediatrics, Chicago, 1984, Year Book Medical Publishers, p 110.]

dix is found at laparotomy or on clinical grounds when the symptoms fail to progress during a period of observation.

Sickle Cell Crisis

The patient with sickle cell anemia will sometimes present with a painful crisis localized to the abdomen, often mimicking acute abdomen. The history of sickle cell disease and previous similar crisis is reassuring but should not lull the physician into a false sense of security. Observation in the hospital allows for both intravenous hydration and serial abdominal examinations.

Torsion of Testis

Torsion of the testis, usually occurring in prepubertal boys, is a result of inadequate attachment of the testis to the intrascrotal subcutaneous tissue. This condition gives the testis the potential to rotate, which may result in infarction of the testis. The patient most often has acute onset of scrotal pain, but the pain often is referred to the abdomen and that abdominal pain may be the chief complaint. In addition, nausea and vomiting are frequently associated with torsion, which may direct attention to the abdomen rather than to the scrotum. The scrotal examination is diagnostic. The involved testicle is swollen and lies higher in the scrotum than its mate. Torsion of the testis is a surgical emergency; when torsion is suspected, consultation should be sought without delay.

Food Poisoning and Dietary Indiscretion

A careful history will help determine whether the child has overeaten or eaten too much of an unfamiliar food. Nausea and vomiting may be present, along with mild, diffuse abdominal pain. Signs of acute abdomen are absent. In the majority of cases laboratory evaluation is not warranted. Treatment consists of support and dietary modification.

Food poisoning can be more difficult to diagnose. The patient may have a history that suggests the diagnosis. For example, consumption of a salad made with mayonnaise or cream points to staphylococcal food intoxication, whereas eating stuffed poultry suggests salmonellosis. More often, however, the dietary history is equivocal. Vomiting, usually the prominent feature of food poisoning, occurs before the onset of maximal abdominal pain. Fever also may be present. The pain is crampy, and signs of acute abdomen are usually not seen, although in occasional patients the pain may be severe enough to require observation in the hospital to rule out significant intra-abdominal disease. Hospitalization also may be required if supportive measures fail to prevent dehydration.

Cholecystitis

Cholecystitis is rare in childhood. It is most often diagnosed in patients who have hemolytic anemia (sickle cell anemia, its variants, or hereditary spherocytosis), but may occasionally be seen in an otherwise normal adolescent. The symptoms of childhood cholecystitis are similar to those in adults: colicky abdominal pain in the right upper quadrant, which is exacerbated by intake of fatty foods. Pain also may be referred to the right scapular region. Nausea and vomiting are frequently reported. Evaluation should proceed with the aid of a surgeon.

Renal Calculus
A renal stone may appear in childhood but is more likely in adolescence. The expected symptom is unilateral flank pain that radiates to the lower abdomen. Radiation to the ipsilateral hemiscrotum in boys is common as well. The pain associated with renal calculus is colicky and severe, and nausea and vomiting are often associated with this disorder. Frank hematuria occurs frequently. Management is aimed at making the patient comfortable until the stone passes and at identifying an underlying cause. Common causes of urolithiasis are urinary tract infection and hypercalcuria; the remainder of stones are idiopathic except for the few caused by rare metabolic diseases.

Pelvic Inflammatory Disease
Pelvic inflammatory disease (PID, acute salpingitis), a disease of sexually active women, causes much diagnostic uncertainty. It may be difficult for the physician to differentiate PID from acute appendicitis. There is usually a history of previous sexually transmitted disease; however, many patients deny sexual activity and deny or are unaware of having a sexually transmitted disease. Other risk factors include multiple sexual partners and use of an intrauterine device. The usual patient is a young woman with abdominal pain that began shortly after the onset of her menstrual period and is associated with vaginal discharge. In severe cases the patient also may have right upper quadrant pain, which suggests FitzHugh-Curtis syndrome, a gonococcal perihepatic inflammation. The physical examination yields variable findings. Signs of peritoneal irritation may be present, but the patient may instead have diffuse abdominal tenderness. On pelvic examination the examiner will often find cervical discharge and adnexal tenderness. In addition to the history and physical examination, a more protracted course of pain may help to differentiate PID from acute appendicitis. Admission to the hospital should be considered for those patients who have fever, severe pain, or recurrent disease and for those in whom the diagnosis of acute abdomen cannot be ruled out.

Ectopic Pregnancy
Any postpubertal female patient with severe acute abdominal pain should have a urine pregnancy test performed, because ectopic pregnancy may cause acute abdomen and is a disease with high mortality if untreated. Ectopic pregnancy is rare, occurring in fewer than 1% of all pregnancies. The history may include symptoms of early pregnancy such as missed or scanty menstrual period, morning sickness, and breast tenderness. Uterine enlargement is a frequent finding. Examination will demonstrate an adnexal mass in approximately half of these patients. Cervical motion tenderness also occurs and may lead to the mistaken diagnosis of PID.

Acute abdominal pain associated with vaginal bleeding should be considered to represent ectopic pregnancy until proved otherwise.

DATA GATHERING

History
Important early clues to serious disease that are useful at all ages include pain that interrupts the child's usual activities, pain that worsens over time, and an ill-appearing patient either lying still or vomiting.

Among the most important signs of abdominal pain or a significant intra-abdominal process in infants are vomiting, diarrhea, anorexia, irritability (particularly paradoxical irritability), and drawing up of the legs.

Vomiting occurs with many childhood illnesses. A careful history of the course of the illness and the quality of the vomitus may help in identification of the cause. Vomiting as a result of acute abdomen usually occurs later in the course of the illness, often after a period of increasing irritability and crying that is pain related. In contrast, vomiting occurs early in the course of infectious gastroenteritis. Vomiting is particularly worrisome if it is bile stained, indicating bowel obstruction, or projectile, indicating obstruction at or near the pylorus.

Diarrhea (ie, increased stool quantity, frequency, water content, or any combination of these features) is most often associated with acute infectious gastroenteritis but may be associated with more serious conditions. Particularly significant is passage of bloody mucus, the "currant jelly" stool of intussusception.

The family will sometimes report that the child's fretfulness seems to increase with rocking or cuddling. This paradoxical irritability usually represents serious disease. Paradoxical irritability occurs in acute abdomen because rocking and cuddling serve to disturb the intra-abdominal contents much as an examiner does when attempting to elicit rebound tenderness. Most infants with serious intra-abdominal disease prefer to lie still in the supine position with the legs flexed to relieve abdominal pressure.

Physical Examination

The physical examination of the infant with symptoms of intra-abdominal disease should not be limited to the abdomen. Most infants have a group of nonspecific symptoms that may suggest an abdominal cause.

The physician should first observe the child and his/her interactions with the caretaker. The active and playful infant is unlikely to have serious disease. Children with significant intra-abdominal disease usually display one of two behaviors: 1) they may lie quietly and become irritable with the slightest movement, which suggests acute abdomen; or 2) they may have periods of near-normal activity punctuated by irritability and writhing, which should lead to consideration of colicky pain such as caused by intussusception.

Infants will be most comfortable if examined in the parent's arms or lap. The examination should proceed slowly, with the invasive or painful portions of the examination deferred to the end. The abdomen should be inspected for distention and for bruises or other signs of trauma. If found, an explanation should be sought from the family and child abuse should be considered. With a warmed stethoscope the examiner first listens for bowel sounds; the child may prefer to have the parent hold the stethoscope. Absent bowel sounds are suggestive of bowel obstruction. After auscultation, the examiner proceeds with very gentle palpation and percussion, focusing on one small area at a time. The physician may discover point tenderness or guarding that seems related more to one area than to others. Depending on location and quality, masses may represent stool in the bowel, appendiceal abscess, the olive of pyloric stenosis, intussusception, or a true

tumor. Paucity of bowel contents in the right lower quadrant (dance sign) suggests intussusception. A child who cries at the physician's slightest touch may be more cooperative if palpation is performed at least partially by a parent or caretaker. The usual test for rebound tenderness can be just as effectively performed by gentle side-to-side rocking or percussion; this method saves the child undue discomfort. With a well-lubricated small finger, rectal examination can be performed without trauma and may yield valuable information.

Examination of the older child and adolescent should be guided by the child's own behavior and desires. Many children and adolescents are more comfortable if a parent or caretaker remains close by during the examination. The child's modesty should be respected insofar as possible without sacrificing a complete examination. The traditional abdominal examination can be performed, although the more gentle tests for peritoneal irritation should be used in place of the rebound tenderness test. Absent bowel sounds, exquisite point tenderness, the presence of peritoneal irritation, abdominal rigidity, involuntary guarding, and abdominal mass are the most significant findings on abdominal examination.

Pain in the right lower quadrant produced by palpation or by rocking or percussion is indicative of appendicitis. Clues to the diagnosis of generalized peritonitis are absent bowel sounds and a rigid abdomen. Voluntary guarding may sometimes be differentiated from involuntary guarding by distracting the child. Colicky abdominal pain associated with right upper quadrant mass suggests cholecystitis. Similar pain in a young girl with a mass in a lower quadrant is likely related to ovarian torsion, tuboovarian abscess, or, rarely, ectopic pregnancy.

Because pneumonia, streptococcal pharyngitis, and urinary tract infection may all cause abdominal symptoms, a complete physical examination is required. The evaluation of abdominal pain in the sexually active adolescent girl should include a pelvic examination. The external genitalia and introitus are first examined for signs of trauma such as tears and bruising. Young women may be unwilling to admit to forcible rape or sexual abuse, but these acts may cause intra-abdominal injury. Purulent cervical discharge, cervical motion tenderness, and adnexal mass are signs of PID. Bloody discharge most likely represents normal menstrual bleeding but may also be seen in ectopic pregnancy or threatened abortion.

Laboratory Evaluation

After a complete history and physical examination the physician will often have to rely on laboratory studies and imaging techniques for a certain diagnosis. Diarrheal stools may be easily evaluated by microscopic examination after staining with methylene blue or Wright stain. Stools that are bloody or contain large numbers of white blood cells should be sent for culture.

The urinalysis is a useful screening device in the patient with somewhat nonspecific symptoms. The physician can quickly identify pyuria and glycosuria, which may be indicative of urinary tract infection and diabetes mellitus, respectively. Hematuria often represents cystitis or renal stone, but may indicate more serious renal disease. In the adolescent girl a urine pregnancy test can be obtained. Finally, the degree to which the urine is concentrated allows the clinician to estimate the patient's state of hydration.

In patients with concomitant pharyngitis and those who have been exposed to streptococcal pharyngitis, a throat culture or a rapid antigen test should be obtained. Abdominal pain can be present prior to the onset of pharyngitis in these patients.

Chest radiographic examination may be helpful in the patient with fever and cough, because lower lobe pneumonias may cause abdominal pain.

Plain radiographs of the abdomen are rarely helpful. Occasionally air-fluid levels or a fecalith may be seen, but unless these studies are immediately available to the physician, obtaining plain films will only serve to delay appropriate referral of the child with suspected acute abdomen.

Serum electrolytes and glucose levels may prove helpful in evaluation of excessive vomiting or diarrhea, but are not routine. More extensive metabolic profiles should be reserved for specific indications.

INDICATIONS FOR CONSULTATION OR REFERRAL

Most acute abdominal pain is related to self-limiting conditions that can be managed easily by the physician in an outpatient setting. A small number of children will benefit from hospitalization. Patients with suspected appendicitis, malrotation, intussusception, ectopic pregnancy, or peritonitis and those who appear to have sustained significant intra-abdominal trauma should be seen by a surgeon early in the course of diagnostic evaluation, because delay in treatment may result in significant morbidity or even death. Likewise, diabetes, sickle cell disease, inflammatory bowel disease, and other such disorders are best managed with the assistance of appropriate subspecialists.

DISCUSSION OF ALGORITHM (FIG. 27-2)

The physician should first ask about trauma and look for evidence of abdominal trauma such as bruising. Inasmuch as significant abdominal trauma is rare in young children, child abuse should be considered unless the history of the event given by the caretakers is plausible and fits with the pattern of injury. When trauma appears to be the cause of abdominal pain, perforated viscus, splenic rupture, bowel wall hematoma, and contusion of the abdominal muscles must be considered in the evaluation. Surgical consultation should be sought early.

In the absence of trauma, the physician should try to fit the symptom complex with a known syndrome. An infant 1 year of age with paroxysms of crying and drawing up of the legs who also has bloody stools may well have intussusception.

When a recognizable pattern cannot be found in a febrile infant, the child should be examined for infections that cause abdominal pain. In the older infant streptococcal pharyngitis can cause abdominal pain, and a throat culture should be considered. Urinalysis, complete blood cell count, chest radiograph, Mono-Spot test, and stool cultures may be diagnostic. When results of these laboratory tests are negative or the child is afebrile, imaging techniques such as abdominal ultrasound may lead to a diagnosis. Surgical consultation should be sought when the diagnosis is unclear.

A dietary history should be included in the evaluation to help identify dietary indiscretion and perhaps to point to common causes of foodborne disease, such as *Salmonella* and *Staphylococcus*.

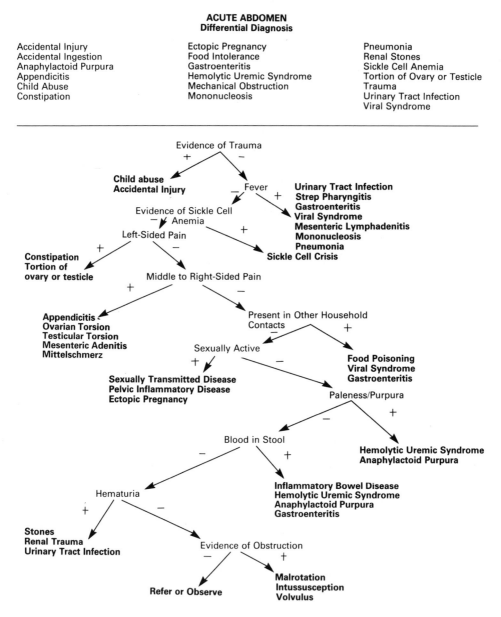

ACUTE ABDOMEN
Differential Diagnosis

Accidental Injury	Ectopic Pregnancy	Pneumonia
Accidental Ingestion	Food Intolerance	Renal Stones
Anaphylactoid Purpura	Gastroenteritis	Sickle Cell Anemia
Appendicitis	Hemolytic Uremic Syndrome	Tortion of Ovary or Testicle
Child Abuse	Mechanical Obstruction	Trauma
Constipation	Mononucleosis	Urinary Tract Infection
		Viral Syndrome

FIG 27-2

Decision tree for differential diagnosis of acute abdominal pain.

Some consideration also should be given to the possibility of sexually transmitted diseases, acquired from sexual abuse or early sexual experimentation.

If no syndrome is recognized, the physician must attempt to differentiate surgical from non-surgical abdomen. Although not infallible, the presence of such signs as rebound or motion tenderness, involuntary guarding, and other signs of peritoneal irritation should lead to prompt surgical consultation.

Urinalysis is useful in the evaluation of pain in those patients who are not thought to have acute abdomen and in whom there is no ready explanation for the symptom. This test is easy to obtain and can quickly rule out diabetic ketoacidosis, urinary tract infection, and renal stone. Hematuria plus abdominal pain may be the result of anaphylactoid purpura or hemolytic uremic syndrome. When urinalysis is also normal, the physician should consider gastrointestinal disorders such as inflammatory bowel disease or constipation.

When the abdominal pain persists without positive physical or laboratory findings, it is wise to enlist the aid of a surgeon before further evaluation.

Adolescents differ from younger children in that they are more independent of their families and are more often involved in sexual exploration and in experimentation with alcohol and other drugs.

Sexually active teenage girls who have abdominal pain should undergo a pelvic examination, because it can be difficult to differentiate PID from other causes of acute abdominal pain in this age group. A urine pregnancy test should be performed in all postmenarcheal girls who have significant abdominal pain, because ectopic pregnancy can mimic appendicitis and other causes of acute abdomen.

Those patients who have acute abdominal pain that persists, have surgical abdomen, or do not have an apparent self-limiting disorder will benefit from consultation with a surgeon. Collaboration with a subspecialist may be necessary to manage sickle cell crisis, hemolytic uremic syndrome, or inflammatory bowel disease. Most other problems related to abdominal pain may be managed by the primary care physician.

BIBLIOGRAPHY

Bongard F, Landers DV, Lewis F: Differential diagnosis of appendicitis and pelvic inflammatory disease: A prospective analysis, *Am J Surg* 150:90–95, 1985.

Dolgin SE, Beck AR, Tartter PI: The risk of perforation when children with possible appendicitis are observed in the hospital, *Surg Gynecol Obstet* 175:320–324, 1992.

Reynolds SL: Missed appendicitis in a pediatric emergency department, *Pediatr Emerg Care* 9:1–3, 1993.

Reynolds SL, Jaffe DM: Diagnosing abdominal pain in a pediatric emergency department, *Pediatr Emerg Care* 8:126–128, 1992.

Rothrock SG, Green SM, Hummel CB: Plain abdominal radiography in the detection of major disease in children: A prospective analysis, *Ann Emerg Med* 21:1423–1429, 1992.

Rothrock SG, Skeoch G, Rush JJ, Johnson NE: Clinical features of misdiagnosed appendicitis in children, *Ann Emerg Med* 20:45–50, 1991.

Ruddy RM: Pain-abdomen. In Fleisher GR, Ludwig S, editors: *Textbook of pediatric emergency medicine,* ed 3, Baltimore, 1993, Williams & Wilkins.

Sivit CJ, Taylor GA, Eichelberger MR: Visceral injury in battered children: A changing perspective, *Radiology* 173:659–661, 1989.

Stevenson RJ: Abdominal pain unrelated to trauma, *Surg Clin North Am* 65:1181–1215, 1985.

CHAPTER 28

Chronic Abdominal Pain

William J. Wenner, Jr.

Abdominal pain that has been present for more than 3 months offers a frequent challenge to the primary care physician. Chronic abdominal pain is common and is estimated to occur in 20% to 30% of the population between ages 5 to 14 years. It is disruptive: only one child in 10 with chronic abdominal pain attends school regularly, and approximately three in 10 miss more than 10% of the school year. The diagnosis can be difficult because there are no pathognomonic findings and no diagnostic test.

Chronic abdominal pain is known by a variety of names, reflecting the confusion regarding the condition. These names include functional abdominal pain, recurrent abdominal pain (RAP), neurovegetative dystonia, nonorganic abdominal pain, and dysfunctional abdominal pain. It occurs mainly in school-aged children, and an onset before 4 years or after 14 years of age is very unusual. The incidence in boys equals that of girls up to 9 years of age, after which age girls predominate. It has been reported that approximately 5% of cases have a discernible organic etiology. However, recent technologic advances, such as endoscopy, have increased the proportion in whom an organic etiology is found.

Chronic abdominal pain is episodic. It lasts for days to weeks, but, in the majority of cases, the episodes last less than 3 hours, and in half of the cases, the pain resolves in 1 hour. Episodes are often clustered. The pain affects the ability to fall asleep but does not wake the child once asleep. Most children have definite pain-free intervals, although in 10% of children the pain may be continuous. The description of the pain is often vague, and the child is unable to describe the nature of the pain. It has a periumbilical or midepigastric location. The pain frequently interrupts normal activity of daily living. It is not relieved with food or bowel movement. It often is associated with headache, nausea, dizziness, and fatigue. Abdominal distention, diarrhea, and constipation can occur but often suggest an organic etiology. Weight loss, growth failure, gastrointestinal bleeding, fever, or other constitutional symptoms are not associated with functional pain. The finding of any of these signs or symptoms must be evaluated.

DIFFERENTIAL DIAGNOSIS

There are more than 100 organic etiologies that present with the symptoms of chronic abdominal pain. Symptoms will frequently allow the practitioner to differentiate organic from functional etiologies (Box 28-1).

Allergy
Celiac disease most frequently is associated with poor growth, a protuberant abdomen, and large bulky stools. Chronic abdominal pain, most likely on the basis of altered motility, may be a component. Other food allergies may have pain as a component. Pain as the only symptom is rare, but the other symptoms may be subtle.

Anatomic
The pain of appendiceal colic is usually in the right lower quadrant, and abdominal pressure often will elicit the pain. Chronic intermittent episodes of this pain have been described as being due to inspissated fecal casts within the appendix. Filling defects are seen on radiographs. The appendix demonstrates distention, and barium is retained, often past 72 hours following the study. Although it is a rare condition, appendiceal colic is seen in children in the same age group as functional pain. Pain is relieved by appendectomy.

BOX 28-1
Functional and Organic Pain Findings

FINDINGS ASSOCIATED WITH FUNCTIONAL PAIN
Normal growth
Nonfocal examination
Diffuse pain
Paraumbilical pain

FINDINGS ASSOCIATED WITH ORGANIC PAIN
Pain that radiates to the back, chest, or hips
Association with meals, defecation
Awakens child from sleep
Growth failure or weight loss
Specific quadrant pain
Mass or fullness
Hepatosplenomegaly
Flank pain
Rectal bleeding
Perianal skin tags or anal fissures
Fever
Joint pain
Vomiting
Fecal incontinence

Differential Diagnosis of Chronic Abdominal Pain

- **Allergy**
  Celiac disease (gluten)
  Individual food allergy
  Mastocytosis
- **Anatomic**
  Appendiceal colic
  Musculoskeletal pain
  Obstruction: intermittent volvulus; duplication cyst; constipation
  Ovarian cyst
  Biliary/pancreatic system: stricture, cholelithiasis/cholecystitis, pancreatic divisum
  Uteropelvic junction obstruction
- **Infection**
  Blastocystis hominis
  Dientamoeba fragilis
  Giardia lamblia
  Helicobacter pylori
  Urinary tract infection
- **Inflammatory**
  Inflammatory bowel disease: Crohn disease (regional enteritis); ulcerative colitis
- **Metabolic**
  Acute intermittent porphyria
  Hyperlipidemia
  Maldigestion
  Fructose
  Lactose
  Oats
  Sorbitol
- **Neurologic**
  Abdominal epilepsy/migraine
- **Toxins**
  Aspirin
  Digitalis
  Erythromycin
  Iron
  Lead poisoning
  Steroids: gastritis/peptic ulcer; pancreatitis
  Theophylline
- **Vascular**
  Vasoocclusive: sickle cell; paroxysmal nocturnal hemoglobinuria
  Vasculitis: polyarteritis nodosa; giant cell arteritis; necrotizing arteritis; Wegener granulomatosis; Takayasu arteritis

Musculoskeletal pain is sharp and well localized. It is associated with exercise or position and is usually located along the ribs, the iliac crest, or the linea alba.

Recurrent episodes of obstruction can cause chronic abdominal pain. The onset is acute, and the pain is crampy, often periumbilical and accompanied by abdominal distension and occasionally by emesis. Radiographs of the abdomen will reveal air-fluid levels and large amounts of gas. In between episodes of obstruction the patient will be asymptomatic. Intussusception, adhesions, and malrotation causing volvulus can cause chronic pain. Chronic constipation is a form of obstruction that may not be evident in the history but can be diagnosed by physical examination. Left lower quadrant fullness and a full rectal vault on digital examination are strongly suggestive of the diagnosis.

Ovarian cysts can cause chronic pain, as can cystic teratoma of the ovary. The pain is in the lower quadrant and may show ascites or a mass. Ultrasound of the pelvis is often diagnostic.

Biliary etiologies such as obstruction, biliary dyskinesia, and an associated ductal divisium are rare causes of chronic abdominal pain. The pain is often in the left upper quadrant, is brought on by meals, and may radiate to the back. However, some biliary pain is nondescript.

Ureteropelvic junction obstruction can cause chronic abdominal pain. The pain occurs in distinct episodes with periumbilical, coliclike pain. Vomiting is often associated, although not in all cases. Serum laboratory tests show no kidney dysfunction. Diagnosis is made by ultrasound at the time of a pain episode.

Infection

Parasitic infections can become chronic. They are often associated with loose stools, bloating, nausea, and weight loss. *Giardia* usually presents as pain only. *Helicobacter,* a cause of gastritis and peptic ulcer disease, is often associated with chronic pain. The pain is located frequently in the epigastric area, but there are no components that confirm the diagnosis. Urinary tract infection, particularly in the young child, also may present as abdominal pain.

Inflammatory

Extraintestinal symptoms such as fever, weight loss, joint pain, and characteristic skin findings of erythema nodosum or pyoderma gangrenosa can be associated with the inflammatory bowel diseases. Colitis is usually found with diarrhea or blood loss. Crohn disease of the upper tract may have no alteration of bowel pattern. The pain is located in the lower abdomen, may be relieved by defecation, and may be associated with a mass effect in the abdomen.

Metabolic

Elevated lipids may be associated with abdominal pain. Frequently, biochemical evidence of pancreatitis accompanies the pain. The pain is located in the epigastric or periumbilical area and may radiate to the back. The pain of pancreatitis may be associated with emesis and abdominal distention. The episodes are distinct and last 1 to 3 days.

Maldigestion is the most frequent organic etiology of chronic abdominal pain. It is often associated with flatulence, diarrhea, and abdominal distension following the ingestion of the nondigestible sugar. Diet history, breath tests, and elimination diets can help distinguish this group of etiologies from functional pain.

Acute intermittent porphyria is a rare cause of chronic abdominal pain in the child or adolescent. It is associated with neurologic and psychologic changes that may be subtle. Most commonly seen in women, it often begins about the time of puberty. It may have an association with the menstrual cycle, because estrogen has an influence on hemoglobin synthesis. The symptoms may be induced by dieting or barbiturate, sulfonamide, or alcohol ingestion.

Neurologic

The pain of abdominal epilepsy or abdominal migraine is not specific in location, is episodic, and may be associated with a variety of neurologic symptoms. These associated symptoms include headache, dizziness, syncope, transient blindness, and memory loss. Sleep electroencephalogram findings include bursts of sharp waves or spikes arising from the temporal lobe. Diagnosis of abdominal epilepsy is supported by resolution with anticonvulsive therapy. Pain, often with nausea or vomiting is associated with migraine. There is suggestion that the pain may be due to delayed gastric emptying. It is difficult to diagnose and, like abdominal epilepsy, is supported by resolution with therapy. The diagnosis of abdominal migraine is controversial and not accepted by all authorities.

Toxins

Many substances can cause abdominal pain. Aspirin ingestion or nonsteroidal anti-inflammatory agents are frequently associated with abdominal pain. Steroids can induce gastritis and pancreatitis. Erythromycin alters intestinal motility. Theophylline, iron, and digitalis have all been associated with abdominal pain. Lead poisoning can have abdominal pain as an early symptom. Lead-induced colic (intermittent pain, constipation, and emesis) has been reported in levels as low as 60 mg/dL of whole blood. Increasing lead levels will lead to emesis, headache, weight loss, and encephalopathy. However, asymptomatic children can be seen with levels of lead as high as 250 mg.

Vascular

Chronic abdominal pain can occur with vasoocclusive diseases such as sickle cell, paroxysmal nocturnal hemoglobinuria, and the multiple forms of vasculitis including polyarteritis nodosa, giant cell arteritis, necrotizing arteritis, Wegener granulomatosis, and Takayasu arteritis.

DATA GATHERING

The importance of a complete history and physical examination cannot be overstressed. The patient should provide a detailed description of the pain including onset, duration, location, resolution, association with activity, and fre-

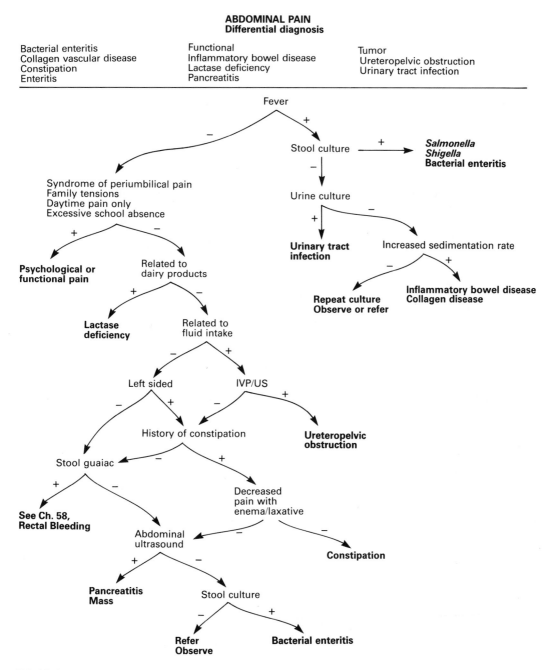

FIG 28-1

Decision tree for differential diagnosis of chronic abdominal pain.

quency of events. Often a pain diary can provide an accurate and complete description. Associated symptoms should be elicited, and attendance at school should be quantified (Fig. 28-1).

Physical examination must include a rectal examination and stool guaiac. The presence of associated physical findings may signal the proper diagnosis.

Laboratory examination should be directed by the physical examination. Important tests include a complete blood count, erythrocyte sedimentation rate, urinalysis, urine culture, stool for ova and parasites (3 samples).

If the history, physical, and laboratory examinations are consistent with functional abdominal pain, this should be considered a positive diagnosis. Therapy can be started for the functional pain without further workup. The goal of therapy should be to restore "normalcy" to the patient's life. The pain is real and often cannot be totally relieved. A concrete explanation of the pain and symptoms should be provided to the patient and parents. Behavioral modification to find and relieve stressors is necessary to lessen the pain. School attendance is mandatory but may require a gradual reintroduction if the child has fallen behind the peer group. Some success has been achieved with dietary manipulation including modified carbohydrates, high fiber, and bulk-producing agents. Drug therapy has not been proven effective and often reinforces the pain-reward cycle of behavior.

INDICATIONS FOR CONSULTATION OR REFERRAL

Although the evaluation and care of chronic abdominal pain can be done by the primary care physician, often the time allocation required results in a referral to a gastroenterologist. Behavioral therapy often will be optimized by consultation with a child psychiatrist or psychologist who is experienced with this entity. Good communication with the consultant is needed to ensure patient compliance and family cooperation.

DISCUSSION OF ALGORITHM

The thrust of the evaluation is to make a positive search for a psychologic cause of the pain, because this will be the final diagnosis in the majority of the cases. The physician should keep in mind a model of this pattern of history, physical examination, and family dynamics. If the patient's condition fits the description of chronic abdominal pain, a modest laboratory examination is necessary. If there are features of the pain that do not fit the description of chronic abdominal pain, then a more detailed evaluation is warranted. Abdominal ultrasonography has changed the approach to the workup because it allows for rapid return of information about the abdominal organs that may be the cause of the pain.

BIBLIOGRAPHY

Apley J: The child with abdominal pains, London, 1975, Blackwell Scientific Publications.

Boyle JT: Chronic abdominal pain. In Walker WA, Durie PR, Hamilton JR, Walker-Smith JA, Watkins JB, editors: *Pediatric gastrointestinal disease,* Philadelphia, 1991, BC Decker.

Chong SK, Lou Q, Asnicar MA, Zimmerman SE, Croffie JM, Lee CH, Fritgerald JF: *Helicobacter pylori* infection in recurrent abdominal pain in childhood: Comparison of diagnostic tests and therapy, *Pediatrics* 96:211–215, 1995.

Oster J: Recurrent abdominal pain, headache and limb pains in children and adolescents, *Pediatrics* 50:429–436, 1972.

Webster RB, DiPalma JA, Cremse DA: Lactose maldigestion and recurrent abdominal pain in children, *Dig Dis Sci* 40:1506–1510, 1995.

CHAPTER 29

Amenorrhea

Liana R. Clark

Menarche, a late event in puberty, normally occurs 2 to 2.5 years after breast budding and 1 year after the growth spurt. The average age of menarche in the United States is 12.8 years, with an age range of 9 to 16 years. By age 16 years, 95% of girls have reached menarche, and 98% have done so by age 18 years.

DIFFERENTIAL DIAGNOSIS

- **Primary Amenorrhea**
    - No breast development/absent uterus (rare)
        - Lack of testosterone
            - 17,20-desmolase deficiency
            - Agodadism
            - 17-α-hydroxylase deficiency with 46, XY karyotype
    - Breast development/absent uterus
        - Testicular feminization
        - Congenital absence of the uterus
    - No breast development/intact uterus
        - Hypogonotrophic hypogonadism
        - Gonadal dysgenesis
            - Turner syndrome and variants
            - Central nervous system lesions—craniopharyngioma, pituitary adenoma
            - Kallmann syndrome
            - Pituitary gonadotrophic deficiencies
                - Chronic diseases, anorexia
    - Normal breast development/intact uterus
        - Structural abnormality—imperforate hymen, disturbance of hypothalamic-pituitary axis (*see* secondary amenorrhea)
- **Secondary Amenorrhea**
    - Stress
    - Anorexia
    - Chemotherapy/radiation
    - Autoimmune disease
    - Exercise

Polycystic ovary syndrome
Ovarian failure
Pituitary lesions

Primary Amenorrhea

Primary amenorrhea, or delayed menarche, is defined as: 1) no episodes of spontaneous uterine bleeding by age 14 to 16 years with an absence of secondary sex characteristics or by age 16 to 18 years with normal secondary sex characteristics; and 2) absence of spontaneous uterine bleeding despite having attained sexual maturity rating 5 for at least 1 year or despite the onset of breast development 4 years previously.

Patients with primary amenorrhea can be divided into four groups based on their breast development and internal genitalia.

No Breast Development/Absent Uterus

The condition of no breast development with absent uterus is extremely rare. It is seen in genetic males (XY) whose gonads produce müllerian inhibiting factor but do not produce enough testosterone to induce development of male internal and external genitalia. Phenotypically these patients are female. This lack of testosterone is due to a gonadal enzyme deficiency or to early gonadal regression ("vanishing testes"). The most common causes are: 1) 17,20-desmolase deficiency; 2) agonadism, including no internal sex organs; and 3) 17-α-hydroxylase deficiency with 46 XY karyotype, whose clinical features include sexual infantilism, absent uterus, and hypertension. Laboratory assessment would include a karyotype, androgen levels, and gonadotropin levels. The karyotype will be male (XY). The testosterone levels are low, and the luteinizing hormone (LH) and follicle-stimulating hormone (FSH) levels are elevated.

Breast Development/Absent Uterus

There are two clinical syndromes which can produce the condition of breast development with absent uterus: testicular feminization and congenital absence of the uterus. Testicular feminization is a syndrome found in chromosomal males caused by an insensitivity to androgens. They have normal male gonads, which produce normal male levels of testosterone. However, there is a genetic X-linked defect in androgen receptor function with resultant end-organ insensitivity to androgen. The wolffian ducts fail to develop, and the external genitalia develop as female in the absence of testosterone stimulation. These male patients do produce müllerian inhibiting factor; therefore, the müllerian ducts regress and there is no development of female internal genitalia. Breast development occurs because of endogenous gonadal and adrenal estrogen unopposed by androgen. The patients have a female phenotype with normal breast development but a lack of axillary or pubic hair because of the androgen insensitivity. They have a blind vaginal pouch with absence of ovaries, uterus, and fallopian tubes.

Congenital absence of the uterus occurs in women with müllerian agenesis (Rokitansky-Küster-Hauser syndrome). This condition accounts for approximately 15% of cases of primary amenorrhea. These patients are phenotypically and chromosomally female but have anomalies in the development of their müllerian system. This condition accounts for the failure of the uterus and vagina to develop normally. The ovaries are present, and the patients' breast development is normal. They have both axillary and pubic hair. Their levels of sex steroids are within the normal female range. Women with this syndrome often have other associated abnormalities. Renal anomalies are found in 15% to 40% of patients, and vertebral anomalies occur in 12%.

No Breast Development/Intact Uterus

Patients in the category of no breast development with intact uterus have a functioning müllerian system but lack ovarian estrogen for normal breast development. The defect in ovarian estrogen production may be related to either the ovary, pituitary, or hypothalamus. Conditions in which the ovary fails to produce estrogen result in hypergonadotropic hypogonadism. The LH and FSH levels are elevated in an attempt to stimulate the ovary to produce estrogen. The most common condition causing hypergonadotropic hypogonadism is gonadal dysgenesis. Hypogonadotropic hypogonadism occurs when either the hypothalamus or pituitary fail to stimulate the ovary to produce estrogen. These conditions include central nervous system (CNS) lesions, Kallman syndrome, and pituitary gonadotropic deficiencies such as chronic diseases or anorexia nervosa.

Approximately 30% of primary amenorrhea is related to a genetic etiology. The types of gonadal dysgenesis include the 45,XO karyotype also known as *Turner syndrome,* other X chromosome variants, pure 46,XX or 46,XY gonadal dysgenesis, and gonadal enzyme deficiencies. These conditions result in failure of the ovaries to develop, leaving remnant fibrous bands called *gonadal streaks.* The most common form of gonadal dysgenesis is Turner syndrome (45,XO karyotype). These individuals have short stature, streak gonads, and sexual infantilism (absent breast development). Associated somatic abnormalities include web neck, short 4th metacarpals, cubitus valgus, and coarctation of the aorta. Individuals with other forms of gonadal dysgenesis that result in structural abnormalities of the X chromosome also have streak gonads and sexual infantilism. Long-arm deletions result in normal stature and no somatic abnormalities, but short-arm deletions cause a phenotype similar to Turner syndrome. Mosaicism (46,X/XX karyotype) causes short stature, somatic abnormality, and sexual infantilism, although 20% of these individuals will have spontaneous menses. Pure gonadal dysgenesis (46,XX karyotype) results in normal stature, streak gonads, and sexual infantilism. The 17-α-hydroxylase deficiency with 46,XX karyotype is an enzyme deficiency that causes hypergonadotropic hypogonadism. These individuals have normal stature, sexual infantilism, hypertension, and hypokalemia. Laboratory tests show an elevated progesterone, low 17-α-hydroxyprogesterone, and elevated serum deoxycorticosterone.

Individuals who have primary amenorrhea due to hypogonadotropic hypogonadism have normal ovaries but lack the hypothalamic or pituitary stimulation of the ovaries to produce estrogen. The FSH and LH levels will be low. Genetically and phenotypically these individuals are female, but they display sexual infantilism.

Lesions of the CNS can cause hypogonadotropic hypogonadism. The most common CNS tumors that cause primary amenorrhea are craniopharyngiomas and pituitary adenomas. Hypothalamic defects in gonadotropin releasing hormone (GnRH) production also will result in hypogonadotropic hypogonadism. These defects occur as a result of abnormal hypothalamic development. One particular syndrome, Kallmann syndrome, occurs when decreased GnRH production occurs in conjunction with anosmia and facial abnormalities. Hypogonadotropic hypogonadism also occurs in cases of chronic illnesses, psychogenic stress, anorexia nervosa, and excessive exercise.

Normal Breast Development/Intact Uterus

Individuals with normal breast development and intact uterus are phenotypically and chromosomally female. They have normal secondary sex characteristics and pubertal milestones. Generally the cause of the amenorrhea can be either a structural abnormality of the vaginal outflow tract or disturbances of the hypothalamic-pituitary-ovarian axis.

Imperforate hymen is a diagnosis that is usually made early in a child's life, but often it is first noted during the evaluation of primary amenorrhea. The patient may have a history of cyclical abdominal pain or may be asymptomatic. Examination reveals a bluish, bulging hymen distended with blood. This mass also can be palpated via rectovaginal examination. The repair of this condition can occur immediately on diagnosis. The finding of a complete transverse vaginal septum is very rare. The septum may be low or high in the vagina, but the external genital examination is usually normal. The vagina appears short, and a mass is palpable above the examining finger. Obstruction with a high transverse septum results in hematometra and endometriosis. Surgical correction of this condition also is necessary.

Disturbances of the hypothalamic-pituitary-ovarian axis that result in primary amenorrhea are identical to the disturbances that occur with secondary amenorrhea. The discussion of these disturbances will be found in the section on secondary amenorrhea.

Secondary Amenorrhea

Secondary amenorrhea occurs in girls who have established menstruation. It is defined as the absence of menses for 6 months or a length of time equal to three previous cycles. It is important to rule out the possibility of pregnancy before beginning an extensive evaluation of secondary amenorrhea.

Menses often are irregular in young girls who have recently begun menarche. The immaturity of the hypothalamic-pituitary-ovarian axis results in frequent anovulation and irregularity of the menstrual cycle. This immaturity usually resolved within 1 to 2 years of menarche. Amenorrhea that begins or persists 18 months after menarche should be investigated.

Stress also is common cause of hypothalamic amenorrhea. The stress causes a eugonadotropic hypogonadism. The LH and FSH levels are normal as is the response to GnRH. The stress may relate to school, family derangements, and peer relationships. Medications and drugs such as phenothiazines, contraceptive steroids, and heroin may cause amenorrhea as well by altering the GnRH secretory patterns.

A unique case of hypothalamic amenorrhea is caused by the polycystic ovary syndrome. This condition is the most common cause of amenorrhea in a postmenarcheal adolescent. This disorder is characterized by oligomenorrhea or amenorrhea, anovulation, infertility, hirsutism, and often obesity. In this condition the pituitary gland has a heightened response to GnRH and displays an exaggerated pulsatile release of LH. The LH levels are often tonically elevated or have an elevated LH:FSH ratio greater than 2 or 3:1. The high LH levels stimulate the ovary to produce androgen from the stromal tissue. The androgens are converted peripherally to estrone and estradiol. Estrogens that are secreted in this tonic manner rather than the usual cyclical pattern are believed to augment pituitary sensitivity to GnRH. This disorder can be diagnosed by the finding of LH:FSH ratio of 2:1 to 3:1, elevated free and/or total testosterone, and a normal to high dehydroepiandosterone sulfate (DHEA-S). A pelvic ultrasound in the older adolescent may reveal multiple small peripheral cysts in both ovaries.

Pituitary causes of secondary amenorrhea include nonneoplastic lesions such as Sheehan's syndrome, Simmonds' syndrome, aneurysm, or empty sella syndrome. Pituitary tumors such as pituitary adenoma or carcinoma also result in amenorrhea.

Premature ovarian failure is sometimes seen in adolescents. It is often associated with autoantibodies directed against ovarian tissue and also is found in association with thyroid or adrenal antibodies. This condition also can occur in individuals who received chemotherapy or radiation therapy for cancer. Patients with gonadal dysgenesis also can occasionally present with secondary amenorrhea. In this case, there may be enough ovarian tissue to cause menarche, but the gonad cannot continue this estrogen production, and ovarian failure results. Uterine synechiae (Asherman syndrome) cause the uterine lining to be unable to proliferate in response to estrogen. This condition will result in amenorrhea.

DATA GATHERING

History

The physician should determine the ages of the pubertal milestones such as breast development and the growth spurt. The neonatal history should include maternal ingestion of hormones that may cause clitoromegaly, birth weight, congenital anomalies, lymphedema (Turner syndrome), and neonatal problems suggestive of hypopituitarism such as hypoglycemia. The family history should include heights of all family members; age of menarche and fertility of sisters, mother, grandmothers, and aunts; and history of gonadal tumors and autoimmune disorders. Any history of surgery, irradiation, or chemotherapy should be noted. A review of systems should be performed to evaluate for chronic illness, abdominal pain, diarrhea, headaches, weight changes, eating disorders, medications, substance abuse, emotional stresses, competitive athletics, and neurologic symptoms.

The first step in assessing secondary amenorrhea should be a detailed assessment of the individual's nutritional status. Many cases of amenorrhea relate to weight loss or failure to gain weight. Because 17% body fat is required for menarche, and 22% body fat is required to have ovulatory cycles, it is important to determine whether the patient is in a nutritional state that would support menstruation. Has she lost weight or failed to gain weight in concordance with her growth? Amenorrhea is one of the presenting signs in adolescents with eating disorders and in those who are competitive athletes. Poor intake, malabsorption, and increased caloric requirements commonly occur in such chronic diseases as cystic fibrosis, sickle cell disease, renal disease, and inflammatory bowel disease. The history should include a diet history with an assessment of caloric intake, weight history with high and low weights, and level of exercise and activity.

Medical assessment should include questions related to chronic illnesses such as history of abdominal pain, diarrhea, headaches, visual changes, fevers, cold intolerance, galactorrhea, and medications being used. These symptoms can relate to many previously undiagnosed medical illnesses. Stress also may be an important factor in amenorrhea. Some patients who are having a prolonged stressful situation occur in their lives, such as being sent to boarding school, may experience prolonged amenorrhea. The causes of secondary amenorrhea relate to abnormalities of the hypothalamic-pituitary-ovarian axis.

Physical Examination

The physical examination should include height, weight (including percentiles), and vital signs. Sexual maturity ratings for breast and pubic hair should be noted. The breasts should be compressed gently to examine for the presence of galactorrhea. Examine closely for congenital anomalies, especially midline facial defects and the stigmata of Turner syndrome. Renal and vertebral abnormalities may be associated with müllerian malformations. The hair, skin, and genitalia should be assessed for evidence of hirsutism, including male hair patterns and clitoromegaly. A neurologic examination should include an assessment of the ability to smell, fundoscopic evaluation, and visual field testing.

The most important aspect of the pelvic examination is the assessment of the external genitalia. The labia majora and minora should be checked for adhesions. The patency of the hymen should then be determined. Digital examination should precede speculum examination to avoid injuring the patient with vaginal agenesis or an outflow obstruction. With the speculum, determine the presence of a normal vagina and cervix. Note the degree of estrogenization of the vaginal mucosa. The finding of a reddened, thin vaginal mucosa is consistent with estrogen deficiency, whereas pink, moist vaginal mucosa reveals appropriate estrogenization. Vaginal smears for degree of estrogenization can confirm this clinical appearance. Bimanual examination either via the vagina or rectovaginally, can determine the presence or absence of the uterus or ovaries. Pelvic ultrasound often is necessary for further delineation of these structures.

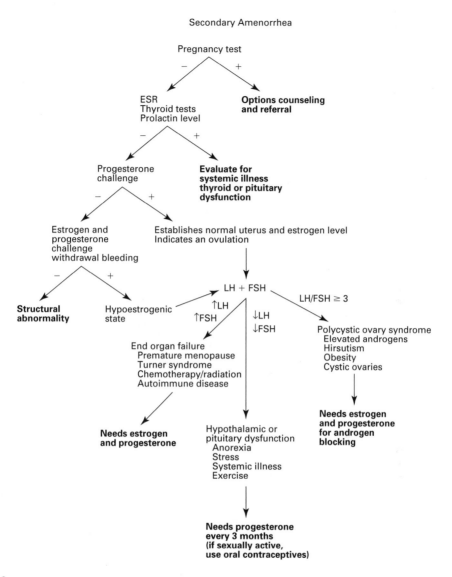

FIG 29-1
Decision tree for differential diagnosis of amenorrhea.

Patients with primary and secondary amenorrhea usually require consultation. The role of the primary care physician includes the organization of the initial workup and follow-up with care of the patient after diagnosis and treatment.

DISCUSSION OF ALGORITHM

It is important to rule out the possibility of pregnancy before beginning an extensive evaluation of secondary amenorrhea. If the pregnancy test is negative, tests should be done to rule out conditions such as hypothyroidism, chronic illness, and pituitary adenoma (Fig. 29-1). Thyroid function tests, erythrocyte sedimentation rate (ESR), and a prolactin level should be performed. It is important to measure prolactin even in the absence of galactorrhea because the majority of patients with elevated prolactin do not have galactorrhea. Often there will be mild elevations of prolactin due to stress, nipple stimulation, hypothyroidism, and certain medications. If the prolactin levels are consistently high, either a computerized tomography or magnetic resonance imaging scan should be performed to rule out a pituitary tumor. Thyroid tests will help determine the presence of hypo- or hyperthyroidism, and appropriate treatment can be started. The ESR often will help identify whether chronic rheumatologic conditions are present such as inflammatory bowel disease.

Progesterone Challenge

After ruling out these other conditions, the next step in the evaluation is the progesterone challenge. Exogenous progesterone given to an amenorrheic adolescent should result in a withdrawal bleeding after the agent is stopped. This withdrawal bleed has two purposes: 1) it establishes the presence of a normal uterus; and 2) it indicates that the uterus has been primed by endogenous estrogen, thus implying ovarian function. Medroxyprogesterone acetate (Provera®) is given in a dose of 10 mg daily for 7 to 10 days. If compliance is an issue, 200 mg of progesterone in oil can be given as a single intramuscular injection. The occurrence of bleeding 2 to 7 days after concluding the progesterone constitutes positive withdrawal bleeding and establishes the presence of anovulation.

If there is no withdrawal bleeding, either there is insufficient endogenous estrogen to prime the endometrium or the uterus is structurally abnormal. A combined estrogen-progestin regimen should then be given. If there remains no withdrawal bleeding, referral should be made for evaluation of Asherman's syndrome. This syndrome consisting of uterine synechiae may occur as a result of uterine instrumentation, trauma, or infection.

If there is withdrawal bleeding after the combined estrogen-progestin regimen, the adolescent can be assumed to be in a hypoestrogenic state. Serum gonadotropins should then be measured. High LH and FSH levels indicate ovarian failure (hypergonadotropic hypogonadism). This ovarian failure may be due to Turner's mosaicism or other chromosomal abnormality. It also may be caused by autoimmune disease, chemotherapy, or radiation. Low LH and FSH levels (hypogonadotropic hypogonadism) result from hypothalamic or pituitary causes of amenorrhea such as anorexia nervosa, systemic illness, or stress.

BIBLIOGRAPHY

Bacon GE, Spencer ML, Hopwood NJ, Kelch RP: *A practical approach to pediatric endocrinology,* ed 3, Littleton, 1990, Year Book Medical Publishers.

Coupey SM, Ahlstrom P: Common menstrual disorders, *Pediatr Clin North Am* 36(3):551–571, 1989.

Emans SJ, Goldstein DP: *Pediatric and adolescent gynecology,* ed 3, Boston, 1990, Little, Brown, and Co.

Golden NH, Shenker IR: *Amenorrhea in anorexia nervosa: Etiology and implications. Adolescent medicine: State of the art review,* Philadelphia, 1992, Hanley & Belfus.

Langman J: *Medical embryology,* ed 4, Baltimore, 1981, Williams & Wilkins.

Neinstein LS: *Adolescent health care: A practical guide,* Baltimore, 1991, Urban & Schwarzenberg.

Polaneczky MM, Slap GB: Menstrual disorders in the adolescent, *Pediatr Rev* 13(2):43–48, 1992.

Rosenfield RL: Puberty and its disorders in girls, *Endocrinol Metab Clin North Am* 20(1):15–42, 1991.

Speroff L, Glass RH, Kase NG: *Clinical gynecologic endocrinology and infertility,* ed 4, Baltimore, 1989, Williams & Wilkins.

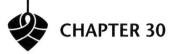

CHAPTER 30

Breast Enlargement

Paulo Ferrez Collett-Solberg
Jerrold S. Olshan
Thomas Moshang, Jr.

The differential diagnosis of breast enlargement ranges from normal changes, such as those seen during puberty or in the newborn, to manifestations of serious systemic illnesses. The purpose of this chapter is to act as a guide for differentiating between common pathologic and physiologic conditions resulting in breast enlargement (Fig. 30-1).

DIFFERENTIAL DIAGNOSIS

Causes of Breast Enlargement
- **Nonglandular breast enlargement**
  Trauma
  Infection, abscess
  Hematoma; lipoma; neurofibroma; lymphangioma
  Neoplasm (sarcoma, carcinoma)
  Obesity
- **Glandular breast enlargement**
  Girls
  Neonatal physiologic breast buds
  Estrogen ingestion
  Feminizing adrenal tumors
  Ovarian tumors (granulosa cell tumors)
  Ovarian cysts (McCune-Albright syndrome)
  Hypothyroidism
  Premature thelarche
  True central precocious puberty
  Boys (gynecomastia)
  Neonatal physiologic breast buds
  Estrogens ingestion
  Feminizing adrenal tumors
  Human chorionic gonadotropin producing tumor
  Testicular tumor

Adolescent gynecomastia
True hermaphroditism
Hypogonadism (Klinefelter syndrome; Kallmann syndrome; congenital or acquired testicular failure)
Thyrotoxicosis
Drugs (antiandrogens; chemotherapeutic agents; digitalis; cimetidine; spironolactone; ketoconazole; marijuana; etc.)
Androgen resistance syndromes
Increased peripheral tissue aromatase

Discussion
Overweight children commonly appear to have increased breast tissue without any real increase in actual glandular tissue, which can be easily mistaken for true glandular hyperplasia. Trauma with subsequent hemorrhage or fat necrosis, inflammation, infection, or other benign masses are common causes of nonglandular breast enlargement that may be mistaken for true increased breast tissue, and usually can be differentiated on thorough physical examination. Malignant neoplasms of the breast in children are exceedingly rare.

Breast enlargement is considered to be part of normal development in newborns and adolescents. Sixty percent to 100% of neonates of both sexes have some degree of physiologic breast hyperplasia. Although this hyperplasia usually lasts only 1 to 3 weeks, it may persist into the second year of life. The rich hormonal milieu in utero responsible for neonatal breast hyperplasia also may result in galactorrhea.

Enlargement of glandular breast tissue, in either sex, can result from increased circulating levels of estrogen or estrogenlike compounds from either endogenous or exogenous sources.

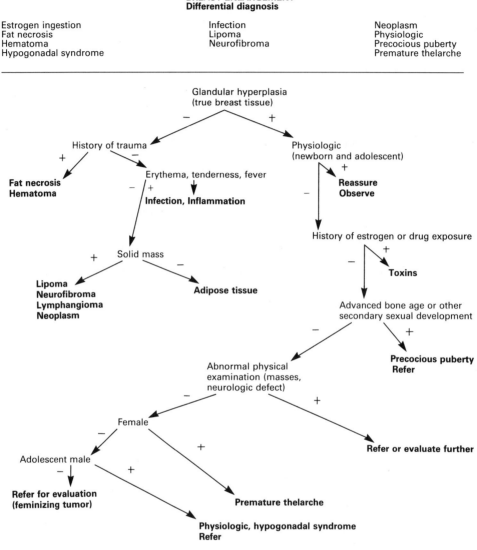

BREAST ENLARGEMENT
Differential diagnosis

Estrogen ingestion	Infection	Neoplasm
Fat necrosis	Lipoma	Physiologic
Hematoma	Neurofibroma	Precocious puberty
Hypogonadal syndrome		Premature thelarche

FIG 30-1
Decision tree for differential diagnosis of breast enlargement.

Endogenous hormones may be responsible in uncommon or rare conditions, such as feminizing tumors of the adrenal gland, liver, or gonads; whereas exogenous hormones can be found in a variety of estrogen-containing products (Box 30-1). Digitalis is thought to be an estrogen precursor and, as such, has effects similar to other estrogen-containing medications. In pubertal boys, drugs that decrease androgen activity, such as ketoconazole and spironolactone, which inhibit testosterone synthesis, or cimetidine, which inhibits androgen binding, can result in breast enlargement. Marijuana use has been linked with breast enlargement as well as galactorrhea. It is believed that other abused street drugs can result in breast enlargement.

In girls, breast development before the age of 8 years requires further investigation. The focus of the evaluation should be to identify girls with precocious puberty from those with the benign condition of premature thelarche (Fig. 30-2). The most common cause of early breast enlarge-

BOX 30-1
Toxins Associated with Breast Enlargement

Estrogens
Estrogen-contaminated food products
Oral contraceptive pills
Diethylstilbestrol
Topical estrogen creams
Digitalis
Antiandrogens
Ketoconazole
Spironolactone
Cimetidine
Hydroxyzine
Unknown mechanism
Isoniazid
Tricyclic antidepressants
Diazepam
Penicillamine
Cannabinoids (marijuana)

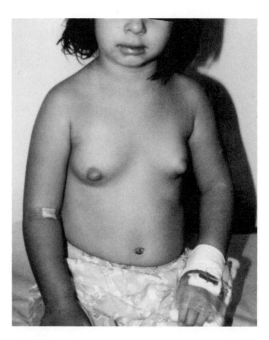

FIG 30-2
Isolated bilateral breast development of unknown cause. This patient has no other secondary sexual development.

ment is premature thelarche, which represents increased end-organ sensitivity to circulating estrogen levels. The estrogen exposure may be maternally derived (such as in breast milk) or possibly may be from exogenous hormones in foods. These girls are otherwise normal, have normal to slightly advanced bone age, and require no treatment. When breast development occurs accompanied by other pubertal changes such as growth spurt, maturation of gonadal-pituitary axis, and advancement of bone age it is considered precocious puberty (*see* Chapter 79). The varied etiology of precocious puberty is shown below. Idiopathic precocious puberty is the diagnosis in the vast majority of cases in this situation but central nervous system tumors can induce precocious production and release of gonadotropins. Hypothyroidism, as well, can cause elevated levels of gonadotropins by mechanisms still not clearly defined. McCune-Albright syndrome is characterized by bone lesions (polyostotic fibrous dysplasia), large café-au-lait skin lesions, and ovarian cysts with gonadotropin-independent production of estrogen.

Precocious Puberty Syndrome
- Idiopathic
- Central nervous system (neoplasms, infection, hydrocephalus)
- Neurofibromatosis
- McCune-Albright syndrome
- Hypothyroidism
- Gonadal tumor
- Congenital adrenal hyperplasia

In boys, breast development (gynecomastia) is due to elevated levels of estrogen or an abnormal ratio of estrogen to androgen levels. Aberrations from the normal ratios of estrogens to androgens may result from decreased testosterone production, decreased end-organ responsiveness to androgens, increased conversion of androgens to estrogen, or increased estrogen production. Adolescent gynecomastia or breast budding seen during puberty is the most common cause of breast enlargement in boys. More than 50% of boys aged 14 to 15 years have some degree of gynecomastia. This condition usually consists of bilateral, although frequently asymmetric, subareolar enlargement that is somewhat tender. In 90% of these adolescent boys, the breast tissue recedes within 2 years without therapy. Obesity may exaggerate the gynecomastia seen in pubertal boys from increased peripheral conversion of androgens to estrogen by excessive adipose tissue. Decreased testosterone production can be seen in any form of hypogonadism. With a frequency of roughly one in 600 live births, Klinefelter's syndrome (XXY) is one of the most common chromosomal abnormalities and is probably one of the more common causes of primary hypogonadism in men. In children with Klinefelter's syndrome often no abnormalities are noted until puberty, when there is evidence of testicular failure, with small testes and poor virilization. Approximately one third of these patients will develop gynecomastia, from both decreased levels of testosterone and increased levels of estrogens. The elevated luteinizing hormone levels in primary hypogonadism stimulates testicular aromatase activity causing increased androgen conversion to estrogen. In true hermaphroditism, in which patients have ovarian and testicular tissue, the elevated levels of estrogen produced by the ovarian tissue can cause gynecomastia. Hyperthyroidism causes increased levels of sex hormone–binding globulin and also increased production of adrenal androstenedione. The former results in decreased levels of free testosterone; the latter increases the substrate for peripheral aromatization to estrogens. The gynecomastia in patients with hyperthyroidism usually resolves with normalization of thyroid hormone levels.

Systemic illnesses such as cirrhosis, renal failure, or AIDS can cause gynecomastia in adolescent boys. In patients with cirrhosis, there is a decrease in the metabolism of estrogen and a decrease in the metabolism of androstenedione, providing extra substrate for estrogen production. In patients with renal failure there is a partial primary hypogonadism caused by the uremia. Testicular function usually returns to normal after renal transplantation but not after hemodialysis. The mechanism is not known in AIDS patients. Malnutrition or substance abuse may be related to the pathogenesis of gynecomastia in AIDS patients.

DATA GATHERING

History
Important information includes a detailed history of the duration of the breast enlargement, any associated signs or symptoms suggesting the onset of puberty, or findings suggestive of nonendocrine systemic illnesses. A careful history of possible trauma or drug ingestion also is important.

Physical Examination
The initial goal of the physical examination is to discern whether there is true glandular hyperplasia. The presence of true breast development is suggested by other findings of estrogenization, such as darkening of the areolar region, protrusion of the areola and nipple above the plane of the breast, or thickening of the vaginal mucosa. It is important to recognize premature breast budding from other breast masses, because surgical removal of breast buds will prevent breast development. Attention should be paid to height, weight, blood pressure, and presence of accompanying secondary sexual characteristics. In boys, determination of testicular volume is essential in assessing pubertal status. The patient should be evaluated for clinical signs of chronic illnesses, drug abuse, and other systemic illnesses, such as thyroid or liver disease.

Laboratory Evaluation
A careful history and physical examination often preclude the need for any further evaluation. Bone age, however, may aid in differentiation of premature thelarche from other disease entities; bone age is normal in premature thelarche and advanced in most cases of true estrogenization.

INDICATIONS FOR REFERRAL OR CONSULTATION

The vast majority of cases of breast enlargement can be dealt with appropriately at the primary care level. The following findings in children after the newborn period would raise concern: gynecomastia in a prepubertal boy, precocious puberty, significantly advanced bone age, or evidence of systemic or central nervous system disease. These children deserve a more complete evaluation, with further laboratory testing or referral.

A more complete endocrinologic evaluation would include determination of circulating levels of estradiol, testosterone, androstenedione, dehydroepiandrosterone, follicle-stimulating hormone, and luteinizing hormone. The new ultrasensitive assays for gonadotropins may indicate premature function of the pituitary-gonad axis. Assessment of the hypothalamic-pituitary axis with a gonadotropin-releasing hormone stimulation test would further clarify the pubertal status. Chromosomal analysis is necessary to exclude the diagnosis of Klinefelter's syndrome in the hypogonadal boy with elevated gonadotropin levels.

Pelvic ultrasonography can show cystic changes or enlargement of the ovaries that can be present during puberty and can be useful in assessing the developmental status of the ovary.

THERAPY

For the adolescent boy, in whom there is rarely pathologic breast enlargement, the psychologic and emotional concerns of the patient are of primary importance and require a dedicated physician to provide the reassurance necessary to support the patient over the usual several years needed for spontaneous regression of gynecomastia.

In other situations of breast enlargement, treatment is usually in the hands of an experienced pediatric endocrinologist and is initially directed toward treating the underlying condition to stop the progression of glandular hyperplasia. In the case of precocious puberty, for example, long-acting gonadotropin-releasing hormone analogues often are used.

In patients with breast enlargement secondary to systemic illnesses, such as renal failure or hyperthyroidism, therapy is directed at the primary illness. In renal failure, kidney transplant is more effective in correcting the hypogonadism than dialysis. In patients with primary hypogonadism, the replacement of testosterone with an improved estrogen:androgen ratio may reduce the gynecomastia in those patients. In other cases of recent-onset gynecomastia, a variety of antiestrogens and weak androgens have been tried, with varied success. Among these, testolactone is one of the more promising agents.

In long-standing breast enlargement, regardless of cause, the initial glandular hyperplasia is replaced by fibrosis and is unresponsive to any medical therapy. If there is enough enlargement to cause serious psychologic or cosmetic concern that cannot be dealt with by appropriate counseling, surgery is the only alternative.

BIBLIOGRAPHY

Braunstein GD: Gynecomastia, *N Engl J Med* 328(7):490–495, 1993.

Glass AR: Gynecomastia, *Endocrinol Metab Clin North Am* 23(4):825–837, 1994.

Kappy MS, Ganong CS: Advances in the treatment of precocious puberty, *Adv Pediatr* 41:223–261, 1994.

Mahoney CP: Adolescent gynecomastia—differential diagnosis and management, *Pediatr Clin North Am* 37(6):1389–1404, 1990.

Plotnick L, Mersey JH: A clinical moment with endocrinology and metabolism: Early breast development in female children, *Maryland Med J* 43(11):987, 1994.

Rosenfield RL: Normal and almost normal precocious variations in pubertal development, premature pubarche and premature thelarche revisited, *Horm Res* 41(suppl 2):7–13, 1994.

CHAPTER 31

Chest Pain

Steven M. Selbst

Chest pain, a fairly common complaint in pediatric practice, occurs in about one in every 300 children who see a doctor because of illness. The pain, often chronic and recurrent, may resemble the syndrome of chronic abdominal pain. Chest pain affects children of all ages, with the highest incidence occurring at age 12 to 13 years. In general, chest pain probably affects boys as often as girls. This chief complaint has considerable importance because it often causes great concern in the patient and family, who fear that the chest pain is a symptom of serious cardiac disease.

DIFFERENTIAL DIAGNOSIS

Common Causes of Chest Pain

- **Trauma**
    Hemothorax
    Pneumothorax
    Fracture
- **Infection**
    Pneumonia
    Upper respiratory tract infection
    Pericarditis
    Myocarditis
- **Toxin/environmental**
    Caustic ingestion
    Foreign body
    Drugs of abuse (cocaine)
- **Allergy–inflammatory**
    Pleurisy
    Costochondritis
    Asthma
    Lupus erythematosus
- **Tumor**
    Metastatic disease
- **Congenital**
    Mitral valve prolapse

    Anomalous coronary arteries
    Sickle cell disease
- **Multiple etiologies**
    Esophagitis
    Pulmonary embolus
    Anxiety
    Hyperventilation
    Arrhythmia
    Acute chest syndrome (sickle cell disease)
    Aortic dissection

The differential diagnosis of childhood chest pain is extensive. In addition to thinking of the problems classified by cause, another approach is to look at each organ system that may be involved in producing pain.

Organ System Involvement in Chest Pain
- **Musculoskeletal**
    Chest wall pain
        Trauma
        Hemothorax
        Pneumothorax
        Rib fractures
        Costochondritis
        Tietze syndrome
- **Gastrointestinal**
    Esophagitis
    Caustic ingestions
    Esophageal foreign bodies
- **Respiratory**
    Asthma
    Pneumonia
    Upper respiratory tract infection
    Pneumothorax
    Pleurisy (*eg,* secondary to systemic lupus erythematosus)
    Pulmonary embolus
- **Cardiac**
    Dysrhythmia
    Mitral valve prolapse

Myocardial infarction
Hypertrophic cardiomyopathy
Pericarditis
Myocarditis
Pneumopericardium
Ischemia (congenital heart disease)
Anomalous coronary arteries
Drugs of abuse (cocaine)
- **Psychogenic**
  Anxiety
  Hyperventilation
- **Miscellaneous**
  Breast tumor
  Sickle cell disease
  Vasoocclusive crisis
  Metastatic disease

Discussion

Studies have shown that young children (younger than 12 years of age) with chest pain are more likely to have cardiorespiratory problems and that older children (more than 12 years of age) are more likely to have psychogenic pain. The broad category of musculoskeletal problems is the most common cause of chest pain in pediatric practice. Usually due to overuse (strain) of chest wall muscles, this pain may occur following extensive exercise or minor trauma (as with wrestling or football) or from direct trauma to the chest, such as from automobile accidents that may result in hemothorax or pneumothorax. Less severe injuries can still cause rib fractures that will produce marked chest pain. In addition, costochondritis is a common cause of chest pain. The cause of this entity is not known, but it is believed that inflammation of the costochondral junctions produces chest pain.

Gastrointestinal problems have been known to cause chest pain because the esophagus is more pain-sensitive in its proximal portion. Esophagitis, or indigestion, often presents as chest pain and should be the presumed cause if there seems to be a definite relationship between the onset of pain and the consumption of certain foods. This pain is often described as a "burning sensation" and may be worse when the individual is in the recumbent position.

Respiratory disease also produces chest pain. Children with an exacerbation of asthma, pneumonia, or other upper respiratory tract infection may complain of intermittent chest pain. These problems are usually associated with coughing or fever, and, in fact, may be due again to overuse of chest wall muscles. Moreover, pneumothorax can cause sudden severe chest pain that is often associated with dyspnea and cyanosis. Such pneumothoraces may occur spontaneously (uncommon) or in association with cystic fibrosis, asthma, or trauma.

Parents and physicians are most concerned about cardiac disease when a child complains of chest pain, although it is an uncommon cause. Supraventricular tachycardia in an older child may cause sudden or intermittent chest pain or palpitations.

Cardiac problems are found in fewer than 5% of children with chest pain. Mitral valve prolapse has been found to cause chest pain in children; however, mitral valve prolapse is no more common in children with chest pain than it is in the general population (*see* Chapter 75).

A myocardial infarction is an exceedingly rare cause of chest pain in children. However, this may occur when anomalous coronary vessels exist. Adolescents who use cocaine may be at risk for myocardial infarction. Cocaine causes tachycardia, increased oxygen demand, hypertension, and coronary artery vasospasm. Children who have had Kawasaki disease may be at risk for future myocardial infarctions because of damage to coronary arteries.

Hypertrophic cardiomyopathy, an uncommon congenital problem that may cause anginalike pain, is often exacerbated by the Valsalva maneuver, which causes decreased venous return to the heart.

Finally, infections of the cardiac structures may cause chest pain. Of these, pericarditis usually precipitates chest pain that may be characterized as dull pressure or sharp pleuritic type pain or even referred to as anginalike pain. This pain seems to be relieved when the child sits up and leans forward. Pericarditis may be caused by a bacterial infection *(Staphylococcus aureus, Hemophilus influenzae, Neisseria meningitidis, Streptococcus pneumoniae)*, viral infection (coxsackievirus and echovirus), tuberculosis, or trauma. Concomitant fever, malaise, and diffuse myalgias are seen with pericarditis that is viral in origin. Pericarditis is often associated with a pericardial effusion. Similarly, myocarditis is most often caused by a virus, usually coxsackievirus B or echovirus. It is also seen secondary to mumps or infectious mononucleosis. With this infection, there is low-grade fever and intermittent, substernal, dull chest pain. Pleuritic type chest pain may be present if there is accompanying pericarditis. Within a few days, the patient with myocarditis may develop dyspnea and chest pain with exertion.

Psychogenic factors or anxiety are among the most common causes of chest pain in the pediatric age group. Many children with chest pain have school phobias, separation anxiety, or fear of illness in association with the symptom of chest pain. With such chest pain, hyperventilation may be obvious or signs of anxiety may be more subtle. Girls and boys are both susceptible to anxiety-induced chest pain, which accounts for approximately 10% of episodes of chest pain in children.

There are other miscellaneous causes of chest pain. For instance, a primary or metastatic intrathoracic tumor is a rare possibility. Also, some adolescent boys will complain of chest pain that is the result of physiologic breast hypertrophy and girls may complain about painful breast cysts. In addition, children with sickle cell disease may have a vasoocclusive crisis that causes chest pain and usually pain in other extremities. Of further interest is the finding that chest pain may be associated with cigarette smoking. One study of adults and adolescents indicated that chest pain was significantly more common in smokers than nonsmokers. This finding was true for all types of chest pain, regardless of coffee and alcohol consumption. More data are needed to assess the role of smoking as a factor in the development of chest pain but parental smoking has been associated with more frequent lower respiratory infections in children. Finally, studies found that in a large number of children (2% to 45%) a specific cause for chest pain could not be found despite a thorough evaluation.

DATA GATHERING

History

In evaluating the specific complaint of chest pain, one must first establish the *severity* of the pain. The primary care physician needs to know if the pain is severe enough to cause limitation of activity or, most notably, school absence. Information about the *frequency* and *duration* of the chest pain is also important. For instance, a child with constant or frequently occurring intermittent chest pain probably has a more serious

problem (not necessarily organic in etiology) than the child with one brief, mild episode of pain. Next, one needs to ascertain the *type* and *location* of the chest pain. This is sometimes difficult to assess because young children often cannot well describe or localize the pain sensation. However, a classic description of sharp, pleuritic chest pain that occurs intermittently and may be relieved by sitting up and leaning forward should lead one to consider pericarditis. Likewise, a "burning" sensation in the sternal area may suggest esophagitis. Furthermore, one needs to learn the *onset* of the chest pain. Chest pain that is acute in onset is more likely to have an organic etiology than pain that has been present for several months. Next, one should question the patient about precipitating factors.

Chest pain that is temporally related to eating meals or particular foods should lead one to consider esophagitis (reflux) as a cause of chest pain. Likewise, one should question the patient and family about any recent choking episodes, because foreign body ingestions may have been forgotten soon after the event. Similarly, it is extremely important to ask about possible trauma to the chest. Although major trauma or direct chest trauma is easily recalled, a history of recent strenuous exercise is often overlooked. Such activity could easily cause chest wall pain as well as rib fractures or more serious injuries such as pneumothorax. Other *precipitating factors* such as anxiety must be questioned. Because chest pain in children is often a manifestation of unrelated stress, it is important to uncover the presence of school phobias, sleep disturbances, and other somatic complaints or the presence of family turmoil that may be temporally related to the onset of chest pain. Teenage girls need to be specifically questioned about the likelihood that they are pregnant, because this may occasionally be the stressful situation that is manifesting itself as chest pain. An adolescent girl should also be asked about the use of birth control pills, which are rarely linked to pulmonary embolism. Any adolescent with sudden onset of pain should be questioned about the possible use of drugs such as cocaine. Chest pain that occurs with exercise may be related to asthma or cardiac pathology.

Although chest pain in children does not have the same ominous prognosis as in adults, the complaint must be taken seriously. One study has found that almost half the children with "psychogenic chest pain" had a positive family history for chest pain. Also, because some congenital problems may be inherited, it is important to find out about heart disease in the patient's family. A previous history of known heart disease in the patient may suggest that the chest pain reflects exacerbation of the long-standing problem. History of smoking in the patient and family may be important.

Finally, a review of systems is needed to see if there are *associated complaints* that may imply that the patient's chest pain is part of a systemic illness, such as infection, collagen vascular disease, acute rheumatic fever, Kawasaki disease, and sickle cell disease. Fever, malaise, and myalgia may indicate that an infection such as pericarditis or myocarditis is responsible for the chest pain. Similarly, an associated cough would lead one to consider pneumonia, asthma, or an upper respiratory tract infection. In addition, chest pain that is associated with palpitations, syncope, or lightheadedness is more often due to anxiety or mitral valve prolapse. One needs to know what treatment has been tried previously and which medicines, positions, or therapeutic regimens seem to relieve the child's chest pain. For example, chest pain that resolves regularly when the child is allowed to sleep with his/her parents suggests an emotional problem.

Physical Examination

It is important to distinguish hyperventilation from true dyspnea so that proper referral and treatment can be instituted. Such hyperventilation is often accompanied by carpopedal spasm, acral paresthesias, headache, and lightheadedness. A general examination may be quite helpful in detecting the cause of the chest pain. For instance, poor growth or cyanosis may suggest serious underlying disease. Also, a rash or joint swelling may indicate the existence of a collagen vascular disease with secondary chest pain. Likewise, the abdominal examination is important, and, at least in one series of chest pain, examination of a teenager's abdomen revealed a large mass that was determined to be an unsuspected uterine pregnancy. Similarly, skin bruising elsewhere on the patient may give a clue to previously inapparent chest trauma. In addition, one should concentrate on additional signs of anxiety during the examination (*eg*, excessive hand wringing, muscle tightness, tics). Although these signs may reflect only the fear of examination, at times they may indicate an underlying stressful situation at home.

Finally, it is necessary to concentrate on examination of the chest itself. Inspection may reveal evidence of trauma or asymmetry due to underlying heart disease or scoliosis. Auscultation may reveal significant cardiac murmurs, tachycardia, or dysrhythmias, or perhaps an apical nonejection systolic click indicating mitral valve prolapse. Also, a friction rub at the left sternal border may suggest pericarditis and muffled heart sounds may suggest an effusion. Moreover, asymmetric breath sounds may indicate a pleural effusion, pneumonia, or, rarely, an intrathoracic tumor. Rales or wheezing implies lower airway disease. Palpation of the chest is useful because musculoskeletal chest pain is frequently reproducible by palpation or movement. For instance, pain induced by palpation of the costochondral junctions is characteristic of costochondritis. This should be distinguished from the extremely rare condition known as Tietze syndrome in which there is actual swelling and tenderness of the costochondral junction. Also, if a pneumothorax is present, subcutaneous emphysema may be palpable at the upper chest or neck.

Laboratory Evaluation

For most children with chest pain, laboratory tests rarely provide positive information to make a diagnosis. Rather, such tests confirm clinical suspicions from the history or physical examination. However, a chest radiograph is indicated if fever is present or if significant trauma has occurred. A chest radiograph is also useful if signs or symptoms suggest cardiac disease or pulmonary pathology, but this is not a useful procedure in diagnosing muscle overuse syndromes or costochondritis.

An electrocardiogram (ECG) may be quite helpful if the results of the history or physical examination suggest an arrhythmia or if chest pain is triggered by exertion. It may also provide confirming evidence of pericarditis if marked elevation of the ST segment is noted or evidence of effusion if there is decreased voltage present. Moreover, an ECG that shows T-wave inversion in the inferior leads may suggest mitral valve prolapse, especially if the results of the history and physical examination are consistent with this. An ECG will indicate the rarely occurring myocardial infarction or strain.

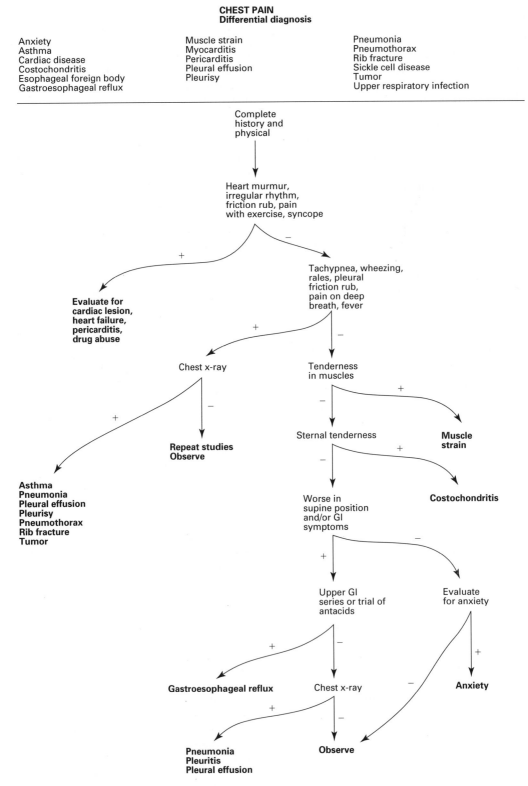

FIG 31-1

Decision tree for differential diagnosis of chest pain.

Additional laboratory tests are rarely needed and should only be ordered if specifically indicated. A complete blood count (CBC) may reveal anemia in the child with tachycardia and palpitations.

A CBC and sedimentation rate may be useful if an infection is suspected but are not of value with common conditions like costochondritis or asthma. A drug screen should be considered in any adolescent with acute severe pain. Finally, most chest pain from esophagitis does not require documentation with radiographs or more invasive studies.

INDICATIONS FOR CONSULTATION OR REFERRAL

Once the cause of chest pain has been established, treatment can be appropriately begun. For the most part, this includes only therapy aimed at relieving symptoms. Heat, analgesics, and rest will suffice for the very common musculoskeletal problems discussed earlier. Likewise, antacids are usually effective for gastrointestinal inflammation with referred chest pain. Antibiotics or bronchodilators may be required if lower airway disease is determined. A pleural effusion should be aspirated while the patient is in the office (or by a consultant) for diagnosis and relief of symptoms.

The rare child in acute severe distress with dyspnea or cyanosis or evidence of major trauma should be immediately referred to an emergency department. Supplemental oxygen may be useful enroute. Also, one should arrange for a hospital admission and rapid referral if a pericardial infection or effusion is suspected. Such an effusion should be aspirated for diagnostic purposes during echocardiography. Likewise, if any evidence of cardiac disease is found at the time of initial evaluation, elective further workup by a pediatric cardiologist would be appropriate. This should include children with chest pain on exertion or those with related syncope, dizzi-

ness, or palpitations. Finally, children found to have significant stress can usually be treated by the primary care physician. However, occasionally chest pain is only a minor symptom of major underlying psychopathology, and referral to an appropriate specialist for counseling would be indicated in these cases.

The child with "idiopathic chest pain" requires additional consideration. There is no evidence that a chest radiograph would be useful for such a patient if the results of the history and physical examination are not revealing. Extensive laboratory tests do not seem to be worthwhile or justified, although an ECG may provide some useful information or reassurance. Certainly, such patients require follow-up care and reevaluation because many have persistent chest pain for several months or years.

Most children and their parents can be reassured that chest pain does not have an ominous prognosis. Long-term follow-up data implies there is little reason to believe that serious cardiac or pulmonary disease will be eventually found if not immediately apparent. However, persistent chest pain may indicate underlying stress or organic disease (such as asthma). Thus the complaint should never be dismissed lightly.

DISCUSSION OF ALGORITHM

A "decision tree" for differential diagnosis of chest pain is presented in Figure 31-1. First, determine if the patient is experiencing acute distress; if so the patient needs emergency care. If there are no major airway problems, the patient should be screened for cardiac problems, pulmonary infection, gastric reflux, or systemic disease. Many patients who have chest pain are under emotional stress, and a careful history of psychosocial concerns may help to make this diagnosis. Still, in one third of patients the evaluations may not yield a diagnosis; these patients need to have close follow-up and be treated symptomatically.

BIBLIOGRAPHY

Asnes R, Santulli R, Bemporad J: Psychogenic chest pain in children, *Clin Pediatr* 20:788–791, 1981.

Brown RT: Recurrent chest pain in adolescents, *Pediatr Ann* 20:194–199, 1991.

Driscoll DJ, Glicklich LP, Gallen WJ: Chest pain in

children: A prospective study, *Pediatrics* 57:648–651, 1976.

Knapp JF, Dowd MD, Tarantino C, Borders V: Case 02-1994: A tall thin 15 year old male with chest pain, *Pediatr Emerg Care* 10:117–120, 1994.

Pantell RH, Goodman BW Jr: Adolescent chest pain, *Pediatrics* 71:881–887, 1983.

Selbst SM: Chest pain in children, *Am Fam Phys* 41:179–186, 1990.

Selbst SM, Ruddy R, Clark BJ: Chest pain in children—follow up of patients previously reported, *Clin Pediatr* 29:374–377, 1990.

Selbst SM, Ruddy RM, Clark BJ, et al: Pediatric chest pain: A prospective study, *Pediatrics* 82:319–323, 1988.

Wien SL, Sabath R, Ewing L, Gowdamarajan R, Portnoy J, Scagliotti D: Chest pain in otherwise healthy children and adolescents is frequently caused by exercise-induced asthma, *Pediatrics* 90:350–353, 1992.

Woodward GA, Selbst SM: Chest pain secondary to cocaine use, *Pediatr Emerg Care* 3:153–154, 1987.

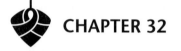

CHAPTER 32

Constipation

Steven M. Altschuler
Maria R. Mascarenhas

Constipation occurs in 5% to 10% of children. Normal defecatory patterns may range from several bowel movements each day to one movement every few days. The diagnosis of constipation is dependent on a history of difficulty passing stools, pain on defecation, a decrease in frequency of passing stools, or the passage of hard stools.

DIFFERENTIAL DIAGNOSIS

Common Causes of Constipation
- **Functional constipation**
- **Anatomic abnormalities**
  Ectopic anus
  Anteriorly displaced anus
  Rectoperineal fistula
  Congenital anal stenosis
- **Inflammatory conditions**
  Proctitis
  Anal fissure

- **Extrinsic lesions causing rectal compression**
  Abscess
  Neoplasm
- **Intrinsic colonic motor disease**
  Hirschsprung disease
- **Extrinsic neurologic disorders**
  Myelomeningocele
  Spinal injury or tumor
- **Metabolic and endocrine disorders**
  Hypothyroidism
  Diabetes mellitus
- **Drugs**
  Opiates
  Phenothiazines

Discussion
In the majority of cases, the cause of constipation is functional or acquired. Functional constipation frequently occurs in infancy after dietary manipulations, such as early introduction of solid food, excessive intake of cow's milk, or a switch from breast feeding to formula feeding.

A history of fussiness, colic, or excessive gas is frequently elicited in addition to the usual symptoms of difficulty passing stool, pain on defecation, or decreased frequency of passing stools. Constipation with the resultant passage of large, hard stool also may lead to fissure formation and result in blood streaking on the outside of the formed stool. The pain from the fissures then can contribute to additional constipation.

During the period of toilet training, constipation may become chronic and lead to impaction and secondary encopresis (fecal soiling). Fecal soiling in a previously toilet-trained child may be the first symptom of severe long-standing constipation. The presence of secondary encopresis also implies there is fecal impaction and abnormal colonic function from chronic constipation and distention. Parents may interpret encopresis as chronic intermittent diarrhea or as a child's weapon in a psychologic conflict.

Important historical information includes urinary frequency, abdominal pain and distention, anorexia, and irritability. The physical examination will frequently reveal abdominal distention, a tubular mass arising in the left pelvis and following the anatomic course of the colon, and normal anal sphincter tone and a dilated rectal vault with a large, soft fecal impaction on digital examination. Treatment of encopresis requires long-term therapy to reverse the chronic distention and return to normal function.

Besides a functional cause, the differential diagnosis of constipation includes a number of organic and anatomic abnormalities. These far less common disorders are conveniently divided into local and anatomic abnormalities, intrinsic colonic motor disorders, and extrinsic neurologic disorders.

Local anatomic abnormalities that may present with constipation include an ectopically placed anus, congenital anal stenosis, rectoperitoneal fistula, external rectal compression from an abscess or neoplasm, and proctitis or colitis. The intrinsic anal rectal abnormalities usually present in early infancy. In fact, they may be evident in the immediate newborn period. These abnormalities may be subtle, thus they can be overlooked unless specifically sought.

Constipation as a result of extrinsic lesions and inflammatory conditions usually occurs in the older child and adolescent. Usually acute in onset, there frequently is a change in stool caliber. When colitis or proctitis is the underlying cause, there may be rectal bleeding without an external anal fissure.

The classic intrinsic colonic motor disorder is Hirschsprung disease, a congenital aganglionosis. The colon in Hirschsprung disease is characterized by an area of transition from normal bowel containing ganglia to aganglionic bowel. The child with Hirschsprung disease usually has a history of constipation from birth. In most patients the disease is diagnosed within the first month of life. Clinical findings in these patients include abdominal distention, bilious vomiting, and failure to pass meconium in the first 24 hours of life. Radiologic evaluation (ie, barium enema) will frequently reveal evidence of intestinal obstruction.

The infant or child with Hirschsprung disease will have a history of intermittent abdominal distention, failure to have a bowel movement without the aid of an enema or laxative, and no history of stool withholding. Encopresis does not occur because the aganglionic segment is at a state of tonic detraction, thus preventing leakage. At the time of the physical examination, the infant or child has abdominal distention and an empty rectum and an apparently long, tight internal sphincter on rectal examination. Thus the history and physical examination are very helpful in distinguishing Hirschsprung disease from functional constipation.

Extrinsic neurologic disorders such as myelomeningocele, spinal injury, or tumors cause constipation by interfering with extrinsic intestinal innervation. The onset of constipation may occur prior to the occurrence of more classic neurologic symptoms. Physical examination may reveal changes in anal sphincter tone, evidence of neurogenic bladder, and subtle changes in lower extremity strength and reflexes.

INDICATIONS FOR CONSULTATION OR REFERRAL

Because most cases of constipation occur as a functional disorder, very few patients require referral to subspecialists or admission to an inpatient facility. Functional constipation (unless complicated by fecal impaction, encopresis, or long-standing duration) can be handled in the outpatient setting. Therapy for constipation includes 1) disimpaction; 2) bowel training; 3) high-fiber diet; and 4) laxatives.

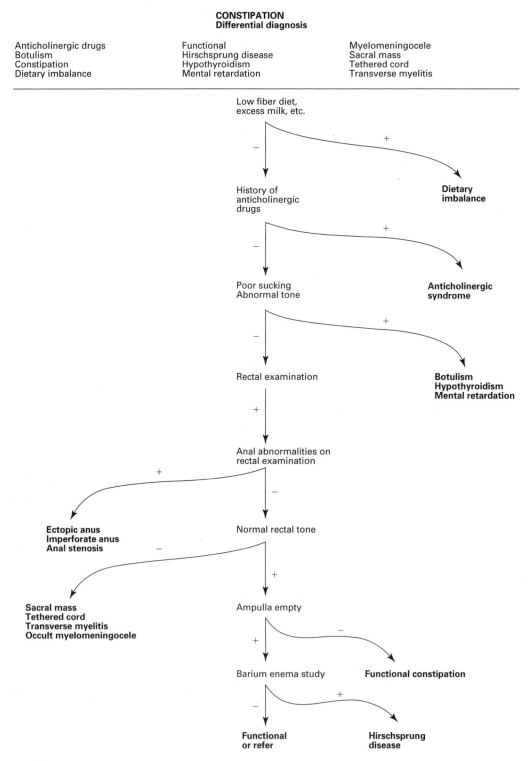

CONSTIPATION
Differential diagnosis

Anticholinergic drugs
Botulism
Constipation
Dietary imbalance

Functional
Hirschsprung disease
Hypothyroidism
Mental retardation

Myelomeningocele
Sacral mass
Tethered cord
Transverse myelitis

Low fiber diet,
excess milk, etc.

History of
anticholinergic
drugs

Dietary
imbalance

Poor sucking
Abnormal tone

Anticholinergic
syndrome

Rectal examination

Botulism
Hypothyroidism
Mental retardation

Anal abnormalities on
rectal examination

Ectopic anus
Imperforate anus
Anal stenosis

Normal rectal tone

Sacral mass
Tethered cord
Transverse myelitis
Occult myelomeningocele

Ampulla empty

Barium enema study   Functional constipation

Functional
or refer

Hirschsprung
disease

FIG 32-1

Decision tree for differential diagnosis of constipation.

Disimpaction

Enemas are included in the treatment protocol to relieve fecal impactions within the rectum. The patient should receive enemas daily for 3 days. On the first day, an adult-size mineral oil enema is given. The next 2 days, adult-size Fleet enemas are given. Parents should be instructed to have children retain enemas for 15 to 20 minutes. Removal of the fecal impactions will immediately end episodes of encopresis.

Administration of a polyethylene glycol solution orally or via a nasogastric tube may be used for disimpaction if enemas fail. However, intestinal obstruction needs to be ruled out prior to its use.

Bowel Training

This part of the program emphasizes bowel retraining. Parents should be instructed to have the child sit on the toilet twice a day for 10 to 20 minutes. Care should be taken to ensure that the child is comfortable and can place his/her feet flat on the floor. Optimal times for toilet sitting are usually in the morning and evening after meals. After the child has had a bowel movement or after 20 minutes, toilet sitting time should be considered over. Over time, daily toilet sitting will develop as a routine.

High-Fiber Diet

A high-fiber diet is instituted to add bulk to the daily diet and thus increase bowel peristalsis. Episodes of bowel spasm and the accompanying pain will also decrease in frequency. In general, fluids should be encouraged in the diets, but milk, apple juice, and tea should be limited to about two 8-oz glasses each day.

Laxative

A nonstimulating laxative is generally used in constipated children. Kondremul, a mixture of mineral oil and Irish moss, acts as a lubricant and bulk-forming agent. This medication softens stools and prevents stool withholding. The initial dose should be 1 to 3 tbsp/day. If there is no response within 4 days, the dose should be increased to effect a response. This dose should be maintained until a leakage of oil occurs or regular bowel movements have occurred for 1 month. Kondremul may decrease the absorption of fat-soluble vitamins, therefore, a multivitamin should be taken while the medication is being received. Alternatively, mineral oil can be used. Lactulose, a nonabsorbed carbohydrate, is frequently used as a stool softener. It acts as a bulk-forming agent. The initial dose is 1 to 3 tbsp/day and can be titrated according to the response. If diarrhea or increased gas occur, the dose needs to be decreased. It is the medication of choice in patients who have the potential of aspirating.

Failure of this regimen generally occurs when the initial "cleanout" with enemas has been ineffective. Occasionally, a constipated child will have to be admitted to the hospital for a closely supervised initial cleanout.

DISCUSSION OF ALGORITHM

An algorithm for the differential diagnosis of constipation is presented in Figure 32-1. The major problems underlying constipation include functional constipation, neurologic defect, Hirschsprung disease, and local problems. First, the rectal area is examined for fissures, fistulae, or abscesses. Next, a rectal examination will detect decreased tone that indicates a problem in the S2–4 innervation. If present, a comprehensive neurologic examination is needed. Otherwise, Hirschsprung disease should be considered. These patients have abdominal distention, poor weight gain, and empty ampulla on rectal examination. For those remaining patients who do not have bleeding, are taking no medication that contains atropine, and may have had decreased bulk or fiber in their diet, a diagnosis of functional constipation can be made.

BIBLIOGRAPHY

Benninga MA, Buller HA, Taminiau JA: Biofeedback training in chronic constipation, *Am J Dis Child* 68:126, 1993.

Clayden GS: Management of chronic constipation, *Arch Dis Child* 67:340, 1992.

Hatch TF: Encopresis and constipation in children, *Pediatr Clin North Am* 35:257–280, 1988.

Loening Baucke V: Factors determining long term outcome in children with chronic constipation and fecal soiling, *Gut* 30:999, 1989.

Seth R, Heyman MB: Management of constipation and encopresis in infants and children, *Gastro Clin North Am* 23:621–636, 1994.

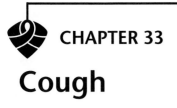

CHAPTER 33

Cough

Robert W. Wilmott

Cough, one of the most common symptoms in pediatrics, has many causes. Recurrent or chronic cough should always be evaluated for underlying conditions such as asthma, sinus disease, or cystic fibrosis, because most normal children do not cough except when they have a respiratory tract infection. Persistent cough is always abnormal in infants and should lead to a search for underlying causes such as cystic fibrosis, gastroesophageal reflux, congestive heart failure, or chlamydial infection. A chronic cough can be defined as one that has lasted for more than 8 weeks, although it may be appropriate to be concerned about a cough that has lasted 3 weeks or more, especially in an infant.

Common Causes of Cough
- **Trauma**
  Foreign body in tracheobronchial tree
- **Infection**
  Pneumonia
  Pharyngitis
  Laryngitis
  Sinusitis
  Pertussis
  Parapertussis
  Influenza
  Tuberculosis
- **Toxin**
  Hydrocarbon ingestion
  Tobacco

  Woodburning stove
- **Inflammatory**
  Asthma
  Allergy
- **Metabolic/genetic**
  Cystic fibrosis
- **Circulatory**
  Congestive heart failure
- **Multiple etiologies**
  Psychogenic
  Gastroesophageal reflux
  Bronchopulmonary dysplasia

Uncommon Causes of Cough
- **Trauma**
  Foreign body in ear or esophagus
- **Infection**
  Pneumocystis
  Cytomegalovirus
  Visceral larva migrans
  Schistosomiasis
  Psittacosis
  Mycosis
  Humidifier fever (protozoa)
  Rickettsiae
  Hydatid cyst
- **Immunologic**
  AIDS
  Congenital immune deficiency
  Vasculitis
  Sarcoidosis

Wegener granulomatosis
- **Tumor**
  T-cell leukemia
  Teratoma
  Lymphoma
- **Congenital**
  Tracheoesophageal fistula
  Vascular ring
  Laryngomalacia
  Bronchogenic cyst
  Pulmonary sequestration
  Pulmonary lymphangiectasia
  Immotile cilia syndrome
- **Multiple Etiologies**
  Bronchiectasis

DIFFERENTIAL DIAGNOSIS

Asthma is the most common cause of chronic cough in children, and wheezing may be unrecognized by parents. The term *cough variant asthma* is used to describe asthma in which coughing is the main complaint. Asthma is relatively common; 8% to 10% of schoolchildren have recurrent coughing and wheezing consistent with this diagnosis (*see* Chapter 102). Other symptoms of asthma include nocturnal coughing and coughing or wheezing after exercise, after laughing, or when exposed to cold air. Physical examination may reveal that the patient has a barrel deformity of the chest from gas trapping or a Harrison sulcus (depression) around the lower chest. The diagnosis of asthma is supported if the chest radiograph shows gas trapping or peribronchial thickening.

Inhalation of a foreign body is a common cause of persistent coughing in children. For example, a young child may choke on a small toy or food such as a peanut or candy, and older children sometimes inhale objects that have been held in the mouth, such as a pen top. A foreign body lodged in the airway usually causes persistent coughing, but there may be no symptoms unless secondary infection develops. Fixed, localized wheezing suggests the diagnosis of an inhaled foreign body, which may require evaluation with bronchoscopy. A retained foreign body or impacted cerumen in the ear also may cause reflex coughing because of stimulation of Arnold's nerve, a sensory branch of the trigeminal nerve.

Infection of the respiratory tract at any level may cause coughing. Pharyngitis is also associated with fever, sore throat, and local erythema. It is usually caused by a viral infection such as parainfluenza, influenza, or adenovirus, although it may be caused by bacteria such as β-hemolytic *Streptococcus* or occasionally by *Staphylococcus aureus*.

Laryngitis is similar in many ways to pharyngitis, except the cough is more noticeable and harsher and the child may lose his/her voice. Supraglottic infection with *Hemophilus influenzae,* or more recently group A streptococcus, can produce acute epiglottitis. Coughing is not a major symptom of this disease, in which rapid onset of toxicity, severe inspiratory stridor, drooling, and sore throat are typical. Inspiratory stridor and coughing are also features of acute laryngotracheobronchitis (croup). Croup is usually caused by parainfluenza, influenza, or respiratory syncytial virus. There is a prodromal upper respiratory tract infection and a harsh, barking cough. The inspiratory stridor and respiratory distress of this disease may not become apparent for 1 or 2 days, usually occurring during the night. Laryngitis does not require specific evaluation unless it persists. Croup may be difficult to distinguish from acute epiglottitis. Lateral radiographic examination of the neck is indicated in children with persistent stridor of acute onset to rule out epiglottitis, which causes a characteristic "thumb sign" due to swelling of the epiglottis and aryepiglottic folds. Patients with severe obstruction should be transferred to a pediatric center for evaluation and consideration of intubation or tracheostomy. In such cases, it is usually best to avoid delaying the referral to obtain studies such as a lateral neck radiograph and to arrange an attended transport as quickly as possible.

Pneumonia produces consolidation of the alveolar spaces and infiltration of the alveolar septae. Fever, respiratory distress, and symptoms of systemic toxicity are found in association with coughing, which is more noticeable in the early stages. Viral pneumonia is more common than bacterial pneumonia in young children. Infants are especially prone to infection with cytomegalovirus and adenovirus. Viruses account for the majority of cases in school-aged children, but pneumonia due to pneumococcus or *Mycoplasma pneumoniae* is more common than in infants. Other causes of pneumonia include *Chlamydia* in infants and pertussis in unimmunized children. The clinical diagnosis of pneumonia is confirmed by the demonstration of consolidation on the chest radiograph, and the specific cause may be sought with appropriate cultures, demonstration of the antigen by ELISA methods, or rapid diagnosis by DNA testing.

Cystic fibrosis is an important cause of persistent coughing. Typical symptoms are recurrent respiratory infection, poor weight gain, wheezing, coughing, and large foul-smelling bowel movements containing excess fat. The diagnosis should also be considered in any child who develops nasal polyps or rectal prolapse. Physical examination in untreated cases may reveal finger clubbing, barrel-shaped deformity of the chest, and signs of poor nutrition. Children with such symptoms should undergo a sweat test.

Bronchopulmonary dysplasia is a chronic lung disease that develops in premature infants who have had mechanical ventilation. The characteristic symptoms are tachypnea, coughing, wheezing, and blue spells from either severe bronchospasm or collapse of the large airways due to an acquired weakness of the airway wall. Physical examination may reveal intercostal retractions and persistent respiratory distress, barrel-shaped deformity of the chest, expiratory wheezes, inspiratory crackles, and poor physical growth. The chest radiograph characteristically shows emphysema, with areas of consolidation, atelectasis, and focal hyperaeration. The diagnosis of bronchopulmonary dysplasia is usually readily apparent from the history; however, sometimes the presence of blue spells can lead to the consideration of other causes, such as gastroesophageal reflux, seizures, and idiopathic apnea.

Chronic sinusitis is difficult to define in children. Typical symptoms are chronic nasal obstruction, persistent nasal discharge, facial pain (or tenderness), and a trickle of infected mucus from the nasopharynx down the posterior pharyngeal wall, associated with a recurrent cough that is especially bad at night. Examination of the throat may reveal mucopurulent secretions or granular mucosa on the posterior pharyngeal wall. Children with chronic sinusitis demonstrate mucosal thickening, air-fluid levels, or opacification on radiographs of the sinuses and appear to have chronic low-grade sinus infection. Many such children also have allergies, which predispose them to infection. Chronic sinusitis is therefore sometimes difficult to distinguish from asthma, with which it may be associated.

Cigarette smoking should always be considered in the older child with respiratory symptoms. It is uncommon for smoking to be the sole cause of symptoms in children, but it may trigger latent airway reactivity. Careful examination may reveal yellow staining of the fingers, teeth, or tongue. Passively inhaled cigarette smoke affects all age groups, especially young children, and it has been reported that infants exposed to such smoke in their homes are significantly more likely to have lower respiratory tract infections. Irritating vapors and odors from paints or insecticide sprays cause coughing and wheezing, particularly in children with asthma.

Psychologic illness may produce a chronic cough without any apparent physical signs or abnormalities on the chest radiograph. Typically these children have a dry foghorn-sounding cough. The cough usually disappears when the child is asleep and is much worse when attention is drawn to it (eg, during a consultation with a physician). If the cough does not resolve with simple reassurance, the child should be evaluated by a pediatric pulmonologist, and if psychogenic cough is suspected, referral to a psychiatrist is recommended.

Less Common Causes of Persistent Cough

Immune deficiency is a serious but uncommon cause of chronic cough. Increased susceptibility to bacterial infections is a feature of immune deficiency syndromes that affect humoral antibody production, bacterial phagocytosis, or bacterial killing. Bronchiectasis or chronic pulmonary infection often develops in patients with these disorders and causes chronic cough with expectoration of infected sputum. AIDS is increasing in frequency in children and may present with persistent coughing and an abnormal chest radiograph due to an opportunistic infection with pneumocystis, cytomegalovirus, atypical mycobacteria, or legionella.

Congenital malformations of the esophagus, larynx, or trachea are rare causes of persistent cough. Diagnoses to be considered include cleft larynx, tracheoesophageal fistula (Fig. 33-1), and a vascular ring (Fig. 33-2). Associated symptoms such as coughing after swallowing, poor feeding, or stridor may suggest the diagnosis.

Mediastinal tumors may produce airway obstruction associated with stridor and a dry cough. Benign tumors include teratomas and cystic hygroma. Malignant tumors such as lymphoma, T-

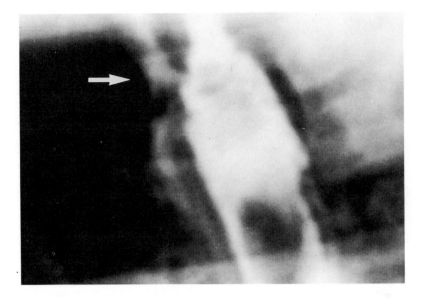

FIG 33-1
The barium swallow study of a child with an H-type tracheoesophageal fistula demonstrating the fistula (arrow) and aspiration of contrast material into the trachea.

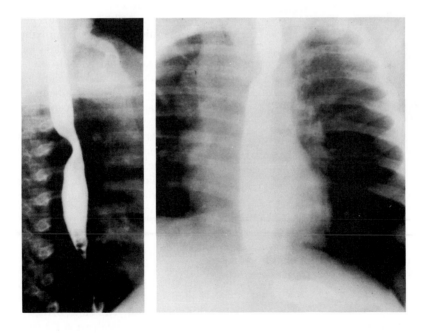

FIG 33-2
The barium swallow study of an infant with stridor demonstrating a vascular ring that makes a bilateral impression on the esophagus in the anteroposterior projection. At surgery, the patient had a double aortic arch.

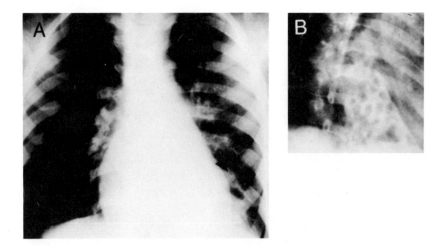

FIG 33-3

A, Atelectasis of the left lower lobe with a dense linear shadow behind the heart (arrow) and inferior displacement of the left hilum. **B,** Cystic lesions due to saccular bronchiectasis in the left lower lobe were demonstrated with an oblique view after chest percussion and postural drainage.

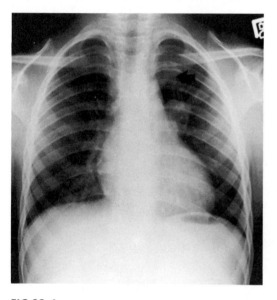

FIG 33-4

A primary tuberculous complex with left hilar adenopathy and a pneumonic infiltrate in the left upper lobe (arrow).

cell leukemia, and thymic neoplasia are rarer and usually lead to additional symptoms. Primary tumors of the lung are extremely rare in children.

Bronchiectasis (Fig. 33-3) and immotile cilia syndrome produce recurrent respiratory infections and persistent cough. The clinical features of a chronic productive cough, finger clubbing, and intercurrent exacerbations are similar to those seen in cystic fibrosis and immune deficiency. In addition, children with immotile cilia syndrome usually have recurrent otitis media and chronic sinusitis. Approximately 50% of those with the dynein arm defect also have situs inversus (Kartagener's syndrome).

Tuberculosis, although relatively uncommon, is an increasing problem affecting economically disadvantaged people, recent immigrants from Southeast Asia, and individuals with AIDS. Children with an undiagnosed persistent cough should therefore undergo a skin test for tuberculosis. The intradermal tuberculin test is more reliable than the tine test. The chest radiograph may show a primary complex (Fig. 33-4), tuberculous pneumonia (Fig. 33-5), or progressive lesions.

Laboratory Evaluation

The chest radiograph is the single most useful tool in the diagnosis of respiratory disorders in general, and is abnormal in many of the conditions described. Two views of the chest should be requested, with evaluation for gas trapping, increased bronchial line shadowing, alveolar infiltrates, reticulonodular shadowing, and localized emphysema. Localized emphysema or a persistent infiltrate should lead to a search for an inhaled foreign body (Fig. 33-6). Right and left

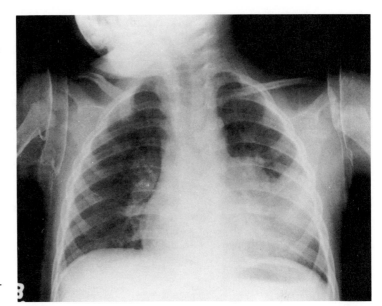

FIG 33-5
Primary tuberculosis with an extensive lingular infiltrate.

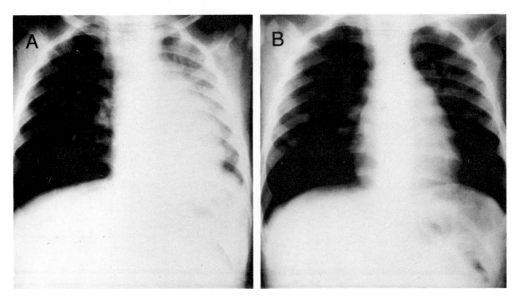

FIG 33-6
A, Atelectasis of the left lung from a peanut in the left main bronchus. **B,** The same patient after bronchoscopy.

lateral decubitus films may help with this diagnosis. If the foreign body is in a main bronchus, there is often gas trapping in the affected lung, which never deflates even if placed in a dependent position. Alternatively, older children may cooperate with inspiratory and expiratory radiographs to assess localized emphysema. The radiograph also should be evaluated for hilar and mediastinal adenopathy, because these may be the only clues to rarer conditions such as tuberculosis and sarcoidosis (Fig. 33-4).

The complete blood count and differential cell count may show eosinophilia in an allergic child with asthma. In young children with cystic

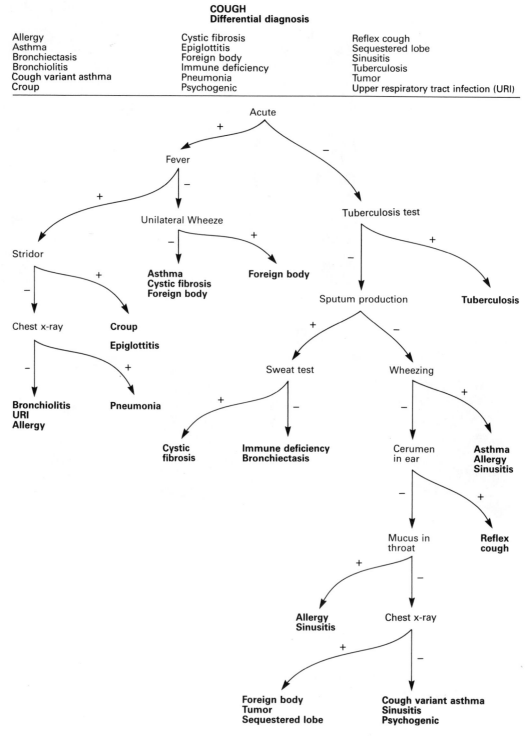

FIG 33-7
Decision tree for differential diagnosis of cough.

fibrosis it may reveal hypochromic anemia or neutrophilia. The white blood cell count is usually increased in bacterial pneumonia, with band forms and toxic granulation. In viral pneumonia there may be lymphocytosis or in severe cases lymphopenia. The most extreme form of lymphocytosis is seen in children with pertussis, although this finding may be absent in the early stages.

Pulmonary function tests before and after administration of bronchodilators often help in the diagnosis of chronic cough. They are most valuable for diagnosing asthma by showing reversible airflow obstruction. If the diagnosis is difficult to establish, most asthmatic children will show exercise-induced bronchospasm if tested before and after a standardized treadmill running test.

A sweat test should be performed in any child who has symptoms that suggest cystic fibrosis. The test should be performed with the pilocarpine iontophoresis method of Gibson and Cooke at an accredited cystic fibrosis center. The selective chloride electrode method is unreliable and is not recommended.

INDICATIONS FOR CONSULTATION OR REFERRAL

The child with severe symptoms, cyanosis, respiratory distress, or stridor, should be evaluated for inpatient care. Cyanosis may indicate incipient respiratory failure, and arterial blood gas measurements are indicated. If the blood gases are abnormal, the child may require specialized care. A referral for evaluation should be considered if the cough is persistent or if the diagnosis is unclear, particularly if there is a possibility of a serious underlying cause, indicated by weight loss, poor general health, or reduced activity.

DISCUSSION OF ALGORITHM

An algorithm for the differential diagnosis of cough is presented in Figure 33-7. In evaluating cough, the first task is to differentiate between acute and chronic disease. Acute cough probably has an infectious cause. Foreign bodies should also be considered, especially if there are unilateral signs or findings on the radiograph.

Patients with chronic cough should be examined for signs of a systemic disease such as wasting, pallor, fever, sputum production, digital clubbing, and wheezing. These findings may lead to the specific tests to make the diagnosis. Coughing may be a sign of asthma, so a careful history of allergic symptoms is important. Because cystic fibrosis may be present even in healthy-looking children, a sweat test should be considered in children with persistent cough. Chest radiographs are helpful, both in establishing a diagnosis and in ruling out organic disease. A psychologic cough is usually "seallike," increases at times of stress, and disappears during sleep.

BIBLIOGRAPHY

Cloutier M: Finding the cause of chronic cough in children, *J Resp Dis* 1:20–28, 1980.

Cloutier M, Loughlin GM: Chronic cough in children: A manifestation of airway hyperreactivity, *Pediatrics* 67:6–12, 1981.

Eigen H: The clinical evaluation of chronic cough, *Pediatr Clin North Am* 29:67–78, 1982.

Gibson LE, Cooke RE: A test for concentration of electrolytes in sweat in cystic fibrosis of the pancreas using pilocarpine by iontophoresis, *Pediatrics* 23:545–549, 1959.

Konig P: Hidden asthma in children, *Am J Dis Child* 135:1053–1055, 1981.

Rachelefsky GS, Katz RM, Siegel SC: Chronic sinus disease with associated reactive airway disease in children, *Pediatrics* 73:526–529, 1984.

Schidlow DV: Primary ciliary dyskinesia (the immotile cilia syndrome) [review], *Ann Allergy* 73:457–468, 1994.

Schuller DE: Persistent cough in childhood, *Immunol Allergy Pract* 8:378–384, 1986.

Sotomayor JL, Douglas SD, Wilmott RW: Pulmonary manifestations of immune deficiency diseases, *Pediatr Pulmonol* 6:275–292, 1989.

Sotomayor JL, Godinez RI, Borden S, et al: Large airway collapse due to acquired tracheobron-

chomalacia in infancy, *Am J Dis Child* 140:367–371, 1986.
Wolf AP, May M, Nuelle O: The tympanic mem-

brane: A source of the cough reflex, *JAMA* 223:1269, 1973.

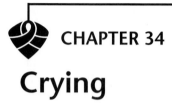

CHAPTER 34

Crying

Kathleen Zsolway
Joel A. Fein

As an infant behavior, crying is often interpreted as the infant's attempt to communicate hunger, discomfort, loneliness, pain, or illness. However, crying also reflects the infant's immature central nervous system. Maturation of the central nervous system control mechanism allows the infant to transition between the various states of arousal: deep sleep, active sleep, alert inactivity, alert active, and crying. As the maturation process continues, the infant begins to filter environmental stimuli, thereby decreasing the time spent in the highest state of arousal, namely crying.

Infant crying typically spurs the parent to seek the cause of the crying. Parents seek the advice of the health care provider when they are unable to identify the cause of their infant's crying, or unable to console their infant such that the crying persists for a longer period than the parents deem "healthy."

DIFFERENTIAL DIAGNOSIS

In his review of the various studies that have looked at normal crying behavior, Barr summarizes five basic propositions on which most experts agree: 1) There is a progressive increase

in crying that peaks in the second month of life and gradually decreases. 2) There is a diurnal rhythm, with clustering in the evening hours. 3) There is considerable between-individual variability. 4) There is a large degree of within-individual variability from day to day. 5) Early crying is not modifiable by differences in caretaking style. Brazelton detailed crying patterns in 80 infants as "average crying lasting 2 hours a day at 2 weeks, increasing to 3 hours a day by 6 weeks and gradually decreasing to 1 hour a day by 3 months." Variations from the anticipated crying time may result from physical problems in the infant. In this situation, historical report of crying usually reveals an abrupt onset that clearly deviates from the infant's normal behavior pattern. A complete history and physical examination by a health care provider is warranted to evaluate for the multiple conditions that may be associated with abrupt, inconsolable crying in infants. Those conditions most often presenting with abrupt crying may be categorized by organ system (Box 34-1).

A final entity that must be included in the differential diagnosis of infant crying is colic. This diagnosis is one of exclusion but does have some discerning features that are discussed in the section on management.

II

BOX 34-1
Conditions Associated with Abrupt Onset of Inconsolable Crying in Young Infants

Discomfort due to identifiable illness
Head and neck
  Meningitis*
  Skull fracture/subdural hematoma*
  Glaucoma
  Foreign body (especially eyelash) in eye†
  Corneal abrasion†
  Otitis media
  Caffey disease (infantile cortical hyperostosis)
  Subdural hemorrhage (shaken impact syndrome)
Gastrointestinal/Cardiac
  Excess air due to improper feeding or burping technique†
  Gastroenteritis†
  Intussusception*
  Anal fissure†
  Milk intolerance
  Anomalous coronary artery
Genitourinary
  Torsion of testis
  Incarcerated hernia*
  Urinary tract infections
Integument
  Open diaper pin
  Burn
  Strangulated finger, toe, penis (often due to an encircling hair)
Musculoskeletal
  Battered child syndrome*
  Fracture or contusion, accidental
  Toe caught in shoe
Toxic/Metabolic
  Drugs: aspirin, antihistamines, atropinics adrenergics,* cocaine, amphetamine
  Metabolic acidosis, hyponatremia, hypocalcemia, hypoglycemia*
  Pertussis vaccine reactions
Colic—Recurrent paroxysmal attacks of crying

*Life-threatening causes.
†Common causes.
Adapted from Henretig FM: Crying and colic in early infancy. In Fleisher G, Ludwig S, editors: *Textbook of Pediatric Emergency Medicine,* ed 3, Baltimore, 1993, Williams & Wilkins.

DATA GATHERING

History

Attention must be paid to securing a complete history of the present complaint. Recent events such as immunization or exposure to new foods should be assessed. An acute change in behavior or the presence of fever may signal a life-threatening illness, and physical examination should be performed promptly in an effort to identify an urgent medical or surgical problem and begin the appropriate interventions.

If historical information reveals that the concern regarding crying is longstanding, a thorough discussion should focus on the perinatal course as well as feeding and sleeping practices. The quality of the crying, the timing of the crying, and the interventions utilized by the parent, both successful and unsuccessful, should be explored in detail. Observation of the methods utilized by the parent to soothe the child during the medical visit may provide more information than direct questioning. Often the problem is not the child crying but the parents' perception of the problem and their fears, insecurities, and stress that do not let them cope with the normal child's activities. The parents should be asked about their interpretation of pain, their coping methods, and outside stresses.

Physical Examination

A complete physical examination is a critical aspect of the evaluation of the chief complaint of crying. A careful assessment of weight, length, and head circumference percentiles will lend insight into the general state of growth and wellness of the patient. The examination must include attention to details such as the possibility of a small foreign body or tourniqueted body part. Fluorescein examination of the eye for corneal abrasion should be performed. A rectal examination may reveal rectal bleeding, an anatomic abnormality, or signs of constipation. Hemoccult positive stool may alert the clinician to acute intra-abdominal processes such as intussusception or infectious gastroenteritis. Vital sign abnormalities may indicate pain or intrinsic cardiac problems such as anomalous left coronary artery. Each part of the body, from head to toe, should be inspected and palpated in a search for swelling, tenderness, or signs of trauma.

Laboratory Studies

Laboratory screening for infants with the complaint of crying should be guided by the history and physical examination. Abnormalities of the complete blood count or electrolytes are rare. Urinalysis and urine culture is suggested by some experts as a screen for occult urinary tract infection in these children. Electrocardiography and chest radiography are useful only if a primary

---

BOX 34-2
Do's and Don'ts of Evaluation of the Crying Patient

Do's	Don'ts
Listen carefully to the history	Make light of parental concerns
Be certain to ask questions and cover all aspects of infant behavior	Hasten your diagnosis prior to obtaining a complete picture of the infant
Perform a complete physical examination	Be short in your discussion of findings/diagnosis
Take the time to explain normal findings to the parent	Appear unsupportive of parental needs for continued reinforcement of the diagnosis
Offer support to the parents and discuss alternative methods to comfort the infant	

---

cardiac problem is suggested by the history or physical examination.

EVALUATION AND DECISION MAKING

If a complete history, physical examination, and laboratory analysis exclude physical illness, then either normal infant behavior or colic is the explanation of episodic crying. Intervention will be based on the delineation between acute and chronic events. The diagnosis of colic is commonly based on recurrent episodes of prolonged crying rather than an acute change in infant behavior.

Wessel and colleagues specify that an infant less than 3 months of age with colic is "one who was otherwise healthy and well fed and experiences paroxysms of irritability, fussing, or crying lasting for a total of more than 3 hours a day and occurring on more than 3 days in any 1 week." As Carey has noted, the entity of colic may be better referred to as "primary excessive crying of infancy," denoting an infant that is otherwise well but experiences crying episodes that fall outside the accepted range of normal behavior. These episodes occur in 10% to 25% of infants less than 3 months of age. Parents witnessing these episodes will commonly express concern that the child is suffering from abdominal pain. Colic almost invariably resolves within 2 to 3 months of onset.

TREATMENT

Acute identifiable problems are treated with the appropriate medical or surgical intervention. If the history and physical examination places the infant's crying pattern into the realm of normal infant behavior, then time must be spent validating the parents' concerns and reassuring them that their infant is displaying normal patterns of crying. Review of parental response to crying may be beneficial. Teaching the parents alternative methods of soothing the infant may provide the desired response if currently implored methods are unsuccessful (Box 34-2).

When recurrent unexplained episodes of crying have been reported and the infant has a normal physical examination, adequate growth parameters, and exclusion of acute illness, then a detailed discussion of colic should ensue. Parents may have the knowledge of some of the proposed theories of colic, such as cow's milk allergy or lactose intolerance. In addition, they may regard the crying as either a failure of their parenting skills or of the medical system. It is advisable to discuss various theories with the parents, noting that they are simply theories and do not offer definite diagnosis unless other clinical signs exist. Studies that have attempted to assess interventions to reduce crying in infants with colic have been inconclusive in demonstrating a reduction in crying with any specific intervention more than reassurance and support offered to the parents. Pharmacologic therapy has been found to be either ineffective or potentially harmful and should be discouraged when discussing interventions with parents.

The clinician should remain in contact with parents to provide support and advice for them as their infant continues to grow and develop. Alternate methods for infant soothing can be assessed, and modification of parental response to infant crying can be encouraged. Continued physical reassessment of the infant during the following months may be necessary to reassure parents that their infant is healthy and developing normally despite episodes of persistent crying.

BIBLIOGRAPHY

Barr RG: The normal crying curve: What do we really know? *Dev Med Child Neurol* 32:356–362, 1990.

Brazleton TB: Crying in infancy, *Pediatrics* 29:579, 1962.

Carey WB: Colic of primary excessive crying in young infants. In Levine MD, Carey WB, Crocker AC, Gross RT, editors: *Developmental-behavioral pediatrics,* ed 2, Philadelphia, 1983, WB Saunders.

Henretig FM: Crying and colic in early infancy. In Fleisher G, Ludwig S, editors: *Textbook of pediatric emergency medicine,* ed 3, Baltimore, 1993, Williams & Wilkins.

Parkin PC, Schwartz CJ, Manuel BA: Randomized controlled trial of three interventions in the management of persistent crying of infancy, *Pediatrics* 92:197–201, 1993.

Poole SR: The infant with acute, unexplained, excessive crying, *Pediatrics* 88:450–455, 1991.

Taubman B: Clinical trial of the treatment of colic by modification of parent-infant interaction, *Pediatrics* 74(6):998–1003, 1984.

Wessel MA, Cobb JC, Jackson EB, et al: Paroxysmal fussing in infancy, sometimes called "colic," *Pediatrics* 14:421, 1954.

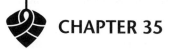

CHAPTER 35

Acute Diarrhea

Linda Arnold

Throughout the world, acute diarrhea claims the lives of more children than any other cause. In the United States, mortality rates from diarrhea are not as high as in developing countries, but the morbidity is still great. After the common cold, diarrhea is the most common chief complaint for children seeking medical care. The average child will have three episodes of infectious diarrhea per year in the first 3 years of life.

Diarrhea is defined as an increase in frequency or decrease in consistency of the stool. Normal stool output varies, but greater than 10 g/kg/day of stool, or greater than 200 g/day in older children, constitutes diarrhea. Infants, malnourished children, and immunocompromised children are at greatest risk for the dehydration and systemic illness that may accompany viral, bacterial, and parasitic gastroenteritis.

DIFFERENTIAL DIAGNOSIS

Common Causes of Diarrhea
- **Infection**
  Viral
  Rotavirus
  Norwalk agent
  Enteric adenovirus
  Astrovirus
  Calcivirus
- **Bacterial**
  Salmonella
  Shigella
  Campylobacter
  Yersinia
  Escherichia coli
  Clostridium difficile
- **Parasitic**
  Giardia lamblia
  Cryptosporidium parvum
  Entamoeba histolytica
  Strongyloides stercoralis
- **Extraintestinal**
  Urinary tract infection
  Otitis media
  Appendicitis
  Encopresis with leakage around fecal mass
- **Toxin**
  Food poisoning
  Staphylococcus aureus
  Clostridium perfringens
  Heavy metals
- **Other**
  Food, milk, or soy protein allergy
  Inflammatory bowel disease
  Protein losing enteropathy
  Laxatives use or abuse

Discussion
The majority of cases of acute diarrhea result from enteric infection. Viral gastroenteritis, in general, is characterized by injury to the proximal small intestine, resulting in vomiting and watery diarrhea. Onset is abrupt, and the duration is limited. Bacterial infections tend to cause colonic inflammation, leading to crampy abdominal pain and stools containing blood or mucous. The distinction is not absolute, because bacterial toxins (eg, *Shigella*, enterotoxigenic *Escherichia coli*) may also induce watery diarrhea.

Rotavirus is the most common cause of diarrhea in infants and children. Rotaviral infection is more common during the winter months in temperate climates, while showing no seasonal variation in tropical regions. It most commonly affects children between the ages of 6 and 24 months. Following a 2- to 3-day incubation period, there is an abrupt onset of vomiting and watery diarrhea, which persists for 2 to 8 days and is often accompanied by respiratory symptoms. Dehydration is a frequent complication, especially in malnourished children. Nosocomial spread of rotavirus has been well documented. Enteric adenoviruses cause diarrhea year round, predominantly in children less than 2 years of age. A brief period of vomiting is followed by up to 14 days of diarrhea, with up to one half of patients developing signs of dehydration. The Norwalk-like agents, conversely, tend to infect older children and adults. Vomiting and diarrhea persist for 12 to 48 hours, and dehydration is rare.

Salmonella is the most common cause of bacterial diarrhea among children in the United States. Estimated to cause between 1 and 2 million episodes of gastroenteritis in this country each year, it is most likely to produce symptoms in infants and young children. Transmission occurs via contaminated food or water or by person-to-person spread. Presentations range from mild gastroenteritis to bloody colitis, with bacteremia developing in 6% of children. Immunocompromised children and those with hematologic disorders are at greater risk for sequelae such as osteomyelitis. Both *Shigella* and *Campylobacter* are frequently implicated in outbreaks of bacterial diarrhea in day care centers. With *Shigella*, fever and malaise progress to crampy abdominal pain and watery diarrhea in which blood and mucous may be seen. Extraintestinal manifestations of infection include seizures and arthritis. *Campylobacter* infection is most commonly seen in children less than 1 year of age and in young adults. As with *Shigella*, symptoms can range from mild diarrhea to dysentery. Complications are rare. *Yersinia* is most likely to cause diarrhea in preschool-aged children. Symptoms of fever, abdominal pain, and diarrhea generally resolve within 5 to 14 days. In older children the abdominal pain associated with *Yersinia* infection may mimic acute appendicitis. Bacteremia, when it occurs, may be fatal. Multiple strains of *E. coli* cause diarrhea, with some infections progressing to dysentery or hemorrhagic colitis. Enterohemorrhagic *E. coli* O157:H7 deserves special mention. It is the organism most frequently cultured from bloody diarrheal stools. Approximately 10% of children with *E. coli*

O157:H7 infection develop hemolytic uremic syndrome (HUS), presumptively as a result of cytotoxin-induced endothelial injury.

Clostridium difficile infection generally follows single or multiple courses of antibiotic therapy. Alterations in bowel flora allow for *C. difficile* overgrowth and the elaboration of cytotoxins A and B. Symptoms of watery diarrhea may last from days to months, with severe cases developing life-threatening pseudomembranous colitis characterized by fever, leukocytosis, hypoalbuminemia, and bloody stools.

Giardia lamblia and *Cryptosporidium* are frequently present in untreated drinking and recreational waters in the United States. Both intestinal parasites have been implicated in outbreaks of diarrhea in day care centers. Infection with *Giardia* is more common and results in nausea, abdominal cramps, and diarrhea that may be self-limited or chronic. Asymptomatic carriers have also been identified. Symptoms from cryptosporidiosis infection are generally mild and self-limited, with cramping abdominal pain and diarrhea the most common complaints. Infants and the elderly are more prone to severe diarrhea and dehydration, as are immunocompromised patients, in whom cryptosporidiosis can become a chronic debilitating illness characterized by copious diarrhea and malabsorption. Amebiasis should be considered in travelers returning from Asia or South and Central America with bloody diarrhea.

Food poisoning results from ingestion of foods contaminated with bacteria or preformed bacterial toxins. *Clostridium perfringens, Staphylococcus aureus,* and *Vibrio parahaemolyticus* are most frequently implicated. Severe crampy abdominal pain is followed by vomiting and watery diarrhea. Symptoms resolve within 24 to 48 hours.

A number of noninfectious causes of diarrhea should be mentioned. Carbohydrate malabsorption commonly leads to diarrhea. Neuroendocrine secreting tumors and thyrotoxicosis frequently present with voluminous stool output. Diarrhea also may be seen in inflammatory conditions such as celiac sprue and inflammatory bowel disease or in the presence of laxative use.

DATA GATHERING

History
The focus of the history should be on the nature and severity of the diarrhea, associated symptoms, and possible sources of exposure. Stools with gross blood and mucus are more typical in bacterial infections, whereas viral gastroenteritis is more apt to produce vomiting and watery diarrhea. Abrupt onset of vomiting after a meal, followed by diarrhea, is common in cases of food poisoning. Foul-smelling stools suggest malabsorption.

Associated symptoms often give clues as to the etiology of diarrhea. Bacterial gastroenteritis is often accompanied by fever, cramping abdominal pain, and tenesmus. Patients with viral syndromes are often afebrile and more likely to present with emesis. Their symptoms are usually of shorter duration, and associated respiratory symptoms or rash are frequently present.

Specific inquiries should be made regarding hydration status. Parents generally have a good recollection of children's intake, whereas output is not as easily assessed. Weight loss should be calculated, if possible, and the number and frequency of diapers should be determined. In infants, the distinction between urine and watery stool may be difficult.

Finally, a history of ill contacts should be sought, with specific references to the home, playmates, school, and daycare. Does the family have pets? Has the child recently visited a farm or petting zoo? Is there a history of travel outside of the country or to areas with an untreated water supply? Has the child been swimming in pools or fresh water subject to fecal contamination?

Physical Examination
The focus of the physical examination should be on assessing the state of hydration. Weight should be checked and compared with premorbid weight, when possible, to determine the amount of fluid lost. In younger children, replacement of ongoing fluid losses can be estimated by weighing diapers. All weights should be plotted on a growth curve; failure to thrive may indicate an underlying chronic disease. The assessment and management of dehydration is presented in Chapter 60.

Examination of the abdomen in cases of diarrhea due to gastroenteritis often reveals mild diffuse tenderness and active bowel sounds. Focal or rebound tenderness warrants further investigation, as do absent bowel sounds or high-pitched rushes, which can be ausculted in cases of bowel obstruction.

Skin rashes may be seen in a number of viral and bacterial illnesses. Arthritis may be a feature of *Shigella* and *Yersinia* infections, as well as inflammatory bowel disease. Discrete loops of bowel may be palpated in cases of intussusception, inflammatory bowel disease, and severe constipation. Intussusception may present with abdominal pain, vomiting, bloody diarrhea, and lethargy. The diarrhea in inflammatory bowel disease often contains gross blood, whereas in constipation a loose, nonbloody stool leaks around the obstructing fecal mass.

Laboratory Evaluation

The nature of the diarrhea and associated symptoms should guide the laboratory evaluation. A history of bloody or tarry stools warrants hemoccult testing. Hemoccult-negative red stools may result from ingestion of fruit juices, popsicles, or gelatin, whereas tarry stools may result from ingestion of iron, bismuth-containing antidiarrheal preparations, or black licorice. Following confirmation of blood in the stool, a complete blood count should be considered to assess the degree of blood loss and to serve as a baseline in the event of ongoing losses. Methylene blue should be added to smears of all bloody or mucoid stools to test for fecal leukocytes, a common finding in bacterial infections. When a bacterial infection is suspected, stool should be sent for culture. A specimen should be sent for *C. difficile* toxin if there is a history of antibiotic use. Although no specific therapies are indicated in cases of viral gastroenteritis, identification of rotaviral and adenoviral infections by immunoassay may be useful in terms of infection control for outbreaks in institutional settings. When a parasitic infection is suspected, three specimens should be submitted for ova and parasite testing; these may be fresh or preserved in formalin. Urine specific gravity and electrolyte testing may be helpful in both the initial and ongoing assessment of hydration status.

MANAGEMENT

The majority of cases of acute diarrhea are self-limiting and can be managed symptomatically. The focus is generally on maintaining hydration. Many physicians advocate a clear liquid diet during the acute phase of illness, followed by advancement to a BRAT type diet (bananas, rice, applesauce, and toast). Clear liquids are especially helpful in those patients with associated vomiting. It is important to remind the caretakers that water should not be used as a maintenance or replacement fluid, but rather "clear" refers to sugar- and salt-containing solutions. A lactose-free diet is often recommended during the convalescent period but is generally necessary only in patients with severe illness or underlying malnutrition.

Antibiotic therapy is seldom indicated in cases of acute diarrhea. Viruses are not susceptible to antibiotics, and food poisoning resolves quickly without therapy. Although patients symptomatic from *Giardia* infection respond to therapy with metronidazole, no effective therapy has been identified for cryptosporidiosis, which fortunately is self-limiting in the immunocompetent patient. Diarrhea caused by *C. difficile* often resolves following discontinuation of antibiotic therapy. Oral vancomycin or metronidazole therapy is effective when symptoms persist, but recurrence rates can be as high as 40%. *Salmonella* infections should be treated with antibiotics in infants less than 3 months of age, in the immunocompromised or functionally asplenic patient, or when bacteremia is suspected. Antibiotic therapy in symptomatic cases of *Shigellosis* shortens both the course of disease and the duration of excretion. Treatment of *Campylobacter* limits shedding to 48 hours, which may be important if a child must return to day care. *Yersinia* should be treated with antibiotics when disease is severe, bacteremia is present, or the patient has an underlying illness. Use of antibiotics in enterohemorrhagic *E. coli* infections is contraindicated, because the resulting release of toxins may actually increase the risk of developing HUS. Extraintestinal infections, such as otitis media and urinary tract infections, that present with diarrhea should receive appropriate antibiotic therapy.

INDICATIONS FOR CONSULTATION OR REFERRAL

Patients with acute diarrhea seldom need referral and can generally be managed as outpatients. Exceptions include patients with severe or progressive dehydration, in whom intravenous hydration and electrolyte monitoring is indicated. Infants and toxic-appearing children also warrant closer observation, as do children with persistently bloody stools. Surgical consultation is

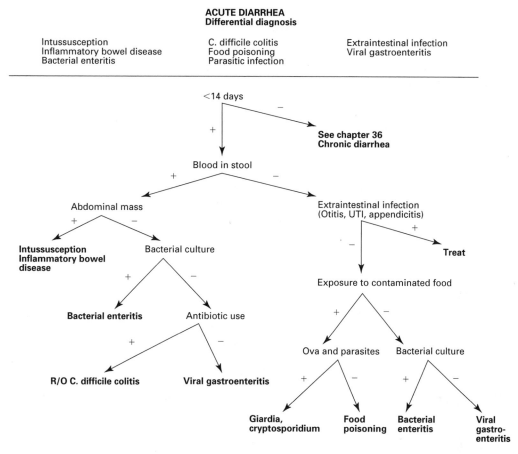

ACUTE DIARRHEA
Differential diagnosis

Intussusception
Inflammatory bowel disease
Bacterial enteritis

C. difficile colitis
Food poisoning
Parasitic infection

Extraintestinal infection
Viral gastroenteritis

FIG 35-1
Decision tree for differential diagnosis of acute diarrhea.

indicated in children presenting with a localizing abdominal examination or peritoneal signs.

DISCUSSION OF ALGORITHM

A "decision tree" for the differential diagnosis of acute diarrhea is presented in Figure 35-1. In patients with nonbloody stools, extraintestinal infections such as otitis media and urinary tract infections should be investigated. Patients with bloody stools should be examined for the presence of an abdominal mass, which may be present in inflammatory bowel disease or intussusception. Stool cultures should be sent to identify bacterial and possibly viral or parasitic pathogens. If there is a history of recent antibiotic use, the stool should also be evaluated for the presence of *C. difficile* toxins. A history of exposure of the patient, family members, or friends to contaminated food should lead to the diagnosis of food poisoning or parasitic infection.

BIBLIOGRAPHY

Bishop WP, Ulshen MH: Bacterial gastroenteritis, *Pediatr Clin North Am* 35:69–87, 1988.

Blacklow NR, Greenberg HB: Viral gastroenteritis, *N Engl J Med* 325:327–340, 1991.

Boyce TG, Swerdlow DL, Griffin PM: *Escherichia coli* O157:H7 and the hemolytic-uremic syndrome, *N Engl J Med* 333:364–368, 1995.

Brown KH, Gastanaduy AS, Saavedra JM, et al: Effect of continued oral feeding on clinical and nutritional outcomes of acute diarrhea in children, *J Pediatr* 112:191–200, 1988.

Brown KH, Peerson JM, Fontaine O: Use of nonhuman milks in the dietary management of young children with acute diarrhea: A meta-analysis of clinical trials, *Pediatrics* 93:17–27, 1994.

Cohen MB: Etiology and mechanisms of acute infectious diarrhea in infants in the United States, *J Pediatr* 4:S34–S39, 1991.

Glass RI, Lew JF, Gangarosa RE, et al: Estimates of morbidity and mortality rates for diarrheal diseases in American children, *J Pediatr* 118: S27–S33, 1991.

Guerant RL, Bobak DA: Bacterial and protozoal gastroenteritis, *N Engl J Med* 325:252–264, 1991.

Ho MS, Glass RI, Pinsky PF, et al: Rotavirus as a cause of diarrheal morbidity and mortality in the United States, *J Infect Dis* 158:1112–1116, 1988.

Pickering LK, Englekirk PG: *Giardia lamblia*, *Pediatr Clin North Am* 35:565–577, 1988.

Williams EK, Lohr JA, Guerrant RL: Acute infectious diarrhea II. Diagnosis, treatment and prevention, *Pediatr Infect Dis J* 5:458–465, 1986.

CHAPTER 36

Chronic Diarrhea

Steven M. Schwarz

Diarrhea occurs as a consequence of a disturbance in the mechanisms that regulate intestinal fluid and electrolyte transport. This disturbance may result from a variety of etiologies, including dietary fluid and carbohydrate excess (particularly during infancy), invasion of the intestinal epithelium by microorganisms, nonspecific inflammatory processes, intestinal atrophy during a period of malnutrition, and the effects of pharmacologic agents. Under normal physiologic conditions, estimates of stool output range from 5 to 10 g/kg/day in children and 100 to 200 g/day in adults. Any increase in stool volume over these levels indicates a diarrheal state. Although the definition of *chronic* diarrhea is controversial, persistence of the diarrheal condition beyond 2-weeks duration indicates the necessity for a diagnostic evaluation.

Although persistent diarrhea may be responsible for significant morbidity (particularly in infants under 3 months of age) characterized by poor growth and weight gain, it may also present as a relatively benign condition associated with normal growth over a period of months to years. Assessment of the nature of any underlying etiology includes attention to any protracted effects of diarrhea, including dehydration and malabsorption leading to malnutrition and growth failure. To fully understand the syndrome and approach it with a rational diagnostic scheme, it is important to consider the major mechanisms responsible for the diarrheal state.

Causes of Chronic Diarrhea

- **Infection**
    - Viral
        - Rotavirus
        - Adenovirus
        - Norwalk agent
    - Bacterial
        - *Salmonella*
        - *Shigella*
        - *Campylobacter*
        - *Yersinia*
        - *Clostridium difficile*
        - *Aeromonas*
    - Parasitic
        - *Giardia*
        - *Cryptosporidium*
        - *Entamoeba*
    - Urinary tract
- **Drugs**
    - Antibiotics
    - Chemotherapy
    - Laxative abuse
- **Allergic–Inflammatory**
    - Crohn disease
    - Ulcerative colitis
    - Protein intolerance in infancy
    - Immunodeficiency
        - IgA deficiency
        - AIDS
        - Combined immunodeficiency
- **Carbohydrate intolerance**
    - Lactase deficiency
        - Late onset
        - Postinfectious
    - Sucrase-isomaltase deficiency
    - Glucose-galactose malabsorption
    - Glucoamylase deficiency
- **Diet related**
    - Excessive fluid intake
    - Sorbitol (fruit juices, dietetic sweets)
- **Pancreatic insufficiency**
    - Cystic fibrosis
    - Schwachman syndrome
    - Enterokinase deficiency
- **Hyperthyroidism**
- **Malnutrition**
- **Malignancy**
    - Ganglioneuroma
    - Graft-vs-host disease
    - Radiation
- **Congenital/anatomic**
    - Congenital microvillus atrophy
    - Blind loop

Partial obstruction—bacterial overgrowth
Fistulas (Crohn disease)
Malrotation
Hirschsprung disease
Celiac disease
Lymphangiectasia
- **Multiple etiologies**
    - Chronic nonspecific diarrhea (irritable bowel syndrome, "toddler's" diarrhea)
    - Secretory diarrhea
        - Enterotoxigenic
        - Tumor related
        - Congenital chloridorrhea
        - Bile salt malabsorption
    - Motility disorders
        - Collagen-vascular disease
        - Pseudoobstruction
        - Constipation—paradoxical diarrhea
        - Diabetes mellitus

DIFFERENTIAL DIAGNOSIS

Chronic diarrhea presents as a perplexing problem because of the long differential diagnosis and the considerable uncertainty regarding the appropriate diagnostic evaluation. Nevertheless, a careful history and physical examination and the use of relatively few readily available diagnostic tests will allow the primary care physician to reach a diagnosis in the majority of cases. This chapter will suggest an initial course of evaluation that may obviate the need for subspecialist intervention in most patients.

Carbohydrate Malabsorption

Certain acute disorders that involve damage to the brush border membrane, such as viral gastroenteritis, result in reduction of hydrolytic activity and malabsorption of carbohydrate, particularly disaccharides. It is now well recognized that this secondary carbohydrate intolerance (most prominently for lactose) may result in persistence of the diarrheal state. Mucosal injury may also result in intestinal glucoamylase deficiency and malabsorption of dietary starch (glucoamylase deficiency can also present as a primary malabsorptive defect). Diarrhea occurring as a consequence of carbohydrate loss is both osmotic and fermentative. The latter results from malabsorbed sugars broken down by colonic bacteria into organic acids, accompanied by H_2 formation. The diarrhea that follows is often explosive, watery, and vinegar-smelling. Because of the massive loss of nonelectrolyte solute molecules during diarrheal conditions associated with carbohydrate malabsorption, osmotic diarrhea can be represented by the formula:

$$2 \times ([Na^+] + [K^+]) < 280 \text{ mOsm}$$

Impaired Intestinal Transport of Nutrient, Water, and Electrolyte Secondary to Mucosal Damage

The apical plasma membrane of the small intestinal epithelial cell, or brush border membrane, is the final common pathway for nutrient and electrolyte uptake across the mucosal surface. Disruption of the structural and functional integrity of this membrane leads to impaired hydrolysis of nutrients and distorted water and electrolyte fluxes. In more severe states of loss of mucosal integrity (such as the celiac syndrome), reduced intestinal surface area and damage to the brush border membrane affects absorption of all nutrient classes and may be associated with luminal excretion of water and electrolytes. Various other insults to mucosal epithelial cells (eg, viral infection) lead to increased cellular turnover and population of the surface epithelium with immature crypt cells containing reduced levels of brush border enzymes. Malabsorption of unhydrolyzed and unabsorbed nutrient molecules, particularly monosaccharides and disaccharides, exert an osmotic effect intraluminally resulting in increased water excretion.

Active Water and Electrolyte Secretion

Secretory diarrheas are characterized clinically by the continuance of large-volume fecal output under fasting conditions. The mechanisms responsible for the secretory state include both malabsorption and secretion of fluid and electrolyte. During health, the gastrointestinal tract absorbs the bulk of an intraluminal fluid load. Most luminal water is absorbed in conjunction with Na^+, by both electrogenic mechanisms (via an epithelial cell ion channel and cotransport of Na^+ with D-sugars and L-amino acids) and electroneutral processes (coupled NaCl uptake). In secretory diarrheas (bacterial toxigenic, tumorogenic), fluid loss is generally mediated by excessive production of the second messengers cyclic adenosine monophosphate (cAMP) and cyclic guanosine monophosphate (cGMP), resulting in active secretion of Cl^- in the crypt regions and inhibition of intestinal villus cell neutral NaCl transport.

Rarely, intestinal hypersecretion occurs as a congenital phenomenon (familial chloridorrhea). In contrast to osmotic diarrheas, stool solute excretion in secretory states is primarily electrolyte, with fecal sodium concentrations typically in excess of 70 mEq/L. Secretory diarrheas may therefore be represented by the formula:

$$2 \times [Na^+] + [K^+] = 280 \text{ mOs}$$

Bile Salt, Fat Malabsorption

Any disorder that damages the terminal ileum may result in bile salt malabsorption. Subsequent bacterial deconjugation of bile salts in the colon leads to fluid and electrolyte secretion induced by bile acid. Fat malabsorption, either consequent to ileal dysfunction and bile salt loss, or secondary to disease of the upper small bowel (eg, celiac) or pancreas (eg, cystic fibrosis) may present with bulky, foul-smelling stools (steatorrhea) or as watery diarrhea induced by bacterial production of hydroxyl-fatty acids in the colon.

Other Mechanisms

Hypermotility states may result from the presence of vasoactive substances (prostaglandins, serotonin). These syndromes are often associated with active secretion (as well as malabsorption) of water and electrolytes. Conversely, decreased motility, often noted in collagen-vascular disorders, and diabetes mellitus lead to secretory and malabsorptive diarrhea secondary to bacterial overgrowth. Dietary-related diarrheal syndromes are less well understood. In recent years, there have been increasing reports of the relationship between chronic diarrhea and ingestion of large quantities of sorbitol. Sorbitol is found in high concentrations in certain fruit juices (apple, pear) and some sugarless candies. The association of the chronic nonspecific diarrhea syndrome ("toddler's" diarrhea) with excessive carbohydrate or fluid intake raises intriguing questions concerning intestinal "thresholds" for fluid and nutrient absorption, particularly in young children, and it additionally suggests altered developmental patterns of colonic motility. In older children, particularly adolescent girls, laxative abuse should be considered a cause of chronic diarrhea when other laboratory studies are normal.

Discussion

For the purposes of evaluation in pediatrics, it is useful to consider the etiologic possibilities in terms of age at presentation rather than diagnostic category. Thus evaluation is divided into cases occurring in three age groups: newborn to 3 months, 3 months to 3 years, and greater than 3 years.

Children in the Age Group of Newborn to 3 Months

Major causes of chronic diarrhea in this age group include:

- Postinfections
- Protein intolerance
- Cystic fibrosis
- Short bowel syndrome
- Transport, enzyme defects
- Malnutrition
- Congenital microvillous atrophy

Here, protracted diarrhea often heralds severe absorptive-secretory defects and is complicated by the development of malnutrition-associated diarrhea. The syndrome of intractable diarrhea of infancy, which may be associated with intestinal microvillous atrophy, necessitates an extensive diagnostic workup and often requires central venous alimentation. Office management of chronic diarrhea in this age group includes a careful clinical assessment to ascertain requirement for hospitalization and an initial workup aimed at confirming or ruling out common diagnostic entities.

The infancy period is most likely one to be complicated by significant morbidity from protracted diarrhea. In the infant who appears to be thriving, however, overfeeding and the passage of normal "breast-milk stools" often present with an associated complaint of diarrhea. In the breast-fed infant, it is not unusual to observe as many as 10 liquid stools per day. This is probably related both to the particular colonic bacterial flora in the infants and the high lactose content of breast milk. Clearly, any newborn who is fed excessive quantities of formula may develop diarrhea secondary to increased fluid intake and demonstrate osmotic effects from malabsorption of nutrients that may exceed normal absorptive capacity.

Postinfections—In a previously well infant, the sudden onset of diarrhea suggests an infectious etiology. When diarrhea is accompanied by heme-positive stools, bacterial pathogens such as *Salmonella, Shigella,* and *Campylobacter* species are suspected. These agents as well as viral pathogens (particularly rotavirus) are often associated with a protracted course secondary to mucosal injury resulting in disaccharide intolerance, confirmed by the presence of Clinitest-positive stools (liquid part) with pH less than 6. Use of a formula free of disaccharides, particularly lactose (eg, Prosobee, disaccharide-free Isomil) in a clinically stable baby may avoid the need for hospitalization secondary to dehydration from an osmotic diarrhea.

Protein intolerance—When diarrhea develops after the introduction of formula feedings at birth or after weaning from the breast, infants may be manifesting cow's milk or soy protein intolerance. Diarrhea is often marked by hemepositive or even grossly bloody stools and the clinical syndrome ranges from a thriving, well baby with some occult gastrointestinal (GI) blood loss to a severely toxic infant with frank enterocolitis. Vomiting may be an associated symptom in more morbid cases. Although the precise mechanism has not been elucidated, absorption of intact macromolecules in the newborn may lead to specific protein sensitization, with subsequent injury to GI mucosa. Recent evidence, in fact, suggests that this sensitization takes place even in breast-fed infants whose mothers ingest cow's milk protein. In the clinically stable child, appearance in the stool of neutrophils or eosinophils (with or without peripheral eosinophilia) suggests the diagnosis after infectious causes have been ruled out. It is important to emphasize that a high percentage of protein-sensitive infants will react to soy and goat's milk as well as cow's milk protein. Therefore, a hydrolyzed protein formula (eg, Nutramigen) should be used in an infant suspected of protein intolerance. In more severe cases, hospitalization for initial parenteral therapy may be required, followed by the institution of an elemental formula (Pregestimil) necessitated by mucosal injury affecting absorption of all nutrient classes. After mucosal recovery, documented by renewed carbohydrate tolerance, gradual reintroduction of the suspected formula (initially in very small amounts) is undertaken as a rechallenge. Recrudescence of symptoms, usually heralded by early carbohydrate malabsorption, confirms the diagnosis.

Cystic fibrosis—When clinically apparent in the first 3 months of life, cystic fibrosis is often complicated by malabsorptive stools secondary to pancreatic insufficiency; the syndrome thus presents with chronic diarrhea and failure to thrive. The physician should suspect cystic fibrosis in any infant with such a clinical course, particularly one with associated pulmonary disease or a positive family history. Although the finding of elevated sweat chloride levels are diagnostic, this test is difficult to perform in small babies because of the inability to obtain adequate quantities of sweat. Until the infant is old enough to be diagnosed specifically, finding a reduced or absent stool trypsin content can be considered presumptive evidence for cystic fibrosis. Under these conditions, a therapeutic trial of pancreatic enzyme replacement is indicated until an adequate sweat test can be performed (*see* Chapter 102).

Short bowel syndrome—With the development of refined surgical techniques and the advent of parenteral nutrition, infants are now surviving catastrophic small-intestinal illnesses resulting in extensive resections. These resections include those for congenital omphalocele and gastroschisis, following resections for small bowel atresias, and the surgical treatment of necrotizing enterocolitis. The primary care provider should be aware of the long-term consequences of these problems, because obviously initial management involves prolonged hospitalization involving both surgeons and gastroenterologists. Thus, despite the intestine's ability to adapt effectively following resections (*eg,* ileum assuming functions of resected jejunum), loss of the terminal ileum invariably leads to bile salt loss with secondary secretory diarrhea and steatorrhea. Therefore, infants will require a formula containing medium-chain triglycerides (*eg,* Pregestimil, Alimentum), which does not require micellar solubilization for absorption. The use of cholestyramine, an anion exchange resin, may be required to treat diarrhea induced by bile acid loss. If the infant with jejunal resection survives the initial postoperative and long recovery period, ileal adaptation will often obviate the need for an elemental diet.

Transport and enzyme defects—Transport and enzyme defects often present with severe, protracted diarrhea leading to inanition. Congenital glucose-galactose malabsorption is manifest by watery, acidic stools after the initial glucose-water feeding at birth; it may be differentiated from mucosal injury-related malabsorption by normal tolerance to fructose. The most common congenital disaccharidase abnormality is sucrase-isomaltase deficiency, which presents with diarrhea after the introduction of sucrose-containing foods (fruits, juices), usually at 3 to 4 months of age. Congenital lactase deficiency is an extremely rare, autosomal recessive disorder.

Children in the Age Group of 3 Months to 3 Years
Major causes of chronic diarrhea in this age group include:

- Postinfections
- Chronic nonspecific diarrhea
- Giardiasis
- Celiac disease
- Protein intolerance
- Sucrase-isomaltase deficiency
- Hirschsprung disease

Diagnoses associated with the development of chronic diarrhea in this age group overlap somewhat with those diagnoses for the age group of birth to 3 months. Although chronic bacterial infections are uncommon, an important disease is protracted diarrhea associated with *Clostridium difficile.* Postinfection carbohydrate intolerance occurs commonly in children up to 1 year of age. Similarly, the onset of protein intolerance often occurs after 3 months (although it rarely persists beyond 2 years), particularly in previously breast-fed infants. A brief comment should be made concerning Hirschsprung disease (intestinal aganglionosis). Although the disorder classically presents with chronic (from birth) constipation, a life-threatening enterocolitis may develop in certain cases, and this may be confused with infections or idiopathic inflammatory bowel disease. In general, however, the majority of children with persistent diarrhea in this age group fall into two broad categories: those with chronic nonspecific diarrhea, who manifest no nutritional deficits, and those with specific malabsorption syndromes associated with steatorrhea.

Chronic nonspecific diarrhea—In the child who presents with a prolonged history of diarrheal stools while continuing to thrive and grow normally, the most likely diagnosis is chronic nonspecific diarrhea (CNSD), or "toddler's diarrhea." These children will have one to as many as 12 loose to watery stools per day, which often appear to contain "undigested" food particles (actually nondigestible cellulose matter that has not undergone disintegration by colonic action), but they are rarely troubled by nighttime diarrhea. In children in whom weight loss or poor weight gain is evident, the cause is invariably caloric deprivation secondary to dietary restrictions. Once caloric intake has been documented and normalized and infection ruled out by adequate cultures, the presence of diarrhea in a well, growing child invariably reflects CNSD. Although the precise mechanisms responsible are not known, some children may benefit from an increase in the fat:carbohydrate ratio in the diet or by a reduction in fluid intake (particularly clear liquids). Antidiarrheal agents are of no value in CNSD, and the syndrome will resolve by the age of 3 to 4 years in almost all children.

Giardiasis—Infection with this protozoal organism represents the most common cause of chronic malabsorption in North America. Although *Giardia lamblia* infestation may present as an acute diarrheal syndrome, the more common course is that of a chronic illness marked by steatorrhea and poor weight gain. Suspicion is particularly high in patients with immunoglobulin deficiency, in whom the infection may be a recurring problem. Although many authors suggest the technique of duodenal aspiration to recover the organism (which resides in the upper small bowel), we have found the culturing of a fresh stool specimen or one preserved for only a short time in formalinized transport medium will lead to a positive diagnosis in well over 90% of cases. At present, the treatment of choice is either Furoxone, 7 mg/kg/day, or metronidazole, 20 mg/kg/day, for a 7-day course.

Celiac disease—Although a common cause of malabsorption in individuals in Europe, the diagnosis of celiac disease is made less frequently in North America. Nevertheless, it is important to consider this diagnosis in appropriate clinical situations, because specific therapy with dietary gluten restriction may be necessary to reduce the occurrence of intestinal lymphoma observed in untreated adult patients. The syndrome occurs as a result of a sensitivity to gliadin, the protein fraction of gluten present in wheat, barley, rye, oats, and malt. The likely etiology of celiac dis-

ease is genetic, manifested by a dominant gene of low penetrance, resulting in incidence figures of roughly 1:3000. Most cases are evident within 1 year of the introduction of gluten-containing products to the diet. The usual clinical course is marked by a falloff in percentile levels from standard growth curves, with the falloff in weight preceding that of height; and it is associated with the presence of foul-smelling, bulky stools resulting from steatorrhea. The physical findings of a protuberant abdomen with wasted buttocks and extremities always raises the possibility of cystic fibrosis and giardiasis as the major differential diagnoses to be considered. The presentation may be considerably more subtle, particularly in older children, and there have been recent reports of cases manifested solely by growth failure without diarrhea. Once the diagnosis is suspected, elevated serum levels of antigliadin antibodies (IgA, IgG), as well as antiendomysial and antireticulin antibodies, strongly suggest the diagnosis. The patient may then be referred for an endoscopic, small intestinal biopsy; a flat villus lesion that responds to gluten withdrawal is diagnostic.

Children in the Age Group of 3 to 18 Years
Major causes of chronic diarrhea in this age group include:

- Giardiasis
- Celiac disease
- Late-onset lactose intolerance
- Inflammatory bowel disease
- Crohn's disease
- Ulcerative colitis

Chronic diarrhea is a less frequent complaint after 3 years of age. Because CNSD invariably resolves by this time, this major nonpathologic cause of diarrhea observed in younger children no longer presents a problem. In fact, the only significant causes of chronic diarrhea after the age of 3 years that do not represent an underlying disease process are chronic constipation resulting in overflow stools, late-onset lactose intolerance, and "adult-type" irritable bowel syndrome. Giardiasis and even celiac disease may become manifest at any age and must be considered in any patient whose course suggests a malabsorptive state.

Late-onset lactose intolerance—With the exception of white persons of Northern European extraction, lactose intolerance is a common, developmentally-related phenomenon in older children and adults, with more than 95% in some ethnic groups being affected. Clinical manifestations result from absent intestinal lactase leading to malabsorption of lactose and an osmotic, fermentative diarrhea. Excessive gas production may cause crampy abdominal pain. When noted by positive breath H_2 testing in a patient under 5 years of age, lactose malabsorption usually reflects underlying small bowel mucosal dysfunction. In older children, however, lactase deficiency usually is a genetically mediated phenomenon without associated gastrointestinal pathologic findings. This diagnosis should be considered in the older patient presenting with diarrhea, abdominal pain, and flatulence, particularly when the child appears otherwise clinically well. A trial of a lactose-free diet is both diagnostic and therapeutic. Long-term management, especially in younger children, may involve treatment of milk with Lact-Aid, a yeast-derived lactase that predigests the offending sugar.

Irritable bowel syndrome—Not to be confused with "toddler's" diarrhea, "adult-type" irritable bowel syndrome (IBS) is a relatively common cause of chronic diarrhea in the adolescent. Passage of frequent, low-volume liquid stools, with concurrent lower abdominal cramping, is often associated with physical and/or emotional stress. Similar to the clinical history in adults with this still poorly understood disorder, diarrheal episodes typically alternate with periods of constipation. As in other chronic diarrheal states of older children and adolescents, the major differential diagnoses include infection, late-onset lactose intolerance, inflammatory bowel disease, and laxative abuse. IBS-related symptoms may improve in response to dietary fiber supplementation (10 to 15 g/day) with either psyllium (Metamucil®) or methylcellulose (Citrucel®), and antispasmodic medications (eg, dicyclomine) have been used in IBS with variable success.

Crohn disease—Crohn disease, or regional enteritis, represents an idiopathic, inflammatory condition that may involve any portion of the digestive tract; however, the terminal ileum and colon are the most frequently affected areas. Malabsorption is an infrequent complication, except in cases in which severe jejunal and ileal involvement results in nutrient and bile salt loss. The most common presenting symptoms include diarrhea (with or without blood), fevers, abdominal pain, and growth failure, with poor growth and weight gain most commonly occurring as a consequence of reduced caloric intake. In fact, Crohn disease, like celiac disease, should be considered in any child manifesting inadequate growth and development, even if the patient is otherwise relatively asymptomatic. Laboratory aids to diagnosis include findings of anemia, thrombocytosis, an elevated erythrocyte sedimentation rate, and hypoproteinemia. Barium studies will often reveal characteristic mucosal abnormalities, but definitive diagnosis requires colonoscopic biopsy evidence of chronic inflammation with granulomas and giant cells (see Chapter 79).

Ulcerative colitis—Evaluation of ulcerative colitis parallels that of Crohn disease, because the presenting signs and symptoms are similar. However, ulcerative colitis may appear in much younger children (with some reported cases in children under 1 year of age), and bloody diarrhea is a more common presentation. Because this disease only affects colonic mucosa ("backwash" ileitis is a relatively uncommon condition in pediatrics), malabsorption is not a problem. Proctosigmoidoscopy with cultures and biopsies should always be performed, because bacterial colitis and amebiasis must be ruled out. Medical treatment, including the use of salicylazosulfapyridine and corticosteroids, is similar to that employed in Crohn disease.

DATA GATHERING

History

Obviously, an attempt to rule out every cause of chronic diarrhea in each patient is a futile and costly exercise. In infants, the most common cause of protracted diarrhea is postinfectious lactose-intolerance. In this group of patients, requirements for inpatient evaluation and treatment are clearly dependent on the infant's state of hydration. In particular, patients who pass large volume, watery stools will require an in-hospital evaluation. Failure to improve while not taking anything by mouth and receiving intravenous (IV) therapy suggests the possibility of a secretory process. In the older infant and child, after a complete dietary and travel history is obtained, the course of diagnostic workup depends largely on the clinical state of the patient. Several screening studies may then direct further workup.

Laboratory Evaluation

Stool Examination
Stool examination is important not only to confirm the diarrheal state but also to give some clues as to the cause. Thus, watery, acidic, explosive stools suggest carbohydrate malabsorption, whereas foul-smelling, bulky ones indicate steatorrhea. Similarly, mucoid stools with or without diarrhea with occult blood (Hemoccult-positive) indicate the possibility of protein intolerance in infants, IBD in older children and adolescents, and infection in all age groups. Specific tests on fecal material should include:

1. pH, reducing substances (to rule out carbohydrate malabsorption)
2. Wright's stain for polymorphonuclear neutrophils, eosinophils (infection, allergy)
3. Hemoccult test for occult blood
4. Cultures for ova and parasites
5. Sudan stain for fat

Growth Curve
The growth curve is the most important single piece of information required to establish the likely nature and chronicity of the problem, and it should include weight, height, and weight-for-height assessments. Thus, a sudden weight falloff while maintaining height percentile suggests a relatively acute process. On the other hand, reduction of both weight and height percentile levels from previous growth points indicates chronic illness and may reflect chronic caloric deprivation (*eg,* in IBD) or malabsorption.

Hematologic Studies
Results of hematologic studies will provide evidence for nutritional deficits (levels of albumin, total protein, folate, vitamin B_{12}) and suggest an infectious or other inflammatory etiology (values for complete blood cell count and erythrocyte sedimentation rate).

Malabsorption Studies
In a case in which chronic malabsorption is suspected, certain screening studies will aid in assessing absorptive function.

Lactose breath H_2—This noninvasive study measures H_2 levels in expired air, formed by colonic bacterial fermentation of unabsorbed lactose. If results are abnormal (*ie,* H_2 >20 ppm above baseline) in patients less than 5 years of age, small bowel disease should be suspected.

Carotene and 1-hour blood D-xylose absorption—These are additional screening studies of small intestinal function. Carotene levels are only useful if dietary carotene intake is adequate; a value of >100 mg/dL is normal. A serum carotene <50 mg/dL suggests malabsorption.

Antigliadin antibodies—These recently developed, serum antibody assays have been shown in several studies to be reliable screening tests for celiac disease. Testing is available in most commercial laboratories, and four antibody titers are currently measured: antigliadin IgA and IgG, antiendomysial, and antireticulin antibodies. Of these tests, the antigliadin IgA, antiendomysial, and antireticulin antibodies are the most specific for celiac disease (when positive, specificity is >95%), whereas an isolated elevation of antigliadin IgG exhibits a high degree of sensitivity in celiac patients but a much lower specificity (*ie,* elevated antigliadin IgG titers are found in a wide range of disorders). A serum antibody screen that suggests celiac disease (most commonly an elevated titer of antigliadin IgA) indicates the need to refer the patient to a pediatric gastroenterologist for small bowel biopsy.

72-hour fecal fat—When properly carried out, this test is the most definitive test for steatorrhea. On a diet containing 100 g of fat, fat excretion should not exceed 7 g/day.

When the workup suggests a malabsorption syndrome, and cystic fibrosis and giardiasis have been ruled out, patients should be referred to a pediatric gastroenterologist.

INDICATIONS FOR CONSULTATION OR REFERRAL

Decisions to hospitalize patients with chronic diarrhea and refer them for subspecialist care are dependent on both the clinical severity and complexity of the problem. The dehydrated infant will obviously require IV hydration. Similarly, the condition of the infant (or even

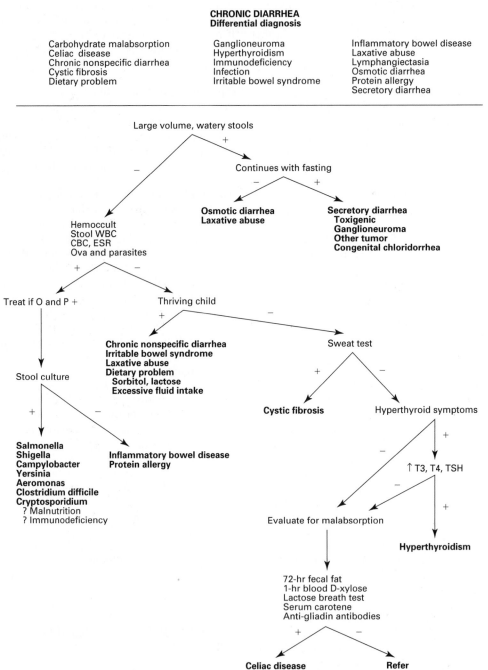

FIG 36-1

Decision tree for differential diagnosis of chronic diarrhea.

older child in some cases) who presents with inanition and severe failure to thrive may be evaluated more rapidly in an inhospital setting, and this patient often requires IV nutrition (central or peripheral) while his/her condition is being evaluated. Figure 36-1 illustrates the basic guidelines for the outpatient evaluation of chronic diarrhea. Obviously, diagnosis of specific entities requiring invasive intervention (eg, celiac disease, IBD) will require consultation by a pediatric gastroenterologist. However, in the majority of cases, workup can be completed by the primary care physician.

DISCUSSION OF ALGORITHM

In patients who present with large-volume, watery stools (often associated with dehydration), hospitalization is frequently required in order to differentiate between an osmotic state (diarrhea abates with fasting) and a secretory condition (diarrhea continues with fasting). Further evaluation according to the "decision tree" includes a careful dietary history, stool culture (bacterial and parasitic), and stool testing for pH, reducing substances, white blood cells (Wright stain) and gross/occult blood (Hemoccult). If the history suggests symptoms in response to dairy product ingestion, a lactose breath test should be performed. Thereafter, patients with infections, specific food intolerances, or suspected IBD can be appropriately treated or referred. If all of these studies are normal, a diagnosis of chronic nonspecific diarrhea (infants and toddlers) or irritable bowel syndrome (older children and adolescents) is reserved for those patients who continue to thrive despite their symptoms. In this group, response to dietary manipulation (eg, increased dietary fat content, reduced fluid intake, fiber supplementation) confirms these diagnoses. If laxative abuse is suspected, certain specific agents may be identified biochemically in the fecal effluent (eg, phenolphthalein). For those patients whose diarrhea is associated with failure to thrive (in association with an appropriate calorie and protein intake), a sweat chloride determination and, if necessary, additional investigations for immunodeficiency states and other malabsorption syndromes should be carried out.

BIBLIOGRAPHY

Ament ME, Barclay GN: Chronic diarrhea, *Pediatr Ann* 11:124, 1982.

Anderson CM: Malabsorption in children. *Clin Gastroenterol* 6:355, 1977.

Baldassano RN, Liacouras CA: Chronic diarrhea: A practical approach for the pediatrician, *Pediatr Clin North Am* 38:667, 1991.

Barr RG, Perman JA, Schoeller DA, et al: Breath tests in pediatric gastrointestinal disorders. *Pediatrics* 62:393, 1978.

Calvin RT, Klish WJ, Nichols BL: Disaccharidase activities, jejunal morphology, and carbohydrate tolerance in children with chronic diarrhea. *J Pediatr Gastroenterol Nutr* 4:949, 1985.

Cohen SA, Hendricks KM, Mathis RK, et al: Chronic nonspecific diarrhea: dietary relationships, *Pediatrics* 64:402, 1979.

Davidson M, Wasserman R: The irritable colon of childhood, *J Pediatr* 69:1027, 1966.

Greene HL, Ghishan FK: Excessive fluid intake as a cause of chronic diarrhea in young children, *J Pediatr* 102:836, 1983.

Hyams JS, Leichtner AM: Apple juice. An unappreciated cause of chronic diarrhea. *Am J Dis Child* 139:503, 1985.

Lebenthal E, Khin-Maung U, Zheng BY, et al: Small intestinal glucoamylase deficiency and starch malabsorption: A newly recognized alpha-glucosidase deficiency in children, *J Pediatr* 124:541, 1994.

Lo CW, Walker WA: Chronic protracted diarrhea of infancy, a nutritional disease. *Pediatrics* 72:786, 1983.

Nichols BL, Carazza F, Nichols VN: Mosaic expression of brush-border enzymes in infants with chronic diarrhea and malnutrition, *J Pediatr Gastroenterol Nutr* 14:371, 1992.

Phillips AD, Schmitz J: Familial microvillous atrophy: A clinicopathological survey of 23 cases, *J Pediatr Gastroenterol Nutr* 14:38, 1992.

Phillips SF: Diarrhea: a current view of the pathophysiology. *Gastroenterology* 63:495, 1972.

San Joaquin VH, Pickett DA: Aeromonas-associated gastroenteritis in children, *Pediatr Infect Dis J* 7:53, 1985.

Sunshine P, Sinatra FR, Mitchell CH: Intractable diarrhea of infancy. *Clin Gastroenterol* 6:445, 1977.

Sutphen JL, Grand RJ, Flores A, et al: Chronic diarrhea associated with *Clostridium difficile* in children. *Am J Dis Child* 137:275, 1983.

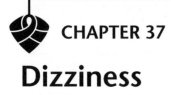

CHAPTER 37

Dizziness

Roger J. Packer

Dizziness is a nonspecific term used to describe diverse symptoms including lightheadedness, weakness, unsteadiness, or the illusion of rotational movement. The significance and proper evaluation of the condition of the dizzy child is dependent on a better understanding of what the patient is actually experiencing when dizziness occurs. If the child complains of feeling a sense of whirling or rotation of himself/herself or the environment, then he/she is suffering from vertigo, which implies dysfunction of the vestibular system.

In this chapter discussion is limited to vertiginous dizziness.

DIFFERENTIAL DIAGNOSIS

Common Causes of Vertiginous Dizziness
- **Infection**
    Otitis media
    Mastoiditis
    Labyrinthitis
- **Toxins**
    Aminoglycosides
    Ethycrynic acid
    Salicylates
    Quinine
- **Trauma**
    Immediate or delayed
- **Tumor**
    Brain stem glioma
    Acoustic neuroma
- **Multiple etiologies**
    Cholesteatoma
    Migraine
    Epilepsy
        Complex partial
        Simple partial
    Benign paroxysmal vertigo
    Benign recurrent vertigo
    Multiple sclerosis
    Ménière disease

Discussion
Vertigo may be conceptualized as occurring either on a peripheral basis, secondary to dysfunction of the vestibular apparatus, or on a central basis, following impairment of the vestibular nuclei or their brain-stem connections.

In childhood, peripheral vertigo is more common than central vertigo and may rarely occur as a complication of acute and chronic otitis media. Mastoiditis and associated suppurative labyrinthitis with vertigo, fever, and pain are rare in the antibiotic era but, when present, cause redness and warmth behind the ear. Variation of the mastoid pneumatization may make diagnosis somewhat difficult. Cholesteatomas, masses of desquamated epithelial cells occurring primarily or associated with chronic otitis media, invade bone and may result in labyrinthitis and vertigo. Small bits of whitish debris in the middle ear are seen extruding from the perforated tympanic membrane. Radiologic studies disclose destruction of the temporal bone.

Vestibular neuronitis (viral labyrinthitis) usually occurs in children over 10 years of age but may occur at any age. It is often associated with intercurrent upper respiratory tract infection or middle ear infection. Viral labyrinthitis is most symptomatic during the first 2 weeks of illness, slowly improving during the following 2 weeks. Results of vestibular function tests are abnormal during the disease, and spontaneous nystagmus is common. Findings of audiologic tests are normal. Two entities frequently confused with vestibular neuronitis, Ménière disease and benign positional vertigo, are rare in childhood. Ménière disease results in recurrent paroxysmal vertigo, tinnitus, and hearing loss. Benign positional vertigo is manifest by intermittent vertiginous episodes associated with rapid changes of head position. Toxic labyrinthitis may occur following the administration of various drugs (most noteworthy, the aminoglycosides). The onset of this illness is usually insidious, and the diagnosis may be missed if a careful history of drug intake is not performed. Other drugs that may rarely cause a similar toxic labyrinthitis include ethacrynic acid, salicylates, and quinine.

Vertigo may occur secondary to trauma. Sudden vestibular damage, occurring immediately after trauma, with resultant vertigo, nausea, vomiting, and spontaneous nystagmus, poses little difficulty in the differential diagnosis. Posttraumatic vertigo occurs days and sometimes weeks following head trauma and is manifest with sudden changes of head position. This condition is associated with abnormal vestibular function as demonstrated by testing. In contrast, dizziness, as a component of the postconcussion syndrome, is rarely associated with vertigo or abnormal vestibular testing.

Benign paroxysmal vertigo, which occurs between the ages of 1 and 3 years, is heralded by acute episodes of imbalance. During the attack, which may occur in clusters, the child seems frightened, becomes pale, and, if standing, either reaches for support or falls but does not lose consciousness. Subjective symptoms are difficult to ascertain. Infrequently, these are associated with upper respiratory tract infection or middle ear infection. The cause of these attacks is unknown, although some believe it to be the equivalent of a migraine attack. Results of radiologic, audiographic, and electroencephalogram (EEG) studies are normal. Findings of tests of vestibular function are usually consistent with peripheral vestibular dysfunction.

Vertigo on a central basis is uncommon in childhood, although it may occur as a component of epilepsy or migraine. Vertiginous symptoms may uncommonly be the sole clinical manifestation of partial complex (temporal lobe) seizures and during these attacks vestibular function is said to be normal. However, usually the vertiginous symptoms are associated with other symptoms referrable to the temporal lobe and abnormalities are noted on EEG. Vertigo may also occur prior to onset of a seizure, and thus be the "aura" of a more complex event. Vertiginous migraine may mimic temporal lobe epilepsy, but the history of associated headaches makes clinical differentiation possible. Similarly, vertigo may occur during a migraine attack.

When vertigo occurs secondary to tumors of the posterior fossa such as brain-stem gliomas, it tends to be overshadowed by associated neurologic deficits. Acoustic neuromas and other tumors of the cerebellopontine angle do present with vertigo but are rare until adulthood. Other rare reported causes of central vertigo are encephalitis, increased intracranial pressure, and syringobulbia. Multiple sclerosis can, in rare cases, present as vertigo in the adolescent.

DATA GATHERING

History
The key to the proper diagnosis and management of the child's complaint is determining what the child or parent means by "dizziness." If the patient's symptoms are that of true vertigo, differentiation between peripheral and central etiologies is of major importance and is often possible. Complaints of tinnitus, hearing loss, pain, or a sensation of fullness in the ear, as well as nausea and vomiting are much more frequent with peripheral lesions. The history of intermittent episodes of severe vertigo is much more

TABLE 37-1
Nylen-Barany Maneuver

TEST	CENTRAL VERTIGO	PERIPHERAL VERTIGO
Nystagmus	Yes	Yes
Latency	Immediate onset	Few seconds delay
Adaption	No	Yes
Fatigue	No	Yes (disappears on repetition)
Subjective vertigo	Usually absent	Present

consistent with peripheral disease, because central vertigo tends to be persistent and somewhat milder.

Physical Examination

Important features on the physical examination include evidence of redness or warmth behind the ear, suggesting mastoiditis, serous labyrinthitis, or bacterial labyrinthitis. Careful cranial nerve examination is mandatory for diagnosis, because involvement of the fifth or seventh cranial nerve implies central vertigo. The fifth cranial nerve supplies sensation to the face and motor innervation to the muscles of mastication. Mass lesions in the pontocerebellar angle may result in paraesthesias of the face with abnormalities of pain, cold, and touch sensation and, less often, in deviation of the jaw to the side of the lesions. The seventh cranial nerve innervates the muscles of the face, and disruption of its fibers causes weakness of the upper and lower portions of the face. The corneal reflex tests for the integrity of both the fifth and seventh cranial nerves; its loss may suggest subtle asymmetries of cranial nerve function. A neural-sensory hearing loss, indicating eighth cranial nerve dysfunction, may be of cochlear or primary eighth nerve origin. Differentiation is often impossible at bedside and requires further audiologic evaluation. Spontaneous nystagmus may result from either central or peripheral vertigo. Nystagmus due to vestibular dysfunction is commonly a jerk nystagmus with a fast and slow component, the fast component being toward the side of the impairment and increasing as one looks toward the lesion. It is primarily horizontal and decreased by fixation. A central basis for the nystagmus is likely if there are vertical or purely rotatory components to the nystagmus and if nystagmus changes direction when the direction of gaze is altered.

Extremely helpful in the diagnosis of vertigo are the inclusions of special tests that simulate the symptom. Not only should the patient's objective responses be evaluated during these procedures, but the child should be asked if these tests reproduce the subjective complaint. If they do not, the importance of any abnormality observed is questionable. The Nylen-Barany maneuver is performed after seating the child on the edge of the examining table. The subject is then asked to quickly lie back, and the head is tilted 45° backward and 45° to one side and maintained in this position for 60 seconds. The eyes are observed for the onset, duration, and direction of nystagmus. The child is then returned to the sitting position, and the maneuver is repeated, with the head turned to the opposite side. If nystagmus occurs, there is evidence for vestibular abnormality that can often be separated into central or peripheral categories (Table 37-1).

Laboratory Evaluation

Performance of additional tests after the initial evaluation is dependent on the clinical impression. These tests should not be done routinely and are included only to help understand what the neurologist or otolaryngologist may do in the evaluation. Caloric testing, which is irrigation of the ear canals with both warm and cold water, may be used to confirm vestibular dysfunction. Electronystagmography is a more sophisticated means of monitoring caloric responses and involves electrorecording the rate, direction, and amplitude of the nystagmus quantitatively with the eye open and closed. Audiometry should be performed if there is a suspicion of hearing loss. Other tests of auditory function, such as auditory recruitment, are useful in differentiating cochlear from eighth nerve dysfunction in the older child.

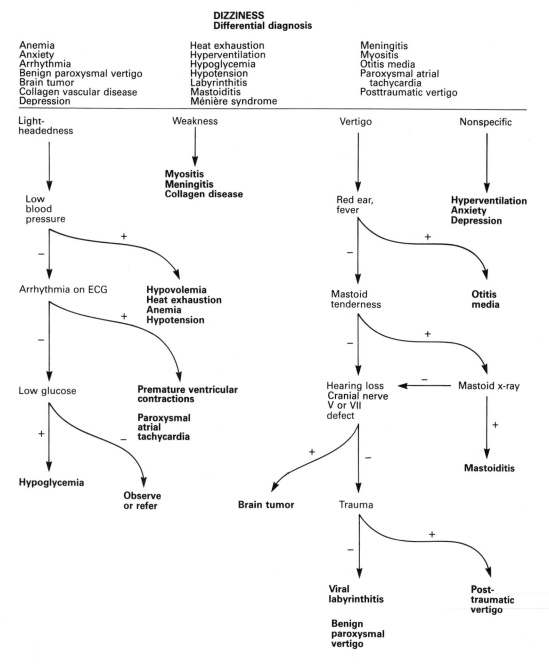

FIG 37-1

Decision tree for differential diagnosis of dizziness.

Radiographic studies are mandatory if one suspects central vestibular disease or labyrinth destruction. Radiographs of the skull and mastoid area, including tomography of the auditory canal, are useful in the detection of infectious or destructive lesions. Computed tomography with contrast enhancement and magnetic resonance imaging are procedures of choice if there is evidence of fifth or seventh nerve involvement. An EEG should be obtained only if there is a high index of suspicion that the vertigo is a seizure equivalent.

Indications for Consultation or Referral

The majority of causes of vertigo are benign, self-limited illnesses, and reassurance is the major aspect of therapy. In most cases, if the etiology is not readily apparent and there is no evidence of associated neurologic dysfunction or labyrinth destruction, the child may be treated symptomatically and the condition reevaluated before proceeding with more specific laboratory studies. In acute labyrinthitis, meclizine (12.5 mg twice a day to 25 mg twice a day for children over 12 years of age) results in symptomatic improvement of nausea and unsteadiness. Treatment of benign paroxysmal vertigo is hard to evaluate because the clinical course is unpredictable.

There may be improvement with the use of diphenhydramine (5 mg/kg/day).

DISCUSSION OF ALGORITHM

A careful history will help develop the further evaluation of dizziness (Fig. 37-1). These symptoms include: lightheadedness, dysequilibrium, weakness, and vertigo. Lightheadedness is usually associated with other systemic problems such as hypertension, hypoglycemia, and drug ingestion. Dysequilibrium and weakness tend to be secondary to neurologic problems. Vertigo should make one consider mastoiditis; deficits of the fifth, seventh, or eighth cranial nerves; or trauma.

BIBLIOGRAPHY

Eviator L: Dizziness in children, *Otolargol Clin North Am* 27(3):557–571, 1994.

Tusa RJ, Saada AA Jr, Niparko JK: Dizziness in children, *J Child Neurol* 9(3):261–274, 1994.

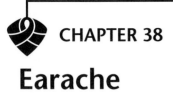

CHAPTER 38

Earache

William P. Potsic

Because earache is one of the most common complaints of pediatric patients, it is important to develop a plan for diagnosis and management. Although the great majority of patients will have an otologic cause for the earache, the diagnosis of earache can be a challenge because pain may be referred to the ear and surrounding structures from multiple areas of the head and neck. These areas are any structures innervated by the cranial nerves (V, VII, IX, X, and XI) and cervical nerves $C_{2,3}$. They include a number of structures that may or may not be visible at the time of direct examination in the office.

Otologic causes of ear pain usually produce severe, constant earache and are associated with fever. Nonotologic pain is usually intermittent, less severe, and not accompanied by fever. In our experience, we found 85% of cases with ear pain are from infection; 7% from referred pain; 5% from eustachian tube dysfunction and serous otitis media; and 3% from miscellaneous causes.

DIFFERENTIAL DIAGNOSIS

Common Causes of Earache
* **Trauma**
    Barotrauma
    Blunt trauma
    Sharp trauma
    Thermal injury
* **Infection**
    External otitis
    Acute supportive otitis media
    Mastoiditis
    Infected preauricular sinus
    Perichondritis
    Lymphadenitis
    Pharyngitis
    Sinusitis
    Aphthous ulcer
* **Allergic–Immunologic**
    Neuralgia
* **Tumor mass**
    Cholesteatoma
    Rhabdomyosarcoma
    Eosinophilic granuloma
    Facial neuroma
    Cystic hygroma
    Arteriovenous malformation
* **Multiple etiologies**
    Eustachian tube dysfunction, effusion
    Referred pain, dental, oropharyngeal
    Temporomandibular
    Psychogenic pain
    Tic
    Migraine
    Myofacial pain
    Parotiditis
    Parotid duct stone

Discussion
The diagnosis of earache involves careful history and examination of the ear by inspection and pneumatic otoscopy. Otologic causes of earache are usually infections but may be from trauma or tumors.

Otologic causes of earache are the most common and present with severe, steady pain. External otitis causes pain with chewing or manipulating the pinna. A foul-smelling discharge

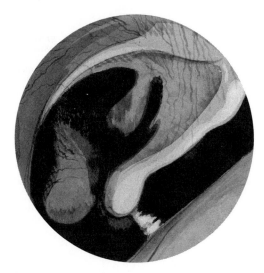

FIG 38-1
Normal eardrum showing translucent tympanic membrane and middle ear structure: malleus in center and incus and stapes above it.

is present in the inflamed, edematous external canal.

Acute suppurative otitis media causes deep, steady, and severe pain that is not aggravated by chewing. Very young children may just be fussy or lethargic but older children either pull at their ear or specifically state that their ears hurt. Otoscopy reveals an inflamed and bulging eardrum. (A normal eardrum is shown in Fig. 38-1).

The earache associated with eustachian tube dysfunction is mild and associated with a steady sensation of fullness. Intermittent acute exacerbations may be present for 30 minutes to 1 hour as the negative pressure fluctuates. Barotrauma usually causes severe sudden pain that resolves spontaneously in 1 hour.

Nonotologic causes of ear pain consist of problems in the head and neck that refer pain to the ear. These include dental and temporomandibular joint pain (trigeminal nerve), Bell palsy, and aphthous ulcers (facial nerve), tonsillitis and adenoiditis (glossopharyngeal nerve), and esophageal foreign body and thyroiditis (vagus nerves). Referred pain from the cervical nerve $C_{2,3}$ include: lymphadenitis, infected cysts, cystic hygroma, hemangioma, and arteriovenous malformation. Cervical spine injury and neuralgia also cause ear pain.

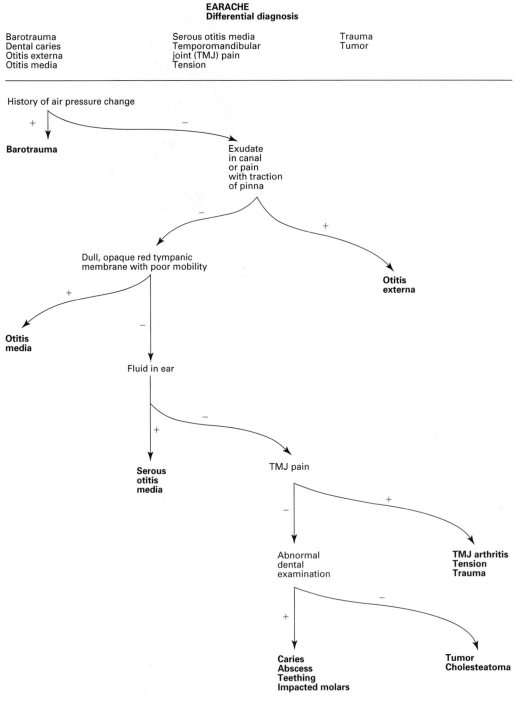

FIG 38-2
Decision tree for differential diagnosis of earache.

DATA GATHERING

History

Because most ear pain is secondary to infection, a careful history should include information about fever and symptoms of upper respiratory tract infection. Traumatic causes should also be excluded. Other important information includes evidence of dental problems, pain on chewing (temporomandibular joint) or after eating food, especially some foods that stimulate saliva flow (parotid pain).

Physical Examination

When the otologic examination is normal, the source of the problem must be searched for by examining the oral cavity, pharynx, and neck region. The signs and symptoms of the primary problem are often overshadowed by ear pain, but they usually cause some difficulty that is detectable to the patient if he/she is asked while the history is taken. The most common reason for referred ear pain in children is dental problems or aphthous ulcerations of the oral cavity. Erupting teeth, caries, or gingivitis may also cause referred pain. The pharynx and nose should be examined carefully to search for pharyngitis, tonsillitis, or evidence of sinusitis. The neck must be palpated for cervical adenitis, thyroiditis, or cysts.

Laboratory Evaluation

When the cause of the referred pain is not apparent, a radiographic sinus series may be helpful to demonstrate the presence of sinusitis. In addition, the complete evaluation of otalgia may need to include a dental examination with dental radiographs and an otolaryngology consultation for a complete head and neck examination including nasopharyngoscopy, hypopharyngoscopy, and laryngoscopy.

Children with severe debilitating pain or severe ear infection may need admission for intravenous antimicrobial therapy and narcotic medication for pain control.

INDICATIONS FOR CONSULTATION OR REFERRAL

Earache of otologic origin usually resolves in 4 to 8 hours after antibiotic therapy is started. If the pain persists after 24 hours, other reasons for the pain should be investigated. The help of an otolaryngologist or neurologist may be needed. If no cause for the pain is apparent by history, physical examination, or laboratory tests, a tension-pain syndrome may be present.

DISCUSSION OF ALGORITHM

An algorithm for differential diagnosis of earache is presented in Figure 38-2. A careful physical examination will detect either external otitis or otitis media, secretory otitis, or cholesteatoma. Neck trauma and dental problems should be excluded. If no diagnosis is made, causes of referred pain from surrounding structures should be considered.

BIBLIOGRAPHY

Bluestone CD, Shurin PA: Middle ear disease in children: Pathogenesis, diagnosis, and management, *Pediatr Clin North Am* 3:15, 1970.

Bluestone CD, Klein JO, Paradise JL, et al: Workshop on effects of otitis media on the child, *Pediatrics* 71:639–652, 1983.

Chasin WO: Otalgia (the ear). In Bluestone CD, Stool SF, editors: *Pediatric otolaryngology,* ed 2, Philadelphia, 1990, WB Saunders.

Potsic WP: Pediatric otorhinolaryngology (the ear). In Rudolph AM, et al: Pediatrics, ed 19, Norwalk, CT, 1991, Appleton & Lange.

Potsic WP, Handler SD: Primary care pediatric otolaryngology, ed 2, Andover, 1995, J. Michael Ryan Publishing.

Tremble GE: Referred pain in the ear, *Arch Otolaryngol* 81:57–63, 1965.

CHAPTER 39

Edema

Michael E. Norman

Edema is the accumulation of excessive salt and water in the extravascular (*eg,* interstitial) spaces. Digital pressure may or may not produce an indentation, and often there is a "doughy" feel to the subcutaneous tissue. Edema may be generalized or localized, but is usually confined to the dependent extremities and the distensible soft tissues, such as the periorbital region, scrotum, and labia majora. Trauma or infection often produces edema at the site of injury. Pathophysiologic causes of edema include decreased plasma oncotic pressure, increased venous or lymphatic hydrostatic pressure, and increased vascular permeability due either to the release of inflammatory mediators, as in an allergic reaction, or to vasculitis, as in collagen vascular disease.

DIFFERENTIAL DIAGNOSIS

The etiology of edema may be divided according to whether the edema is localized, especially if asymmetric, or generalized.

Common Causes of Edema

- **Localized**
  - Trauma
  - Infection
  - Lymphatic obstruction
    - Lymphedema praecox
  - Venous obstruction
  - Allergic reaction
  - Immediate-type hypersensitivity
- **Generalized**
  - Toxins
  - Drugs
  - Contraceptives
- **Metabolic/genetic**
  - Malnutrition
  - Protein-losing enteropathy

Premenstrual swelling
Inappropriate level of antidiuretic hormone (ADH)
- **Congenital**
  - Biliary atresia
  - Lymphedema praecox
- **Multiple etiologies**
  - Cardiac
    - Congestive heart failure
    - Pericardial tamponade
    - Constrictive pericarditis
  - Hepatic-biliary
    - Hepatitis
    - Cirrhosis
  - Renal disease
    - Nephrotic syndrome
    - Glomerulonephritis
    - Renal failure
  - Gastrointestinal
    - Protein-losing enteropathy
    - Cirrhosis
  - Endocrine
    - Hypothyroidism
    - Mineralocorticoid excess

DATA GATHERING

History

Indolent localized edema such as "puffy eyes" on awakening is usually due to an infection such as periorbital cellulitis, an allergic reaction, or nephrotic syndrome. Traumatic edema is usually apparent from the history. Allergic reactions may or may not be evident, either on the basis of past medical or family history or exposure to a known allergen. In such cases the presence of pruritus, urticaria, laryngeal obstruction, or abdominal pain suggests the diagnosis. Lymphatic obstruction is almost always unilateral and provides a "woody" feeling to the affected extremity.

EDEMA
Differential diagnosis

Allergy	Hepatic disease	Pregnancy
Cellulitis, infection	Lymphatic obstruction	Premenstrual swelling
Collagen disease	Lymphedema praecox	Renal failure
Glomerulonephritis	Nephrotic syndrome	Trauma
Heart failure	Pericardial effusion	Vasculitis

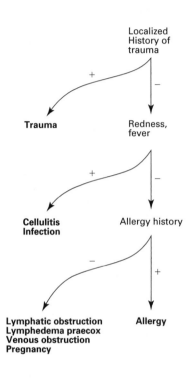

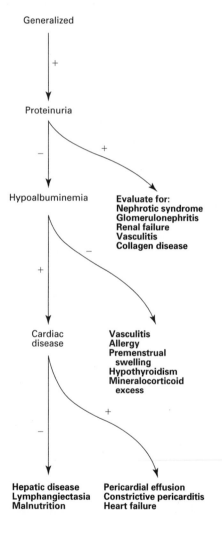

FIG 39-1
Decision tree for differential diagnosis of edema.

Physical Examination

Generalized edema may be insidious, with only progressive weight gain offering a clue to the diagnosis. This is particularly true in lean, muscular individuals. Careful attention must be paid to sudden changes in shoe or belt size. Pitting edema may become apparent only after firm direct pressure with the fingertips; the forehead and shin are favored places to perform this examination. An examination for ascites should be done with palpation and percussion.   In edema secondary to particular organ system involvement, the symptoms and physical signs are referable to that particular system and are usually obvious; they are not discussed here. Bloating and cyclical symptoms point to premenstrual edema in the menstruating girl. Occasionally a severe allergic reaction will cause generalized edema, which is often associated with acute laryngeal edema and/or acute abdominal pain, secondary to edema of the gastrointestinal tract.

Laboratory Evaluation

The presence of localized edema other than bilateral periorbital edema rarely requires any investigation other than bacterial cultures for suspected primary infection (*eg,* cellulitis) or urticaria secondary to infection (*eg,* strep throat). Bilateral periorbital edema or generalized edema always necessitates a complete urinalysis, unless there are obvious symptoms and signs of congestive heart failure, constrictive pericarditis, or pericardial tamponade. Proteinuria indicates the need for further investigations to differentiate idiopathic nephrotic syndrome (levels of serum albumin and cholesterol, 24-hour urine sample for measurement of total protein excretion) from glomerulonephritis (determination of antistreptolysin O, C3 complement, antinuclear antibody [ANA] titer).   The absence of proteinuria is compatible with hepatobiliary disease or vasculitis. A low level of serum albumin without proteinuria indicates protein-losing enteropathy, cirrhosis, or malnutrition. Determinations of erythrocyte sedimentation rate, ANA titer, and

anti-DNA antibodies are often helpful in vasculitis. Edema with associated hyponatremia but inappropriately concentrated urine suggests antidiuretic hormone excess.

INDICATIONS FOR CONSULTATION OR REFERRAL

Patients who should be considered for referral or consultation include those with suspected anaphylaxis with laryngeal edema or edema of the abdominal viscera, unexplained generalized edema, and specific disease such as protein-losing enteropathy or cirrhosis.

DISCUSSION OF ALGORITHM

A "decision tree" for differential diagnosis of edema is presented in Figure 39-1. The first task is to determine if the edema is localized or generalized to more than one area of the body. Localized edema is likely secondary to trauma, infection, allergy, or lymphatic obstruction (lymphangiectasia or tumor). Generalized edema is usually secondary to heart failure, increased protein loss, or decreased protein production. The patient should be examined for heart failure, the urine tested for protein, and the serum albumin level measured. If the diagnosis cannot be confirmed by these investigations, the patient may have vasculitis, serum sickness or allergy, premenstrual swelling, or generalized lymphangiectasia.

BIBLIOGRAPHY

Baglia R, Levy JE: Pathogenesis and treatment of edema, *Pediatr Clin North Am* 34:639, 1987.
Dixon BS, Berl T: Pathogenesis of edema in renal disease. In Edelmann CM Jr, editor: *Pediatric kidney disease,* ed 2, Boston, 1992, Little, Brown, and Co.

Gauthier B: Edema. In Gauthier B, Edelman CM, editors: *Nephrology and urology for the pediatrician,* Boston, 1982, Little, Brown, and Co.
Lewis JM, Wald ER: Lymphedema praecox, *J Pediatr* 104:641, 1984.

CHAPTER 40

Enuresis

Jeffrey C. Weiss

Enuresis, the involuntary passage of urine, is a poorly understood symptom with several possible causes and corresponding treatments. To evaluate and treat this common and annoying problem, the primary care physician should follow a logical stepwise approach of first defining the problem, screening for infection, and developing a reasonable treatment plan.

The term *primary nocturnal enuresis* means that the child has never kept a bed dry for a continuous period of several months. In contrast, secondary enuresis implies that nighttime bladder control was achieved for at least a 3-month period before the wetting resumed. Approximately 85% of all cases of enuresis fall into the primary class. Both primary and secondary enuresis can be caused by maturational, organic, or psychosocial problems, but many authorities think that secondary enuresis is less likely to be due to a simple maturational factor.

DIFFERENTIAL DIAGNOSIS

Common Causes of Nocturnal Enuresis
- **Maturational**
  Small bladder capacity
  Immature sleep arousal pattern
- **Organic**
  Urinary tract infection
  Urinary tract structural abnormality
  Bladder innervation disorder
  Myelomeningocele
  Diabetes mellitus
  Diabetes insipidus
  Hyposthenuria (inability to concentrate urine)
  Constipation (compression of bladder)
  Lack of nighttime antidiuretic hormone spike
  Chronic upper airway obstruction

Sickle cell anemia and trait
Sensitivity to certain foods (milk, eggs, orange juice)
- **Emotional**
  Temporary stress
  Regressive behavior (birth of a sibling)
  Severe emotional disturbance

Discussion
Most nocturnal enuresis is due to maturational factors. Boys are affected twice as often as girls, and nearly 75% of patients have a positive family history. The underlying pathogenesis may be an immature sleep pattern or small urinary bladder capacity. Studies correlating the electroencephalogram with enuresis indicate that these children are actually asleep when wetting occurs, usually shortly after bedtime. Children with maturational enuresis show little evidence of emotional maladjustment. Organic causes of bedwetting account for less than 5% of all cases. Most of those are due to a urinary tract infection. An organic cause should be considered likely if the child had previously been dry at night for a prolonged period or if daytime wetting accompanies the nocturnal enuresis. Temporary stress and regressive behavior commonly cause bedwetting, especially in preschool-aged children. However, in rare cases enuresis is a symptom of severe emotional disturbance. These children tend to be older than most enuretics, and wetting may occur just prior to morning awakening; other behavior problems are often obvious.

DATA COLLECTION

History
When asking about the wetting pattern, determine if the enuresis is primary or secondary, whether it is associated with diurnal enuresis,

whether the wetting is constant or sporadic, and at what time of the night wetting usually occurs. Daytime frequency can be due to the small bladder capacity found in maturational enuresis; however, the presence of dysuria or an abnormal urinary stream suggests urinary tract infection.

The physician must know which treatments have already been attempted, how successful these were, and whether a punitive approach had been tried. This information will be particularly important in planning the future management.

The family history should focus on enuresis in other family members. Questioning about sickle-cell disease, food allergy, diabetes, constipation, and upper airway problems is occasionally helpful. Although a review of systems is part of any thorough evaluation, significant information is rarely obtained in cases of nocturnal enuresis. Because enuresis is probably not related to coercive toilet training, lengthy discussions of this topic may serve only to generate parental guilt.

The child's behavior patterns should be discussed in detail. Specific attention should be paid to how he/she feels about the enuresis and whether this problem is affecting self-image and limiting the child's social activities. Asking about family dynamics and stresses is necessary to uncover hidden psychologic factors. Even with maturational or organic enuresis, an understanding of how the family is responding to the problem is important. Parents should be asked why they are seeking help at this particular time and what bothers them the most about their child's problem.

Physical Examination
Because organic problems rarely are the cause of enuresis, the physical examination is not usually diagnostic. However, the external genitalia should be examined carefully, especially for abnormalities of the urethral meatus. To detect urinary tract problems, the physician should observe the urinary stream and examine the child for costovertebral-angle tenderness and bladder distention. If a child has the urge to void, an estimation of bladder capacity can be made by measuring the urine volume. Because one study found tonsillectomy cured some children of nocturnal enuresis, the pharynx should be examined and upper airway obstruction should be ruled out. A neurologic examination (to look for bladder innervation disorders) should include an evaluation of lower extremity muscle strength,

deep tendon reflexes, and sensory functioning. Children with a history of constipation should be checked for stool impaction (which may cause enuresis by compressing the bladder). In addition, rectal sphincter tone and the anal wink reflex should be assessed because both the bladder and the rectal area are innervated by sacral nerves II to IV.

Laboratory Evaluation
In most cases of nocturnal enuresis, a urinalysis with a screening test for infection (such as the nitrite-reaction or Uricult) is the only test needed. Even this test rarely adds much information to a carefully obtained history and physical examination. Routine sickle-cell testing in black children with enuresis is often recommended. Urine culture, pyelography, cystourethrography, and renal ultrasonography should be reserved for children whose symptoms suggest organic disorders.

TREATMENT

At present there is no treatment modality that is 100% successful for eliminating enuresis. As summarized below, the methods most commonly used include counseling, medication, and behavior modification with buzzer alarms.

Summary of Treatment
- Counseling
    Child and parent education
    Active role for child
    Motivation: physician interest, star charts, rewards
- Bladder exercises
    Stretching bladder
    Urine stream interruption
- Elimination diet
    Avoid milk, eggs, citrus fruits, and corn
- Hypnosis and imagery
- Medication (for special circumstances)
    Imipramine (Tofranil)
    Desmopressin (DDAVP)
    Oxybutynin (Ditropan)
- Buzzer-alarm conditioning

Before any successful treatment can begin, the family must understand that enuresis is a problem that is out of the child's conscious control. It is important that the child's enuresis is not perceived as bad behavior. Parents should realize that not only is enuresis a very common problem, but that it usually resolves spontaneously. Because scolding, restricting fluids, and waking the child generally do not help (and may actually delay the eventual cure), these methods should be discouraged.

The child must take an active role in the treatment process, taking responsibility for the symptoms himself/herself. Therefore, the physician should communicate directly with the child during office visits and phone contacts. The enuretic child must understand that he/she will be responsible for all aspects of his/her problem, including changing and washing the pajamas and sheets.

With motivational counseling, positive reinforcement should be given when the child stays dry. Keeping a calendar with stars and using small rewards can be quite helpful. Interest from a strongly optimistic physician can be a strong reinforcement factor to keep the child's motivation high. Although the cure rate with motivational counseling itself is not well known, many experts believe that this safe approach is quite useful as an adjunct to other forms of treatment.

Dry All Night by Alison Mack is a book that uses imagery to help young children learn nighttime bladder control. In a small study, reading *Dry All Night* every evening helped 40% of the children have a decrease in wetting of at least 2 nights per week. The book, available in paperback, contains much practical information and advice for parents.

Many children with nocturnal enuresis have been found to have a small functional bladder capacity (less than 4 oz in children who are 6 years of age). Starfield and Mellits have described a method to stretch the bladder, in which the child is told to postpone voiding as long as possible and the urge to urinate is gone. When sensing an uncomfortable feeling, the child is instructed to void into a measuring cup. The goal is to increase the bladder capacity steadily so that the child can get through the night without wetting. A second exercise, known as stream interruption, is designed to increase the child's ability to withstand bladder spasms. Here, the child starts to void and then stops the urine flow for a 10-second count before emptying his/her bladder. In Starfield's studies, approximately 35% of the children were successfully treated when bladder stretching exercises were used for

6 months. The successful treatment occurred in children with the greatest increases in bladder capacity.

Some children stopped wetting the bed when certain foods were eliminated from their diet. One study showed that milk, eggs, citrus fruits, and corn were most frequently found to be associated with enuresis. A 2-week trial of dietary therapy places little burden on the child or the family and may occasionally be worthwhile.

Imipramine is the medication most commonly used in the treatment of enuresis. It may work by anticholinergic action on the bladder or by altering the sleep cycle so as to improve arousal. Cure may occur rapidly, but there are frequent relapses. This medication may be a common cause of serious accidental ingestion or may even produce pulse rate and blood pressure changes when appropriate amounts are given. The dose ranges between 25 and 75 mg, depending on the child's age. Some children do better when the medication is given at supper rather than at bedtime. Imipramine should not be given to children younger than 5 or 6 years of age.

Oxybutynin (Ditropan), a smooth muscle relaxant, is not generally effective for primary nocturnal enuresis. It may, however, be of benefit for some children with associated diurnal enuresis.

Because some children do not have an increase in antidiuretic hormone levels at night, they produce a higher than normal urine volume. No study has shown exactly what percentage of enuretic children actually have this problem. Nevertheless, desmopressin (DDAVP) nasal spray, a vasopressin analogue, has recently been approved for the treatment of enuresis. Although a decrease in the number of wet nights has been shown, few children become completely dry, and when the medicine is withdrawn, the relapse rates are 60% to 100%. Side effects are uncommon, but the medication is extremely expensive.

In recent years, enuresis alarms have been shown to be the most effective treatment for bedwetting. The old bell-and-pad systems (which woke the family, were difficult to use, and occasionally caused skin ulcers) have been replaced by inexpensive (approximately $50) alarms that work on hearing-aid batteries. Small sensitive electrodes attach to the child's underwear and generally do not cause skin irritation. The two most popular models are the Wet Stop and Nytone buzzers. A new device, the Potty

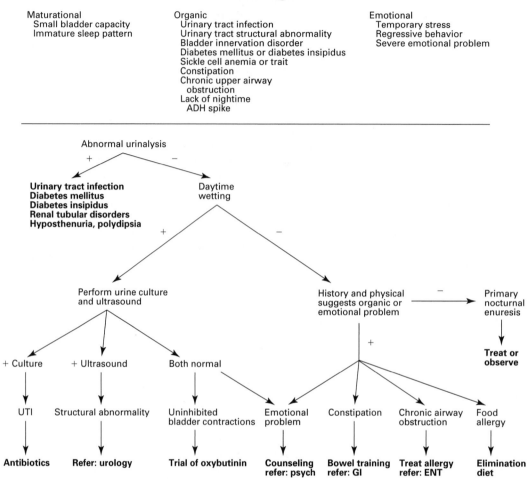

FIG 40-1

Decision tree for differential diagnosis of nocturnal enuresis.

Pager, uses vibration, rather than an auditory alarm, to wake the child. The physician will find it helpful to have a demonstration model, with detailed instruction sheets, in the office.

The buzzer-alarm conditioning method works slowly, but approximately 75% of enuretics are dry within 4 months after the initiation of therapy. By the end of the first month, the "puddles" in the bed are smaller each night. Some dry nights occur in the second month, and cure is seen by the third or fourth month. The alarm is used until there are no nights with wetting for 3 weeks. Some children get up to go to the bathroom at night; others learn to inhibit their micturition reflex until bladder contractions subside. Approximately 10% to 15% of children have relapses, but reconditioning is usually easy. Symptom substitution (the appearance of new emotional symptoms that replace the enuresis) has not been a problem with buzzer conditioning techniques. The motivation and cooperation needed to utilize the buzzer-alarm system usually requires that the child be at least 8 years of age. If the child is older than this, failure is most often associated with either family difficulties or behavior problems.

INDICATIONS FOR CONSULTATION OR REFERRAL

Most cases of nocturnal enuresis can be managed by the primary care physician. At the time of the initial evaluation, a combination of motivational counseling, bladder stretching exercise, and elimination diet can be tried. If significant improvement has not occurred within 2 weeks and the child is at least 8 years of age, a buzzer-alarm system is the next step. Use of medications depends on the physician, who must be aware of the potential side effects and relapse rates.

Referral to a urologist is indicated if the child has repeated urinary tract infections, urethral reflux, constant daytime dribbling, or an abnormal urinary stream. Children with severe family or behavioral problems require psychiatric consultation.

DISCUSSION OF ALGORITHM

An algorithm for the differential diagnosis of nocturnal enuresis is presented in Figure 40-1. In the vast majority of children only a careful history, physical examination, and urinalysis are required. Some experts recommend a urine culture for all enuretic children, but the yield is extremely low. It is probably more cost efficient to reserve urine culture and sensitivity for patients in whom the problem likely is organic, such as secondary or diurnal enuresis. Ultrasound and radiologic studies are very rarely necessary.

BIBLIOGRAPHY

Alon US: Nocturnal enuresis, *Pediatr Nephrol* 9:94–103, 1995.

Dische S, Yule W, Corbett J, et al: Childhood nocturnal enuresis: Factors associated with outcome of treatment with enuresis alarm, *Dev Med Child Neurol* 25:67–80, 1983.

Maizels M, Gandhik K, Keating B, Rosenbaum D: Diagnosis and treatment for children who cannot control urination, *Curr Prob Pediatr* 23: 402–450, 1993.

Olness K: The use of self-hypnosis in the treatment of childhood nocturnal enuresis, *Clin Pediatr* 14:273–279, 1975.

Ritvo ER, Ornitz EM, Gottlieb F, et al: Arousal and nonarousal types of enuretic events, *Am J Psychiat* 126:1, 1969.

Shelov SP, Gundy J, Weiss JC, et al: Enuresis: A contrast of attitudes of parents and physicians, *Pediatrics* 67:707–710, 1981.

Starfield B, Mellits ED: Increase in functional bladder capacity and improvements in enuresis, *J Pediatr* 72:483–487, 1968.

SUGGESTED READING FOR PARENTS

Mack A: *Dry all night,* Boston, 1989, Little, Brown, and Co.

Scharf M: *Waking up dry: How to end bedwetting forever,* Cincinnati, 1986, Writer's Digest Books.

Schmitt BD: Nocturnal enuresis: Finding the treatment that fits the child, *Contemp Pediatr* 7:70–97, 1990. Contains parent instruction sheets.

CHAPTER 41

Facial Weakness

Roger J. Packer

Acute facial paralysis is usually marked by either weakness in eyelids and/or facial expression, including furrowing of the brow and upward or downward movement of the corner of the lips. There may also be decreased lacrimal and salivary gland secretions as well as diminished taste sensation on the anterior two thirds of the tongue. Weakness in only the lower portion of the face (central) results from contralateral upper motor neuron damage, whereas weakness in the upper and lower portion of the face (peripheral) results from lower motor neuron damage of the seventh cranial nerve.

DIFFERENTIAL DIAGNOSIS

Common Causes of Facial Weakness
- **Congenital**
  Möbius syndrome
  Hypoplasia angulus oris
- **Trauma**
- **Infection**
  Meningitis
  Encephalitis
  Lyme disease
  Mastoiditis
  Otitis (acute and chronic)
  Herpes reactivation (Ramsay Hunt syndrome)
  Sarcoid
- **Neoplastic**
  Intrinsic pontine brain tumor
  Posterior fossa tumor
  Leptomeningeal dissemination
  Bone (mastoid) tumor
  Cholesteatoma
  Rhabdomyosarcoma
- **Autoimmune**
  Guillain-Barré syndrome

Myasthenia gravis
- **Miscellaneous**
  Bell palsy (possibly viral)
  Myotonic dystrophy
  Muscular dystrophy
  Congenital myopathy
  Melkersson-Rosenthal syndrome

Discussion

Facial weakness recognized immediately after birth is most likely traumatic in origin. This condition is usually secondary to intrauterine sacral pressure on the peripheral portion of the seventh nerve, although it may occur in traumatic deliveries with or without the application of forceps. These traumatic etiologies are clinically distinguishable from the Möbius syndrome, which is usually bilateral and involves other cranial nerves (especially the sixth cranial nerve nuclei, bilaterally). An often misdiagnosed condition is congenital hypoplasia of the depressor angulus oris muscle, resulting in an inability to depress the lower lip. Children with this condition are often referred for evaluation of facial weakness of the other side of the face, because parents note that the child's mouth pulls to the opposite side when crying (which is in reality an inability to depress the lip on the aplastic side). The importance of the recognition of this condition is not only its distinction from a more extensive cranial nerve involvement but the association of hypoplasia of the angulus oris with other congenital anomalies, especially cardiac anomalies.

The next major distinction in the diagnostic process is whether the acquired facial weakness is secondary to interruption of cortical input to the facial nerve nucleus or from direct nuclear nerve damage. Although interruption of cortical control of the facial nerve is relatively uncommon, its recognition is mandatory. Etiologies of so-called central facial weakness are similar to those of acute hemiplegia of childhood, including cerebrovascular accidents, primary central nervous system and metastatic tumors, traumatic injury, and a postseizure state.

Peripheral or lower motor neuron weakness is the common cause of facial weakness and the most common etiology is Bell palsy, which is a unilateral process.

Idiopathic or Bell palsy was initially believed to be secondary to primary or secondary ischemia of the facial nerve as it exits through the facial canal. There is now increasing evidence that Bell palsy is not a result of ischemia but rather is an acute cranial polyneuritis secondary to reactivation of herpes simplex virus.

Other causes of seventh nerve dysfunction are more frequent in children than they are in adults. Conditions that may mimic Bell palsy include lesions within the brain stem such as infiltrating pontine tumors, tumors that may secondarily infiltrate or arise on the surface of the brainstem (ependymomas and medulloblastomas), and demyelinating disease. Meningitis of bacterial, fungal, or neoplastic origin may selectively cause facial nerve dysfunction.

Isolated facial nerve palsy has recently been associated with central nervous system Lyme disease.

A rare variant (the Fisher variant) of acute postinfectious polyradiculitis (Guillain-Barré syndrome) may initially present with facial weakness. Rarely a child may have idiopathic cranial nerve neuropathies. Infections or neoplastic lesions (cholesteatomas, rhabdomyosarcomas) may compress the facial nerve outside of the brain stem. Acute and chronic otitis media may result in facial nerve dysfunction, although this complication is much less frequent in the antibiotic era. Herpetic involvement of the geniculate ganglion (Ramsay Hunt syndrome) may selectively cause facial weakness. Traumatic injury, especially to the base of the brain or the side of the face, may result in disruption of the facial nerve. Muscular causes of facial weakness are bilateral and slower in evolution. Rarely, a child may suffer from the Melkersson-Rosenthal syndrome, which is a triad of recurrent facial paralysis, facial edema, and furrowing of the tongue of unknown etiology.

DATA GATHERING

History
The basis of appropriate management of acute acquired facial palsy is careful clinical evaluation. Patients with idiopathic (Bell palsy usually suffer a paralysis of one side of the face that has evolved over a few hours. The child's face may have suddenly pulled to one side or the child could not close one of his/her eyes while sleeping. Another presentation is difficulty in eating or drinking, as substances in the mouth fall out of the involved side. If the child is old enough, however, there is frequently the complaint of a dull ache or sharp pain behind the ear for 1 to 2 days prior to the onset of the weakness. Information concerning recent headaches, fever, or rashes should be obtained at the initial evaluation. In addition, the child should be questioned about recent tick bites or tick exposure, which might suggest Lyme disease.

Physical Examination
A careful neurologic examination for the extent of weakness and associated neurologic deficits is mandatory in all cases of acquired facial palsy. The presence of greater involvement of the lower face suggests a supranuclear lesion and is usually associated with evidence of hemiparesis on the involved side. More extensive brain stem dysfunction is suggested by the presence of associated cranial nerve deficits, such as the inability to completely abduct the eye on the side of weakness (abduction of the eye controlled by the sixth cranial nerve), sensory loss in the face or the absence of the corneal reflex (sensation conveyed by the sensory component of the fifth cranial nerve), jaw muscle weakness (innervated by the motor portion of the fifth cranial nerve), abnormal palatal movements (innervated by the ninth and tenth cranial nerves), or abnormal tongue movement (innervated by the twelfth cranial nerve). It should be remembered that in idiopathic Bell palsy there are frequently mild sensory alterations to touch and pin sensation that often may confuse the diagnosis. The presence of bilateral facial weakness, ataxia, or systemic illness suggests meningeal involvement or the Guillain-Barré syndrome.

Obviously, it also is necessary to complete a careful otolaryngolic examination for signs of inner ear or mastoid bone involvement. The presence of a vesicular eruption in the outer ear suggests herpetic involvement of the geniculate ganglion.

If after careful clinical evaluation there is no other evidence for other sites of neurologic or otolaryngolic involvement, a diagnosis of Bell palsy is likely. The yield from additional tests such as complete blood cell count or glucose is quite low in children and probably need not be obtained in an otherwise well child. In a child with a history of recent tick exposure, especially in areas where Lyme disease is endemic, blood should be drawn at the time of presentation for determination of Lyme titers. If these titers are consistent with recent infection, a spinal tap should be performed. At present there is no evidence to support the routine need for cerebrospinal fluid evaluation in children with facial palsy who are otherwise well. Similarly, computed tomography or magnetic resonance imaging is not indicated in children with isolated, unilateral facial weakness. Skull radiographs with special views of the internal auditory meatus and formal audiologic evaluation are often recommended for all patients with acquired facial palsy, but in the otherwise asymptomatic patient for whom follow-up can be assured, this test can probably be delayed. Electrodiagnostic tests such as measurements of nerve conduction velocity and muscular denervation are unreliable in the first 72 hours of illness. These evaluations can be carried out later in the course of illness, if necessary, to confirm the diagnosis and supply prognostic information.

INDICATIONS FOR CONSULTATION OR REFERRAL

The management of acute facial nerve paresis of any specific cause is appropriate neurologic, neurosurgical, or otolaryngologic referral. Neurologic consultation should be immediately obtained if there is evidence of disruption of cortical control of seventh nerve function or associated cranial nerve deficits. Otolaryngologic consultation should be immediately obtained in children with signs of inner ear or mastoid bone involvement. If there is any evidence of meningitis of whatever cause, the patient should be immediately hospitalized and appropriately treated. Facial weakness secondary to trauma usually requires careful radiologic evaluation and appropriate neurosurgical or oto-

laryngologic consultation. We recommend that any patient without any recovery between 5 and 7 days of the active onset of paresis be referred for neurologic evaluation and electrodiagnostic studies. It is also reasonable to obtain otolaryngologic consultation in such patients for consideration of decompression of the facial nerve within the facial canal.

Most children with idiopathic (Bell) palsy can be treated by their primary physician, and we presently recommend a 10-day course of oral prednisone (60 mg/m^2/day) in divided doses for 7 days, tapered over the next 3 days. The effects of such therapy are hard to document, because the natural history of idiopathic Bell palsy is improvement in most cases. This is especially true in children with only partial paralysis at diagnosis. However, because there does seem to be some benefit for early steroid therapy in patients with severe involvement and the potential side effects of a short course of treatment are minimal, we recommend treatment for all children with acute Bell palsy. If a child is seen after the first few days of illness (arbitrarily 4 days), there is little evidence that steroids are beneficial. In such patients, we do not recommend the use of prednisone. The role of surgical decompression for acute Bell palsy is controversial and, by and large, we do not refer patients for surgical decompression.

During the period of facial weakness, if the patient cannot close his/her eyes, artificial tears (three times daily and at night) should be applied to the eye. Eye patches can be used to protect the cornea but are usually unnecessary except during sleep.

The prognosis for the vast majority of patients is excellent, and most patients recover fully. In children, the muscle weakness is usually partial at onset, and these patients uniformly do well. In those patients with complete paralysis at onset, some recovery also can be expected, but it is within this group of patients that partial or delayed recovery occurs.

All patients with idiopathic (Bell) palsy should be seen within 5 days following the initial diagnosis. If at this point there is evidence for some facial movement, chances for full recovery are excellent within the next 2 to 3 weeks. In those patients with no evidence of facial movement at this point, the chances of residual weakness is greater, and nerve conduction velocity measurements are prognostically helpful.

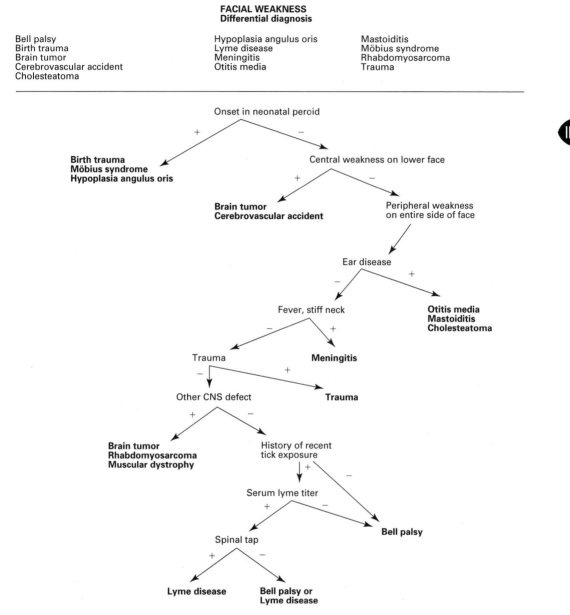

FIG 41-1
Decision tree for differential diagnosis of facial weakness.

DISCUSSION OF ALGORITHM

An algorithm for the differential diagnosis of facial weakness is presented in Figure 41-1. If the condition is not congenital, a differentia-

tion should be made between central or peripheral weakness. Those with a central cause most likely have a brain tumor or a cerebral vascular accident. Next, systemic problems such as brain tumor, meningitis, rhabdomyosarcoma, encephalitis, or ear abnormalities should be considered. Those who have none of these problems most likely have Bell palsy.

BIBLIOGRAPHY

Adour KK: Diagnosis and management of facial paralysis. *N Engl J Med* 307:348–351, 1982.

Kansu T, Us O, Sarpel A, et al: Recurrent multiple cranial nerve palsies. *J Clin Neuro Ophthalmol* 3:263–268, 1983.

Pachner AR, Steere AC: Neurological manifestations of Lyme disease: Meningitis, cranial neuritis and radiculoneuritis. *Neurology* 35:47–53, 1985.

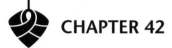

CHAPTER 42

Growth Problems

Stuart Alan Weinzimer
M. William Schwartz

Problems with growth, either poor weight gain or short stature, present an opportunity for an interesting diagnostic evaluation. Many solutions become apparent after the initial assessment; others require special laboratory tests. In some situations, observation and the proper setting will help make the diagnosis. The designation failure to thrive serves as a convenient diagnosis in those children who do not gain weight or grow linearly. It is not a final diagnosis but a label for a problem that needs further definition.

DIFFERENTIAL DIAGNOSIS

The majority of patients with growth problems will be found to have inadequate nutrition, social interaction problems, gastrointestinal disease, or neurologic disorders. A number of studies have outlined what diagnoses are made after evaluation. Box 42-1 shows the cause of failure to thrive in a series of patients from one center. The following list includes the major problems that affect growth. Many unusual problems are not included because of rarity or because the children usually have symptoms other than growth problems.

Common Causes of Growth Problems
- **Infection**
   AIDS
   Urinary tract infection
   Tuberculosis
- **Congenital/anatomic**
   Congenital heart disease
   Gastroesophageal reflux
   Pyloric stenosis
   Posterior urethral valves

BOX 42-1
Etiology of Failure to Thrive in a Series of Patients*

> Constitutional short stature, 56%
> Isolated human growth hormone deficiency, 7%
> Intrauterine growth retardation, 6%
> Maternal deprivation syndrome, 3%
> Chromosomal anomalies, 3%
> Hypothyroidism, 3%
> Central nervous system disease, 6%
> Skeletal disease, 4%
> Congenital heart disease, 2%
> Respiratory disease, 2%
> Gastrointestinal disease, 2%
> Renal disease, 1%
> Immune deficiency, 1%
> Other metabolic disease, 3%

*From Horner JM, Thorsson A, Hintz R: Growth deceleration patterns in children with constitutional short stature: An aid to diagnosis, *Pediatrics* 62:59, 1978. Used by permission.

> Sequestrated lobe of lung
> Diaphragmatic hernia
> Aspiration pneumonia
- **Metabolic/nutritional**
> Malabsorption
> Malnutrition
> Diabetes mellitus
> Diabetes insipidus
> Growth hormone deficiency
> Hypothyroidism
> Renal tubular acidosis
> Short bowel syndrome
- **Genetic**
> Cystic fibrosis
> Chromosomal anomaly (*eg,* Turner syndrome)
> Genetic short stature
> Sickle cell anemia
- **Immunologic**
> Inflammatory bowel disease
> Immune deficiency
- **Miscellaneous**
> Constitutional growth delay
> Cerebral palsy
> Cocaine abuse by mother
> Fetal alcohol syndrome
> Genetic short stature
> Liver disease
> Placental insufficiency
> Renal failure

Discussion

Most of the problems listed previously are discussed throughout this text (*see* index). A few of the more common problems are presented here.

Insufficient Nutrition

Usually detected with a careful history, most cases of poor growth result from inadequate caloric intake. The families may give an initial history that lacks sufficient detail or contains unreliable information. Infants require at least 80 to 125 kcal/kg for growth in the first year, then 70 to 115 kcal/kg for the next 3 years. Sometimes asking the parent to complete a diary of food intake will document that the child's actual caloric intake is insufficient for good growth.

Family Dysfunction

Often family dysfunction and social problems contribute to poor caloric intake. The families expend most of their energy coping with daily problems and conflicts, with the result that the child does not get sufficient feeding. Observations made through a one-way mirror in a family therapy unit showed the variance between the history and what actually transpired at feeding time. This is not a conscious effort to deceive the physician but another symptom of the distracted, disorganized caretaker saying what he/she believes rather than what happened.

Constitutional Delay

Constitutional delay describes a growth pattern in which there is normal size at birth followed by delayed growth velocity for 1 to 2 years. After the third year the child is small but has normal growth velocity. Puberty often develops late in these children, but when it does occur it results in a normal growth spurt and final adult height. The clues to this diagnosis are the growth record, growth velocity calculations, family history of delayed maturation, and bone age radiographs. The bone age is less than the chronologic age and is equal to the height age (Fig. 42-1). Delayed bone age indicates more potential for growth.

Genetic Short Stature

The child with the familial trait of short stature differs from one with constitutional delay by having a family history of short adult stature and a bone age equal to the chronologic age. These patients will be short adults, whereas those with constitutional delay will be taller.

Height   0–36 months

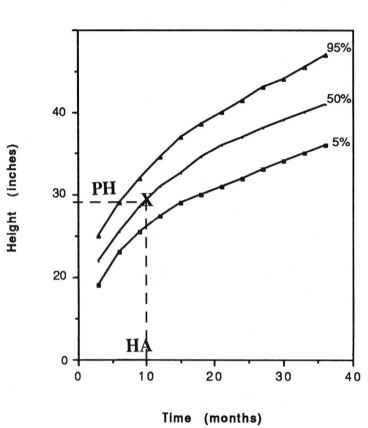

FIG 42-1

Calculation of height age. Intersect patient height (PH—29″) with 50% line (X) on growth chart. Read down the age marks to determine the age that corresponds with this height (HA—10 months).

DATA GATHERING

History

Obtaining a record of previous growth patterns will help establish the onset of the problem and allow calculation of growth velocity or the amount of growth in a year (*see* Chapter 79). Some children whose parents are concerned about short stature are really in the 3rd or 10th percentile and have normal growth velocity. The family history also may reveal information about other members who had growth delay suggestive of genetic short stature or constitutional short stature.

Because family problems are often the basis for growth problems, obtaining a reliable history requires skill and time. Often the patient will give answers to questions to satisfy the interviewer rather than accurately describe what is going on at home. More time and concentration are required to allow the patient to feel comfortable and give details to a nonjudgmental listener so that the child can be helped. A day history (*see* Chapter 4) in which the parent gives a detailed account of a typical day provides information about the details of feeding plus an indication of the family interactions and support systems. After hearing that the underweight patient eats "a good balance of meat, vegetables, and fruit," press for details of favorite and least favorite foods to document the caloric intake. If it seems as if the intake is good, inquire about stool problems, which are seen in malabsorption or cystic fibrosis. Other symptoms, such as cough (cystic fibrosis), developmental delay, change in stool pattern, or weak urinary stream (posterior urethral valves), will lead to possible diagnoses.

Decreased intake or increased losses are common causes of poor growth. A complete dietary history can detect a problem with inadequate caloric intake or suggest a malabsorption problem when the patient has not grown despite a large intake. For those with a good nutritional and social history, look for the problem of increased losses, either gastrointestinal or urinary. An increased number of loose stools leads to consideration of cystic fibrosis, steatorrhea, short bowel syndrome, and food intolerance. Urinary losses, characterized by polyuria, lead to consideration of diabetes mellitus, diabetes insipidus, renal tubular disorders, or chronic glomerulonephritis. Vomiting suggests gastroesophageal reflux, pyloric stenosis, or metabolic diseases.

The birth history, including duration of gestation and birth weight, may yield clues to the diagnosis. A full-term infant with a low birth weight suggests placental insufficiency, or cocaine or alcohol abuse by the mother. Patients with placental insufficiency may have persistent small size; those small infants exposed to cocaine usually grow normally if the family provides adequate calories.

Physical Examination

The physical examination should emphasize careful assessment of the chest, because conditions such as aspiration pneumonia or pulmonary anomalies such as diaphragmatic hernia may escape early detection. Heart murmurs are sometimes undetected prior to evaluation because of growth problems. A protuberant abdomen and wasted buttocks suggests malabsorption, such as with gluten sensitivity or cystic fibrosis. In a short teenaged girl with an increased carrying angle and webbed neck, Turner syndrome may explain the growth problem.

Laboratory Evaluation

In the majority of cases, the laboratory tests are limited. Because the two major causes of poor growth, poor intake and social problems, are detected with the history, laboratory tests should be reserved for confirming specific diseases suggested by the history or physical examination or

GROWTH FAILURE
Differential Diagnosis

AIDS	Genetic short stature	Posterior urethral valve
Aspiration pneumonia	Growth hormone deficiency	Pyloric stenosis
Celiac disease	Fetal alcohol syndrome	Pulmonary problems
Cocaine abuse	Hypothyroidism	Sequestration
Congenital heart disease	Immune deficiency	Diaphragmatic hernia
Constitutional short stature	Inflammatory bowel disease	Renal failure
Cystic fibrosis	Liver disease	Renal tubular acidosis
Cerebral palsy	Malabsorption	Sickle cell anemia
Chromosomal anomaly	Malnutrition	Social problems
Diabetes mellitus	Metabolic disease	Tuberculosis
Diabetes insipidus	Neurogenic bladder	Turner syndrome
Gastroesophageal reflux	Placental Insufficiency	Urinary tract infection

A. Poor growth

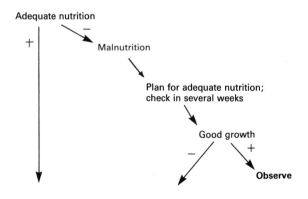

FIG 42-2
Decision tree for differential diagnosis of growth failure.

Continued.

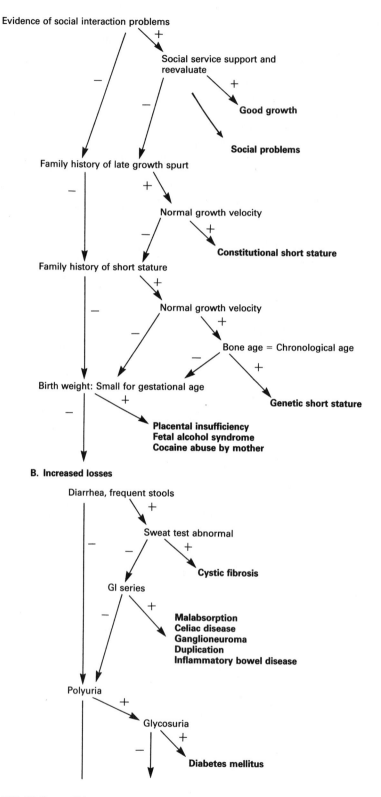

FIG 42-2, cont'd.
For legend, *see* p. 265.

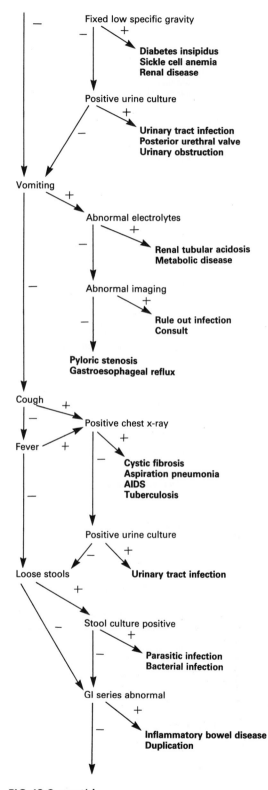

FIG 42-2, cont'd.
For legend, *see* p. 265.

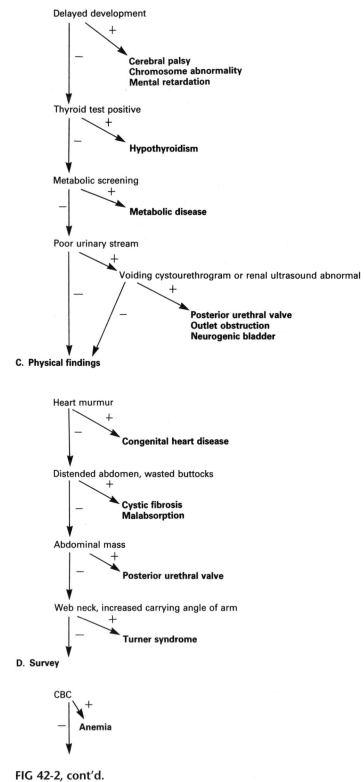

FIG 42-2, cont'd.
For legend, *see* p. 265.

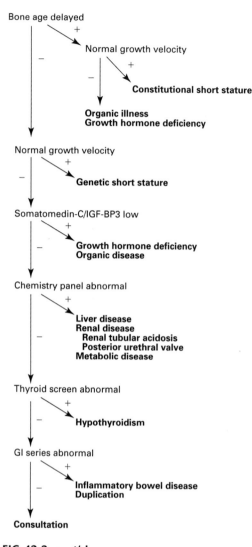

FIG 42-2, cont'd.
For legend, *see* p. 265.

for screening those patients in whom the initial assessment does not suggest a specific problem. Screening tests that are most helpful include bone age, urinalysis, thyroid function tests, and chemistry panel. The insulin-like growth factor binding protein binding protein-3 (IGFBP-3) and somatomedin-C (IGF-1) levels, which are screening tests for growth hormone function, are helpful in specific patients without chronic illness, thyroid disease, or malnutrition, in whom growth hormone deficiency is suspected.

INDICATIONS FOR CONSULTATION OR REFERRAL

Usually a careful history with special attention for nutrition and family interaction problems, documentation of growth velocity, and bone age will suffice to make a diagnosis. If after working through the flow sheet the diagnosis is unclear, or if results of a laboratory test conflict with the history, consultation may help to detect a rare cause of growth failure.

DISCUSSION OF ALGORITHM

The first phase follows the scheme of determining the major causes of growth problems in infants, which are poor nutrition and dysfunctional parenting (Fig. 42-2). If these problems are detected, counseling and support followed by observation are sufficient treatment in the majority of the children.

For those patients with a good nutritional and social history, look for increased losses, either gastrointestinal or urinary. Increased or loose stools lead to consideration of cystic fibrosis and other diseases in which malabsorption is the major feature. Urinary losses, characterized by polyuria, lead to consideration of diabetes mellitus if there is glycosuria or renal disease or diabetes insipidus if there is low specific gravity or osmolarity. Vomiting suggests gastroesophageal reflux, pyloric stenosis, sepsis, or metabolic disease.

Next, ask a series of questions about symptoms that may lead you to consider specific diseases, *eg*, cough (cystic fibrosis or other pulmonary problems), diarrhea (malabsorption, fever, delayed development), and poor urinary stream (posterior urethral valves).

Physical findings may detect such problems as congenital heart disease (murmur), cerebral palsy (neurologic deficit), abdominal mass (posterior urethral valves), and increased carrying angle of the arm and webbed neck (Turner syndrome).

Family history may detect the familial short adult stature seen in genetic short stature or the growth delay seen in constitutional delay of growth and development. Neonatal history may reveal that the infant was small for gestational age or had neonatal complications resulting in short bowel syndrome. The latter should be known from a general history.

If this general screen does not help suggest a diagnosis, a general survey may. Laboratory tests include bone age determination, chemistry panel, thyroid function tests, and somatomedin-C/IGFBP-3 levels. Because this system helps detect the cause of the growth problem in the majority of cases, any cases that remain undiagnosed require either another pass through the system or referral to a consultant.

BIBLIOGRAPHY

Barbero GJ, Shaheen E: Environmental failure to thrive: A clinical view, *J Pediatr* 71:639–644, 1967.

Berwick DM, Levy JC, Leinerman R: Failure to thrive: Diagnostic yield of hospitalization, *Arch Dis Child* 57:347–351, 1982.

Goldbloom R: Growth failure in infancy, *Pediatr Rev* 9:57, 1987.

Horner JM, Thorsson A, Hintz R: Growth deceleration patterns in children with constitu-tional short stature: An aid to diagnosis, *Pediatrics* 62:59, 1978.

Mahoney CP: Evaluating the child with short stature, *Pediatr Clin North Am* 34(4):825–846, 1987.

Saenger P: Use of growth hormone therapy for short stature: Boon or abuse? *Pediatr Rev* 12:355, 1991.

Stickler GB: "Failure to thrive" or the failure to define, *Pediatrics* 74:559, 1984. 43

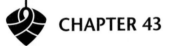

CHAPTER 43

Headache

Lawrence W. Brown
Edward B. Charney

The primary care physician is frequently asked to assess the child complaining of headaches. Only rarely does the child present with a first severe headache; typically, the complaint is intermittent or progressive over many weeks or months. Although headaches are benign in the vast majority of children, parents are often concerned that their child may have a brain tumor or other serious medical problem. Assessment of the child within the office setting often can help to establish the cause of the headache and provide guidance for therapeutic management.

DIFFERENTIAL DIAGNOSIS

- **Acute generalized headache**
  Acute febrile illness
  Meningitis, encephalitis
  Hypertension
  Intracranial hemorrhage
  Postlumbar puncture
  New onset migraine
- **Acute localized headache**
  Sinusitis
  Dental caries

Temporomandibular joint dysfunction
Trauma
New onset migraine
- **Acute intermittent headache**
  Migraine
  Seizure equivalent
- **Chronic progressive headache**
  Mass lesion (tumor, brain abscess, subdural
  hematoma)
  Hydrocephalus
  Pseudotumor cerebri
- **Chronic nonprogressive headache**
  Postconcussive syndrome
  Muscular contraction-tension headache
  Psychogenic (depression, conversion reac-
  tion, school phobia)

DISCUSSION

Fever associated with any infectious process, from viral syndrome to bacterial meningitis, is the most common cause of acute headache in children. Vasodilatation of intracranial and superficial vessels leads to generalized or frontotemporal pounding headache. Central nervous system (CNS) infection including bacterial meningitis and viral meningoencephalitis also can produce headache by inflammation of pain-sensitive structures at the base of the brain and over the convexity. Primary CNS involvement usually is associated with altered mental status, seizures, and nuchal rigidity. Headache from a brain abscess may result from the increased intracranial pressure and traction on neighboring pain-sensitive vessels and dura; focal motor weakness and cranial nerve palsies often are seen on neurologic examination. Dental abscess from caries or gingivitis can lead to generalized head pain, or it can be referred to distant points with frontal, temporal, or retroauricular localization. Sinusitis with inflammation of the pain-sensitive sinusoidal ostia is usually associated with localized pain and tenderness over the affected sinuses, in addition to a steady, dull headache. Chronic sinusitis may present with nonspecific headaches without the typical signs of acute involvement such as purulent rhinorrhea, nasal congestion, and fever.

Trauma-related headaches usually are seen with severe injury associated with prolonged loss of consciousness, fractures, and structural intracranial disease (*eg*, hematoma, contusion). They likely result from irritation of extracranial and intracranial pain-sensitive structures by small hemorrhages, edema, or anatomic disruption. They often occur soon after return of consciousness, and prolonged persistence for weeks to months may be associated with a history of multiple psychogenic and somatic complaints.

Migraine is the most common cause of recurrent headaches in childhood. They often are characterized by intermittent severe, unilateral, pounding headaches with nausea, vomiting, photophobia, and relief from sleep in an otherwise healthy child. General medical history is usually benign. Family history is frequently positive for similar "sick" headaches. Attacks of migraine with aura (classic migraine) start with neurologic complaints. Visual disturbances are most common with scintillations, scotomas, fortification fields, or hemianopsia. Sensory disturbances, motor deficits (hemiplegic migraine), brain stem findings and ataxia (basilar migraine), or cognitive impairment may be seen. Distortion of body image (Alice in Wonderland headaches) is associated with acute confusion. Migraine without aura (common migraine) does not have the neurologic phase, but the characteristics of the headache are identical. Rarely, migraine may present with neurologic deficits without prominent headache (complicated migraine). All types of migraine may be precipitated by a variety of factors including specific food intolerance or chemical sensitivity, fasting, inadequate or excessive sleep, weather changes, psychologic stress, or hormonal changes (*eg*, menses or oral contraceptives).

Migraine headaches are typically marked by unilateral frontal or temporal onset, although they may spread bilaterally or start with generalized pain. During acute migraine attacks, the child often tries to avoid bright lights and noise. Relief may be provided by rest or analgesics; most migraine sufferers find that sleep is the most effective treatment. There is a late stage of migraine, usually after partial recovery with sleep, characterized by a steady, dull headache. The pathophysiology of migraine is not completely understood, although it appears to involve functional disturbance of serotonin on a familial basis. The vascular hypothesis, which described vasoconstriction leading to neurologic symptoms followed by vasodilation leading to pounding headaches followed by leakage of vasoactive compounds leading to the lingering, dull pain, has been shown to be wrong. Rather, it appears that migraine is more closely related to epilepsy in terms of a primary neurophysiologic disturbance that progresses in the brain with a spreading wave of depression. Symptoms usually cannot be explained by discrete vascular involvement. However, vascular effects are clearly important in the manifestations of some neurologic symptoms. Treatment is based on prevention of precipitating causes, acute pharmacologic management of the acute attack, and prophylactic medication. Maintenance of a headache diary can reveal dietary or other provoking causes. Analgesics should be used as needed, but narcotics should be avoided. Specific serotonin receptor drugs can be used in older children and teenagers (sumatriptin and dihydroergotamine tartrate) for severe attacks. When headaches are frequent and disabling, consideration should be given to prophylactic treatment. Younger children often respond to cyproheptadine, but older children often complain of excessive sedation or appetite stimulation. Amitryptiline, propanolol, and verapimil are other treatment considerations.

Systemic hypertension is an unusual cause of headaches in children, and when it occurs it is often associated with diastolic pressures greater than 100 mm Hg. It is frequently a sign of acute glomerulonephritis or other renal disease such as systemic lupus erythematosus (SLE). SLE and other forms of cerebral vasculitis also can produce headaches directly in the absence of systemic hypertension. Postlumbar puncture headache is caused by intracranial hypotension. This headache is characteristically worse on sitting up and relieved by lying down. Conservative treatment with bed rest and analgesics for up to several days usually is effective. Persistence of headache can be treated with an isologous blood patch administered into the subarachnoid space.

Tension headaches result primarily from sustained contraction of the skeletal musculature of the head and neck. Emotional stress or fatigue frequently can precipitate pain that is localized most often to the occipital region or posterior neck, although generalized head pain can be noted. These headaches tend to be more common in the adolescent than in the younger child. Psychogenic headaches often are precipitated by stress in the environment. They also may represent depression, somatization, or function as a mechanism for secondary gain such as school

avoidance. Ocular abnormalities such as refractive errors, astigmatism, strabismus, and impaired convergence also may cause headaches. Typically, eyestrain produces periorbital pain that occurs late in the day and is relieved by rest. Ocular headaches should be responsive to proper corrective lenses. Headaches associated with a seizure disorder may occur either as an aura of a partial or generalized seizure, during the postictal state, and rarely as the only manifestation of the seizure. In the absence of a definite seizure history, a clearly epileptiform electroencephalogram is necessary to establish this diagnosis.

Chronic progressive headaches indicate a persistent pathologic condition with symptoms generally caused by increased intracranial pressure or direct involvement of pain-sensitive structures (stretching or infiltration). Although these headaches may present with milder and briefer attacks than migraines or headaches of other etiologies, they are significant because of their early morning timing, postural features, and associated neurologic abnormalities with papilledema and cranial nerve dysfunction. Brain tumors, although relatively uncommon causes of headaches, are often the major fear of parents bringing their child for evaluation of a headache complaint. Brain tumor headaches often are accompanied by neurologic disturbances such as ataxia, head tilt, diplopia, strabismus, decreased visual acuity, and motor deficit. These headaches also may be associated with vomiting, exacerbation with positional change, and arousal from sleep.

DATA GATHERING

History

An adequate history is the most critical portion of the evaluation of headache. However, children often are unable to describe their pain. They often point to their forehead or occiput and complain only that it hurts. Children over the age of 8 years often can be coaxed to put their headaches into words, or even into drawings. Gently offering a variety of possible descriptions, such as sharp, dull, steady, knifelike, throbbing, pounding, squeezing, or bandlike, may allow the child to define the pain. The examiner can allow younger children to choose between "steady" or "pounding" by taking the child's finger in his/her hand and pressing steadily or intermittently. Severity can be assessed by how often headaches interfere with activities or how often the child prefers to lie down or sleep with attacks. Frequency of the headaches is best determined by having the child or parent keep a headache diary. Another way to arrive at the frequency of severe headaches is to ask about the number of school absences or visits to the school nurse for headaches. It is important to distinguish the patterns of intermittent pain in the otherwise normal child (most likely migraine) from fluctuating daily pain (psychogenic) or chronic progressive headaches (increased intracranial pressure). Although migraine often causes unilateral pain, any child who can point to one precise spot where headaches always start should be evaluated for an intracranial process. Time of onset also may provide a clue to the cause of headache. Rarely is the time of onset as obvious as always occurring on gym day or on school mornings only, but specific precipitants can be demonstrated if carefully evaluated. Early morning headaches may suggest brain tumor, and periorbital pain late in the day points to eye strain.

Physical Examination

Whether or not fever is present often is the critical feature that helps to direct the physician's initial office assessment. Nonspecific headache with fever may result from increased cerebral blood flow producing a vascular headache. Nuchal rigidity, changes in sensorium, and Kernig or Brudzinski sign are characteristic of bacterial meningitis or subarachnoid hemorrhage, whereas fever with delirium suggests encephalomyelitis. Cranial nerve palsies or focal weakness may be signs of a brain abscess. For the febrile child with headache and a normal neurologic examination, attention should be directed at examination of the sinuses and dentition. Localized tenderness and pain to gentle finger tapping over the sinuses in a child with nasal mucosa congestion suggests sinusitis. Dental caries with localized tenderness and pain over the teeth or gums may suggest a dental abscess. If the neurologic examination and evaluation of sinuses and mouth are unremarkable, physical evidence for other infectious processes should be vigorously pursued. In the majority of cases, results of the comprehensive examination are unrevealing, and the acute headache in the febrile child is part of a nonspecific viral syndrome.

Although a detailed history often is the most important part of the assessment of the afebrile child with headache as a chief complaint, particular attention also must be directed toward vital signs including blood pressure and growth parameters, a complete physical examination, careful ophthalmologic testing, and full neurologic assessment. Children with nonneurologic disease such as acute glomeronephritis may present with headaches secondary to hypertension, but other objective findings such as hematuria or edema are usually present. Persistent abnormalities such as ataxia, hemiparesis, or strabismus in association with a headache complaint strongly suggest an underlying brain tumor. Headaches in a child with evidence of deceleration in linear growth and a history of polyuria and polydypsia specifically suggests a craniopharyngioma. Although bitemporal hemianopsia is common, most children are unaware of any visual limitation. Transient neurologic deficits suggest seizures or migraine. A sudden severe headache with stiff neck and decreased level of responsiveness is characteristic of intracranial hemorrhage most often secondary to ruptured arteriovenous malformation.

LABORATORY EVALUATION

When there is a suggestive history and normal neurologic examination, laboratory investigations often are unnecessary in the outpatient office setting. A suggestive history or specific abnormal findings may lead to complete blood count, urinalysis, sinus films, magnetic resonance imaging (MRI), or lumbar puncture. Additional laboratory diagnostic studies may be ordered by consultants.

INDICATIONS FOR CONSULTATION OR REFERRAL

Any child with persistent neurologic abnormalities should be referred to a child neurologist or pediatric neurosurgeon for further diagnostic work-up including MRI. The child with suspected eye abnormalities should be referred for formal ophthalmologic consultation. Children with suspected migraine would benefit from referral to a child neurologist to confirm the diagnosis as well as for specific management. The child with intractable psychogenic headaches should be referred for individual and family counseling.

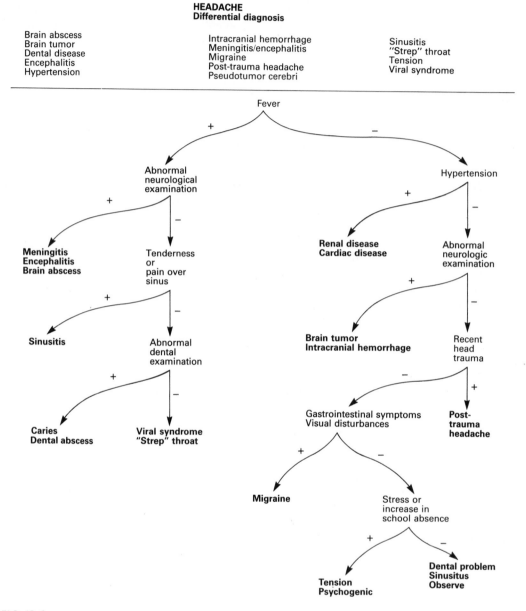

FIG 43-1
Decision tree for differential diagnosis of headache.

DISCUSSION OF ALGORITHM

An algorithm for differential diagnosis of headaches is presented in Figure 43-1. The first step in the evaluation is to evaluate for the possibility of meningitis, hypertension, or brain tumor. Next, dental and vision problems should be considered. A careful history will allow for the proper diagnosis of migraine. If these considerations are not productive, the most likely cause of recurrent headaches in the neurologically normal child is tension or stress.

BIBLIOGRAPHY

Casey R, Ludwig S, McCormick MC: Morbidity following minor head trauma in children, *Pediatrics* 78:497, 1986.

Chu ML, Shinnar S: Headache in children younger than 7 years of age, *Arch Neurol* 49:79, 1992.

Faleck H, Rothner AD, Erenberg G, et al: Headache and subacute sinusitis in children and adolescents, *Headache* 28:96, 1988.

Honig P, Charney EB: Children with brain tumor headaches, *Am J Dis Child* 136:121, 1982.

Igarachi M, May WN, Golden GS: Pharmacologic treatment of childhood migraine, *J Pediatr* 120:653, 1992.

Prensky AL, Sommer D: Diagnosis and treatment of migraine in children, *Neurology* 29:506, 1978.

Rothner AD: Classification, pathogenesis, evaluation and management of headaches in children and adolescents, *Curr Opin Pediatr* 4:949, 1992.

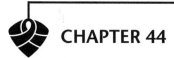

CHAPTER 44

Hematuria

Michael E. Norman

Hematuria in children presents in two ways: the accidental discovery of asymptomatic microhematuria on routine urinalysis or a complaint of abnormal color of the urine (red, brown, or cola-colored). Discolored urine can be due to either a variety of diseases (eg, myoglobinuria) or the ingestion of various foods or drugs (eg, beets, desferrioxamine, Rifampin). In considering the differential diagnosis and the indication for a workup, an operational definition of significant hematuria is required: 10 or more red blood cells (RBCs) in a freshly voided urine specimen is convenient, though arbitrary. Confirmation may then be obtained by documenting hematuria in several early morning urine specimens examined over several days. Hematuria should be differentiated from hemoglobinuria or myoglobinuria, which presents with a dipstick-positive finding for blood but few if any RBCs in the corresponding urine sediment. Conditions that rule out lysis of RBCs include a freshly voided urine specimen that is suitably acid (pH < 7.0) and concentrated (specific gravity > 1.015). Early morning urine specimens yield the best results. Urine specimens that test falsely positive for blood by the commonly used reagent-impregnated dipsticks include the following: 1) highly concentrated specimens, 2) the presence of ascorbic acid at concentrations greater than 5 mg/dL, or 3) the presence of other oxidizing agents such as common household bleach. A positive dipstick examination should always be followed-up by the microscopic examination of a freshly voided urine sediment.

Prevalence figures suggest that 4% to 6% of children will have at least one episode of hematuria sometime during childhood. Persistent or recurrent asymptomatic microhematuria is found in 0.1% to 0.5% of school-aged children.

DIFFERENTIAL DIAGNOSIS

Common Causes of Hematuria
- **Trauma**
- **Infection**
    Pyelonephritis
    Cystitis
    Sepsis
- **Toxin**
    Penicillin and derivatives
    Cyclophosphamide
    Phenacetin
- **Inflammatory**
    Glomerulonephritis
    Collagen disease
    Subacute bacterial endocarditis
    Anaphylactoid purpura (vasculitis)
    Hemolytic uremic syndrome
    IgA nephropathy
- **Metabolic–Endocrine**
    Cystinuria
    Kidney stone
    Idiopathic hypercalciuria
- **Bleeding disorders**
    Hemophilia
    von Willebrand disease
- **Tumor**
    Wilms tumor
    Leukemia
- **Congenital**
    Obstruction
        Ureteropelvic
        Stricture
    Medullary sponge kidney
- **Multiple etiologies**
    Renal vein thrombosis
    Benign recurrent hematuria: familial or non-familial

Discussion
Although the differential diagnosis of hematuria is extensive, relatively few causes are seen in clinical practice. These causes are listed below in decreasing order of frequency:

1. Urinary tract infection
    a. Bacterial
    b. Viral (*eg*, cystitis)
2. Trauma
    a. Kidney
    b. Bladder
    c. Local (*eg*, urethral, meatal)
3. Benign recurrent hematuria
4. Glomerulonephritis
    a. Poststreptococcal infection
    b. Berger disease
    c. Henoch-Schönlein purpura

Perhaps 5% of children will have nephrolithiasis or hypercalciuria, sickle cell trait or anemia, tumor, a bleeding diathesis, or postexercise hematuria. It is useful when commencing an evaluation of hematuria to determine whether the bleeding is coming from the upper or lower urinary tract. This determination is likely to reduce the number of diagnostic investigations required.

Differentiating Between Lower and Upper Tract Hematuria

- **Upper urinary tract**
    No terminal hematuria
    No clots
    Red, brown, cola-colored
    Proteinuria (> 2+)*
    RBC casts
- **Lower urinary tract**
    Terminal hematuria
    Clots
    Red
    Proteinuria (< 2+)*
    No RBC casts

Benign Recurrent Hematuria
Benign recurrent hematuria is an idiopathic disorder, more common in boys than in girls, and the most frequent cause of referral to a nephrologist. It typically occurs in an asymptomatic child with normal findings on physical examination. The hematuria is usually microscopic and may be persistent or intermittent. Episodes of gross bleeding may occur but are not a prominent part of the history. Family history may be positive for similar findings. The hematuria may subside over time. Prognosis for preservation of renal function is excellent.

---

*With dipsticks, the maximum readable protein concentration in grossly bloody urine that is due to RBCs and plasma proteins is 2+.

Immunoglobulin A Nephropathy (Berger Disease)

IgA nephropathy may produce either persistent or intermittent hematuria. The characteristic feature, proved with renal biopsy results, shows deposition of IgA in the mesangium of all glomeruli. These glomeruli may be otherwise normal or show focal nephritis. In many cases, gross hematuria and RBC casts occur. Those patients with IgA nephropathy plus proteinuria have a less favorable prognosis than those without proteinuria. Approximately 10% to 20% of patients with IgA deposition may develop renal failure. These patients have marked glomerular disease compared with the majority of patients who maintain good renal function.

Hypercalciuria

Many patients who have hematuria may have hypercalciuria, defined as the excretion of more than 4 mg of calcium per kilogram of body weight per day. This problem, commonly seen in adults with kidney stones, is being recognized more frequently in children, reaching 40% to 60% in some series. The characteristics include greater than 4 mg/kg of calcium in a 24-hour urine collection or a spot urine calcium/creatinine ratio greater than 0.2; family history of kidney or gallbladder stones; absence of other signs of renal disease, such as proteinuria or azotemia; and calcium oxalate crystals. The condition is rare in blacks. Many patients will develop renal stones in adulthood. The hypercalciuria may develop from either increased absorption of calcium in the intestine or increased excretion in the renal tubules. Good hydration to maintain high urine volume plus dietary restriction of sodium seem to decrease the hematuria. Reduction of calcium intake and use of hydrochlorothiazide are helpful in some patients.

Poststreptococcal glomerulonephritis or the nephritis of Henoch-Schönlein purpura is more likely to present with a history of upper respiratory tract infection, strep throat or pyodermia, hypertension, edema, and oliguria. Children with severe abdominal pain, vomiting, pallor, and diaphoresis should be suspected of having renal colic. Black children should undergo sickle cell screening tests. Children with hematuria due to hydronephrosis or a kidney tumor may have a palpable flank mass. Hematuria due to a clotting defect is virtually always associated with a positive finding of a medical or family history of bleeding or hemorrhage elsewhere in the body.

DATA GATHERING

History

Children with urinary tract infections usually have other signs and symptoms, such as fever; abdominal, flank, or suprapubic pain; and urinary urgency, frequency, or dysuria. It should be noted, however, that the passage of gross blood is irritating to the bladder and urethra and may mimic the symptoms of urinary tract infection. Some patients may have local irritation of the urethra from trauma, masturbation, or chemicals such as a bubble bath. A family history of stones may be the initial clue to the detection of hypercalciuria.

Physical Examination

The external genitalia should be examined for signs of trauma. A careful abdominal examination can help detect flank masses consistent with Wilms tumor, renal vein thrombosis, or obstruction. Blood pressure measurements are also important.

Laboratory Evaluation

Because certain dyes, hemoglobin, myoglobin, and beets can cause the urine to appear bloody, the urine should be examined microscopically to find RBCs. Tests to determine the presence of myoglobin and hemoglobin also will give false positive results for blood with the dipstick method. Relatively few laboratory or radiologic investigations are required to diagnose the cause of hematuria in children. In 70% to 80% of children with gross hematuria a specific cause is usually found. The urine sediment is the key to initiating a workup. Heavy pyuria and positive gram staining suggest bacterial infection; urine culture is then mandatory, whether the results of gram staining are positive or negative. Patients with glomerular bleeding are likely to have proteinuria (>2+), and those with RBC casts are assumed to have some form of glomerulonephritis until proved otherwise. Sometimes several urine sediments must be carefully scanned to find casts. After urinalysis, two approaches can be taken:

(1) For suspected trauma, obstruction with or without kidney stones, or tumor, a renal ultra-

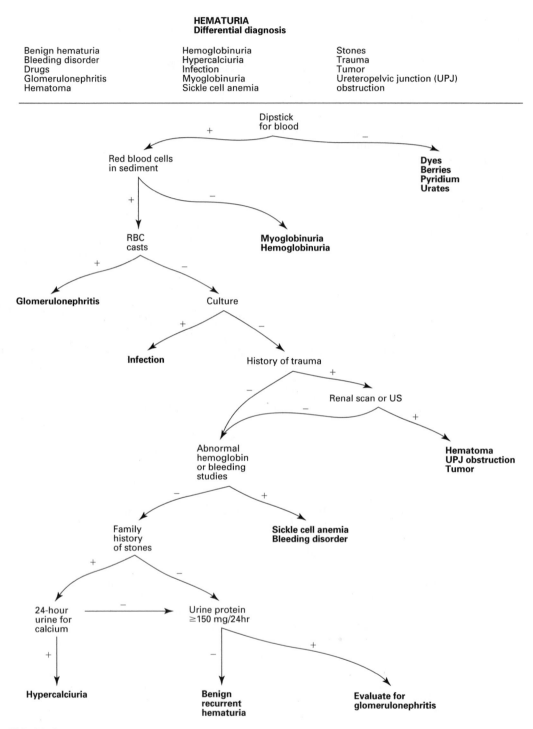

FIG 44–1

Decision tree for differential diagnosis of hematuria.
*With dipsticks, the maximum readable protein concen-
tration in grossly bloody urine that is due to RBCs and
plasma proteins is 2+.

sound is useful and noninvasive. An isotope renogram (*ie,* renal scan) will demonstrate structural details by documenting the site of obstruction, confirming extravasation of blood or urine outside the kidney, or revealing compromised or absent renal perfusion. If trauma to the lower urinary tract is suspected, voiding cystourethrography should be performed.

(2) If glomerulonephritis is suspected, a test to measure the serum creatinine level to estimate glomerular filtration rate and determination of antistreptolysin O and C3 to document poststreptococcal glomerulonephritis should be performed. Occasionally the history of vague musculoskeletal complaints is elicited, suggesting the need to screen for lupus nephritis with an antinuclear antibody titer. A family history of nephritis should prompt a search for visual abnormalities and sensorineural hearing loss.

In general, renal biopsy should be considered when significant proteinuria accompanies hematuria.

INDICATIONS FOR CONSULTATION OR REFERRAL

Consultation or referral is necessary when the following symptoms or conditions are present:

1. Fever, systemic toxicity, severe abdominal colic
2. Persistent (> 48 hours) gross hematuria
3. Gross hematuria after significant abdominal or perineal trauma
4. Gross hematuria followed by urinary retention
5. Hypertension, oliguria, edema
6. Coexistent heavy proteinuria
7. Azotemia

DISCUSSION OF ALGORITHM

An algorithm for the differential diagnosis of hematuria is presented in Figure 44–1. Keep in mind the common causes of hematuria will help guide the explanation of this problem. First, the presence of blood rather than hemoglobin or myoglobin should be established by looking at the sediment rather than relying on the dipstick detection of blood. A history of trauma should make the physician consider renal ultrasound or intravenous pyelography to delineate renal hematoma, laceration, or blood clots in the bladder. The urinary sediment should be examined for RBC casts, which if present will lead to evaluation for glomerulonephritis. A positive urine culture will confirm a urinary tract infection.

BIBLIOGRAPHY

Fleischer GR: Hematuria. In Fleisher GR, Ludwig S, editors: *Textbook of pediatric emergency medicine,* ed 3, Baltimore, 1992, Williams & Wilkins.

Gauthier B: Asymptomatic hematuria. In Gauthier B, Edelman CM, editors: *Nephrology and urology for the pediatrician,* Boston, 1982, Little, Brown, and Co.

Gauthier B: Gross hematuria. In Gauthier B, Edelman CM, editors: *Nephrology and urology for the pediatrician,* Boston, 1982, Little, Brown, and Co.

Hogg RJ, Silva F, Walker P, et al: A multicenter study of IgA nephropathy in children, *Kidney Int* 22:643, 1982.

Houston IB: Recurrent hematuria syndrome. In, Edelmann CM Jr, editor: *Pediatric kidney disease,* ed 2, Boston, 1992, Little, Brown, and Co.

Kalia A, Travis LB: Hematuria, leukocyturia, and cylindruria. In Edelmann CM Jr, editor: *Pediatric kidney disease,* ed 2, Boston, 1992, Little, Brown, and Co.

Kitagawa T: Lessons learned from the Japanese nephritis screening study, *Pediatr Nephrol* 2:256, 1988.

Norman ME: An office approach to hematuria and proteinuria, *Pediatr Clin North Am* 34:545, 1987.

Stapleton FB, Roy S, Nue HN, et al: Hypercalciuria children with hematuria, *N Engl J Med* 310:1345, 1984.

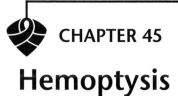

CHAPTER 45

Hemoptysis

Richard M. Kravitz

Hemoptysis, a serious and potentially life-threatening problem, is defined as blood originating from the pulmonary system. Hemoptysis must be distinguished from other sources of bleeding, such as the nasopharynx or the gastrointestinal (GI) tract. Unlike in adults, hemoptysis is uncommon in the pediatric age range. Most cases of hemoptysis are mild in quantity and occur as isolated events. Massive hemoptysis (> 200–300 mL/24 hrs), however, can quickly cause death either through exsanguination or, more commonly, profound hypoxia. The presence of hemoptysis usually heralds significant underlying lung disease. This etiology needs to be identified quickly so that appropriate treatment may be instituted to control the bleeding and prevent its recurrence.

DIFFERENTIAL DIAGNOSIS

Common Causes of Hemoptysis

- **Infectious etiology**
  Pneumonia
  Pulmonary abscess
  Tuberculosis
- **Pulmonary diseases**
  Cystic fibrosis
  Bronchiectasis
  Foreign body
  Arteriovenous malformation
  Congenital lung malformation
- **Cardiovascular diseases**
  Congenital heart disease
  Pulmonary hypertension
  Pulmonary embolus
- **Connective tissue diseases**
  Goodpasture syndrome
  Wegener granulomatosis
  Systemic lupus erythematosus
  Systemic vasculitis

- **Miscellaneous**
  Pulmonary hemosiderosis
  Trauma
  Coagulopathy
  Munchausen syndrome by proxy

Discussion

Hemoptysis is not frequently encountered in pediatric patients. Initially, the more common sources of bleeding need to be ruled out, including the nasopharynx (epistaxis), oropharynx (gingivitis, tooth abscess), and the GI tract (hematemesis). Bleeding from the nasopharynx and oropharynx can be easily identified on visual inspection. However, bleeding from the GI tract can be more difficult to distinguish. Young children frequently do not expectorate their sputum; rather, they swallow it. Thus, blood in a child's emesis does not always imply it is from the GI tract. Similarly, the lack of a cough productive for blood does not rule out its presence in the lung. In general, blood from the lungs is usually bright red in color and frothy in its consistency with an alkaline pH, whereas blood from the GI tract is usually dark brown and has an acidic pH.

Infectious diseases are the most common cause of hemoptysis in children. Necrotizing pneumonitis or pulmonary abscesses can frequently erode into the bronchial arterial supply and can cause bleeding.

Bronchiectasis can occur after numerous recurrent insults to the lung, including recurrent pneumonia, recurrent aspiration, cystic fibrosis, allergic bronchopulmonary aspergillosis, and immotile cilia syndrome. Although bronchiectatic changes frequently are reversible if discovered early enough, repeated damage to the bronchial tree leads to permanent changes. Bronchiectatic changes to the lungs cause bronchial arterial hypertrophy and the formation of fragile, tortuous blood vessels, which can rupture causing hemoptysis.

In cystic fibrosis, a defect in the chloride channel is present, which results in abnormally thickened secretions. This defect allows for colonization with a variety of unusual organisms such as *Staphylococcus aureus* and *Pseudomonas aeruginosa*. Recurrent infections with these organisms during pulmonary exacerbations damage the bronchi, ultimately causing the development of bronchiectasis and subsequent hemoptysis.

Many times, aspiration of foreign bodies goes unrecorded or unremembered. Patients usually present with acute onset of coughing and/or wheezing with asymmetric breath sounds. Hemoptysis does not occur in the immediate postaspiration phase. If the foreign body remains in the bronchi for a long enough period of time, however, inflammation will occur, eventually leading to bronchiectasis. Also, the foreign body itself can erode through the bronchial wall and into a vessel, allowing easy access of blood into the bronchi.

Abnormalities of the pulmonary arterial system can arise from abnormal formation of alveolar capillaries. Rupture of these arteriovenous malformations (AVMs) can lead to hemoptysis, although it is rarely massive. Connections that can occur between the bronchial and pulmonary arterial systems are sites for potential bleeding. These connections can be associated with congenital lung malformations such as pulmonary sequestrations, hemangiomas, and hereditary hemorrhagic telangiectasia (Osler-Weber-Rendu syndrome).

Congenital cardiovascular disease associated with pulmonary hypertension can cause hemoptysis. Common diseases include mitral valve stenosis and Eisenmenger complex. Tetralogy of Fallot and other diseases with right ventricular outflow tract obstruction (such as pulmonary artery hypoplasia) can cause hemoptysis secondary to the development of bronchial arterial hypertrophy with eventual rupture. A pulmonary embolus also may cause hemoptysis, although infarction of the pulmonary parenchymal tissue is rare.

Goodpasture syndrome presents with hemoptysis and glomerulonephritis. The disease is caused by circulating autoimmune antibodies that attach to the alveolar or glomerular basement membrane. Renal involvement may precede, follow, or be concomitant with the pulmonary disease. In Wegener granulomatosis, necrotizing lesions appear in the upper and lower respiratory tract as well as the kidney. Systemic lupus erythematosus (SLE) and systemic vasculitis are other collagen vascular diseases that can cause hemoptysis.

In pulmonary hemosiderosis, alveolar hemorrhage frequently presents as recurrent pneumonia with iron-deficient anemia. In severe cases, the hemoglobin can get as low as 2 to 3 gm/dL. In the majority of cases, the underlying etiology remains unknown. Many times, however, the condition is associated with milk-protein allergy (Heiner syndrome), renal disease (Goodpasture syndrome), collagen vascular disease (SLE), or immunodeficiency.

Trauma also can lead to hemoptysis. Penetrating trauma such as knife or bullet wounds may rupture blood vessels and cause intraparenchymal bleeding. Blunt trauma, such as motor vehicle collisions with deceleration injuries, may cause tearing or shearing of the bronchial or pulmonary arteries.

DATA GATHERING

History

The initial history of a patient with the complaint of hemoptysis should assess the severity, timing, and source of the bleeding, as well as a prior history of similar complaints. Patients may occasionally be able to localize the site of the bleeding by describing a gurgling sensation at the site of the bleed prior to having hemoptysis. A history of recurrent pulmonary infections increases the likelihood that bronchiectasis has developed and is now the cause of the hemoptysis. In a previously healthy patient who now is experiencing systemic symptoms such as weight loss, night sweats, increased fatigue, or symptoms of recurrent infections, more serious systemic illness needs to be considered, such as malignancy, connective tissue diseases, or immunodeficiency (especially HIV-related infections). In patients with no previous medical problems, recent changes in their health could prove important. Symptoms such as fevers, coughing, and shortness of breath suggest an infectious etiology for the bleeding, such as a pneumonia or abscess. In addition, a history of throat pain may lead to the diagnosis of severe pharyngitis as a nonpulmonary cause of bleeding. A previous history of choking, especially with subsequent wheezing, suggests a foreign body aspiration. If the bleeding was sudden in onset but not preceded by any illness, an AVM should be considered.

Family history also can be important in assessing the patient with hemoptysis. A family history of cystic fibrosis or a connective tissue disease increases the possibility of an undiagnosed chronic illness. A history of environmental exposures also can prove useful. Ask if the patient had been exposed to anyone with tuberculosis in the past weeks to months. Strong solvents, chemicals, or hydrocarbon products in the house might have been inhaled or aspirated by younger patients causing lung damage. In teenagers, one needs to always consider the possibilities of illicit drug use, such as the smoking of crack cocaine or paraquat-laced marijuana.

Physical Examination

The initial physical examination of a patient with hemoptysis should be directed toward assessing the patient's vital signs and any abnormalities of oxygenation or circulation.

Inspection of the nasopharyngeal cavity can identify other sites of bleeding such as epistaxis. The presence of nasal polyps raises the possibility of cystic fibrosis. The presence of rales, especially with associated fever and tachypnea, suggests pneumonia. Decreased breath sounds can be noted over the area of a pulmonary abscess. Wheezing, especially if monophonic and unilateral, suggests a foreign body. Rales with evidence of peripheral edema can implicate associated cardiac or renal disease. Cardiac examination should emphasize the search for murmurs. An accentuated second heart sound can be detected in the presence of pulmonary hypertension. Cyanosis of the lips or extremities suggests the presence of hypoxia, either from the underlying cause of the hemoptysis (eg, pneumonia) or from the presence of blood in the alveoli interfering with gas exchange. The presence of clubbing, especially with other pulmonary findings, is associated with cardiac disease, cystic fibrosis, or bronchiectasis. Rashes or joint findings, especially in conjunction with any of the previously mentioned associated signs, raise the possibility of a connective tissue disease.

Laboratory Evaluation

All patients with hemoptysis should have a chest radiograph performed. Many of the infectious causes of hemoptysis (pneumonia, pulmonary abscess, bronchiectasis) can be identified on routine chest film. Often the site of the bleeding will be identified on the radiograph. A hemoglobin and hematocrit are useful in assessing the extent of the blood loss. If iron-deficient anemia is seen, pulmonary hemosiderosis should be considered. An elevated white blood cell count, especially with many immature neutrophils present in the differential count, raises the possibility of an infection as a cause of the bleeding.

Bronchoscopy can be used to localize the site of bleeding, to instill iced saline at the site of hemoptysis to help control or stop the bleeding or to search for a foreign body and remove it. A pulmonologist or otolaryngologist should be consulted to perform this procedure and to choose the correct methods of treatment. A computed tomographic (CT) scan of the chest may discover areas of bronchiectasis, granulomas, or congenital lung malformations. If done with contrast, the CT scan may possibly aid in localizing the site of the bleeding. However, a CT scan with contrast may not be helpful in the initial 24 to 48 hours after the bleed because the blood present in the lungs may be difficult to differentiate from the contrast media. The "gold standard" for assessing the site of pulmonary bleeding (especially in cases of AVMs) is an angiogram. This study also allows the radiologist to inject material into the affected vessel in an attempt to embolize the bleeding artery.

Other diagnostic studies should be obtained as dictated by the differential diagnosis. Sputum cultures should be obtained in cases of infection and a purified protein derivative skin test performed if tuberculosis is suspected. A sweat test can be done to rule out cystic fibrosis. A urinalysis, blood urea nitrogen and creatinine, and serologic markers (eg, ABMA or antineutrophil cytoplasmic antibody) should be obtained if Goodpasture syndrome or Wegener granulomatosis are being considered. An immunologic profile, such as quantitative immunoglobulins (IgG, IgA, and IgM), complement levels (C3, C4, and CH_{50}), and other serologic markers (antinuclear antibody, RF, erythrocyte sedimentation rate) should be considered as part of a connective tissue disease evaluation. Sinus films, as well as CT scans, can be used to look for the necrotizing granulomas seen in Wegener granulomatosis. Finally, a drug screen should be conducted if illicit drug use is suspected.

Differential diagnosis

Abscess
Arteriovenous malformation (AVM)
Bronchiectasis
Cardiac disease
Congenital lung malformation
Connective tissue disease
Cystic fibrosis
Foreign body
Pneumonia
Pulmonary hemosiderosis
Trauma
Tuberculosis

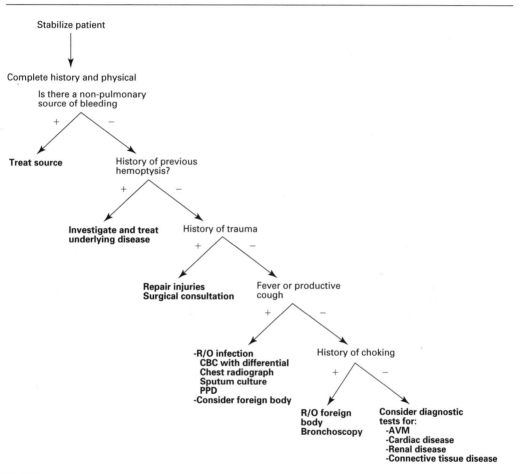

FIG 45-1

Decision tree for differential diagnosis of hemoptysis.

MANAGEMENT

The treatment of hemoptysis should be directed toward the stabilizing of the patient prior to diagnosing and treating the underlying cause. In cases of massive hemoptysis (> 300 mL/24 hrs), maintaining adequate gas exchange and perfusion are critical to patient stabilization. Bronchoscopy may identify the site of the bleeding. Although bleeding is usually self-limited, excessive bleeding may need to be stopped with bronchoscopy-directed saline lavage, the use of an intravenous vasoactive substance, or selective embolization of the bleeding vessel. In life-threatening cases, lobectomy may be necessary.

INDICATIONS FOR CONSULTATION OR REFERRAL

Initial evaluation of most patients with hemoptysis can be performed by the primary care physician. A pediatric pulmonologist can prove useful in helping perform the evaluation, especially if bronchoscopy is indicated. Consultation with a critical care physician should be made early in the course of the illness to aid in providing optimal management of a potentially unstable patient. If a foreign body is suspected, consultation with an otolaryngologist should be made. An interventional radiologist should be consulted if embolization therapy is required. Once the underlying cause of the bleeding is identified, the appropriate subspecialty service should be involved for the patient's long-term management.

DISCUSSION OF THE ALGORITHM

An approach to the child with hemoptysis is presented in Figure 45-1. Patient stabilization should be done before anything else. If necessary, an artificial airway should be established and supplemental oxygen administered. Hypotension and hypovolemia should be corrected with volume expanders (preferably blood). Once patient stabilization is obtained, a diagnostic evaluation based on a detailed history should be undertaken. Nonpulmonary sources of bleeding should be excluded. Early bronchoscopy, especially while the patient is still bleeding, should be considered to determine the site of bleeding and to institute localized therapeutic measures to bring the bleeding under control. Ultimate treatment of the hemoptysis will be based on treating the underlying cause of the bleeding.

BIBLIOGRAPHY

Bowman CM: *Respiratory disease in children: Diagnosis and management,* Baltimore, 1994, Williams and Wilkins.

Cahill BC, Ingbar DH: Massive hemoptysis: Assessment and management, *Clin Chest Med* 15:147–168, 1994.

Camacho JR, Prakash UBS: 46-Year old Man with chronic hemoptysis, *Mayo Clin Proc* 70:83–86, 1995.

Firth JR, McGeady SJ, Smith DS: *Kendig's disorders of the respiratory tract in children,* Philadelphia, 1990, WB Saunders.

Levy J, Wilmott RW: Pulmonary hemosiderosis, *Pediatr Pulmon* 2:384–391, 1986.

Rosenstein BJ: *Hillman's pediatric respiratory diseases: Diagnosis and treatment,* Philadelphia, 1993, WB Saunders.

Thompson AB, Teschler H, Rennard SI: Pathogenesis, evaluation, and therapy for massive hemoptysis, *Clin Chest Med* 13:69–82, 1992.

Zhang JS, Cui ZP, Wang MQ, Yang L: Bronchial arteriography and transcatheter embolization in the management of hemoptysis, *Cardiovasc Intervent Radiol* 17:276–279, 1994.

CHAPTER 46

Hoarseness

William P. Potsic

Chronic hoarseness, a common complaint, is brought to the attention of the primary care physician when the voice is husky, breathy, or weak.

Acute onset of hoarseness is most commonly (90% of cases) associated with inflammation that occurs with viral infections of the upper respiratory tract. Croup and epiglottitis also are accompanied by hoarseness but the parents and patients are more concerned by the stridor or respiratory insufficiency. Acute voice abuse from shouting or smoking are other frequent causes of hoarseness.

DIFFERENTIAL DIAGNOSIS

Common Causes of Hoarseness

- **Trauma**
  Blunt neck trauma
  Arytenoid dislocation from intubation
  Postoperative recurrent nerve injury
    Cervical
    Mediastinal
    Thoracic
  Recurrent laryngeal nerve trauma
  Vocal cord nodules
  Vocal polyps
  Intubation granuloma
  Scar formation
- **Infection**
  Viral
  Bacterial
  Diphtheria
  Bulbar polio
  Botulism
- **Drug–Toxin**
  Lead

- **Allergy–Inflammation**
  Allergic laryngitis
  Rheumatoid arthritis
  Guillain-Barré syndrome
  Gastroesophageal reflux
- **Laryngeal tumors**
  Benign
    Laryngeal papilloma
  Malignant (rare)
    Rhabdomyosarcoma
    Myeloma
  Mediastinal masses
    Tumors
    Cysts
- **Congenital laryngeal disorders**
  Webs
    Glottic
    Subglottic
  Laryngoesophageal cleft
  Cysts
    Mucocele (mucus retention cyst)
    Laryngocele
  Vascular lesions
    Subglottic hemangioma
    Lymphangioma
    Cri-du-chat syndrome
  Unilateral vocal cord paralysis
  Arnold-Chiari malformation
  Gastroesophageal reflux–chronic laryngitis

Discussion

In the neonate, congenital lesions such as laryngeal webs of the larynx may cause hoarseness. This condition is always of concern, and if it is associated with difficulty breathing or feeding, it requires immediate referral to an otolaryngologist for evaluation by laryngoscopy and bronchoscopy. If there is no respiratory distress or

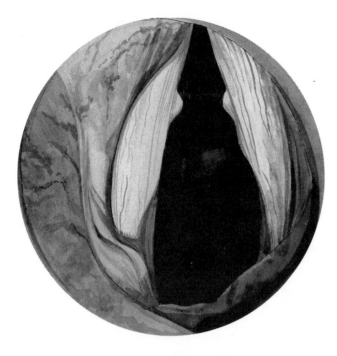

FIG 46-1
Vocal cord nodules.

feeding difficulty, a lateral neck radiograph and barium swallow should be done to rule out mass lesions. If no masses are identified, laryngoscopy should be postponed until the infant is 10 to 12 weeks of age if the problem has not resolved. Laryngoscopy should be done if there is any worsening of the hoarseness in the infant prior to 12 weeks of age.

Children, aged 18 months and older, often develop progressive hoarseness. The most common cause is vocal nodules from vocal misuse and abuse. Nodules are usually indicated by hoarseness that is progressive and worse in the afternoon or evening in a child who screams or shouts frequently. Laryngeal nodules (Fig. 46-1) may resolve with resting of the voice, speech therapy, or changes in vocal behavior. However, any other cause of hoarseness that may be progressive also requires a specific diagnosis.

Papillomas on the vocal cords cause increasing hoarseness and, if severe, respiratory distress. These wartlike lesions are easily visualized by laryngoscopy. Although removal of the papilloma can be carried out under direct visualization, they recur, necessitating numerous procedures. At puberty, the papillomas may regress.

Rarely, unusual conditions like hypothyroidism, botulism, traumatic recurrent nerve paralysis, blunt laryngeal trauma, or mycotic infection of the larynx may cause a weak or hoarse voice.

DATA GATHERING

History
Hoarseness of acute onset suggests infection or trauma, including trauma from both direct injury and overuse from screaming. Often documentation of trauma is difficult but indirect evidence of hoarseness in an enthusiastic sports participant or fan may be enough to suggest the diagnosis.

Botulism is suggested in infants who are breast-fed or offered honey in their feedings. Hoarseness appearing in the neonate should suggest laryngeal anomalies.

Physical Examination
The physical examination requires direct visualization of the cords to make a definite diagnosis. Not all patients need this procedure if an obvious cause of hoarseness is detected on the general physical examination. The most likely

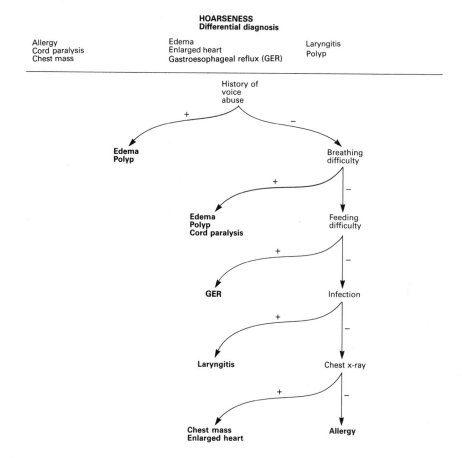

FIG 46-2
Decision tree for differential diagnosis of hoarseness.

positive physical finding will be evidence of upper airway infection. Other entities suggested by the physical examination include botulism with decreased or absent reflexes, hypotonia, and a weak cry. Hypothyroidism also causes hypotonia and decreased reflexes, but characteristic facies.

Laboratory Evaluation
The laboratory tests required by the primary care physician are few because visualization of the larynx is required. This procedure can usually be done by an otolaryngologist with a mirror or flexible fiberoptic instruments. Other tests such as lateral neck radiography, barium swallow, and chest radiography are ordered before or after laryngoscopy as indicated.

INDICATIONS FOR CONSULTATION OR REFERRAL

Patients who do not respond to treatment of infection or voice rest should be seen by someone experienced in visualization of the larynx.

DISCUSSION OF ALGORITHM

An algorithm for differential diagnosis of hoarseness is presented in Figure 46-2. The patient should be assessed for respiratory distress or feeding difficulty. If these symptoms are present, the patient's airway should be evaluated by ordering lateral neck radiographs, if needed, and consulting with an otolaryngologist.

Next, the condition of the patient should be evaluated for infection and voice abuse. If these are not present, these patients need visualization of the vocal cords by a specialist.

BIBLIOGRAPHY

Ferguson CF: Congenital abnormalities of the infant larynx, *Otolaryngol Clin North Am* 3:185–200, 1970.

Hander SD: Trauma to the larynx and upper trachea, *Int Anesthesiol Clin* 26:39–41, 1987.

Holinger PH, Brown WT: Congenital webs, cysts, laryngoceles and other anomalies of the larynx, *Ann Otol Rhinol Laryngol* 76:744–753, 1967.

Holinger PH, Schild JA, Weprin L: Pediatric laryngology, *Otolaryngol Clin North Am* Oct: 625–637, 1970.

Kenna MA: Consultation with the specialist: Hoarseness, *Pediatr Rev* 16(2):69–72, 1995.

Potsic WP, Handler SD: *Primary Care Pediatric Otolaryngology,* ed 2, Andover, 1995, J. Michael Ryan Publishing.

Senturia BH, Wilson FE: Otorhinolaryngic findings in children with voice deviation, *Ann Otol Rhinol Laryngol* 77:1027–1041, 1968.

Silverman E, Zimmer CH: Incidence of chronic hoarseness among school-age children, *J Speech Hear Disord* 2:211–214, 1975.

Yairi E, Currin LH, Bulian N: Incidence of hoarseness in school children over a one year period, *J Commun Dis* 7:321–328, 1974.

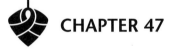

CHAPTER 47

Hypertension

Michael E. Norman

Hypertension is now known to be common in children; as in adults, it is often asymptomatic even when severe. Diagnosis is usually unsuspected and made during a routine examination rather than because of specific signs or symptoms related to elevated blood pressure (BP). The diagnosis of hypertension always depends on the physician's interpretation of the patient's measurements relative to published normal values; therefore, a definition of the upper limit of normal for both the systolic and diastolic values is required (Table 47-1).

Symptoms, when present, are generally nonspecific, such as nausea, vomiting, headache, epistaxis, and abdominal pain. Blurred vision and diplopia occur with prolonged hypertension. On the other hand, frequently overlooked as related to hypertension are complaints of facial palsy, altered personality, sudden onset of deteriorating school performance, and confusion. In any child with catastrophic symptoms such as sudden blindness, seizures, cerebrovascular accident, or coma, malignant hypertensive encephalopathy must be considered.

TABLE 47-1
Definition of Upper Limit of Normal Blood Pressure (mm Hg)

| | BOYS | | | | GIRLS | | | |
| | 95TH PERCENTILE | | HYPERTENSION | | 95TH PERCENTILE | | HYPERTENSION | |
AGE (YR)	SYSTOLIC	DIASTOLIC	MODERATE	SEVERE	SYSTOLIC	DIASTOLIC	MODERATE	SEVERE
0–2	110	65	>125/80	>140/90	110	65	>125/80	>140/95
3–6	112	78	>125/95	>140/100	112	80	>125/90	>140/100
7–10	124	84	>140/95	>160/105	124	84	>144/95	>170/110
11–15	140	90	>155/105	>165/110	138	88	>144/94	>170/110

DIFFERENTIAL DIAGNOSIS

Few major diagnoses need be considered in the child with asymptomatic hypertension. Common causes vary with age. Renal parenchymal diseases occur more frequently in the younger child, 1 to 12 years of age, whereas essential hypertension is most often seen in the teenager, 12 to 18 years of age. Overall, 95% have primary or essential hypertension; the other 5% have secondary hypertension due to renal (4%), renovascular (0.5%), or miscellaneous (0.5%) causes.

Common Causes of Hypertension

- **Infection**
  Pyelonephritis
  Reflux nephropathy
- **Toxin–Drugs**
  Corticosteroids
  Sympathomimetic drugs
  Licorice
- **Metabolic**
  Hyperthyroidism
  Hyperaldosteronism
  Hypercalcemia
- **Allergic–Immunologic**
  Glomerulonephritis
  Serum sickness
- **Vascular**
  Hemolytic uremic syndrome
  Coarctation of the aorta
  Renal artery stenosis
- **Urologic**
  Ureteropelvic junction obstruction
- **Tumor**
  Wilms tumor
  Pheochromocytoma
  Neurofibromatosis
  Brain tumors

- **Multiple etiologies**
  Primary (essential)
  Traction-immobilization (orthopedic surgery)
  Burns
  Bronchopulmonary dysplasia
  Increased intracranial pressure
  Guillain-Barré syndrome

DATA GATHERING

History
Approximately 50% of children with essential hypertension have a positive family history of hypertension and are obese. Although essential hypertension is more common in black adults than in white adults, the same is not true for children. Children with secondary hypertension are more likely to have symptoms referable to elevated BP such as headache and irritability. Clues to the cause may be a history of prior urinary tract infections (*eg,* reflux nephropathy), red or cola-colored urine (*eg,* glomerulonephritis), or the use of excessive cold remedies containing sympathomimetic amines.

Physical Examination
The BP cuff should cover two thirds of the upper arm length, and the inflatable bladder should encircle the arm. Repeated measurements are required before making the diagnosis, both for accuracy and to reduce the impact of initial patient anxiety on the observed values (*see* Report to the Task Force on Blood Pressure Control for details). In the physical examination, pay particular attention to the presence or absence of a cardiac murmur (*eg,* coarctation of the aorta), bruits over the flanks (*eg,* renal artery stenosis), the external genitalia (*eg,* evidence of distal uri-

nary tract obstruction), and evidence of target organ damage from the hypertension itself (eg, retinopathy, cardiomegaly). Any child with severe diastolic hypertension must be considered to have renal parenchymal renovascular hypertension until proved otherwise. In any girl with severe diastolic hypertension, reflux nephropathy must be ruled out with a renal (radionuclide) scan and voiding cystourethrography unless another diagnosis is obvious. Finally, always remember that severe hypertension, especially with marked diastolic elevations, may present with encephalopathy mimicking intracranial disease or congestive heart failure mimicking primary cardiac disease. A search for underlying renal or renovascular disease must be made in such cases.

Laboratory Evaluation

The urinalysis will often point toward primary glomerulonephritis. Subsequent studies would include a complete blood cell count (CBC), serum blood urea nitrogen (BUN) and creatinine levels, and electrolytes, including calcium, C3, antistreptolysin O, and antinuclear antibody titer. Occasionally the urine culture will be positive, but often in reflux nephropathy the urine is sterile when hypertension is discovered. In these cases, renal scarring seen on renal scan suggests prior infection. In some patients reflux is inferred because voiding cystourethrography does not show it. Some experts prefer to begin the radiologic workup with renal ultrasound (US) rather than a renal scan to diagnose obstruction or scarring of the kidney. An electrocardiogram (ECG) and chest radiograph are helpful to screen for coarctation of the aorta and to evaluate the heart for signs of hypertensive effects. Cardiac abnormalities should then be followed up with an echocardiogram. Renal arteriography is recommended when the hypertension is severe, the child is young (less than 10 years of age), and the cause is obscure after urinalysis and urine culture, renal US or renal scan, and voiding cystourethrography. A renal scan, even when combined with oral captopril, is often not sensitive enough to rule out renal artery stenosis. A workup for pheochromocytoma should be done only when symptoms and signs suggest excess circulating catecholamines (eg, palpitations, sweating, pallor). These tumors are rare. The neurologic, orthopedic, and drug-related causes of hypertension are obvious from the history and physical examination and few laboratory investigations are needed. Finally, although some investigators favor measuring a random serum renin level to distinguish between primary and secondary hypertension, I do not believe that it is a particularly useful test in primary practice.

INDICATIONS FOR HOSPITAL ADMISSION

Patients should be admitted to the hospital if the following conditions are present:

1. Severe hypertension at any age, as determined by repeated BP measurements during the examination.
2. Symptomatic hypertension, whatever the BP, particularly if newly discovered.
3. Hypertension associated with a renal bruit or a nephritic urine sediment (eg, hematuria, proteinuria, red blood cell casts).

A pediatric nephrologist should be consulted regarding treatment and workup. If the patient has encephalopathy or congestive heart failure, emergency intravenous therapy either with diazoxide (5 mg/kg by rapid or intravenous injection) or intravenous nitroprusside (0.5 to 0.8 µg/kg/min) may be given even before the cause is determined.

DISCUSSION OF ALGORITHM

An algorithm for the differential diagnosis of hypertension is presented in Figure 47-1. The first task in the evaluation is to confirm the diagnosis of hypertension by determining the BP on at least three occasions, while trying to minimize the patient's excitement and worry. If the BP reading just exceeds the 95th percentile, the hypertension is considered mild. In this group of patients urinalysis should be done to screen for renal disease. If results of urinalysis are normal, other predisposing factors (eg, family history, salt intake, obesity) should be identified and appropriate counseling about weight, diet, and exercise should be given.

Patients with higher BP readings require examination for renovascular disease, including arteriography if the patient is younger than 10 years of age and no other disease to explain hypertension is found.

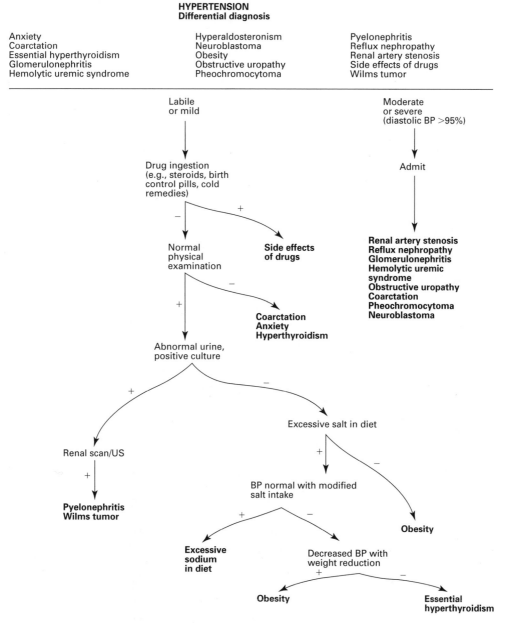

FIG 47-1
Decision tree for differential diagnosis of hypertension.

BIBLIOGRAPHY

Dillon MJ: Clinical aspects of hypertension. In Holiday MA, Barratt TU, Vernier RL, editors: *Pediatric nephrology*, ed 2, Baltimore, 1987, Williams & Wilkins.

Gauthier B, Edelmann CM, Barnett H: *Nephrol-ogy and urology for the pediatrician*, Boston, 1982, Little, Brown, and Co.

Ingelfinger JR: Hypertension. In Edlemann CM Jr, editor: *Pediatric Kidney Disease*, ed 2, Boston, 1992, Little, Brown, and Co.

Norman ME: Renal and electrolyte emergencies. In Fleisher G, Ludwig S, editors: *Textbook of pediatric emergency medicine,* ed 3, Baltimore, 1993, Williams & Wilkins.

Report of the Second Task Force on Blood Pressure Control in Children, 1987, *Pediatrics* 79:1, 1987.

CHAPTER 48

Jaundice

William J. Wenner, Jr.

Jaundice in the pediatric population occurs with a frequency sufficient to instill an appropriate degree of confidence in the primary care physician. The majority of the diseases associated with jaundice should be managed by the primary physician. However, serious consequences and the documented need for timely diagnosis create an absolute need for a correct diagnostic approach.

Jaundice, specifically the yellow discoloration of the skin, is visible in infants with a total bilirubin concentration of greater than 5 mg/dL and in the older child at a level greater than 2.5 mg/dL. The yellow color can be most easily noticed in the conjunctiva. It also is more noticeable under the tongue, on the palate, and in compressed nail beds. Jaundice is caused by excessive levels of serum bilirubin, the waste product of the degeneration of hemoglobin. It may be due to enhanced production or decreased clearance.

DIFFERENTIAL DIAGNOSIS

Commmon Causes of Hyperbilirubinemia

* **Increased production**
    Excess hemoglobin volume
        Adrenal hyperplasia
        Polycythemia
        Delayed clamping of the umbilical cord

Maternal or sibling transfusion
        Maternal diabetes
    Hemolysis
        Infection: Clostridium perfringens; group B streptococci; *Escherichia coli*
        Maternal-fetal incompatibility: ABO; Rh; Others
        Red blood cell defects
            Enzyme deficiencies: G6PD; pyruvate kinase; hexokinase; etc.
            Membrane defects: hereditary spherocytosis; elliptocytosis
    Internal bleeding
        Cephalhematoma
        Central nervous system bleeding
        Cutaneous bruising
        Hemangiomas
        Swallowed blood
* **Decreased clearance**
    Anatomic obstruction
        Alagille syndrome (arteriohepatic dysplasia)
        Biliary atresia
        Choledochal cyst
        Cystic fibrosis
    Drugs: vitamin K; oxytocin
    Hormones
        Hypopituitarism
        Hypothyroidism
    Infections *E. coli; Listeria monocytogenes;*

syphilis; tuberculosis; toxoplasmosis; cytomegalovirus; Epstein-Barr virus; hepatitis A, B, C; herpes; HIV; rubella; and other viral infections

Metabolic

Alpha-1 antitrypsin deficiency

Bile acid synthesis disorders

Crigler-Najjar

Disorders of amino acid; fat, lipid, carbohydrate metabolism: galactosemia; hereditary fructose intolerance; type IV glycogenosis; Niemann-Pick; Gaucher; Wolman disease; urea cycle disorders; etc.

Gilbert disease

Peroxisomal disorders: Zellweger

Tyrosinemia

Increased enterohepatic circulation

Bowel obstruction: pyloric stenosis; atresia; ileus; breast milk jaundice

Increased Bilirubin Production

Excess Hemoglobin Volume

Found most often in the newborn population, the jaundice of this group of etiologies is a result of an excess of hemoglobin that degenerates in the postnatal period. The degradative pathway for hemoglobin is overwhelmed, and an unconjugated hyperbilirubinemia develops. Often, the etiologies that are found in this category can be diagnosed with blood tests. Following equilibration, the hemoglobin will be elevated and the reticulocyte count will be normal. Determining the etiology of the hemoglobin elevation may be more of a challenge, because delayed clamping of the cord, prenatal transfusion, or adrenal hyperplasia may not be readily evident.

Hemolysis

Hemolysis, confirmed by blood tests, should be evaluated by a complete blood count (CBC), blood smear, reticulocyte count, Coombs tests, and blood cultures. Jaundice may be the only symptom at presentation of serious infection. These infections can be rapidly fatal, and this etiology must be considered, evaluated, and treated in a timely manner. Urinary tract infection, often in the second week of life, may demonstrate bilirubin levels greater than 10 mg/dL, mild elevation of serum transaminases, and either a conjugated or unconjugated predominance. *Clostridium perfringens* can directly cause a hemolysis that will manifest mild jaundice early but will progress to severe anemia and

death. An entry site such as an abrasion or scalp monitor wound is often found.

The most common hemolytic cause is ABO incompatibility. It is diagnosed by a positive Coombs test (anti-A or -B). The presence of microspherocytes on a blood smear is suggestive of ABO incompatibility. Rh incompatibility is suggested by a positive Coombs test, maternal anti-Rh titer, an elevated reticulocyte count, and nucleated red blood cells. Red cell defects such as membrane or enzyme defects are considered when a normal white count, negative Coombs and APT tests, or an enlarged liver or spleen are found. Family or maternal history of recent exposure to oxidant in food or drugs is suggestive of a red cell defect.

Extravascular Blood

Blood located outside of the vascular system is slowly broken down and may overload the already challenged system of an infant. It usually is seen approximately 3 days following the blood loss and can require 2 or more weeks to resolve. Cephalhematoma or bruising are easily recognized but internal blood, such as a central nervous system or gastrointestinal bleed, or swallowed blood requires evaluation for diagnosis.

Decreased Clearance

Anatomic Obstruction

A paucity of bile ducts is associated with and is the probable cause of the jaundice of Alagille syndrome. The syndrome is associated with cardiac, musculoskeletal, ocular, facial, renal, and neurologic abnormalities. It occurs in one of 100,000 births and is autosomal dominant, and the defect has been located on chromosome 20p12. The clinical presentation is extremely variable. Often cholestasis is the primary complaint. Older children may have pruritis, but it is rarely seen before 5 months of age. Chronic liver disease, xanthomas, poor growth, and fat-soluble vitamin deficiency appear after the neonatal period. Hepatomegaly is seen in almost all patients, and splenic enlargement is rare in the infant. The cardiovascular findings demonstrate a wide range of defects, with pulmonary vascular defects, usually stenotic lesions, being the most common. Teratology of Fallot, truncus arteriosus, secundum atrial septal defects, and systemic vascular anomalies have been noted. The majority are of minimal clinical significance, but serious anomalies do occur. The musculoskeletal lesions are usually vertebral, with failure of fusion of the anterior arches (butterfly verte-bra) the most common lesion. The ocular find-ings include posterior embryotoxon, Axenfeld anomaly, and other minor findings. Facial find-ings are characteristic, including a small pointed chin, a prominent forehead, deep eyes with hy-pertelorism, and a nose that is in the same plane as the forehead when viewed in profile.

Biliary atresia holds a unique position in the differential diagnosis of jaundice. This illness, which occurs in one of 25,000 infants, usually is an acquired, progressive process. The jaundice usually appears at 3 to 6 weeks of age, during which time a child usually is not seen by the pe-diatrician. Because corrective surgery is most ef-fective if performed prior to 8 to 12 weeks of age, failure to promptly evaluate jaundice could have a devastating outcome. The classic presentation of acholic stools occurs only after the disease has progressed. An enlarged liver, term gestation, healthy appearance, and a total bilirubin of 6 to 12 mg/dL and a conjugated fraction of less than 7 mg/dL are associated findings. Any jaundice that is present after 2 weeks of age should not be pre-sumed to be physiologic. Biliary atresia is associ-ated with congenital defects in 15% of the af-fected infants, including asplenia, polysplenia, and cardiovascular and intestinal anomalies.

Other anatomic obstructions include chole-dochal cyst, congenital segmental cystic dilation of the biliary ducts, and miscellaneous other ductal anomalies. These obstructions most often are diagnosed by ultrasound or hepatoiminodi-acetic acid nuclear isotope scan but may not be noted until exploratory surgery.

Cystic fibrosis, inspissated bile ducts, gall stones, and parenteral nutrition can obstruct bile flow and result in jaundice.

Drugs
Many medications have some effect on bile flow. Cholestasis further influences drug metabolism by interfering with enzyme systems. This result has been reported with appropriate doses of cimetidine, erythromycin, estrogens, nitrofuran-toin, phenobarbital, phenytoin, phenothiazine, trimethoprim-sulfamethoxazole, and large doses of vitamin K and oxytocin.

Hormones
Prior to newborn screening, more than 25% of cases of congenital hypothyroidism presented with jaundice. The jaundice may persist for several weeks following replacement therapy. Hyperthyroidism can be associated with jaun-dice, but it is due to the associated high-out-put cardiac failure. Intrauterine hypopituitarism can present with prolonged jaundice, hypo-glycemia, and micropenis and undescended testis.

Infections
In addition to the hemolysis that occurs in some infections, certain infections interfere with the excretion of bilirubin. *Escherichia coli* is the pro-totype infection, and it is postulated that endo-toxin interferes with the excretion of conjugated bilirubin into the canaliculi. *Listeria* can directly invade the liver parenchyma causing hepatitis and microabscesses. Tuberculosis, *Mycobacte-rium avium-intracellulare,* and other bacteria have been associated with jaundice. The infec-tions highlighted in the acronym TORCH (toxo-plasmosis, rubella, cytomegalovirus, herpes sim-plex) can have jaundice as a component of the clinical presentation. Other viral etiologies such as hepatitis A, B, C; Epstein-Barr virus; and HIV also may have jaundice in their presentation.

Metabolic
Because the liver plays a unique and crucial role in metabolism, jaundice and other forms of liver disease are often the consequence of meta-bolic disorders. Some metabolic disorders di-rectly affect the metabolism of bilirubin. These disorders include Crigler-Najjar syndrome in the infant and Gilbert disease in the older child, both of which with an unconjugated hyperbili-rubinemia. Jaundice is a particular finding in those entities with a cholestatic component such as alpha-1 antitrypsin deficiency and in those with severe hepatic damage such as tyrosinemia. The presentation of emesis, poor feeding, diar-rhea, lethargy, or failure to thrive with associated jaundice should suggest metabolic disease. Urine organic and amino acids and serum amino acids should be analyzed. Urine should be checked for reducing substances in infants with jaundice who have been fed lactose-containing formula, because this condition is part of the clinical presentation of galactosemia.

Increased Enterohepatic Circulation
In the adult, conjugated bilirubin is broken down by the bowel bacterial flora. However, in the newborn, without the adult flora, conjugated bilirubin is hydrolyzed by intestinal enzymes to lipophilic unconjugated bilirubin, which can

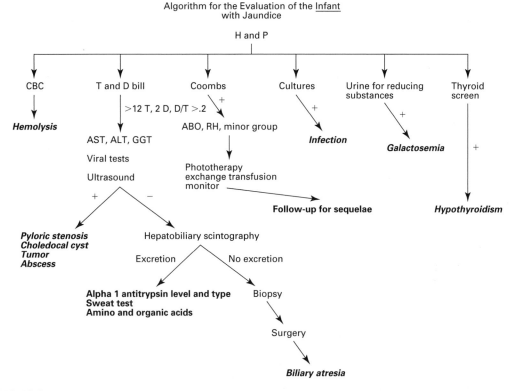

FIG 48-1
Decision tree for differential diagnosis of jaundice in infants.

diffuse across the enterocyte into the blood. Increased enterohepatic circulation can cause jaundice when intestinal obstruction is present, such as pyloric stenosis, atresia, and small bowel ileus. It has been postulated that the emesis and starvation of these conditions contribute to the hyperbilirubinemia by interfering with the uptake and conjugation of bilirubin. Any child with emesis, abdominal distension, or feeding difficulty associated with jaundice should be evaluated for intestinal obstruction.

Breast milk–associated jaundice has been estimated to occur in up to 12% of breast-fed infants. Most cases have early onset and probably are due to caloric deprivation and dehydration interfering with uptake and conjugation of bilirubin. Late onset occurs in up to 3% of breast-fed infants and begins on approximately the fourth day of life and peaks at approximately 14 days of life. Jaundice over 15 mg/dL occurs in 2% of all breast-fed infants. Frank kernicterus is not associated with breast

milk jaundice. The etiology is not clear. Early studies suggested an inhibition of hepatic glucuronyl transferase. More recent studies suggest increased enterohepatic circulation of bilirubin as the etiology. Breast milk usually inhibits the absorption of bilirubin by the intestine, however, breast milk from mothers of infants with jaundice promotes the absorption.

DATA GATHERING

History and Physical Examination
The critical aspects of the evaluation of the patient with jaundice are those that indicate the severity of liver disease and those that indicate other organ involvement. Liver status can be evaluated by obtaining a history of acholic stools, bleeding from mucous membranes, petechiae, emesis, failure to thrive, and edema. Physical examination of liver status includes assessing liver size and texture, bruising, or pete-

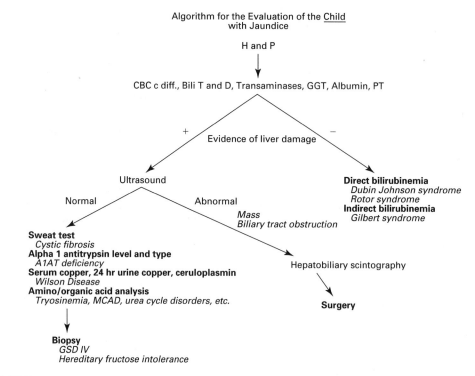

FIG 48-2
Decision tree for differential diagnosis of jaundice in children.

chiae. Extrahepatic involvement is evaluated by obtaining a history of the pregnancy and gestation, family history, feeding history, medication history, and history of exposure to infections.

LABORATORY EVALUATION

Initial evaluation should include a CBC with differential, blood smear, transaminases, gamma-glutamyl transferase, albumin and total and direct bilirubin, urine analysis, and urine reducing substances (Figs. 48-1 and 48-2). Blood and urine cultures should be obtained if there is any suspicion of infection, especially in patients with fever or under 8 weeks of age. A total bilirubin of greater than 13 mg/dL should not be considered physiologic until evaluated. A direct bilirubin greater than 2 mg/dL or when the direct component is >20% of the total bilirubin should be evaluated for the etiology. Jaundice persisting for more than 2 weeks should be evaluated, and any

jaundice presenting at 4 to 8 weeks of age should be evaluated expeditiously.

Further evaluation will be guided by laboratory results and physical findings. Ultrasound should be considered when the liver is enlarged or any anatomic abnormality is suspected. The liver is easily evaluated in its entirety. The size and texture of the liver, pancreas, kidneys, and spleen can be evaluated by ultrasound. Tests for hepatic excretion are valuable in the evaluation of jaundice because they provide information on the patency of the biliary drainage system. Hepatobiliary scintigraphy has been shown to be useful in differentiating extrahepatic obstruction as the cause of jaundice from those cases with no obstruction. This differentiation is improved if the patient is prepped with phenobarbital for 5 days prior to the injection of the marker. Because some etiologies of jaundice, such as biliary atresia, are progressive, early studies (before 5 to 7 weeks of age) may show excretion, and the patient must be followed-up and reevaluated. Elevated levels of bilirubin can interfere with the uptake of the marker and excretion by the liver into the ducts. Bowel activity of the marker, diagnostic of excretion, still may be achieved with direct bilirubin levels greater than 20 mg/dL.

INDICATIONS FOR CONSULTATION OR REFERRAL

Most causes of jaundice can be evaluated, diagnosed, and treated by the primary care pediatrician. Preliminary tests can discriminate between the self-limited, easily diagnosed causes of jaundice from those that cause progressive damage and require expedient therapy. If the tests needed to evaluate conjugated hyperbilirubinemia are not quickly available, or if experience with these diseases is limited, referral to a pediatric gastroenterologist is indicated. Persistent elevation for more than 2 weeks without an etiology should be referred for evaluation.

DISCUSSION OF ALGORITHM

Algorithmic approaches to diagnosis offer the advantages of linear flow and logical process. An algorithmic approach to jaundice (Figs. 48-1 and 48-2) has three critical decision points. The first is the age of the child. The diseases that cause jaundice during infancy (0 to 12 months of age) (Fig. 48-1) differ from those of the older child (Fig. 48-2). The second decision point is following a comprehensive history and physical examination. Often the history and physical examination will allow the physician to bypass a linear algorithm and proceed directly to finding specific tests for diagnosis. The third decision point is the preliminary laboratory tests. These broad-based tests direct the clinician to the proper path to diagnosis. Algorithms can be valuable, but no algorithm can replace the functioning intellect of the primary care physician.

BIBLIOGRAPHY

Andres JM: Congenital infections of the liver. In Walker WA, Durie PR, Hamilton JR, Walker-Smith JA, Watkins JB, editors: *Pediatric gastrointestinal disease,* Philadelphia, 1991, BC Decker.

Gremse DA, Balistreri WF: Neonatal cholestasis. In Lebenthal E, editor: *Textbook of gastroenterology and nutrition in infancy,* ed 2, New York, 1989, Raven Press.

Moyer MS, Balistreri WF: Prolonged neonatal obstructive jaundice. In Walker WA, Durie PR, Hamilton JR, Walker-Smith JA, Watkins JB, editors: *Pediatric gastrointestinal disease.* Philadelphia, 1991, BC Decker.

Newman TB, Maisels MJ: Evaluation and treatment of jaundice in the term newborn, *Pediatrics* 89:809, 1992.

Piccoli DA, Witzleben CL: Disorders of the extrahepatic bile ducts. In Walker WA, Durie PR, Hamilton JR, Walker-Smith JA, Watkins JB, editors: *Pediatric gastrointestinal disease,* Philadelphia, 1991, BC Decker.

Spivak W: Disorders of bilirubin metabolism. In Walker WA, Durie PR, Hamilton JR, Walker-Smith JA, Watkins JB, editors: *Pediatric gastrointestinal disease,* Philadelphia, 1991, BC Decker.

Zipursky A: Isoimmune hemolytic diseases. In Nathan DG, Oski FA, editors: *Hematology of infancy and childhood,* ed 2, Philadelphia, 1981, WB Saunders.

CHAPTER 49

Large Liver

William R. Treem

An enlarged liver is found in many diverse disease processes in infancy and childhood; thus the primary care physician must direct the workup toward the most fruitful areas of investigation and make a decision to follow-up, refer, or hospitalize the child. This chapter offers guidelines for that decision process based on the pathophysiology of hepatomegaly, review of selected diseases, careful history, physical examination, and selected screening laboratory tests.

DIFFERENTIAL DIAGNOSIS

Common Causes of Large Liver

- **Infection**
    Hepatitis types A through E
    Sepsis
    Epstein-Barr virus
    Syphilis
    Enteroviruses
    TORCH infections (toxoplasmosis, rubella, cytomegalovirus, herpes)
    Parasites
    Hepatic abscess
    Tuberculosis, histoplasmosis
    AIDS
- **Trauma**
    Traumatic cyst
    Hematoma
- **Tumor**
    Leukemia
    Lymphoma
    Neuroblastoma
    Hepatoblastoma
    Hemangioma
    Adenoma
- **Toxin**
    Drug-induced hepatitis

Hypervitaminosis A
- **Metabolic**
    Glycogen storage disease
    Galactosemia
    Tyrosinemia
    Hereditary fructose intolerance
    Sphingolipidosis (Gaucher disease, Niemann-Pick disease)
    Mucolipidosis (I-cell disease)
    GM_1 gangliosidosis
    Mucopolysaccharidoses (Hurler syndrome, Hunter syndrome)
    α_1-Antitrypsin deficiency
    Wilson disease
    Urea cycle disorders
    Diabetes
    Disorders of fatty acid oxidation
    Cystic fibrosis
- **Inflammatory**
    Chronic active hepatitis
    Sclerosing cholangitis
    Sarcoidosis
- **Multiple etiologies**
    Malnutrition
    Hyperalimentation
    Obesity
- **Vascular**
    Budd-Chiari syndrome
    Venoocclusive disease
    Congestive heart failure
    Constrictive pericarditis
- **Congenital**
    Cyst
    Hamartoma
    Congenital hepatic fibrosis
- **Biliary obstruction**
    Common duct stones, stricture
    Pancreatitis, cystic fibrosis
    Choledochal cyst, tumors of biliary tract (rhabdomyosarcoma)

Discussion

Pathophysiologic mechanisms involved in liver enlargement include 1) congestion secondary to elevated central venous pressure or localized vascular obstruction, as in congestive heart failure or Budd-Chiari syndrome; 2) inflammation with expansion of portal tracts by inflammatory cells, as in viral hepatitis; 3) storage of materials that are accumulating because of metabolic enzyme deficiencies as in glycogen storage disease; 4) accumulation of fat, as seen in malnutrition, diabetes mellitus, Reye syndrome, and disorders of fatty acid oxidation; 5) intrinsic expanding masses such as adenomas, hemangiomas, and hepatoblastomas; and 6) biliary obstruction with accompanying jaundice, as seen with common duct stones or strictures, choledochal cysts, or lesions in the head of the pancreas. Subsequent chapters cover hepatomegaly with jaundice, especially in infancy, and acute viral hepatitis. The following discussion is limited to some of the differential diagnoses of chronic hepatomegaly and chronic hepatitis in the older child who is asymptomatic or subacutely ill. A reasonable definition of "chronic hepatitis" is persistence or relapse of features of acute hepatitis beyond 3 months including elevated aminotransferase levels, hepatomegaly, hard liver, splenomegaly, ascites, anorexia, weight loss, muscle wasting, persistent fever, or jaundice.

Infections Causing Chronic Hepatitis

Although hepatitis A almost always causes an acute self-limited hepatitis, other viruses can cause a more prolonged indolent disease with chronic hepatomegaly and elevated liver enzymes (see Chapter 80, Viral Hepatitis).

Extrahepatic manifestations of hepatitis B virus (HBV) infection are common in children. HBV is found in up to 20% of cases of membranous glomerulonephropathy in early childhood. A specific erythematous nonpruritic papular eruption of the skin of the face and extremities has been described in children with acute or chronic HBV infection. This condition is called papular acrodermatitis of childhood or Gianotti-Crosti disease.

Cytomegalovirus (CMV) infection also must be considered in the differential diagnosis of unexplained hepatomegaly in older children usually accompanied by only mild abnormalities in aminotransferase levels. CMV can be isolated from fresh urine or from liver tissue obtained via needle biopsy. Liver histologic findings vary from minimal chronic persistent hepatitis to granulomatous hepatitis.

AIDS secondary to HIV infection frequently results in hepatosplenomegaly, especially in infants. These findings often occur in the setting of failure to thrive, lymphadenopathy, persistent thrush, chronic pulmonary infiltrates, and diarrhea. Biochemical tests of liver function, including hyperbilirubinemia and prolonged prothrombin time (PT), frequently yield abnormal results.

Chronic Active Hepatitis

After the first few months of life, when liver disease is primarily caused by neonatal hepatitis or anatomic aberrations of the biliary system, the leading cause of persistent jaundice and chronic liver disease in the pediatric population is chronic active hepatitis. This clinicopathologic entity is defined by chronic elevations of liver enzyme levels, hepatomegaly, and a histologic lesion of periportal inflammation, piecemeal necrosis, and portal, septal, and intralobular bridging fibrosis or cirrhosis. Known associations include hepatitis B (but not hepatitis A) Epstein-Barr virus (EBV), and most other viral causes of acute hepatitis), hepatitis C, hepatitis D, a positive antinuclear antibody (ANA) test, or other markers of autoimmune phenomena, ulcerative colitis or Crohn disease, Sjögren syndrome, thyroiditis, diabetes, or immunodeficiency syndromes. Girls are affected more often than boys, and patients usually have hepatosplenomegaly and jaundice. A significant proportion of patients will not have had an identifiable episode of acute hepatitis preceding the insidious onset and may show physical stigmata of chronic liver disease, such as spider angiomas, clubbing, ascites, and palmar erythema. Accompanying extrahepatic signs and symptoms may be prominent and may include epistaxis, easy bruising, urticaria, vitiligo, amenorrhea, arthralgia, arthritis, pleural effusions, iridocyclitis, and laboratory evidence of glomerulonephritis and Coombs-positive hemolytic anemia.

Chronic active hepatitis often can be distinguished from the less serious chronic persistent hepatitis only by liver biopsy. There are two major differences: 1) The inflammatory infiltrate is confined to the portal areas of the liver in chronic, persistent hepatitis and does not spread into the lobule. 2) Chronic, persistent hepatitis usually is self-limited and does not progress to either cirrhosis or liver failure. The differential diagnosis is similar to that of chronic active hepatitis except that it includes other viruses, such as cytomegalovirus (CMV) or even hepatitis A, which rarely cause chronic active hepatitis.

Drug-Induced Hepatitis

Drugs and toxins can cause severe hepatic damage resulting in hepatomegaly, "hepatitis," cholestasis, jaundice, and even hepatic failure. Some agents produce liver damage in a predictable dose-related fashion, usually starting at a predictable time after exposure to the drug. Other agents are unpredictable, causing an idiosyncratic reaction in only a small proportion of patients taking the drug. The list of drugs that may cause liver injury is vast, but some of the more commonly used agents are erythromycin salts, trimethoprim-sulfamethoxazole, isoniazid, ketoconazole, methotrexate, azathioprine, cyclosporine, halothane, sodium valproate, phenytoin, phenothiazines, acetaminophen, aspirin, hydralazine, anabolic steroids, oral contraceptives, vitamin A, and cimetidine. Erythromycin, anabolic steroids, and phenothiazines cause a predominantly cholestatic injury pattern with clinical jaundice; phenytoin and sulfa drugs can cause hepatocellular necrosis with features of a generalized hypersensitivity reaction, such as fever, arthralgia, rash, lymphadenopathy, and eosinophilia. Fatty infiltration of the liver can be seen with the use of corticosteroids, tetracycline, and also sodium valproate, which has also been associated with hyperammonemia and a Reye-like syndrome. Drugs such as isoniazid used in therapeutic doses predictably cause hepatotoxicity in approximately 10% of patients based on the accelerated rate of metabolism of the drug. Acetaminophen, iron, vitamin A, and salicylates are only toxic when taken in massive overdoses.

The essential clinical feature in establishing the diagnosis is a history of exposure to the drug or toxin, knowledge of the dose ingested, and the timing between ingestion and onset of symptoms. Other possible causes for liver dysfunction must be excluded. The simultaneous appearance of rash, fever, arthralgia, or eosinophilia can be helpful. Disappearance of the symptoms on discontinuation of the drug is strong confirmatory evidence. Most drug-induced hepatic injury is completely reversible with removal of the offending agent.

Wilson Disease

A rare but treatable cause of hepatomegaly in children older than 3 years of age is Wilson disease, an autosomal recessive disorder characterized by defective biliary copper excretion and accumulation of toxic amounts of copper in the liver, brain, kidney, and cornea. This entity frequently presents during childhood, either as asymptomatic hepatomegaly, insidious cirrhosis, or with biochemical and laboratory features that may mimic chronic active hepatitis. More than 50% of all patients with Wilson disease have symptoms before 15 years of age, and more than 50% have overt hepatic involvement.

The absence of more classic manifestations of the disease, such as tremor, dysarthria, muscular rigidity, Kayser-Fleisher rings in the cornea, and renal tubular disturbance, is common in childhood and should not prohibit consideration of the diagnosis. Neurologic abnormalities associated with Wilson disease in childhood may be subtle and include deteriorating school performance, behavior problems, clumsiness, and particular difficulty in fine motor skills such as handwriting.

It is important, therefore, for physicians to think of Wilson disease when evaluating hepatomegaly in the school-aged child, because prompt and specific therapy with D-penicillamine affords a favorable prognosis for many and subsequent identification and treatment of asymptomatic homozygote siblings can be accomplished. The best screening tests are an ophthalmologic examination for Kayser-Fleischer rings and measurements of serum ceruloplasmin and 24-hour urinary copper excretion. Often a quantitative measure of liver copper content is necessary for definitive diagnosis.

α_1-Antitrypsin Deficiency

In addition to presenting as a neonatal cholestatic syndrome, α_1-antitrypsin deficiency may be serendipitously discovered later in infancy or childhood during evaluation because of hepatomegaly or failure to thrive, or progress insidiously through anicteric hepatitis to cirrhosis with accompanying splenomegaly and portal hypertension. The incidence of this defect ranges from one in 1500 live births in Sweden to one in 7000 in the United States. Only 5% to 15% of homozygote PiZZ individuals will manifest neonatal jaundice, but 25% to 50% will continue to show either clinical or biochemical abnormalities of liver function, suggesting hepatic damage. Diagnosis is made by quantitation of circulating α_1-antitrypsin levels and protease inhibitor (Pi) typing to determine if the patients' phenotype corresponds to PiZZ, the only phenotype definitely associated with liver disease.

Liver transplantation has been successful in many children with cirrhosis due to α_1-antitrypsin deficiency, with conversion to the normal donor phenotype of PiMM and restoration of normal circulating levels of the protein. No other specific treatment exists at this time, but the importance of diagnosis may be in the early institution of monitoring, prevention of exposure to hepatotoxins (alcohol), avoidance of smoking, and identification and counseling of PiMZ heterozygotes.

Other Metabolic Liver Diseases

Many metabolic liver diseases present in the neonatal period or within the first year of life and are accompanied by hepatomegaly, jaundice, and often other signs and symptoms such as vomiting, failure to thrive, seizures, hypotonia, abnormal facies, and neurologic or visual impairment. However, a few of these entities can develop later in childhood, primarily with asymptomatic hepatosplenomegaly, thrombocytopenia, bone pain, or even cirrhosis, severe liver dysfunction, and portal hypertension. Glycogen storage disease, type IV (deficiency of amylo-1,4-1,6-transglucosidase–branching enzyme) is a rare cause of early childhood cirrhosis in which neither fasting hypoglycemia nor acidosis is likely to be found. Type VIa and type IX glycogenoses are milder forms, both resulting in hepatomegaly in which the liver fluctuates in size, being enlarged during periods of well-being and often normal during intercurrent illnesses.

Of the sphingolipidoses, a predominantly visceral form of Gaucher disease without neurologic involvement may develop in late childhood or adolescence, with hepatosplenomegaly and slow progression to cirrhosis. The presence of vacuolated lymphocytes in the peripheral smear, radiologic abnormalities in long bones, and an elevated acid phosphatase level are suggestive of Gaucher disease. Bone marrow examination will show foam cells, and the diagnosis is confirmed by peripheral leukocyte lipid enzyme studies.

Portal Hypertension

Many liver diseases can progress to cirrhosis and present with primary splenomegaly, hematologic evidence of hypersplenism (thrombocytopenia, neutropenia), upper gastrointestinal bleeding from esophageal and gastric varices, or ascites. At this stage the liver may be of normal size or small, hard, and nodular on palpation. Two causes of portal hypertension without cirrhosis peculiar to the pediatric population are cavernous transformation of the portal vein and congenital hepatic fibrosis. Cavernous transformation of the portal vein usually presents with asymptomatic splenomegaly or upper gastrointestinal bleeding as the initial manifestation, between the ages of 1 and 10 years. The lesion consists of replacement of a stenotic, thrombosed, or fibrous portal vein with a collection of small portoportal recanalized collateral vessels and is a prehepatic or presinusoidal obstruction. Therefore the liver is usually normal in size or only mildly enlarged, and the determinations of aminotransferase levels, bilirubin levels, and PT are normal. The liver is histologically normal. Although the cause of this condition remains obscure, a history of neonatal illness (respiratory distress syndrome, sepsis, omphalitis, dehydration) or umbilical vein catheterization is obtained in one third of patients. Ultrasonography can facilitate making the diagnosis, and abdominal angiography will give the clearest picture of the portal venous system.

Congenital hepatic fibrosis is an intrahepatic disorder characterized by a pathologic lesion of broad bands of mature connective tissue in portal and periportal distribution. These fibrous bands surround increased numbers of ectatic and dysplastic bile ducts within portal areas. Regenerative nodules are lacking, individual hepatocytes are normal, and cholestasis and inflammatory cells are seldom observed except in a rare variant complicated by bacterial cholangitis. Half the cases occur sporadically; the other half are associated with a family history of portal hypertension, splenomegaly, gastrointestinal bleeding, or renal disease, including polycystic kidney disease in infancy or adulthood. The coexistence of hypertension, mild azotemia, decreased urinary concentrating ability, or abnormal results of in-

II

travenous pyelography, with hepatomegaly in the young child, should alert the physician to the diagnosis.

Portal hypertension is regularly accompanied by splenomegaly and gradual reductions in the platelet account to less than 100,000/mm³ and the white blood cell count to less than 4000/mm³. This result has been attributed to trapping and sequestration of platelets and white blood cells in the markedly enlarged spleen and is called *hypersplenism*. Often this finding prompts consideration of a hematologic malignancy as the primary diagnosis and deflects attention from the possibility of primary liver disease, cirrhosis, and portal hypertension.

Intrahepatic Tumors and Space-Occupying Lesions

Benign and malignant intrahepatic tumors are exceedingly rare in childhood, but focal or asymmetric liver enlargement should alert the clinician to this possibility. Vascular lesions (hemangiomas and hemangioendotheliomas) are the most common primary benign tumors of childhood, usually presenting within the first year of life with hepatomegaly with or without cutaneous hemangiomas, or systemic symptoms such as congestive heart failure, petechiae, and thrombocytopenia. Hamartomas contain normal hepatic elements of an embryonic nature in disorderly array, tend to be solid, and present as an abdominal mass, with the only symptoms related to the pressure effects and resulting disturbances in the function of neighboring structures. The prevalence of a third benign liver tumor, the highly vascular liver cell adenoma, has increased since the advent of oral contraceptives. Other nontumorous causes of asymmetric liver enlargement or abdominal masses include local abscess, hepatic trauma and resulting parenchymal hemorrhage, solitary or multiple cysts, congenital hepatic fibrosis, echinococcal cysts, and focal nodular hyperplasia.

Hepatoblastoma is the most common primary malignant liver tumor in children. Most lesions present as enlarged livers or masses and are greater than 10 cm in diameter at the time of diagnosis. Hepatocellular carcinoma, seen frequently complicating the later stages of chronic HBV infection or α_1-antitrypsin deficiency in adults, has been reported as early as the age of 7 years in a congenital carrier of HBV, in cirrhosis induced following intravenous hyperalimentation in a young child, and in children requiring long-term anabolic androgen therapy for aplastic anemia.

DATA GATHERING

The clinical disease states and the age at presentation of hepatomegaly are summarized in Table 49-1. The clinical questions for the primary pediatrician are: Is the apparent hepatomegaly pathologic? If so, is it representative of an acute or chronic process? Does the patient's condition require immediate extensive evaluation or hospitalization? Is evaluation best accomplished by a consultant? After initial screening, can the patient be safely observed over time for any progression in liver abnormality? The preliminary evaluation should include an accurate evaluation of liver size, consistency, and contour as well as a complete history and physical examination.

History

The history is invaluable in differentiating acute from chronic processes. Careful questioning is essential about exposure to jaundiced or ill persons, possible contact with carriers of HBV or animal vectors of hepatotropic infections, previous blood transfusions, shellfish exposure, intravenous drug use, and travel history. Exposure to potentially hepatotoxic drugs such as acetaminophen, salicylate, phenytoin, sulfonamides, erythromycin, valproic acid, iron, halothane, or vitamin A should be ruled out, as should poisonings with tetrachlorethanes, carbon tetrachloride, mushrooms *(Amanita phalloides),* phosphorus, or arsenic.

The evolution of symptoms must be accurately understood and the rapidity of their development assessed. Disease of acute onset is more likely to be infectious, toxic, or congestive rather than infiltrative, obstructive, or metabolic (with the exceptions of the acute presentation of galactosemia and hereditary fructose intolerance in infancy or of Wilson disease in later childhood). Characteristic prodromal symptoms facilitate diagnosis. Acute hepatitis associated with EBV is preceded by fever and pharyngitis; hepatitis A infection is commonly associated with a prodrome of nausea, vomiting, anorexia, and fever; and HBV infection usually has a more gradual onset with associated malaise, arthalgia, occa-

TABLE 49-1
Clinical Disease States and Age of Presentation of Hepatomegaly*

AGE	CLINICAL DISEASE STATES
Newborn (Birth–2 mo)	Intrauterine and intrapartum acquired infection (TORCH, syphilis, other)
	Erythroblastosis fetalis
	Neonatal hepatitis, α_1-antitrypsin, Alagille syndrome
	Biliary atresia
	Congestive heart failure
	Congenital paroxysmal atrial tachycardia
	Sepsis
Infant (2–12 mo)	Cystic fibrosis
	Metabolic disease: glycogen storage, α_1-antitrypsin deficiency, galactosemia, tyrosinemia, hereditary fructose intolerance, other
	Neonatal hepatitis, hepatitis B
	HIV infection (AIDS)
	Histiocytosis
	Malnutrition
	Tumors (intrinsic, metastatic)
	Cholelithiasis
	Choledochal cyst
Young child (1–6 yrs)	Viral hepatitis
	Drug-toxic hepatitis
	Parasitic
	Tumor
	Leukemia, lymphoma
Older child, adolescent (7–20 yrs)	Viral hepatitis
	Drug-toxic hepatitis
	Wilson disease
	Chronic active hepatitis
	Congenital hepatic fibrosis
	Focal nodular hyperplasia, adenoma
	α_1-Antitrypsin deficiency
	Reye syndrome
	Sickle cell anemia
	Cholelithiasis
	Juvenile rheumatoid arthritis, lupus erythematous, sarcoidosis
	Leukemia, lymphoma
	Gonococcal perihepatitis
	Cystic fibrosis
	Diabetes

*Adapted from Walker WA, Mathia RK: *Pediatr Clin North Am* 22:929, 1975.

sional arthritis, an urticarial or maculopapular rash, or hematuria and proteinuria.

Clues to the cause of more chronic liver disease can be obtained by careful family history, past medical history, and review of systems. Patients and families should be questioned about a history of liver or lung disease, jaundice, gastrointestinal bleeding, neurologic or psychiatric disease, mental retardation, infantile renal disease, and early infant deaths. A search should be made for a medical history of prolonged neonatal jaundice and failure to thrive. Review of systems specifically focuses on dietary intake, chronic diarrhea or vomiting, chronic pulmonary problems, developmental delay, easy bruising, frequent nosebleeds, and pruritus. Pruritus is an important symptom of cholestasis, and its relationship to the appearance of jaundice should be defined. In general, pruritus before jaundice suggests extrahepatic obstruction; jaundice before pruritus is more typical of intrahepatic disease.

Physical Examination

A palpable liver is not synonymous with an enlarged liver, particularly in infants or young children. During the first 6 months of life, the palpable edge of the liver extends from 1 to 3 cm below the right costal margin in the midclavicular line. It seldom exceeds 2 cm in the child from

TABLE 49-2
Expected Liver Span of Infants and Children*

AGE (YR)	BOYS		GIRLS	
	MEAN ESTIMATED LIVER SPAN	STANDARD ERROR OF MEAN	MEAN ESTIMATED LIVER SPAN	STANDARD ERROR OF MEAN
0.5	2.4	2.5	2.8	2.6
1	2.8	2.0	3.1	2.1
2	3.5	1.6	3.6	1.7
3	4.0	1.6	4.0	1.7
4	4.4	1.6	4.3	1.6
5	4.8	1.5	4.5	1.6
6	5.1	1.5	4.8	1.6
8	5.6	1.5	5.1	1.6
10	6.1	1.6	5.4	1.7
12	6.5	1.8	5.6	1.8
14	6.8	2.0	5.8	2.1
16	7.1	2.2	6.0	2.3
18	7.4	2.5	6.1	2.6
20	7.7	2.8	6.3	2.9

*From Lawson EE, Grand RJ, Neff RK, et al.: Am J Dis Child 132:475, 1978. Used by permission.

6 months to 4 years of age. In older children the liver edge should not be palpable 1 to 2 cm below the thoracic cage unless the upper edge is percussible below the sixth intercostal space. The normal adult liver extends from the right fifth intercostal space in the midclavicular line to the right costal margin and may descend 1 to 3 cm with deep inspiration. Liver span (height in the right midclavicular line) is obtained by percussing the upper border and palpating the lower border and is the only reliable measure of liver size. Table 49-2 offers guidelines for liver span in children aged 6 months to 20 years. Great variation is present in infants, making interpretation difficult. Epigastric palpation revealing a liver edge below the xiphoid may be a good indication of hepatomegaly.

Perception of hepatomegaly is influenced by the relationship between the liver and adjacent structures. Anatomic variations such as narrow costal angle, pectus excavatum, flared costal margins, and Riedel lobe (downward prolongation of the right liver lobe caused by an adhesion to the mesocolon) lead to overestimation or underestimation of liver size based solely on palpation of the lower edge. Other pathologic states such as obstructive lung disease, retroperitoneal mass, perihepatic abscess, or pneumothorax may be associated with apparent hepatic enlargement.

In addition to the size of the liver, evaluation should include shape (symmetry or asymmetry), consistency (soft, firm, rock-hard), presence or absence of tenderness, and surface contour (smooth, irregular, nodular). Asymmetry suggests an intrinsic space-occupying lesion, although a choledochal cyst or hydropic gallbladder can simulate focal enlargement. Firm symmetric hepatomegaly with a rounded edge is consistent with infiltration, fibrosis, or congestion and connotes a more chronic process. Rock-hard hepatomegaly with a sharp, nontender edge favors cirrhosis or malignancy. Diffuse liver tenderness implies generalized capsular distention from acute parenchymal inflammation or congestion. Rubs and bruits should be auscultated to rule out infectious or traumatic inflammation of the liver capsule or intrahepatic vascular tumors.

Serial examinations are important to assess changes in liver size. A rapidly enlarging liver may indicate congestion associated with congestive heart failure or cardiomyopathy, or massive rapid infiltration with fat seen in malnutrition, cystic fibrosis, diabetes mellitus, and metabolic disorders of fatty acid oxidation or branched-chain amino acid oxidation. A rapidly shrinking liver may signal a resolving problem but also may indicate hepatic necrosis and collapse of hepatic parenchymal architecture, especially if accompanied by a rising bilirubin level and PT.

Careful physical examination reveals diagnostic clues in the evaluation of hepatomegaly.

Some, such as spider angiomas, clubbing, and gynecomastia, indicate chronicity of liver dysfunction. Rickets or pathologic fractures, multiple ecchymoses, decreased or absent reflexes, and glossitis or gingival inflammation reflect the malabsorption of fat-soluble vitamins and malnutrition that at times accompany chronic cholestatic liver disease. Conjugated hyperbilirubinemia and jaundice characterize extrahepatic biliary tract obstruction and inflammatory hepatitis secondary to drugs, toxins, and infectious agents and are seen in the later stages of many chronic processes (eg, Wilson disease, chronic active hepatitis, cystic fibrosis). However, jaundice is unusual in infiltrative processes (malignancies), storage diseases, or chronic congestive syndromes. The evaluation of jaundice, especially in the infant, is more fully discussed in Chapter 48.

Splenomegaly associated with hepatomegaly is an important sign in the differential diagnosis. In the presence of other symptoms and signs such as fever, malaise, pharyngitis, or adenopathy, splenomegaly suggests acute viral infection such as mononucleosis or CMV. However, in the absence of systemic symptoms, a large spleen connotes chronic liver disease and portal hypertension. Massive enlargement justifies concern over storage diseases such as Gaucher disease or Niemann-Pick disease with stored material in both liver and spleen, or infiltrative disease with stored material in both liver and spleen, or infiltrative disease such as histiocytosis or hematologic malignancy.

Ascites is a manifestation of chronic liver disease secondary to increased portal vein pressure and low circulating serum albumin levels. It also is found in hepatic venous obstruction (Budd-Chiari syndrome), constrictive pericarditis, or congestive heart failure. The cardiopulmonary examination, including a search for jugular vein distention, peripheral edema, pulmonary rales, or a gallop rhythm will help exclude cardiac causes of hepatomegaly or ascites.

Careful mental status examination is particularly important in assessing the severity of liver dysfunction. The early findings of hepatic encephalopathy seen in Reye syndrome, acute severe viral or drug-induced hepatitis, or severe chronic liver disease with cirrhosis are subtle and often missed. These include inversion in the sleep-wake cycle, hypersomnia or insomnia, impaired computation, shortened attention span, euphoria or depression, irritability, impaired handwriting, muscular incoordination, and hyperventilation. In the older patient, the physician should look for asterixis or liver flap. Fetor hepaticus, a sweetish odor described as fruity or musty, can occasionally be detected on the breath and urine of such patients.

Laboratory Evaluation

Patterns of laboratory abnormalities permit rough classification of liver disease as inflammatory, obstructive, and infiltrative and allow assessment of the extent of compromise of liver function. In conjunction with the physical findings, these tests influence the decisions about hospitalization or referral versus office follow-up. The following studies should be performed in all infants and children with hepatomegaly: aspartate aminotransferase (AST) level, alanine aminotransferase (ALT) level, total and direct bilirubin levels, PT, partial thromboplastin time (PTT), total protein and albumin levels, alkaline phosphatase level, complete blood cell (CBC) count, sedimentation rate, differential cell count, platelet count, electrolyte levels, glucose level, and blood urea nitrogen (BUN). Inflammatory diseases resulting in hepatocyte necrosis produce dramatic elevations of AST and ALT levels, usually proportional to the extent of the damage. Extreme elevation of AST, greater than 1000 U/L, implies severe acute viral, drug, or ischemic injury. An elevated alkaline phosphatase level (of confirmed hepatic origin) or γ-glutamyl transpeptidase (GGT) level out of proportion to elevations of aminotransferases indicates an obstructive or infiltrative disorder, the latter being more likely in the absence of jaundice and pruritus. Serum albumin levels and clotting studies more accurately reflect hepatocellular synthetic function and yield abnormal results only after profound liver injury. End-stage liver disease may occur with normal levels of serum enzyme levels and subclinical jaundice but abnormal results of serum albumin levels and clotting studies. Derangements of PT and PTT can occur with severe acute hepatitis, but when found with a low albumin level, more chronic liver disease is suggested. An attempt at correction of PT by parenteral administration of vitamin K is valuable in assessing the severity of hepatocyte synthetic dysfunction.

Hypergammaglobulinemia is characteristic of the entities that cause chronic active hepatitis.

The serum IgG is usually elevated above 1.6 g/dL. Non-organ-specific IgG autoantibodies to internal components of cells are present in nearly every case of chronic active hepatitis. These include, in various combinations, ANA, smooth muscle antibody (SMA), and liver/kidney microsomal antibody (also called *endoplasmic reticulum antibody*).

Depending on the prodromal illness and presenting symptoms and signs, tests for hepatitis A antibody, hepatitis B surface antigen, and infectious mononucleosis (Mono-spot test) should be performed. In a child younger than 3 years of age, the Mono-spot test has a very high false-negative rate; thus an EBV titer is the only confirmatory test. If acholic stools, asymmetric enlargement, hepatic bruit, or abdominal mass is present, abdominal ultrasound should be performed, provided an experienced ultrasonographer is available.

Further laboratory evaluation, including technetium-99m sulfur colloid or DISIDA nuclear medicine scans, computed tomography of the abdomen, endoscopic retrograde cholangiopancreatography, percutaneous transhepatic cholangiography, selective angiography, and closed-needle liver biopsy, should only be performed at referral centers under the direction of trained pediatric gastroenterologists. Urine and blood metabolic screens, serum α_1-antitrypsin level, serum and urinary copper determinations, ophthalmologic slit-lamp examination, ANA titer, immunoglobulin levels, α-fetoprotein, and values for fasting serum bile acids are all part of the evaluation of chronic liver disease undertaken by the consultant.

INDICATIONS FOR CONSULTATION OR REFERRAL

Patients with an enlarged liver can be divided into three groups. The first group manifests signs, symptoms, and laboratory values that dictate immediate hospitalization and consultation:

1. Persistent anorexia or vomiting
2. Mental status changes, hyperventilation, respiratory alkalosis, fetor hepaticus
3. Persistent or deepening jaundice
4. Relapse of initial symptoms after a period of improvement

5. Known toxin or hepatotoxic drug ingestion
6. Prolonged PT
7. Depressed serum albumin and fibrinogen levels
8. Bilirubin >20 mg/dL
9. AST level >2000 IU
10. Development of ascites
11. Hypoglycemia
12. Leukocytosis and thrombocytopenia

The second group has evidence of chronic liver disease or chronic multisystem disease that requires a more extensive evaluation by a pediatric gastroenterologist but does not call for immediate hospitalization. The third group seems to have benign self-limited acute liver disease or asymptomatic hepatomegaly discovered on physical examination. These children can be observed safely, with monthly physical examinations and determinations of bilirubin, AST, ALT, and GGT levels, until liver size and chemical parameters have normalized, provided they completely recover, remain asymptomatic, liver size does not increase, and there is no development of splenomegaly or stigmata of chronic liver disease. If after 3 months hepatomegaly persists, with or without elevated transaminase levels, they should be referred to a consultant for workup of potential chronic liver disease. The decision to observe the patient may be difficult, but in the asymptomatic patient, perhaps recovering from an intercurrent viral illness, good clinical judgment and careful serial follow-up examinations may save the child and the parents many expensive and traumatic procedures.

DISCUSSION OF ALGORITHM

An algorithm for differential diagnosis of hepatomegaly is presented in Figure 49-1. The first task of the evaluation requires the primary care physician to determine if the palpable liver is really enlarged. Next, a physical examination should reveal if there is any irregularity of the liver margins. Patients with asymmetric liver require an abdominal ultrasound study; those with a smooth and large liver require blood tests to detect hepatitis or chronic liver disease. Those with asymptomatic hepatomegaly can be observed for 3 months; if the liver is still large, referral is indicated.

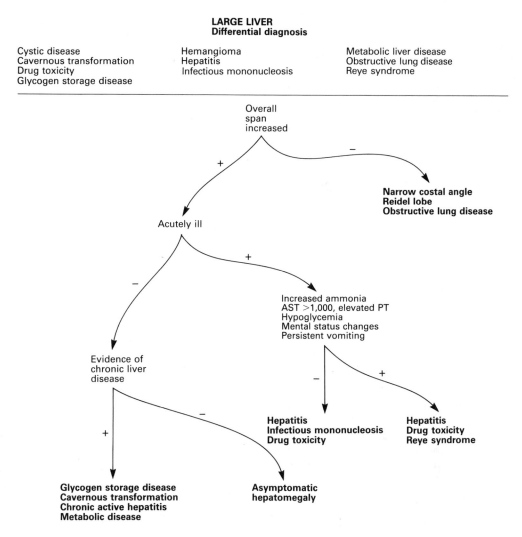

LARGE LIVER
Differential diagnosis

Cystic disease
Cavernous transformation
Drug toxicity
Glycogen storage disease

Hemangioma
Hepatitis
Infectious mononucleosis

Metabolic liver disease
Obstructive lung disease
Reye syndrome

Overall
span
increased

+   −

Narrow costal angle
Reidel lobe
Obstructive lung disease

Acutely ill

+

Increased ammonia
AST >1,000, elevated PT
Hypoglycemia
Mental status changes
Persistent vomiting

−

−   +

Evidence of
chronic liver
disease

−

Hepatitis
Infectious mononucleosis
Drug toxicity

Hepatitis
Drug toxicity
Reye syndrome

+

Glycogen storage disease
Cavernous transformation
Chronic active hepatitis
Metabolic disease

Asymptomatic
hepatomegaly

FIG 49-1
Decision tree for differential diagnosis of large liver.

BIBLIOGRAPHY

Mews C, Sinatra F: Chronic liver disease in children, *Ped Rev* 14:436–444, 1993.

Schwartz MZ, Shaul DB: Abdominal masses in the newborn, *Pediatr Rev* 11:172–179, 1989.

Walker WA, Mathis RK: Hepatomegaly: An approach to differential diagnosis, *Pediatr Clin North Am* 22:929–942, 1975.

Yarze JC, Martin P, Munoz SJ, Friedman LS: Wilson's disease: Current status, *Am J Med* 92:643–654, 1992.

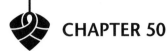

CHAPTER 50

Large Spleen

Maria R. Mascarenhas
Steven M. Altschuler

Splenomegaly is detected when the spleen is increased two to three times its normal size. A palpable spleen is not always abnormal. Of normal neonates, 15% to 30% will have a palpable spleen on examination. Additionally, a palpable nonenlarged spleen can be found in children with chronic pulmonary disease secondary to increased lung volume and flattening of the diaphragm. Abdominal masses can displace an abnormal spleen to a position below the left costal margin. Massive hepatic enlargement may result in the left hepatic lobe being palpable in the left upper quadrant and mistaken for an enlarged spleen. The physician must remember, however, that palpation of a normal-sized spleen is not common. Therefore, a palpable spleen is usually a significant physical finding and warrants further work-up.

Functionally, the spleen plays a role in the body's immune system with the presence of lymphoid tissue and reticuloendothelial cells. Normally, the spleen produces antibodies against blood-borne antigens and acts as a filtering system removing damaged and altered blood elements. The spleen is a vascular organ, anatomically part of the liver's portal circulation. Disturbance to any splenic function or alteration in portal circulation can result in an enlarged spleen.

DIFFERENTIAL DIAGNOSIS

Common Causes of Large Spleen

- **Trauma**
  Hematoma
  Cyst
- **Infection**
  Bacterial

  Acute
    Sepsis
    Salmonella
  Chronic
    Subacute bacterial endocarditis
    Tuberculosis
    Rickettsial infections
    Spirochetal infections
  Viral
    Sepsis
    Cytomegalovirus
    Epstein-Barr virus
    Hepatitis virus A, B
    Coxsackievirus
    HIV
  Parasite
    Malaria
    Toxoplasmosis
    Schistosomiasis
  Fungal
    Histoplasmosis
- **Allergic–Immunologic**
  Collagen vascular disease
    Rheumatoid arthritis
    Systemic lupus erythematosus
    Rheumatic fever
  Serum sickness
  Immunodeficiency
    Severe combined immunodeficiency syndrome
    Chronic granulomatous disease
    Hypogammaglobulinemia
- **Hematologic**
  Iron-deficiency anemia
  Hemolytic anemia
    Sickle cell disease
    Thalassemia
    Hereditary spherocytosis
  ABO incompatibility

- **Infiltrative**
    Malignancy
    Gaucher disease
    Neimann-Pick disease
- **Disordered blood flow**
    Cirrhosis with portal hypertension
    Cavernous transformation of the portal vein
- **Miscellaneous**
    Splenic cyst
    Budd-Chiari syndrome
    Storage disease
      Gaucher disease
      Niemann-Pick disease
      Wolman disease
      Mucopolysaccharidoses
      Glycogen storage disease, type IV

Discussion

Detection of splenomegaly requires a careful examination of the left upper abdominal quadrant. Ideally, the examination should be carried out with a patient relaxed in a supine and right lateral decubitus position. If this is impossible, as in the case of a crying infant, palpation during deep inspiration between cries is helpful. Occasionally, percussing along the anterior axillary line will reveal an enlarged spleen when palpation is unsuccessful. Abdominal radiography, ultrasound, computed tomography (CT), or a Tc-99m sulfur colloid liver-spleen scan can be used to confirm splenomegaly.

Splenomegaly is usually indicative of a systemic illness and rarely the result of a localized process within the spleen. Splenomegaly can result from five basic mechanisms: 1) activation of the immune response as occurs in infection, autoimmune disease, and immune defects; 2) increased filtering of blood-borne elements found in hemolytic anemias; 3) vascular congestion from an obstructed portal venous system in liver disease; 4) proliferative malignancy as occurs in acute leukemias and lymphoma; 5) infiltration of reticuloendothelial cells, as occurs in storage diseases. Extremely rare causes of splenomegaly include cysts and trauma resulting in splenic hematoma or rupture.

In the newborn period, splenomegaly is most commonly found in association with the syndrome of neonatal hepatitis. Neonatal hepatitis can result from many etiologies, infection being the most common. Neonates with infection will classically present with fever, hepatosplenomeg-

aly, and direct hyperbilirubinemia. The congenital TORCH (toxoplasmosis, rubella, cytomegalovirus, herpes virus) and hepatitis A and B infections and bacterial sepsis are the most common causes of splenomegaly. Bacterial sepsis is diagnosed by appropriate culturing of the blood, urine, and spinal fluid. Definite diagnosis of viral infections requires serologic methods; however, the prenatal history and thorough physical examination will strongly suggest these infections. Hepatic dysfunction will be prominent in these disorders. Additional causes of neonatal hepatitis and splenomegaly include metabolic disorders such as α_1-antitrypsin deficiency, galactosemia, cystic fibrosis, and fructosemia. Storage diseases, such as Niemann-Pick disease and Wolman disease, present in later infancy. Neonatal hepatitis must always be differentiated from obstructive lesions of the liver. These include biliary atresia, congenital hepatic fibrosis, infantile polycystic disease, and congenital cirrhosis.

Thus, isolated splenomegaly is rare in the neonatal period. Splenomegaly is usually seen simultaneously with hepatomegaly and direct hyperbilirubinemia. This triad of findings requires immediate workup for etiology and, usually, admission to the hospital.

Splenomegaly in older infants, children, and adolescents usually results from a viral infection. Common viral infections include infectious mononucleosis, hepatitis A, coxsackie virus A5 or A6, and measles. Transient enlargement of the spleen occurs in these cases. Infectious mononucleosis is characterized by fever, easy fatigability, exudative tonsillitis, and diffuse adenopathy in addition to the splenomegaly. Rarely, hepatomegaly and hepatitis will be found. Diagnosis is confirmed by appropriate laboratory studies. A complete blood cell (CBC) count will show an elevated white blood cell count and an absolute lymphocytosis, with a differential cell count revealing greater than 10% atypical lymphocytes. In the patient over 10 years of age, the heterophile titer will be positive. Specific serologic methods, now available for detecting antibody against Epstein-Barr virus, provide the best means of diagnosis.

Infection with hepatitis A virus will classically present with fever, nausea, vomiting, and jaundice as indicated by the presence of scleral icterus. Both splenomegaly and hepatomegaly will be quite evident. Splenomegaly will rarely last longer than 1 to 2 months (*see* Chapter 49).

Splenomegaly in the older child and adolescent can occur secondary to chronic urinary tract infections. Therefore, the workup of any child with splenomegaly should usually include urinalysis and culture. The older child with heart disease who develops splenomegaly also must have his condition evaluated for bacterial endocarditis. Workup for this should include a CBC count, blood cultures, and echocardiographic examination for evidence of vegetations within the heart. Other less-common causes of splenomegaly in children include tuberculosis, fungal infection, rickettsial infection, protozoal infection, and parasitic infections.

Generally, any child with splenomegaly of duration greater than 2 months who has relapsing fevers, associated hepatomegaly, failure to thrive, or evidence of anemia, neutropenia, and thrombocytopenia needs additional workup and possible referral. The presence of anemia, neutropenia, or thrombocytopenia can occur secondary to infiltration of the bone marrow from a malignancy or other infiltrative process or secondary to hypersplenism. Hypersplenism implies increased work by the spleen and removal of normal elements from the bloodstream. Hypersplenism can occur in any process in which the spleen is enlarged or in which there is an increased destruction of bloodborne elements. Common causes of hypersplenism in infancy include hemolytic anemias. In black children, the most common hemolytic anemia is sickle cell disease. Splenomegaly commonly develops within the first year of life.

Infiltrating diseases of bone marrow such as leukemia, neuroblastoma, and storage diseases may also present with evidence of anemia, thrombocytopenia, and neutropenia, in addition to splenomegaly. The basis of the cytopenia in these patients is decreased production of these elements within the bone marrow. The child with a malignancy also may present with a history of recurrent fevers, failure to thrive, and episodes of bleeding.

Immune defects may be present in the child who has a history of failure to thrive, recurrent infections, and fever in addition to splenomegaly. Common immune defects include severe combined immunodeficiency, chronic granulomatous disease, and hypogammaglobulinemia.

In children of Mediterranean descent, thalas-semia is a common hemolytic anemia. Most children with hemolytic anemias will present with hemoglobins in the 7 to 8 g/dL range. Further evaluation of these cases and chronic therapy for these children should be carried out in a center with experience.

Hypersplenism is also a common finding in any condition that affects the liver. The child with a history of neonatal umbilical vein catheterization needs appropriate workup for cavernous transformation of the portal vein. Cavernous transformation of the portal vein results in portal hypertension and secondary splenomegaly. Approximately 25% of these children present between 2 and 5 years of age with splenomegaly. Usually, there is evidence of anemia, thrombocytopenia, and, uncommonly, neutropenia. Diagnosis can usually be made with ultrasound. Additional studies that may be considered are a barium swallow study or cautious endoscopy looking for evidence of esophageal varices.

DATA GATHERING

History
The history items have been mentioned in the discussion. Important information should include history of trauma, exposure to infectious disease, any medical events that predispose to liver disease such as umbilical catheters or familial liver disease such as polycystic disease of the liver and kidney.

Physical Examination
Detection of splenomegaly requires a careful examination of the left upper quadrant. Ideally the examination should be carried out with the patient relaxed in a supine and right lateral decubitus position. If the infant is crying, a bottle or pacifier will help to relax the abdominal muscles. Occasionally, percussing along the anterior axillary line will reveal an enlarged spleen when palpation is unsuccessful.

Laboratory Evaluation
Laboratory aids will depend on the diagnostic pathway. A CBC count with platelet and reticulocyte count will begin the evaluation of viral illness, infectious mononucleosis, hemolytic anemia, or leukemia. More definitive testing should follow any positive screening. If there is a history of trauma, abdominal ultrasound or CT

LARGE SPLEEN
Differential diagnosis

Bacterial endocarditis
Chronic pulmonary disease
Collagen vascular disease
CMV
Cystic fibrosis

Hemolytic anemia
Immune deficiency
Infiltrative disease
Infectious mononucleosis
Leukemia

Neoplasm
Ruptured spleen
Sepsis
Viral syndrome

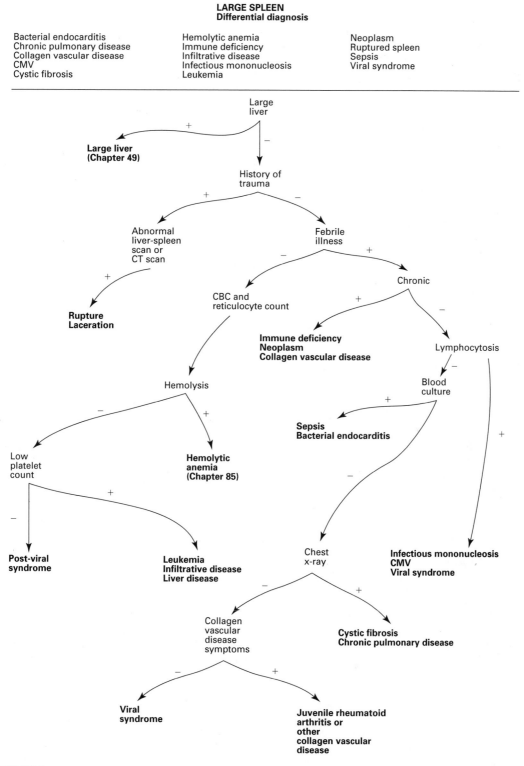

FIG 50-1
Decision tree for differential diagnosis of large spleen.

will be helpful. If the liver is also enlarged, hepatitis testing and liver function testing are indicated as the initial assessment. An elevated sedimentation rate may be seen with infectious causes as well as with connective tissue disorders.

INDICATIONS FOR CONSULTATION OR REFERRAL

Children with cavernous transformation of the portal vein and hypersplenism have a high instance of upper gastrointestinal bleeding from ruptured varices; thus, when this diagnosis is suspected, referral to an appropriate center is advisable. Other chronic active hepatitis or cirrhosis of undefined etiology can lead to portal hypertension and hypersplenism. As with the patient with cavernous transformation, these patients also require additional workup and referral.

The child with recurrent fevers, arthralgias, and fleeting rashes, in addition to splenomegaly, should have his/her condition evaluated for evidence of connective tissue disease. Common disorders presenting in childhood include juvenile rheumatoid arthritis (JRA), rheumatic fever, and systemic lupus erythematosus. Workup of these patients may reveal anemia of chronic disease, an elevated erythrocyte sedimentation rate, and thrombocytosis.

Any child who presents with acute onset of left upper quadrant pain and splenomegaly may have an acute splenic hematoma or rupture. The most common cause of acute splenic rupture or hematoma is trauma. Other less common causes of splenic rupture or hematoma include an infectious etiology. Infectious mononucleosis would be the most common infectious cause encountered by the practitioner. When splenic rupture or hematoma is contemplated, workup and evaluation must be expedited. Effort should be made to have the patient transferred to a center where a pediatric surgeon experienced in surgery of the spleen is available. The child who presents with anemia, thrombocytopenia and anemia in addition to recurrent fevers, failure to thrive, and bleeding should be evaluated for malignancy.

DISCUSSION OF ALGORITHM

An algorithm for differential diagnosis of splenomegaly is presented in Figure 50-1. First the patients with an enlarged spleen should be differentiated from those with a normal-sized palpable spleen. The next task in evaluating an enlarged spleen includes detecting the spleen with an associated large liver, a recent trauma episode, or fever. If these factors are not positive, then anemia should be ruled out. Finally, either a search for rare diseases should be undertaken or, if the patient is making a recovery or looks well, a tentative diagnosis of viral syndrome can be made, and the patient observed for improvement or development of new problems.

BIBLIOGRAPHY

Balistreri WF: Viral hepatitis, *Emerg Clin North Am* 9:365–399, 1991.

Barkun AN, Camus M, Green L, et al: The bedside assessment of splenic enlargement, *Am J Med* 91:512, 1991.

Mieli-Vergani G, Howard ER, Mowat AP: Liver disease in infancy: A 20 year perspective, *Gut* 32(suppl):S123–128, 1991.

Okano M, Thiele GM, Davis JR, et al: Epstein-Barr virus and human diseases: Recent advances in diagnosis, *Clin Microbiol Rev* 1:300, 1988.

Sills RH: The spleen and lymph nodes. In Oski FA, DeAngeles CD, Feigin RD, McMillan JA,

Warshaw JB, editors: *Principles and practice of pediatrics,* ed 2, Philadelphia, 1994, JB Lippincott.

Sumaya CV, Ench Y: Epstein-Barr virus infectious mononucleosis in children: I. Clinical and general laboratory findings, *Pediatrics* 75: 1003, 1985.

Sumaya CV, Ench Y: Epstein-Barr virus infectious mononucleosis in children: II. Heterophil antibody and viral specific responses, *Pediatrics* 75:1011, 1985.

Yang JC, Rickman LS, Bosser SY: The clinical diagnosis of splenomegaly, *West J Med* 155:47, 1991.

CHAPTER 51

Limb Pain

Gregory F. Keenan
Andrew Eichenfield
Robert Doughty

Aches and pains in the extremities are among the commonest childhood complaints. The vast majority of these painful episodes are self-limited and probably are related to minor trauma, physical overexertion, or intercurrent systemic illness. When limb pain becomes recurrent or when a child suddenly develops a limp or is reluctant to bear weight, medical attention frequently is sought. The primary care physician can effectively evaluate such problems through careful questioning of the parent and child, physical examination, and a few simple laboratory evaluations. This chapter outlines the differential diagnosis of limb pain in childhood and an approach to its evaluation.

DIFFERENTIAL DIAGNOSIS

Common Causes of Limb Pain

- **Trauma**
  Muscle or bone contusion: sprains and strains
  Fractures, subluxations, internal derangements
  Hyperextensibility
  Overuse syndromes: tendonitis
  Superficial irritation
  Muscle injection
  Child abuse
- **Infection**
  Osteomyelitis
  Septic arthritis
  Lyme disease
  *Acute myositis
  *Neuritis

---

*Less common.

*Pyogenic sacroiliitis and/or diskitis
*Retroperitoneal or pelvic infection
- **Toxins**
  *Hypervitaminosis A
  *Acrodynia
- **Allergic–Immunologic**
  "Postinfectious" arthritides or toxic synovitis
  Hypersensitivity vasculitides
  Juvenile rheumatoid arthritis
  Inflammatory bowel disease
  Kawasaki syndrome
  *Systemic lupus erythematosus
  *Dermatomyositis or polymyositis
  *Polyarteritis nodosa
- **Endocrine–Metabolic**
  Sickle cell disease
  Rickets caused by vitamin D deficiency
  Renal osteodystrophy
  Hypothyroidism
  *Hyperlipidemias
  *Fabry disease
  *Gaucher disease
- **Tumor**
  Leukemia and/or lymphoma
  Metastatic neuroblastoma
  Malignant bone tumors
    Osteogenic sarcoma
    Ewing sarcoma
  Benign bone tumors
    Osteoid osteoma
    Benign osteoblastoma
- **Localized orthopedic**
  Slipped capital femoral epiphysis
  Avascular necrosis (osteonecrosis)
  Legg-Calvé-Perthes disease
  Osgood-Schlatter disease
  Osteochondritis dissecans

*Blount's disease
*Freiberg disease
*Kohler disease
*Sever disease
Chondromalacia patellae
- **Multiple etiologies**
Growing pains
Raynaud phenomenon
Reflex sympathetic dystrophy
Fibromyalgia

Discussion

Trauma

The most common causes of limb pain in childhood are related to trauma. The major concern will be differentiating soft-tissue injuries from fractures and subluxations in an anxious child in pain. Children whose extremities are hyperextensible are more prone to soft-tissue injury and may present with recurrent extremity pain and swelling, usually with only minor injury.

"Overuse" syndromes are seen in increasing numbers of school-aged children involved in organized sports activities. Localized tendonitides such as "Little League shoulder" and tennis elbow are not uncommon. Another consideration that may be elucidated through careful history-taking is superficial irritation secondary to muscle injections. Child abuse should be suspected if the degree of injury seems out of proportion to the history or if it is recurrent.

Infection

Bacterial infections of the bone or joint present with the acute onset of localized pain associated with fever. *Staphylococcus aureus* is the most common organism in children over the age of 2 years. *Haemophilus influenzae* previously was a common cause in younger children; however, since the advent of routine early vaccination with *H. influenzae* type B, this bacterium is now a rare causative agent. Adolescents are at risk for gonorrhea and chlamydial infections, with assorted joint manifestations. Radiographs and bone scans assist in diagnosis of bacterial infections. Failure to recognize septic arthritis or osteomyelitis early can result in a prolonged and complicated course and residual dysfunction. Myalgia associated with viral infections such as influenza and with parasitic infections should be considered when pain appears to be diffuse and localized to muscle. Herpes zoster can present as exquisite neuritic limb pain, which precedes the appearance of vesicles. Pyogenic sacroiliitis and diskitis may present insidiously with back pain, which may be referred to the hip. These diagnoses are notoriously difficult to document and may require serial bone scans to be confirmed. Retroperitoneal or pelvic infection may present with hip pain as well, and ultrasonography is invaluable in such cases. In endemic areas, Lyme disease also is a common infectious cause of limb pain and limp. Most importantly, children may not have a history of known tick bite or erythema chronicum migrans–type rash.

Toxins

Toxins are rare causes of limb pain. Chronic excessive ingestion of vitamin A can result in cortical hyperostosis and limb pain. Children with chronic mercury poisoning suffer from acrodynia, which is characterized by excruciating pain in the hands and feet an unusual cutaneous manifestation.

Allergic–Immunologic

Arthralgia and arthritis may follow bacterial or viral infections, immunizations, or other antigenic stimulation (*eg,* drug exposure). Toxic synovitis of the hip or other joints is probably the most common form of postinfectious arthritis in childhood. It usually is not associated with fever or systemic illness. Other well-characterized postinfectious syndromes include acute rheumatic fever and the "reactive" arthritides associated with enteric infections and parvovirus. Hypersensitivity vasculitides (serum sickness) and Henoch-Schönlein purpura are similar pathophysiologically and may present with myalgia, arthralgia, or arthritis, usually with typical rashes.

Rheumatologic diseases that commonly present with inflammatory arthropathy include juvenile rheumatoid arthritis and systemic lupus erythematosus. Muscle pain is frequently the presenting feature of dermatomyositis, polymyositis, and polyarteritis nodosa. Inflammatory bowel disease can be preceded by arthralgia and arthritis for months to years. Kawasaki syndrome can occasionally occur with extremity changes (*eg,* indurative edema and extremity pain) as the predominant physical findings, but usually the constellation of associated symptoms will be present.

Endocrine–Metabolic

Symmetric painful swelling of the hands and feet in a black toddler suggests the hand-foot syndrome of sickle cell disease. The swelling and painful extremity occur mainly in patients under 2 years of age. Radiographic findings such as periosteal reaction take approximately 2 weeks to appear. Extremity pain may be the presenting sign of sickle cell crisis in a previously undiagnosed case.

Bone abnormalities arising from rickets caused by vitamin D deficiency and renal osteodystrophy can lead to bone pain. Hypothyroidism may result in a proximal myopathy of the extremities and, rarely, an arthritis that can be uncomfortable.

Tendon xanthomas associated with hyperlipidemias may result in tendonitis of the Achilles tendon and other tendons. The bone lesions of Gaucher disease are frequently symptomatic. Fabry disease "crises" are characterized by severe burning pain in the hands and feet.

Tumor

Bone pain is a frequent early manifestation of systemic malignancy such as leukemia, lymphoma, and metastatic neuroblastoma. Pain is frequently excruciating, is worse at night, and may awaken the child from sleep. Systemic signs may not be appreciated early in the disease course; exquisite night pain should provoke an appropriate workup for malignancy.

Tumors of the bone itself present with persistent, increasing pain. Osteogenic and Ewing sarcomas commonly occur in adolescents and are diagnosed radiographically. Benign osseous tumors that can cause pain include osteoid osteoma and osteoblastoma. The former should be suspected when night pain is relieved by a nonsteroidal anti-inflammatory drug.

Localized Orthopedic Problems

Slipped capital femoral epiphysis (Fig. 51-1) occurs in adolescents from 10 to 17 years of age and results in a painful limp and loss of hip abduction and internal rotation. Because the pain of hip disease may be referred to the knee, radiographs of the hips should be performed in all patients with knee pain. Affected children should not bear weight because further weight bearing on the hip may result in greater deformity. Prompt orthopedic consultation should be sought.

Avascular necroses of bone (osteochondroses) result in localized tenderness and pain and are known by their eponyms. Legg-Calvé-Perthes disease involves the femoral head, is more com-mon in boys than girls, and affects younger children more often than does slipped epiphysis. Other osteochondroses include Osgood-Schlatter disease, which affects the tibial tubercle; Frieberg disease, which affects the second metatarsal head; Kohler disease, which affects the tarsal navicular; Sever disease, which affects the calcaneal apophysis; and osteochondritis dissecans, which usually affects the medial femoral condyle.

Chondromalacia patellae is common in adolescent girls and is the result of softening and roughening of the articulating surface of the patellar cartilage. This results in an ill-defined aching within the knee. Descending stairs and prolonged knee flexion tends to aggravate the condition. Patellofemoral crepitus may be present on physical examination, and occasionally a small, bland effusion may be noted. Compressing the patella against the distal femur with the knee in extension while the patient contracts the quadriceps usually will reproduce the pain. This entity needs to be distinguished from internal derangements of the knee.

Multiple Etiologies

Growing pains is an idiopathic symptom complex that affects 10% to 20% of school-aged children. The pain probably originates from muscle use by active children. Pain is intermittent and most frequently affects the lower extremities, most commonly localized deep within the thighs or calves. Joint pain is rare. Symptoms tend to occur at night and may awaken the child from sleep. The pains last from 30 minutes to several hours and generally respond to analgesics, massage, and local heat. There are no associated physical or laboratory abnormalities. Although attacks may be precipitated by overexertion, emotional factors may play a role as well.

Raynaud phenomenon, characterized by the triad of pallor, cyanosis, and rubor, is frequently associated with pain, particularly during the reflex vasodilatation phase on rewarming. The hands and feet can be swollen, reddened, and extremely tender to palpation.

Reflex sympathetic dystrophy as it affects pediatric patients is a disorder characterized by complaints of severe limb pain that follows seemingly trivial trauma. The child refuses to move the affected extremity, setting up a "pain-disuse" cycle, in which disuse leads to further pain on attempted movement. With time, vasomotor

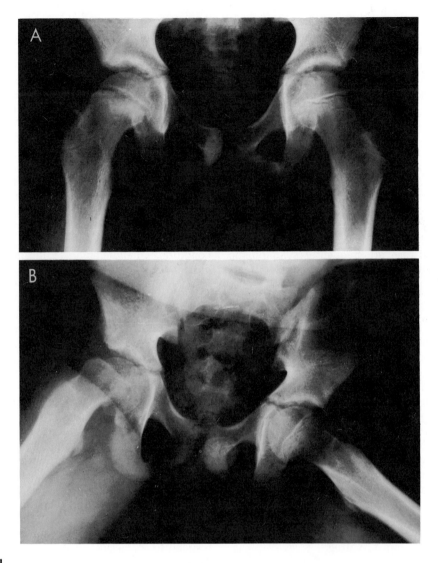

FIG 51-1

Slipped capital femoral epiphysis. **A,** This film of the hip was taken in neutral position and shows asymmetry in the physis of the femoral heads. The right appears wider, and the head appears somewhat medially displaced. In all suspected cases of slipped capital femoral epihyses, a frog-leg lateral film is taken. **B,** Frog-leg lateral film shows complete separation of the right femoral head. This will require pinning of the head to the neck. [From Haller JO, Slovis TL: Introduction to Radiology in Clinical Pediatrics, Chicago, 1984, Year Book Medical Publishers, p. 159. Used by permission.]

changes occur with mild acrocyanosis, coolness to palpation, and hyperhydrosis. The hyperesthesia may be exquisite, virtually neuritic in nature. Disuse can result in marked muscle wasting. Many of these children have psychologic problems that contribute to the condition. Laboratory investigations fail to reveal evidence of inflammation. Bone scanning may show deceased or, less commonly, increased uptake over affected areas, and mild osteopenia may be seen on radiographs. Successful treatment consists of positive reinforcement, graded physical therapy, and judicious use of transcutaneous electronic nerve stimulation, with remarkable relief of pain and return of function in a majority of cases.

Fibromyalgia is an increasingly recognized entity in adolescent girls. They may have numerous complaints, but the most important is non-restorative sleep and typical tender points on examination with normal pain sensation at control points.

DATA GATHERING

History

Careful history taking is of paramount importance in the evaluation of the child with limb pain. A history of trauma should always be sought but may be exceedingly difficult to document in the younger child. New hobbies and other physical activities may predispose to tendonitis. A history of "double-jointedness" should be noted. The character of the child's pain may provide clues to diagnosis: the pain of acute bone and joint infection or malignancy is most severe; the pain of osteochondritides and juvenile arthritis is more aching in nature; the child with reflex sympathetic dystrophy may complain of pain out of proportion to objective physical findings. Night pain that does not allow sleep is suggestive of malignancy unless it is dramatically relieved by aspirin, in which case osteoid osteoma is likely. Night pain that is poorly localized and responds to massage and heat is suggestive of growing pains. Stiffness, rather than pain, is more characteristic of chronic joint inflammation, particularly when it is worse in the morning. Other significant historical features include the presence of antecedent illness, fever, or malaise that makes infection, malignancy, and collagen-vascular disease more likely considerations. Sleep patterns should be addressed because children with fibromyalgia will not feel refreshed in the morning, and children with growing pains will be asymptomatic in the morning.

Physical Examination

The general demeanor of the child should be noted. A patient who will absolutely not allow an extremity to be touched or moved may very well be suffering from a septic arthritis or osteomyelitis. Other foci of bacterial infection (eg, otitis, cellulitis) may be present in such cases. Rashes, generalized lymphadenopathy, and hepatosplenomegaly should be noted as markers of systemic inflammation associated with malignancy, chronic infection, or rheumatic disease. The musculoskeletal system should be exam-

ined in detail, noting any swelling, tenderness, loss of range of motion, or other asymmetry. Subtle muscle wasting may become apparent on careful measurement of the thighs and calves. The examination should include assessment of the child's gait, and the examiner should note if ambulation elicits pain or a limp.

Hyperextensibility is often associated with recurrent limb pain and swelling (the benign hypermobile joint syndrome of childhood) presumably secondary to trivial trauma of which patient and parent are not aware. Hyperextensibility may be documented by attempting to approximate the thumb to the volar forearm, extending the metacarpophalangeal joints so that they parallel the forearm, and noting hyperextension at the elbows and knees. These may be the only abnormal findings in the child with recurrent pain of seemingly obscure etiology. Tender points present in patients with fibromyalgia should be palpated over the occiput, trapezius, and paraspinal muscles, buttocks, greater trochanters, anserine bursae, and humeral epicondyles.

Laboratory Evaluation

If after the history and physical examination the diagnosis is unclear, appropriate radiographs may be obtained of the affected extremity and, especially in the younger child, of the opposite side for comparison. The radiographs will effectively demonstrate fractures, dislocations, and traumatic effusions. In the absence of a clear-cut history of trauma, a complete blood cell (CBC) count and erythrocyte sedimentation rate (ESR) should be obtained. The latter is a sensitive, though nonspecific, screening test for ongoing inflammation. The CBC count is helpful in revealing anemia (suggesting malignancy, chronic disease, or hemoglobinopathy), leukocytosis (acute infection or inflammation), or thrombocytopenia (malignancy or severe infection). The peripheral smear is invaluable in suggesting acute infection and malignancy. If fever, systemic signs or symptoms, and/or abnormal laboratory findings are present, hospitalization should be strongly considered to rule out bone and/or joint infection, malignancy, or collagen-vascular disease. Imaging studies including radiographs, computed tomography (CT), magnetic resonance imaging (MRI), and bone scan may be helpful in differentiating among these disease states.

In the absence of a history of trauma, systemic

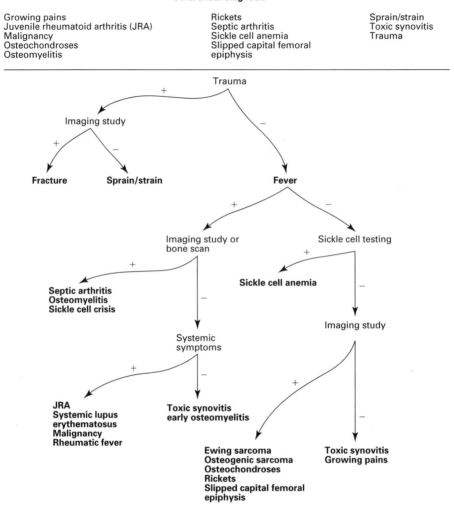

FIG 51-2
Decision tree for differential diagnosis of leg pain.

illness, or abnormal laboratory findings, the musculoskeletal examination should be carefully repeated over time to reveal any focal abnormalities. CT scan and/or MRI may prove helpful in revealing occult bone tumors, osteonecrosis, or slipped epiphysis. Orthopedic consultation may prove helpful at this point. If no abnormality can be documented on careful physical examination or radiographs, then growing pains or muscle or tendon strain remain the most likely diagnosis of exclusion. Other entities to be considered include fibromyalgia and benign hypermobile joint syndrome. Persistent or recurrent complaints of pain should be investigated with repeated physical examination and laboratory investigations as indicated depending on the duration and severity of the problem.

INDICATIONS FOR CONSULTATION OR REFERRAL

The majority of limb pain problems resolve with rest, analgesics, and time. When the pain is more severe or when symptoms of systemic disease, anemia, or fever is present, the limb pain requires additional evaluation.

DISCUSSION OF ALGORITHM

An algorithm for differential diagnosis of limb pain is presented in Figure 51-2. Because trauma is the cause of most limb pain, this possibility should be ruled out first. Next, bone or joint infection should be considered as well as malignancy and rheumatic disease. Bone scans, radiographs, and possibly needle aspiration will be needed to explore these possibilities.

For the patient without fever or systemic illness, the overuse syndrome or growing pains need to be considered. If the clinical picture does not fit, imaging studies should be performed to rule out avascular necrosis, bone tumor, slipped epiphysis, or chondromalacia.

BIBLIOGRAPHY

Bernstein BH, Singsen BH, Kent JT, et al: Reflex neurovascular dystrophy in childhood, *J Pediatr* 93:211, 1978.

Buskila D, Press J, Gedalia A, et al: Assessment of nonarticular tenderness and prevalence of fibromyalgia in children, *J Rheumatol* 20:368, 1993.

Committee on Sports Medicine: *Sports medicine: Health care for young athletes,* Evanston, 1983, American Academy of Pediatrics.

Gedalia A, Person DA, Brewer EJ, et al: Hypermobility of the joints in juvenile episodic arthritis/arthralgia, *J Pediatr* 107:873, 1985.

Kunnamo I, Kallio P, Pelkonen P, et al: Clinical signs and laboratory findings in the differential diagnosis of arthritis in children, *Am J Dis Child* 141:34, 1987.

Naish JM, Apley J: 'Growing pains': A clinical study of non-arthritic limb pain in children, *Arch Dis Child* 26:134, 1951.

Passo MH: Aches and limb pain, *Pediatr Clin North Am* 29:209, 1982.

Rivara FP, Parish RA, Mueller BA: Extremity injuries in children: Predictive value of clinical findings, *Pediatrics* 78:803, 1986.

ter Meuten DC, Majd M: Bone scintigraphy in the evaluation of children with obscure skeletal pain, *Pediatrics* 79:589, 1987.

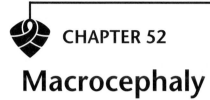

CHAPTER 52

Macrocephaly

Carol Carraccio
Karen Miller

The child with a large head represents a diagnostic dilemma because of the spectrum of etiologies and clinical outcomes. The possibilities range from a normal familial trait to the life-threatening case of a child with increased intracranial pressure. In some cases, there is apparent head enlargement because of a small body. The evaluation of a large head requires the physician to be familiar with a standard of normal head circumferences, the concept of growth velocity, and an approach to evaluation that identifies those patients who can be safely observed versus those needing a diagnostic workup or immediate intervention.

DIFFERENTIAL DIAGNOSIS

Because parents rarely complain about large head size, the problem is detected by measuring and recording head circumference. The primary task in pursuing the differential diagnosis is to identify those children who need immediate workup and treatment. The causes of macrocephaly are listed below. Although the list is large, certain causes, such as hydrocephalus, mass lesions, congenital malformations, and intracranial hemorrhage, are more common and deserve more attention here.

Common Causes of Macrocephaly

- **Trauma**
  Subdural hematoma or hemorrhage leading to hydrocephalus
- **Infection**
  Congenital
  Postmeningitis hydrocephalus
- **Metabolic–Endocrine**

Metachromatic leukodystrophy
Infantile leukodystrophy
Tay-Sachs disease
Mucopolysaccharidosis
Gangliosidoses
Rickets
Hyperphosphatasia
- **Mass lesions**
  Brain tumors
  Brain abscess
  Cysts
  Arteriovenous malformation
- **Congenital**
  Malformations associated with hydrocephalus
    Dandy-Walker syndrome
    Vein of Galen aneurysm
    Aqueductal stenosis
    Hydranencephaly
    Myelomeningocele with Arnold-Chiari malformation
  Neurocutaneous syndromes
    Neurofibromatosis
    Tuberous sclerosis
    Sturge-Weber disease
    Klippel-Trénaunay-Weber syndrome
  Skeletal and cranial dysplasia
    Achondroplasia
    Camptomelic dwarfism
    Osteogenesis imperfecta
    Craniosynostosis
    Cleidocranial dysostosis
    Osteopetrosis
- **Other**
  Severe chronic anemia
  Beckwith-Weidemann syndrome
  Cerebral gigantism
  Histiocytosis X

Pseudotumor cerebri

Megalencephaly as a normal variant

Discussion

Hydrocephalus

Hydrocephalus results from either excessive production of spinal fluid, obstruction to flow, or decreased ability to resorb the fluid into the circulation. The causes range from congenital malformations, trauma, and intracranial hemorrhages to infection and tumors. Although some of the patients will present at birth with an obviously large head and full fontanelle, in others the condition will develop insidiously. Especially suspect are patients who recover from neonatal ventricular hemorrhage or meningitis.

Mass lesions—Enlarging head circumference is most likely due to primary brain lesions rather than metastatic spread. Common primary tumors include astrocytoma, ependymona, glioma and glioblastoma, medulloblastoma, meningioma, and craniopharyngioma. Neurologic deficits are usually the presenting signs. Other mass lesions such as cysts, abscesses, and vascular malformation also require consideration.

Intracranial hemorrhage—Intracranial hemorrhage may result from congenital defects such as arteriovenous malformations, intraventricular hemorrhage—seen in premature infants—or trauma. The latter should raise a suspicion of child abuse.

Dysplasias of the Cranium and Skeleton

Craniosynostosis or premature closure of cranial sutures distorts the normal shape of the skull and makes the head appear enlarged. Careful inspection of the sutures should identify this problem.

Skeletal dysplasias will be obvious on inspection. The most common of these conditions is achondroplasia, which results in limb shortening as well as an enlarged head. Macrocephaly also is associated with camptomelic dwarfism and Conradi syndrome.

Systemic Diseases

Macrocephaly may be a feature of a variety of systemic conditions. The neurocutaneous syndromes will be easily recognizable by their peculiar skin manifestations: the port-wine stain of Sturge-Weber syndrome, the hypopigmented macules and ash-leaf patches of tuberous sclerosus, and the café-au-lait spots and neurofibromas of neurofibromatosis. Seizures also are a common manifestation of these disorders.

Children with metabolic causes of macrocephaly also will have other features of these disease entities on physical examination. The mucopolysaccharidoses and gangliosidoses cause characteristic coarse facial features. Tay-Sachs disease and the leukodystrophies are associated with progressive neurologic impairment. Hypophosphatasia and rickets will manifest with other deformities of the long bones and ribs.

Pseudomotor cerebri—Pseudotumor cerebri manifests as increased intracranial pressure without obstruction to cerebrospinal fluid flow. It may be idiopathic or secondary to such drugs and toxins as steroids, excessive amounts of vitamin A, and lead. Association with certain endocrine conditions, such as hypoparathyroidism and adrenal insufficiency, has also been found.

Megalencephaly as a normal variant—This condition is a diagnosis of exclusion made in a child with a negative history and normal physical examination, including developmental and neurologic assessments. It may be familial, so head circumference measurements in other family members are helpful.

DATA GATHERING

History

The age of the child is an important historical factor in the evaluation. Congenital causes of hydrocephalus as well as some cranial and skeletal abnormalities present at birth or very early in life. The neurocutaneous, metabolic, and degenerative diseases may not manifest themselves until late infancy and early childhood. Other etiologies such as mass lesions, infection, hemorrhage, and toxins may occur at any age. It is important to find out whether associated symptoms of headache, vomiting, or abnormal motor activity are present.

Developmental delay has been associated with many of the diseases that cause macrocephaly. Careful developmental assessment should be part of the evaluation.

Family history of anemia such as thalassemia

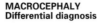

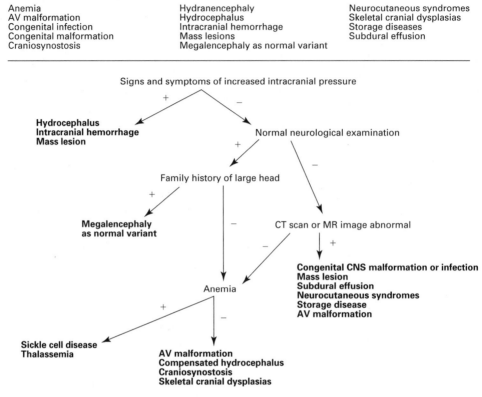

FIG 52-1
Decision tree for differential diagnosis of macrocephaly.

or sickle cell anemia may help explain the presence of a large head secondary to increased bone marrow activity. Primary megalencephaly tends to run in families. A history of large heads in other family members should be sought.

Physical Examination

Because many of the diseases that present with a large head also may manifest signs and symptoms of increased intracranial pressure, a rapid assessment of neurologic status is necessary to differentiate the child who needs immediate treatment and referral from the child who can be approached in a more systematic fashion. Hypertension accompanied by bradycardia, change in mental status, asymmetry of pupil size, decrease in pupil reactivity, papilledema, and focal neurologic findings are all signs associated with increased intracranial pressure.

The head should be measured carefully. The

measuring tape is placed from the glabella and supraorbital ridge to the most prominent part of the occiput. This circumference should be compared to that of previous measurements, if available. Head size that crosses two main percentile curves of the head growth chart raises great concern. The head size also should be compared with the height and weight percentiles. In cases of malnutrition, the normal head size may appear large in comparison with a small torso. A child with weight, length, and head circumference all greater than the 95th percentile on the growth curve is likely to be normal. A clue that hydrocephalus is the cause of macrocephaly is that the head is disproportionately large with respect to the face. A complete physical examination will reveal other signs that will be helpful in generating a differential diagnosis. This is particularly true of the congenital and metabolic causes of macrocephaly. A detailed developmental and neurologic examination must be performed.

Laboratory Evaluation

Children with macrocephaly who have a positive family history of large head size, a normal head growth velocity, and normal physical examination (including developmental and neurologic) do not require additional evaluation. By contrast, children with signs of increased intracranial pressure should be referred directly to a neurologist or neurosurgeon for diagnostic workup and therapeutic intervention.

Skull radiographs are helpful in determining the status of the sutures as well as calcifications that may indicate tumor, congenital infection, or a neurocutaneous syndrome. Ultrasound examination in young infants will detect hydrocephalus.

Computed tomography or magnetic resonance imaging of the head are the most sensitive tests for the detection of mass lesions. Examination of the cerebrospinal fluid will aid in determining an infectious or metabolic etiology. Determination of the hemoglobin level is important when hemorrhage or a hemoglobinopathy is suspected. Arteriograms are indicated in the evaluation of vascular anomalies and certain tumors.

INDICATIONS FOR CONSULTATION OR REFERRAL

A child with symptoms or signs of increased intracranial pressure requires immediate hospitalization for workup and treatment. The child who has a large head as part of a more global systemic process may benefit from a genetic or neurologic consultation.

DISCUSSION OF ALGORITHM

An algorithm for differential diagnosis of macrocephaly is presented in Figure 52-1. The major task in evaluating a child with a large head is determining if there is increased intracranial pressure, which requires immediate referral for therapy. If there are no signs of increased pressure, the history and physical, developmental, and neurologic examinations can be pursued in a systematic fashion. These measures will provide clues to distinguish those patients who require additional laboratory tests from those who can be observed with close follow-up.

BIBLIOGRAPHY

Aicardi J: *Diseases of the nervous system in childhood,* London, 1992 MacKeith Press.

Bodensteiner JB, Chung EO: Macrocrania and megalencephaly in the neonate, *Semin Neurol* 13:84–91, 1993.

Dykes FD, Dunbar B, Lazarra A, Ahmann PA: Posthemorrhagic hydrocephalus in high-risk preterm infants: Natural history management and long-term outcome, *J Pediatr* 114:611–618, 1989.

Ferry P: Pediatric neurodiagnostic tests: A modern perspective, *Pediatr Rev* 3:248–255, 1992.

Horton WA, Rotter JI, Rimoin DL, et al: Standard growth curves for achondroplasia, *J Pediatr* 93:435–438, 1978.

Lemieux BG, Wright FS, Swaiman KF: Genetic and congenital structural defects of the brain and spinal cord. In Swaiman KF, Wright FS, editors: *The practice of pediatric neurology,* St. Louis, 1982, CV Mosby.

Nellhaus G: Head circumference from birth to 18 years, *Pediatrics* 41:106, 1968.

Page RB: Hydrocephalus. In Hoekelman R, Friedman S, Nelson N, Seidel H, editors: *Primary pediatric care,* ed 2, St. Louis, 1992, Mosby–Year Book.

Tunnessen WW: *Signs and symptoms in pediatrics,* Philadelphia, 1988, JB Lippincott.

CHAPTER 53

Neck Masses

William P. Potsic

Children often present to the primary care physician with the complaint of a neck mass. A systematic approach is helpful, combining the history, physical findings, and location to lead to a diagnosis. It must also be remembered that neck masses that are congenital may not be evident until the child is several years old or even a teenager.

DIFFERENTIAL DIAGNOSIS OF NECK MASSES

Common Causes of Neck Masses

- **Trauma**
  Hematoma
  Sternocleidomastoid fibrosis in neonate
- **Inflammatory and infection**
  Lymphadenitis viral
  Bacterial lymphadenitis
  Staphylococcus
  Haemophilus influenzae
  Tuberculosis
  Atypical myobacteria
  Actinomycosis
  Kawasaki syndrome
  Cat scratch disease
  Sialadenitis, parotitis
- **Drug-induced**
  Dilantin-induced lymphoid hyperplasia
- **Neoplasms**
  Benign
    Benign salivary gland tumor
    Thyroid tumors
    Parathyroid tumors
    Juvenile fibromatosis
    Neurilemoma
    Carotid body tumor
    Lipoma
  Malignant
    Lymphoma

  Metastatic carcinoma or sarcoma
  Salivary gland carcinoma
  Neuroblastoma
- **Congenital masses**
  First, second, or third branchial cleft cysts
  Thyroglossal duct cyst
  Cystic hygroma
  Hemangioma
  Dermoid cyst
  Vernous malformation

Discussion

A history of trauma should suggest a hematoma or fibrosis following ecchymosis. Rapidly enlarging masses cause concern about malignancy or an acute inflammatory process. Inflammatory masses are usually painful, and a history of recent head and neck infection can be elicited. Soft and fluctuant masses are usually cysts, vascular lesions, or secondary to inflammation. Firm neck masses suggest a possible malignant process. A mobile mass is most often benign, but malignant masses as well as recently infected nodes or cysts may become fixed. Any mass associated with regional cranial nerve paralysis should immediately bring to mind a malignant process. Vascular lesions enlarge with crying, and salivary lesions may enlarge with eating. Vascular lesions (i.e., hemangioma) may also cause a reddish-blue discoloration of the skin. Presence of cutaneous hemangiomas are often associated with a second lesion in the head and neck including the aerodigestive tract. Café-au-lait spots may be found on the trunk or limbs of patients with neurilemoma. Most of the lesions of the neck are inflammatory or infections. The incidence of neck masses is as follows: lymph nodes, 95% (with hyperplastic nodes constituting 90% and cervical adenitis, 10%); congenital masses, 3%; and others, 2% (Fig. 53-1).

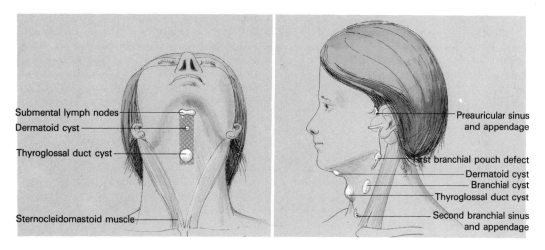

FIG 53-1
Common neck masses and their lesions.

DATA GATHERING

When a neck mass is evaluated, attention to a careful history and physical examination in conjunction with the location of the mass may lead to the diagnosis. Additional diagnostic studies such as a complete blood cell count, skin tests, and radiographic studies should be obtained. Computed tomography (CT) of the head and neck may be useful to determine the character of a neck mass. If the mass is in or around a salivary gland (Fig. 53-2), CT can be combined with sialography to demonstrate the mass.

Inflammatory masses such as cervical adenitis that are painful, erythematous, and fluctuant can be aspirated with a needle. Drainage aspiration is both diagnostic for material to culture and to obtain sensitivities, but it also hastens the resolution of the infection. Incision and drainage should be reserved for abscesses that are about to drain spontaneously.

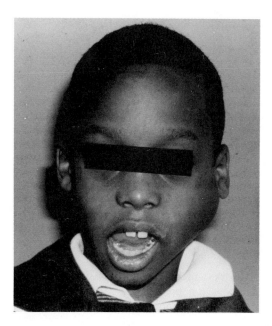

FIG 53-2
Parotid swelling, secondary to parotitis.

INDICATIONS FOR CONSULTATION OR REFERRAL

Neck masses that do not appear to be inflammatory and do not resolve with antibiotic therapy should be evaluated by an otolaryngologist who will perform a complete head and neck examination including pharyngoscopy. Aspiration of masses near or in the salivary glands should be left to an otolaryngology consultant because of the potential for facial nerve injury and paralysis.

DISCUSSION OF ALGORITHM

An algorithm, or "decision tree," for differential diagnosis of neck mass is presented in Figure 53-3. The evaluation of a neck mass initially is determined by the presence or absence of the findings associated with inflammation. If the lesion is not tender or erythematous, then the differential diagnosis is focused on congenital structure, hematomas, and neoplastic disease.

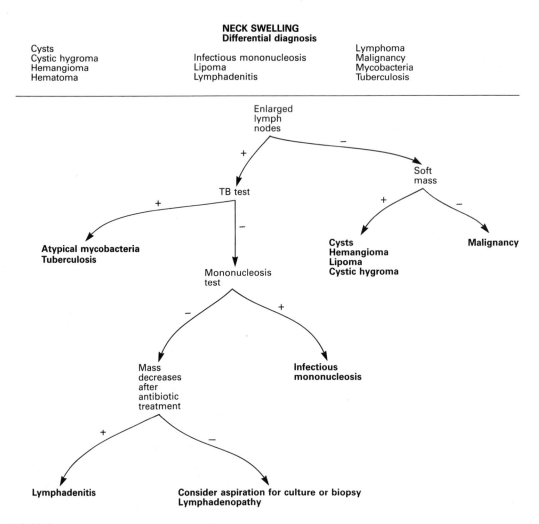

FIG 53-3
Decision tree for differential diagnosis of neck swelling.

The patient with an inflamed, tender mass that does not involve the salivary gland may have the mass evaluated with needle aspiration and receive treatment with antibiotics. It is important to recall that congenital structures such as branchial cleft cysts may present with signs of infection.

BIBLIOGRAPHY

Handler S, Raney RB: Management of neoplasms of the head and neck in children. I. Benign tumors, *Head Neck Surg* 3:395–405, 1981.

Lane RJ, Keane WM, Potsic WP: Pediatric infectious cervical lymphadenitis, *Otolaryngol Head Neck Surg* 88:332–335, 1980.

Mair JW: Cervical myobacterial infection, *J Laryngol Otol* 89:933–939, 1975.

Marcy S: Infections of the lymph nodes of the head and neck, *Pediatr Infect Dis J* 2:397–405, 1983.

Park YW: Evaluation of neck masses in children, *Am Fam Physician* 51(8):1904–1912, 1995.

Raney R, Handler SD: Management of neoplasms of the head and neck in children. II. Malignant tumors, *Head Neck Surg* 3:500–507, 1981.

Tom LWC, Handler SD, Wetmore RF, et al: The sternocleidomastoid tumor of infancy, *Int J Pediatr Otorhinolaryngol* 13:245–255, 1987.

Torsiglieri AJ, Tom LWC, Ross AJ, et al: Pediatric neck masses: guidelines for evaluation, *Int J Pediatr Otorhinolaryngol* 16:199–210, 1988.

Traggis D: Non-Hodgkin's lymphoma of the head and neck in children, *Arch Otolaryngol* 102:244–247, 1976.

Waggoner-Fountain LA, Hayden GF, Hendley JO: Kawasaki syndrome masquerading as bacterial lymphadenitis, *Clin Pediatr* 34(4):185–189, 1995.

CHAPTER 54

Nosebleeds

William P. Potsic

Epistaxis, a common pediatric problem, is intermittent, minor, and usually occurs during the winter when humidity is low and nasal hyperemia is present from viral upper respiratory tract infections. The vast majority of cases of epistaxis are treated at home without medical consultation.

Recurrent epistaxis is reported because it is a frightening experience. Life-threatening epistaxis is rarely a problem in otherwise normal children because it almost always occurs in hospitalized patients with disturbed coagulation from chemotherapy.

DIFFERENTIAL DIAGNOSIS

Common Causes of Nosebleeds
- **Trauma**
    - Dry mucosa (low humidity)
    - Digital trauma (nose-picking)
    - Blunt trauma
    - Foreign body
    - Postsurgical bleeding
    - Barotrauma (self-limited hemorrhage into a sinus)
- **Infection and inflammation**
    - Viral upper respiratory tract infection
    - Bacterial rhinosinusitis
    - Rare fungal infection in immune-suppressed host
        - Mucormycosis
        - *Aspergillus*
    - Parasitic infection
    - Nasal syphilis
    - Allergic rhinosinusitis
- **Neoplasms**
    - Benign
        - Hemangioma (Osler-Weber-Rendu disease)
        - Nasopharyngeal angiofibroma
        - Nasal granuloma
        - Nasal glioma
    - Malignant
        - Rhabdomyosarcoma
        - Lymphoma
        - Nasopharyngeal carcinoma
        - Leukemia
- **Coagulopathy**
    - Thrombocytopenia
        - Idiopathic
        - Drug-induced (chemotherapy)
    - Thrombosthenia
    - von Willebrand disease
    - Aspirin ingestion
    - Hemophilia

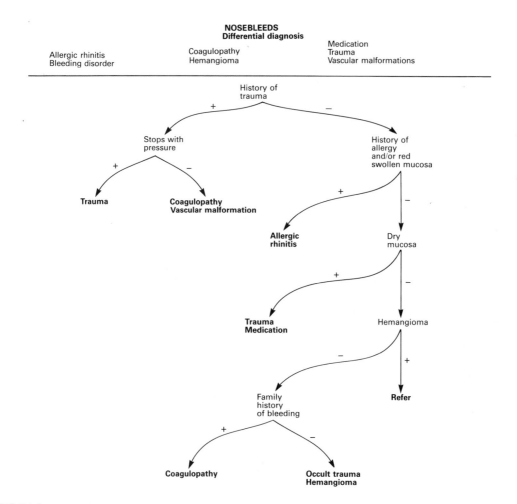

FIG 54-1
Decision tree for differential diagnosis of nosebleeds.

Discussion

An algorithm for differential diagnosis of epistaxis is presented in Figure 54-1. Recurrent epistaxis can be evaluated carefully and healed by the primary care physician. The etiology of the vast majority of recurrent epistaxis is obvious after a history and an examination of the nose. One usually sees an excoriated area with crusted mucus on the anterior septum either on both sides or even more often on the side of the dominant hand (nose-picking).

Most bleeding usually can be stopped with 1.5 minutes of digital compression of the soft part of the nose between the index finger and thumb. Nasal vasoconstrictor drops (Neosynephrine or

Afrin) or spray can be introduced to shrink the mucosa and assist in attaining hemostasis and direct visualization. The involved area usually is near the mucocutaneous junction of the nose (Little's area). If needed, the excoriated surface can be cauterized by application of silver nitrate with a stick but this is usually not necessary. Occasionally, but rarely, a light packing of the nostril with oxidized cellulose (surgical or Oxycel) is needed to stop the bleeding (Fig. 54-2).

Management of uncomplicated epistaxis is directed toward increasing humidity and reducing trauma. Humidity can be improved at home by placing a humidifier on the heating system and in

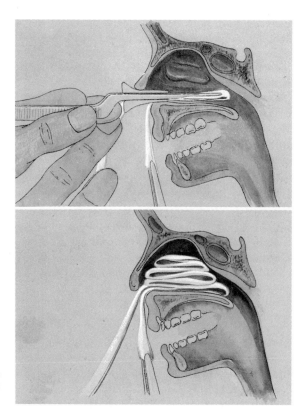

FIG 54-2
The nasal packing technique. One end of packing is held by the hemostat, while the remainder is passed through the speculum with forceps.

the child's room. Antibiotic ointment or petroleum jelly should be applied to the nasal septum bilaterally twice daily by the child. This application heals the excoriated areas and gives the child something to do with his/her finger. Commercially prepared nonprescription saline nasal sprays also are helpful and should be used before bedtime.

DATA GATHERING

History
The best screening for a coagulopathy is a carefully obtained family history of bleeding problems. Usually inquiry about trauma is unrevealing because the most common trauma is secondary to an exploring finger, which, for social reasons, the child will deny. Rather than asking if the child picks his/her nose, the patient could be asked "which finger do you use?" The physician should perform a general review of systems, including looking for medication that might depress the bone marrow and cause epistaxis and evidence of allergy.

Physical Examination
The major task of the physical examination concerns the location of the bleeding so that treatment can be planned if direct pressure to the nose is not successful in stopping the bleeding.

Laboratory Evaluation
No laboratory tests are needed if there is no family history of bleeding and direct pressure stops the problem. If a bleeding disorder is suspected, a coagulation profile, including value of platelets, prothrombin time, and partial thromboplastin time should be ordered. On review of the other causes of epistaxis listed earlier, it is apparent that other problems require subspecialist evaluation.

INDICATIONS FOR CONSULTATION OR REFERRAL

Several factors will identify the patient whose condition needs further investigation: 1) if pressure and/or packing do not stop the problem; 2) if there is a family history of bleeding disorder, physical findings of systemic bleeding, or other symptoms of malignancy; and 3) when the cause of recurrent epistaxis is found to be more complex, as in a nasal foreign body or Osler-Weber-Rendu syndrome, the child should be referred to an otolaryngologist. However, when the cause of recurrent epistaxis is not identified or is unresponsive to therapy, additional data must be gathered.

BIBLIOGRAPHY

Culbertson MC: Epistaxis. In Bluestone CD, Stool SE, editors: *Pediatric otolaryngology,* vol 1, ed 3, Philadelphia, in press, WB Saunders.

Guarisco JL, Graham HD III: Epistaxis in children: Causes, diagnosis, and treatment. *Ear Nose Throat J* 68:522–538, 1989.

Handler SD: Epistaxis. In Gellis S, Kagan B, editors: *Current pediatric therapy,* ed 15, Philadelphia, in press, WB Saunders.

Leslie J, Ingram GI: The diagnosis of long-standing bleeding disorders, *Semin Hematol* 8:440, 1971.

Mulbury PE: Recurrent epistaxis. *Pediatr Rev* 12:213–217, 1991.

Murray AB, Milner RA: Allergic rhinitis and recurrent epistaxis in children, *Ann Allerg Asthma Immunol* 74(1):30–33, 1995.

Potsic WP, Handler SD: *Primary Care Pediatric Otolaryngology,* ed 2, Andover, 1995, Michael Ryan Publishing.

Potsic WP, Wetmore RF: Pediatric Rhinology. In Goldman J, editor: *The Principles and Practice of Rhinology,* New York, 1987, John Wiley.

Quick AJ: Telangiectasia: Its relationship to the Minot-von Willebrand syndrome, *Am J Med Sci* 154:585, 1967.

Randall DA, Freeman SB: Management of anterior and posterior epistaxis, *Am Fam Phys* 43(6):2007–2014, 1991.

Saunder WH: Septal dermoplasty: Its many uses, *Laryngoscopy* 80:1342, 1970.

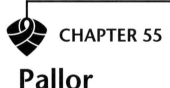

CHAPTER 55

Pallor

Mortimer Poncz

Pallor or paleness, a common parental concern, may be related to a child's fair skin or reflect a significant illness in the child that can be elucidated by an orderly diagnostic approach.

Significant pallor in a child often reflects an underlying anemia but also may indicate a circulation disorder. A brief review of the normal physiology of blood flow in the skin will illustrate these other clinical conditions associated with pallor. Besides providing nutrients and removing wastes, blood flow to the skin helps regulate body heat and acts as a blood volume reservoir. When needed, the body can shift blood flow away from the skin to conserve heat or to increase the supply of blood to essential internal organs.

The thin infant with a large surface area and little substaneous fat will; in a cool environment, have more vasoconstriction in order to conserve body heat. Pallor secondary to peripheral vasoconstriction can be seen with intravascular volume loss as in acute blood loss, vomiting or diarrhea, and disseminated intravascular coagulopathy (DIC). Atropinic ingestions also will cause peripheral vasoconstriction (and loss of sweating) leading to an inability to dissipate heat. At times, pallor may be due to more than one factor. For example, a child with recurrent severe epistaxis may be pale secondary to the volume of blood lost and peripheral vasoconstriction as well as from anemia due to chronic loss of blood.

DIFFERENTIAL DIAGNOSIS

Common Causes of Pallor

- **Trauma**
    Blood loss
    Infection
    Sepsis
- **Toxin**
    Atropine
    Lead poisoning
    Aplastic anemia
- **Metabolic–Inherited**
    Iron deficiency
    Thalassemia
    Sideroblastic anemia
    Sickle cell anemia
    Hereditary spherocytosis
    Glucose-6-phosphate dehydrogenase
        (G-6-PD) deficiency
    Allegic-immunologic
    Autoimmune hemolytic anemia
    Goodpasture syndrome
    Hemolytic-uremic syndrome
    Systemic lupus erythematosus
- **Tumor**
    Leukemia
    Marrow infiltration
- **Congenital**
    Diamond-Blackfan syndrome
- **Multiple etiologies**
    Acute blood loss
    Anemia of chronic illness
    Recurrent blood loss (*eg,* menorrhagia)

Pulmonary hemosiderosis
Pallor also can be considered in relationship
    to the hemoglobin level:

- **Normal hemoglobin level**
    Acute intravascular volume loss
    Atropine exposure
    Cold exposure
    Fair-skinned
- **Anemia (low hemoglobin level)**
    Microcytic anemia
        Iron deficiency
        Lead poisoning
        Thalassemia
        Sideroblastic anemia
    Normocytic anemia
        Low reticulocyte count
            Anemia of chronic disease
            Transient erythroblastopenia of childhood (TEC)
            Diamond-Blackfan syndrome
            Leukemia
            Marrow infiltration
            Aplastic anemia
        Elevated reticulocyte count
            External blood loss
            Pulmonary hemosiderosis
            Goodpasture syndrome
            Intraerythrocyte defects
            Hemolytic uremic syndrome
            Sickle cell disease
            Hereditary spherocytosis
            G-6-PD deficiency
    Macrocytic anemia
        Low reticulocyte count
            Folate or vitamin B_{12} deficiency
            Preleukemia
            Aplastic anemia
            Diamond-Blackfan syndrome
        Elevated reticulocyte count
            Hemolytic anemia and high reticulocyte count
            Autoimmune hemolytic anemia
            Secondary folate deficiency in chronic hemolytic anemia

Discussion

As can be seen in the previous lists, the differential diagnosis of pallor in childhood covers many aspects of pediatrics. The most common cause of significant pallor in children is iron deficiency anemia. This microcytic hypochromic anemia is most commonly seen in children under the age of

3 years and in adolescent girls. These two periods of life involve rapid growth and poor dietary iron intake. Adolescent girls also might be losing blood from menstruation. Outside of these two age groups, iron deficiency anemia is unusual, and an underlying cause of blood loss should be considered if iron deficiency anemia occurs.

Microcytic anemia also can be due to lead poisoning or thalassemia. Thalassemia is found predominantly in populations from the malarial belt of the world (Mediterranean, Africa, and East Asia). Lead poisoning tends to occur in toddlers. The potential risk for environmental exposure to lead should be explored in a child with an unexplained mild microcytic anemia.

Normocytic anemias also are common causes of childhood pallor. These anemias can be divided into those associated with increased blood destruction or blood loss and those associated with decreased blood production. The most common cause of these disorders is increased blood loss. Two caveats need be remembered about blood loss. Initially the hemoglobin level may remain high, only to fall later as volume is replaced. Initial pallor often is due to peripheral vasoconstriction. The second caveat is that significant blood loss can be occult. The child who has recurrent iron deficiency anemia despite adequate iron supplementation may have occult gastrointestinal blood loss (and needs a guaiac stool test) or internal bleeding in a site where iron cannot be efficiently reutilized as in pulmonary hemosiderosis.

Other causes of increased blood destruction leading to a normocytic anemia include autoimmune disorders, DIC, and intraerythrocytic disorders. The first two causes may have other signs and symptoms besides pallor, whereas ethnic background (*eg,* sickle cell disease) and family history (*eg,* hereditary spherocytosis) may be of value in diagnosing the intracellular disorders.

Normocytic anemias may be due to decreased production. Most often these anemias are secondary to either an anemia of chronic disease or marrow failure. Pallor secondary to decreased red blood cell (RBC) production may be the presenting symptom of a chronic illness. Hypothyroidism and inflammatory bowel disease can present in this fashion, although the latter anemia often is due to a combination of iron deficiency from recurrent blood loss and anemia

of chronic disease. Marrow failure in leukemia or aplastic anemia involves other cell lines besides the RBCs, although rarely only the RBC line can be predominantly affected.

An increasingly common cause of pallor in the first years of life is transient erythroblastopenia of childhood (TEC). This disorder of transient loss of RBC production is associated with a slow onset of anemia and pallor in an otherwise well child. Often the diagnosis is made on a routine blood count or when the child is noticeably pale.

Macrocytic anemias are uncommon. Most often the macrocytosis is secondary to a high number of reticulocytes. True macrocytic anemia in childhood often is due to folate or vitamin B_{12} dietary deficiency. A thorough history of the dietary habits of the child (and of the mother in a breast-fed child) may reveal an unusual diet. For example, a baby aged 1 year fed only goat's milk may become folate deficient, whereas the breast-fed baby of a mother who is a strict vegetarian may become vitamin B_{12} deficient.

DATA GATHERING

History

In a child aged 1 year, a detailed birth history as well as a dietary history can help in assessing the risk of iron deficiency, whereas in an adolescent girl the menstrual and dietary histories are of value. The acuteness of the pallor as well as the presence of other symptoms such as fever, weight loss, cough, rash, pica, change in activity, bruising, obvious blood loss, or jaundice can be of value. The child's ethnic background should be obtained as well as a family history for anemia, jaundice, splenectomy, or cholecystectomy. The latter three conditions can be found in families with inherited hemolytic anemias.

Physical Examination

The physical examination should first determine whether the child is acutely ill. The presence of tachycardia or postural changes in pulse and blood pressure with pallor might be due to loss of significant intravascular volume, DIC, or severe anemia. If the child is stable, the degree of anemia can roughly be assessed by examining the mucosal surfaces and plamar creases. Other physical signs can suggest the cause of the pallor. Scleral icterus can be present in a hemolytic anemia, pigmented gums in lead ingestion, rales and wheezes in pulmonary hemosiderosis, spooning of nails in iron deficiency, a malar rash in lupus erythematosus, and adenopathy and hepatosplenomegaly in malignancy. Petechiae, bruising, and mouth ulcers can be seen when more than just the erythroid cell line is affected by an underlying disorder.

Laboratory Evaluation

The single most important laboratory test to be done in evaluating pallor is the complete blood cell (CBC) count, which is preferably done by an electronic counter. The counter not only gives values for hemoglobin and hematocrit but also provides information about RBC size and size distribution (mean corpuscular volume and red cell distribution width, respectively) and the hemoglobin content of the RBC (mean corpuscular hemoglobin and mean corpuscular hemoglobin concentration). In addition, most counters give a platelet count and a white blood cell count and differential. Thus from a single determination, information is provided about whether the child is anemic (for his/her age) as well as providing accurate additional information that is of significant aid in the differential diagnosis.

A child with a microcytic hypochromic anemia should have serum iron and iron-binding capacity determined. This test is highly specific for iron deficiency. If iron deficiency is confirmed, a 2- to 4-month therapeutic trial of iron at 6 mg of elemental iron per kg per day should be instituted. In most cases further evaluation such as determination of levels of serum ferritin and serum iron and iron-binding capacity can be avoided.

If determination of available iron is normal, a microcytic hypochromic anemia can be due to thalassemia. In β-thalassemia, β-globin peptides are underproduced. Hemoglobin electrophoresis with quantitation of the various hemoglobins present should confirm the diagnosis. α-Thalassemia trait does not have any abnormalities demonstrable on hemoglobin electrophoresis. In a child of appropriate ethnic background with microcytic anemia not due to any other cause, α-thalassemia trait is a diagnosis of exclusion best made by a pediatric hematologist.

Normocytic anemia can be divided into those conditions predominantly due to increased destruction of RBCs with an elevated reticulocyte count and those due to decreased production of RBCs and a low reticulocyte count. In both categories, examination of the blood smear often can lead to a diagnosis. In anemias secondary to a hemolytic process, examination of the smear can show abnormal RBC morphology as, for example, sickle forms, spherocytes, or schistocytes. Decreased platelet numbers can be present along with a hemolytic anemia in lupus erythematosus, hemolytic uremic syndrome (Fig. 55-1), and DIC. In normocytic anemias with low reticulocyte counts, malignant cells (as in leukemias) and increased number of neutrophils with a shift to immature forms or toxic granulation (as in infection) can lead to the proper diagnosis.

If the blood smear is benign and there is a reticulocytosis, the most common diagnosis is acute blood loss. Internal blood sequestration such as pulmonary hemosiderosis also can cause pallor with reticulocytosis and a normal smear. Less commonly, an intraerythrocytic defect can be the cause and needs diagnostic evaluation by a hematologist.

Normocytic anemia with a low reticulocyte count and no abnormality seen on the peripheral smear may be due to TEC or to an anemia of chronic disease. Determination of values for serum iron and iron-binding capacity can be done to support this diagnosis. A bone marrow examination may be required to document a malignant or a congenital or acquired erythrocytic stem cell failure.

Occasionally, children with hemolytic anemias can first present in an aplastic crisis in which the reticulocyte count is low. Often a personal or family history of splenectomy or early cholecystectomy suggestive of a hemolytic anemia can be obtained. Examination of the blood smear can be of diagnostic value. However, repeated evaluation of the patient's condition and his/her blood smear after recovery from the aplastic crisis may be necessary to confirm the diagnosis.

Rarely, pallor is due to a macrocytic anemia. If the dietary history supports folate or vitamin B_{12} deficiency and serum levels confirm the diagnosis, appropriate supplementation and dietary manipulation can be done. Juvenile pernicious anemia and congenital folate and vitamin B_{12} malabsorptions can rarely occur. Proper evaluation of these and other causes of macro-

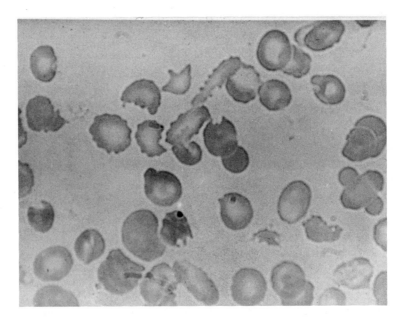

FIG 55-1
Example of red blood cell abnormalities.   Hemolytic uremic syndrome with burr cells, fragmented cells, and a low platelet count.

cytic anemia shown in the second list usually requires consultation with the appropriate pediatric subspecialist.

INDICATIONS FOR CONSULTATION OR REFERRAL

The child with pallor should, in general, be hospitalized for one of three reasons: 1) The anemia is associated with congestive heart failure or shock. This association is most commonly seen with acute blood loss and secondary hypovolemia. The child with a chronic anemia that has slowly developed can tolerate a very low hemoglobin level without congestive heart failure and rarely requires a blood transfusion. 2) The cause of an anemia cannot be easily determined in the office. The majority of cases due to iron deficiency anemia, thalassemia trait, sickle-cell disease, and a number of other disorders can be diagnosed on the basis of the CBC count and blood smear. However, a number of disorders require specialized tests. 3) An anemia associated with a severe underlying disor-

der may require hospitalization to confirm and treat the underlying disease.

DISCUSSION OF ALGORITHM

An algorithm for differential diagnosis of pallor is presented in Figure 55-2. In the evaluation of pallor, after documentation that the patient is anemic, the differential diagnosis is dependent on determination of RBC size. The condition of the patient with microcytic anemia and decreased available iron is evaluated for iron deficiency. In these cases, the cause of anemia should be determined. If there is no evidence for a dietary cause, then blood loss from the gastrointestinal tract should be investigated.

Those patients with microcytic anemia and a normal available iron should have their conditions evaluated for thalassemia, sideroblastic anemia, and lead poisoning. If a normocytic or macrocytic anemia is present, further study by reticulocyte count aids in the differential diagnosis.

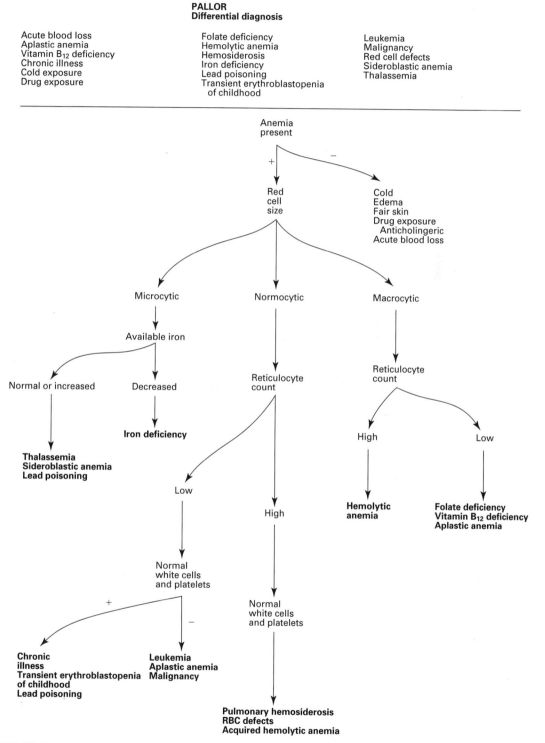

FIG 55-2

Decision tree for differential diagnosis of pallor.

BIBLIOGRAPHY

Baehner RI, editor: Pediatric hematology, *Pediatr Clin North Am* 27:217–292, 403–486, 1980.

Crosby WH, Herbert V, Forget BG, et al: A new clinical strategy series—the anemia, *Hosp Pract,* vol 15, Feb-June 1980.

Kahn R, Romslo I, Lamuik J: Anemia in general practice, *Scand J Clin Invest* 50(suppl):41, 1990.

Romslo I, Lamuik J, Kahn R: Anemia in general practice. Which laboratory tests are requested—how are the result interpreted and what are the consequences to patient care, *Scand J Clin Invest* 50(suppl):46, 1990.

(*Also see* references for Chapter 60.)

CHAPTER 56

Polyuria

Andrew M. Tershakovec

Parents often complain that their child urinates frequently, which means voiding has increased from its usual pattern. The number of times a child normally urinates varies with age: an infant may urinate 20 or more times a day, whereas an adolescent urinates approximately five times a day. This developmental progression can make the recognition of what is normal difficult. Frequency in children rarely stems from organic disease.

Polyuria, the production of an abnormally large amount of urine, is an unusual cause of frequency. A child who consistently produces more than 30 mL of urine per kilogram of body weight per day (with a urine specific gravity of less than 1.010 in most cases) has some pathologic condition.

When evaluating urinary frequency, the primary care physician must first determine if true frequency or polyuria exists. Although a wide variety of causes for these conditions is known, an organized approach allows for differentiation between the majority of benign complaints of frequency and those resulting from serious conditions.

DIFFERENTIAL DIAGNOSIS

Common Causes of Urinary Frequency
- **Trauma**
  Urethral trauma or irritation (masturbation, sexual abuse)
  Chemical irritation (bubble bath)
- **Infection**
  Cystitis
  Urethritis
- **Endocrine**
  Neurogenic or central diabetes insipidus
    Idiopathic or familial
  Diabetes mellitus
  Primary aldosteronism
  Adrenogenital syndrome
  Bartter syndrome
  Catecholamine excess
    Pheochromocytoma
    Neuroblastoma/ganglioneuroblastoma
- **Multiple etiologies**
  Anxiety/behavioral
    Nephrogenic diabetes insipidus
  Familial/idiopathic
    Sickle-cell disease

Medullary cystic kidney disease
Renal tubular acidosis
Fanconi syndrome
Hypokalemia
Hypercalcemia
Cystinosis
Partial urinary tract obstruction/hydro-
    nephrosis
Sarcoidosis
- **Primary polydipsia**

Discussion

Trauma

Manipulation of the urethra with a variety of instruments may cause irritation and symptoms of frequency. Boys commonly induce irritation with sexual play and exploration. However, sexual abuse should always be considered a possibility in a child with irritative urethritis. Examination of the urethral meatus may show signs of trauma or irritation, which can produce hematuria. Although a child will rarely admit self-manipulation, this may be assumed if other causes are ruled out.

Infection

Cystitis is one of the most common causes of frequency. The child and parent may note any combination of the classic symptoms of frequency, dysuria, and cloudy, malodorous urine. Viral cystitis presents with gross hematuria and fever and lasts less than a week. Bacterial cystitis also may cause hematuria and systemic signs (eg, diarrhea, vomiting), but fever is less likely unless the infection has progressed to pyelonephritis. *Neisseria gonorrhoeae* (gonococcus), *Chlamydia trachomatis, Ureaplasma urealyticum, Tricho-monas vaginalis,* and herpes simplex virus have been identified as causes of urethritis in children. Although a child may be infected by innocent means, culture should be performed in all cases of suspected infectious urethritis and the cause considered to be sexual abuse until proved otherwise.

Endocrine

The basic types of neurogenic or central diabetes insipidus are familial and acquired. The uncommon familial forms occur as both autosomal dominant and X-linked recessive conditions. Most cases of acquired diabetes insipidus can be attributed to a specific cause, involving some injury to the pituitary region. Intracranial injury (*eg,* head trauma, surgery, intracranial hemorrhage, meningitis, encephalitis, tumor) can cause immediate or delayed onset diabetes insipidus through direct injury to the pituitary region or indirectly by increasing intracranial pressure. After the primary process causing the increased pressure or inflammation resolves, most of these cases remit spontaneously. Idiopathic cases of central diabetes insipidus also occur. Care must be exercised in making this diagnosis, because diabetes insipidus may be the first manifestation of an intracranial tumor, preceding the onset of other signs or symptoms by many years. Of the tumors that cause diabetes insipidus, craniopharyngiomas, histiocytomas, and optic gliomas most often are found. The examining physician must carefully evaluate the child for signs of papilledema, optic atrophy, or other neurologic deficits induced by the malignant process. Chemotherapeutic agents also may induce central and nephrogenic diabetes insipidus in children receiving treatment of a malignant disease.

Hyperglycemia associated with diabetes mellitus causes osmotic diuresis, the most frequent cause of true polyuria that the primary care physician will see. The physician should screen all such cases for the classic history of the three "polys" (polyuria, polydipsia, and polyphagia), weight loss, and a family history of diabetes mellitus.

Multiple Etiologies

Anxiety/behavioral—Anxiety and behavioral problems can cause intermittent frequency, as in the child who is overcome by a need to urinate when entering the physician's examining room. When a child complains of frequency unrelated to a urinary tract infection, the physician should investigate the timing and setting of the complaints and recent changes in the child's life or environment. The cause of most cases of behavioral frequency are thus identified. More obscure cases and those involving more significant psychopathology (such as daytime wetting) may require psychiatric evaluation and intervention. School teachers will attest to the high number of young children who have brief episodes of frequency that are secondary to mild anxiety or pressure.

Nephrogenic diabetes insipidus—By a broad definition of the term, all children with polyuria due to an inadequate renal response to antidiuretic hormone (ADH) have nephrogenic diabetes insipidus. Familial forms occur, but acquired forms are much more common. Familial nephrogenic diabetes insipidus usually presents in infancy or early childhood. Although it seems to be inherited as an X-linked recessive trait, the disorder has been reported in girls.

Chronic pyelonephritis can significantly alter renal function, especially concentrating ability and tubular reabsorption. Affected children produce a large volume of dilute urine containing increased amounts of electrolytes and glucose.

Drugs may contribute to tubular dysfunction through a variety of mechanisms. Methicillin and related penicillin antibiotics, analgesics, and mercury poisoning can induce interstitial nephritis. Other agents (eg, diuretics) directly affect tubular function. Such drugs as lithium and demeclocycline interfere with ADH-stimulated cyclic adenosine monophosphate production, indirectly influencing tubular function. Drug-induced tubular dysfunction may be transient, as with diuretics, whereas agents such as analgesics and mercury cause permanent dysfunction. Amphotericin can cause permanent tubular dysfunction that is significantly worsened when the agent is administered and transient dysfunction, that remits when the amphotericin is stopped.

Electrolyte abnormalities may cause tubular dysfunction and polyuria. Hypercalcemia inhibits adenyl cyclase activity, which interferes with the response to ADH. Hypokalemia also alters renal response to ADH. The polyuria independently seen in some conditions (eg, diabetic ketoacidosis, Bartter syndrome, primary aldosteronism, Fanconi syndrome) may be exacerbated by the hypokalemia also common in these conditions.

Interstitial nephritis may be idiopathic or related to conditions such as autoimmune diseases, ureteral reflux, and drug reactions. Acute cases ordinarily present with oliguria and progress to polyuria when permanent tubular damage occurs. Hypokalemia and hypercalcemia also may cause interstitial nephritis when allowed to continue for an extended time.

Children with sickle cell disease acquire renal concentrating defects after the age of 5 years. The poorly oxygenated medullary region of the kidney is predisposed to recurrent local sickling crises and infarcts, significantly altering concentrating ability.

Urinary tract obstruction and hydronephrosis also damage renal concentrating ability. Neonates with polyuria should be examined for the presence of posterior urethral valves or other obstructions. It should be noted that significant urinary tract dilatation has been seen in children with polyuria in the absence of any anatomic obstruction.

Medullary cystic kidney disease, an autosomal recessive condition, presents in early childhood with polyuria, renal loss of sodium and calcium, and anemia. Renal failure usually develops over a period of years.

Primary polydipsia—The diagnosis of primary polydipsia is sometimes difficult to make. Infants develop primary polydipsia in response to an inappropriate feeding pattern (eg, the child who displays any signs of distress is given a bottle of water instead of having his/her needs appropriately assessed). In older children, the search for recent changes or disturbances in the child's life may yield precipitating factors for psychogenic polydipsia. Some cases have been reported in households in which family members have true diabetes insipidus or a history of polydipsia or polyuria. A slightly low serum sodium level may be a clue to the diagnosis. Rare cases of primary polydipsia have been reported secondary to a reset osmolality control mechanism. Affected persons continue to be thirsty until serum osmolality drops to their new "normal" value.

Long-standing polyuria dilutes renal medullary solute concentration, limiting the concentrating ability of the otherwise intact kidney and ADH system. As a result, laboratory evaluation of primary polydipsia (eg, water deprivation test) may not be diagnostic and is potentially dangerous. If considered, this evaluation should be performed in a hospital under carefully monitored conditions.

Miscellaneous—Conditions causing urinary tract irritability (eg, bladder masses, renal calculi) can cause urinary tract spasm and feelings of urgency and dysuria.

DATA GATHERING

When evaluating a child because of frequent urination, the primary care physician should initially focus on the most common causes, including frequency associated with anxiety and behavioral factors, urinary tract infection, mucosal irritation, and diabetes mellitus. If indicated, the physician should then study the information obtained for clues leading to a more obscure diagnosis.

History

As a first step it must be determined if the child has frequency or if the parent misinterpreted a normal pattern of urination. Specifically asking how many times the child goes to the bathroom to urinate (or has episodes of enuresis) per night and estimating the volume produced at each void is useful. Although it is difficult to estimate urinary volume unless the child regularly urinates into a small container, the physician can ask if the urinary stream is strong for a significant length of time. Frequency unrelated to polyuria presents with small volumes of urine and a weak stream. Dysuria, darkened or cloudy urine, hematuria, or a change in odor of the urine are consistent findings of a urinary tract infection.

Variations in the pattern of urination associated with behavior or activity may indicate psychologic influences. However, even children with frequency due to organic causes urinate more frequently at times of stress or excitement. Significant changes in the child's life and behavior should be investigated, along with the reaction of the child and family to the problem. Extremes in response may be indicative of psychopathology. For example, if the parent makes a major issue of the child's enuresis, a disturbed parent-child relationship may exist.

Children with frequency and fever may have an infection (cystitis or pyelonephritis), but central temperature instability (associated with hypothalamic-pituitary dysfunction) or severe dehydration related to large free water losses in the urine should be considered. The latter condition occurs in young children with diabetes insipidus who do not have adequate access to drinking water.

Historic evidence of diabetes mellitus should be explored; a history of polyphagia or weight loss and a family history of diabetes mellitus may be diagnostic.

Physical Examination

Although the physical examination is rarely diagnostic in cases of frequency, a thorough examination should be performed. Specific attention should be directed toward neurologic defects and the presence of irritation or injury at the urethral meatus.

Laboratory Evaluation

The examination begins with urinalysis and urine culture. The urinalysis provides evidence of concentrating ability (specific gravity), diabetes mellitus (glycosuria, ketonuria), urinary tract infection (pyuria, hematuria), urinary tract abnormalities (hematuria), and renal disease (eg, glycosuria, hematuria, proteinuria). A serum glucose level should be determined if glycosuria is present. Serum electrolyte levels may provide evidence for metabolic, endocrinologic, renal, neurologic, or emotional disease but are not a necessary part of the initial evaluation.

If a child is suspected of having frequency related to polyuria, a 24-hour urine sample can be collected. A child normally produces less than 30 mL of urine per kilogram of body weight per day (2 L in adults). However, because accurate 24-hour samples are difficult to obtain in children, this collection should not be undertaken initially. Measuring the specific gravity of a first morning urine sample is the most useful test to grossly evaluate renal concentrating ability. Normally this sample will have a specific gravity greater than 1.010. It would be unusual to have true polyuria and a urine specific gravity above 1.010.

Any child suspected of having diabetes insipidus must have free access to water at all times. A water deprivation test should be undertaken only in a controlled and monitored environment.

INDICATIONS FOR REFERRAL OR CONSULTATION

The primary care physician should refer children with true polyuria or an inability to concentrate urine for renal or endocrinologic evaluation. Children with frequency unrelated to cystitis or urethritis may have a urinary tract abnormality that is causing bladder irritation. If urinalysis yields normal results, however, most cases of frequency are related to mild trauma, behavior, or anxiety. If the problem persists, urologic or psychologic evaluation may be considered.

DISCUSSION OF ALGORITHM

An algorithm for the differential diagnosis of frequency is presented in Figure 56-1. The outlined method seeks to eliminate common

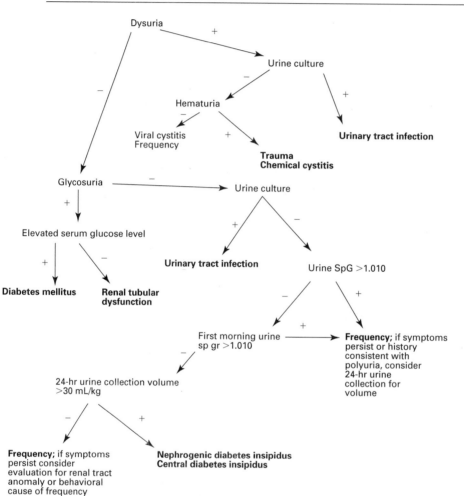

FIG 56-1

Decision tree for differential diagnosis of polyuria.

causes of frequency with screening tests that are readily available to primary care physicians. This method begins with the evaluation of dysuria.

After eliminating dysuria, the physician should identify those children with glycosuria associated with diabetes mellitus or renal tubular dysfunction. In the absence of glycosuria, the urine sample should be cultured. (Although the steps are listed separately in the flow chart, urinalysis and urine culture should be performed simultaneously as part of the initial evaluation). As a urinary tract infection is being eliminated, the specific gravity of the urine should be evaluated as a gross screen of renal concentrating ability. A first morning urine sample is more indicative of true concentrating ability. Those children with continued dilute urine samples should have a 24-hour urine collection completed. Those children with polyuria should then be referred for evaluation of nephrogenic or neurogenic diabetes insipidus. In most cases,

children with urine specific gravity above 1.010 do not have polyuria.

With this protocol, most causes of urinary tract infections, diabetes mellitus, and diabetes insipidus will be identified. In the face of persistent signs or symptoms, other causes of frequency, such as trauma, anxiety, and primary polydipsia, should be considered. If the cause still is not evident, more obscure causes involving neurologic, endocrinologic, renal, or psychologic disease may be present.

BIBLIOGRAPHY

Leiken S, Caplan H: Psychogenic polydipsia, *Am J Psychiatry* 123:1573–1576, 1967.

Linshaw M, Hipp T, Gruskin A: Infantile psychogenic water drinking, *J Pediatr* 85:520–522, 1974.

McMillan JA, Nieburg PI, Oski FA: *The whole pediatrician catalog,* Philadelphia, 1977, WB Saunders.

Robertson GL: Differential diagnosis of polyuria, *Ann Rev Med* 39:425–442, 1988.

Siegel N, Gaudio K: Disorders of urine volume in the critically ill child, *Yale J Biol Med* 57:29–47, 1984.

Vaamonde CA: Differential diagnosis of polyuria, *Pediatr Nephrol* 1:261–175, 1974.

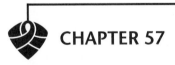

CHAPTER 57

Purpura

Mortimer Poncz

Purpura or bruising represents the presence of extravasated blood in the superficial layers of the skin. Excessive bruising is a common complaint seen in children in the primary care office and often simply reflects their high level of physical activity. Because purpura also might be the first sign of a significant systemic illness, proper office evaluation is of great importance in the diagnosis and management of the child with purpura.

The integrity of the vascular system depends

on three interacting factors: platelets, the plasma coagulation factors, and the vessels and their supporting tissues. Decreased platelet counts or defective platelets can lead to extravasation of blood, resulting in either extensive hemorrhages, called *ecchymosis,* or fine pinpoint hemorrhages, called *petechiae.* Defects in the serum coagulation pathway and in the vascular system also can present with ecchymosis, although petechiae are rarely seen.

In addition, to properly understand the pathophysiology of a patient's purpura, the degree and the nature of the trauma suffered by the child must be taken into account. An infant aged 1 month with severe thrombocytopenia may have no ecchymosis or petechiae because the infant spends most of his/her time quietly in the horizontal position. In contrast, a child aged 2 years with the same degree of thrombocytopenia will have multiple bruises as a result of his/her active lifestyle.

DIFFERENTIAL DIAGNOSIS

Common Causes of Purpura

- **Trauma**
    - Child abuse
    - Self-inflicted
    - Easy bruisability
- **Infection**
    - Congenital infections
    - AIDS
- **Toxin**
    - Aspirin exposure
    - Drug-induced platelet count depression
- **Metabolic–Genetic**
    - von Willebrand disease
    - Hemophilia
    - Inherited platelet defects
    - Scurvy
    - Uremia
    - Cushing disease
- **Allergic–Immunologic**
    - Idiopathic thrombocytopenic purpura
    - Lupus erythematosus
    - Henoch-Schönlein purpura
    - Vasculitis
- **Tumor**
    - Bone marrow infiltration
- **Congenital**
    - Kasabach-Merritt syndrome
    - Thrombocytopenia, absent radii
- **Multiple etiologies**
    - Hemolytic-uremic syndrome
    - Thrombotic thrombocytopenic purpura
    - Aplastic anemia
    - Disseminated intravascular coagulation

Discussion

The major cause of excessive unprovoked purpura in childhood is thrombocytopenia. The normal range of platelet counts is 150,000 to 400,000 mm^3. Increased bruising can be seen with a count below 100,000 mm^3, whereas significant purpura is seen when the count is under 20,000 mm^3. Thrombocytopenia can be due to either increased destruction, decreased production, or both. The most common cause of increased destruction is immune thrombocytopenic purpura (ITP) in which the platelets are destroyed secondary to an autoimmune antiplatelet antibody. Frequently ITP occurs after a viral illness or the taking of certain medications (*eg*, a sulfa drug). It must be distinguished from the often more virulent autoimmune disorder, Evans syndrome, in which other hematologic cell lines are involved. Most frequently ITP occurs in younger children. In older children, especially in girls, an autoimmune-based thrombocytopenia may represent the onset of systemic lupus erythematosus (SLE). Hemolytic-uremic syndrome also may present with purpura in which there is increased platelet destruction. Often the purpura and other bleeding manifestations are excessive for the degree of thrombocytopenia reflecting the effect of the uremia on platelet function. In Kasabach-Merritt syndrome increased platelet destruction occurs within a large hemangioma. Disseminated intravascular coagulation (DIC) and hypersplenism represent other medical conditions associated with increased platelet destruction and potential bruising. DIC is a complicated syndrome, and the bleeding manifestations not only reflect thrombocytopenia but also consumption of the plasma coagulation factors and loss of vascular integrity.

In neonates, sepsis should be considered whenever thrombocytopenia is present. In an otherwise well newborn, thrombocytopenia may be due to increased destruction secondary to transplacental transmitted antiplatelet antibodies. These acquired antibodies can be secondary to an isoimmune disorder, maternal SLE, or maternal ITP. Decreased platelet production also can underlie neonatal purpura. Congenital infections such as cytomegalovirus or rubella can cause thrombocytopenia due to decreased production ("blueberry muffin baby").

AIDS may present with thrombocytopenia. Often the degree of thrombocytopenia is moderate, but it can be severe. The decrease in platelets is due to the combination of decreased production of HIV-infected megakaryocytes and an immune-related increased destruction.

In older children, decreased platelet production can be seen when the marrow is infiltrated with another cell line as in leukemias and neuroblastoma. Decreased production also can be seen when there is defective production of megakaryocytes, as can occur following a viral illness or in aplastic anemia and in congenital disorders such as thrombocytopenia absent radii syndrome.

Platelet dysfunction can account for excessive bruising. Platelet counts are normal or near normal. The platelet dysfunction may be intrinsic to the platelet as in the congenital disorder of Bernard-Soulier syndrome, which also is associated with giant platelets. It may be extrinsic to the platelet as in von Willebrand disease, uremia, or aspirin ingestion. In addition, hemophilia and related inherited plasma coagulation factor defects, while rare, can present with purpura.

Vasculitis and other causes of decreased vascular integrity can result in purpura. In Henoch-Schönlein purpura, there can be recurrent waves of purpura often confined to the lower extremities and buttocks. The diagnosis depends on the history, the characteristic rash, and the other signs of arthritis, nephritis, and intestinal vasculitis. Purpura fulminans is a rare, often postviral, vasculitis of the skin, leading to large purpuric areas of skin associated with systemic DIC. Vascular integrity also can be decreased either secondary to scurvy, excessive steroids (Cushing syndrome), or due to an inherited elastic defect (such as that seen in pseudoxanthoma elasticum, osteogenesis imperfecta, and Marfan syndrome).

Unusual trauma may underlie the purpuric lesions in a child. Petechiae limited to the face and chest of a child with a cough may be secondary to the intravascular pressure exerted during the accompanying Valsalva maneuver. Purpuric lesions that are inconsistent with the described trauma or that have an unusual distribution may be secondary to child abuse. Occasionally, in the older child, self-inflicted bruises can be seen. These, too, tend to be associated with an unusual history or physical distribution. Finally, easy bruisability after minor trauma with no underlying disorder is seen fairly frequently in adolescent women. Extensive evaluation of bruises in these patients when there is no other history of a bleeding disorder is not often productive.

DATA GATHERING

History

A thorough history and physical examination is important for the proper evaluation of purpura. Questions should be asked concerning the dura-tion, severity, and location of the purpura; recent viral illness; the occurrence of any significant trauma; and the presence of any other symptoms such as fever, weight loss, or joint involvement. A history of drug ingestion (such as aspirin) and a family history of bleeding manifestations or drug abuse by a parent are also important.

Physical Examination

Physical examination should be directed first to determining how acutely ill the child is. Next, the location and severity of ecchymosis and petechiae should be noted. The fundi and mucosal surfaces should be examined for hemorrhages. Signs of associated illness such as pallor, adenopathy, or hepatosplenomegaly should be sought.

Laboratory Evaluation

In the child with excessive unprovoked purpura, the most important single test is a complete blood cell (CBC) count including a quantitative platelet count and examination of the peripheral smear by experienced personnel. If the platelet count is low and values for the rest of the CBC count and smear are normal, ITP is the most likely diagnosis. However, because other diseases such as leukemia and SLE are still possible, the patient should be referred to a pediatric hematologist for further evaluation of the purpura, possibly including a bone marrow aspiration. If other abnormalities are present on the peripheral blood smear, further appropriate diagnostic workup based on the given abnormality should be done.

When the platelet count is normal, a bleeding time test should be performed. This test should be done by an experienced laboratory so that it can be relied on as a true indicator of both platelet function and vascular integrity. A prolonged bleeding time can be found in von Willebrand disease and in other inherited or acquired defects of platelet function. Several medical disorders affecting subcutaneous tissue such as Cushing syndrome, scurvy, and Marfan syndrome can prolong bleeding time. Usually the history and physical examination will help establish these diagnoses.

INDICATIONS FOR CONSULTATION OR REFERRAL

Purpura associated with a normal platelet count and a normal bleeding time can be seen in Henoch-Schönlein purpura and in inherited or

PURPURA
Differential diagnosis

Thrombotic thrombocytopenic purpura (TTP)
Anaphylactoid purpura
Aplastic anemia
Child abuse
Drug reaction
Hemolytic anemia

Hemolytic uremic syndrome
Hemophilia
Hypersplenism
Idiopathic thrombocytopenic purpura (ITP)

Disseminated intravascular coagulation (DIC)
Leukemia
Lupus
Malignancy
Trauma
von Willebrand disease

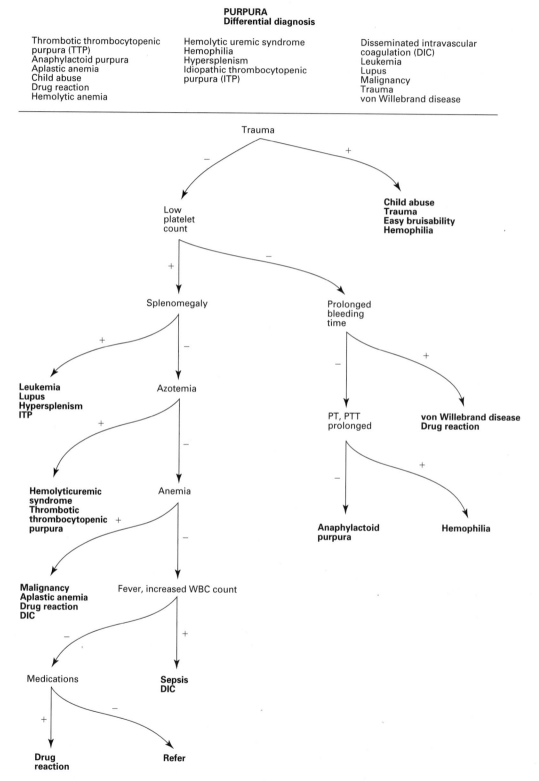

FIG 57-1

Decision tree for differential diagnosis of purpura.

acquired coagulation disorder. Usually the characteristic history and physical examination together with plasma coagulation studies will lead to an appropriate diagnosis. If the evaluation does not produce a diagnosis, consultation with a pediatric hematologist may be of value, as a number of the previously mentioned diagnoses such as von Willebrand disease may require either special laboratory tests or repeat testing.

Patients with purpura associated with low platelet counts may require evaluation within the hospital, often under the care of a pediatric hematologist. The patient with thrombocytopenia may require a bone marrow aspiration depending on the history, physical examination, degree of thrombocytopenia, and the blood count results.

In addition, the child is at increased risk of significant internal bleeding, and his/her condition should be carefully monitored at least until the diagnosis is established, the child's clinical course understood, and the parents educated to the potential risks associated with thrombocytopenia.

Patients without thrombocytopenia but with excessive bruising should be hospitalized if there is a possibility of child abuse. In addition, patients with abnormal coagulation studies (either a prolonged bleeding time or prothrombin time or partial thromboplastin time) should have the purpura evaluated by a hematologist. They

may or may not need hospitalization depending on the clinical state.

Purpura also may represent one symptom of a life-threatening presentation. Thus, patients with either hemolytic urea syndrome or thrombotic thrombocytopenia purpura may have concurrent azotemia. Patients with overwhelming sepsis will have concurrent signs of infection and multiorgan failure.

DISCUSSION OF ALGORITHM

An algorithm for differential diagnosis of purpura is presented in Figure 57-1. If the physician evaluating purpura is assured that trauma has not played a significant role, the cause of the condition is frequently defined by use of the platelet count. The child with purpura who has a low platelet count in association with other hematologic abnormalities of the CBC count needs to have the purpura evaluated for malignancy, hemolytic-uremic syndrome, DIC, or other conditions listed under differential diagnosis.

If a patient has a low platelet count without other hematologic abnormalities, ITP is most likely. The patient with a normal platelet count requires determination of bleeding time and other laboratory studies to rule out von Willebrand disease, uremia, or congenital platelet or plasma coagulant dysfunction.

BIBLIOGRAPHY

Eden OB, Lilleyman JS: Guidelines for management of idiopathic thrombocytopenic purpura, *Arch Dis Child* 67:1056, 1992.

CHAPTER 58

Rectal Bleeding

David A. Piccoli

Rectal bleeding, a common manifestation of gastrointestinal (GI) disease, is the final pathway of hemorrhage from any site along the GI tract or nasopharynx and may, in the neonate, represent blood of foreign origin. A common, and often unsuspected cause of rectal bleeding is an upper GI tract hemorrhage, originating above the ligament of Treitz. Factors such as volume of the hemorrhage and intestinal transit time may lead to the mistaken clinical impression of lower GI tract bleeding. Lower GI tract bleeding that originates from sites below the ligament of Treitz, most frequently from the distal ileum and colon, may result from a discrete anatomic lesion or diffuse mucosal disease. The degree of rectal bleeding depends on the site and severity of the lesion.

DIFFERENTIAL DIAGNOSIS

Common Causes of Rectal Bleeding

- **All causes of upper GI tract bleeding**
- **Lower GI tract bleeding**
- **Trauma**
  Anal fissure
  Child abuse
  Foreign body
- **Infection**
  Bacterial: *Salmonella; Shigella; Yersinia; Campylobacter; Aeromonas;* enteropathogenic *Escherichia coli; Clostridium difficile* (antibiotic-associated colitis)
  Protozoal: amebiasis *(Entamoeba histolytica)*
  Parasitic: *Trichuris;* hookworm
  Viral (rarely)
- **Inflammatory**
  Necrotizing enterocolitis

Ischemic colitis
Acute colitis
Ulcerative colitis
Crohn disease
Henoch-Schönlein syndrome
Hemolytic-uremic syndrome
Nodular lymphoid hyperplasia
- **Vascular–Tumor**
  Hemangiomas
  Arteriovenous malformations
  Telangiectasias
  Hemorrhoids
- **Congenital**
  Meckel diverticulum
  Duplications
- **Structural**
  Intussusception
  Juvenile polyp
  Polyposis syndromes
  Midgut volvulus
- **Allergic**
  Cow milk (soy milk) protein allergy

Discussion

Pseudoblood

It is important in the well child to verify rectal bleeding biochemically. A number of substances can be mistaken for blood in its various states including food coloring, fruit-flavored drinks, beets, grapes, colored antibiotics, iron, and other medications. Even the most dramatic diaper should be tested for heme positivity. Several biochemical tests are currently available for the detection of blood in feces.

The guaiac reagent in cards or paper strips (*eg*, Hemoccult) utilizes a heme-catalyzed color change in a phenolic compound for detection. This reagent has good sensitivity, excellent reproducibility, and rare false-positive results. There is only minimal effect of specimen storage, and iron will not cause a false-positive result. An added advantage of the guaiac cards is the ability to test the stool specimen that is obtained by the parent or patient at home and delivered or sent to the physician's office. This not only improves the detection of intermittent bleeding but also may obviate the need for repeated rectal examinations. The tablet tests utilizing the peroxidation of the chromogen orthotoluidine (eg, Hematest) have higher false-positive rates.

Foodstuffs causing false-positive reactions in various tests include iron, high-meat diets, bananas, horseradish, turnips, and tomato skins. Black stools that give a negative guaiac reaction may result from ingestion of iron preparations, bismuth (Pepto-Bismol), lead, licorice, charcoal, coal, or dirt. False-negative reactions may occur with prolonged storage in some reactions, and with high vitamin C intake that interferes with the color change normally produced by peroxidase.

"Red diaper syndrome" may occur with storage of soiled diapers for 24 to 36 hours and is due to *Serratia marcescens,* which produces the red pigmentation. The stools give a negative guaiac reaction.

Type and Color of Bleeding

A description of the color, location, and amount of blood in feces may provide valuable information. Bright red blood or blood streaking of the stool most often is due to distal lesions such as fissures or polyps. In the newborn, an upper GI tract hemorrhage may present with bright red rectal bleeding. The bleeding of a Meckel diverticulum may produce red or dark bleeding. An ileocolic intussusception classically produces a "currant jelly" stool.

Mucus-associated bloody stools may be due to infection, milk and/or soy protein allergy, ischemia, hemolytic-uremic syndrome, or Hirschsprung enterocolitis. Melena is generally a sign of upper GI tract bleeding but may rarely occur with a Meckel diverticulum.

A comprehensive list of the causes of GI bleeding in all pediatric age groups was provided under differential diagnosis. The more frequent etiologies are listed by age group in the following sections. The focus of the initial evaluation should be guided by the patient's age, associated symptoms, and the magnitude of blood loss (Table 58-1).

MOST FREQUENT CAUSES OF RECTAL BLEEDING

Newborn to Infants Aged 3 Months

- Swallowed maternal blood
- Nasopharyngeal trauma
- Anal fissure
- Upper GI tract sources
- Hemorrhagic disease of the newborn
- Anatomic abnormalities

Swallowed Maternal Blood

A well newborn or breast-fed infant with red or tarry rectal bleeding but no other signs of hypovolemia or systemic disease may have swallowed maternal blood from the time of delivery or from breast feeding. The Apt-Downey alkali denaturation test should be performed to determine if the blood is of maternal origin. A specimen of emesis, nasogastric aspirate, or stool is mixed with five to 10 parts water to lyse the red blood cells. Black coffee-grounds material or melena cannot be used because the hemoglobin has been changed to hematin. The pink suspension is then centrifuged and decanted or filtered.

A specimen from the infant's blood and a control (child or adult) blood lysate also is prepared. One milliliter of 0.25N (1% solution) NaOH is mixed with five parts hemoglobin solution. Adult hemoglobin changes from pink to brown-yellow over 2 minutes, whereas fetal hemoglobin remains pink (undenatured).

Nasopharyngeal Trauma

Suctioning following delivery of the newborn or nasopharyngeal trauma may cause upper GI tract bleeding that can manifest itself as rectal bleeding. A careful physical examination will be useful, and history in the older child is helpful.

Anal Fissure

Anal fissure is the most common cause of rectal bleeding in children less than 2 years of age. It presents with recurrent small amounts of bright red blood coating the stool. It may be associated with hard stools or pain during defecation. Visual inspection or anoscopy will identify the lesion. In the older child a fissure or fistula may be associated with systemic symptoms in inflammatory bowel disease.

TABLE 58-1
Etiologies of Rectal Bleeding Based on Age and Common Clinical Presentation

SIGNS	NEONATAL	INFANCY	CHILDHOOD	ADOLESCENCE
Occult blood	Milk or soy allergy; gastric outlet obstruction; oropharyngeal trauma	Milk/soy allergy; esophagitis; peptic disease; gastric outlet obstruction	Esophagitis; peptic disease; gastric outlet obstruction; hemangiomas/ telangiectasias	Peptic disease; esophagitis; vascular malformations
Visible blood, well child	Anal fissure; swallowed maternal blood; fissure; milk/ soy allergy; bleeding disorders	Anal fissure; colonic polyp; swallowed epistaxis; foreign body; nodular lymphoid hyperplasia; gastric heterotopia in ileum	Anal fissure; polyps; foreign body; epistaxis; nodular lymphoid hyperplasia	Polyps; anal fissure; hemorrhoids; foreign body; epistaxis
Evidence of systemic disease	Infections; sepsis; necrotizing enterocolitis; gangrenous bowel; midgut volvulus; intussusception; hemorrhagic disease of the newborn; Hirschsprung disease enterocolitis; tumor; colitis with immune deficiency	Infections; milk/soy allergy; esophagitis; intussusception; gangrenous bowel; antibiotics; parasites; Henoch-Schönlein syndrome; acute colitis	Infections; parasites; antibiotics; esophagitis; Crohn disease; intussusception; hemolytic uremic syndrome; Henoch-Schönlein syndrome; ulcerative colitis; acute colitis	Infection; ulcerative colitis; Crohn disease; acute colitis; parasites
Massive hemorrhage	Hemorrhagic gastritis; peptic ulcer; Meckel diverticulum; duplications; vascular malformations	Meckel diverticulum; gastritis; peptic ulcer; vascular malformations; duplications	Meckel diverticulum; gastritis; peptic ulcer; varices; vascular malformations	Meckel diverticulum; varices; peptic ulcer; gastritis; vascular malformations

Upper Gastrointestinal Tract Sources

The newborn is susceptible to a variety of perinatal stresses that may result in gastric ulceration or hemorrhagic gastritis. Although the usual presentation is hematemesis and hypovolemia, rectal bleeding may be the only symptom. The diagnosis is suggested by prolonged labor, fetal bradycardia, meconium staining, hypoxemia, acidosis, sepsis, or low Apgar scores. Primary central nervous system disease has been associated with peptic ulcers, as have trauma, systemic illness, and burns. A nasogastric tube should always be placed to identify the site of bleeding and to provide accurate ongoing assessment of the extent of current hemorrhages. In older children and adolescents, an upper hemorrhage may present with occult heme positivity or melena without hematemesis. There may be associated nausea, heartburn, or epigastric pain.

A history of aspirin ingestion should be aggressively pursued. All over-the-counter preparations should be reviewed, because the patient and parent may be unaware of the salicylate content in decongestant and cold preparations.

Hemorrhagic Disease of the Newborn

Deficiency of vitamin K results in the most commonly acquired coagulation abnormality in the newborn. There is a normal transient depression of the four clotting factors dependent on vitamin K. Newborns and especially premature infants are at risk. Vitamin K is routinely given in delivery rooms but may be neglected in some situations and in home deliveries. Breast feeding also has been implicated because of the lower concentration of vitamin K in human milk. The GI tract hemorrhage may be large and is associated with other signs of bleeding or bruising. The neonate generally appears well unless there are signs of hemodynamic compromise.

Other acquired coagulopathies occur in sepsis with disseminated intravascular coagulation in an ill-appearing infant. Coagulation abnormalities may be secondary to fat malabsorption in the older child but rarely present with GI tract bleeding.

Hereditary coagulopathies are less common but must be considered in a well-appearing child with GI tract bleeding and abnormal prothrombin and partial thromboplastin times.

Anatomic Abnormalities

Structural lesions of the GI tract may present as rectal bleeding, often with catastrophic results. A midgut volvulus may produce red or tarry stools in an irritable or lethargic infant with a distended abdomen, who appears to be in shock. Volvulus is frequently secondary to an intestinal malrotation with malfixation of the mesentery. Prompt diagnosis based on examination and radiographs is critical for the preservation of viable bowel.

Another structural abnormality is intestinal duplication, which usually presents early in life. The stool may be red to tarry, in variable amounts, and a mass or obstruction may be suspected on examination. Diagnosis is made by upper GI tract series, isotope scans, ultrasound, or laparotomy.

Children—3 Months to 3 Years of Age

- Infection
- Anal fissure
- Milk or soy protein allergy
- Colonic polyp
- Intussusception
- Antibiotic-related colitis
- Meckel diverticulum
- Esophagitis
- Lymphoid hyperplasia
- Peptic ulcer or gastritis
- Structural abnormalities
- Hemolytic uremic syndrome
- Vascular abnormalities

Infection

Infection of the GI tract is common at all ages and frequently presents with bloody stool, often associated with mucus. Culturing for *Salmonella* and *Shigella* alone is inadequate for diagnosis. *Campylobacter* is increasingly recognized as a cause of bloody diarrhea and requires special microbiologic techniques for its isolation. *Yersinia, Aeromonas,* and enteropathogenic *Escherichia coli* may produce a colitis and require special isolation techniques. Parasitic infections such as amebiasis may cause a colitis, mimicking a bacterial infection. Multiple fresh ova and

parasite examinations and specific serum counterimmunoelectrophoresis establish the diagnosis. Viruses may cause heme-positive diarrhea, especially in infancy and in AIDS. Nematode parasites (hookworms, *Trichuris,* or *Strongyloides*) cause occult heme positivity without mucus and are associated with anemia and eosinophilia.

Milk or Soy Protein Allergy

Protein allergy can cause occult or small amounts of visible rectal bleeding and may be associated with mucus in the stool. The onset of disease occurs from the first week of life to 2 years of age. Associated symptoms may include colic, chronic diarrhea, vomiting, rhinitis, wheezing, rash, eczema, or edema. Up to 30% of atopic children may have formula protein allergies. A family history of atopy, early exposure to cow milk protein, or a recent enteritis may be predisposing factors. In younger infants, the syndrome includes severe diarrhea with enteric bleeding, distention, and emesis following exposure to milk protein antigens. Symptoms resolve with elimination of the offending antigens. Because soy and goat milk can have cross-reactivity, an elemental protein formula may be necessary. Other infants present only with chronic mucoid heme-positive diarrhea. Anemia, iron deficiency, hypoproteinemia, and failure to thrive may occur. No laboratory test is totally diagnostic and the clinical response to withdrawal and rechallenge is frequently employed, with clinical remission followed by a recrudescence within 48 hours of rechallenge on repeated trials. Lactose intolerance may simulate diarrheal aspects, but does not cause protein or blood loss in the stool.

Polyp

Juvenile polyps are the most common cause of enteric bleeding in children 2 to 5 years of age (Fig. 58-1). They frequently present with intermittent, mild-to-moderate, bright or dark red blood. This bleeding may persist over months to years and is usually unassociated with pain or failure to thrive. The juvenile polyp is a benign colonic lesion that rarely causes significant bleeding and may undergo spontaneous autoamputation. Chronic significant bleeding or associated symptoms may necessitate colonoscopic polypectomy. The majority are solitary and located in the rectum or sigmoid. Diagnosis is made on rectal examination, via air contrast

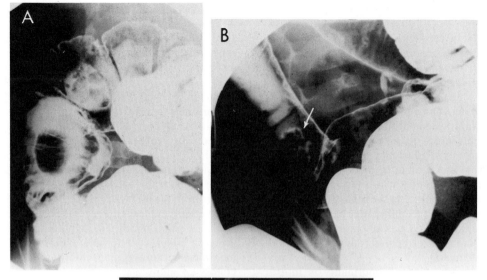

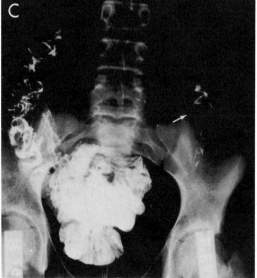

FIG 58-1

Juvenile polyp of the colon. **A,** Coned-down view of the ascending colon reveals a large lesion, well outlined by contrast medium. **B,** When the patient is positioned so that there is contrast material in this portion of the colon. The lesion (arrow) is seen with its irregular margins. **C,** Evacuation film are most helpful to show polypoid lesions. Note how a large juvenile polyp (on another patient) distends the otherwise collapsed descending colon (arrow). [From Haller JO, Slovis TL: Introduction to Radiology in Clinical Pediatrics, Chicago, 1984, Year Book Medical Publishers. Used by permission.]

barium enema in a well-prepared colon or via colonoscopy. All resected polyps should be examined microscopically because of the very rare occurrence of adenomatous change.

Other polyposis syndromes present in child-hood. Peutz-Jeghers syndrome consists of diffuse polyposis of the GI tract and is associated with melanotic areas on the buccal mucosa and lips. The polyps are hamartomas and most frequently occur in the small intestine but may be found from the stomach to the rectum. A small number of the polyps may undergo malignant transformation. The polyps may cause obstruction or serve as a lead point for intussusception.

The autosomal dominant familial polyposis coli, with a late childhood onset, is clearly a premalignant lesion. The majority of polyps, which may number up to thousands per patient, are in the colon. Therapy is colectomy, and genetic counseling is advised.

Gardner syndrome is familial adenomatous polyposis associated with subcutaneous tumors, cysts, and bone lesions. Inheritance is autosomal dominant. The polyps have a high frequency of malignant transformation in early adulthood and colectomy is advised.

Intussusception

Intussusception occurs most commonly during the first 2 years of life. It occurs three times as frequently in boys and is usually ileocolic. Only rarely is there a specific lesion (Meckel diverticulum, polyp, hematoma, or tumor) initiating the intussusception. Gastroduodenal, ileoileal, and colocolic intussusceptions are rare and may present atypically. Intussusception is the most common cause of intestinal obstruction in infants. There may be recurrent attacks of abdominal pain, colic, crying, and drawing up the knees that can progress to vomiting, lethargy, irritability, and "red currant-jelly" stools late in the course. Examination may demonstrate a mass or an empty right lower quadrant. Abdominal tenderness may proceed to peritonitis with perforation. Hydrostatic reduction, the initial treatment of choice, is successful in three fourths of cases. Failure of hydrostatic reduction, significant bleeding, obstruction, peritonitis, or recurrent intussusception necessitates surgery.

Meckel Diverticulum

Usually asymptomatic, Meckel diverticulum, the remnant of the omphalomesenteric duct, is the most common anomaly of the GI tract. Less than half actually contain gastric mucosa. Significant bleeding is more frequent in boys and usually presents in children less than 2 years of age. The bleeding is painless, may be massive, and is usually red or maroon. Meckel diverticulum may lead to obstruction, intussusception, or volvulus. Diagnosis may be suggested by a radionuclide scan with ^{99}Tc pertechnetate that is taken up by

gastric and heterotopic gastric mucosa. Surgery is indicated for a bleeding Meckel diverticulum.

Children and Adolescents—3 to 18 Years of Age

- Infection
- Polyps
- Anal fissure
- Inflammatory bowel disease
- Peptic ulcer disease and/or gastritis
- Varices
- Lymphoid hyperplasia
- Vascular lesions

Inflammatory Bowel Disease (see Chapter 79)

Crohn disease or ulcerative colitis may present with occult or visible rectal bleeding. There are frequently associated systemic complaints including diarrhea, abdominal pain, tenderness, weight loss, anorexia, malaise, fatigue, joint pain, or reduction in linear growth velocity. Family history is positive in about one sixth of cases. Laboratory signs include a microcytic anemia, thrombocytosis, elevated erythrocyte sedimentation rate, hypoalbuminemia, low levels of serum minerals (zinc, magnesium, copper, iron), and water-soluble (folate) and fat-soluble (carotene) vitamins. The final diagnosis will be based on specific colonoscopic and radiographic findings (Fig. 58-2).

Vascular Lesions of the Intestine

Telangiectasias, angiodysplasia, and hemangiomas of the GI tract are rare causes of rectal bleeding in pediatric populations but may be responsible for occasional significant bleeding episodes undiagnosed by other testing. Arterial aneurysms may be seen on arteriography. Several syndromes, including Turner, Osler-Weber-Rendu, blue rubber nevus, and Ehlers-Danlos, may have GI vascular abnormalities with associated bleeding.

DATA GATHERING

History

The most useful diagnostic test in the evaluation of rectal bleeding is a careful history and physical examination. The age of the patient and the associated symptoms will guide the investigation. The initial evaluation should determine if the child has had cardiovascular compromise or

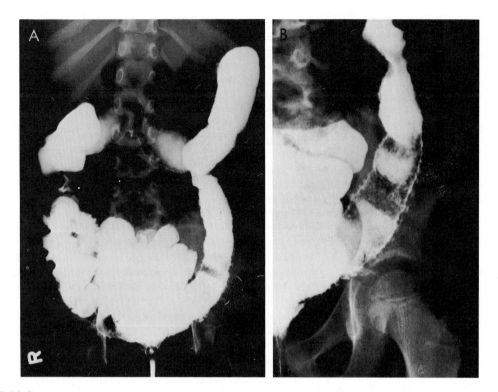

FIG 58-2

Ulcerative colitis. **A,** Frontal film from a barium enema reveals contrast material outside the lumen and in the wall, particularly evident in the descending colon. Note "collar button" ulcerations. **B,** Close-up shows the "collar-button" ulcerations to advantage. The key to diagnosis in this case is the abnormal contour of the bowel. [From Haller JO, Slovis TL: Introduction to Radiology in Clinical Pediatrics, Chicago, 1984, Year Book Medical Publishers.]

if a surgical condition may exist, which would necessitate immediate hospitalization and consultation. The association of bleeding with systemic symptoms such as abdominal pain, diarrhea, weight loss, or fever may be due to infectious or inflammatory conditions of short duration or secondary to inflammatory bowel disease over months or years. Terminal pain with defecation unassociated with abdominal pain suggests fissure or hemorrhoids. Bleeding from a Meckel diverticulum, juvenile polyp, or vascular malformation is nonpainful. Massive bleeding suggests a Meckel diverticulum, vascular anomaly, or upper GI tract hemorrhage.

The presence of other child care or family members with similar concurrent illness suggests an infectious etiology. A family history of polyps, colitis (but not irritable or "spastic" colitis), bleeding disorders, or severe food allergy is useful. Patients with chronic constipation may have a fissure or Hirschsprung enterocolitis (a very rare but serious complication of Hirschsprung disease). Increasingly, an adolescent's sexual activity must be considered in cases of infectious proctitis or anorectal trauma. Anorectal or perineal trauma in a younger child mandates a careful evaluation for child abuse by family or nonfamily caretakers.

All prescription and over-the-counter medications should be reviewed. Antecedent viral infections may not only be treated with aspirin or antibiotic-containing medications leading to GI bleeding, but also may be the prodromal phase of diseases that may present with a colitis (hemolytic-uremic syndrome). Recent anorexia, hypoglycemia, hypoperfusion, or intrinsic cardiac disease may result in ischemic colitis.

The following information should be gathered at history-taking:

- Age of patient
- Estimation of the quantity of blood loss
- Condition of the patient
- Character of blood
- Association with abdominal or rectal pain
- Association with diarrhea or mucus
- Association with fever
- Association with other systemic symptoms (arthritis or uveitis)
- Failure to thrive or to grow
- Recent illnesses
- Family history of GI diseases
- Family history of bleeding disorders
- Travel history
- Drinking water

Physical Examination

The initial assessment should determine the extent and duration of recent and ongoing blood losses. Attention to vital signs is more reliable than estimation of blood loss, which may be exaggerated. Evidence of skin lesions or bruising may support coagulopathy, vasculitis (Henoch-Schönlein syndrome), or inflammatory bowel disease (pyoderma gangrenosum, erythema nodosum). Pallor may be due to decreased perfusion or anemia. Abdominal pain, distention, or an "acute" abdomen may be present in intussusception or midgut volvulus, or may indicate infection or inflammatory bowel disease. A careful perirectal examination will reveal fissures or fistulae. The digital rectal examination will confirm the presence of blood and may reveal a distal polyp. Physical examination should include determination or evaluation of the following:

- Vital signs (heart rate, blood pressure, temperature)
- General condition
- Skin vascular lesions, pallor, or bruising
- Evidence of oropharyngeal trauma or epistaxis
- Cardiac abnormalities
- Abdominal pain
- Organomegaly
- Rectal examination to verify blood in stools and identify fissures, fistulae, and distal polyps

Laboratory Evaluation

The laboratory tests, outlined in this section, help organize an evaluation. The first stage, guided by the history and physical examination, contains hematology tests and cultures. The second stage involves direct observation or imaging. The sulfur colloid test or tagged red blood cell scans may demonstrate active bleeding. The technetium scan will be concentrated in gastric mucosa, which will help identify a Meckel diverticulum.

Laboratory Evaluation

First stage (guided by history and physical examination)
- Complete blood cell count, differential cell count, platelet count
- Reticulocyte count
- Erythrocyte sedimentation rate
- Stool cultures
- Stool ova and parasites
- Apt-Downey test
- Serologic evidence of chronic malnutrition
Second stage
- Nasogastric aspiration to rule out upper GI tract bleeding
- Sigmoidoscopy or colonoscopy
- Sulfur colloid or red blood cell bleeding scan
- Technetium Meckel scan
- Abdominal radiograph for "thumbprinting," obstruction
- Barium enema with air contrast
- Pentagastrin-stimulated scan for Meckel diverticulum
- Upper GI tract barium series with small bowel follow-through
Third stage
- Arteriography
- Surgical exploration

INDICATIONS FOR CONSULTATION OR REFERRAL

The evaluation of rectal bleeding can usually be coordinated in the outpatient setting. Screening serologic studies and stool cultures should be performed before an advanced evaluation is performed. Radiographic, sigmoidoscopic, and nuclear medicine scans can be performed on most patients on an ambulatory basis.

DISCUSSION OF ALGORITHM

The evaluation of rectal bleeding is guided by the age of the patient in association with the particular symptoms and signs. The "decision tree"

RECTAL BLEEDING
Differential diagnosis

Arteriovenous (AV) malformation	Inflammatory bowel disease	Polyp
Colitis	Intussusception	Swallowed blood
Constipation	Meckel diverticulum	Stricture
Duplication	Milk protein allergy	Viral enteritis
Fissures	Necrotizing enterocolitis (NEC)	Volvulus
Enteritis		

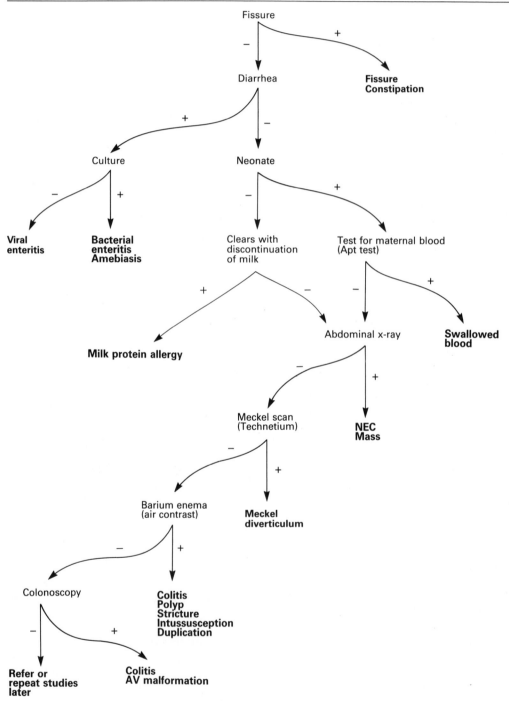

FIG 58-3

Decision tree for differential diagnosis of rectal bleeding.

(Fig. 58-3) stresses a differential diagnosis based on the age of the patient and knowledge of the circumstances under which the blood loss is identified. Table 58-1 stresses the large number of conditions that may result in rectal bleeding.

Categorization based on whether blood loss is occult, visible but in a well child, associated with systemic findings, or a result of massive hemorrhage will aid narrowing the diagnostic consideration.

BIBLIOGRAPHY

Hyams JS, Leitner AM, Schwartz AN: Recent advances in the diagnosis and treatment of gastrointestinal hemorrhage in infants and children, *J Pediatr* 106:1–9, 1985.

Nagita A, Amemoto K, Yoden A, Yamazaki T, Mino M, Miyoshi H: Ultrasonographic diagnosis of juvenile colonic polyps, *J Pediatr* 124(4):535–540, 1994.

Silber G: Lower gastrointestinal bleeding, *Pediatr Rev* 12:85–93, 1990.

Teach SJ, Fleisher GR: Rectal bleeding the pediatric emergency department, *Ann Emerg Med* 23(6):1252–1258, 1994.

Vinton NE: Gastrointestinal bleeding in infancy and childhood, *Gastroenterol Clin North Am* 23(1):93–122, 1944.

CHAPTER 59

Red Eye

Stephen D. Kronwith
David B. Schaffer

The term "red eye" is used to denote a myriad of ocular entities, including trauma, infection, allergy, and underlying systemic processes. Parents of children with discoloration, swelling, itching, pain, excessive tearing, photophobia, decreased vision, and frank trauma all seek medical advice and help. The purpose of this chapter is to help the clinician recognize and identify the specific location and probable cause of the eye disorder, understand its immediate significance and potential complications, institute appropriate initial and even definitive therapy, or refer the patient to an ophthalmologist for more involved diagnostic techniques and treatment.

DIFFERENTIAL DIAGNOSIS

Common Causes of Red Eye
Ocular adnexa
- **Trauma**
  Blunt
  Lid swelling or discoloration
  Hyphema
  Ruptured globe
  Iris or lens abnormality
  Retinal abnormality
  Orbital bone fracture
  Suspected child abuse or neglect
  Sharp

Lacerations of lid
Underlying lacerations of globe
- **Inflammation**
  Localized
  Blepharitis
  Hordeolums and chalazions
  Dacryocystitis
  Generalized
  Periorbital (preseptal) cellulitis
  Orbital cellulitis
  Other
  Viral
  Allergic
  Insect bites
  Contact dermatitis
  Systemic
  Reactive blepharospasm
Conjunctiva
- **Trauma**
  Subconjunctival hemorrhage
  Foreign body
- **Inflammation**
  Conjunctivitis
  Neonatal (ophthalmia neonatorum)
  Chemical
  Bacterial
  Viral
  Obstructed nasolacrimal duct
  Older children
  Bacterial
  Viral
  Allergic
  Vernal catarrh
  Limbal catarrh
- **Systemic reaction**
  Phlyctenular
  Other systemic disease
  Physical or chemical irritant
Cornea
- **Trauma**
  Foreign body
  Abrasions
  Physical or chemical irritant
- **Inflammation**
  Ulceration
  Keratitis
Anterior segment
- **Trauma**
- **Inflammation**
Posterior eye
- **Decreased visual acuity**
- **Abnormal findings on ophthalmoscopy**

Discussion

Ocular Adnexa (Orbit and Lids)

Nonpenetrating trauma to the ocular adnexa may belie its seriousness. Under a swollen, intact but discolored, traumatized lid could be a ruptured globe, painful iridocyclitis, anterior chamber bleeding (hyphema), retinal detachment, or a blowout fracture of one of the orbital bones. If the eye is intact, visual acuity and pupillary size and reactivity should be compared with those of the uninjured eye. Patients who have obviously decreased vision, a hyphema, an unresponsive pupil, restricted motility, inferior orbital skin anesthesia, periorbital crepitus, or lack of visualization of a normal posterior fundus on ophthalmoscopy should be referred.

If there is even suspicion that the integrity of the brain or the eye has been violated, the child should not ingest any food or liquids and should be transported for definitive care. Both eyes should be taped closed under soft eye pads, with a protective hard shield over the injured eye.

Inflammatory discoloration and swelling of the adnexal structures also can denote trivial or significant disease. Scaling at the lid margins, styes (hordeolums) or chalazions, dacryocystitis, allergic reactions, and superficial or deep orbital cellulitis are collectively more common adnexal problems than is trauma.

Inflammation of the lid margins (blepharitis) frequently is seen in the pediatric population. The typical findings consist of waxy scaling at the base of the lashes (Fig. 59-1); red, irritated, slightly swollen lid margins; loss of lashes; and even lid margin ulceration in the more severe forms. Mild to moderate conjunctivitis is common, and occasionally there is corneal involvement (keratitis). Treatment consists of daily cleansing of the lid margins with baby shampoo and warm water. If needed, an antimicrobial ophthalmic ointment also is massaged onto the lid margins. Once resolved, the medication is titrated to the least frequent application that keeps the condition quiescent. Recurrence is common.

Rarely, pediculosis can mimic seborrheic blepharitis. With proper magnification, visualization of black lice eggs attached to the cilia confirms the diagnosis. Manual removal of the lice and their eggs is required.

Styes are acute, often painful, localized bacterial infections arising in either a gland of the lid's

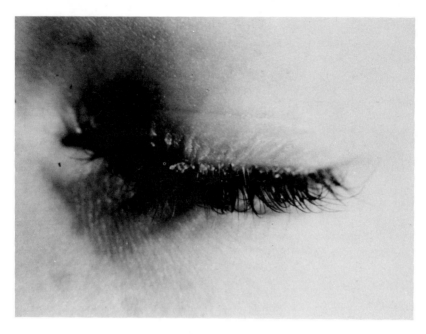

FIG 59-1
Encrustations at base of lashes and wrinkling of the eyelid.

fibrous tarsal plate or in the glands located around the eyelashes. The causal organisms are usually *Staphylococcus aureus* or nonhemolytic *Streptococcus*. Most styes cause erythematous swelling of the involved lid, with a localized tender mass that may point, rupture, and drain through the palpebral conjunctival surface, at the lid margin, or through the external skin (Fig. 59-2). Treatment consists of frequent application of hot compresses.

The oil secreted by each meibomian gland may break out of the gland into the lid tissue and produce a granuloma called a *chalazion*. Although acute meibomitis is painful, the chronic granulomatous chalazion slowly undergoes painless enlargement and can be palpated as a firm, nonmovable nodule, often presenting on the palpebral surface of the lid as a yellowish-white area (Fig. 59-3). In time, large chalazions may produce significant astigmatism because of chronic pressure on the cornea. Although hot compresses decrease its size, a chalazion usually must be surgically incised.

In neonates and very young infants, acute dacryocystitis also can produce inflamed, tender, localized swelling in the lid, typically at the inferonasal border of the bony orbital rim (Fig. 59-4). These abscesses can be associated with fever and elevated white blood cell (WBC) counts. The abscessed sac can be decompressed by aspiration of its purulent contents with a fine needle, which relieves symptoms and produces a specimen for culture and sensitivity tests. Appropriate intravenous antibiotics should be started. Once under control, definitive irrigation and probing of the lacrimal drainage system must be performed.

By far the most serious inflammatory processes involving the ocular adnexa are preorbital and orbital cellulitis, both of which are almost invariably unilateral. Either condition may result in a number of significant complications (eg, orbital or subperiosteal abscesses, cavernous sinus thrombosis, extradural brain abscess, meningitis, and osteomyelitis of the skull) and therefore requires hospitalization. Predisposing factors for either disease include sinusitis (most commonly ethmoid and maxillary), coryza, otitis media, local trauma, and local skin infections. Many patients have a history of a recent cold that was partially treated. The most frequent causal organisms are *Haemophilus*, parainfluenza virus,

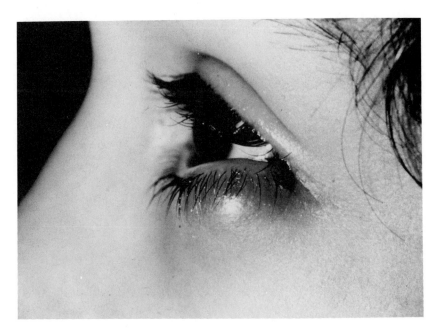

FIG 59-2
External hordeolum (stye) of the inferior lid just before spontaneous rupture and drainage.

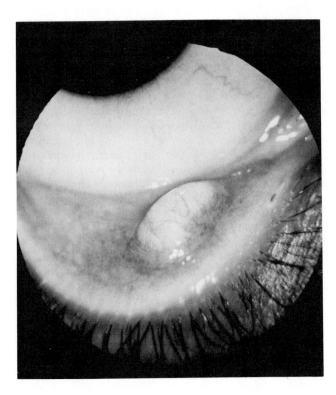

FIG 59-3
Chronic chalazion. Note the large, raised, yellowish granuloma on the internal aspect of the lower eyelid.

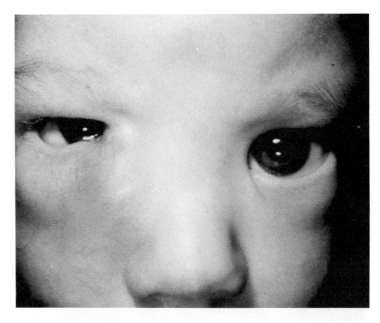

FIG 59-4
Swollen, inflamed lacrimal sac (dacryocystitis) at the inferonasal border of the orbit. Courtesy of Dr. James A Katowitz.

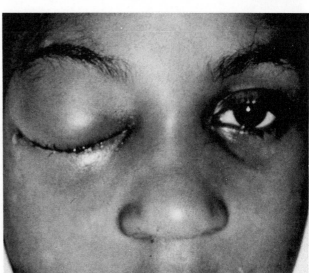

FIG 59-5
Preorbital cellulitis. Note that the child appears alert and the eye is not proptosed.

S. aureus, β-hemolytic *Streptococcus,* and *Streptococcus pneumonia.*

Local findings of periorbital (preseptal) cellulitis consist of painless erythema and edema of the eyelids (Fig. 59-5). The conjunctiva usually is not congested or chemotic, there is little to no discharge, and ocular motility and vision are normal. Rhinorrhea is frequent; the patient is often alert, irritable, febrile, and has significant leukocytosis. There often is a previous history of recent trauma to the involved lid.

In contrast, orbital cellulitis presents with marked pain, redness, and swelling of the lids, with marked conjunctival injection, chemosis, and obviously decreased ocular motility. Proptosis may be present (Fig. 59-6). A dilated pupil with abnormal responsiveness and decreased visual acuity may occur from inflammation surrounding the eye and from compression of the optic nerve. The fundus may reveal retinal vascular engorgement and low-grade papilledema, both grave findings heralding the begin-

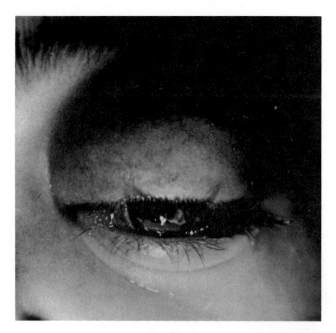

FIG 59-6
Orbital cellulitis. Lids are swollen but eye is proptosed. Conjunctiva is chemotic and engorged, and the cornea is exposed.

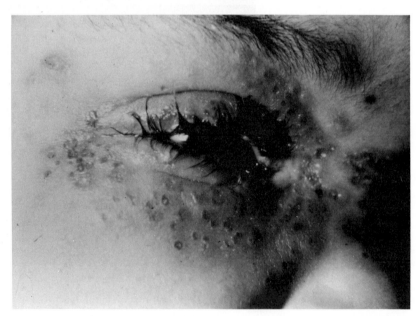

FIG 59-7
Primary herpes simplex causing periorbital cellulitis. Secondary bacterial invasion is causing purulent discharge, and the eye itself is not involved.

ning of cavernous sinus thrombosis. The patient is not always alert, is very irritable, may have a stiff neck, is febrile, and has a markedly elevated WBC count.

Not all swollen or erythematous eyelids are due to trauma or cellulitis. Insect bites, contact dermatitis, varicella-zoster reactions, and primary herpes simplex (Fig. 59-7) can all present with swollen lids. However, the possible underlying ocular involvement is a far more important

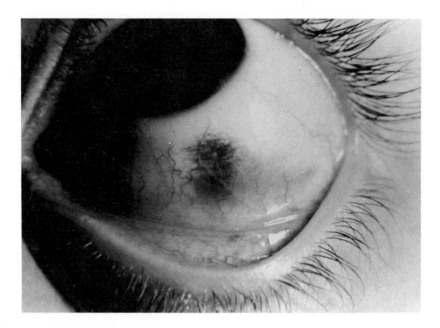

FIG 59-8
Subconjunctival hemorrhage from sneezing.

consideration. If the eye itself is involved, referral is necessary.

Recurrent painless ecchymosis of the lids may occur in children with hemophilia and can even be the hallmark of a nonpalpable orbital neuroblastoma. Furthermore, any recurrent traumatic finding around the eye must suggest child abuse or neglect.

Conjunctiva

Rupture of a small bulbar conjunctival vessel can result in extravasation of blood (Fig. 59-8) between the transparent conjunctiva and the sclera. This bright red subconjunctival hemorrhage frequently is caused by hard coughing, sneezing, vomiting, or other action that produces a Valsalva-like maneuver. It also can occur from the innocent rubbing of the eye, from foreign bodies on the conjunctiva, and from more serious injuries. Simple subconjunctival hemorrhage is asymptomatic, requires no treatment, and will absorb spontaneously in days to weeks, depending on its extent. Recurrent subconjunctival hemorrhages may be a sign of a blood dyscrasia or hypertension.

Foreign bodies in the conjunctiva cause various degrees of discomfort, congestion, lacrimation, and photophobia. If a foreign body is suspected and not immediately visible, the upper lid should be everted and its surface inspected. Once located, a foreign body is usually easily removed with a sterile, moist cotton swab. After removal of the foreign body the cornea should be checked with fluorescein. If staining is noted, local antibiotic drops should be used until the cornea heals (1 to 2 days). Topical anesthetics should never be prescribed, because they retard healing and mask the pain of either a worsening condition or incidental injury.

Conjunctivitis (pink eye) is the commonest ophthalmologic problem. It consists of a minimally painful conjunctival hyperemia associated with some type of discharge. The cornea is clear, the pupil is normal, and the vision is only slightly, if at all, decreased. Conjunctivitis is caused by many infectious agents, allergy, or chemical or gaseous irritants.

Newborn infants are prone to a few particular types of potentially serious conjunctividities, grouped under the term *ophthalmia neonatorum*. Chemical ophthalmia neonatorium results from silver nitrate (Credé ointment). Frequently unilateral, it occurs on the first day of life and is characterized by blepharospasm and injected, swollen conjunctiva and lids with occasional rapidly clearing corneal haze. In the absence of any secondary bacterial infection, this

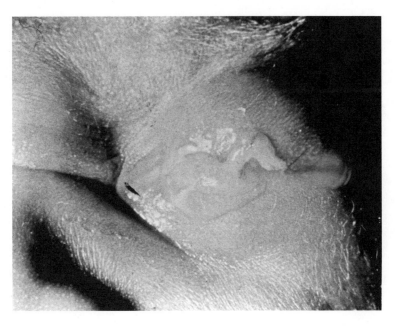

FIG 59-9
Marked lid edema and massive purulent discharge common with gonococcal ophthalmia neonatorum.

common conjunctivitis resolves rapidly and is rarely seen in an outpatient office.

In children between 2 days and 1 month of age, ophthalmia neonatorum usually presents with markedly swollen eyelids, hemorrhagic chemotic conjunctiva, and a purulent discharge (Fig. 59-9). This appearance can be caused by any acute bacterial infection, by *Chlamydia trachomatis,* and by the herpes simplex viruses (HSV)-1 or -2. The most immediate need is to rule out *Neisseria gonorrhoeae,* which can penetrate an intact cornea and rapidly result in destruction of the eye. The heavy purulent discharge should be rinsed away, followed by a rigorous scraping of the palpebral conjunctival epithelium for specimens to be smeared with both Gram and Giemsa stains and inoculated directly onto Thayer-Martin medium or chocolate agar. Viral cultures for HSV and *Chlamydia* also should be obtained.

The finding of intraepithelial gram-negative diplococci on the smear is enough for a presumptive diagnosis of gonococcal conjunctivitis, and topical gentamycin or bacitracin should be applied every 2 hours until the results of the culture and sensitivity test are known. More important, saline lavage of the infected area should be done as often as needed to remove purulent discharge.

Hospitalization is mandatory, along with intravenous administration of appropriate antibodies.

C. trachomatis is the most frequent cause of ophthalmia neonatorum. Although its onset is usually later than gonococcal infections (5 to 30 days postpartum), it can produce a purulent hemorrhagic picture (Fig. 59-10) similar to any acute bacterial involvement or milder variant. Treatment consists of local sulfonamides, erythromycin, or tetracycline given four times daily for 2 weeks. Chlamydial pneumonitis occurs occasionally, and some clinicians use systemic erythromycin along with topical drugs. Gonococcal and chlamydial conjunctivitis can occur concomitantly, and treatment for one organism may not be effective against the other.

Severe ophthalmia neonatorum occurs in more than 5% of neonates infected with HSV. Onset begins between 3 to 14 days after birth. Unilateral or bilateral, it starts with lid edema, followed quickly by conjunctival hyperemia and swelling with a serosanguineous exudate. Early HSV is indistinguishable from chlamydial infections, and secondary bacterial invasion causes a heavy purulent discharge similar to gonorrhea. Keratitis is a common complication, ending in corneal scarring. Availability of specific antiviral drugs

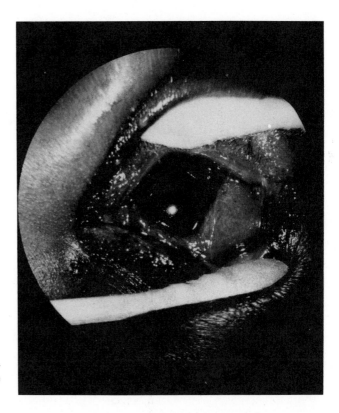

FIG 59-10
An infant, aged 9 days, with a severe hemorrhagic chemotic ophthalmia neonatorum from *C. trachomatis.*

makes it imperative to establish the presence of the virus as well as its type. Because of the frequency of corneal involvement, HSV infections should be followed up by an ophthalmologist.

Persistent or recurrent conjunctivitis in the newborn should raise the question of an obstructed nasolacrimal system. Tearing (epiphora) and a mucopurulent discharge may be present without obvious swelling of the lacrimal sac. Simple pressure on the sac usually causes the expulsion of purulent material. The discharge should be cultured and appropriate local antibiotics started; frequent, firm downward massage of the sac often results in opening of the obstructed tear duct without the need for surgical probing. If symptoms persist to 1 year of age, probing is recommended.

In contrast to ophthalmia neonatorum, bacterial conjunctivitis in older children rarely requires a workup. Most clear within 48 to 72 hours with antibacterial preparations. Bacterial conjunctivitis often is unilateral and not associated with fever. The palpebral conjunctiva is more injected than the bulbar conjunctiva, and there

usually is a mucopurulent or purulent discharge (Fig. 59-11). The lashes are often matted, especially in the morning, and both preauricular and submandibular lymph node swelling can occur. There should be no pain or photophobia, no corneal involvement, no change in pupillary size or response, and no decrease in vision beyond that thought reasonable as secondary to the blurring caused by the purulent discharge.

Viral conjunctivitis occurs more frequently than bacterial conjunctivitis, is often bilateral with a watery discharge, and is frequently associated with upper respiratory tract symptoms and fever. Resistant to treatment, the infection usually lasts longer than bacterial disease. The lack of response to therapy, the annoying tearing and gritty sensation, and the prolonged course are often the reasons these patients are improperly given local steroid-antimicrobial preparations, with the hope of symptomatic relief. Except for a local pure decongestant or antibiotic, no medication is indicated for viral conjunctivitis. Local steroids can have serious ocular side effects, and the antiviral agents are usually saved for specific viruses (HSV). Some strains of ade-

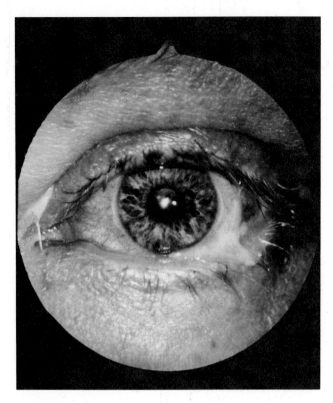

FIG 59-11
Diffuse conjunctival injection and heavy purulent discharge in a child, aged 10 years, with acute *H. influenzae* conjunctivitis.

noviruses can cause corneal scarring, and viral conjunctivitis with obvious corneal opacities or a decrease in visual acuity not seemingly attributable to tearing should be referred to an ophthalmologist.

Allergic reactions are often seasonal or associated with a particular contact. The itching and tearing are often disproportionate to the findings, which consist of pale, edematous bilateral conjunctival and lid swelling. In its mildest form, the lower lids are most involved (Fig. 59-12). However, severe allergic conjunctivitis (vernal catarrh) can have large cobblestone-like papillary hypertrophy, best seen by everting the upper lids. There also may be pronounced photophobia and circumcorneal injection. A third type of allergic conjunctivitis is limbal vernal catarrh, in which the palpebral reaction may be minimal, but there are white infiltrates within the limbus (Fig. 59-13). Mild allergic conjunctivitis may respond to local and systemic antihistamines; the more severe forms usually require referral to both an allergist and an ophthalmologist, because systemic desensitization is needed as well as rather extensive use of local steroids.

A somewhat similar reaction is phlyctenular conjunctivitis, a localized allergic response in the conjunctiva at or close to the limbus. The phlyctenule results from an antigenic stimulus arising somewhere in the body. In the past it was almost synonymous with tuberculosis, but in the United States today it most often occurs as an allergy to some underlying bacterial infection, usually *S. aureus.* Topical steroids are indicated.

Chemical and gaseous conjunctivitis also occur commonly. The principal and most important treatment is immediate irrigation with water. Contact lenses, if present, should be removed immediately. Once the patient reaches any medical facility, further irrigation must be continued. This is best accomplished by instilling a local anesthetic, retracting the lid, and pouring 1 to 2 L of sterile saline solution directly onto the eye. The upper lid and lower fornix should be inverted and swept with a cotton swab to remove any particulate matter. Never try to neutralize acids with bases or vice versa. These patients should be referred to an ophthalmologist.

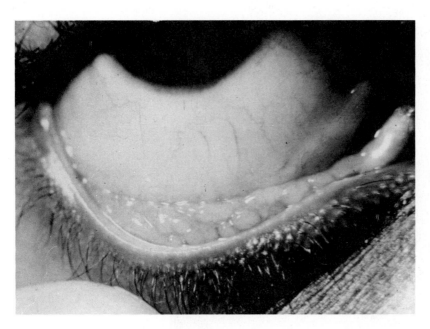

FIG 59-12
Allergic papillary response of lower palpebral conjunctiva.

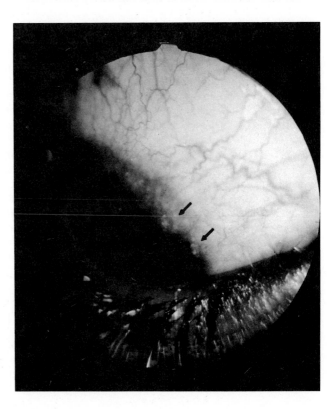

FIG 59-13
Limbal vernal catarrh. The white dots (arrows) in the superior limbal area are focal collections of degenerated eosinophils.

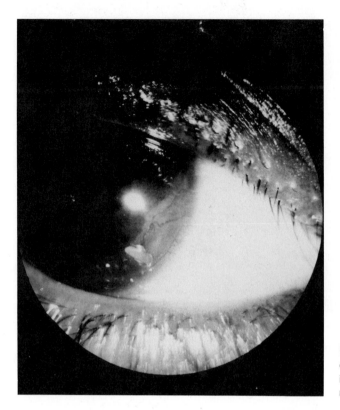

FIG 59-14
Chronic foreign body of the cornea producing hazy white edema as well as early corneal neovascularization.

Cornea and Anterior Segment

Trauma to the cornea most commonly results from small airborne particles, and includes blepharospasm, tearing, local sharp pain, and photophobia. Conjunctival congestion is rapid and followed by a deeper circumcorneal (limbal) flush. Secondary spasm of the muscles of the iris and ciliary body causes pupillary constriction and even severe headache. If not removed, the foreign body can cause edematous clouding and even vascularization of the cornea (Fig. 59-14). Removal of corneal foreign bodies requires a local anesthetic to break the blepharospasm. A sterile, moist cotton swab should be tried first, and sharp instrumentation (sterile metal spud or syringe needle) used only if the swab fails. After removal, there will always be a residual corneal defect that stains with fluorescein, so prophylactic local antibiotic drops should be used until the abrasion heals. A simple soft eye patch can be taped over closed lids to promote comfort, but if there is marked ciliary spasm, a cycloplegic agent is needed to stop the pain.

Continued use of a local anesthetic for comfort while healing takes place should never be prescribed.

Primary corneal abrasions and scratches from fingernails, pets, branches, cigarette burns, and other objects can be treated as for a foreign body. However, these abrasions tend to be large and more contaminated, and healing can take several days. Any evidence of corneal clouding during the acute or healing phase of an abrasion should warrant referral, because it is the earliest sign of onset of a corneal ulcer. Repeated trauma, especially cigarette burns, should alert the clinician to the possibility of child abuse.

Exposure to excessive ultraviolet light, chlorine in swimming pools, many aerosol sprays, tear gas, and other noxious gases can all cause diffuse superficial punctate corneal abrasions that are painful. The history, severe pain, photophobia, excessive lacrimation, and circumlimbal flush are diagnostic; immediate relief with a drop of local anesthetic helps confirm the diagnosis. Once the eyes are irrigated with sterile saline

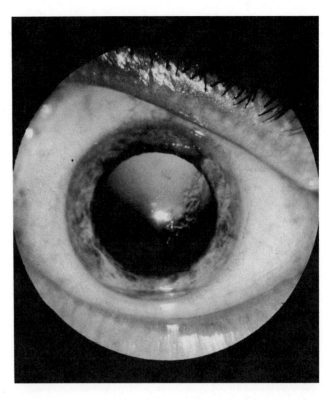

FIG 59-15
Fine circumcorneal (limbal) flush with acute herpes simplex keratitis. The dendritic nature of the acute herpes lesion can be seen within the dilated pupil by using the red reflex as viewed through a direct ophthalmoscope.

solution, periodic instillation of a cycloplegic agent combined with patching of both eyes should allow enough comfort during healing (less than 24 hours).

Inflammation of the cornea (keratitis) may not be quite so symptomatic as trauma, but decreased vision, photophobia, and especially limbal flush (Fig. 59-15) associated with any visible corneal lesion are reason enough for referral.

Anterior segment (aqueous, iris, lens, ciliary body) disorders mimic symptoms and signs of corneal disease, and once detected demand appropriate consultation. Irritation of the iris and ciliary body (iridocyclitis) can result from trauma or infection; the telltale sign is ciliary flush (Figs. 59-16 and 59-17).

Posterior Segment
Purely posterior (vitreous, retina, optic nerve) problems commonly cause decreased vision. Without obvious anterior trauma or inflammation, the eye is usually asymptomatic. The patient who has unexplained decreased vi-

sion in one or both eyes should see an ophthalmologist.

DATA GATHERING

For any acute eye problem, history taking is often quickly accomplished and usually governed by the immediate appearance of the child as he/she enters the office. First, was there trauma? Was it physical, chemical (acid or alkali), or thermal? Is there decreased vision, foreign body sensation, or pain? The answers to the questions can tell the examiner at once if the child needs direct referral. In the absence of trauma, history taking can be accomplished more leisurely and in more detail. Is there decreased vision, pain, or other uncomfortable sensation (photophobia, tearing, itching)? Is it acute, chronic, or recurrent; unilateral or bilateral? Are there associated acute systemic findings such as fever, irritability, or upper respiratory tract or gastrointestinal tract symptoms? Does the child have any primary disease or syn-

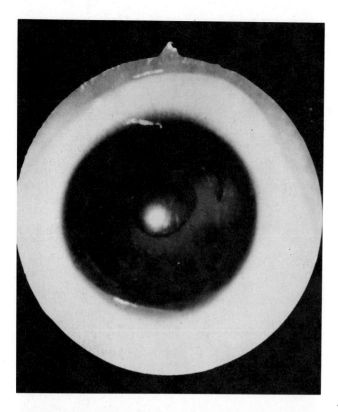

FIG 59-16
Layered hyphema (blood) in the anterior chamber. Note the corneal lesion (by fluorescein staining) and irregular pupil. The eye was struck while open.

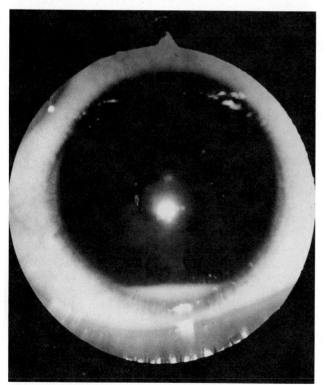

FIG 59-17
Red ciliary flush, irregular pupil, and layer of white blood cells (hypopyon).

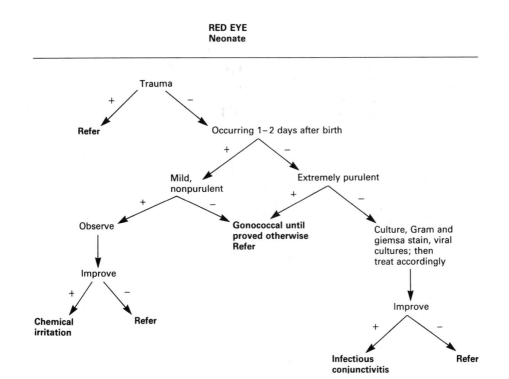

FIG 59-18
Decision tree for red eye in the neonate.

drome associated with ocular changes (*eg*, prematurity, juvenile rheumatoid arthritis, Marfan syndrome, homocystinuria, phakomatosis, tuberculosis, sarcoidosis, allergic or immunologic disorder)?

INDICATIONS FOR REFERRAL OR CONSULTATION

The following causes of red eye require that the patient be referred to an ophthalmologist (compare with the differential diagnosis).

Ocular Problems Requiring Referral
Ocular adnexa
- **Trauma**
  Punctures and lacerations
  Orbital blow-out fractures
- **Inflammation**
  Persistent chalazions
  Acute dacryocystitis
  Periorbital cellulitis
  Orbital cellulitis
- **Intractable blepharospasm**
Conjunctiva
- **Trauma**
  Lacerations >5 mm
  Chemical or gaseous burns
- **Inflammation**
  Ophthalmia neonatorum
    Gonococcal
    Herpes simplex
  Recurrent conjunctivitis
Cornea
- **Trauma**
  Large abrasions (more than one fourth
    corneal diameter)
  All lacerations
  Chemical burns
  Thermal burns
- **Inflammation**
  All keratitis
  All cloudy corneas
Anterior segment
- **Trauma**
  Hyphema
  Torn iris
  Dislocated lens
  Steamy cornea (glaucoma)
- **Inflammation**
  Hypopion

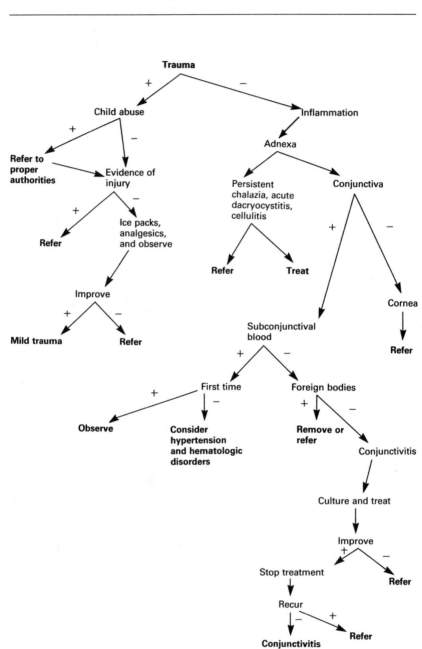

RED EYE
Older child

FIG 59-19
Decision tree for red eye in the older child.

Bound-down pupil
Hazy cornea (endothelial debris)
Posterior eye
   Unexplained decrease in vision
   Abnormal findings on ophthalmoscopy

SUMMARY

It is important to realize the extreme range of diagnoses that red eye brings to mind (Figs. 59-18 and 59-19). An orderly approach involves proper history taking, rapid in instances of obvious trauma and in-depth when time allows. Attention to all the symptoms, an accurate assessment of the visual acuity, a logical step-by-step examination of the ocular adnexa and thorough and gentle evaluation of the globe should afford most clinicians with sufficient and appropriate data to identify the cause and location of the ocular irritant. Once done, the ability to treat or the need to refer should be immediately clear.

BIBLIOGRAPHY

Katowitz JA: Trauma to the eye and adnexa. In Kelly VC, editor: *Practice of pediatrics,* vol 10, Philadelphia, 1983, Harper & Row.

Katowitz JA: Lacrimal drainage surgery. In Duane TD, editor: *Clinical ophthalmology,* vol 5, Philadelphia, 1983, Harper & Row.

Raucher RS, Newton MJ: New issues in the prevention and treatment of ophthalmia neonatorum, *Ann Ophthalmol* 15:1004–1009, 1983.

Rubenstein JB, Handler DS: Orbital and periorbital cellulitis in children, *Head Neck Surg* 5:15–21, 1982.

Schaffer DB: Eye findings in intrauterine infections. In Plotkin SA, Starr SE, editors: *Clinical perinatology,* Philadelphia, 1981, WB Saunders.

Schaffer DB: Pediatric ophthalmology. In Scheie HG, Albert DM, editors: *Textbook of ophthalmology,* ed 9, Philadelphia, 1977, WB Saunders.

Scheie HG, Albert DM, editors: Ophthalmic overview: An introduction to ophthalmic diseases and their terminology. In *Textbook of ophthalmology,* ed 9, Philadelphia, 1977, WB Saunders.

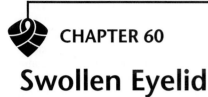

CHAPTER 60

Swollen Eyelid

Nicholas Tsarouhas

Because of the very thin skin of the eyelid and the loose subcutaneous periorbital tissues, dramatic swelling frequently occurs. The physician must consider a broad differential diagnosis before embarking on a therapeutic course of action.

DIFFERENTIAL DIAGNOSIS

Common Causes of Swollen Eyelid

- **Infectious**
  - Periorbital cellulitis
  - Orbital cellulitis
  - Conjunctivitis
  - Sinusitis
  - Cavernous sinus thrombosis
  - Dacryocystitis
  - Hordeolum
- **Allergic**
  - Insect stings
  - Contact dermatitis
  - Medications
  - Foods
  - Inhalants
  - Serum sickness
- **Traumatic**
  - Injuries
  - Foreign bodies
- **Malignant**
  - Retinoblastoma
  - Neuroblastoma
  - Leukemia/lymphoma
  - Rhabdomyosarcoma
- **Systemic**
  - Cardiac
  - Renal
  - Thyroid
  - Gastrointestinal/hepatic
  - Collagen-vascular

Discussion

Periorbital Cellulitis

The preseptal space is defined as the area between the eyelid skin and the orbital septum. The orbital septum is a continuation of the periosteum and is bounded by dense connective tissue attachments at the superior and inferior orbital rims (Fig. 60-1). Inflammatory edema anterior to this orbital septum leads to marked periorbital swelling.

Tender, erythematous, periorbital edema in a febrile child may indicate periorbital cellulitis. The key question to answer is whether the skin was breached by some traumatic event. If this is the case, then *Staphylococcus* or *Streptococcus* species are the likely microbial culprits. A bug bite, abrasion, laceration, or excoriated rash is often an important clue (Fig. 60-2).

If no obvious skin breach is detected, hematogenous dissemination may be a possibility. In this event, *Hemophilus influenzae* type b (HIB) must be considered in children less than 5 years of age. Fortunately, the incidence of invasive HIB disease has been declining since immunization began against this pathogen. If at least two HIB vaccines have been administered, the likelihood of hematogenous periorbital cellulitis is low. A violaceous hue has been touted as a good indicator of HIB disease, but this finding is neither sensitive nor specific.

In the "prevaccination" literature, up to 25% of blood cultures in children younger than 5 years of age with periorbital cellulitis were positive. A lumbar puncture should be considered if a breach in the periorbital skin cannot be found but may be omitted in well-appearing children without meningeal signs. A computed tomography (CT) scan of the orbits is necessary only in severe cases of periorbital cellulitis when the

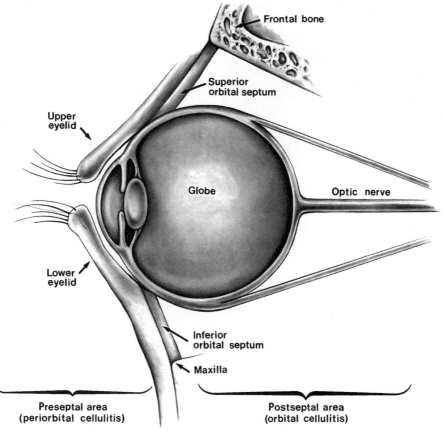

FIG 60-1
The orbit and its septum.

distinction between orbital cellulitis (discussed below) is in doubt.

The majority of children with periorbital cellulitis should be hospitalized and treated with intravenous antibiotics against *Staphylococcus,* *Streptococcus,* and *H. influenzae,* especially if HIB is suspected. Most hospitalized children can be discharged after 2 to 3 days when the physical examination has improved and they have been afebrile for at least 24 hours. Well-appearing children who are older than 5 years of age and have only mild periorbital inflammation may be managed as outpatients. These children should receive oral antibiotics effective against *Staphylococcus* and *Streptococcus* and daily follow-up to ensure steady improvement. A 10-day total course of antibiotics is recommended.

Orbital Cellulitis

Orbital cellulitis is an infection that occurs posterior to the orbital septum. Infiltration of orbital fat and extraocular muscles cause the classic findings of proptosis and ophthalmoplegia, which distinguish orbital from periorbital cellulitis. Visual disturbances also are suggestive of this diagnosis. Most orbital cellulitis results from a spread from an adjacent sinus infection, although dental infections are sometimes implicated. Patients with suspected orbital cellulitis should have a CT scan of the head to delineate the extent of their orbital disease. All children with orbital cellulitis should have a blood culture drawn and be admitted for several days of high-dose intravenous antibiotics active against *Staphylococcus, Streptococcus,* *H. influenzae,* and anaerobes. Fortunately, or-

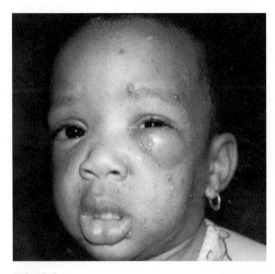

FIG 60-2
Periorbital cellulitis secondary to infected varicella.

bital cellulitis is much less common than periorbital cellulitis.

Conjunctivitis

Severe conjunctivitis is often difficult to distinguish from periorbital cellulitis. Marked lid edema may obscure the underlying conjunctival injection and chemosis (swelling of the conjunctiva), which also may be present in orbital and periorbital cellulitis. Bilateral periorbital swelling with a history of eye discharge (especially in the morning on awakening) is most commonly infectious conjunctivitis. A thick, mucupurulent discharge is suggestive of bacterial disease.

A history of sexually transmitted infections in the mother of a newborn should heighten the suspicion for gonoccocal, chlamydial, or herpetic conjunctivitis. In the neonate, gonococcal conjunctivitis may lead to severe corneal ulceration. Herpes virus is not only vision threatening but also life threatening to the untreated neonate. Grouped vesicles around the eye or "dendritic" staining on fluorescein examination should suggest possible herpes infection. Chlamydial conjunctivitis, if not recognized and treated in the neonate, may progress to pneumonia.

Other bacterial etiologies of conjunctivitis include *Staphylococcus, Streptococcus, H. influenzae* (often seen with a coexisting otitis media), and *Moraxella catarrhalis*. Adenovirus, notori-

ous for causing a prolonged, painful conjunctivitis, frequently is seen in older children with pharyngitis. Allergic conjunctivitis often is associated with a thin, watery discharge, along with papules of the palpebral conjunctivae ("cobblestoning"). Chemical conjunctivitis, due to silver nitrate or erythromycin neonatal prophylaxis, is benign, self-limited, and usually appears 1 to 3 days after its chemoprophylactic instillation. Neonates with conjunctivitis should have the appropriate stains and cultures done to rule out the serious infectious etiologies discussed previously. Diagnosis and treatment of infants and children with conjunctivitis are discussed fully in Chapter 59.

Sinusitis

Sinusitis can produce eye and facial swelling even without a complicating orbital cellulitis. A history of upper respiratory symptoms for more than 10 days, unilateral purulent nasal discharge, and/or tenderness to percussion over the sinuses should suggest the diagnosis. Plain radiographs of the sinuses are sometimes helpful in children older than 2 years of age, but many practitioners will initiate a 14- to 21-day course of oral antibiotics empirically when clinical evidence is supportive.

Cavernous Sinus Thrombosis

A cavernous sinus thrombosis usually is caused by spread of a bacterial sinusitis into the cavernous sinus but also may occur after surgical or accidental trauma. Proptosis, limitation in extraocular muscle movement, problems with visual acuity, papilledema, and especially mental status changes are suggestive of this diagnosis. Magnetic resonance imaging is the study of choice when cavernous sinus thrombosis is a concern.

Dacryocystitis

Dacryocystitis is a lacrimal sac infection, which commonly occurs in infants with dacryostenosis (congenital obstruction of the drainage system of the eye). Tender, warm edema develops at the medical lid margins in babies who have a long history of tearing, discharge, and crusting of the eyes. Nasolacrimal massage, warm soaks, and sometimes antibacterial drops are used for simple dacryostenosis. Treatment for dacryocystitis, however, includes systemic antibiotics and occasionally surgical intervention.

Hordeola

Hordeola are classified as styes (external) and chalazia (internal). They produce eyelid swelling secondary to blocked or infected meibomian glands. The common stye is readily visible on the surface of an eyelid. A chalazion can be discerned as a pea-sized, mobile nodule within the lid. Hordeola usually respond to baby shampoo scrubs at the eyelash bases, warm compresses, and topical antibiotics.

Allergic Reactions

Allergic reactions often cause the most impressive cases of eyelid edema. The classic example is a bee sting to the periorbit. Other causes of allergic reactions include medications, foods, inhalants, and plant (poison ivy) hypersensitivity reactions. Afebrile, well children with bilateral eyelid edema should be suspected to have an allergic cause of their periorbital edema. Serum sickness, an immune complex–mediated reaction, usually appears 7 to 14 days after a given medication, but viral infections also may be responsible. Elimination of the offending antigen is paramount in the management of allergic disorders. Additionally, antihistamines such as hydroxyzine and diphenhydramine are usually palliative. Topical and/or systemic steroids are necessary in some allergic reactions.

Trauma

Traumatic injuries commonly lead to eyelid edema. The child with periorbital ecchymosis, better known as a "black eye," must be evaluated for the presence of visual deficits, eyelid lacerations, orbital fractures, corneal abrasions, globe injuries, and retinal injuries. Conjunctival foreign bodies may be an occult cause of eyelid edema. Exquisite orbital rim tenderness may indicate an orbital rim fracture. Furthermore, if orbital rim tenderness is associated with limited eye movement, an orbital rim fracture with muscle entrapment is likely. The traumatized, tightly swollen eyelid should be shielded (not patched) and the patient transported to the nearest medical facility for ophthalmologic evaluation. Any attempt to aggressively open the eye could result in serious disruption to the globe, especially in a resisting child. Ominous indicators of severe eye trauma include visual deficits, pupillary irregularity, hyphema (blood in the anterior chamber), and any evidence of prolapsed eye contents, usually recognized as a dark tissue protruding through the white sclera.

Malignancies

Malignancies are an uncommon, but obviously important, diagnostic consideration in the swollen eyelid. Retinoblastoma is the hallmark primary eye malignancy and usually is diagnosed prior to age 2 years. Although periorbital edema and conjunctivitis may be present, leukocoria ("white pupil") and strabismus are the most common findings at presentation. Neuroblastoma is notorious for its orbital and periorbital metastases, which cause proptosis and periorbital ecchymoses. Opsoclonus ("dancing eyes") is another indicator of neuroblastoma. Leukemia and lymphoma also may produce eyelid edema. Rhabdomyosarcoma may present anywhere in the head or neck, including the orbit, nasopharynx, middle ear, or mastoid.

Systemic Disease

Systemic disease always should be considered as a possible underlying cause for eyelid edema. Congestive heart failure, glomerulonephritis, and nephrosis can all cause generalized edema. Eyelid edema can be seen with hypo- or hyperthyroidism. The exophthalmos of hyperthyroidism easily can be mistaken for true proptosis. Liver disease with or without hypoalbuminemia can be the cause of bilateral eyelid edema. Finally, collagen-vascular diseases including dermatomyositis, systemic lupus erythematosus (SLE), and scleroderma have all been associated with periorbital swelling.

DATA GATHERING

History

Fever and upper respiratory and constitutional symptoms support an infectious etiology. The immunization history is important when HIB is in the differential diagnosis. A history of insect bite is important for both infectious (periorbital cellulitis) as well as allergic diagnoses. Recent changes in diet, medications, cosmetic use, and other environmental exposures or a past medical history or family history positive for atopy support the diagnosis of allergic reaction. In cases of eye trauma, the immediate history should include the time elapsed since injury, blunt versus penetrating trauma, type of foreign body or chemical, and current as well as premorbid visual acuity.

Symptoms such as fever, anorexia, weight loss, malaise, irritability, bone pain, limp, easy bruising, and pallor can be signals of malignancies. Additionally, one type of retinoblastoma is transmitted in an autosomal dominant fashion, therefore family history is crucial. A thorough past medical history, as well as complete review of systems, also should be obtained. Urinary abnormalities suggest kidney disease, whereas trouble feeding or sweating with eating suggest cardiac disease. Poor feeding, as well as constipation, also are seen with hypothyroidism. Conversely, children with hyperthyroidism are nervous and emotionally labile and may have a history of heat intolerance, palpitations, or weight loss.

Physical Examination

Inspection of the swollen eyelid should include determining the color and degree of swelling. Erythema is a common finding with infections. Eye discharge may suggest conjunctivitis or dacryocystitis. The associated finding of a rash is very important because it may be the clue to the etiology of a periorbital cellulitis, allergic reaction, or rarely, a collagen-vascular disorder, such as dermatomyositis or SLE. Periorbital swelling that is *bilateral* is most commonly infectious conjunctivitis or allergic edema but also may be a malignancy or systemic disorder. Lid lacerations, periorbital ecchymoses, and external foreign bodies are obvious indicators of trauma.

Tenderness on palpation of the periorbital edema usually denotes infection or trauma. The safest way to visualize the globe of a low-risk eye trauma patient is to place the thumbs over the supraorbital and infraorbital rims and exert gentle upward and downward traction, respectively. If any of the severe indicators of eye trauma previously discussed are revealed, the examination should be terminated, the eye shielded, and the patient referred. Conjunctival injection or chemosis, extraocular muscles function, and visual acuity should be assessed, and a fundoscopic examination should be performed.

A *complete* physical examination should be done in all patients with eyelid swelling. Meningismus heralding meningitis may be seen in a patient with orbital and periorbital cellulitis, as well as with cavernous sinus thrombosis. Mental status changes or neurologic abnormalities point to a complicated orbital cellulitis or cavernous sinus thrombosis. Diffuse rash, arthralgia, and adenopathy are seen in serum sickness. Lymphadenopathy also should raise the suspicion of malignancies, especially when associated with findings of pallor, ecchymoses, petechiae, bony tenderness, hepatosplenomegaly, or other abdominal masses.

Thorough examination of the heart, lungs, and abdomen should detect signs of congestive heart failure or hepatic disease, whereas hypertension and edema raise the concern of renal disease. Goiter and other signs of thyroid disease also should be excluded. Finally, the acute as well as chronic manifestations of collagen-vascular disorders, which commonly have multisystem organ involvement, should be considered.

Laboratory Evaluation

As with most diseases, the history and physical examination are usually all that is needed to diagnose most causes of eyelid swelling. However, in some instances, laboratory evaluation may be helpful. The complete blood cell (CBC) count is the most useful diagnostic tool. Most commonly, children with sinusitis and orbital and periorbital cellulitis will have high white blood cell counts, but children with infectious conjunctivitis, dacryocystitis, and chalazia also can have leukocytosis. Extreme leukocytosis, as well as leukopenia, anemia, and/or thrombocytopenia are ominous findings of malignancy.

Plain radiographs may be helpful, but a CT scan is more definitive in suspected cases of orbital cellulitis, severe eye trauma, and eye malignancies. Bone marrow aspirate and biopsy are crucial in patients with suspected malignancies. Electrolytes, blood urea nitrogen, creatinine, and urinalyses should be done in patients suspected of having renal disease and, in some cases, serum sickness. Thyroid studies and liver enzyme studies should be obtained when thyroid and hepatic disease, respectively, are considered. Chest radiograph, electrocardiogram, and echocardiogram are important tests when cardiac disease is a concern. Ultrasound and abdominal CT should be considered for suspected renal or hepatic disease.

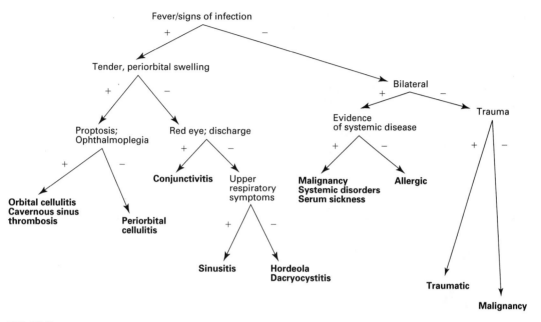

FIG 60-3
Decision tree for differential diagnosis of swollen eyelid.

INDICATIONS FOR CONSULTATION OR REFERRAL

Ophthalmology consultation is indicated for all cases of orbital cellulitis and some patients with complicated periorbital cellulitis. Suspected gonococcal or herpetic conjunctivitis, recurrent or persistent conjunctivitis, and conjunctivitis in contact lens wearers also should be referred. Patients with hordeola should be referred if the styes are painful, cosmetically displeasing, or persist despite therapy. Patients with trauma to the eye, unless minor and uncomplicated, also should be referred. Referral is especially important in cases of possible globe disruption or when visual acuity is altered. Thyroid orbitopathy or malignancy requires urgent, but not emergent, ophthalmology consultation.

Otorhinolaryngology referral is indicated in some severe cases of sinusitis, especially if orbital cellulitis is a possibility. Neurosurgical consultation should be obtained in cases of suspected cavernous sinus thrombosis.

DISCUSSION OF ALGORITHM

A decision tree for the differential diagnosis of the swollen eye is presented in Fig. 60-3. The first consideration always should be to rule out infection. Tenderness of the skin suggests some form of cellulitis. Bilateral, noninfectious disease commonly suggests allergic edema, although malignancies and other systemic diseases also are possible. Unilateral, noninfectious disease is usually traumatic, but malignancy is again possible.

BIBLIOGRAPHY

Catalano RA: Eye injuries and prevention, *Pediatr Ophthalmol* 20(4):827–839, 1993.
Ciarallo LR, Rowe PC: Lumbar puncture in children with periorbital and orbital cellulitis, *J Pediatr* 122(3):355–359, 1993.

Fisher MC: Conjunctivitis in children, *Pediatr Clin North Am* 34(6):1447–1455, 1987.
Fleisher GR, Ludwig S, editors: *Textbook of pediatric emergency medicine,* ed 3, Baltimore, 1993, Williams & Wilkins.

Isreale V, Nelson JD: Periorbital and orbital cellulitis, *Pediatr Infect Dis J* 6(4):404–410, 1987.

King RA: Common ocular signs and symptoms in childhood, *Pediatr Clin North Am* 40:753, 1993.

Lessner A, Stern GA: Preseptal and orbital cellulitis, *Infect Dis Clin North Am* 6(4):933–952, 1992.

O'Hara MA: Ophthalmia neonatorum, *Pediatr Clin North Am* 40(4):715–725, 1993.

Pownall KR: Periorbital and orbital cellulitis, *Pediatr Rev* 16(5):163–167, 1995.

Shields JA, Shields CL, Suvarnamani C, et al: Retinoblastoma manifesting as orbital cellulitis, *Am J Ophthalmol* 112(4):442–449, 1991.

Tunnessen WW: *Signs and symptoms in pediatrics,* ed 2, Philadelphia, 1988, JB Lippincott.

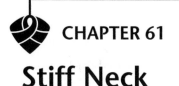

CHAPTER 61

Stiff Neck

Carol Carraccio
Karen Miller

Stiff neck may be either a presenting complaint or an accompanying sign of a more generalized illness. The diagnostic possibilities make it a challenge for the primary care physician, because some cases run a self-limited course, whereas others require immediate intervention.

DIFFERENTIAL DIAGNOSIS

Common Causes of Stiff Neck
- **Trauma**
  - Vertebral
    - Subluxation
    - Dislocation
    - Fracture
  - Intracranial hemorrhage
  - Muscle spasm
- **Infection**
  - Cervical adenitis
  - Meningitis
  - Brain abscess
  - Epidural abscess
  - Encephalitis
  - Epiglottitis
  - Retropharyngeal abscess
  - Tonsillitis
  - Cervical osteomyelitis
  - Diskitis
  - Pneumonia
  - Otitis media
  - Poliomyelitis
  - Tetanus
  - Other systemic infections
    - Infectious mononucleosis
    - Influenza
- **Immunologic**
  - Collagen diseases
- **Intoxications**
  - Phenothiazines
- **Tumor**
  - Brain or spinal cord
  - Meningeal
  - Vertebral
- **Congenital**
  - Bony deformities of the spine
  - Spastic cerebral palsy
  - Congenital torticollis
  - Cerebral aneurysms

Discussion

The differential diagnosis of neck stiffness includes such benign conditions as muscle spasm and such life-threatening conditions as meningitis. Typically, the more serious causes of neck stiffness, such as significant trauma, epiglottitis, and central nervous system (CNS) disease will present with other historical and physical features suggestive of the cause.

Any infection that causes significant cervical adenopathy also may cause a patient to present with a chief complaint of neck stiffness. Included in this category would be streptococcal pharyngitis manifested by fever, tonsillar exudate, and cervical adenopathy and also infectious mononucleosis manifested by fever, generalized adenopathy, pharyngitis, and, possibly, hepatosplenomegaly. Cat scratch disease also may cause neck stiffness on the basis of cervical adenitis or the myeloradiculopathy that may be part of its clinical spectrum. The scratch should be visible on physical examination. There may be a pustule at the site of the scratch with involvement of the regional lymph nodes. The atypical mycobacteria cause cervical adenopathy that is oftentimes suppurative. Other local infectious processes such as upper lobe pneumonia, cervical osteomyelitis, and dental abscess may be associated with neck stiffness. The child with osteomyelitis usually has low-grade fever and point tenderness over the involved cervical vertebra. Dental abscess may be detected by examination of the oral cavity for erythema and swelling of the alveolar ridge or sensitivity to percussion of the involved tooth. Viral infections, particularly influenza, have been associated with neck stiffness. Children with these infections usually will have other respiratory signs as well as fever and myalgias to go along with this stiffness.

Children with a complaint of stiff neck secondary to drug reactions usually have severe nuchal rigidity and often opisthotonic posturing and facial grimacing. Reactions to phenothiazine may be treated with intravenous diphenhydramine.

Nuchal rigidity secondary to cervical arthritis is one of the findings in juvenile rheumatoid arthritis and also in ankylosing spondylitis. Because neck stiffness usually is not a presenting complaint in these diseases, a past history of joint involvement with limitation of motion are consistent with the diagnosis. Likewise, most congenital causes of neck stiffness will be readily diagnosed on the basis of history and physical examination.

DATA GATHERING

History

Typically, with the more serious injuries, the acute onset of pain immediately follows the injury. The type of activity in which the child was engaged when the injury occurred also will be helpful in determining the sequelae of the injury. For children with Down syndrome, ligamentous laxity involving the upper cervical spine causes atlantoaxial instability. A number of these children will go on to develop symptoms after neck injury. Minor trauma leading to muscle strain or spasm is usually more insidious in onset and thus more difficult to relate to a specific traumatic event. In the young infant, a history of birth trauma is important because a hematoma may form within the sternocleidomastoid muscle. Irritation of the meninges by blood, as occurs in a subarachnoid hemorrhage, causes nuchal rigidity. Likewise, tumor cells can cause similar meningeal irritation.

Once a history of serious injury has been explored, symptoms of serious infections must be addressed. Fever and stiff neck with change in mental status or seizure activity suggests meningitis, encephalitis, or brain abscess. Fever and stiff neck with respiratory difficulty suggests epiglottitis, retropharyngeal abscess, or pneumonia.

There are numerous other less severe infections that may be associated with neck stiffness, and specific complaints must be sought. Does the child have a sore throat? Cervical adenitis associated with pharyngitis, whether bacterial (as in streptococcal infection) or viral (as in Epstein-Barr virus infection), may cause neck stiffness. Cervical adenitis unassociated with pharyngitis also may cause neck stiffness. Multiple pathogens may be implicated. These include bacteria such as *Staphylococcus aureus* and *Streptococcus* as well as mycobacteria, especially the atypical types, and *Bartonella henselae,* the etiologic agent of cat scratch disease. Mouth pain and cervical adenopathy are seen with dental abscesses. Upper respiratory tract symptoms accompanied by fever and headache suggest influenza infection. Back pain accompanying the neck stiffness may be indicative of diskitis, cervical osteomyelitis, or a vertebral tumor such as osteoid osteoma. Other tumors associated with stiff neck are those that infiltrate the meninges by local spread or metastasize to the meninges, as occurs with leukemia. Joint involvement with a history of pain and stiffness should alert the physician to explore other features consistent with collagen diseases.

A medication history also is important because drugs such as phenothiazines and metoclopramide may cause dystonic reactions of which neck stiffness is a major manifestation. Because ingestions are not always witnessed, the acute onset of nuchal rigidity associated with facial grimacing and, oftentimes, opisthotonic posturing in an otherwise healthy child should alert the physician to the possibility of drug toxicity. Phenothiazine derivatives are a common ingredient in cough medications. Metoclopramide, an antiemetic drug, also has been implicated in causing these reactions. Lead poisoning may cause an encephalopathy characterized by cerebral edema that has neck stiffness as one of its manifestations. A history of pica as well as associated symptoms of ataxia and change in mental status should be sought.

Physical Examination

A rapid assessment for signs of respiratory distress, significant traumatic injury, and change in mental status is indicated. In these cases, immediate diagnostic and/or therapeutic procedures should be initiated. A child with epiglottitis or a retropharyngeal abscess will present in respiratory distress. Classically, patients with these disorders have difficulty swallowing; thus, drooling is a classic sign of these diseases. The neck is rigidly held in a position that allows maximal air entry into the trachea.

If significant traumatic injury to the head and/or neck is suspected, physical examination of this area should be deferred. Neck immobilization is indicated while appropriate radiographic studies are obtained.

Children who have a stiff neck secondary to CNS pathologic conditions usually have other signs on physical examination. There may be an altered mental status as well as abnormal neurologic findings or seizure activity.

Cervical adenitis is manifested by erythematous, swollen, hot, tender lymph nodes. Children with cervical adenitis are typically febrile. Cervical adenopathy may accompany systemic illnesses such as infectious mononucleosis or influenza; generalized adenopathy, pharyngitis, and splenomegaly should be sought in the former and other signs of respiratory infection in the latter. Cervical lymph nodes, providing lymphatic drainage to the pharynx, will respond to an infection in this area by becoming swollen and tender.

Because neck stiffness secondary to cervical arthritis in the rheumatologic disorders is typically not a presenting complaint but a later manifestation, the physical examination will usually reveal stiffness in other joints and possibly joint deformity with some limitation of motion.

Neck stiffness as a result of congenital anomalies is quite evident on physical examination. Klippel-Feil syndrome, which is characterized by failure of segmentation of the cervical spine, usually is associated with other skeletal anomalies. Likewise, Arnold-Chiari malformations, which consist of abnormal development and displacement of cerebellar and medullary tissue, are usually associated with aqueductal stenosis and thus hydrocephalus. Spastic cerebral palsy will be evident by a generalized increase in tone, not just neck stiffness, and possibly contractures resulting in significant impairment of motor skills. Congenital torticollis is, however, usually found in otherwise healthy infants. It is associated with unilateral shortening of the sternocleidomastoid muscle with subsequent tilting of the head to the shortened side.

Laboratory Evaluation

For some patients, such as those suffering from minor trauma or minor infectious processes, laboratory tests may not be indicated. However, for more severe pathologic conditions, laboratory tests may be quite helpful in diagnosis.

When indicated, the most useful laboratory aid in establishing a diagnosis is radiography of the neck. Radiographic studies are useful in determining the severity of a traumatic injury. They also will be helpful in diagnosing epiglottitis, retropharyngeal abscess, some tumors, arthritic changes, osteomyelitis, pneumonia, and congenital anomalies. A bone scan is more sensitive in detecting osteomyelitis and diskitis.

Computed tomography (CT) provides excellent resolution of bone and the paraspinal soft

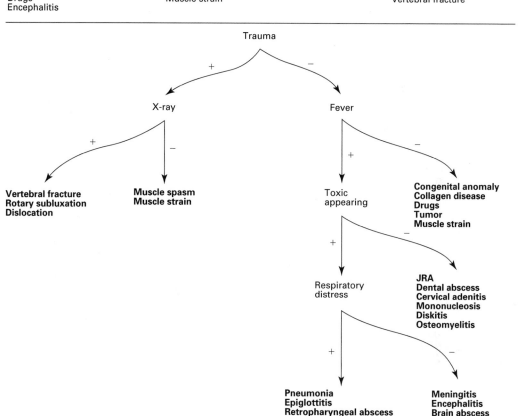

STIFF NECK
Differential diagnosis

Brain abscess	Epiglottitis	Osteomyelitis
Cervical adenitis	Intracranial hemorrhage	Pneumonia
Collagen disease	Juvenile rheumatoid arthritis (JRA)	Retropharyngeal abscess
Congenital anomaly	Lumphadenitis	Rotary subluxation
Dental abscess	Meningitis	Trauma
Diskitis	Mononucleosis	Tumor
Drugs	Muscle strain	Vertebral fracture
Encephalitis		

FIG 61-1
Decision tree for differential diagnosis of stiff neck.

tissues, making it a useful diagnostic tool for injuries, congenital malformations, and tumors. The ability of magnetic resonance imaging to complement CT with excellent resolution of processes involving the marrow and soft tissues allows detection of lesions within the spinal cord.

A high white blood cell count and sedimentation rate will support the suspicion of an infectious cause of neck stiffness. Examination of the cerebrospinal fluid is critical when CNS infection is considered. Screening tests for toxins are useful when such an ingestion is suspected.

DISCUSSION OF ALGORITHM

An algorithm for differential diagnosis of stiff neck is presented in Figure 61-1. After documentation of the absence of trauma as a causation of neck stiffness, signs of fever and toxicity should be sought.

The febrile, toxic-appearing patient demands prompt evaluation so that treatment of such medical emergencies as meningitis, epiglottitis, and retropharyngeal abscess may be initiated.

In the afebrile patient who appears toxic, consideration centers on drug reaction and intracranial catastrophies.

The febrile patient who is not toxic-appearing can be evaluated for the less serious infections associated with neck stiffness.

BIBLIOGRAPHY

Barnes PD: Imaging of the central nervous system in pediatrics and adolescence, *Pediatr Clin North Am* 39:743–776, 1992.

Doughty RA, Rose C: Stiff neck. In Fleisher G, Ludwig S, Henretig F, et al, editors: *Textbook of pediatric emergency medicine,* ed 3, Baltimore, 1993, Williams & Wilkins.

Fitz CR: Diagnostic imaging in children with spinal disorders, *Pediatr Clin North Am* 32: 1537–1558, 1985.

Menkes J: *Textbook of child neurology,* ed 5, Baltimore, 1995, Williams & Wilkins.

Pueschel SM, Scola FH, Pezzullo JC: A longitudinal study of atlanto-dens relationships in asymptomatic individuals with Down syndrome, *Pediatrics* 89:1194–1198, 1992.

Weiner HL, Urion DK, Levitt LP: *Pediatric neurology for the house officer,* ed 3, Baltimore, 1988, Williams & Wilkins.

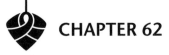

CHAPTER 62

Syncope

Lawrence W. Brown
Edward B. Charney

Brief, sudden loss of muscle tone and abrupt unresponsiveness is a frightening complaint with a broad differential diagnosis. Syncope is loss of awareness due to a transient reduction in cerebral blood flow due to irregular activity, reduced blood volume, or redistribution. Fainting is synonymous with syncope. The major condition to be distinguished is an epileptic seizure, which can present in a similar fashion, but symptoms are caused by a disruption of normal electrical activity of the brain.

During the syncopal event the child is often limp, unresponsive, and diaphoretic with decreased blood pressure, diminished deep tendon reflexes, slow pulse, and dilated pupils. The period of unresponsiveness generally lasts for only a few seconds and is followed by rapid return to full mental alertness. Longer episodes may be harder to distinguish from epileptic seizures and other causes because headache, prolonged lethargy, and confusion usually occur more often.

DIFFERENTIAL DIAGNOSIS

Common Causes of Syncope
- Congenital
- Structural heart lesions
- Arrhythmias

- Metabolic
- Anemia
- Hypoglycemia
- Miscellaneous
- Vasovagal syncope
- Breath-holding spells
- Hyperventilation syndrome
- Orthostatic hypotension
- Cough syncope

Discussion

Congenital heart disease, particularly severe aortic or pulmonic stenosis and tetralogy of Fallot, may result in fainting episodes. These episodes are most common during or immediately following strenuous physical activity. Cardiac arrhythmias may lead to inadequate cardiac output with inadequate cerebral blood flow from mechanisms such as atrial fibrillation, complete atrioventricular block (Stokes-Adams disease), or the prolonged QT interval syndrome. The latter can be associated with autosomal recessive deafness (surdocardiac syndrome) or as an autosomal dominant trait in families with normal hearing (Romano-Ward syndrome).

Metabolic causes of fainting include anemia and hypoglycemia. Children with orthostatic hypotension are frequently syncopal. Severe coughing spells can be caused by a variety of conditions including asthma, cystic fibrosis and pertussis-like acute respiratory infections. Rarely, psychogenic causes or tic disorders may present with severe cough leading to fainting spells. Tussive syncope results from hypoxia and reduced cardiac return from the Valsalva maneuver or respiratory spasm experienced after completion of strenuous coughing.

The majority of cases of fainting in children are caused by a wide variety of conditions listed as miscellaneous. Vasovagal syncope, the most common cause of fainting, results in a sudden loss of resistance in the peripheral circulation. Attacks usually are precipitated by emotional upsets. Orthostatic hypotension is associated with an excessive and prolonged fall in blood pressure on sitting or standing. Although this condition is uncommon in children, it may occur from prolonged bed rest, dehydration, anorexia, excessive use of diuretics, and familial dysautonomia.

Breath-holding spells frequently are precipitated in an infant or toddler by emotional upset or pain. Cyanotic spells are the most common

type of breath holding, often beginning at 6 months to 3 years of age. They are characterized by an initial crying event provoked by pain, fear, or surprise. After several breaths, there is respiratory arrest, opisthotonus, cyanosis, loss of responsiveness, and an abrupt return to awareness after a few seconds. Long spells may be associated with a few generalized clonic jerks of all extremities, suggesting an epileptic seizure. However, the history is characteristic of a preceding environmental event, and ictal electroencephalogram (EEG) confirmation of spells provoked by stimulation such as ocular compression shows only generalized slowing of background without epileptiform activity. Pallid breath holding is a form of vagovagal syncope caused by reflex asystole, which is most often provoked by sudden minor trauma rather than anger or fright. The first manifestation usually is not loud crying followed by arching of the back, but rather sudden pallor, limpness, and loss of responsiveness. Stiffening and clonic movement typically occur at the end of the event. Any tonic or clonic activity represents the effects of cerebral hypoxia rather than an epileptic mechanism. Treatment of both cyanotic and pallid breath holding includes reassurance of the benign nature of the attacks and prevention of secondary gain. It is possible to block reflex asystole by anticholinergic medications or cardiac pacemaker when pallid spells are frequent and prolonged, but this treatment is rarely necessary.

Hyperventilation with fainting often is precipitated by anxiety and may be associated with chest pain, palpitations, numbness, carpopedal spasm, and breathlessness prior to loss of responsiveness. Often patients are unaware of overbreathing, and it is therefore necessary to carefully define the circumstances and associated features to determine the nature of the event. Hyperventilation produces fainting by its powerful effect on reducing cerebral blood flow. Fainting also can be induced consciously when hyperventilation is coupled with the Valsalva maneuver during play.

DATA GATHERING

Physical Examination

The physical examination is generally normal in children who have experienced a fainting episode. Particular attention should be directed to

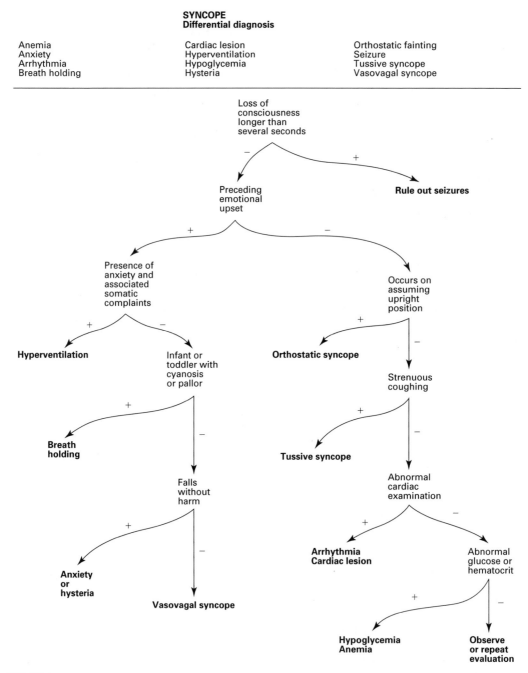

SYNCOPE
Differential diagnosis

Anemia	Cardiac lesion	Orthostatic fainting
Anxiety	Hyperventilation	Seizure
Arrhythmia	Hypoglycemia	Tussive syncope
Breath holding	Hysteria	Vasovagal syncope

FIG 62-1

Decision tree for differential diagnosis of syncope.

the cardiac examination including arrhythmias and the systolic murmurs of aortic or pulmonic stenosis. Clinical cyanosis at rest may suggest congenital heart disease, and pallor may indicate anemia.

Laboratory Evaluation

An electrocardiogram (ECG) rhythm trip and corrected QT interval should be obtained. Serum glucose and hematocrit are also worthwhile screening studies. An EEG should be performed if seizure or breath-holding spells are a consideration. Ocular compression with simultaneous EEG and ECG monitoring should be performed under the supervision of trained professionals because prolonged asystole can be induced in sensitive individuals even when mild pressure is maintained for only 10 seconds.

INDICATIONS FOR CONSULTATION OR REFERRAL

Children with recognized or suspected cardiac lesions should be referred to a cardiologist for further evaluation and management. Patients with hyperventilation or hysterical fainting require referral for professional counseling.

DISCUSSION OF ALGORITHM

An algorithm for differential diagnosis of syncope is presented in Figure 62-1. The two major tasks in the evaluation of fainting are to exclude the major pathophysiologic causes of heart disease and epilepsy in addition to hypoglycemia and cough syncope. Once these problems are eliminated, other causes can be carefully explored. There are many occasions when the cause of fainting cannot be determined. These patients should be followed up with repeated examinations. Persistent complaints should be referred to a cardiologist for full physiologic testing including Holter monitoring and tilt table testing.

BIBLIOGRAPHY

Gospe SM, Choy M: Hereditary long Q-T interval syndrome presenting as epilepsy: Electroencephalography laboratory diagnosis, *Ann Neurol* 25:514, 1989.

Herman SP, Stickler GB, Lucas AR: Hyperventilation syndrome in children and adolescents: Long term follow up, *Pediatrics* 67:183, 1981.

Katz RM: Cough syncope in children with asthma, *J Pediatr* 77:48, 1970.

Lombroso C, LernLan P: Breathholding spells (cyanotic and pallid infantile syncope), *Pediatrics* 39:563, 1967.

Strieper MJ, Auld DO, Hulse JE, Campbell RM: Evaluation of recurrent pediatric syncope: Role of tilt table testing, *Pediatrics* 93:660, 1994.

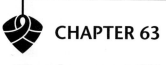

CHAPTER 63

Tachycardia

Marie M. Gleason

Tachycardia may be defined as a heart rate that exceeds the normal range for age or clinical condition (Table 63-1). The primary care physician should be familiar with the evaluation of tachycardia in infants and children. The most common type of tachycardia in children is sinus tachycardia. Although primary cardiac tachydysrhythmias are less common, they are not rare and may have important cardiovascular consequences if undetected and untreated.

TABLE 63-1
Heart Rate Ranges*

AGE	BEATS PER MINUTE
0–3 days	90–160
3–30 days	90–180
1–6 months	105–185
6–12 months	110–170
1–3 years	90–150
3–5 years	70–140
5–8 years	65–135
8–12 years	60–130
12–16 years	60–120

*Adapted from Dauvignon A, et al: ECG standards for children, *Ped Cardiol* 1:133–152, 1979.

DIFFERENTIAL DIAGNOSIS

Common Causes of Sinus Tachycardia
- **Pain**
- **Anxiety**
- **Infectious illness (with and without fever)**
  Bacterial (noncardiac)
  Viral (noncardiac)
  Myocarditis
  Pericarditis/pericardial effusion
  Endocarditis
- **Systemic inflammatory disease**
  Inflammatory bowel disease
  Juvenile rheumatoid arthritis
- **Altered fluid status**
  Intravascular volume depletion
  Intravascular volume overload
- **Trauma/acute blood loss**
  Chest injury/pneumothorax
  Myocardial contusion
  Pleural or pericardial effusion
  Abdominal injury
- **Cardiac**
  Congenital heart disease
  Acquired heart disease
    Congestive cardiomyopathy
    Kawasaki disease
    Rheumatic fever
  Physical deconditioning
- **Metabolic/pharmacologic**
  Metabolic acidosis
  Drug-induced
    Amphetamines
    Cocaine
    Caffeine
    β-Agonists/bronchodilators

Tricyclic antidepressants
Cough and cold preparations with pseudoephedrine and/or phenylpropanolamine
- **Endocrine**
  Thyrotoxicosis
  Pheochromocytoma
  Catecholamine secreting lesions
  Diabetes mellitus or insipidus with dehydration

Cardiac Tachydysrhythmias (With or Without Heart Disease)
- **Narrow-complex tachycardias**
  Supraventricular tachycardia (SVT)
    Re-entrant SVT
    Automatic ectopic atrial tachycardia
  Atrial flutter
  Junctional tachycardia
- **Wide-complex tachycardia**
  Ventricular tachycardia
  Supraventricular tachycardia with aberrant conduction

Discussion

Sinus tachycardia frequently is associated with febrile illness, pain, anxiety, or trauma. In the obviously ill child, it may be difficult to determine if the elevated heart rate is secondary to the illness or a primary tachydysrhythmia. For example, an infant with septic shock and sinus tachycardia shows similar clinical findings to an infant with previously undiagnosed, protracted supraventricular tachycardia (SVT) with congestive heart failure and systemic hypoperfusion. Under extreme stress or fever, some infants can develop sinus tachycardia to levels as high as 220 to 240 beats per minute (Fig. 63-1). More commonly, the rate ranges from 180 to 200 beats per minute.

In the otherwise well child with resting tachycardia or complaints of intermittent palpitations, the differential diagnosis will focus less on infectious, inflammatory, or traumatic etiologies and more on metabolic, endocrinologic, and primary cardiac causes. It is not unusual for older children to perceive a "rapid heart rate" during sinus tachycardia, which is usually at or below 130 to 140 beats per minute.

Supraventricular tachycardia accounts for greater than 80% of the cardiac arrhythmias in childhood and occurs in approximately one per 250 to 1000 children. By definition, the rhythm

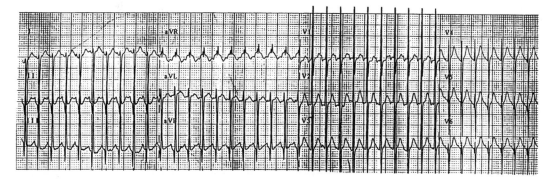

FIG 63-1

12-Lead electrocardiogram showing extreme sinus tachycardia, at a rate of 220 to 230 beats per minute, in an infant 3 days of age. Note the presence of a P wave prior to each narrow QRS complex. Upright P waves in limb leads II, III, and AVF are consistent with rhythm of sinus origin.

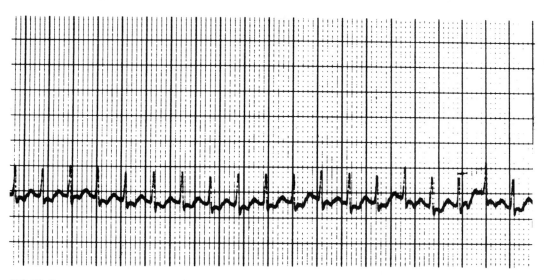

FIG 63-2

Rhythm strip showing re-entrant supraventricular tachycardia at a rate of 250 beats per minute. Note the presence of a retrograde (inverted) P wave after each narrow QRS complex.

arises from above the His bundle in the heart. The rate of most re-entrant SVT in older children exceeds 160 to 180 beats per minute and often exceeds 200 beats per minute. In newborns and young infants, SVT generally ranges from 240 to 300 beats per minute (Fig. 63-2). When sustained for protracted periods, congestive heart failure can result. In older children, rapid heart rates may cause the patient to experience discomfort, shortness of breath, pallor, or dizziness. The older child usually will bring his or her condition to the attention of an adult. Obtaining a pulse rate at the time of onset of symptoms can be extremely helpful in the diagnosis. Supraventricular arrhythmias generally are better tolerated clinically than ventricular arrhythmias, because the latter are more likely to result in symptoms of dizziness or syncope after a shorter period of time.

Ventricular tachycardia (VT) is rare in well children. It is defined as three or more premature ventricular contractions, at a rate greater than 100 beats per minute, usually with atrioventricular dissociation. The wide QRS complex is of a different morphology than the QRS in sinus rhythm. VT may have a metabolic or drug-related etiology or be related to congenital heart disease or cardiomyopathies. Tachydysrhythmias may occur with almost any congenital heart defect, but the postoperative patient is at special risk. The practitioner's index of suspicion should be very high if presented with symptoms of palpitations, chest pain, and dizzy or syncopal spells in such children and adolescents.

DATA GATHERING

History
When a child is noted to be tachycardic, the present illness must be characterized, with particular attention to a history of fever, rash, pain, or respiratory or gastrointestinal illness. Evaluation of fluid status is important, especially if emesis, diarrhea, decreased oral intake, or decreased urine output is noted. Cardiac dysfunction may manifest as change in appetite, tachypnea, shortness of breath, or irritability. Sometimes, a rapid heart rate is an incidental finding. Knowledge of the patient's other significant medical issues such as congenital heart disease or prior arrhythmia or chronic conditions such as inflammatory bowel disease, juvenile rheumatoid arthritis, diabetes, asthma, hemoglobinopathy, or immune disorder is important in considering causes of tachycardia.

Pharmacologic Agents
Several drugs with sympathomimetic activity can stimulate heart rate, and a careful history regarding their use should be obtained. These drugs include bronchodilators (β-agonists and xanthine derivatives), cough and cold preparations (pseudoephedrine, phenylpropanolamine), and hyperactivity or behavior-modifying drugs (methylphenidate, tricyclic antidepressants). Excessive intake of chocolate and caffein-

ated beverages is associated with palpitations in some sensitive patients. The use of illicit stimulant drugs also should be considered in older children and adolescents.

If SVT or VT is suspected, the patient should be questioned carefully about the circumstances surrounding the tachycardic events: 1) Does the rapid heart rate occur at rest, with exercise, or both? 2) How long does it last, and what, if anything, makes it go away? 3) Is there any chest pain, dizziness, nausea, shortness of breath, or syncope that accompanies the tachycardia? 4) When did these episodes begin and with what frequency do they occur? 5) Has anyone ever counted the heart rate during an occurrence?

Family history is quite important in patients with palpitations and documented or suspected SVT or VT. Are there known dysrhythmias (*eg,* Wolff-Parkinson-White syndrome, long QT syndrome) or sudden death in children or adults under 40 years of age? Are there close relatives with mitral valve prolapse or familial hypertrophic cardiomyopathy or relatives who require cardiac medications?

Physical Examination
Accurate vital signs should be obtained with the patient as quiet as possible.

Assessment of heart rate variability may be helpful in identifying whether a tachycardia is of sinus or nonsinus origin. The rate of sinus tachycardia should change with the patient's respiratory pattern and level of agitation. "Sinus arrhythmia" is a normal variant, with repetitive slowing during exhalation and acceleration during inspiration, which may be misinterpreted as an "irregular" heartbeat. Conversely, abrupt onset and termination of a rapid heart rate is more likely with primary cardiac tachydysrhythmias.

In febrile patients, the primary care physician is well acquainted with the problem of identifying the sites and severity of viral or bacterial infectious illnesses, and the noncardiac issues will not be discussed further. It is very important to assess whether the heart, and hence the cardiac output, is directly affected by the infectious agent or whether it is compensating for other causes of poor perfusion. The presence of a rub, gallop, or cardiac murmur might suggest pericarditis, myocarditis, or endocarditis, respectively. Muffled heart sounds with thready pulses may suggest a pericardial effusion. Primary cardiac tachycardias also may result in congestive heart failure symptoms.

Cardiac murmurs of the "innocent" type are very common in children and may be exaggerated by systemic illness or fever. These vibratory systolic murmurs are best heard at the left lower sternal border, radiate to the base of the heart in older children and adolescents, and increase in intensity in the supine position. Innocent murmurs, in general, do *not* radiate to the back, with the exception of branch pulmonary artery flow murmurs, which can be heard in the back and axillae of infants less than 6 months of age. These murmurs should not be confused with heart murmurs suggestive of endocarditis, such as the harsh holosystolic murmurs of mitral or tricuspid insufficiency or a new diastolic murmur consistent with aortic insufficiency. Tricuspid insufficiency associated with endocarditis may be related to ventricular septal defects, intravascular line sepsis, or intravenous drug use. Although endocarditis usually is associated with congenital heart disease, immunocompromised patients may be at risk even with structurally normal hearts.

Tachycardia in the afebrile, nontraumatized patient takes on a different connotation. A goiter, tremulousness, weight loss, and exophthalmos suggest thyroid disease. A pathologic heart murmur, gallop, systemic hypertension, or abnormal pulses suggest congenital or acquired cardiac disease. Eyelid or peripheral edema and changed quality and quantity of urine suggest renal disease.

Laboratory Evaluation

The pediatrician's decision to obtain laboratory information is influenced by the patient's age, severity of clinical illness or fever, and degree of tachycardia.

A clinically ill, febrile patient may require a complete blood cell count with white blood cell differential and blood culture if sepsis or endocarditis is suspected. This test especially is warranted if underlying congenital heart disease or relative immune deficiency is present. Electrolyte abnormalities can be associated with ventricular dysrhythmias: VT may be seen with hyperkalemia, or with hypokalemia if the patient is taking digoxin preparations. Patients taking chronic antiarrhythmic medication (in particu-

lar, digoxin, procainamide, quinidine, or flecainide) should have a trough drug level checked if there is a worsening in their arrhythmia status. If respiratory symptoms are prominent or a cardiac problem is suspected, evaluating the cardiac silhouette, pulmonary vasculature, and pulmonary parenchyma on chest radiography may be helpful.

Electrocardiography (ECG) should be performed if the heart rate is so rapid that auscultation alone is insufficient to differentiate between sinus tachycardia and a primary cardiac dysrhythmia. Any patient with hemodynamic compromise and significant tachycardia should be considered for an ECG to determine the underlying rhythm mechanism and to assess ST segment and T-wave abnormalities. Such abnormalities could suggest myocarditis (T-wave inversions, low voltages), pericarditis (diffuse ST segment elevations), or ischemia (ST segment depressions and T-wave abnormalities). The 12-lead ECG may demonstrate the presence of premature atrial or ventricular ectopic beats or abnormal conduction intervals, such as short PR interval with delta waves consistent with Wolff-Parkinson-White syndrome (Fig. 63-3), or prolongation of the QTc interval greater than 0.44 seconds.

Most patients who have demonstrated irregular heart rates or complain of palpitations should undergo ambulatory ECG (Holter) monitoring. This procedure provides additional information, including heart rate variability through the day and night, assessment of QT interval at slow and fast heart rates, and documentation of tachycardia episodes both with and without symptoms. Intermittent Holter monitoring is useful in adjusting patient medications when an arrhythmia is known. Some patients, however, have quite sporadic symptoms that are unlikely to be captured with 24 or 48 hours of ambulatory monitoring. In these specific cases, transtelephonic "event monitoring" devices are available to capture recordings of intermittent events.

Echocardiography has advanced greatly in recent years, is widely available, and provides comprehensive assessment of cardiac anatomy and physiology in skilled hands. Although not all tachycardic patients require an echocardiogram, any patient with tachycardia and severe hemodynamic compromise should be considered a candidate for this procedure. Echocardi-

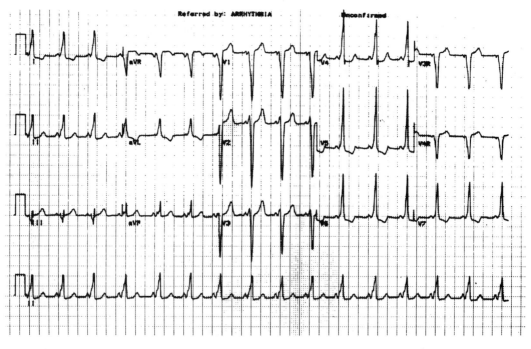

FIG 63-3

12-Lead electrocardiogram showing multiple leads with short PR interval and slurred QRS upstroke (delta waves) consistent with Wolff-Parkinson-White syndrome. This condition results in a widened QRS complex at rest, but most tachycardia is narrow QRS complex.

ography will document overall cardiac contractility, effusions, valve vegetations, or large left-to-right shunt lesions (ventricular septal defect, atrioventricular canal defect) where patients often present with tachycardia, heart murmur, and failure to thrive in the first months of life. In addition, if a cardiac tachydysrhythmia is documented by ECG or ambulatory monitoring, echocardiography is performed to evaluate the presence of cardiac lesions.

Additional laboratory studies may be needed for specific clinical conditions. An erythrocyte sedimentation rate may be informative in patients suspected of having Kawasaki disease, rheumatic fever, acute or subacute bacterial endocarditis, and exacerbation of collagen vascular disorders. In almost any patient with tachycardia, it is important to rule out hyperthyroidism by checking thyroid functions (T3, T4, thyroid-stimulating hormone). A urinanalysis for glucosuria and ketonuria should be performed in

---

BOX 63-1
When to Refer a Tachycardic Patient

Clinical congestive heart failure
Documented SVT or VT
Known congenital heart disease (pre- or post-operative)
Tachycardia/palpitations with chest pain or syncope
Exercise-related palpitations or syncope
Family history of arrhythmias
Unexplained sinus tachycardia

---

patients with suspected diabetes with dehydration. A urine or serum drug screen should be done in older children or adolescents with suspected substance abuse or in younger children with possible ingestion. Patients who are tachycardic and hypertensive may need a 24-hour urine catecholamine screen if a catecholamine-secreting tumor is suspected.

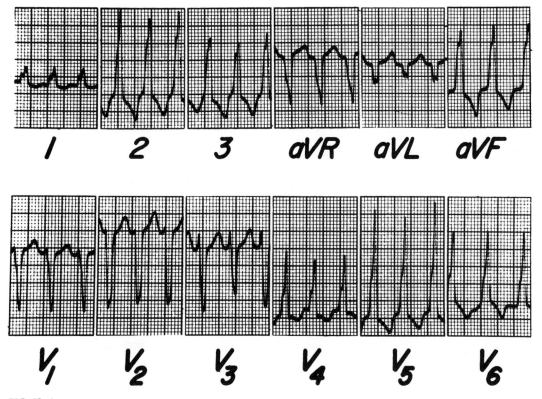

FIG 63-4

12-Lead electrocardiogram showing widened QRS complex with a rapid heart rate of 160 to 170 beats per minute. P waves are not clearly seen, and ventricular tachycardia must be assumed. The presence of atrioventricular dissociation on rhythm strip supports the diagnosis of ventricular tachycardia. [Courtesy of Dr. V. Vetter.]

INDICATIONS FOR CONSULTATION OR REFERRAL

In most instances, tachycardia may be successfully evaluated and treated by the primary care physician, but on occasion, referral of a patient with tachycardia (sinus or nonsinus) to a subspecialist is indicated (Box 63-1 and Fig. 63-5).

The tachycardic child with congestive heart failure, respiratory distress, or cardiomegaly should be referred to a pediatric cardiologist. The primary care physician, however, may be required to emergently stabilize a child with a tachydysrhythmia prior to transport. After vital signs are obtained and the airway is secured, a 12-lead ECG and chest radiography should be performed and intravenous access obtained. If a cardiac dysrhythmia is demonstrated, the physician needs to determine if it is SVT or VT. If a rapid, narrow complex tachycardia is noted, a trial of intravenous adenosine is indicated, even in an unstable patient while preparing for cardioversion. Adenosine interrupts SVT by slowing conduction in the atrioventricular node. Bradycardia is a side effect, therefore its use is contraindicated in patients with known high-degree atrioventricular block without an electronic pacemaker. Adenosine's half-life is only 10 seconds, therefore side effects, such as bradycardia, flushing, chest pain, or shortness of breath, are short lived. An initial dose of 50 to 100 µg/kg is rapidly pushed and followed by a quick saline flush, while blood pressure and heart rate are monitored continuously. The dose may be increased by 50-µg/kg increments every 2 to 3 minutes to a maximum of 250 µg/kg (the starting

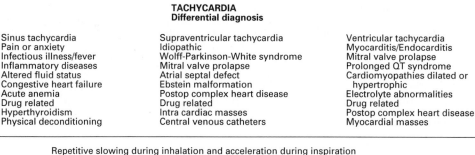

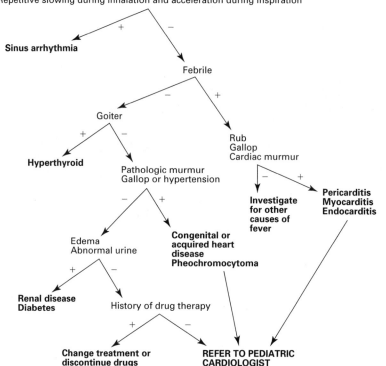

FIG 63-5

Decision tree for differential diagnosis of tachycardia.

adult dose is 3 mg with a maximum of 12 mg). If the patient remains hemodynamically unstable after a trial of adenosine, then direct-current synchronized cardioversion (0.5–1 J/kg) may be indicated. Stable patients with SVT may undergo vagal maneuvers prior to the use of adenosine or electrical cardioversion. Long-term medical management of SVT usually includes digoxin, β-blockers such as propranolol or nadolol, and occasionally flecainide.

A wide complex regular tachcardia on ECG should be considered VT until proven otherwise (Fig. 63-4). Hemodynamic compromise is more likely with VT than SVT, and accurate assessment of blood pressure, pulses, and perfusion is mandatory. If the patient's pulses are weak or absent, then referral to an emergency department for emergent cardioversion is required. Lidocaine (1 mg/kg) given intravenously can be used initially if VT is relatively slow and the patient is hemodynamically stable. Long-term medical management generally includes β-blockers, mexilitine, or procainamide. Patients with documented SVT or VT should be evaluated by a pediatric cardiologist.

Patients who report tachycardia with dizziness

or syncopal events, especially associated with activity or stress, should be evaluated by a cardiologist, because this condition may represent a ventricular tachydysrhythmia. Chest pain is a common complaint in the pediatric population with many underlying causes. However, if a patient describes a rapid heart rate preceding chest discomfort, then the possibility of a cardiac arryhthmia exists, and further evaluation and/or referral is warranted.

Most importantly, the successful management of a patient with a tachydysrhythmia requires a collaborative effort between the primary doctor and the appropriate subspecialist to educate and work with the family.

DISCUSSION OF THE ALGORITHM

An algorithm for the differential diagnosis of tachycardia is presented in Figure 63-5. After determining whether the heart rate varies with the respiratory cycle, the physician should assess the patient for intercurrent illness or pain. If the patient is febrile, specific physical findings that suggest cardiac infection or inflammation should be sought, with subsequent referral to a pediatric cardiologist. The afebrile patient should be evaluated for physical findings of congestive heart failure, hyperthyroidism, or altered fluid status, including supine and erect heart rates and blood pressure measurements. An accurate history of both prescription and over-the-counter medications, available in either the home or day care settings, should also be obtained.

If no obvious physical cause for the tachycardia is found, an electrocardiogram should be obtained and referral to a pediatric cardiologist should be made. With referral, a more comprehensive evaluation for supraventricular or ventricular arrhythmias can be pursued. If the patient has associated chest pain, dizziness, or syncope when the tachycardia is noted, referral to a cardiologist should be expedited.

BIBLIOGRAPHY

Hesslein P: Noninvasive arrhythmia diagnosis. In Garson A, Bricker J, McNamara D, editors: *The science and practice of pediatric cardiology,* Philadelphia, 1990, Lea & Febiger.

Ludomirsky A, Garson A: Supraventricular tachycardia. In Garson A, Bricker J, McNamara D, editors: *The science and practice of pediatric cardiology,* Philadelphia, 1990, Lea & Febiger.

O'Connor B, Dick M II: What every pediatrician should know about supraventricular tachycardia, *Pediatr Ann* 20:368, 1991.

Vetter V: What every pediatrician needs to know about arrhythmias in children who have had cardiac surgery, *Pediatr Ann* 20:378, 1991.

Vetter V: Ventricular arrhythmias in pediatric patients with and without congenital heart disease. In Horowitz LN, editor: *Current management of arrhythmias,* Ontario, 1991, BC Decker.

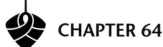

CHAPTER 64

Vaginal Discharge in the Pediatric Patient

Steven D. Spandorfer

Vaginal discharge, often as a result of a primary vaginal infection, is the most common gynecologic symptom in the pediatric patient. Accompanying symptoms often include dysuria, vaginal odor, vulvar burning, and dyspareunia.

VAGINAL ECOSYSTEM

It is very important to distinguish the premenstrual and the postmenarchal patient because the vaginal ecosystem in each is very different. The prepubertal vaginal epithelium appears redder and thinner, and the secretions are of a neutral pH. The prepubertal child lacks glycogen and lactobacilli to help fight infection. The postmenarchal patient has a vaginal pH of 3.8 to 4.2. The increased estrogen stimulates an increased glycogen content of vaginal epithelial cells. The glycogen is metabolized to lactic acid principally by lactobacilli. This acidic environment limits the potential pathogenic bacteria and protozoa.

A normal physiologic vaginal discharge consists of cervical and vaginal epithelium, normal bacterial flora, water electrolytes, and other chemicals.

Bacterial counts of approximately 109 are found in vaginal fluid. Anaerobic bacteria are found in higher concentrations than aerobic bacteria, up to five times as high. These normal vaginal secretions are described as white, floccular or curdy, and odorless.

The normal vaginal ecosystem is in a delicate balance. Perturbations of the ecosystem may lead to pathologic changes and create a vaginal discharge.

DIFFERENTIAL DIAGNOSIS

Common Causes of Vaginal Discharge
- **Infection**
   Bacterial vaginosis
   Trichomonas vaginalis
   Candida
   Herpes simplex virus
   Cervical or pelvic infection
      Neisseria gonorrhoeae
      Chlamydia trachomatis
   Pinworms *(Enterobius vermicularis)*
   Shigella
   Staphylococcus aureus
   Group A β-hemolytic streptococci
- **Trauma**
   Foreign body
   Sexual abuse
- **Carcinoma**
   Sarcoma botryoides
   Granulosa cell tumor
- **Endocrine–Metabolic**
   Normal physiologic discharge
   Pregnancy related
   Physiologic discharge of the newborn
- **Congenital**
   Ectopic ureter
- **Others**
   Primary vulvar skin disease
   Chemical disorders

Discussion

Physiologic Discharge
Physiologic discharge frequently is noted in various stages of female development. In the newborn, due to the intrauterine exposure to maternal estrogens, a discharge often is noted that lasts approximately 1 week. The discharge is odorless

and white with mucoid features. Some bloody discharge may be noted as the estrogen levels begin to fall, resulting in estrogen withdrawal and shedding of the endometrium.

During the 6- to 12-month period before menarche, as the levels of estrogen are increasing, girls often develop a physiologic discharge, which is usually gray and nonirritating. On microscopic evaluation the clinician will note many epithelial cells.

Both of these physiologic discharges are common and completely benign. Reassurance of the patient is the only treatment required.

Foreign Bodies

Vaginal foreign bodies account for approximately one in 25 gynecologic problems in children. A foreign body may present as a foul-smelling, bloody discharge. The principal complaint is often the odiferous discharge. Patients with foreign bodies generally are more likely to note a bloody discharge than a patient with an infectious cause of her vaginitis. The history often is not helpful because it is rare that the child will actually describe placing an object in her vagina. Items most commonly found in the vagina include toilet paper, sand, and toy parts.

A recent study found an association between vaginal foreign bodies in pediatric patients and sexual abuse. Eight of 12 girls evaluated for vaginal foreign bodies in this study were found to have been sexually abused. Thus, any child presenting with a foreign body should be evaluated closely for possible sexual abuse.

Removing the item with forceps and/or irrigating the vagina with a small foley is often sufficient. Occasionally, using viscous xylocaine or lubricant facilitates removal. Instruction on good hygiene is paramount.

Bacterial Vaginosis

Patients with bacterial vaginosis (BV) often will complain of a "musty, fishy" odor and a thin, gray-white discharge. The discharge is mildly adherent to the vaginal walls. A 10-fold increase in anaerobic bacteria associated with a decrease in lactobacilli also is noted.

The patient usually has an increased vaginal pH. A recent prospective study noted a specificity of 87% when the vaginal pH is greater than 5.0. A wet mount (normal saline) slide of the discharge demonstrates vaginal epithelial cells with clusters of bacteria adherent to the external surfaces and partially obscuring the border of the epithelial cells (clue cells). The wet mount also reveals no white blood cells and decreased lactobacilli.

A positive whiff test is noted, which refers to the release of aromatic amines when potassium hydroxide (KOH) is added to the vaginal discharge. This result is due to the increased (10-fold) anaerobic metabolism noted in a BV infection.

Treatment of BV is with Flagyl (metronidazole), 500 mg twice a day for 7 days. Other treatment options include clindamycin, 450 mg every 6 hours for 1 week, or Augmentin (amoxicillin and clavulaunic acid), 500 mg every 8 hours for 1 week.

Candida Infections

Candida infections commonly occur in postmenarchal women but rarely in the prepubertal girl. Candida vaginitis is produced by a fungus, and most are secondary to Candida albicans. Patients often will note a thick, white, cottage cheese–like discharge. The patient will complain of severe vaginal burning and itching. She also may report dysuria. The discharge is odorless, and the pH is normal (4.0). KOH preparation reveals hyphae and spores.

Candida infections are opportunistic infections related to a change in the vaginal ecosystem. Risk factors for Candida infections include pregnancy, use of diapers, recent ingestion of antibiotics, immunocompromised status, or diabetes.

Treatment consists of an antifungal topical cream such as mycostatin, miconazole, or clotrimazole applied to the vulva and intravaginally.

Cervical Infections

Cervical infections, including Chlamydia trachomatis, Neisseria gonorrhoeae, and pelvic inflammatory disease may first present as a vaginal discharge noted by the patient. The sexually active adolescent is at least 10 times as likely to develop pelvic inflammatory disease as a woman aged 25 years. Early coitus is a risk factor for developing a sexually transmitted disease. In the young adolescent patient, sexual abuse must always be suspected. Unfortunately, sexual abuse is very common, with an estimated one in four girls having been the victim of sexual assault.

N. gonorrhoeae may present in the prepubertal girl simply as vaginitis. Gonococcal vaginitis usually is manifested by a copious, purulent vaginal discharge. Cultures should be obtained and confirmed by a qualified laboratory because

TABLE 64-1
Possible Causes of Vaginal Discharge

ETIOLOGY	ODOR	COLOR	pH	SLIDES (KOH OR NORMAL SALINE)
Bacterial vaginosis	Yes	Gray	5–6	Clue cells
Candida	No	White	4–5	Hyphae
Trichomonas	Some	Cream	6–7	Motile Trichomonas
Cervical infection	No	Variable	Variable	Many white blood cells
Normal	No	White/clear	4	Lactobacilli
Pregnancy	No	White/clear	4	Lactobacilli

false-positive results can have very detrimental results. Treatment of *N. gonorrhoeae* is a single muscular injection of ceftriaxone (125 mg for children less than 45 kg and 250 mg for children weighing more than 45 kg). Children older than 8 years of age also should receive doxycycline, 100 mg every 12 hours for 7 to 10 days.

C. trachomatis often is acquired by perinatal exposure, sexual abuse, or consensual sexual contact. The diagnosis of *C. trachomatis* infection should be confirmed by culture. The recommended treatment is oral erythromycin for a child less than 8 years of age (12.5 mg/kg four times a day for 10 days). For children over 8 years of age, oral doxycycline should be administered as 100 mg twice a day for 7 days.

Patients with pelvic inflammatory disease, if suspected, should be referred for hospitalization and started on intravenous antibiotics, which is the best measure to preserve a patient's fertility.

Trichomonas vaginalis

Trichomonas vaginalis is an infection caused by a flagellated protozoa. Many patients with *T. vaginalis* are asymptomatic. The diagnosis generally is made on a wet mount detecting motile, unicellular trichomonads slightly larger than a white blood cell. Although wet-mount examination is the most commonly used method to diagnose *T. vaginalis*, cultures are more sensitive.

These hardy organisms can survive up to 24 hours on a wet towel and up to 6 hours on a hard surface. However, human experimental evidence indicates that patients need a large inoculum, therefore, infection from bath towels or pools is unlikely.

Patients often will complain of a thin, profuse discharge. On examination, the cervix appears erythematous with a frothy discharge. Patients also will note a foul odor.

Treatment is Flagyl (metronidazole) as a one-time dose of 2 g, or 250 mg every 8 hours for 7 days.

DATA GATHERING

History

The patient should be asked to describe the discharge. Is there an odor? Is any color noted? The patient should describe the amount of the discharge. She also should be asked about related pruritis of the vagina and vulva. The patient should be asked if she is sexually active. Healthcare providers should inquire about anal intercourse. Penile-vaginal penetration after anal intercourse may cause vaginal discharge secondary to contamination.

In any child with a sexually transmitted disease, a careful examination for evidence of sexual abuse should be made. The younger patient should be asked if anyone has touched her in her "private parts." The patient also should be asked about possible placement of foreign bodies in her vagina.

Physical Examination

A physical examination includes a careful general examination for evidence of systemic illnesses or possible sexual abuse. A thorough abdominal examination should be performed to evaluate peritoneal signs, particularly in the patient with suspected pelvic inflammatory disease.

The pelvic examination should begin with a close inspection of the vagina and genital areas. The color, odor, consistency, and amount of the discharge should be noted. The cervix should be examined, and a swab of cervical secretions should be obtained for microscopic review. A pelvic examination should include a determination of possible cervical motion tenderness and adnexal tenderness to rule out the possibility of pelvic inflammatory disease.

Laboratory examination includes evaluating the pH of the discharge and performing a whiff test. Slides of vaginal discharge (normal saline and KOH) should be evaluated. Cultures of the cervix should be obtained. In addition, a pregnancy test should never be overlooked.

INDICATIONS FOR REFERRAL

- Suspect child abuse
- Suspect pelvic inflammatory disease
- Persistent vaginal discharge despite conventional treatment
- Pregnancy
- Suspect ectopic ureter

BIBLIOGRAPHY

Arsenault PS, Gerbie AB: Vulvovaginitis in the preadolescent girl, *Pediatr Ann* 15(8):577–785, 1986.

Cohall AT, Warren A: Persistent vaginal discharge in a sexually active adolescent female, *J Adolesc Health* 12(1):58–59, 1991.

Herman-Giddens ME: Vaginal foreign bodies and child sexual abuse, *Arch Pediatr Adolesc Med* 148(2):195–200, 1994.

Larsen B: Vaginal flora in health and disease, *Clin Obstet Gynecol* 36(1):107–121, 1993.

Nelson MS: Clinical diagnosis of bacterial vaginosis, *Am J Emerg Med* 5(6):488–491, 1987.

Paradise JE, Willis ED: Probability of foreign body in girls with genital complaints, *Am J Dis Child* 139(5):472–476, 1985.

Pokorny SF: Prepubertal vulvovaginopathies, *Obstet Gynecol Clin North Am* 19(1):39–58, 1992.

Rimsza ME: An illustrated guide to adolescent gynecology, *Pediatr Clin North Am* 36(3):639–663, 1989.

Sanfillippo JS: Adolescent girls with vaginal discharge, *Pediatr Ann* 15(7):509–519, 1986.

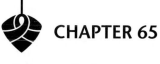

CHAPTER 65

Vomiting

Jeffrey R. Avner

Vomiting is defined as forceful expulsion of matter from the stomach through the mouth. This action is often preceded by nausea and accompanied by gastric and abdominal contractions. These various components are coordinated by a vomiting center located in the reticular formation of the medulla. Physicians must differentiate true vomiting from spitting up or regurgitation, which is common in young infants. Unlike the rhythmic and coordinated action of

vomiting, regurgitation refers to nonforceful reflux of stomach contents, which tend to roll out
rather than being expelled from the mouth, and is
usually of little significance.

The clinical findings in a child with acute vomiting relate to both the underlying cause and the
duration of the vomiting. For example, fever, diarrhea, abdominal pain, headache, and other systemic complaints may predominate initially, but
as the vomiting continues, the signs and symptoms of dehydration, such as lethargy, tachycardia, and poor skin turgor, become increasingly
apparent. Associated symptoms that should
serve as warning signs of more serious illness include age of less than 6 months, intractable or
projectile vomiting, bloody or bilious emesis, severe abdominal pain, and abdominal distention.

DIFFERENTIAL DIAGNOSIS

Common Causes of Vomiting
* **Infectious**
  Gastroenteritis
  Otitis media
  Upper respiratory tract infection
  Sepsis
  Meningitis
  Urinary tract infection or pyelonephritis
  Pneumonia
  Pertussis
  Appendicitis
  Hepatitis
* **Gastrointestinal**
  Esophageal
    Innocent vomiting
    Gastroesophageal reflux
    Chalasia
    Hiatus hernia
    Esophageal stricture
  Gastric
    Pyloric stenosis
    Peptic ulcer disease
    Gastric bezoar
  Intestinal
    Intussusception
    Incarcerated hernia
    Postoperative adhesions
    Malrotation
    Volvulus
    Cholelithiasis
* **Central nervous system**
  Head trauma

  Increased intracranial pressure
  Brain tumor
  Hydrocephalus
  Migraine
  Seizure
  Shaken baby syndrome
* **Metabolic–Endocrine**
  Inborn errors of metabolism
  Diabetic ketoacidosis
  Congenital adrenal hyperplasia
  Hypercalcemia
  Renal tubular acidosis
  Reye syndrome
* **Genitourinary–Renal**
  Urinary tract obstruction
  Renal stones
  Renal failure
  Pregnancy
* **Allergic–Immunologic**
  Cow's milk allergy
  Celiac disease
* **Toxic**
  Drugs
  Toxins
  Food poisoning
* **Psychosocial**
  Inappropriate feeding
  Nervous vomiting
  Psychogenic vomiting
  Cyclic vomiting

Discussion

Infection
Viral infection of the GI tract is the most common
cause of acute vomiting. There may be associated
low-grade fever and diarrhea, but the child usually appears well unless the vomiting is prolonged and signs of dehydration ensue. Bacterial
gastroenteritis is more abrupt and is accompanied by abdominal pain, fever, anorexia, and
bloody diarrhea. *Salmonella, Shigella,* and *Yersinia* are the common bacterial agents. Vomiting
may be a symptom of parasitic infection, such as
giardiasis, amebiasis, ascariasis, and hookworm;
other symptoms include abdominal pain, poor
weight gain, and bloody diarrhea.

Infections that occur outside the GI system may
present with vomiting. Otitis media, for example, is one of the most common causes of
vomiting. Upper respiratory tract infections may
produce vomiting when postnasal drip or swallowed mucus cause gastric irritation. However,
in the young child, in whom clinical signs are

often absent or difficult to ascertain, vomiting may herald the onset of a more serious underlying infection. A child with meningitis often presents with vomiting, irritability, and lethargy before other meningeal signs appear. Urinary tract infection and pyelonephritis often present with the same constellation of findings seen in gastroenteritis (vomiting, fever, abdominal pain, back pain) and may not include urinary tract symptoms. A young child with pneumonia may have vomiting and dehydration as a result of fever and tachypnea. The child with paroxysmal cough and posttussive emesis should alert the physician to the possibility of pertussis.

Infection of the abdominal organs usually begins with anorexia and vomiting and may progress to severe abdominal pain and peritonitis. Appendicitis may occur at any age, and typically begins with nausea, vomiting, periumbilical abdominal pain, and low-grade fever. As the inflammation of the appendix progresses, peritoneal irritation occurs and the abdominal pain shifts to the right lower quadrant. There is marked tenderness at McBurney's point (one third the distance from the right iliac crest to the umbilicus), but this tenderness varies depending on the position of the appendix (eg, retrocecal, pelvic, retroileal). Prompt diagnosis of appendicitis is important because appendiceal abscess or perforation may occur.

Hepatitis usually presents with jaundice in addition to nausea, vomiting, and right upper quadrant tenderness. In the infant, hepatitis is usually caused by congenital infection, whereas in the older child viruses and toxins predominate.

Gastrointestinal

GI disorders that lead to vomiting are related to abnormal anatomy in the GI tract that interferes with normal peristalsis. It is useful to think of these disorders based on the presence or absence of intestinal obstruction.

An abnormality of esophageal or gastric motility usually presents in the first few months of life with recurrent vomiting or regurgitation after feeding. Chalasia is poor tone in the lower esophageal sphincter and may be accompanied by physiologic gastroesophageal reflux in as many as one half of all healthy newborns. Often called functional gastroesophageal reflux, some physicians prefer the term "innocent vomiting," because the latter implies a normal variant rather than an abnormal state. Innocent vomiting often begins in the newborn period and usually resolves within the first year of life as the child spends more time upright and esophageal sphincter tone increases. Vomiting episodes, although as frequent as several times an hour, are not accompanied by nausea, retching, or pain. Anything that increases intraabdominal pressure, and thus intragastric pressure, will exaggerate this condition. Thus, it is common for an infant to vomit or regurgitate after eating, coughing, or exercising. The position of an infant in an infant seat also tends to increase intraabdominal pressure and lead to reflux. Innocent vomiting almost always occurs during the wakeful state. Infants with innocent vomiting have normal growth and development; if the infant fails to thrive, there is likely to be a more severe case of gastroesophageal reflux associated with aspiration, pneumonia, or esophagitis.

Hiatal and paraesophageal hernias, which involve prolapse of a portion of the stomach into the thoracic cavity, present with recurrent gastroesophageal reflux. Intermittent colicky abdominal pain, often associated with fatty foods, point to cholelithiasis, especially in children with risk factors for the development of biliary stones (eg, patients with sickle cell disease and recurrent hemolysis develop bilirubin stones).

Any projectile, nonbilious vomiting should raise a high suspicion of pyloric stenosis. The infant usually has an unremarkable birth history, but episodes of vomiting begin by the first month of life. The vomiting is at first intermittent, but soon becomes projectile (often described as "shooting across the room"). The symptoms depend on the duration of the vomiting. Initially the infant appears well, but as the illness progresses, may appear irritable or lethargic. With prolonged vomiting, metabolic changes (hyponatremia, hypochloremia, hypokalemia, alkalosis) become evident. On physical examination, there may be a palpable olive, the hypertrophied muscle, just to the right of the midline above the umbilicus. Visible abdominal peristaltic waves may also be seen.

Intussusception is the telescoping of an intestinal segment and usually involves invagination of the ileum through the ileocecal valve into the colon. It is characteristically seen in children between 3 and 24 months of age and begins with the sudden onset of crampy abdominal pain during which the child screams and pulls the knees up to the abdomen. Vomiting follows shortly thereafter, and the child becomes increasingly lethargic or demonstrates paradoxic irritability. An abdominal mass, usually in the right lower quadrant, and heme-positive or currant jelly stools may be seen later in the course of the disease. Intussusception may also occur in an older child, in which case there is usually a lead point in the intestine, such as a polyp or mesenteric adenitis.

Gastric bezoars can present with intermittent vomiting, an abdominal mass, and weight loss. In children the bezoar usually consists of large quantities of matted hair in the stomach. Other causes of vomiting associated with small bowel obstruction include inguinal hernia, intestinal volvulus, or if there was previous abdominal surgery, intestinal adhesions.

Central Nervous System

Any process that causes irritation of the central nervous system (CNS) may result in vomiting. Cerebral edema, increased intracranial pressure, or changes in cerebral vascular flow may cause hypersensitivity of the vomiting center. The vomiting is often forceful, at times projectile, and may not be preceded by nausea.

It is common for head trauma to cause vomiting. Even minor head trauma, without any loss of consciousness, may cause vomiting for 6 to 8 hours after the initial injury. However, persistent vomiting or any associated neurologic change should alert the physician to the possibility of more serious intracranial injury (ie, epidural, subdural, or subarachnoid bleed).

The vomiting associated with increased intracranial pressure from brain tumors, hydrocephalus, or pseudotumor cerebri is usually worse in the morning or when the patient is lying down and is accompanied by headache. Over time, other signs of increased intracranial pressure develop, such as increasing head circumference, bulging fontanelle, sunsetting, cranial nerve palsies, ataxia, or papilledema.

Certain types of headache, especially migraine, have vomiting as a prominent symptom. The classic migraine headache is pulsatile, preceded by an aura, and accompanied by nausea, vomiting, abdominal pain, and the desire to rest or sleep. Common migraine headache, the most frequent type of migraine in children, typically lacks the preceding aura but is accompanied by nausea, vomiting, and pallor. Vomiting is occa-

sionally seen with seizures, either during the acute event or in the early postictal period.

Shaken baby syndrome, or shaken impact syndrome, is a particular type of closed head injury resulting from child abuse. When a baby is violently shaken and the baby's head hits a wall or crib/changing table mattress, significant acceleration and deceleration forces cause shearing of the long axonal fibers, tearing of venous sinusoids, and brain deformation. Several types of intracranial injuries may result (eg, diffuse axonal injury, subdural hematoma). Because the history from the parent is often vague or nonspecific, the physician should be acutely aware of this presenting signs of this syndrome, which include vomiting, lethargy, and irritability.

Metabolic-Endocrine

Recurrent or persistent vomiting may be a sign of an underlying defect in amino acid, organic acid, or carbohydrate metabolism. These inborn errors of metabolism usually present as either acute decompensation or failure to thrive. In the acute setting, there is often a mild preceding illness, which is followed by rapid production of a metabolic acidosis or hyperammonemia. These metabolic derangements are accompanied by persistent, forceful vomiting. The child becomes progressively lethargic, and seizures or coma may ensue. On a more chronic basis, there is growth retardation and slowly progressive neurologic deterioration.

Diabetic ketoacidosis often presents with nausea, vomiting, and abdominal pain, although there is usually a history of tiredness, polyuria, polydipsia, and anorexia. As the vomiting, osmotic diuresis, and acidosis proceed, the child becomes more dehydrated and shock may ensue. The fruity smell of ketones on the breath reflect ketoacidosis.

Vomiting can be seen in acute adrenal insufficiency, which may be precipitated in a child with congenital adrenal hyperplasia who is under stress, noncompliant with medication, or undiagnosed. Hypercalcemia usually produces anorexia, vomiting, dehydration, headache, polydipsia, and polyuria.

The abrupt onset of protracted vomiting, lethargy, and sleepiness after varicella or a flulike illness should immediately alert the physician to the possibility of Reye syndrome. The vomiting usually starts within 1 week of the prodrome and is present in more than 80% of cases. Rapidly progressive encephalopathy and increased intracranial pressure can lead to altered mental status, stupor, and coma. Rapid evaluation and immediate referral to an intensive care unit should be the rule.

Genitourinary-Renal

Infections of the genitourinary system, such as pelvic inflammatory disease, urethritis, cystitis, and pyelonephritis, are often accompanied by vomiting. In addition, any process that causes urinary obstruction usually has vomiting in association with abdominal pain. Obstruction in the urinary tract can be caused by a variety of problems including posterior urethral valves, congenital or anatomic anomalies, calculi, or trauma. Typically there is nausea, vomiting, abdominal pain, and flank pain that is colicky in nature. Overflow incontinence and poor urinary stream may be noted as well. Obstructive renal insufficiency can lead to vomiting, diarrhea, and failure to thrive. Other causes of acute renal failure may be accompanied by anemia, edema, hypertension, and lethargy.

Pregnancy is a commonly overlooked diagnosis when an adolescent girl complains of nausea, vomiting, or morning sickness. A teenage girl should be questioned (without her parents present) about sexual activity, and a urine pregnancy test performed if there is the slightest suspicion of pregnancy.

Allergic-Immunologic

Cow's milk allergy usually manifests itself within the first 2 months of life, and is more common in boys and children with a family history of allergies. There is an abnormal GI response probably related to the protein in cow's milk. Vomiting, diarrhea, and abdominal pain predominate, and may progress to gastric outlet obstruction. In addition, there is often GI blood loss and protein malabsorption leading to anemia, edema, and failure to thrive.

Toxins

Several drugs may cause vomiting when toxic levels are achieved either by inappropriate dosing, accidental ingestion, or suicide attempt. Theophylline is a medication used for reversible bronchospasm in the pediatric age group. The recommended oral dose is 16 to 24 mg/kg/day to maintain a serum concentration of 10 to 20 mg/L. Changes in theophylline metabolism are com-

monly seen in children during certain illnesses or when used in combination with certain drugs (eg, erythromycin). As the toxic level is approached, nausea, vomiting, and abdominal cramping become apparent, and at high levels seizures may ensue.

Digitalis toxicity is often first manifested by nausea and vomiting, and may progress to weakness, worsening heart failure, and cardiac arrhythmias. With aspirin and iron toxicity, GI upset usually predominates the clinical picture and may be severe enough to cause GI hemorrhage. Lead poisoning is classically seen in children younger than 6 years old who often have a history of pica. As blood lead levels rise, there is the onset of forceful vomiting, irritability, and weight loss. At very high levels the signs of increased intracranial pressure and encephalopathy (personality change, seizures, coma) become more apparent.

Food poisoning usually presents with the abrupt onset of vomiting, cramps, and diarrhea. These symptoms are mediated by emetic and necrotizing toxins produced by bacteria in contaminated food. Staphylococci are found in dairy and cream preparation; Vibrio is associated with fish, shellfish, and crabs; toxigenic *Escherichia coli, Clostridium,* and *Bacillus* are found in a variety of contaminated meats and food.

Psychosocial

Overfeeding and inappropriate feeding are common causes of regurgitation and vomiting during the first year of life. Excessive amounts of formula given at each feeding or given too frequently will result in gastric distention and lead to vomiting of small amounts of formula. High-fat diets result in delayed gastric emptying, causing vomiting, distention, and discomfort. Inappropriately mixed formula resulting in a high caloric content can cause gastric irritation, vomiting, and diarrhea.

Nervous vomiting is a disorder that can begin as early as the newborn period. Heightened parental anxiety causes the infant to have an exaggerated response to external stimuli. When the infant vomits, the parent becomes overly distressed by an inability to calm the infant. If repeated, this tension is sensed by the infant who then becomes nervous, emotional, and anxious. The infant can become tense to even the slightest stimulus, and often vomits with an accompanying expression of pain and discomfort. Prolonged nervous vomiting can lead to the infant's failure to thrive.

Psychogenic vomiting is related to stress, fear, depression, or anticipation of unpleasant events. In these situations, the medullary vomiting center probably receives afferent stimuli from the sensory organs. Cyclic vomiting is recurrent episodes of forceful vomiting without an apparent cause. There may be associated nausea, headache, and abdominal pain as well as a family history of migraine.

DATA GATHERING

The most common diagnosis in a child with vomiting is gastritis or gastroenteritis, often viral. However, this diagnosis is usually a result of exclusion. A careful history and physical examination are necessary to narrow the long list of differential diagnoses and rule out more serious illness.

History

The history should concentrate on several areas: age of the child, time course and characteristics of the vomiting, associated abdominal and extraabdominal symptoms, and state of hydration. First, it is necessary to ascertain that the complaint is truly one of vomiting and not simply regurgitation. The age of the child will help narrow the diagnosis, because many disorders are seen almost exclusively in certain age groups. A detailed history about the vomiting should be sought. Is the vomiting nonforceful or is it projectile? When did it begin? How many times a day? Is it related to eating? Vomiting immediately after eating leads to a diagnosis of infection. Recurrent vomiting 1 to 4 hours after eating is consistent with intrinsic gastric or duodenal lesions. When during the day is the vomiting worse? Early morning vomiting is usually seen with increased intracranial pressure, pregnancy, uremia, or postnasal drip. Is there associated nausea? Vomiting without nausea is common in CNS lesions. The characteristics of the vomiting are important. Blood or bile in the vomitus may be related to prolonged vomiting or to obstruction. Is there vomiting of mucus or food particles?

Associated symptoms may help further define the cause of the vomiting. Abdominal pain, obstipation, and abdominal distention are seen in intestinal obstruction. Diarrhea is consistent with gastroenteritis. Headache, stiff neck, blurred vision, mental status change, or a history of head trauma are suggestive of a CNS injury. Irritability, a high-pitched cry, and convulsions suggest meningitis. A sore throat, cough, or earache point to other infectious causes.

Finally, a detailed dietary history should be obtained. Is the child tolerating clear fluids? Does the child have normal urine output? Is the child taking any medicines or have any predisposing illness?

Physical Examination

The general appearance of the child often reflects the severity of the underlying illness. A toxic-appearing or inconsolable child usually has a serious infection. Paradoxical irritability (ie, the child cries more when held by parent) is commonly seen with meningitis or intussusception. A chronically ill child may have metabolic or renal disease.

A careful and thorough examination is necessary to detect a source of infection. Next, attention should be directed to an orderly and complete abdominal examination. Inspection of the abdomen for distention and visible peristalsis may help diagnose an intestinal obstruction. Auscultation of all four quadrants is necessary to assess bowel sounds. Percussion should be used to determine liver size. Tenderness to percussion is often used as a clinical predictor for rebound tenderness. Finally, the abdominal examination should concentrate on palpation. It is helpful to identify which quadrant has guarding, tenderness, or rebound. A patient with jaundice may have hepatitis or cholelithiasis. A palpable olive in the right upper quadrant just to the right of midline above the umbilicus suggests pyloric stenosis (Fig. 65-1). Intussusception often presents with a palpable mass in the right lower or right upper quadrant. Finally, a rectal examination and stool heme test should be performed.

Assessment of hydration is best done by serial weights, but in their absence, clinical parameters are often helpful. Tachycardia, rapid respirations, poor skin turgor, dry mucous membranes, and sunken eyes are indicators of dehydration.

Finally, observation of how the child is fed and the parent-infant interaction may be a clue as to the diagnosis of overfeeding or nervous vomiting.

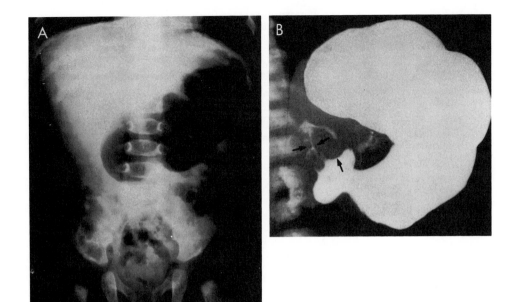

FIG 65-1

Pyloric stenosis. **A,** Supine film of the abdomen reveals distension of the stomach. Multiple peristaltic waves (contractions) are visible. This is one of the plain-film findings of gastric outlet obstruction. **B,** Oblique view of this patient shows the elongated upturned pyloric channel with a single track (contrast in a compressed lumen) above the arrows, and a double, or railroad track, configuration (contrast in two asymmetric lumens) below the arrows. In addition, there is an impression of the pyloric muscle on the base of the duodenal bulb and on the antral surface of the stomach (single arrow). [From Haller JO, Slovis TL: Introduction to Radiology in Clinical Pediatrics, Chicago, 1984, Year Book Medical Publishers. Used by permission.]

Laboratory Evaluation

The majority of cases of vomiting are benign; the child usually appears well, and no further laboratory tests are required. Otherwise, the physician should direct the workup based on the history and physical examination. If the child is febrile and ill-appearing, it may be necessary to sample blood, urine, stool, or cerebrospinal fluid to identify a source of infection. Upright and supine abdominal x-ray films are the first step in evaluation of intraabdominal disease. Ultrasound is useful in diagnosing pyloric stenosis, and a barium enema study is often both diagnostic and therapeutic for intussusception. Other specific tests should follow from positive assessment. Any child in whom the status of hydration is in question should undergo tests for urine specific gravity and serum electrolyte levels.

Management Issues

Most vomiting is caused by an underlying disease. Therefore, prompt treatment of the primary illness is the most effective therapy. In addition, appropriate symptomatic treatment will stop most vomiting within 8 to 12 hours.

The basic treatment is frequent small feedings, which produce less distention and stress on the stomach. At first, all feedings, including formula, liquids, and solids, should be stopped. When no vomiting has occurred for 2 hours, a clear liquid diet should be initiated. The child should be allowed only 1 ounce of liquid every hour. This approach is often difficult, because the child usually wants more fluid; but if allowed, the vicious cycle—gastric distention causing vomiting causing hunger causing increased intake causing gastric distention—will ensue. Commercial rehydration solutions may be given to infants; flat soda, juices, tea, or popsicles are appropriate for the older child. Plain water should be avoided. If there is no vomiting for 8 to 12 hours, a BRAT (bananas, rice, applesauce, toast) diet may be started. If no vomiting occurs after 24 hours, breast-feeding, formula, and milk products may be added slowly.

The parent should understand the importance

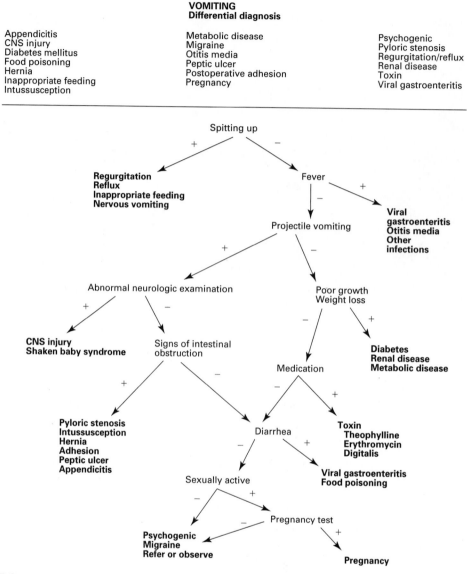

VOMITING
Differential diagnosis

Appendicitis	Metabolic disease	Psychogenic
CNS injury	Migraine	Pyloric stenosis
Diabetes mellitus	Otitis media	Regurgitation/reflux
Food poisoning	Peptic ulcer	Renal disease
Hernia	Postoperative adhesion	Toxin
Inappropriate feeding	Pregnancy	Viral gastroenteritis
Intussusception		

FIG 65-2
Decision tree for differential diagnosis of vomiting.

of these guidelines and not be tempted to give the child large amounts to drink; this will only increase the vomiting. It should also be stressed that a clear liquid diet should not be given for more than 2 days, because reactive loose stools or starvation stools may result.

Antiemetic therapy in the form of antihistamines and anticholinergics is occasionally used, but the associated side effects are often more troubling than any relief it offers and may mask

intraabdominal disease. Furthermore, antiemetics should be avoided in the young or ill-appearing child. Proper hygiene and handwashing techniques should be stressed to help prevent spread of disease.

Parents of infants diagnosed with innocent vomiting or function gastroesophageal reflux should be reassured that the child is growing and developing normally and that the regurgitation is expected to resolve within a few months. For infants with nervous vomiting, parents should be counseled to decrease excessive stimulation and attempt to reduce the tension that developed in the parent-infant interaction.

INDICATIONS FOR CONSULTATION OR REFERRAL

Most vomiting can be treated in the outpatient setting by frequent telephone follow-up calls or office visits. If the child is ill-appearing or has signs of moderate-to-severe dehydration, referral for IV fluids and assessment of acid-base status is indicated. Any child with projectile vomiting or an abnormal abdominal examination should be seen by a surgeon. In addition, bloody, feculant, or bilious vomiting suggests an anatomic etiology.

Children with persistent vomiting for more than 12 hours and infants younger than 6 months are at high risk for rapid development of dehydration and may need in-hospital observation.

Finally, any child with a severe underlying illness, such as serious infection, CNS injury, a suspected metabolic disorder, as well as a child with persistent vomiting for 4 to 6 hours in the absence of any oral intake during that time, should be admitted to the hospital and appropriate consultation sought.

DISCUSSION OF ALGORITHM

An algorithm for the differential diagnosis of vomiting is presented in Figure 65-2. The first step is to make sure that the problem is not just "spitting up" or regurgitation. Next, a careful history will help differentiate acute and chronic causes. If the vomiting is acute then infectious, CNS, and intraabdominal causes should be ruled out. Recurrent vomiting associated with failure to thrive suggests chronic disease. Finally, if these pathways are not productive, viral gastroenteritis, food poisoning, or psychogenic vomiting are the more likely causes.

BIBLIOGRAPHY

Fleisher DR: Functional vomiting disorders of infancy: Innocent vomiting, nervous vomiting, and infant rumination syndrome, *J Pediatr* 125:S84-S94, 1994.

Hyman PE: Gastroesophageal reflux: One reason why baby won't eat, *J Pediatr* 125:S103-S109, 1994.

Ramos AG, Tuchman DN: Persistent vomiting, *Pediatr Rev* 15:24-31, 1994.

Roy CC, Silverman A, Cozzetto FJ: *Pediatr Clin Gastroenterol,* St. Louis, 1995, CV Mosby.

Walker WA, Durie PR, Hamilton JR, et al: *Pediatric Gastrointestinal Disease,* Philadelphia, 1991, BC Decker.

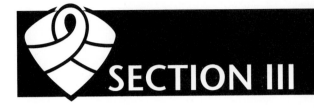

SECTION III

The Ill or Injured Child

Section III offers information on the treatment of the ill or injured child. It includes chapters that detail the management of childhood illness and injuries: acute and chronic, biomolecular and psychosocial, self-limiting and life-threatening. The goal of this section is to provide the primary care physician with clinical information that will be useful in the office setting. A limited amount of background information has been included with the expectation that this section will be used as an immediate practical desk reference rather than as a shelved volume used for interest reading. Obviously, in a book of this size, we could not include every rare condition and syndrome. Thus, we have limited ourselves to the most common illnesses (*eg*, fever, pneumonia, minor trauma) and the ones that bring the primary care provider and subspecialist in frequent communication (*eg*, epilepsy, hemophilia, diabetes).

We also have limited the scope of management guidelines to what can be done in the office. The authors have provided clear indications for when and in what situations a referral to the hospital or to the specialist should be made. Many of the chapters in this section have been written by primary care providers. Other chapters, written by pediatric subspecialists or pediatric surgeons, stress not what the subspecialist knows but what the primary care provider may want to know and be able to do.

The chapters are arranged in alphabetic order for easy reference. There are two major chapter clusters; one having to do with infections and the other with traumatic injuries. These two areas consume the greatest percentage of the primary care physician's time beyond that devoted to well-child care.

PART ONE

General Concerns

CHAPTER 66

Dehydration

John Loiselle
Marc Gorelick

INTRODUCTION

Dehydration resulting from gastroenteritis or other acute illness is one of the most common problems encountered in pediatric patients, leading to significant utilization of health resources and morbidity. In the United States, diarrheal illness accounts for an estimated 2 to 3.5 million healthcare visits annually among children less than 5 years of age alone. However, more than 90% of these cases are successfully managed on an outpatient basis. This chapter will address the diagnosis and management of dehydration in children, with emphasis on clinical evaluation and oral rehydration, which can be accomplished in the primary care setting.

BACKGROUND

Normal Fluid and Electrolyte Metabolism
Water constitutes 60% to 70% of a child's body weight. Of this total body water, approximately one third is extracellular (including intravascular and interstitial fluid) and the remainder is intracellular. The predominant extracellular anion is sodium, with a normal concentration of 144

mmol/L. Intracellular fluid, conversely, contains very little sodium but is rich in potassium (154 mmol/L). There is a regular turnover of body fluids, related to metabolic activity. Under normal circumstances, fluid intake replaces the water and electrolytes lost through respiration and evaporation from the skin (together known as *insensible losses*), urinary excretion, and the gastrointestinal tract. The water required for maintenance of homeostasis can be estimated in several ways. The simplest formula is based on the child's weight: for the first 10 kg of body mass, 100 mL/kg/day of water is needed; add 50 mL/day for each of the next 10 kg, and 20 mL/day for each subsequent kg. Regardless of weight, the daily maintenance requirement for sodium is 3 to 4 mmol/kg, and 2 to 3 mmol/kg for potassium.

Dehydration
Circumstances leading to increased loss of fluid, or decreased intake, can produce a deficiency of water and electrolytes. In children, the most common cause of dehydration is acute gastroenteritis. Poor oral fluid intake in children with pharyngitis, stomatitis, oral trauma, or a variety of other acute illnesses also may lead to dehydra-

tion. The fluid deficit usually is defined in terms of the percentage of body weight lost. Ideally, the fluid deficit is calculated from the child's weight before illness, if it is known:

Fluid deficit (%) =

$$\frac{\text{Pre-illness weight} - \text{Weight on presentation}}{\text{Pre-illness weight}} \times 100\%$$

Mild dehydration is defined as a loss of 3% to 5% of body weight, moderate dehydration is a loss of 6% to 10%, and a deficit in excess of 10% constitutes severe dehydration. Because the pre-illness weight often is not reliably known, an estimate of the fluid deficit is made using other clinical parameters as described below.

Under most circumstances, water and electrolyte losses are roughly proportional, and serum sodium concentration remains normal. This condition is referred to as isonatremic, or isotonic, dehydration. Hyponatremia, defined as a serum sodium concentration less than 130 mmol/L, results when sodium is lost in excess of water, or when replacement fluids contain too little sodium. Conversely, a proportionately greater loss of water compared with sodium, or inadequate free water replacement, produces hypernatremia (serum sodium concentration greater than 150 mmol/L). The incidence of hypo- and hypernatremia reported in the literature varies widely. Among children with mild to moderate dehydration, however, significant abnormality of the serum sodium is quite unusual.

Although either hyponatremia or hypernatremia may occur in simple gastroenteritis, depending on the electrolyte content of the fluids lost, certain factors increase the risk of these complications. Young infants, whose renal regulatory function is immature, are at special risk of electrolyte imbalance. In addition, a common clinical scenario leading to hyponatremic dehydration is feeding of excess plain water to young infants with vomiting or diarrhea. Less common conditions that may cause hyponatremia include cystic fibrosis with abnormal sodium losses in sweat, renal salt wasting, adrenal insufficiency, and excessive gastrostomy tube output. Hypernatremia accompanies excessive sodium replacement and may occur if infant formula is improperly prepared or water intake is inadequate, the latter being more common in neurologically impaired children. Illnesses associated with fever or tachypnea, which lead to increased insensible losses of free water, also can cause hypernatremic dehydration.

CLINICAL EVALUATION

History
The history can provide clues to the presence of dehydration and to the possibility of an associated electrolyte imbalance. The duration of the illness is important, because dehydration usually develops over a period of 1 to several days, rather than a few hours. The primary care physician should question the child's caretaker about the presence, frequency, and volume of vomiting or diarrhea and whether the child is able to keep down any liquids. The physician should keep in mind that the actual volume of emesis is difficult to quantify accurately. The amount and type of fluids taken by the child during the illness should be noted. For bottle-fed infants, the physician should ask specifically about how the formula is prepared, whether the child has been given plain water, or if the child has high fever and tachypnea, which may be associated with hypernatremia.

It is important to get an estimate of the child's urine output by asking about frequency and quantity of urination. The caretaker may report that the urine appears concentrated. Oliguria is a very sensitive indicator of dehydration. However, because it is one of the earliest findings to appear, many children without a significant fluid deficit will report decreased urine output. Urine output also may be difficult to quantify in children with severe diarrhea who are in diapers.

Physical Examination
The physical examination should begin with a careful measurement of the patient's weight without clothing, or in a dry diaper. If the pre-illness weight is known from the office records, the fluid deficit can be calculated. In addition, weight gain will be a very useful indicator of progress during treatment.

Physical findings in dehydration reflect primarily losses of intravascular volume and interstitial fluid. Signs indicative of dehydration include mental status changes, tachycardia, decreased tears, dry mucous membranes, sunken eyes, prolonged capillary refill, decreased skin elasticity, sunken anterior fontanelle, weak radial pulse, and hyperpnea (Table 66-1). Skin

TABLE 66-1
Clinical Signs of Dehydration

FINDING	NORMAL	5% OR MORE DEHYDRATION
Mental status	Alert, may be thirsty	Lethargic, drowsy
Mucous membranes	Moist	Dry
Tears	Present	Absent
Capillary refill time	Less than 2 seconds	Greater than 2 seconds
Skin elasticity	Pinch retracts immediately	Pinch retracts slowly
Eyes	Normal	Sunken
Anterior fontanelle	Flat	Sunken
Heart rate	Normal	Increased
Respirations	Normal	Deep or rapid
Radial pulse	Normal strength	Weak or thready

elasticity is examined by pinching the skin on the side of the abdomen, which should retract immediately. When measuring capillary refill time, the physician holds the child's hand at approximately the level of the heart, applies moderate pressure to a fingertip, and counts the time until return of normal color. When determined in this way, a time of greater than 2 seconds is abnormal. The normal capillary refill on the foot is longer than at the fingertip, so 2 seconds may not be a reliable indicator of decreased skin perfusion. Also, even moderately cool ambient temperature may falsely prolong capillary refill time. Other physical signs may be similarly affected by extraneous factors. Dry mucous membranes may be seen in children with mouth breathing, for example, and fever may increase heart rate even in the absence of dehydration.

In general, patients without clinically important dehydration will not manifest any of these signs, although they may have diminished urine output. By the time the fluid deficit reaches 4% to 5% of body weight, several of these findings will be apparent. No single individual sign is pathognomonic for the presence of dehydration. A reasonable guideline is that three or more findings indicate a deficit of 5% or more. As dehydration becomes more severe, the number and severity of the findings will increase. Children with a deficit of greater than 10% often will show signs of cardiovascular instability such as severe tachycardia, mottled skin, or hypotension.

Children with hyponatremia have a relatively greater loss of extracellular than intracellular fluid. Consequently, the physical findings in such patients may be more marked, and the actual fluid deficit will be somewhat less than estimated on the basis of the clinical assessment.

Conversely, in hypernatremic dehydration, intravascular volume is relatively preserved, moderating the clinical picture and leading to underestimation of the deficit. Certain findings are particularly suggestive of electrolyte imbalance. Hyponatremia is associated with muscle cramps, weakness, extreme lethargy, hyporeflexia, and seizures. Hypothermia is also commonly seen. Doughy skin, irritability, hypertonicity, hyperreflexia, and high-pitched cry are characteristic of hypernatremia.

Laboratory Studies

Serum sodium concentration is the most useful laboratory test in children with dehydration, because it allows classification of the type of dehydration. However, in the child with clinically mild or moderate disease, a significant abnormality that would alter the patient's management is unlikely in the absence of suggestive features in the history or physical examination. Electrolytes should be obtained in the child with clinically severe dehydration, or if hyponatremia or hypernatremia is suspected on the basis of the history or physical examination.

Other laboratory tests are not generally helpful in the diagnosis and management of dehydration in children. Elevated urine specific gravity, like diminished urine output, is an early finding and is frequently seen even with a small fluid deficit. Conversely, blood urea nitrogen does not typically become abnormally increased until the dehydration is advanced and clinically obvious. The serum bicarbonate concentration is often low in children with dehydration, and the level correlates inversely with the magnitude of the fluid deficit. However, decreased serum bicarbonate is common in children with gastroenteritis with or without dehydration due to loss of bicarbonate ion in the stool. Thus, these tests are unlikely to affect the management of a child with a clinical picture of mild or moderate dehydration.

MANAGEMENT

Oral Rehydration

The management most readily available to the primary care physician when faced with a mild to moderately dehydrated child is oral rehydration therapy. Rehydration of the child within the office setting offers several advantages. Foremost among these is the empowerment of the parents. Rather than promoting a feeling of helplessness, it instills confidence in the parents because the care of their ill child remains within their means. High-technology therapy, in the majority of cases, is not necessary to treat this condition. Parents may utilize this knowledge in the future to properly manage or even avoid similar episodes.

Experience has proven oral rehydration to be safe and medically effective regardless of the underlying cause of dehydration. It eliminates the need for emergency department visits, intravenous (IV) line placement, and admission to the hospital in more than 90% of cases. Equipment required to institute this approach is easily stocked in the office, and training of personnel in its administration is not difficult.

There are also some inherent disadvantages to this approach. Some parents may be reluctant to try something they feel is no different from what has already failed at home. Oral rehydration therapy involves an investment of time by both the parent and staff to provide the continuous observation, repeated evaluations, and positive reinforcement necessary in this approach. Further constraints arise when therapy is limited to the daily working hours of the staff. In the majority of cases the potential for success and its associated benefits, as well as the avoidance of painful procedures and hospital admission, almost always outweigh the disadvantages.

In approaching management it is important to remember that dehydration is not a disease, but a disease state with multiple etiologies. Each patient must be carefully evaluated prior to instituting therapy to ensure that he/she is a candidate for oral rehydration therapy (Box 66-1).

BOX 66-1
Contraindications to Oral Rehydration Therapy

- Etiology requiring further evaluation
- Shock
- Poor gag reflex
- Poor sucking reflex
- Unresponsiveness or significantly depressed mental status
- Intractable vomiting
- Preterm infant
- Stool output >15 cc/kg/hr
- No capable family member

Sepsis, intestinal obstruction, appendicitis, pyloric stenosis, and diabetic ketoacidosis are only a few of the causes of dehydration in children that require further evaluation or urgent therapy and must be considered prior to initiating oral fluids. Oral rehydration therapy is reserved for the child meeting the following criteria: 1) mild to moderate dehydration, 2) stable vital signs, 3) the ability to protect his/her airway, and 4) accompanied by a capable family member. Severe dehydration, shock, unresponsiveness, or a depressed mental status are absolute contraindications to oral rehydration therapy. Ongoing fluid losses may be too extreme to initiate oral rehydration therapy. Stool output greater than 15 cc/kg/hr has been associated with only a 15% success rate with oral rehydration therapy, whereas stool output below this has an 80% chance of success. Intractable vomiting is considered a contraindication, although vomiting in and of itself is not and can be overcome in 90% of cases. The preterm infant generally is considered a poor candidate, as are infants with a poor suck or gag reflex.

Electrolyte Disturbances

The possibility of coexisting electrolyte disturbances and the difficulty in detecting these without the ability to measure serum sodium is a concern of many physicians caring for the dehydrated child. The presence of a sodium imbalance is not a contraindication to oral rehydration therapy and can be corrected with this therapy. As noted previously, a sodium imbalance is more commonly associated with one of the previously listed contraindications to oral rehydration therapy or is suspected based on characteristics of the presenting history or findings on the physical examination.

TABLE 66-2
Electrolyte Composition of Oral Solutions

	SUGAR (g/L)	SODIUM (meq/L)	OSMOLARITY (mOsm/L)
Rehydration solutions:			
Rehydralyte	25	75	305
World Health Organization packet	20	90	330
Maintenance solutions:			
Pedialyte	25	45	250
Infalyte	30	50	200
Commercial products:			
Apple juice	104–112	1.7–4.4	700
Orange juice	100	4.4	675
Cola	104	4.4–6.0	>500
Kool Aid®	64	0	—
Ginger ale	100	4.4	>500
Gatorade®	19	56	350
Chicken noodle soup	4	167	—

III

Physiology

The management of dehydration requires the replacement of water and electrolytes in the same quantities as they are lost. The intestinal epithelium contains an active glucose/sodium cotransport process so that the addition of glucose to sodium-containing solutions facilitates movement of both water and sodium across the intestinal wall and into the bloodstream.

Rehydration solutions contain isoosmolar concentrations of glucose and sodium, which best promote the rapid absorption of fluids and electrolytes (Table 66-2). These concentrations are based on the active glucose absorption and passive sodium absorption in the intestine. Maintenance solutions, used to prevent dehydration or to maintain hydration following rehydration, differ mainly in having a lower sodium concentration.

Solutions in which the sodium and glucose concentrations are not optimal may result in electrolyte imbalances or increased water loss. Solutions containing glucose in concentrations greater than 3% will exceed the absorptive capacity of the intestines. The unabsorbed glucose remaining in the lumen forms an osmotic gradient across the intestines, resulting in the loss of intravascular water, which may exacerbate diarrhea and produce a hypernatremic state. This condition occurs with commonly available commercial products such as juices and sodas, all of which contain excessively high concentrations of glucose. Hypernatremia also may be induced by hyperosmolar solutions containing an excessively high sodium content. Alternatively, administration of free water or diluted commercial products results in a reversed osmotic gradient with excess water absorption contributing to a hyponatremic state. For these reasons it is important that replacement fluids with the appropriate concentration of solutes be used in oral rehydration therapy.

Rehydration Phase

There are two phases in the treatment of dehydration: the rehydration phase and the maintenance phase. The goal of the replacement phase is to correct the incurred deficit while providing maintenance requirements and keeping up with ongoing losses. The replacement phase takes place over a 4-hour period while the child remains under observation in the office. A few calculations are necessary to determine the optimum rate of fluid administration for the individual patient suffering from dehydration. Sample replacement calculations for an infant weighing 10 kg who has become 5% dehydrated as the result of a 3-day course of vomiting and diarrhea is demonstrated below:

	DAILY	OVER 4 HOURS
Deficit	500 cc	500 cc
Maintenance	1000 cc	167 cc
Losses	300 cc*	50 cc
	Total	717 cc

*The estimated losses of 30 cc/kg/day are based on the average losses from common causes of acute gastroenteritis in the United States.

This patient would require the administration of 717 cc over the first 4-hour period. This treatment could be accomplished by delivering approximately 1 tablespoon of rehydration solution every 5 minutes. Administration of 5 cc each minute by teaspoon or syringe is frequently advocated. This rate is frequently successful even in the vomiting infant because these solutions pass rapidly through the stomach. Delivery of small, frequent aliquots over time is better tolerated and results in increased absorption in a vomiting infant. It is essential to place strict limits on the speed of administration and to have the parent, rather than the child, control the intake. This is the most common mistake resulting in failure at home. Fluid administration should be performed by the parent and not the nurse in order to instill confidence in the parent. Education regarding fluid replacement and signs of dehydration can occur during this time.

A rehydration solution is the preferred fluid for this phase. As stated previously, the goal is to match the composition of the replacement fluid with that of the losses. Rehydration solutions initially were designed to replace fluids lost in victims of cholera. In the United States common causes of diarrhea and dehydration do not result in such high sodium losses. The sodium concentration in current rehydration solutions is a compromise between these conditions. In the United States and other developed countries where cholera is uncommon, the lower sodium-containing maintenance solutions have been used successfully for the rehydration phase. Future oral rehydration solutions containing proteins and complex carbohydrates are being developed with the goal of reducing the severity and duration of the vomiting and diarrhea.

Monitoring

Monitoring consists of hourly recordings of intake and output, serial weights, vital signs, and clinical condition. Treatment failure occurs if the child clinically deteriorates, becomes further dehydrated during the time of observation, or develops a persistently negative fluid balance or if the parent refuses to continue with the therapy (Table 66-2). These children then will require IV therapy.

Intravenous Therapy

Normal saline or lactated Ringer's solution are the initial fluids used in IV therapy for the dehydrated infant or child. These solutions are administered as a 20-cc/kg bolus over 20 to 30 minutes. A sodium level should be obtained at the time of IV placement if a sodium abnormality is suspected. A dextrostick also should be obtained. Calculations for IV fluid corrections generally are not carried out in the primary care practitioner's office and are beyond the scope of this chapter.

Maintenance Therapy

A maintenance solution such as Pedialyte® or Infalyte® is used for the prevention of dehydration in the presence of vomiting or diarrhea or for the maintenance of hydration following the rehydration phase. This phase is carried out by the parents at home. Calculations for fluid requirements during this phase should take into account maintenance needs as well as ongoing losses and should be conveyed to the parents in terms of ounces per day.

Maintenance solutions should not be used exclusively for periods greater than 24 hours. A return to breast feeding should begin following the rehydration phase while offering maintenance fluids between feedings. High glucose-containing foods and fluids should be avoided especially in children with diarrhea. The need for lactose-free formulas or half-strength lactose-containing formulas, diluted 1:1 with water, remains controversial, but they frequently are recommended following rehydration. In addition, the physician has to be cautious when recommending "clear liquids" because this may be interpreted to mean water alone, which can induce hyponatremia in the presence of ongoing losses.

The parent should be encouraged to carefully record the child's intake and output, including assessing the volume of food and liquids ingested, estimates of emesis losses, and weighing of diapers to determine stool and urine output. The previously discussed signs of dehydration should be reinforced. The primary care physician will want to reevaluate any child requiring replacement therapy. This reevaluation generally is in the form of a phone call or follow-up visit within 24 hours.

BIBLIOGRAPHY

American Academy of Pediatrics Committee on Nutrition: Use of oral fluid therapy and post-treatment feeding following enteritis in children in a developed country, *Pediatrics* 75: 358–361, 1985.

Goepp JG, Katz SA: Oral rehydration therapy, *Am Fam Phys* 47(4):843–848, 1993.

Santosham M, Greenough WB: Oral rehydration therapy: A global perspective, *J Pediatr* 118(4): S44–S51, 1991.

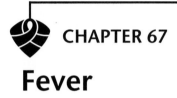

CHAPTER 67

Fever

William J. Malone

Fever is the most common sign of disease that causes parents to seek medical evaluation and advice. Because children with high fevers may appear uncomfortable, many parents worry that fever may harm their children, particularly that brain damage may result. The physician, knowing that a variety of treatable diseases are accompanied by fever, often determines whether and how soon a patient needs to be seen on the basis of the presence and height of fever, thereby adding, perhaps inadvertently, to parental anxiety about fever. Every parent of every child will eventually have to confront problems caused by fever: What has caused the fever? Will my child be harmed by the fever? How can I help my child to feel better and get rid of the fever for good (or at least until next time)? The care with which the physician responds to these concerns at the time of a febrile illness often affects not only the level of trust that parents develop for the physician, but also the level of confidence that parents develop in their own ability to cope with their children's illnesses.

BACKGROUND

Body temperature is regulated by the hypothalamus. "Normal" temperature varies diurnally, with the high temperature occurring in the early evening and low in the early morning. Children show even more variability than adults, 0.9° C (1.6° F) between the ages of 2 and 6 years and 1.1° C (2° F) in children over 6 years of age. There is also variability of "normal" set point temperature among individuals. In the appropriately clothed child, a rectal temperature greater than 38.0° C (100.4° F) is defined as fever.

To provide appropriate therapy, it is useful to distinguish between fever and heat illness when considering the pathophysiology of elevated body temperature. Heat illness (heat prostration, heat stroke) occurs when the normal temperature-regulating mechanisms are overwhelmed, usually by extraordinary environmental conditions such as strenuous exercise in hot, humid weather, prolonged sauna exposure, or accidental enclosure in hot automobiles.

TABLE 67-1
Predictive Model: Six Observation Items and Their Scales*

OBSERVATION ITEM	1 NORMAL	3 MODERATE IMPAIRMENT	5 SEVERE IMPAIRMENT
Quality of cry	Strong with normal tone *or* content and not crying	Whimpering *or* sobbing	Weak *or* moaning *or* high-pitched
Reaction to parent stimulation	Cries briefly then stops *or* content and not crying	Cries off and on	Continual cry *or* hardly responds
State variation	If awake → stays awake *or* if asleep and stimulated → wakes up quickly	Eyes close briefly → awake *or* awakes with prolonged stimulation	Falls to sleep *or* will not rouse
Color	Pink	Pale extremities *or* acrocyanosis	Pale *or* cyanotic *or* mottled *or* ashen
Hydration	Skin normal, eyes normal *and* mucous membranes moist	Skin, eyes-normal *and* mouth slightly dry	Skin doughy *or* tented *and* dry mucous membranes *and/or* sunken eyes
Response (talk, smile) to social overtures	Smiles *or* alerts (≤2 mo)	No smile, face anxious, dull, expressionless *or* no alerting (≤2 mo)	

*From McCarthy PL, et al: *Pediatrics* 70:802, 1982. Used by permission.

In contrast, fever is a regulated elevation of body temperature. A variety of infectious agents, such as bacteria and viruses, as well as other substances such as antigen-antibody complexes and etiocholanolone act as exogenous pyrogens. These exogenous pyrogens stimulate both fixed and mobile phagocytic leukocytes to produce endogenous pyrogen, a small molecular weight protein, now thought to be identical to interleukin-1, which promotes lymphocyte proliferation as part of the inflammatory process. Endogenous pyrogen acts on thermoregulatory areas in the preoptic area of the hypothalamus, perhaps by stimulating production of prostaglandins of the E series. These thermoregulatory areas can be conceptualized as a thermostat that, when reset, causes physiologic and behavioral responses that change the core body temperature. When the thermostat is "reset" at a higher temperature, the organism suddenly "feels cold" and a variety of physiologic and behavioral responses occur. Metabolic rate and oxygen consumption increase. Mammals shiver and seek warmer environmental conditions. While these changes are occurring, the organism is developing a fever. Because they are regulated, febrile temperatures rarely, if ever, reach levels that are hazardous to the organism. In humans, fevers rarely reach 41.7° C (107° F).

APPROACH TO THE FEBRILE PATIENT

There is an extensive differential diagnosis for acute onset of fever. Before considering individual diagnoses, the primary care physician must access the child's overall clinical appearance or "toxicity" and ascertain the immune status. These determinations will affect both the diagnostic focus and the management plan.

Toxicity

No single clinical skill is more important for the management of acute febrile illness than the ability to recognize ill-appearing, or "toxic," children. Because observational skills are subjective and based mainly on the examiner's clinical experience, there have been several recent attempts to develop quantitative observation scales to assist in initial assessment. The Acute Illness Observation Scale (AIOS) uses the following six variables: 1) quality of cry, 2) reaction to parent stimulation, 3) state variation, 4) color, 5) hydration, and 6) responses to social overtures (Table 67-1). Because toxic-appearing febrile children are likely to have life-threatening infections (Box 67-1), the physician must respond rapidly. In addition to a physical examination, a toxic patient requires a complete blood cell

BOX 67-1
Selected Life-Threatening Conditions Associated With Fever*

Central nervous system
  Bacterial meningitis
  Encephalitis
  Brain abscess
Upper airway
  Acute epiglottitis
  Retropharyngeal abscess
  Laryngeal diphtheria (rare)
  Croup (severe)
Pulmonary
  Pneumonia (severe)
  Tuberculosis (miliary)
  Bronchiolitis (severe)
Cardiac
  Myocarditis
  Bacterial endocarditis
  Suppurative pericarditis
Gastrointestinal tract
  Acute gastroenteritis (fluid/electrolyte
    losses)
  Appendicitis
  Peritonitis (other causes)
Systemic
  Meningococcemia
  Other bacterial sepsis
  Rocky Mountain spotted fever
  Toxic shock syndrome
Collagen-vascular
  Acute rheumatic fever
  Systemic lupus erythematosus
  Polyarteritis nodosa
  Polymyositis
  Kawasaki disease
  Stevens-Johnson syndrome
Miscellaneous
  Thyrotoxicosis
  Heat stroke
  Acute poisoning: atropine, aspirin, amphetamine

*Adapted from Henretig F: Fever. In Fleisher G, Ludwig S, editors: *Textbook of pediatric emergency medicine,* Baltimore 1983, Williams & Wilkins, pp 149-158.

BOX 67-2
Common Infectious Causes of Fever in Children Seen in the Emergency Department*

Central nervous system
  Acute bacterial meningitis
  Viral meningoencephalitis
Oral cavity
  Dental abscess
  Herpangina
  Herpetic gingivostomatitis
  Mumps
Upper respiratory tract
  Common cold
  Pharyngitis
  Cervical adenitis
  Epiglottitis
  Croup
  Sinusitis
  Otitis media
Pulmonary
  Bronchiolitis
  Pneumonia
Gastrointestinal tract
  Acute gastroenteritis
  Appendicitis
Genitourinary
  Urinary tract infection
  Acute salpingitis
Musculoskeletal
  Septic arthritis
  Osteomyelitis
Cutaneous or systemic with prominent rash
  Cellulitis
  Scarlet fever
  Viral exanthems
  Rocky Mountain spotted fever
  Meningococcemia

*Adapted from Henretig F: Fever. In Fleisher G, Ludwig S, editors: *Textbook of pediatric emergency medicine,* Baltimore, 1983, Williams & Wilkins, pp 149-158.

(CBC), differential, and platelet count; blood culture, and, when appropriate, chest radiograph and cultures of urine and cerebrospinal fluid. Assessment of arterial blood gases and of the status of the coagulation system also may be needed. Subsequently, these children should be admitted to the hospital. In general, broad-spectrum intravenous (IV) antibiotic therapy is initiated until cultures either reveal a specific organism or are negative after 48 to 72 hours.

DATA GATHERING

Assessment
The vast majority of children with acute onset of fever will not be toxic-appearing. Box 67-2 contains a list of the common infectious conditions causing acute fever in children.

History
The history should include information about the duration and pattern of fever and associated symptoms such as cough, vomiting, and diarrhea. The volume of urine output will help estimate adequacy of fluid intake. Alteration in the child's activity level (*ie,* sleeping, eating, and

playing patterns) provides clues to the severity of illness. If old enough, the child may be able to provide specific information about ear pain, sore throat, or dysuria. In younger children, paradoxic irritability, manifest as increased irritability during attempts to rock or comfort the child, is a particularly important symptom suggesting meningitis. A history of exposure to others with similar illness may be useful. The physician also should inquire about recent immunizations, because fever can be caused by diptheria-pertussis-tetanus vaccine for 24 to 48 hours and by measles-mumps-rubella vaccine 7 to 10 days after immunization.

Toxic ingestions also can cause acute onset of fever, especially salicylates, atropine, phenothiazines, amphetamine, and tricyclic antidepressants. Generally, the child's caretaker discovers an ingestion; however, when fever and altered mental status are present, ingestion should be suspected even in the absence of a positive history.

The physician may use the time during the history taking to observe the child for both overall toxicity and specific signs of illness. The respiratory rate is best counted prior to touching the child. To correct a respiratory rate, for every 1° C of temperature elevated, subtract 3.7 breaths per minute. Similarly, the presence and color of a rash can be observed. Also, notice peculiar postures assumed by the child that might indicate the presence of localized pain or airway compromise.

Physical Examination

The physical examination, already begun during the observation period, must then focus on specific important areas. Because otitis media frequently is found in febrile infants, the tympanic membranes must be examined. Mild redness of the tympanic membrane may be erythema secondary to the fever, but in boys less than 6 months and girls less than 3 years of age, with temperature greater than 39° C, urinary tract infection must be ruled out. In addition to redness, there should be dullness and poor mobility. The mouth may contain characteristic signs: anterior ulcers suggesting herpes stomatitis, posterior ulcers suggesting herpangina caused by coxsackie virus, Koplik spots suggesting measles, and so forth. Evidence of pus on the tonsil does not always indicate a *Streptococcus* infection. Examination of the chest may be surprisingly benign in the presence of pneumonia, especially in children under 12 months of age. Often, tachypnea and cough will be the only signs of pneumonia. The triad of tachypnea, flaring of the alae nasi, and end-expiratory grunting are signs of more advanced pneumonia. Meningism and/or a bulging anterior fontanelle are obviously important signs, but infants with meningitis who are under 12 to 18 months of age may have neither of these signs. The abdomen should be examined for distention, localized rigidity, or tenderness. Again, appendicitis in the child aged 2 to 3 years may present with few abdominal signs. The extremities should be inspected thoroughly for rashes, redness, and/or bony tenderness suggesting cellulitis, arthritis, or osteomyelitis.

If the history and physical examination fail to reveal a focus of infection, several possibilities remain:

1. A clinically silent focal bacterial infection exists, which will be discovered with appropriate laboratory tests. Examples include urinary tract infections, pneumonia, sinusitis, and subacute bacterial endocarditis.
2. The patient has a nonspecific, self-limited viral syndrome. This category accounts for 85% to 98% (depending on age of patient and height of fever) of patients with acute onset of fever who have no discernible focal infection.
3. The patient does not have an infectious disease but rather is manifesting early signs of other entities associated with chronic fever such as collagen vascular disease, cancer, or drug fever.
4. The patient has occult bacteremia.

Laboratory Evaluation

There are no universally established indications for use of the various laboratory investigations that may assist in diagnosis of febrile illness. The younger or more ill-appearing the child and the higher the fever, the stronger are the indications to order laboratory tests. Many children will require no laboratory tests, either because the physical examination yields a specific diagnosis, or because, despite the failure to reach a specific diagnosis, the children appear relatively well, have exposure histories, and have rectal temperatures less than 40° C.

Complete Blood Count

On average, children with bacterial disease have higher total white blood cell (WBC) counts than do those with viral disease. Indeed, the phenomenon of transient bone marrow suppression by viral disease has been well described. However, the problem for the clinician arises when trying to interpret the meaning of the total WBC count in an individual child. Although the child with an elevated WBC count is more likely than one with a low WBC count to have bacterial disease, that same child is still even more likely to have self-limited disease with no detectable bacterial pathogen than to have bacterial disease. A common cutoff number used in saying a WBC is elevated is 15,000/μL. One study showed that of bacteremia patients, 79% had WBC counts greater than 15,000/μL. The same study showed that 67% of the nonbacteremia patients had WBC counts less than 15,000/μL. However, the positive predictive value of a count greater than 15,000/μL is only 7%.

Radiology

Several studies have shown that using a chest radiograph as a screening test without symptoms is not helpful in the acute evaluation of fever.

Cultures

Cultures of blood, urine, cerebral spinal fluid, oropharynx, and stool will yield definitive diagnosis when positive. However, most cultures require 1 to 3 days to incubate. Positivity rates are fairly low and seem to depend to some extent on age of the patient and degree of fever. When no apparent focus of infection is present, but the child appears ill enough to obtain cultures, the blood and urine will yield bacterial pathogens approximately 3% to 5% of the time.

Special Situations

Young Children Without Localizing Signs of Infection

Neonate (birth to 1 month of age)—Neonates have maturational deficiencies in immune function that render them susceptible to serious infections. Nonspecific immune mechanisms such as chemotaxis and opsonization for gram-negative organisms are developmentally immature. Neonates often manifest fevers and more subtle signs of serious infections than do older

children. When fever occurs, the possibility of infection must be seriously considered.

Mottling of the skin, temperature instability, lethargy, and altered feeding patterns are clues to serious infection. Fever in this age range if associated with only subtle findings at most institutions necessitates a complete work-up for sepsis and empiric treatment with broad spectrum antibiotics. The choice of antibiotics must cover the most likely organisms in this age group (group B *Streptococcus,* enteric gram-negatives, and *Listeria*). A common combination for empiric treatment includes an aminoglycoside plus ampicillin if the patient has not left the hospital. If a neonate is readmitted during the first month of life, a third-generation cephalosporin usually replaces the aminoglycoside.

Young infant (1 to 3 months of age)—Until recently all young infants with fever were handled in the same manner as the neonate. Studies have shown that when strict criteria are used, many of these infants can be handled as outpatients. The Rochester Criteria for the Evaluation of Febrile Infants (Box 67-3) commonly is used to screen febrile infants to identify which ones can be sent home on therapy. In most instances, when the young infants are sent home, they are placed on ceftriaxone therapy after a complete sepsis work-up has been performed and reevaluated within 24 hours and given a second dose of ceftriaxone. In many cases after a total of 48 hours, if the cultures are negative and the child is doing well, no further therapy is needed. In all instances, the examiner must feel confident in the parents' ability to reliably observe their child and bring the child back for reexamination. A recent study has even used close observation of these children as outpatients without antibiotics and may be considered in the future if the studies can be substantiated.

Older infants and children (3 months to 3 years of age)—In contrast to the 38° C threshold used to evaluate infants less than 3 months of age, occult bacteremia is not usually considered in a nontoxic-appearing child in this age group until temperature is greater than 39° C. Using the AIOS, the toxicity of the child is assessed. Most physicians then use the guidelines that appeared in the July 1993 issue of *Pediatrics* (Fig. 67-1) to decide on treatment as an outpatient or to observe

---

**Rochester Criteria for the Evaluation
of Febrile Infants***

A febrile (temperature ≥38°C) infant 60 days of age or younger is at low risk for serious bacterial infections if the infant:

- Appears generally well
- Has been previously healthy, defined as:
  Born at term (≥37 weeks gestation)
  Did not receive perinatal antimicrobial therapy
  Was not hospitalized longer than the mother
  Was not treated for unexplained hyperbilirubinemia
  Had not received and was not receiving antimicrobial agents
  Had not been hospitalized previously
  Has no chronic or underlying illness
- Has no evidence of skin, soft-tissue, bone, joint, or ear infection on physical examination
- Has the following laboratory values:
  Peripheral white blood cell count between 5000 and 15,000 cells/mm³
  Absolute band form count <1500/mm³
  ≤10 white blood cells per high-power field (× 40) on microscopic examination of a spun urine sediment
  ≤5 white blood cells per high-power field (× 40) on microscopic examination of a stool smear (for infants with diarrhea)

---

*From Evaluation and management of the febrile infant 60 days of age and younger, *Pediatr Ann* 22:480, 1993.
SBI—serious bacterial infections.

carefully as an outpatient without antibiotics. When treatment is selected, most physicians currently use ceftriaxone, but in the immunized child with *Haemophilis influenzae* B vaccine, treatment with amoxicillin may be a reasonable choice.

Immunocompromised

Splenectomized Patients

Loss of splenic function is most common in the child with sickle cell anemia due to autosplenectomy but may be due to surgical removal for heredity spherocytosis, cancer staging, or congenital asplenia. No matter what the etiology, these patients are susceptible to overwhelming infections with encapsulated organisms such as *Streptococcus pneumoniae* and *Haemophilus influenzae* B. For this reason, a thorough investigation for source of fever and admission to hospital for antibiotics is warranted in most circumstances. A study by Wilimas and colleagues using strict criteria demonstrated that

some of these patients could be treated safely as outpatients.

Children With Cancer

Children undergoing intensive chemotherapy for cancer are often put at high risk for infection. The immunosuppression may be manifest in any of three common ways: granulocytopenia, B-cell hypofunction, and T-cell suppression. The patients with granulocytopenia especially are vulnerable to overwhelming infection, so the presence of fever in these patients requires a thorough evaluation and inpatient treatment with broad-spectrum antibiotics. The therapy should cover gram-positive and enteric pathogens including *Pseudomonas.* One combination commonly used is cephalosporin, ticarcillin, and tobramycin, but many other regimes have been used successfully.

Other diseases that require aggressive therapy with acute fever due to immunosuppression are HIV disease, nephrotic syndrome, and the child undergoing steroid treatment. In general, careful history, physical examination, judicious use of laboratory studies, and aggressive therapy are needed.

Management

Treating the Source of Fever

If the source of fever is known in the febrile child, appropriate antibiotics can be chosen on the basis of the most likely organisms to cause this problem. It also may be feasible to treat some viral infections (*eg,* respiratory syncytial virus with ribavarin and herpes simplex and varicella-zoster infections with acyclovir). Most viral infections, however, are treated symptomatically only. Other causes of acute fever such as cancer and collagen vascular disease may be treated specifically also.

Treating the Fever

In addition to treating the underlying cause of fever, the pediatrician should develop an approach to the treatment of fever itself. Three issues arise: 1) establishing a threshold temperature above which antipyretic therapy is instituted, 2) determining the best antipyretic regimen, and 3) managing parental concerns about fever.

There is some disagreement in the pediatric literature about when and whether to provide antipyretic therapy for fever. Proponents of early and vigorous treatment cite patient comfort and

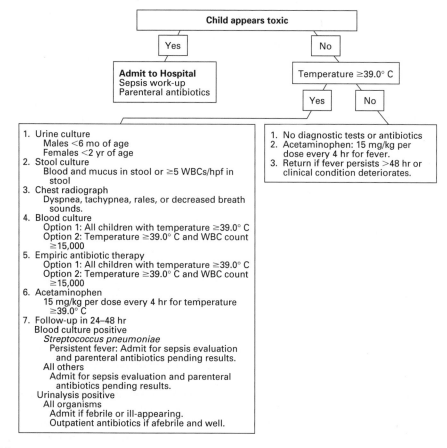

FIG 67-1

Decision tree for management of a previously healthy child 91 days to 36 months of age, with a fever of unknown origin.   (From Practice Guidelines for the Management of Infants and Children 0 to 36 Months of Age With Fever Without Source, Pediatrics, 92:9, 1993.)

prevention of febrile seizures as reasons for treatment.   Opponents of this approach refer first to the phylogenetic argument that fever represents an adaptation of the organism to fight infection. Some animal research has shown improved response to experimentally induced infection at higher body temperatures; however, neither the application of these findings nor the precise mechanism of action has been established. Another hazard of vigorous therapy is potential overdosage with any of the antipyretic drugs by well-intentioned, but overzealous, parents. There is also concern that pharmacologic fever control will mask important signs of illness and obscure diagnosis.

A middle course between the two extreme positions seems reasonable.   Low fevers (less than 38.5° C) unaccompanied by apparent discomfort may be left untreated.   Children with temperatures of greater than 38.5° C or any child appearing uncomfortable may be treated.   Aspirin or acetaminophen will lower the hypothalamic set point temperature effectively for 4 hours and ibuprofen for 6 hours.   Epidemiologic data linking aspirin use to Reye syndrome has led the American Academy of Pediatrics to recommend against the use of aspirin for treating fever associated with varicella or influenza.

Sponge bathing in tepid water will reduce body temperature. If no antipyretic medication is provided, however, the child will experience discomfort and the benefit will be temporary. Alcohol bathing is hazardous because intoxication and hypoglycemia may result.

Finally, parental concerns about fever must be addressed.   Many parents believe that fever may harm their children. It is often useful for the physician to explore parental concerns specifically. Discussion then can begin with a review of the diagnostic effort that has occurred. If a specific cause of the fever has been discovered, then, of course, its nature, course, and management should be discussed. Those antipyretic measures selected should be explained. Most important, parents often require specific reassurance that fever is a transient state that will not cause any permanent harm to their children.

Fever of Unknown Origin

In some instances, fever may persist and cause parents to be concerned about the presence of serious underlying disorder. The physician must be certain to detect and treat serious infections or potential life-threatening disease, while at the same time recognizing that many children with fever of unknown origin have a benign self-limiting process and should not be subject to extensive, painful, or unnecessary laboratory investigation.

The most commonly used definition for fever of unknown origin in childhood was expounded by Dechovitz and Moffett. This definition includes a fever of 100° F or more for 2 weeks without a recognized site of infection. Many physicians add to this definition that routine outpatient investigations are unrevealing of the source of fever (history; physical examination; CBC count with differential, blood, and urine cultures; chest and sinus radiographs; and sedimentation rate).

Broad categories of disease processes frequently found in children with fever of unknown origin include infections, collagen vascular disease, malignancies, miscellaneous conditions, and undiagnosed illnesses. The most extensive study in children with fever of unknown origin is that of Pizzo and colleagues. (Table 67-2). If one adds to this list the newly recognized diseases HIV, cat scratch disease, ehrlichiosis, and Kawasaki disease, most potential diagnoses will be found. One can see that at all ages, infections cause a majority of these fevers.

In evaluating children with fever of unknown origin, it is important for the physician to remember that 75% or more patients will have common pediatric diagnoses. An extensive history is required to begin sifting through the various diagnostic possibilities. The early events in the disease process should be sought, including

signs and symptoms, the epidemiology setting, and season of the year (eg, Lyme disease, ehrlichiosis). It is important to determine other past diseases that the child may have encountered such as a urinary tract infection or previously investigated fevers or febrile illness treated with antibiotics without a specific diagnosis, which might indicate a relatively clinically silent source of infection (eg, vesicoureteral reflux with urinary tract infections). Previous behavioral or psychiatric difficulties might indicate the possibility of a factitious fever. Reservoirs of infection must be ascertained, such as an undiagnosed contagious case of tuberculosis, a grandparent who might be a typhoid carrier, attendance in a daycare center that might be sustaining an unrecognized outbreak of hepatitis, unusual food habits in the family such as preference to raw meat (a potential source of toxoplasmosis), or a pet bird that might harbor *Chlamydia psittaci,* the etiologic agent of psittacosis. If pica is present, the physician should consider the diagnosis of *Toxocara canis* or *Toxocara cati.* Because many children with regional enteritis have absent or vague gastrointestinal tract symptoms, the physician must inquire specifically about anorexia, changes in bowel habit, weight loss, or intermittent abdominal pain. Certainly in this day and age, risk factors for HIV also should be sought.

The most important elements of the physical examination are the observation of the general appearance of the child and the comparison of current weight with previous weight. Weight loss should be viewed as a serious sign that mandates a comprehensive evaluation with laboratory and radiologic studies. Examination of each organ system is frequently rewarding. Tenderness of the sinuses may be detected, although this is not an invariable sign of sinusitis. It is particularly important to observe the skin for evidence of a heliotrope rash, suggestive of dermatomyositis, or a facial rash that might indicate systemic lupus erythematosus or a mixed collagen vascular disease. Heart murmurs must be sought to detect the occasional case of endocarditis. Examination of the abdomen may reveal splenic enlargement, which may indicate malignancy or unrecognized mononucleosis. Pain or a mass in the right lower quadrant of the abdomen suggests the possibility of inflammatory bowel disease. There may be generalized lymphadenopathy with a lymphoma or with an infectious process such as cytomegalovirus, toxoplasmosis,

TABLE 67-2
Final Diagnoses in 100 Patients With Fever of Unknown Origin*

<6 YRS OF AGE (n = 52)		≥6 YRS OF AGE (n = 48)	
DIAGNOSIS	NO. OF PATIENTS	DIAGNOSIS	NO. OF PATIENTS
Infectious	34	Infectious	18
Viral syndrome	13	Viral syndrome	4
Urinary tract infection	3	Endocarditis	3
Bacterial meningitis	3	Infectious mononucleosis	2
Pneumonia	3	Streptococcosis	2
Tonsillitis	3	Osteomyelitis	1
Septicemia	2	Sinusitis	1
Sinusitis	2	Tonsillitis	1
Generalized herpes simplex	1	Tuberculosis	1
Malaria	1	Typhoid fever	1
Peritonsillar abscess	1	Urinary tract infection	1
Osteomyelitis	1	Pneumonia	1
Enteric fever	1		
Collagen-inflammatory	4	Collagen-inflammatory	16
Rheumatoid arthritis	3	Rheumatoid arthritis	7
Henoch-Schönlein purpura	1	Lupus erythematosus	3
		Regional enteritis	4
		Ulcerative colitis	1
		Vasculitis (undefined)	1
Malignancy	4	Malignancy	2
Leukemia	3	Lymphosarcoma	1
Reticulum cell sarcoma	1	Leukemia	1
Miscellaneous	7	Miscellaneous	3
Central nervous system fever	2	Behçet syndrome	1
Agranulocytosis	1	Hepatitis, anicteric	1
Lamellar ichthyosis	1	Ruptured appendix	1
Milk allergy	1		
Aspiration pneumonia	1		
Agammaglobulinemia	1		
Undiagnosed	3	Undiagnosed	9

*From Pizzo PA, et al: *Pediatrics* 55:468–473, 1975. Used by permission.

or some other viral pathogen. Muscle pain may indicate polymyositis. Bone pain may be seen with osteomyelitis or tumor infiltration.

After completion of the history and physical examination, the physician must make an assessment about the likelihood of making a definite diagnosis and whether a treatable or life-threatening condition is present. If the patient appears chronically ill or has sustained weight loss, hospitalization and a full diagnostic evaluation should be considered. If, on the other hand, the child appears healthy, has little or no weight loss, and has normal findings on physical examination, the likelihood of serious illness or a treatable bacterial disease is diminished, and a less extensive outpatient evaluation is appropriate. Other tests can be added, depending on the history. For example, if mononucleosis is occurring in the community, then rapid test for hetero-

phil antibodies (Mono-spot test) and, in patients less than 3 years of age, Epstein-Barr virus titers should be done.

For more worrisome signs or symptoms, the same screening tests as for an acute evaluation need to be done, probably as an inpatient, along with some or all of the following procedures:

1. Bone scan
2. Gallium scan
3. Abdominal ultrasound
4. Upper and lower gastrointestinal tract series
5. Blood cultures
6. Stool cultures
7. Antinuclear antibody titers
8. Rheumatoid factor determination
9. C3, C4, and total hemolytic complement measurement

The sequence in which tests are performed will be determined by the physician, depending on leads from the history, physical, and laboratory studies. For example, if the child is having vague abdominal complaints and/or diarrhea, gastrointestinal contrast radiography should be performed early in the investigation. If, on the other hand, the history and physical examination are totally unhelpful in pointing to a diagnosis, then the tests should be done in whatever order is convenient. Many studies have shown that ordering laboratory or imaging tests in a "shotgun" manner is unrewarding. If all tests are nondiagnostic, the physician may wish to consider a bone marrow aspiration, both for cytologic examination and bacterial culture.

After the laboratory and radiologic evaluations are completed, most life-threatening or treatable disease will have been detected. Most of the remaining children will either have a self-limited infectious process or remain undiagnosed with ultimate resolution of the febrile process. For children who continue to be febrile but appear healthy on examination with no focal physical signs, it is appropriate to reassure the parents and not pursue test after test. These children, however, must be carefully followed up with additional tests (or previously ordered tests redone) as the clinical condition changes.

The emotional state of the parents of children with fever of unknown origin must be recognized. In general, these parents are anxious and frustrated because of the unknown diagnosis. The physician should explain to the parents that they are not the only ones to have faced this problem and that as long as the child looks well and does not develop a new sign or symptom, he/she can be observed. This will serve to reassure the parents by indicating that they are undergoing the same emotional responses as other parents. The physician must continue to see these patients frequently, both to ensure that no previously unrecognized disease process is becoming clinically manifest and to continue to reassure the parents and the child that the child is not seriously ill.

At times, getting a second opinion is helpful not only in coming to a diagnosis but is reassuring to the parents and the physician that all possibilities are being assessed.

BIBLIOGRAPHY

Baker MD, Bell LM, Avner JR: Outpatient management of selected 29-56 day old febrile infants without antibiotics: A variable alternative, *N Engl J Med* 329:1437–1441, 1993.

Baraff LJ, Bass JW, Flesscher GR, et al: Evaluation and management of infants and children 0 to 36 months of age with fever without source, *Pediatrics* 92:1–12, 1993.

Baskin MN, O'Rourke EJ, Fleisher GR: Outpatient management of febrile infants 28-89 days of age with intramuscular administration of ceftriaxine, *J Pediatr* 120:22–27, 1992.

Bellanti JA, Boner AL: Immunology of the fetus and the newborn. In Avery GB, editor: *Neonatology: Pathophysiology and management of the newborn,* Philadelphia, 1991, JB Lippincott.

Carroll WL, Farrell MK, Singer JI, et al: Treatment of occult bacteremia: A prospective randomized clinical trial, *Pediatrics* 72:608, 1981.

Caspe WB, Chamudes O, Louis B: The evaluation and treatment of the febrile infant, *Pediatr Infect Dis* 2:131, 1983.

Committee on Infectious Diseases of the American Academy of Pediatrics: Aspirin and Reye's syndrome, *Pediatrics* 69:810, 1982.

Crain EF, Bulas D, Bijur PE, et al: Is a chest radiograph necessary in the evaluation of every febrile infant less than 8 weeks of age? *Pediatrics* 88:821–824, 1991.

DeAngelis C, Jaffe A, Wilson M, et al: Iatrogenic risks and financial costs of hospitalizing febrile infants, *Am J Dis Child* 137:1146, 1983.

Dechovitz AB, Moffett HL: Classification of acute febrile illnesses in childhood, *Clin Pediatr* 7:649, 1968.

Jaffe DM, Tanz RR, Davis AT, et al: Antibiotic administration to treat possible occult bacteremia in febrile children, *N Engl J Med* 317: 1175–1180, 1987.

Jaskiewicz JA, McCarthy CA: Evaluation and management of the febrile infant 60 days of age or younger, *Pediatr Ann* 22:477–483, 1993.

Kauffman RE, Sawyer LA, Scheinbaum ML: Antipyretic efficiency of ibuprofen vs. acetaminophen, *Am J Dis Child* 146:622–625, 1992.

Kleinman MD: The complaint of persistent fever: Recognition and management of pseudo fever of unknown origin, *Pediatr Clin North Am* 29:201, 1982.

Kluger MJ: Fever, *Pediatrics* 66:720, 1980.

Marshall R, Teele DW, Klein JO: Unsuspected bacteremia due to *Haemophilus influenzae:* Outcome of children not initially admitted to the hospital, *J Pediatr* 95:690, 1979.

McCarthy PL: Controversies in pediatrics: What tests are indicated for the child under 2 with fever? *Pediatr Rev* 1:51, 1979.

McCarthy PL, Sharpe MR, Spiesel SZ, et al: Observation scales to identify serious illness in febrile children, *Pediatrics* 70:802, 1982.

McCarthy PM, Jekel JF, Dolan TF: Temperature greater than or equal to 40°C in children less than 24 months of age: A prospective study, *Pediatrics* 59:663, 1977.

O'Dempsey TJD, Laurence BE, McArdle TF, et al: The effect of temperature reduction on respiratory rate in febrile illness, *Arch Dis Child* 68:492–495, 1993.

Oshman D: Diagnostic imaging procedures in the evaluation of fever of unknown origin, *Semin Pediatr Infect Dis* 4:43–47, 1993.

Pearson HA: Splenectomy: Its risks and its roles, *Hosp Pract* 15:85, 1980.

Pizzo PA, Lovejoy FH Jr, Smith DH: Prolonged fever in children: Review of 100 cases, *Pediatrics* 55:468, 1975.

Roberts KB: Blood cultures in pediatric practice, *Am J Dis Child* 133:996, 1979.

Stern RC: Pathophysiologic basis for symptomatic treatment of fever, *Pediatrics* 59:92, 1977.

Teele DW, Marshall R, Klein JO: Unsuspected bacteremia in young children: A common and important problem, *Pediatr Clin North Am* 26:773, 1979.

Wiliams JA, Flynn PM, Harris S, et al: A randomized study of outpatient treatment with ceftriaxone for selected febrile children with sickle cell disease, *N Engl J Med* 329:472–476, 1993.

CHAPTER 68

Lumps and Bumps

Joseph A. Cox
Moritz M. Ziegler

Superficial visible masses, commonly detected by parents, require prompt recognition and appropriate treatment and disposition. The major task for the primary care physician is to decide how serious the problem is and how quickly evaluation and treatment should be initiated. Fortunately, malignancy is not a common cause of visible lumps and not all lesions need to be removed. The following discussion is based on the location of the mass and is written to help the physician make the appropriate diagnosis and initiate the proper treatment.

HEAD AND FACE MASSES

Sebaceous or epidermoid cysts are soft masses usually found on the scalp, face, or back. Epidermoid cysts vary from 0.2 to 5 cm, are nontender, and may be mobile. The contents are thick and cheesy epithelial debris. These cysts may become infected, requiring excision or drainage. Pilomatrixomas are firm, calcified cystic lesions, which also occur over the face, neck, and supraclavicular region. They usually have a bluish discoloration, and the etiology is unclear. They usually are removed to prevent infection and confirm the diagnosis.

Inclusion or dermoid cysts, located either in the midline of the face, scalp, or over the lateral aspect of the eyebrow, are subcutaneous, vary in diameter from several millimeters to more than a centimeter, and are mobile and nontender. These lesions should be removed to establish a diagnosis and prevent possible infection. Rarely they are characterized by dumbbell extension through the tables of the skull. The lesions do not recur; providing they are totally excised.

Preauricular lesions may be classified as a simple pit with a cutaneous orifice, a sinus tract with an associated subcutaneous cyst, a tract extending to the auditory canal or to the base of the skull, or as a cutaneous tag with or without a cartilaginous component. Unilateral or bilateral, they are quite common in the population at large. The sinus and cysts do require removal to prevent secondary infection if there is a palpable cystic component in the subcutaneous tissue lying below the sinus.

NECK MASSES

Midline Neck Lesions

These lesions include submental lymph nodes in the upper midline of the neck. These lymph nodes, which are normally present, may become enlarged following an infection in the floor of the mouth or the perioral area. Dermoid cysts, located anywhere within the midline of the neck from the mandible to the supraclavicular fossa, most commonly are nontender, mobile, and in the subcutaneous tissue. A thyroglossal duct cyst originates from the normal descent of the thyroid gland and occurs anywhere along the tract from the base of the tongue down the midline (although they may be eccentric) of the neck to just above the thyroid cartilage. The lesions, usually painless, move with swallowing and protrusion of the tongue.

If a patient consults a physician because of the discovery of an undiagnosed but asymptomatic mass on the neck, then referral for elective surgery is appropriate. A patient who has tenderness and redness of the neck should be treated with antibiotics. A limited incision and drainage is appropriate for an acute abscess; but with the diagnosis of an infected thyroglossal duct cyst, such an incision should be followed by a delayed definitive operation after clearing of the infection to remove the cyst and its associated tract that penetrates the central portion of the hyoid bone. This removal will prevent recurrent infections and will prevent the rare occurrence of carcinoma in cyst remnants in adults.

Lesions of the thyroid gland include goiters due to hyperthyroidism (toxic goiters) or hypothyroidism (nontoxic goiters) or solitary or multiple nodules. Thyroid neoplasms usually are solitary, nonfunctioning nodules, whereas thyroiditis may produce nodules, diffuse enlargement, or no change in thyroid size.

Lateral Neck Lesions

Cervical lymphadenitis, the most common neck lesion, is characterized by the onset of swelling and tenderness in the neck followed by heat and redness of the overlying area, a sequence that often follows an episode of pharyngitis or otitis. If these lymph nodes have a hard texture and are in the location of a known lymph node group, a course of antistaphylococcal antibiotic therapy is indicated. With progression of the infection and suppuration, the inflamed lymph nodes demonstrate central softening as abscess formation occurs. Such suppurative lymphadenitis is best treated with drainage in addition to the antistaphylococcal antibiotics. Needle aspiration with Gram stain and culture of the aspirate will help in the choice of antibiotics. Aspiration plus antibiotics is often the only treatment necessary for controlling suppurative lymphadenitis. If repeated aspiration is necessary or if systemic toxicity exists, then surgical drainage and parenteral antibiotics are the preferred method of treatment.

Tuberculosis lymphadenitis (scrofula), a chronic lymphadenopathy with tenderness and enlargement suggesting an inflammatory process, is best evaluated with a diagnostic chest radiograph and tuberculin skin test, although a negative skin test may occur with an infection by an atypical mycobacterium. The rubbery, woody lymph nodes are treated best with surgical excision (with culture and histologic examination), because fistulae may result from needle aspiration or simple incision and drainage.

Malignant neoplasms of the neck include a lymph node affected by leukemia or lymphoma or a lymph node enlarged from metastatic disease. The most common solid tumor in childhood that causes lymph node metastases is neuroblastoma. Definitive histologic diagnoses of neoplastic involvement of cervical lymph nodes require an excisional biopsy, proper specimen handling for touch preparation and lymphocyte markers, histologic studies, and proper staining and culturing for bacteria, fungi, and acid-fast organisms. Only needle aspiration is safe in the realm of the primary care physician, whereas formal excisional biopsies and drainage procedures require the skills of a surgeon.

Salivary glands most commonly are affected by a stricture of the duct system, collagen diseases, sarcoidosis, or vascular lesions such as hemangioendotheliomas. Salivary gland infection in the lateral neck induces inflammation of the submandibular gland or parotid gland with or without secondary abscess formation. These processes are unusual, result in systemic symptoms of infection and sepsis, and require prompt antibiotic therapy and/or operative drainage.

Branchial cleft cysts and sinus tracts in the lateral neck occur either along the anterior border of the sternocleidomastoid muscle from the upper to the lower neck (branchial pouch II cysts and sinus tracts), or they occur in the submandibular triangle up onto the anterior face (branchial pouch I cleft deformities). Such lesions range from a pore in the skin, to a subcutaneous cyst associated with that pore, to a proximally ascending sinus tract. Additionally, there may be only a subcutaneous cystic component or a subcutaneous cartilaginous remnant.

Elective surgical referral for branchial cleft lesions is done to establish the histologic diagnosis of a subcutaneous nodule, to excise a skin-communicating cystic mass that would be prone to infectious problems requiring interval drainage and subsequent excision, or to prevent the statistically increased likelihood of an in situ carcinoma forming in a branchial cleft remnant.

Lymphangiomas are congenital aberrant lymphatic system tumors varying from a single cyst to a cluster of grapes multicystic lesion due to an abnormal continuity in or dilatation of lymphatic channels. Such lymphangiomas or cystic hygromas most commonly are located in the neck, although they can be found throughout the child's body especially on the chest wall, axilla, and the extremities. These spongy, soft-tissue tumors are variable in size and filled with clear yellow or hemorrhagic fluid. Aspiration of fluid from the mass usually will confirm the diagnosis. Lymphangiomas are not characterized by spontaneous regression, but they do demonstrate a gradual coalescence with restriction of their boundaries and better definition of their margins. Patients with lymphangiomas frequently have a history of recurrent lymphangitis with associated acute swelling, tenderness, and erythema of the overlying skin; these lesions require broad-spectrum antibiotic therapy. Hospital admission is indicated if the acute inflammatory swelling might compromise the airway or if there is evidence of a proximal lymphangitis or systemic infection. Surgical referral is indicated electively or urgently depending on the clinical spectrum displayed.

VASCULAR MALFORMATIONS

These lesions range from mild skin discoloration to large soft-tissue masses. There are three general types: port-wine stain, strawberry hemangioma, and cavernous hemangioma. The port-wine stain (nevus flammeus) is a purplish discoloration usually found around the face and neck. These lesions, consisting of mature capillaries, may need cosmetic coverage because conventional surgery or sclerosing therapy is less effective. Laser therapy has been used effectively. Capillary hemangiomas (nevus vasculosus), a raised reddish lesion, also is known as a strawberry hemangioma. After an initial proliferative phase (the peak of the growth period occurring when the child is 1.5 to 3 years of age), these lesions spontaneously regress. As regression begins, the central portion begins to undergo an ischemic change. This change is followed by the development of an irregular surface with a whitish sheen, and then there may be occasional ulceration and crust formation. During this involution, the hemangioma may become infected. Hemangioendotheliomas are characterized by a discolored cutaneous involvement associated with a soft-tissue swelling beneath the surface of the skin. If untreated, these lesions will regress. Large hemangiomatous lesions may cause complications that include platelet trapping with a secondary bleeding diathesis or cardiac failure. Cavernous hemangiomas consist of large lakes of vascular channels, and they are not characterized by spontaneous regression. Many lesions are true mixed hemangiomas with capillary, port-wine, and cavernous components, and the treatment needs to be individualized. Venous lakes, in the head and neck area, especially in the supraclavicular fossa, are most visible when children increase their intrathoracic pressure. During a Valsalva maneuver, a bulge anterior to the sternocleidomastoid muscle or in the supraclavicular space may appear representing a venous lake of the jugular system.

Pyogenic granulomas, particularly over the head and neck region, can be confused with vascular malformations. These granulomas will be pedunculated and bleed intermittently. They consist of granulation tissue, may represent reaction to a foreign body, and require removal or local treatment with a caustic agent, such as silver nitrate.

THORACIC MASSES

Breast
Breast lesions that require emergency treatment are infectious in nature and include a breast abscess in a neonate or an older child. These swellings, usually secondary to staphylcocci, are tender, red, and warm. If antibiotic therapy does not clear the lesion or if central fluctuation develops, careful drainage is necessary, avoiding injury to the underlying breast bud.

Gynecomastia, or breast enlargement in boys, may be unilateral or bilateral and frequently presents as a tender breast enlargement with a palpable subareolar nodule. Enlargement may persist for up to 2 years before regression occurs. Only in the case of unusual signs or symptoms, excessive size change, or with chronicity is surgical referral indicated.

Breast tumors are usually benign in adolescents, and carcinoma of the breast in a young girl is very rare. Most breast tumors in girls are fibroadenomas characterized by a discrete, firm, nontender nodule. Such palpable fibroadenomas may vary in size with menstruation, and they may be especially sensitive to growth hormones. A breast tumor associated with a nipple discharge most commonly will be an intraductal papilloma. Adolescents also may develop breast

lesions that are secondary to true fibrocystic disease.

The rapidity with which one proceeds to surgery for a breast mass should be tempered in the young girl. A dominant nodule ideally is managed with serial examinations over one or two menstrual cycles to confirm the persistent presence of the mass before proceeding to biopsy. In a child less than 5 years of age, an inappropriately performed biopsy may damage the breast bud and subsequently limit breast development; therefore, biopsies should rarely be performed in that age group.

Chest Wall
Chest wall deformities either protrude as a pigeon chest (pectus carinatum) or retract as a funnel chest (pectus excavatum). Other costochondral and sternocostal abnormalities exist including the absence of the second, third, and fourth ribs along with the overlying pectoralis muscle (Poland syndrome) or even the absence of a part of the sternum with the exposure of the underlying heart or its surrounding membranes (ectopia cordis). These lesions produce cosmetic abnormalities and may produce functional limitations as well, and elective surgery is indicated.

ABDOMINAL MASSES

Abdominal wall lesions may occur in the midline, the lateral abdominal wall, and the inguinoscrotal region.

Midline Abdominal Wall Lesions
These lesions may be localized to the area around the umbilicus or above and below that region. A weeping umbilicus may be due to either a granuloma at the site of the previous umbilical cord attachment, a patent urachus secondary to a persistence of the urachal remnant connected to the dome of the bladder, or a patent omphalomesenteric duct, an epithelialized remnant extending from the antemesenteric border of the distal ileum to the umbilicus. A granuloma is best treated with topical cauterization with silver nitrate, and usually no further difficulties occur. A patent urachus requires surgery after a study for the presence of bladder neck or posterior urethral valve distal urinary tract obstruction. A patent omphalomesenteric duct represents an extension of the area of the ileum from a Meckel

diverticulum and requires formal laparotomy with excision of the bowel with the draining sinus.

Umbilical hernias are an extremely common developmental anomaly. Such hernias represent a failure of closure of the abdominal wall at the body stalk or umbilical cord. Umbilical hernias are characterized by a fascial defect through which a true peritoneal sac bulges. The more common course of a neonatal umbilical hernia is gradual contracture of the fascial ring with spontaneous closure of the defect after months to several years. Elective surgery is deferred in boys until the age of 4 or 5 years and in girls until the age of 2 or 3 years. Strangulation of the hernia or skin rupture with evisceration is rare. Supraumbilical hernias, fascial defects located just above the umbilicus with associated protrusion of intra-abdominal contents, are not characterized by spontaneous regression, and the detection of a supraumbilical hernia is an indication for elective surgery. A midline fascial attenuation extending from the umbilicus to the xiphoid process of the sternum with prominent rectus muscle margins on either side is a normal anatomic variant termed *diastasis recti*. This finding is best demonstrated by a Valsalva maneuver or by having the patient lie supine with subsequent lifting of the head to tense the abdominal wall musculature. A midline 1.0- to 1.5-cm subcutaneous abdominal wall nodule between the xiphoid process and umbilicus most likely represents an epiplocele or epigastric hernia. An epiplocele, in contrast to a true ventral hernia, is a protrusion of preperitoneal fat through a small midline fascial defect. Epiploceles may present as an acute abdomen because of incarceration and strangulation of the fat, and in that circumstance the patient requires a prompt surgical evaluation. Most often these epigastric hernias present as an undiagnosed soft-tissue nodule; for those lesions that are symptomatic or that seem to be enlarging, we recommend elective surgical excision with closure of the fascial defect.

Lateral Abdominal Wall Lesions

Lateral abdominal wall protrusions include the very rare lumbar hernia located in the posterior lateral lumbar triangle. A spigelian hernia is similarly rare and occurs along the lateral border of the rectus abdominus muscle where it interdigitates with the oblique musculature. Both lumbar and spigelian hernias may require elective and, rarely, urgent surgical repair of the fascial weakness, but their major interest is their very infrequent occurrence and peculiar presentation.

Inguinal hernia follows the failure of closure of the processus vaginalis, a developmental obliteration that occurs in the last trimester of pregnancy and that occurs later on the fetal right side. Patency of the processus vaginalis may result in a physiologic hydrocele in which case the proximal processus has been obliterated, but fluid has been trapped in the distal scrotum. It may produce a hydrocele of the spermatic cord in which there is a loculation of fluid in the mid-processus vaginalis with a proximal patency, or it may produce a frank communicating or hernia-hydrocele in which the entire processus is patent and is filled either with fluid from the abdominal cavity or with other intra-abdominal contents, depending on the diameter of the neck of the hydrocele sac. A physiologic hydrocele is characterized by a mild scrotal swelling that has been present since birth, and there is neither a history of a suprapubic bulging nor of intermittent scrotal size change. A hydrocele of the spermatic cord is represented by a swelling confined to the midinguinal canal with an empty space in the area of the deep inguinal ring. It is at times impossible to make a distinction between this lesion and an incarcerated inguinal hernia. If an ancillary rectal examination does not exclude an incarcerated inguinal hernia, then prompt surgical review and surgical exploration are indicated. A communicating hydrocele also may be noted in the newborn period, but it is characterized by an intermittent scrotal size change. It is more appropriate to designate these lesions as an indirect inguinal hernia when the diameter of the neck of the patent processus vaginalis is large enough to accommodate other intraabdominal contents such as omentum, the intestine, or an ovary. Inguinal hernias are more common in the premature child, on the right side, in boys, and in children with a family history of such hernias. An inguinal hernia should be electively repaired to prevent the potential complications of incarceration and strangulation. Although this complication is not common, occurring in only 5% to 10% of children, it is a devastating event that complicates the operative safety and repair of such a hernia.

The differential diagnosis of an inguinal canal swelling in the presence of a normally placed scrotal testis includes the following: an inguinal hernia, a hydrocele of the spermatic cord, or ilioinguinal lymphadenopathy, the latter being suggested especially in the presence of an infected distal extremity lesion. If the swelling is sudden in onset, if the child seems irritable with signs and symptoms of a partial bowel obstruction, and if the mass is tubular in nature, extending out of the area of the deep inguinal ring, then an incarcerated inguinal hernia is the likely diagnosis. Emergency hernia reduction is best accomplished by the examiner applying simultaneous V-shaped distal traction with the upper hand at the area of the deep inguinal ring while performing a distal-to-proximal transscrotal compression of the hernia contents with the lower hand. After reducing such an incarcerated hernia, hospital admission may be necessary and early elective surgical repair is indicated; but if the hernia cannot be reduced, then prompt surgical exploration is necessary to avoid strangulation of the contents of the hernia.

PERINEAL MASSES

Scrotum

The normal physiologic descent of the testis may arrest at any stage within the abdomen, the inguinal canal, the medial-to-lateral thigh, or most commonly, the suprapubic pouch. It is also possible that the empty scrotum represents agenesis of the testis. The diagnosis of an undescended testicle requires a clear understanding of embryology and a relaxed child examined in a comfortable and warm environment. Undescended testicles most commonly need to be differentiated from the retractile testis in which the gonad can be identified, grasped, and pulled to the bottom of the scrotum. With this maneuver, the physician ensures the normal location of the testis, regardless of where it resides when released. True undescended testes require elective surgical evaluation. However, the child presenting with pain and an acutely tender groin mass with the absence of a palpable testis in the scrotum on that side should be suspected of having either incarceration of a hernia associated with that undescended testis or torsion of the undescended testis. Testicular torsion itself is an uncommon event, but torsion of an undescended testis is statistically more likely. Such a diagnosis represents a true surgical emergency, and testicu-

lar salvage is possible only by rapid surgical intervention.

Testicular torsion also may occur in the intrascrotal testis in which the gonad is twisted either extravaginally or intravaginally, and the twisted and foreshortened spermatic cord pulls the testis to the top of the scrotum. These suddenly tender scrotal masses usually are associated with pain, nausea, and vomiting and are absolute surgical emergencies requiring rapid differential diagnosis by physical examination. Urinalysis and use of Doppler ultrasound or nuclear medicine scanning to evaluate testicular blood flow may be of value in the differential diagnosis. The differential diagnosis of a painful scrotal mass includes an incarcerated hernia, testicular torsion, acute epididymitis, and torsion of the appendix testis. The latter diagnosis is made by localizing a discrete tender blue spot on the spermatic cord–testis surface in a patient in whom scrotal pain is not severe. This is referred to as the *blue dot sign*. Epididymitis may produce abnormal results on a urinalysis, and it will produce an increased vascularity by either ultrasound or flow scanning techniques. Still another cause of the acutely tender scrotum is acute hemorrhage into a testicular tumor. Occasionally severe trauma to the scrotum can produce rupture of an otherwise normal testis.

Anorectum

Anal fissures most often occur secondary to local anal canal trauma secondary to constipation. Fissures are the most common cause of bright red rectal bleeding in childhood and are best diagnosed either by direct physical inspection or with the use of limited proctoscopy with a proctoscope. These fissures frequently are accompanied by a perianal hypertrophied skin tag. Acute fissures are best treated by stool softeners, sitz baths, and rectal lubricants such as glycerin suppositories. Chronic fissures require elective surgery. Perianal abscesses require drainage and adequate decompression, a procedure best performed in the operating room. Drainage of a small abscess in an infant in the emergency room is also appropriate. Sitz baths help treat the acute inflammatory response and keep the area clean. A late appearing anal fistula extending from the crypts of the rectal glands through perianal soft tissue to the skin rarely requires elective surgery. Most of these fistulas heal spontaneously within 6 weeks to 2 months. Perianal fistulas, fissures, and abscesses in older children may herald the presence of underlying inflammatory bowel disease.

Rectal prolapse may be without apparent cause, or it may be associated with underlying chronic constipation, cystic fibrosis, hookworm infestation, or neuromuscular disorders such as myelomeningocele. Usually the prolapsed rectum can be reduced with gentle compression. Efforts should be made to soften the stool, add a lubricant to the diet, and limit the time a child spends on the toilet. Surgery is rarely necessary.

Pilonidal dimples are common congenital variations in children. Such dimples may present only as a skin lesion over the sacrococcygeal area, or there might also be a subcutaneous sinus leading to a cyst beneath the skin. The acute pilonidal abscess may require incision and drainage, and elective surgical removal of such chronically infected areas is then indicated. For the shallow broad-based noninfected dimple, surgical referral or prophylactic excision is not indicated.

MASSES ON THE EXTREMITIES

Cysts

A wrist ganglion, which is a synovial sheath cyst, is a common cystic lesion of the extremities. These usually are located on the dorsum of the wrist, although they can be located in any joint or tendon synovial sheath area. These tense, spongy subcutaneous masses may produce discomfort that is treated best by splinting or joint rest, and a surgical referral can then be made to decide whether or not aspiration or excision is indicated. A Baker cyst represents a ganglionic type of synovial sheath cyst located in the popliteal space. These lesions may produce a mass as well as discomfort, and elective surgery is indicated.

Vascular Malformations

Enlarged extremities (whether an arm or a leg) may occur over an entire half of the body, or it may involve only one extremity. Such enlargement may be due to hemihypertrophy or to other vascular or lymphatic anomalies of the extremities. Hemihypertrophy should raise the suspicion of possible associated problems including a higher incidence of Wilms tumor; and such children with diagnosed hemihypertrophy should be screened with serial renal ultrasound. Vascular extremity anomalies represent a tremendous challenge in treatment, and usually they represent hemangioendotheliomas or mixed lymph-hemangiomas. Arteriovenous malformations may also be a part of such vascular hamartomas. Such vascular extremity lesions carry the same complications as vascular lesions elsewhere in the body (platelet trapping, high-output cardiac failure, bleeding following traumatic injury). An additional problem unique to the extremity vascular malformation is overgrowth of the hyperemic limb. All of these lesions require elective surgical review. At times the multidisciplinary approach of a surgeon and radiologic interventionalist is optimum to assess the potential role of operative or embolization therapy.

Lymphangiomas of the extremities are characterized by recurrent episodes of lymphangitis and cellulitis secondary to bacterial trapping in aberrant lymphatic channels. These lesions require repeated courses of antibiotic therapy, and there may be some benefit in utilizing chronic prophylactic antibiotics to suppress such infections. Lymphatic anomalies also include congenital lymphedema (Milroy disease) or traumatic lymphedema. Such abnormalities characterized by an intact arterial and venous system on examination require elective referral.

Skin Lesions

Integumentary lesions seen on the extremities of children include viral warts or verruca vulgaris producing local pain and discomfort or cosmetic problems only. Symptomatic plantar warts on the ventral surface of the feet can cause significant discomfort, and such children are best referred for elective treatment by the topical application of epidermal exfoliatives, electrodessication, cryotherapy, or excision.

Nevi are classified as raised or flat, pigmented or nonpigmented, and are hair-bearing or hair-free. Spider nevi or spider angiomas represent true vascular hamartomas and are not true nevi. Nevi that are congenital do have a documented increased incidence of malignant degeneration, and such patients should be referred for either prolonged follow-up or for surgical excision. The presence of irritation and erythema, bleeding, growth, or darkening are all warning signs that biopsy and surgical excision should be considered. The location of a nevus on the plantar surface of the foot, the palm of the hand, or the genitalia are, per se, not indications to consider surgery.

BIBLIOGRAPHY

Filston HC: Common lumps and bumps of the head and neck in infants and children, *Pediatr Ann* 18:180–186, 1989.

Gauderer MWL, Rajput A: A simple classification of neck lesions in children, *Surg Rounds* 599–602, Oct. 1994.

Gellis SE: Warts and molluscum contagiosum in children, *Pediatr Ann* 16:69–76, 1987.

Knight PJ, Reiner CB: Superficial lumps in children. What, When, and Why? *Pediatrics* 72: 147–153, 1983.

Koop CE: *Visible and palpable lesions in children,* New York, 1976, Grune & Stratton.

Putnam TC: Lumps and bumps in children, *Pediatr Rev* 13:371–378, 1992.

Sherman NH, Rosenberg HK, Heyman S, Templeton J: Ultrasound evaluation of neck masses in children, *J Ultrasound Med* 4:127–134, 1985.

Slap GB, Brooks JSJ, Schwartz JS: When to perform biopsies of enlarged peripheral lymph nodes in young patients, *JAMA* 252:1321–1326, 1984.

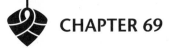

CHAPTER 69

Orthodontics

James L. Ackerman

The several million children receiving orthodontic care in the United States today represent only approximately 15% of patients who could benefit from this therapy. The purpose of this chapter is to help the primary care practitioner recognize orthodontic problems, make the necessary referral to an orthodontist, and have a basic understanding of the rationale of orthodontic treatment. More specifically, this chapter will discuss how the patient's medical history impacts on orthodontic treatment and how orthodontics can affect the patient's overall health.

MALOCCLUSIONS

In the transition from the edentulous state of the neonate to the complete primary dentition at approximately 3 years of age to the complete permanent dentition (with the exception of the permanent third molars) at age 12 years, environmental influences on the development of the dentition and heritable factors lead to a variety of abnormalities that require orthodontic consultation. In the normal anteroposterior relationship of the gum pads in the neonate, the mandible

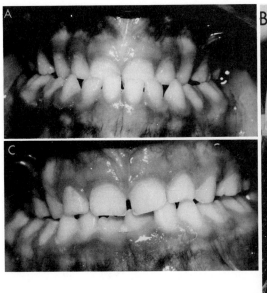

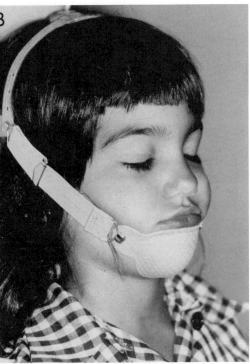

FIG 69-1

A, Anterior crossbite in the primary dentition. Note that the mandibular primary incisors are anterior to the maxillary primary incisors. **B,** In some cases, a chin cup is effective in treating anterior crossbite in the primary dentition. **C,** The same patient as in (A) 1 year after chin cup wear. Note that mandibular permanent central incisors have erupted. Chin cups are used when mild mandibular prognathism is the cause of the anterior crossbite.

is somewhat posterior to the maxilla. Parents rarely recognize this anteroposterior disproportion between the maxilla and the mandible because it causes no symptoms, unless it is severe as in the case of the Pierre Robin syndrome. Occasionally, when the maxillary and mandibular primary incisors have fully erupted by age 1 year, the parent might note that when the child closes the jaws the mandibular incisors bite in front of the maxillary incisors (anterior crossbite or underbite) (Fig. 69-1). Although in an older child an anterior crossbite is justification for seeking an orthodontic consultation, at this early phase it is often merely a habit or imitative of a parent. It is wise to ask the parents if anyone in the family, including older siblings, has an anterior crossbite. This often offers a clue as to whether this trait is an early manifestation of mandibular prognathism or maxillary hypoplasia that will require orthodontic or even surgical

correction at a later date. Abnormal bite relationships in the primary dentition do not occur with great frequency, so it is unusual to have to seek an orthodontic consultation for a child under 3 years of age unless there is a severe craniofacial abnormality.

Crowding of the permanent teeth is the most common form of malocclusion (Fig. 69-2). When the primary teeth emerge, spacing between the primary teeth is normal. If interdental spacing does not exist, the permanent teeth, which are much larger, will emerge in a crowded and overlapped position. The primary care physician should be wary of the patient whose primary dentition looks "too perfect," whose mother admiringly notes that her child has "beautiful baby teeth." Perfectly aligned and nonspaced primary teeth are often a clue that there will be crowding problems later in the development of the permanent dentition. Other factors involved in attain-

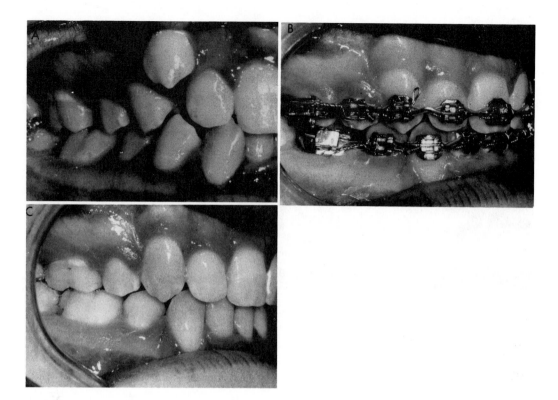

FIG 69-2

A, Crowding occurs when there is insufficient arch perimeter available in the dental arch to accommodate all of the permanent teeth. In this example of a common problem, the maxillary permanent canine is completely blocked out of the dental arch and has erupted ectopically. **B,** In this patient, first premolar teeth were extracted to relieve the crowding. Permanent canine teeth, no matter how badly malaligned, are rarely extracted for orthodontic purposes. **C,** Alignment of teeth after the orthodontic appliances were removed. Treatment time was approximately 2 years.

ing good alignment of the permanent teeth include the comparison between the widths of the primary teeth (Fig. 69-3) and their permanent successors as well as jaw growth. There is little increase in the transverse dimension of the dental arches once the permanent first molars erupt at approximately age 6 years. The greatest dimensional arch changes that take place are when the accessional teeth erupt (permanent teeth without primary tooth counterparts, *ie,* the permanent first and second molars) adding arch length at the posterior portion of the dentition. Because bone does not grow interstitially, there is no increase in the length of the anterior portion of the dental arches due to growth once the primary molar teeth emerge.

Crossbite problems (either anterior or posterior) in the primary dentition should be referred to an orthodontist, because early correction of these problems is sometimes quite simple and can prevent the development of more serious problems at a later date (Fig. 69-4). It is unlikely that the primary care physician would have much need to consult an orthodontist about a patient until the patient is approximately 6 or 7 years of age. A question often asked of the primary care physician relates to the eruption of the mandibular permanent incisors, which normally develop lingually to the mandibular primary incisors and often erupt in this position prior to exfoliation of the primary incisors. Commonly, the primary care physician or dentist receives a call from a mother who has discovered that her child has a "double row of teeth." Often in this circumstance, it is necessary to extract the overretained primary teeth. If there is sufficient

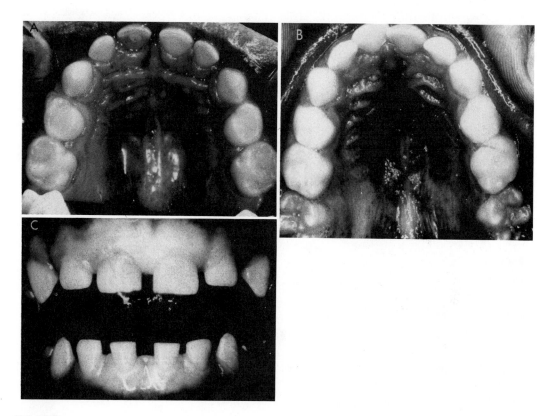

FIG 69-3

A, Interdental spacing of maxillary primary anterior teeth is prerequisite for well-aligned successional permanent incisor teeth. **B,** The patient with no interdental spacing of the maxillary primary anterior teeth. One can predict with some assurance that this patient will have crowding of the permanent incisor teeth when they emerge. **C,** A patient with excessive interdental spacing of the primary teeth. Depending on the size of the succedaneous permanent incisors, this patient may also have spacing in the permanent dentition.

space, normal tongue pressure alone usually guides the lingually displaced permanent teeth into their positions in the dental arch (Fig. 69-5). If there is sufficient space for the erupting permanent incisors, additional primary teeth may have to be removed, more or less "robbing Peter to pay Paul." This procedure should only be done after careful evaluation by an orthodontist, because this procedure of "serial extraction" often leads to the necessity of extracting permanent teeth at a later date to establish the desired esthetic and functional goals of the orthodontic treatment (Fig. 69-6).

During the ages of approximately 7 to 9 years, the primary care physician might be queried most by the mothers about developing orthodontic problems, because it is at this point that malocclusion is first easily recognized by the parent. When maxillary permanent lateral incisors erupt, the crowns of these teeth may appear displaced because the developing unerupted maxillary permanent canines normally press on the lateral portion of the roots of the erupted permanent lateral incisors, causing the teeth to tip. This stage of dental development, the "ugly duckling" phase, often corrects itself as the rest of the permanent teeth emerge. Maxillary permanent canines sometimes become impacted and simply do not emerge at age 12 or 13 years when they are due to erupt. These teeth can become impacted in the palate or also can be impacted on the facial side of the alveolar ridge. Permanent canine teeth are important teeth, from an esthetic as well as functional point of view. As a result, orthodontists generally recommend that these teeth be surgically exposed and an orthodontic

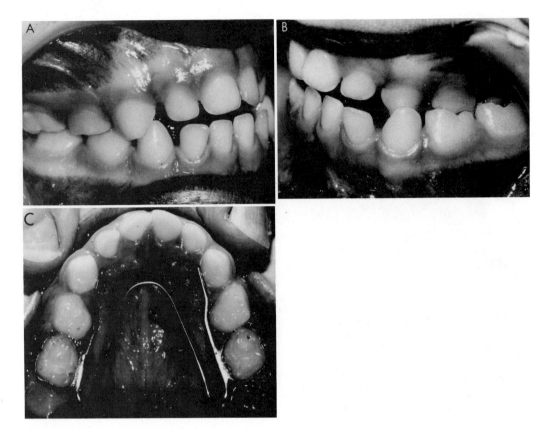

FIG 69-4

A, A 5-year-old patient with normal occlusion of primary teeth on the right side. Note that the maxillary molar teeth occlude to the buccal side of the mandibular teeth. **B,** On the left side, note that the maxillary posterior teeth are occluding to the palatal side of the mandibular teeth.

The patient shifts the lower jaw to the left on closure. This is a maxillary palatal crossbite caused by bilateral constriction of the maxillary dental arch. **C,** Fixed expansion in place attached to the maxillary primary second molars.

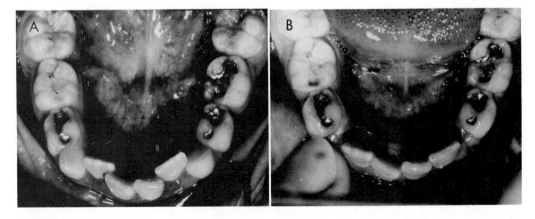

FIG 69-5

A, Anterior arch perimeter deficiency in the early transitional dentition. When there is insufficient space, mandibular permanent lateral incisors erupt ectopically to the lingual side. **B,** Mandibular primary canine teeth have been removed and autoalignment of these teeth has

occurred because of the molding effect of the tongue and lip pressure. This approach amounts to "robbing Peter to pay Paul," because ultimately there will be insufficient space for the mandibular permanent canines.

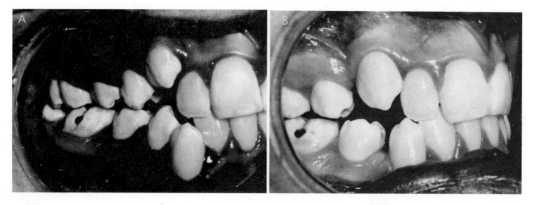

FIG 69-6

A, An example of serial extraction shows that if the first premolar teeth are extracted at the propitious time, the ectopically erupting canines often spontaneously drift into the correct position. **B,** Note the absence of the first premolars and the nearly complete extraction space closure from the result of serial extractions without orthodontic appliance therapy. The vast majority of serial extraction cases do require fixed orthodontic appliance therapy to achieve optimal tooth positions.

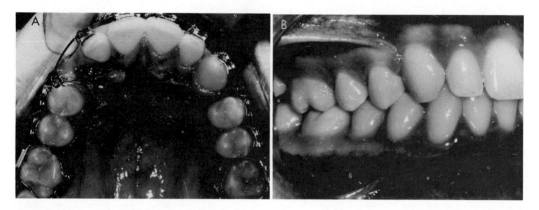

FIG 69-7

A, A palatally impacted permanent canine surgically exposed and orthodontic appliances applying traction to the tooth to bring it into the dental arch. **B,** Orthodontic appliances are removed when the permanent canine has achieved a good aesthetic and functional position.

attachment be bonded to the tooth (Fig. 69-7). With orthodontic traction, the tooth gradually can be brought into its normal position in the dental arch.

Another common concern among parents of children in the transitional or mixed-dentition stage (some primary and some permanent teeth) relates to the space, or diastema, which occurs normally between the newly emerged maxillary permanent central incisors. Unless there is an exceptionally thick band of tissue (frenum) that is preventing the natural mesial drift of the permanent incisor teeth (Fig. 69-8), or unless the maxillary permanent incisors are unusually small, this space will close naturally, particularly when the maxillary permanent canines emerge at approximately age 11.5 years of age in girls and 12.5 years of age in boys.

There is a wide range of variation in terms of the timing of tooth eruption. In general, girls are somewhat more advanced than boys in terms of their dental age. Dental age may vary by as much as a year or two when compared with the chronologic age, giving a very low correlation between dental age and skeletal age.

In general, if the child's orthodontic problem relates to a disproportion in the size or position of the jaws, the referral to an orthodontist should be

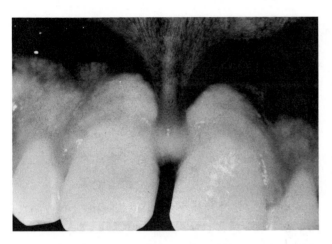

FIG 69-8

In this patient, a hypertrophied maxillary labial frenum has prevented the natural closure of a midline diastema. When the maxillary permanent canines erupt, they usually exert a mesial force, which closes this space. Frenectomies are rarely performed for hypertrophied maxillary labial frenum unless it is in conjunction with orthodontic treatment.

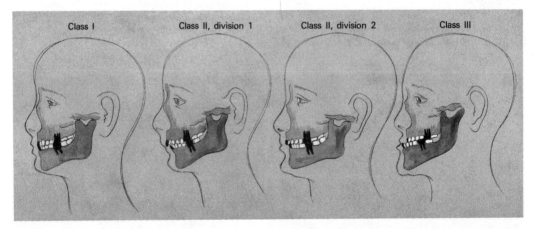

FIG 69-9

Malocclusion is classified according to the anteroposterior relationships of the teeth (*ie,* the relationship of the permanent first molars). Angle (1898) described three major types of malocclusion: Class I, normal occlusion but crowding of teeth; Class II, upper teeth forward; Class III, lower teeth forward. [Courtesy of TM Graber.]

made on the basis of skeletal age, because part of the treatment may involve an attempt to achieve facial growth modification. On the other hand, if the orthodontic problem is one relating to tooth position and either intra-arch spacing or crowding, the orthodontic referral perhaps should be made on the basis of the dental age.

Just as the maxillary posterior teeth can be occluding palatally in relationship to the mandibular molar teeth, the opposite condition, whereby the mandibular molars are occluding too far lingually in relationship to the maxillary molars, can also occur. Thus, there are a number of different types of crossbites that can occur unilaterally or bilaterally and can occur between individual antagonist teeth or can include entire segments of the dental arch. Long-term crossbites cause abnormal loading forces on the teeth, which can ultimately cause stresses within the supporting structures of the teeth leading to periodontal problems. Crossbites also can cause deflection of the mandible while biting, which can cause stress on the temporomandibular joints. This problem ultimately can lead to pain and dysfunction in the jaw joints. Many individuals maintain excellent oral health throughout life with severe crossbites, and the judgment of whether these problems should be corrected requires careful analysis of the problem. The common, easily recognizable orthodontic problems are those that relate to the anteroposterior dimension or the sagittal plane (Fig. 69-9).

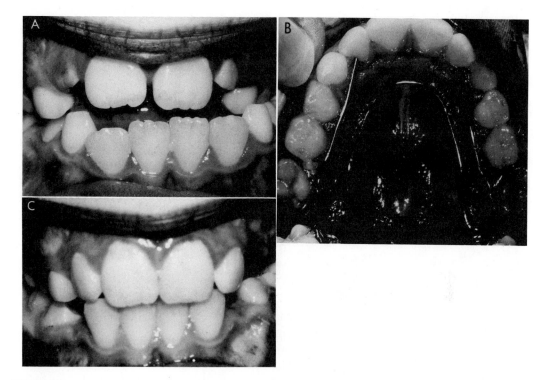

FIG 69-10

A, A patient with anterior open bite (insufficient overlap of anterior teeth) in early transitional dentition, caused by thumb sucking, immature oral and pharyngeal function, and unfavorable tongue posture at rest, while swallowing, and during speech. **B,** Crossbite was corrected with an expansion appliance, which also served as a thumb-sucking habit reminder. **C,** Corrected crossbite. There was simultaneous maturation of oral-pharyngeal function.

The vertical dimension must be considered when defining malocclusion. The major categories of bite problems in the vertical dimension are anterior open bite (Fig. 69-10), in which there is insufficient vertical overlap of the anterior teeth, and anterior deep bite, in which the mandibular incisors are biting too deeply toward the palate, often impinging on the palatal mucosa (Fig. 69-11). It is also possible to have a posterior open bite, in which the maxillary and mandibular teeth are not in contact. Problems in the vertical dimension can be caused by skeletal disproportion or merely insufficient dental compensation for an underlying skeletal dysplasia.

There is an enormous range of variations for jaw positions and some patients who are at the outer limits of the normal range of jaw disproportion often have quite normal dentition based on natural dental compensation that can occur from the positions and inclinations of the teeth. On the other hand, some patients whose jaw proportions are seemingly more harmonious and proportional can have severe malocclusion based on the malpositions of the teeth themselves in all three planes of space. From an epidemiologic point of view, only a small segment of the population has ideal occlusion. Thus, in many respects, malocclusion must be considered as the usual rather than the unusual finding in a pediatric population, and the decision as to whether orthodontic treatment is indicated is based on dentofacial esthetics, psychosocial factors, and functional considerations.

Treatment

There are three basic modalities for treating malocclusion and dentofacial deformity. The first of these is orthodontic tooth movement alone, the second is redirecting the growth of the jaws as well as regulating the positions of the teeth, and the third is the utilization of surgical techniques for repositioning the jaws in conjunc-

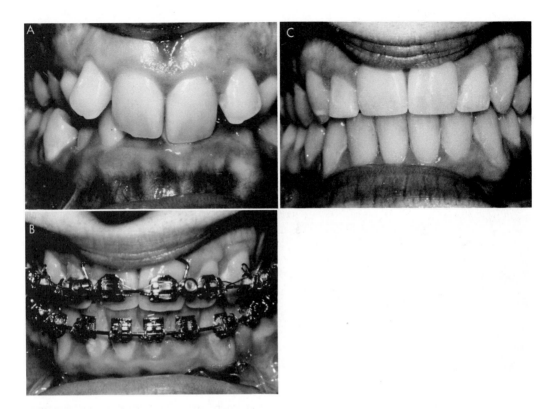

FIG 69-11

A, This patient, in the late transitional stage of dentition, had a severe anterior deep bite (increased vertical overlap of the incisor teeth). Note that the maxillary incisors are impinging on the labial gingiva of the mandibular incisors. The lower incisors are also impinging on the palatal mucosa posterior to the maxillary incisors. **B,** Through differential eruption (inhibiting incisor eruption and encouraging molar eruption) the "bite" is opened. **C,** After fixed orthodontic appliances are removed, note the correct vertical and horizontal overlap of the anterior teeth. This patient will wear retainers at night for several years to maintain this correction.

tion with orthodontic tooth movement. The nature and degree of the deformity and the age of the patient (growth potential) help determine which mode of treatment is selected.

The simplest type of treatment, preventive and interceptive orthodontics, is utilized when there is some event or insult to the developing dentition that, if not modified, will certainly lead to a malocclusion. A good example of such an event is the early loss of a primary molar tooth, which would allow the mesial drift of the posterior teeth, leaving insufficient space for eruption of the successional tooth. If indicated, an appliance called a *space maintainer* can be placed on the adjacent teeth to hold the space where the primary tooth was lost. On the other hand, if a primary tooth has been lost prematurely and some of these unfavorable sequelae have already

occurred, a simple appliance can sometimes be utilized to regain the space. This mode of treatment is called *interceptive orthodontics*. Once the early treatment is performed, no further therapy will be required on the remaining permanent teeth. Thus, preventive and interceptive orthodontic treatment usually is performed in the primary and transitional dentitions, and its goal is to achieve a substantial result with minimal effort.

Orthodontic tooth movement is based on the principle that the force applied to the crown of a tooth is transmitted to the periodontal ligament, which is interposed between the root surface (cementum) and the lamina dura of the dentoalveolus. Because all these tissues are cellular, the resulting differential apposition and resorption that takes place within the tooth socket is medi-

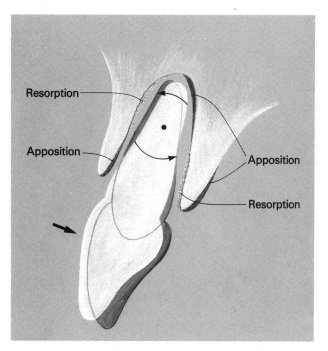

FIG 69-12

A diagram of the tissue reaction to orthodontic tooth movement, where differential apposition and resorption at the tension and pressure sites causes the tooth socket to "drift" slowly along with the movement of the tooth. [Courtesy of TM Graber.]

ated by cellular responses. The periodontal ligament consists of fluid plus fibers that connect the root of the tooth to the alveolar bone. Thus, the periodontal ligament acts as a type of "shock absorber," which is both suspensory and hydraulic in nature. The periodontal ligament and the suspensory apparatus of the tooth seems particularly well-designed to resist the normal type of forces that are applied to the teeth, which is along their long axis during mastication. The forces of mastication are usually quite strong but are of an intermittent nature. If, on the other hand, a light, continuous force is applied to the tooth, particularly if it is in an eccentric direction, adaptive changes take place within the alveolar bone and the tooth drifts along with the tooth socket (Fig. 69-12). Cells in the cementum of the root cause resorption of the tooth root, but the cellular activity on the alveolar bone surface is much more labile and the osteoclastic and osteoblastic activity at the alveolar bone level operates at a more rapid rate than does the resorption of the root. If the opposite were true, it is obvious that orthodontic tooth movement would not be a possibility. In the most simple type of orthodontic tooth movement, which is the tipping of a tooth, there is a center of resistance; along the alveolar wall on the compression side of a peri-

odontal ligament there is osteoclastic activity, and on the tension side there is osteoblastic activity. This is the mechanism whereby the suspensory mechanism of the tooth in the alveolar bone remains intact during orthodontic tooth movement. The most biologic manner for orthodontically moving a tooth results from the application of light, continuous force. These pressures can be applied to the teeth through either removable appliances or fixed appliances. The removable appliances are constructed of acrylic and wire and can incorporate a variety of springs and levers to apply the light, continuous forces to the teeth. Because the forces of removable appliances only can be applied to a single point on each tooth, one is only able to tip the teeth. With this method, there is only a minimal amount of control of individual tooth movement.

Because the patient must be willing to wear the appliance on a full-time basis, patient compliance is a major consideration with this treatment. Fixed appliances, the major type of orthodontic treatment, consist of bands usually constructed of stainless steel that are fitted and adapted to the tooth and cemented with a luting medium such as zinc phosphate cement. These bands have welded attachments consisting of tubes or brackets in which wires can be engaged for applying

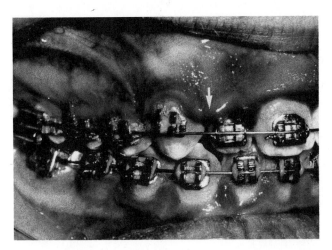

FIG 69-13
Gingivitis, partly attributable to mouth breathing. The additional gingival irritation from the appliance and space closure compressing and gingiva leads to further inflammation and hypertrophy of the tissues.

more controlled force to the tooth. The other method of attaching brackets to teeth is direct bonding, in which an adhesive is used to directly adhere the bracket to the tooth. With fixed appliances, arch wires of stainless steel or titanium alloys are used to apply controlled forces to the teeth. It is the relative strength, stiffness, and range of these wire elements that allow the orthodontist to control the magnitude, direction, and distance over which these forces operate.

Complications

These mechanical devices can be quite physically irritating to the oral mucosa. If a patient has a predilection for aphthous ulcers he/she can have considerable discomfort during the first 7 to 10 days that he/she is wearing orthodontic appliances. Palliative treatment such as warm saline rinses, the use of benzocaine in Orabase, and the use of soft wax over any element of the appliance that is particularly sharp can minimize the discomfort to the oral soft tissues. Within several weeks, almost all patients adapt to even the most complex types of orthodontic appliances. When the appliances are placed, particularly when small elastomeric units called *separators* are placed between the teeth to gain room for applying the orthodontic bands, and when the bands themselves are fitted, a transient bacteremia occurs due to the trauma to the teeth. If a patient has a health history of rheumatic fever or congenital heart disease, which places him/her at risk to this type of transient bacteremia, prophylactic antibiotics should be prescribed.

Root resorption is another hazard of orthodontic treatment. Almost all patients who have had orthodontic tooth movement do demonstrate minor signs of root resorption on radiographs. In some cases, as much as a quarter to a third of the root can be lost through root resorption. Appliances make maintenance of good oral hygiene difficult. Decalcification of the enamel adjacent to the orthodontic band or bracket may occur if the plaque and debris are not removed thoroughly at least once a day. Many orthodontists prescribe a fluoride mouth rinse, which is used daily for 1 minute after the patient has brushed the teeth to further prevent decalcification of the enamel. If this decalcification proceeds sufficiently, cavitation of the enamel surface may actually occur, which requires restoration of the tooth after the orthodontic appliances are removed. The gingiva can become hypertrophied and inflamed during treatment (Fig. 69-13). Although this particular sequela usually resolves spontaneously once the orthodontic appliances are removed, under some circumstances the gingival inflammation can cause increased resorption of the alveolar bone and can, under unusual circumstances, lead to periodontal defects. Patients at puberty, particularly girls, seem more prone to this type of gingival hypertrophy.

When orthodontic appliances are placed and forces applied to the teeth, the patient initially experiences a great deal of tooth tenderness, particularly on palpation (such as during mastication). As a result, for the first few days after orthodontic appliances are placed, the patient should eat a soft diet and take acetaminophen or aspirin.

Forces applied to the teeth also are transmitted through the jaws to growth sites considerably removed from the teeth themselves and, as a result, orthodontic force systems can have an effect on facial sutures, synchondroses, the mandibular condyle, and other growth sites. When an orthodontist is attempting to accomplish this type of growth redirection, usually stronger forces are used, and often the anchors for such forces are extraoral (such as headgear, facial masks, and chin cups). If the maxilla is extremely constricted, under some circumstances an orthodontist might use a fixed appliance with a screw in the midline of the palate, which causes rapid separation of the two halves of the maxilla. Over a period of several weeks after this rapid separation, bone fills in the midpalatine suture. This type of orthopedic device often sounds quite radical to parents, and frequently they will consult with their primary care physician about the wisdom and efficacy of such an appliance.

In a late adolescent sometimes there is a skeletal disproportion and facial imbalance that is sufficiently great to warrant surgical repositioning of one or both jaws to improve both facial esthetics and oral function.

Myofunctional Therapy and Orthodontics

Because form and function in the oral-pharyngeal area is important in the development of the dentition and the overall growth of the craniofacial complex, it is not surprising that the issue of swallowing and speech has received considerable attention as it relates to oral architecture. It is currently believed that the infantile pattern of swallowing and speech in which the tongue is placed in a forward position, interposed between the anterior teeth and in approximation with the lip, is an early maturational feature. At some point, the child goes through a transition in which a more adult pattern of tongue posture both at rest and in swallowing and speech is adopted. The adult pattern is thought to be with the tongue tip posterior and superior to the maxillary anterior teeth, without the tongue protruding or thrusting between incisor teeth during speech or swallowing. The more immature pattern has been called *tongue thrusting,* and speech therapists and orthodontists over the past two decades have developed an approach that attempts to correct this immature oral-pharyngeal function. The method is called *myofunctional therapy* and consists of a series of exercises that the child practices to overcome this "habit." Both the American Speech and Hearing Association and the American Association of Orthodontists have taken the position that there is little evidence that myofunctional therapy is efficacious and that more research is required before this method can be embraced as a clinical tool that should be widely used. Surely, there are patients for whom myofunctional therapy is useful, and those patients are usually ones whose speech problems are also the result of immature oral and pharyngeal function. At the present time, the view of the orthodontist is that the best approach to these patients is to change the architecture of the mouth so that the improved function will follow the new form. Because there has been greater utilization of surgical correction of jaw position in severe malocclusions, the clinical results have led orthodontists to the expectation that, in many patients, function can follow form of the jaw.

On the other hand, American orthodontists have begun to use removable orthodontic appliances, which have been popular in Europe for nearly 50 years and are called *functional appliances.* The purpose of these appliances is to alter oral function in an attempt to redirect the growth of the jaws. Unlike the heavy forces used with orthopedic devices to inhibit growth, these appliances attempt to alter muscle activity and jaw posture in such a way as to stimulate and redirect jaw growth. Because most of these appliances are toothborne, they also, obviously, cause considerable orthodontic tooth movement; over the years there has been considerable debate as to whether their greatest effect is as tooth-moving devices or in redirecting growth of the jaws. There is some evidence that over a short time interval, such as 1 or 2 years, there can be changes in skeletal proportions created by these appliances. Whether these changes are permanent and what the implication is for the ultimate configuration of the craniofacial complex in these children is yet to be determined. Nonetheless, these appliances have become popular in the United States and, unfortunately, there are more extravagant claims being made about the efficacy of these appliances than the evidence would support.

When patients are using removable orthodontic appliances, these appliances should not be worn during active play and sports. As well, if fixed appliances are being worn, a special mouth

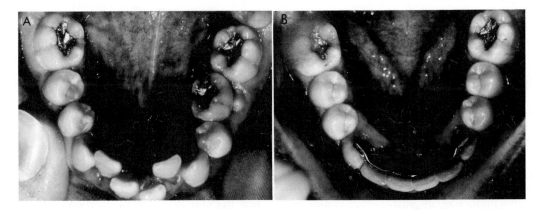

FIG 69-14

A, Malaligned mandibular incisors. **B,** After orthodontic correction, it is not uncommon for the patient to wear a bonded mandibular canine-to-canine fixed retainer. There is a greater tendency for mandibular incisor teeth to become crowded, and these fixed retainers are sometimes left in place until the fate of the mandibular third molars (wisdom teeth) is determined, which usually occurs during college years.

guard to protect the lips from trauma should be used while playing active sports.

When orthodontic appliances are removed, there is a tendency for physiologic rebound or recovery (relapse) to occur, and the teeth have a tendency to move in the direction of their original positions. As a result, retaining devices (which are made of acrylic and wire) are worn either full-time or just at night for some period of time after the fixed orthodontic appliances are removed. These devices hold the teeth in their corrected positions and serve as a template to ascertain whether the teeth are shifting. Very little relapse is required before a retainer becomes tight and, as a result, the patient has an early warning signal that his/her teeth are not maintaining their original corrections. In some instances, fixed retainers are used rather than removable retainers (Fig. 69-14).

THE VISIT

When a patient is referred to an orthodontist, the first visit usually consists of an initial evaluation during which the orthodontist performs an oral examination and thoroughly reviews the medical/dental history. Based on these initial findings, the orthodontist usually recommends that orthodontic records be taken, which consist of impressions of the teeth to make plaster models that carefully reproduce the anatomy of the oral

structures, facial and intraoral photographs, intraoral radiographs, and a cephalometric radiograph. The cephalometric radiograph is taken in norma lateralis at a fixed anode-to-target distance and can be used for ascertaining the nature of the orthodontic problem based on skeletal proportions. These radiographs can be taken at intervals, and the patient's craniofacial growth and development can be studied by superimposing tracings of the radiographs. The results of treatment and growth also can be ascertained using the same clinical tool.

With increasing concern of the public regarding diagnostic radiographs, the orthodontist is being asked more frequently whether it is necessary to take radiographs as part of the diagnostic regimen. Because of the complex nature of the developing dentition and the fact that many patients can profit from early treatment, there is no alternative at the present time other than to take a survey series of dental radiographs to establish a proper orthodontic diagnosis and treatment plan. Issues such as congenital absence of teeth, supernumerary teeth, impacted teeth, cysts, and other pathologic conditions, as well as just the normal sequence, position, and timing of eruption of teeth, are factors that cannot be ascertained in any other way other than with radiographs.

In all of the health sciences, the risks of treatment must be weighed against the benefits. Orthodontics is no exception. When orthodontic treatment is elective, it may be decided that it is inadvisable due to one or more aspects of the patient's health history. For some patients orthodontics is mandatory, such as those with craniofacial and dentofacial anomalies as well as those with other handicapping orthodontic conditions. For these patients, especially those with other health problems, close cooperation between the primary care physician and various specialists can reduce the complications of orthodontic treatment.

BIBLIOGRAPHY

Epker BN, Fish LC: *Dentofacial deformities: Integrated orthodontic and surgical correction,* St Louis, 1986, CV Mosby.

Forrester DJ, Wagner ML, Fleming J: *Pediatric dental medicine,* Philadelphia, 1981, Lea & Febiger.

Graber TM, Swain BF: *Orthodontics: Current principles and techniques,* St Louis, 1986, CV Mosby.

Proffit WR: *Contemporary orthodontics,* St Louis, 1986, CV Mosby.

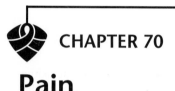

CHAPTER 70

Pain

Joel A. Fein

DEFINITION OF PAIN

Pain is defined as "an unpleasant sensory and emotional experience associated with actual or potential tissue damage, or described in terms of that damage." This rather broad definition generates from the notion that an individual's interpretation of painful stimuli is modified by a number of factors (Fig. 70-1). In this sense, pain is a psychological state rather than a physical one. The goal of the primary care physician is not to uncover the exact contributions of each of these factors but rather to understand and treat each individual's pain as a real and unique culmination of these components.

Pain in children may be categorized into acute pain and chronic pain. Chronic pain may be of a persistent or recurrent nature, the latter being more common in children. Examples of chronic pain include recurrent headaches, abdominal pain, or limb pain. Acute pain, on the other hand, is persistent, has its origin within days to weeks of presentation rather than months or years, and commonly wanes within a few days of tissue injury. Another distinction between acute and chronic pain is the greater potential for chronic pain to render the child dysfunctional with regard to school, home life, and friendships.

NEUROPHYSIOLOGY OF PAIN

The neurophysiologic mechanisms that result in the perception of pain are complex, consisting of excitatory and inhibitory neural pathways and neurotransmitters. Sensory pain fibers, called

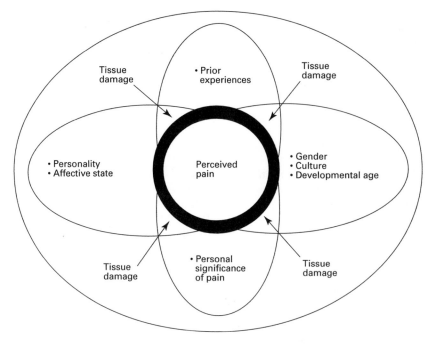

FIG 70-1
Factors involved in the perception of pain.

nociceptors, can transmit sharp pain rapidly (A delta fibers) or more slowly and persistently (C fibers). The afferent transmission from sensory receptors can be influenced by other neuronal transmissions from the cerebral cortex, diencephalon, or spinal cord. Various neuropeptides either can enhance (substance P) or inhibit (endorphins, enkephalins, serotonin) the transmission of pain. In addition, concurrent stimulation of "nonpainful" sensory fibers by touching, rubbing, or transcutaneous nerve stimulation can exert an inhibitory effect on painful sensory input. Finally, the involvement of the cerebral cortex can alter pain perception based on prior pain experiences, cultural norms, and the significance of the pain to the individual. For example, an individual who perceives pain as signifying "cancer" might regard the same sensory stimulation differently than if it signifies "food poisoning." Interestingly, tissue damage need not be apparent for pain to exist: phantom limb pain and neuropathic pain can result from ongoing neuronal excitability in the absence of ongoing tissue damage.

One does not need to understand the intricate details of pain transmission to treat pain successfully. However, it is important to recognize how to modulate the aforementioned control mechanisms to manage the individual with painful symptoms.

ASSESSMENT OF PAIN IN CHILDREN

Environment, context, and prior experiences influence the interpretation of painful stimuli and create a difficult task of assessing pain in children. The practitioner initially should question the location, timing, character, and severity of the pain as described by the child or the parents. A mnemonic for the descriptive characteristics of pain is "REACTS" (Box 70-1).

Pain assessment must take into consideration the child's level of development. In infants and toddlers, practitioners rely mostly on the behavioral manifestations of pain, whereas preschool and school-aged children may add self-report to this body of information. Younger, nonverbal children may require interpretation of their symptoms by their parents. Parents may provide information about the timing and location of the pain but are less likely to accurately describe

Historical Characteristics of Painful Symptoms

Relief	What makes the pain go away?
Exacerbation	What makes the pain worse?
Area of pain	Where is the pain? Does it radiate anywhere?
Character	Is the pain sharp, burning, throbbing, etc.?
Timing	When was the initial onset of the pain? What time of day is it worse? Is it intermittent or constant?
Severity	Is the pain mild, moderate, or severe? (May use pain scale.)

character or severity. Nevertheless, parents are valuable sources of information regarding observations of "distress," using facial and motor cues, behavioral state, and quality of cry. In particular, parents provide much needed information regarding their child's usual pain behaviors and previous pain experiences, which help to individualize the approach to a particular child's pain relief. For health care professionals, observation scales such as the Children's Hospital of Eastern Ontario Pain Scale (CHEOPS) or the Observational Scale of Behavioral Distress (OSBD) have been used with success in quantifying these behaviors. Physiologic changes such as heart rate, blood pressure, and palmar sweating may be used adjunctively. It is notably difficult to separate issues of pain, anxiety, fear, and sadness in younger children; however, it can be argued that the overall management goals are to alleviate all of these experiences rather than just one component.

Children 2 years of age and older frequently can express "hurt," although details of the painful experience will be sketchy. These children frequently will identify the location and timing of their pain but usually do not have the skills to describe its character. Because toddlers are preoperational and cannot fully understand comparisons, description of pain intensity is often limited to "hurts a little" or "hurts a lot."

In children over the age of 3 years, simple graphic scales, such as the "oucher" scale, which uses faces in various stages of painful expression, may be helpful in the assessment and reassessment of pain. In addition, these children can more easily discern the varying intensity and severity of pain in different locations.

In school-aged children, more accurate mea-surement of pain intensity can be obtained using graphic scales such as the pain thermometer (Fig. 70-2A). Visual analog scales also may be used to distinguish and separate pain, anxiety, and sadness (Fig. 70-2B). These scales require some level of abstract thinking and have been validated for children older than 7 years of age.

INTERVENTIONS IN PAIN MANAGEMENT

Most children experiencing acute pain require simple pharmacologic management and, if possible, alleviation of the underlying illness. However, the child experiencing chronic pain requires a multidimensional approach that includes pharmacologic therapy, psychological counseling, and patient and parent education regarding appropriate expectations. Adjuvant therapies, both pharmacologic and nonpharmacologic, may require consultation with a pain specialist.

Pharmacologic Agents

Efficient and effective use of analgesics stems from knowledge of the pharmacologic and neurochemical aspects of each agent, including their onset of action, duration of action, and potential side effects. The following general guidelines may be helpful in the practitioner's approach to pain management:

1. *Maintain a steady state of analgesia.* The dosage required to initially abolish pain is greater than the dose needed to prevent re-emergence of that pain. Therefore, medication should be administered frequently and persistently enough to prevent the pain from returning to its full intensity. The "as needed" or "PRN" approach to prescribing pain medication is therefore counterintuitive. Rather than waiting for the patient to recognize the presence of pain severe enough to require medication, it is better to administer an appropriate standing dose at an interval concomitant with the known duration of the medication's effects. Alternatively, older children may be offered pain medication at given intervals and allowed the right to refuse ("reverse PRN"). This approach allows the child to reassess his/her pain intensity just prior to the expected lapse of medication effect. It also

III

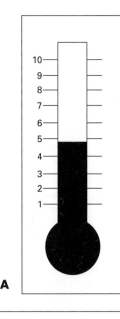

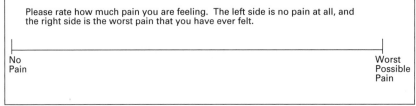

FIG 70-2

A, A pain thermometer. **B,** The visual analog scale used for rating pain intensity in children more than 7 years of age.

prevents the patient from exhibiting "drug seeking" behavior.

2. *Use combinations of agents that are synergistic for analgesia.* Combinations of opioid and nonopioid analgesics frequently result in greater pain relief than either agent used alone. Because lower doses of each agent can be used to achieve the same analgesic effects, there is less potential for adverse effects. Conversely, combinations of opioids and sedative/anxiolytics may elicit more severe side effects than either medication taken alone.

3. *Address and clarify the patient's concern about "addiction."* Addiction or *psychological dependence* is manifest as compulsive drug-seeking behavior leading to an obsessive quest for procurement of the drug. As opposed to persons who self-administer drugs for pleasure, patients who are treated for painful symptoms will stop seeking the drug after the pain is relieved or resolved. Psychological dependence rarely occurs as a result of appropriate administration of analgesics for pain. Psychological dependence differs from *physical dependence,* which is the presence of withdrawal symptoms after cessation of the drug. Physical dependence is common after long-term narcotic use and resolves easily with the administration of tapering doses of medication. *Tolerance* occurs when an increased dose of a medication is required to produce an equal analgesic effect and duration compared with previous doses. Tolerance must be distinguished clinically from increasing pain caused by a worsening pathologic process.

The pharmacologic agents used for pain relief may be divided into opioid analgesics, nonopioid analgesics, and adjuvant therapies such as antidepressants and anticonvulsants. Management of specific situations such as procedural pain, acute pain, and chronic pain will be covered in following sections.

Nonopioid Analgesia

The most commonly used nonopioid analgesic is acetaminophen. Acetaminophen has both analgesic and antipyretic properties. It is not effective for chronic inflammatory disease, however it may exhibit anti-inflammatory effects in acutely injured tissues. The dose is 10 to 15 mg/kg every 4 hours; however, single doses of 15 to 20 mg/kg are appropriate if the total daily dose does not exceed 120 mg/kg. Side effects are rare with appropriate dosing. Single ingestions of greater than 140 mg/kg or chronic therapy using greater than 150 mg/kg per day have been associated with serious hepatic injury and subsequent death.

The nonsteroidal anti-inflammatory drugs (NSAIDs) that are approved for use in the pediatric population include aspirin, tolmetin (Tolectin™), naproxen (Naprosyn®), choline magnesium trisalicylate (Trilisate®), and ibuprofen (Motrin™, Advil™). The NSAIDs act via inhibition of prostaglandin synthesis and have antipyretic, anti-inflammatory, and analgesic properties. Aspirin use has decreased secondary to its association with Reye syndrome; however, it is still the drug of choice for patients with Kawasaki disease and juvenile rheumatoid arthritis. The doses, indications, and side effects of these agents are presented in Table 70-1. To minimize gastric and lower intestinal symptoms, these agents should be taken with food. Antacids may be required in severe cases of NSAID-induced gastritis. Ketorolac (Toradol™) is a new parenteral NSAID approved for children over the age of 12 years. It can be used intravenously, intramuscularly, or orally for pain that might otherwise require an opiate analgesic. Ketorolac has been used in place of or as an adjunct to morphine in the management of postoperative pain, sickle cell vaso-occlusive crisis, and other acute causes of musculoskeletal pain. Ketorolac should not be administered to patients with coagulation disorders, renal disease, or pregnancy and should not be used in any patient for more than 5 days.

Opioid Analgesia

Although most painful symptoms can be alleviated successfully without the use of opiate medication, the most severe cases do require the adjunctive use of this class of medications. In contrast to the nonopiate medications, the opiate medications cause varied effects depending on the class of neuronal receptors that are activated. At high doses, these agents produce a sedative effect, albeit with possible loss of airway reflexes. The major differences between opiate classes lie in their relative affinity for mu (μ), kappa (κ), delta (δ), and sigma (σ) opioid receptors (Box 70-2). The pure agonists have more μ activity than κ activity. They are effective analgesics, are sedatives at higher doses, and cause decreased gastrointestinal motility and difficult urination. In addition, both morphine and fentanyl can cause pruritis, particularly nasal or facial. The agonist-antagonist nalbuphine (Nubain®) has strong σ effects and *partial* κ effects and is an antagonist to μ effects. For this reason, analgesia is at the spinal level, gastrointestinal effects are minimized, and sedation is increased. Other agents that have pure κ and σ effects are not used in the pediatric age group. Naloxone is antagonistic to all opioid receptor subtypes.

Medication classes and equianalgesic doses of the most commonly prescribed opiates are presented in Table 70-2. The opiate most often prescribed for pain in the outpatient setting is codeine. It is most effective when used in conjunction with a nonopiate analgesic such as acetaminophen and is available as combination-preparations in both elixir and tablet form. Although in many parts of the United States codeine with acetaminophen tablets can be ordered without a Drug Enforcement Agency (DEA) number, many pharmacies still require this license to dispense the drug. Hydromorphone (Dilaudid®) is also commonly used in the outpatient setting, especially in patients with recurrent or persistent pain syndromes caused by chronic illnesses such as sickle cell disease.

Adverse effects from opiates are common but can be minimized in most cases. If sedation occurs, decreasing the dose of the medication while increasing the frequency of administration may help. Stool softeners and cathartics help to alleviate the constipation associated with these medications. If nausea or vomiting occur, switching to a different medication at equianal-

TABLE 70-1
Frequently Prescribed NSAIDs in the Pediatric Population

AGENT	DOSE	ROUTE	INDICATIONS	SIDE EFFECTS	COMMENTS
Aspirin (Generic, Ecotrin™, Bufferin™, Zorprin™)	*Low dose* 10–20 mg/kg per dose every 4–6 hrs *High dose* 75–90 mg/kg/day given every 4–6 hrs	po	Analgesia Antipyresis Kawasaki disease Anti-inflammatory	Gastric irritation Reye syndrome Toxic levels produce tinnitus, hyperpnea, lethargy	Enteric coated form (Ecotrin™) and controlled release form (Zorprin™) are available
Choline magnesium trisalicylate (Trilisate®)	50 mg/kg/day given BID or TID	po	Anti-inflammatory, analgesia, antipyresis		Available as 500 mg/5 cc
Ibuprofen (Motrin™, Advil™)	10 mg/kg per dose given every 6 hrs	po	Analgesia, anti-inflammatory, antipyresis	*All of the NSAIDs may cause the following side effects:* Abdominal pain, nausea, diarrhea, renal insufficiency (lowered glomerular filtration rate), mild anemia, increased LFTs	Available as 100 mg/5 cc suspension
Naproxen (Naprosyn®)	10–20 mg/kg/day given BID or TID	po	Analgesia, anti-inflammatory, juvenile rheumatoid arthritis (higher dose)		Available as 125 mg/5 cc suspension
Tolmetin (Tolectin™)	20–50 mg/kg/day given TID or QID	po	Rheumatic disease (juvenile rheumatoid arthritis)	Tolmetin may rarely cause hypersensitivity (asthma, nasal polyps, anaphylaxis)	Not approved for children <2 yrs of age
Ketorolac (Toradol™)	*IV/IM:* <50 kg: 15 mg every 6 hrs >50 kg: 30–60 mg every 6 hrs *po:* 10 mg every 6 hrs (May double first doses in patients >50 kg)	IV, IM, po	Short-term management of moderate to severe musculoskeletal/visceral pain	Gastritis, platelet dysfunction, renal insufficiency, hypersensitivity Do not exceed a total of 5 days of use	Not approved for children <12 yrs of age

BID—twice a day; IM—intramuscular; IV—intravenous; po—oral; QID—four times a day; TID—three times a day.

BOX 70-2
Effects of Opioid Classes

mu (μ)	kappa (κ)	delta (δ)	sigma (σ)
• Supraspinal analgesia	• Spinal analgesia	• Analgesia	• Hallucinations
• ↓ Smooth muscle motility	• Sedation	• Euphoria	• Dysphoria
• Bradycardia	• Miosis		• Psychomotor stimulation
• Sedation (high dose)	• ↓ Antidiuretic hormone		
• Dependence	release		

gesic doses may be successful. Similarly, switching medications may prevent tolerance to that medication from occurring.

Adjuvant Medications

Medications such as anxiolytics, antidepressants, psychostimulants, antihistamines, or neuroleptics may be indicated for use in the management of pain. Given the potentially severe adverse effects of these agents, the primary care physician should consult a neurologist or pain specialist to guide their use. In addition, some baseline laboratory values are required prior to administering antidepressant or neuroleptic medications.

The most commonly used anxiolytic medications are the benzodiazepines midazolam (Versed®, 0.05–0.1 mg/kg), lorazepam (Ativan®, 0.05–0.1 mg/kg), and diazepam (Valium®, 0.1–0.2 mg/kg). The anxiolytic and sedative effects of these medications reduce the amount of opiate required to appropriately treat procedure-related pain. Midazolam has the added advantage of providing transient amnesia as well. These medications can be administered orally, intranasally (midazolam), or intravenously. Antidepressants act through the serotonergic pathway to treat rheumatic, postherpetic, and denervation pain, as well as chronic headaches. Psychostimulant medications such as methylphenidate (Ritalin®) or dextroamphetamine may be useful in decreasing the sedation associated with narcotic administration. In addition, there is some evidence that they also potentiate analgesia in patients already receiving opiate medications. Antihistamine medications such as diphenhydramine (Benadryl®) and hydroxyzine (Atarax®, Vistaril®) can provide an additive effect to the opioid analgesics. In addition, antihistamines have antiemetic properties that combat some of the adverse effects of the opioid medications. Neuroleptic medications have limited use due to the severe adverse effects, sedation, and dysphoria associated with long-term use.

Nonpharmacologic Techniques

The decision to use pharmacologic agents for the management of pain does not preclude other nonpharmacologic modalities. Psychological support should be provided by the patient's family and the practitioner regardless of the source of the child's pain. Family members might require detailed and specific advice about their participation, especially during painful procedures.

Specific psychological techniques may be useful in these situations; however, the appropriateness of these modalities vary with the developmental age of the child. Muscle relaxation, hypnosis, and biofeedback may be best suited for children over the age of 3 years. Play therapy and distraction techniques are suitable for even younger children. The depth of teaching involved in these techniques depends on the nature of the pain. For example, it may be sufficient for children undergoing a short, painful procedure to be quickly taught how to "blow bubbles" as a distracting maneuver. Children with cancer or sickle cell pain, on the other hand, may benefit from several sessions learning how to create distracting and relaxing mental imagery or even hypnotic fantasies for use during painful exacerbations of their illness. Children with musculoskeletal or neuropathic pain may benefit from the local application of a transcutaneous electrical nerve stimulator (TENS) unit, which provides "countercurrent stimulation" to the pain fibers in the area of injury. With the exception of the TENS unit and hypnosis, the nonpharmacologic techniques for pain management may be utilized by any practitioner with the interest and creativity to individualize these therapies. Detailed descriptions of these techniques can be found in the comprehensive textbook on pain management in children by Schechter, Berde, and Yaster (1993).

TABLE 70-2
Frequently Prescribed Opiate Medications in the Pediatric Population

AGENT (CLASS/NAME)	TRADE NAME (EXAMPLES)	ROUTE	EQUIANALGESIC DOSE	ONSET (MIN)	PEAK EFFECT (MIN)	DURATION (HRS)	COMMENTS
Agonists (+μ, +κ, ±σ)							
Codeine	(codeine/Tylenol™) Elixir (12 mg/120 mg) Tylenol #2 (15/300), #3 (30/300), #4 (60/300)	po	1.0 mg/kg every 3–4 hrs	10–30	30–60	4–6	Also has antitussive properties
Hydromorphone	Dilaudid®	IM po	0.015 mg/kg every 3–4 hrs 0.06 mg/kg every 3–4 hrs	N/A	15–30 30–60	3–4	
Oxycodone	Roxicodone™ With *acetaminophen:* Roxicet™, Percocet® (5/325), Tylox® (5/500) With *aspirin:* Percodan® (4.5/325)	po	0.2 mg/kg every 3–4 hrs	15–30	60	3–4	
Morphine	Roxanol™	IV	0.1 mg/kg every 3–4 hrs	5–10	30–60	3–4	• May cause seizures at high doses or in newborns • Dosing is based on requirements of prior forms of morphine
	MS Contin®	po	0.3 mg/kg every 8–12 hrs Six times total in 24 hrs	60	60–120	8–12	
Fentanyl	Sublimaze®	IV, IM	1–2 μg/kg, (may repeat dose one time) IV dose, given twice a day	Immediately	1–3	0.5–1	• Procedural pain/sedation (possible chest wall rigidity, laryngospasm)
	Duragesic™ patch (2.5, 5.0, 7.5, and 10 mg)	TD	See *Physician's Desk Reference* for conversion from MSO4 to fentanyl			72	Chronic pain management
Methadone	Dolophine®	po	0.2 mg/kg every 6–8 hrs	30–60	30–60	6–24	
Meperidine	Demerol®	IV, IM	0.75 mg/kg every 2–3 hrs	10–45	30–60	3–4	Neuroleptic malignant sxn if used with tricyclic antidepressants
Agonist/antagonist (–μ, ±κ, –σ)							
Nalbuphine	Nubain®	IV	0.1 mg/kg every 3–4 hrs	5–10	30–60	1–2	Less gastrointestinal motility problems
		IM		60	60–120	4–7	Less sphincter of Oddi spasm
Antagonist (–μ, –κ, –σ)							
Naloxone	Narcan®	IV, IM, SQ, ET	Acute overdose: 1–2 mg Medication reversal: 0.01–0.1 mg/kg	1		20–30	For slow reversal, may dilute in 100 cc of saline and titrate dose to effect

ET = endotracheal; IM = intramuscular; IV = intravenous; po = oral; SQ = subcutaneous; TD = transdermal.

MANAGEMENT OF PAIN IN THE PRIMARY CARE SETTING

The following sections address some of the more common scenarios involving pain in the pediatric practice setting. These scenarios can be categorized as the pain associated with procedures, acute illness, or chronic illness.

Procedural Pain

Most of the procedures that children undergo in the ambulatory pediatric setting involve needle punctures. In some offices, more invasive procedures also are performed. A number of techniques are available to diminish the amount of pain perceived by the child during these procedures. The easiest and perhaps the most important of these techniques includes preparation of the child for the procedure. Prior and detailed disclosure of the forthcoming events allows the child to trust the health care professionals who are performing the procedure. This trusting relationship serves to lower the total anxiety of this and subsequent visits to the office, in that the child realizes that he/she will never be "surprised" with painful stimuli in that setting. It is helpful to ask the parents how much time their child requires to enlist coping skills prior to the procedure. For many children, disclosure should occur as close to the event as possible in order to minimize anxiety time. Distraction techniques such as singing or "blowing bubbles" during the procedure may be successful as well. Because younger children may perceive painful procedures as a form of punishment, the physician should have the parent address this issue by stating out loud, in simple terms, that this is absolutely not the case. In addition, struggling or screaming should not be treated as a negative behavior, nor should the child be threatened or embarrassed into cooperating. Instead, positive reinforcement, such as praise for calm behavior or colorful stickers, should be used.

Local Anesthesia

Any procedure involving the manipulation of skin tissue such as laceration repairs, incision and drainage, and foreign body removal requires local anesthesia. In general, the subcutaneous injection of 1% lidocaine, with or without epinephrine, into the area achieves excellent anesthesia within minutes of application. Box 70-3 suggests some methods of reducing the pain associated with this procedure. Topically admin-

---

BOX 70-3

Suggested Methods to Reduce the Pain of Local Anesthetic Administration

- Use the longest, smallest needle available
- Mix 1 part sodium bicarbonate with 9 parts lidocaine ("buffered lidocaine")
- Warm the anesthetic solution
- Inject into already anesthetized portions of tissue
- Inject slowly
- Have the parent provide "counter-stimulation" by rubbing an area adjacent to the injection site

---

istered liquids or gels such as TAC (tetracaine, adrenaline, cocaine) or LET (lidocaine, epinephrine, tetracaine) have been used successfully in lieu of subcutaneous injection prior to laceration repair. TAC or LET require approximately 10 to 20 minutes to work and are best used for repair of lacerations with limited depth of penetration. They should not be used in areas where epinephrine is contraindicated (mucous membranes or poorly vascularized areas).

Regional anesthetic techniques such as peripheral nerve blocks may be helpful in complicated injuries such as nailbed lacerations or drainage of a felon; however, the details of these procedures are beyond the scope of this chapter. The routine use of a dorsal penile block for neonatal circumcisions has gained recent favor, but its universal use remains controversial.

For intravenous needle insertion, phlebotomy, and lumbar punctures, recently developed products such as eutectic mixture of local anesthetics (EMLA) have been successful in reducing the amount of pain perceived during subcutaneous injections. EMLA must be administered at least 1 hour prior to needle stick and has the additional disadvantage of being expensive. This form of topical anesthesia may be a useful adjunct in the management of select children who do not respond to psychological support or who encounter frequent painful procedures.

Systemic Analgesia

Some children may also benefit from the administration of oral or parenteral analgesics, especially if it is known that the procedure will be lengthy or painful, such as the treatment of second-degree burns. In such cases, acetaminophen plus codeine may be administered approximately 30 minutes prior to the procedure. If rapid effects, easy titration, or conscious sedation are required, the intravenous route should be used.

TABLE 70-3
Analgesia for Common Pediatric Illnesses

	PRIMARY TREATMENT	SECONDARY TREATMENTS	COMMENTS
Otitis media	Acetaminophen	Ibuprofen Acetaminophen + codeine	No strong evidence for topical treatment
Stomatitis (herpetic, coxsackie)	"Magic mouthwash" (1:1 ratio of diphenhydramine/Maalox™)	Acetaminophen	May add viscous lidocaine in older children, especially those who can spit out the remainder
Pharyngitis	Ibuprofen	Acetaminophen	Efficacy of salt water gargles or anesthetic sprays not formally studied
Burns	Ibuprofen/other NSAIDs (if coagulation is normal)	Opiates for dressing changes Acetaminophen	Allow enough time for peak action of agent prior to procedure
Minor trauma	Ibuprofen	Acetaminophen (± codeine)	RICE (rest, ice, compression, elevation)
Urinary tract infection	Phenazopyridine (100 mg) (contraindicated in patients <6 yrs of age or those with glucose-6-phosphate dehydrogenase deficiency)	Acetaminophen (± codeine)	Child may urinate into warm bath to decrease pain of urethritis

The parenteral opiates most commonly prescribed in the ambulatory setting include morphine, fentanyl, and meperidine. Combinations of opiates and benzodiazepines work well to allay both pain and anxiety. Oral or intranasal administration of sedative/anxiolytics such as midazolam have been shown to reduce the overall distress associated with painful procedures. The dosage is 0.3 to 0.4 mg/kg intranasally and 0.5 mg/kg orally. Continuous monitoring of these patients is imperative, and discharge should be delayed until the patient regains his/her premedication level of awareness.

Thankfully, the intramuscular administration of pain medication has justifiably fallen out of favor and is discouraged by the American Academy of Pediatrics. The most commonly used of these medication was the DPT (also known as MPC, or the "lytic cocktail"), which contains meperidine, promethazine, and chlorpromazine (Demerol®, Phenergan®, Thorazine®). Because children will do almost anything to avoid a needle, many patients would rather hide their pain than receive this medication. Other, more humane forms of analgesia and sedation are available without enlisting the intramuscular route.

Pain Associated With Acute Illness

The common illnesses that present to the pediatric practitioner frequently have pain as a primary or associated symptom. Although arriving at a specific diagnosis and treatment targeted at the cause of the illness is the mainstay of modern medical teaching, it is the removal of symptoms that may interest the patient most. Table 70-3 lists some effective analgesic approaches to the most common pediatric diagnoses.

Chronic Pain

Most acute illnesses that cause pain will resolve within 1 or 2 months of onset of symptoms, and many will resolve within weeks. Chronic pain may be categorized as pain that is of a persistent (greater than 3 months) or recurrent nature, the latter being more common in children. Although the physician's focus may be well aimed at eradicating the source of the child's symptoms, this task is not always clear or simple. It is useful, therefore, for the physician to consider how the pain affects the child's lifestyle and to institute pharmacological and/or psychological therapy early in the course of the evaluation if the pain interferes with the child's daily activities. The degree to which pain deters the child from his/

TABLE 70-4
Functional Categorization of Chronic Pain

ORGANIC PAIN	DYSFUNCTIONAL PAIN	PSYCHOGENIC PAIN
Identifiable tissue injury	No apparent tissue injury	Vague description of pain
Constant pain	Patient aware of physiologic "problem"	Secondary gain
Awakens child from sleep	No underlying disease process	Family psychopathology
Well-localized pain	Interferes with daily life	Personality disorder

her routine activities is a valid measurement of severity of illness. Restricted ability to perform an activity is termed a *disability.* When this disability alters a social role within the child's former lifestyle, it is termed a *handicap.* Sometimes this altered social role may be the first clue to the practitioner that the child is experiencing pain.

As most pediatric practitioners realize, an organic cause of a child's pain may not be obvious during the initial evaluation. In children with vague painful symptoms, an organic etiology may never be discovered. It is wise for the practitioner to invest time and energy into discovering environmental factors that affect painful symptoms or coping mechanisms. A "pain diary" helps to define patterns of symptoms and behavior. These patterns may suggest an organic etiology or, more commonly, clarify appropriate coping skills. This information also empowers the patient and the family to aid in the assessment of the problem. Information about the timing, location, exacerbation, and relief of pain should be part of any pain diary. Activities prior to and after the episode, as well as those missed because of the pain also should be listed. Parents may help their child describe the intensity and quality of pain in terms that are familiar to the child or in comparison to other, more common painful experiences. Other helpful information depends on the location of the pain. For example, the child with chronic abdominal pain should write down the timing and content of meals, as well as his/her stooling patterns. On the other hand, patients with chronic headaches may want to describe phenomena such as associated visual disturbances. The approaches to abdominal pain and headaches are discussed in Chapters 28 and 43.

During the assessment of a child with persistent or recurrent pain, it is important to avoid categorizing the pain as "in the child's head."

This categorization would most likely alienate both the child and the family and hinder the therapeutic relationship that is necessary to manage the patient with chronic pain. Instead, management should focus on creating an accurate and complete definition of the problem, enlisting the methods previously mentioned in this chapter. Detailed information obtained about the pain syndrome, as well as the relative positions of the child and family members on the stage of the pain drama, may aid in its characterization as organic, dysfunctional, or psychogenic pain (Table 70-4). Nonpharmacologic techniques such as visualization, hypnosis, biofeedback, and muscle relaxation have been used with varied success in cases of chronic pain. More invasive methods such as regional nerve blocks, sympathetic nerve blocks, or epidural anesthesia should be performed by pain specialists or anesthesiologists. Frequently, the help of a psychologist or family therapist is required and may be introduced to the child and family as one of many methods of coping with a pain syndrome.

REFERRAL

The primary care physician can successfully apply the pharmacologic techniques described in this chapter in the majority of patients. In cases in which monitoring of cardiopulmonary parameters is not available for patients requiring invasive procedures, referral to an emergency medicine facility is appropriate. The nonpharmacologic management of painful symptoms in children also can be successfully applied in the primary care setting. The practitioner's relationship with the patient and family is most conducive to the assessment and manipulation of environmental factors that impact on the patient's pain. However, referral may be indicated if symptoms persist or are worsening and if they interfere with the child's function at school or at home. Most tertiary care centers are affiliated with a pain management center, which can provide a comprehensive approach to these difficult situations. In addition, community services such as psychologists, family therapists, and physical therapists are frequently available in closer proximity to the patient's home. The primary care physician should coordinate these interventions, remain available to the family, and reassess the patient at regular intervals.

BIBLIOGRAPHY

Anand KJS, Phil D, Carr DB: The neuroanatomy, neurophysiology, and neurochemistry of pain, stress, and analgesia in newborns and children, *Pediatr Clin North Am* 36:795–823, 1989.

Drugs for pain, *Med Let* 35(887):1–6, 1993.

International Association for the Study of Pain, Subcommittee on Taxonomy: Pain terms: A list with definitions and notes on usage, *Pain* 6:1609–1613, 1979.

McGrath PJ: An assessment of children's pain: A review of behavioral, physiological, and direct scaling techniques, *Pain* 31:147–176, 1987.

McGrath PJ, Johnson G, Goodman JT, Schillinger J, Dunn J, Chapman J: The CHEOPS: A behavioral scale to measure postoperative pain in children. In Fields HL, Dubner R, Cervero F, editors: *Advances in pain research and therapy,* New York, 1985, Raven Press.

Schecter NL: *Pain and pain control in children: Current problems in pediatrics,* Chicago, 1985, Year Book Medical Publishers.

Schechter NL, Berde CB, Yaster M, editors: *Pain in infants, children, and adolescents,* Baltimore, 1993, Williams & Wilkins.

Yaster M, Tobin JR, Fisher QA, Maxwell LG: Local anesthetics in the management of acute pain in children, *J Pediatr* 124:165–176, 1994.

CHAPTER 71

The Poisoned Child

James F. Wiley II

Children under 6 years of age accounted for more than half of the 2 million poisonings reported to regional poison centers in 1994. In most instances, pediatric poisonings are unintentional and involve one substance. Factors predisposing to ingestions in this group include pica, behavioral disturbance in the child that makes him/her difficult to supervise, stressful social environment with unintentional neglect (*eg,* new baby in the home, recent move), and willful parental neglect. Children over 6 years of age are more likely to ingest a toxic substance intentionally or to be exposed to drugs through substance abuse. Thus, intoxication in older children and adolescents resembles many of the patterns seen in adults. Poisoning prevention efforts have helped reduce the morbidity and mortality of childhood ingestions through legislation requiring safety enclosures on prescription medication, voluntary industry measures to reduce the toxicity of their products through repackaging, improved education of physicians and patients, and the establishment of regional poison control centers to help manage acute toxic exposures. Nevertheless, management of the poisoned child remains a common pediatric problem for the practitioner. This chapter provides an approach to the poisoned patient with attention to the use of the regional poison control center, principles of gastric decontamination, emergency care of the poisoned child, and definitive care of the poisoned child. In addition, initial management strategies for selected common poisonings are presented.

GENERAL PRINCIPLES

Use of the Regional Poison Control Center

The first step in caring for a poisoned child is to determine the seriousness of the toxic exposure. Regional poison control centers are available to help identify toxic exposures based on clinical findings, distinguish drug ingested based on pill color and identification number, and provide resources for classification of ingested plants or mushrooms based on submitted specimens. Centers are staffed 24 hours a day, 7 days a week, by poison control specialists who have passed stringent training requirements and who give advice based on written protocols with physician backup. Available resources include the Poisindex, a computerized database updated quarterly with more than 1 million poison entries, books and journals dealing with a variety of topics in toxicology, and physician consultants who are boarded in medical toxicology or have specific training. Regional poison centers are accessible by telephone, and many have toll-free numbers.

When calling a poison center, useful information includes the patient's name, age, race, past medical history (if pertinent), time of ingestion or exposure, suspected poison, estimated dosage, and the current status of the patient (if available). When identifying potential toxicity from a specific product, the specialist needs to know the *exact* brand name, the manufacturer, any ingredients listed on the container, and any warnings listed on the container. With this information,

---

BOX 71-1

Agents with Limited or Uncertain Binding to Activated Charcoal

Iron
Lithium
Heavy metals (arsenic, mercury, lead, thallium)
Alcohols (methanol, ethanol, isopropanol, ethylene glycol)
Hydrocarbons (kerosene, gasoline, mineral seal oil)
Caustics (sodium hydroxide, potassium hydroxide, hydrochloride, H_2SO_4)*
Low molecular weight compounds (cyanide)
Pesticides (organophosphates, carbamates)

*Administration of activated charcoal also may impede further management.

the poison center can help identify the poison, determine the seriousness of exposure, and give recommended steps for management, including specific instructions on the use of antidotes. Regional poison centers also provide educational outreach such as recommended readings for educational purposes, poison prevention literature for the public, and poison prevention programs for school children.

Gastric Decontamination

Gastric decontamination refers to the attempted removal of an ingested poison from the stomach or gastrointestinal (GI) tract. Recently, the administration of activated charcoal, which binds many ingested poisons and prevents absorption, or the institution of whole bowel irrigation, which forces the ingested substance through the GI tract before significant absorption can occur has become the preferred method of decontamination. Gastric lavage and syrup of ipecac play a much lesser role in the emergent management of the poisoned child but may still be of benefit in selected patients, particularly as a method of decontamination at home when indicated.

Activated charcoal is a steam-treated carbonaceous material, which has a large surface area for binding ingested poisons. The optimal ratio for binding occurs with 10 g of activated charcoal for 1 g of ingestant. Efficacy approaches 60% binding of poison when activated charcoal is given 30 to 60 minutes after ingestion. Activated charcoal is of limited usefulness following large overdoses in which a 10:1 binding ratio cannot be achieved or after ingestion of small molecular weight poisons (Box 71-1).

Activated charcoal is indicated for any potentially toxic ingestion unless specifically contraindicated. Activated charcoal should not be used in patients who have an unprotected airway (aspiration risk), GI bleeding, GI perforation, caustic ingestions (impedes endoscopic visualization), or aliphatic hydrocarbon ingestion (may promote vomiting and aspiration). The dose is 1 g/kg, up to 100 g total, of activated charcoal alone or premixed with 1 g/kg of 35% sorbitol. Mixing the charcoal with flavored syrups and putting it in a covered cup with a straw facilitates oral administration. Nasogastric intubation and charcoal administration is required in patients with altered mental status and in alert, uncooperative patients. Complications of activated charcoal use include vomiting, pulmonary aspiration, obstipation/constipation, and desorption of poison from charcoal with the potential for late toxicity if delayed GI motility exists following ingestion (eg, drugs with anticholinergic properties).

Whole bowel irrigation involves the copious irrigation of the GI tract via nasogastric tube to force the poisons rapidly through the tract prior to significant absorption, using polyethylene glycol 3500 MW isoosmotic bowel solution (Golytely®). This solution causes no net fluid or electrolyte loss in the gut. Indications, to date, have been limited to agents that do not adsorb well to charcoal or have potential for absorption distally in the GI tract, such as iron, heavy metals, lithium, sustained release products (many antiarrhythmics, theophylline), and "body packers" (people who ingest large numbers of packets of cocaine or heroin wrapped in latex condoms). Other drugs may be amenable to whole bowel irrigation as an adjunct to activated charcoal administration. Contraindications include ileus or bowel perforation. Whole bowel irrigation is administered in a dose of 500 mL/hr in young children up to a maximum of 2 L/hr in adolescents and adults, usually via nasogastric tube. The endpoint for stopping whole bowel irrigation consists of a clear rectal effluent and evidence of decreasing or absent poisoning signs and symptoms. Vomiting and abdominal pain are the major complications reported from this procedure.

Gastric lavage removes 10% to 25% of ingested toxin when performed within 30 to 60 minutes of ingestion. It has been shown to improve outcome in patients who are comatose and receive gastric lavage within 60 minutes. In other patients, the potential risks of gastric lavage must be weighed heavily against its benefit. This procedure should be reserved for the critically ill poison patient or a patient who is likely to undergo rapid decompensation. In addition, patients who ingest large amounts of a strong acid, such as toilet bowl cleaner, should receive gastric lavage with a small flexible nasogastric tube. Patients who ingest liquid medicines may benefit from lavage if it is performed within 30 to 60 minutes. Gastric lavage should not be performed in patients with airway compromise prior to endotracheal intubation. Other contraindications include caustic ingestions, hydrocarbon ingestions, and patients with abnormal esophageal anatomy or bleeding diatheses. Gastric lavage may not be useful more than 1 hour after ingestion unless the ingested poison delays gastric emptying. Gastric lavage requires the placement of a large bore (24 to 36 French) orogastric tube followed by repeated infusion and withdrawal of room-temperature normal saline in 50- to 200-mL aliquots. Prior to lavage, one must ensure a protected airway, position the patient on the left side with the head below the feet, and determine correct gastric tube position. Complications include vomiting with pulmonary aspiration, gastric or esophageal perforation, hypopharyngeal and airway trauma with bleeding, laryngospasm, and accidental tracheal intubation with inadvertent pulmonary lavage.

Syrup of ipecac comes from the Ipecuana plant. It causes vomiting by direct gastric irritation and through a direct central effect at the chemotactic trigger zone in the medulla. Up to 93% of patients who receive ipecac vomit within 30 to 60 minutes. Indications for syrup of ipecac administration are now limited to ingestion of toxic plant material and to home decontamination on the advice of a physician or poison control specialist. Contraindications consist of altered mental status (lethargy, coma, convulsions either existing or impending), caustic ingestions, aliphatic hydrocarbon ingestion, and ingestion of drugs with a high likelihood of rapid serious effects, such as cyclic antidepressants, antidysrhythmics, clonidine, isoniazid, lithium, and alcohols. In addition, patients who have already spontaneously vomited will not receive any further benefit from syrup of ipecac administration. The dose varies by age as follows: for children 6 months to 1 year of age, 10 mL (2 tsp); 1 to 12 years of age, 15 mL (1 tbs); and greater than

12 years of age, 30 mL (2 tbs). Syrup of ipecac is followed by 10 mL/kg of water, up to 8 oz. The dose should be repeated if no vomiting occurs within 30 minutes. Complications consist of excessive vomiting, Mallory-Weiss tear of the esophagus, pneumomediastinum, and delayed delivery of activated charcoal. Chronic use of syrup of ipecac or inadvertent administration of the much more concentrated *extract* of ipecac has caused myocardial and neuromuscular toxicity.

Cathartics have no demonstrated efficacy in poisoning treatment, but they are frequently recommended to hasten the passage of activated charcoal. Multiple doses of cathartics should be avoided except as outlined under elimination enhancement with multiple dose activated charcoal. Sorbitol is preferred because it has a more rapid onset of catharsis. Patients with bowel perforation, ileus, or diarrhea should not receive cathartics. Sorbitol is given in a concentration of 35% and a dose of 1 g/kg (3 cc/kg). Complications include electrolyte imbalance and dehydration with death reported in infants who received four to 6 doses of sorbitol over 24 hours.

Emergency Care of the Poisoned Child

Stabilization of the poisoned child should proceed with the same general approach as any critically ill patient. Airway, breathing, circulation, and disability must be assessed in order, and compromise in any of these areas requires prompt attention. Exposure of the patient accompanies the rapid assessment. Vital signs, including a rectal temperature, should be performed, and continuous monitoring of heart rate, respiratory rate, and blood pressure should ensue.

Issues specific to the poisoned patient during this period of care comprise emergency administration of substrates and antidotes, gastric and external decontamination of the patient, presumptive diagnosis based on the clinical presentation, bedside tests, and institution of supportive and expectant care.

Any potentially poisoned child with a depressed level of responsiveness requires a rapid reagent strip determination of glucose and consideration of naloxone administration. Hypoglycemia suggests exposure to ethanol, oral hypoglycemic agents, salicylates, or propranolol and requires correction with 0.5 to 1 g/kg intravenous (IV) dextrose bolus followed by a 6 to 8 mg/kg/min dextrose infusion. Thiamine, 100 mg intramuscularly (IM) or IV, should proceed dextrose infusion in a patient who is suspected to be alcoholic.

Naloxone, 2 mg IV, IM, or via endotracheal tube, will reverse coma caused by opiates. It also may help some patients who have ingested clonidine. It has few adverse effects and may prevent the need for aggressive intervention, such as endotracheal intubation. Children who have ingested codeine, dextromethorphan, propoxyphene, pentazocine, butorphanol, diphenoxylate, or methadone may require up to 10 mg of naloxone to fully reverse the narcotic effects. Response to naloxone occurs within 1 to 2 minutes of administration. By 30 minutes, naloxone has worn off, and resedation may appear. Repeated naloxone administration or continuous intravenous naloxone infusion is often required to prevent further depressed mental status.

Flumazenil is a benzodiazepine antagonist, which has reversed lethargy and coma in adult benzodiazepine overdose patients. Flumazenil may cause seizures in patients who have coingested cyclic antidepressants or in patients with a seizure disorder controlled by benzodiazepines and may cause cardiac dysrhythmias in poisoned patients who have coingested chloral hydrate. Other side effects include vomiting and anxiety. Flumazenil administration may help differentiate benzodiazepine overdose from other causes of coma in children. Given its potential risks, flumazenil only should be given to children with severe symptoms of benzodiazepine ingestion and only if no signs of significant cyclic antidepressant overdose are present. The currently recommended dose is 0.01 mg/kg over 1 minute up to 0.5 mg and a total maximum dose of 1 mg. Response occurs within 1 minute in most cases, and resedation may occur 2 hours after administration.

Physostigmine, a cholinesterase inhibitor, is indicated for severe central anticholinergic effects, such as severe agitation with hyperthermia or seizures caused by antihistamines (*eg*, diphenhydramine, doxylamine, scopolamine), certain plants (jimson weed, deadly nightshade, henbane), anti-Parkinson medications, dilating eye drops, and skeletal muscle relaxants. Physostigmine administration has preceded asystole and death in patients who ingested cyclic antidepressants and should be avoided in these patients as well as in patients with asthma, GI obstruction, or genitourinary obstruction. The dose of physostigmine for children is 0.5 to 1 mg IV, given

TABLE 71-1
Common Toxidromes in Children*

AGENT	VITAL SIGNS	CENTRAL NERVOUS SYSTEM	PUPILS	SKIN	ODOR	OTHER
			TOXIDROME			
Narcotics	Hypothermia, brady-pnea, bradycardia, hypotension	Flaccid coma	Miotic to pinpoint	—	—	Extraocular paralysis, delayed GI motility
Sedatives	Hypothermia, brady-pnea, bradycardia, hypotension	Coma, often prolonged or cyclical, nystagmus	Miotic (early barbiturate), dilated (late barbiturate, glutethimide)	—	—	Delayed GI motility
Ethanol	Hypothermia, brady-pnea, bradycardia	Coma, nystagmus	Miotic	Flushed	Sickly sweet breath odor	Hypoglycemia, in-creased osmolal gap
Anticholinergic agents	Hyperthermia, tachy-cardia, hypertension	Agitation, delirium, seizures	Dilated	Flushed, dry, warm	—	Decreased GI motility, urinary retention, cardiac tachydys-rhythmias
Sympathomimetic agents	Hyperthermia, tachy-cardia, hypertension (bradycardia if pure α adrenergic)	Agitation, delirium, seizures	Dilated	Diaphoretic, cool and clammy	—	Increased GI motility, piloerection
Cholinergic agents	Bradycardia or tachy-cardia, hypotension, tachypnea with bronchospasm	Coma, seizures	Miotic	Diaphoretic	—	Muscle fasciculation, weakness, paralysis, salivation, lacrima-tion, vomiting, uri-nary and fecal incon-tinence

Adapted from Henretig FM, Shannon M: Toxicologic emergencies. In *Textbook of pediatric medicine*, ed 3, Baltimore, 1993, Williams & Wilkins; and Mofenson HC, Greensher J: *Pediatrics* 54:336, 1974.
*Toxidromes represent a collection of clinical findings often associated with poisoning by a specific class of drugs. However, a poisoned child may not display all physical findings commonly associated with a specific drug, or the child may have findings not usually associated with a specific drug. Toxidromes alone cannot be used to exclude or confirm ingestion of a particular drug.
GI—gastrointestinal.

slowly over 5 minutes, with atropine immediately available for administration should cholinergic symptoms develop. Response to physostigmine occurs within minutes, and beneficial effects may persist longer than expected based on physostigmine's half-life of 60 minutes.

Pyridoxine, vitamin B$_6$, stops seizures due to ingestion of isoniazid by reversing gamma-aminobutyric acid depletion. The dose is 3 to 5 g or the equivalent dose of isoniazid ingested, in grams. This dose is much larger than the therapeutic dose and requires the administration of multiple vials of pyridoxine.

Gastric decontamination should only be performed after stabilization of the patient has been accomplished as previously discussed. External decontamination of the patient requires removal of any clothing and copious irrigation of the skin and eyes with room-temperature normal saline. Certain toxins such as organophosphate pesticides can diffuse through the skin and poison health care providers unless appropriate precautions are taken to avoid contact—usually gowns, gloves, and masks are sufficient. Radioactive toxins and severely toxic chemicals require special hazardous materials handling but are rarely seen in pediatric overdoses. Care should be taken to monitor a child undergoing external irrigation so that hypothermia does not occur.

Presumptive diagnosis of the type of agent causing poison symptoms can guide further treatment until a definitive diagnosis is made. Many times the exact toxin is known from the outset by the patient's history. However, with very ill children, the first history is often not the best, and the practitioner must look for specific clues on physical examination. Combinations of physical findings, or toxidromes, indicate specific classes of drugs with effects on vital signs, pupillary response, neurologic status, breath and body odors, and skin changes (Table 71-1 and Box 71-2).

Bedside tests give further information as to the poison ingested but require definitive laboratory studies for confirmation. As previously mentioned, the rapid glucose reagent stick detects hypoglycemia and suggests a limited list of potential toxins if present. Two to three drops of ferric chloride 10% turns 1 mL of urine purple in the presence of salicylates. Positive results require a quantitative serum level. The nitroprusside reaction (ketone square on the urine dipstick) turns purple in the presence of acetoacetic acid. Urinary ketones are commonly seen after

---

BOX 71-2
Common Causes of Toxidromes in Children

Narcotics
  Cough syrups (dextromethorphan)
  Codeine
  Propoxyphene (Darvon®)
  Methadone (child of a heroin addict)
Sedatives
  Benzodiazepines
  Barbiturates
Anticholinergic agents
  Antihistamines
  Antidepressant drugs*
  Antipsychotic drugs*
  Plants (jimson weed, *Amanita muscaria* mushrooms, henbane, *Atropa belladonna*)
  Skeletal muscle relaxants (cyclobenzaprine)
Sympathomimetic agents
  Decongestants (pure α-adrenergic drugs)
  Cocaine
  Amphetamines
Cholinergic agents
  Pesticides (organophosphate, carbamate)
  Mushrooms

*Significant potential for cardiotoxicity.

---

ingestion of salicylates and isopropanol. A chocolate brown or persistent dark color of venous blood that is exposed to air on a piece of filter paper suggests methemoglobinemia.

Institution of supportive care is the most important aspect of managing the poisoned patient. The patient's clinical course is altered by administration of specific antidotes in only 3% of toxic exposures. Good outcome for the remainder of patients depends on adherence to general principles in toxicology and good general medical care.

Definitive Care of the Poisoned Patient

Definitive care encompasses definitive evaluation, diagnosis, and management. Specific components essential to ongoing care of the poisoned patient include a comprehensive history, physical examination, laboratory evaluation with appropriate diagnostic studies, and consideration of the benefit of and indications for elimination enhancement and antidote administration.

The following historical information is essential: the ingestant(s) or list of possible ingestants, estimated poison dose, time of toxic exposure, preceding events and details of poisoning, recent trauma, and recent fever or illness. Past medical history should be explored with attention to presence of seizure disorder, respiratory illness such as asthma, and cardiac disease. Social

---

BOX 71-3
Initial Laboratory and Diagnostic Studies of Use in the Poisoned Child

Arterial blood gas
Cooximetry
Serum
    Electrolytes
    Blood urea nitrogen
    Creatinine
    Glucose
    Osmolarity (freezing point depression method)
Urine
    Dipstick
    Microscopic evaluation
12-Lead electrocardiogram
Abdominal radiograph (if ingestion of radiopaque
    toxin suspected)
Abdominal ultrasound (to evaluate for presence of
    gastric pills)

BOX 71-4
Poisons Causing an Abnormal Anion Gap*

Increased anion gap with metabolic acidosis
    Carbon monoxide[†‡]
    Cyanide[‡]
    Ethanol[†]
    Ethylene glycol[†]
    Iron[†‡]
    Isoniazid[‡]
    Methanol[†]
    Salicylates[†]
    Theophylline[†]
Decreased anion gap
    Bromide
    Lithium[†]
    Hypermagnesiumia[†]
    Hypercalcemia[†]

---

*Partial list of representative poisons.
[†]Specific levels rapidly available.
[‡]Antidote available.

---

history should be reviewed with emphasis on current stress in the household and previous injuries including previous history of poisoning suggestive of possible neglect. All available sources of history should be used such as parents, other caretakers, friends, and paramedics.

History and physical examination provide the diagnosis in one third or more of pediatric poisonings. The physical examination can provide valuable clues to the possible ingestant even when the patient does not display all components of a toxidrome. Drugs that commonly cause coma and respiratory depression in children include barbiturates, clonidine, cyclic antidepressants, ethanol, narcotics, carbon monoxide, and atropine/diphenoxylate (Lomotil). Tachycardia with hypotension may be caused by β_2-adrenergic agonists, iron, phenothiazines, or theophylline. Tachycardia with hypertension suggest amphetamines, antihistamines, cocaine, LSD, or phencyclidine (PCP). Bradycardia with atrioventricular block occurs after ingestions of β-blockers, calcium channel blockers, and digoxin. Ventricular dysrhythmias are seen following poisoning with cyclic antidepressants, chlorinated hydrocarbons, astemizole, terfenadine, and many antidysrhythmic agents. Seizures develop after ingestion of amphetamines, cocaine, cyclic antidepressants, antihistamines, camphor, isoniazid, and theophylline.

Laboratory evaluation in patients with suspected poisoning should progress from less specific to more specific testing with emphasis on clearly identifying the presence of toxins that require antidotes or other specific management procedures to prevent morbidity or mortality. Box 71-3 lists laboratory and diagnostic studies that may be helpful in the poisoned child.

Arterial blood gases determine the presence of hypoxemia, hypercapnia, or metabolic acidosis, which often accompanies serious poisoning. The anion gap is calculated using the following equation:

$$\text{Anion gap} = \text{Na} - (\text{Cl} + \text{CO}_2)$$

A normal anion gap varies from 12 to 16 meq/L and reflects the electrostatic balance of unmeasured cations and unmeasured anions. Abnormalities in the anion gap suggest certain poisons, many of which require specific serum levels to determine toxicity and treatment (Box 71-4).

The osmolar gap is calculated by taking the difference between measured osmolarity, determined by freezing point depression and calculated osmolarity based on electrolyte measurements as follows:

$$\text{Osmolar gap} = \text{Measured osmolarity}$$
$$\text{(freezing point depression)} -$$
$$[(2 \times \text{Na}) + \text{BUN}/2.8 + \text{glucose}/18]$$

The normal osmolar gap is less than 10 mOsm. An elevated osmolar gap suggests the presence of ethanol, isopropanol, methanol, ethylene glycol, mannitol, or acetone. A normal osmolar gap does

TABLE 71-2
Helpful Specific Drug Levels

DRUG	TIME TO PEAK BLOOD LEVEL (HOURS POSTINGESTION)	POTENTIAL INTERVENTION
Acetaminophen	4	N-Acetylcysteine administration
Carbamazepine	2–4*	Predictive of toxicity and clinical course
Carboxyhemoglobin	Immediately	Hyperbaric oxygen therapy
Digoxin	2–4	Fab (digoxin antibody) fragment
Ethanol	0.5–1	Predictive of toxicity and clinical course
Ethylene glycol	0.5–1	Ethanol infusion and hemodialysis
Iron	2–4	Deferoxamine administration
Isopropanol	0.5–1	Predictive of toxicity and clinical course
Lead	5 weeks*	Chelation and environmental abatement
Lithium	2–4	Hemodialysis
Methanol	0.5–1	Ethanol infusion and hemodialysis
Methemoglobinemia	Immediately	Methylene blue administration
Phenobarbital	2–4	Alkaline diuresis, multiple-dose activated charcoal
Phenytoin	1–2*	Multiple-dose activated charcoal
Salicylates	6–12*	Alkaline diuresis, multiple-dose activated charcoal, hemodialysis
Theophylline	1–36*	Multiple-dose activated charcoal, whole bowel irrigation, charcoal hemoperfusion, hemodialysis

*Repeated levels necessary due to significant variation in time to peak level.
Adapted from Weisman RS, Howland MA, Flomenbaum NE: The toxicology laboratory. In Goldfrank LR, Flomenbaum N, Lewin LN, Weisman RS, editors: *Toxicologic emergencies*, ed 4, Norwalk, 1990, Appleton & Lange.

not rule out the potential for a serious ethylene glycol poisoning. Cooximetry is the direct measurement of oxygen saturation. A discrepancy between cooximetry and pulse oximetry or between oxygen saturation by cooximetry and calculated oxygen saturation (what one typically gets on an arterial blood gas sample) suggests the presence of abnormal hemoglobins; most commonly, carboxyhemoglobin, methemoglobin, or sulfhemoglobin.

Specific drug levels are helpful for management when the poison shows a dose-dependent toxicity or has an antidote or when a specific intervention such as extracorporeal removal is helpful. Table 71-2 lists many of the important quantitative tests for the poisoned child.

The Comprehensive Drug Screen, or "tox screen," has limited usefulness in the management of the poisoned child. In most cases of pediatric poisoning, the potential poison can be elicited by history, physical examination, and a combination of the laboratory studies previously discussed. Results of comprehensive drug screens typically take 6 to 24 hours and rarely change immediate management of the patient. False-positive and false-negative drug screens can lead to misinterpretation of the patient's signs and symptoms. Toxicologic screening may be warranted to confirm the diagnosis of poisoning as opposed to other conditions such as central nervous system infection or trauma or to investigate for intentional ingestion or child abuse. However, evaluation for other clinical problems besides poisoning should not be delayed while awaiting drug screen results. When interpreting drug screen results, the practitioner must remember that some hospitals and laboratories vary in the number of drugs tested from as few as 3 to more than 60. Also, many common ingestants are not detected on the comprehensive drug screen (Box 71-5).

Certain diagnostic studies may be very useful in evaluating the poisoned child (Box 71-3). A 12-lead electrocardiogram with attention to rhythm, QRS interval, and QT interval can provide presumptive evidence of serious toxicity and predict potential morbidity. Atrioventricular blocks suggest ingestion of specific drugs, such as β-blockers, calcium channel blockers, and digoxin. Widening of the QRS interval to ≥0.10 msec indicates an increased risk of ventricular tachycardia; prolongation of the QT interval as indicated by a prolonged corrected QT interval (QT [msec]/$\sqrt{RR}$ [msec]) predicts an increased risk of torsades de pointes due to drugs such as cyclic antidepressants, lithium, astemizole, terfenadine, quinidine, and sotalol.

An abdominal radiograph will detect the presence of some toxic agents, such as iron, calcium salts, potassium salts, heavy metals, and chlorinated hydrocarbons. The absence of radiopaque pills or fragments does not rule out the possibility of ingestion if the film is taken after the substance has been absorbed. Ultrasound of the stomach can detect the presence of some types of pills and could be helpful in deciding the usefulness of gastric emptying in selected patients. However, ultrasound currently is not available in many hospitals on an emergency basis for this indication.

Once a specific toxin is identified as present, the next step is to evaluate the potential for enhancing drug removal. Elimination enhancement refers to a group of procedures that can increase the extracorporeal clearance of toxin: multiple-dose activated charcoal, whole bowel irrigation, alkaline diuresis, hemodialysis, charcoal hemoperfusion, and exchange transfusion.

Multiple doses of activated charcoal can increase clearance of theophylline, carbamazepine, phenytoin, phenobarbital, and acetaminophen. With these drugs, there is support for enteroenteric dialysis, which means the movement of toxin from the microvillous blood vessels into the gut lumen, where it is bound to the activated charcoal and subsequently passed out of the body. Multiple-dose activated charcoal also may decrease toxicity in patients who ingest drugs with enterohepatic circulation of active metabolites (*eg*, some cyclic antidepressants).

The dose of activated charcoal is 1 g/kg with cathartic as an initial dose followed by 0.5 to 1 g/kg of activated charcoal without cathartic every 4 hours. Cathartic may be repeated every 12 hours as needed. Contraindications to multiple-dose activated charcoal include ileus, bowel perforation, or compromised airway. The end points for this therapy are nontoxic blood levels, clinical improvement, and the passage of charcoal-laden stool.

Alkaline diuresis refers to the administration of sodium bicarbonate in order to raise the urine pH to 8.0. This procedure converts renally excreted toxins, which are weak acids, to their ionized form within the proximal renal tubules and thereby prevents reabsorption in the distal tubules (ion trapping). This technique is most useful for enhancing the excretion of salicylates and phenobarbital (but not other barbiturates). The dose of sodium bicarbonate necessary to achieve this change in urine pH is 1 to 2 meq/kg given over 3 to 4 hours. Urine alkalinization cannot occur in the presence of hypokalemia due to the potassium-sparing effect of aldosterone with subsequent hydrogen ion excretion. Any potassium deficits must be corrected. Urinary alkalinization has caused pulmonary and cerebral edema, especially when combined with forced diuresis (large volume fluid infusions with diuretic administration). For this reason, severe salicylate poisoning should be managed with hemodialysis rather than urinary alkalinization. Electrolyte and acid-base disturbances can result from sodium bicarbonate administration and require frequent (every 4 to 6 hours) monitoring of blood pH and serum sodium, potassium, calcium, and magnesium.

Forced diuresis and urinary acidification are no longer recommended for elimination enhancement because risks of these procedures (pulmonary and cerebral edema with forced diuresis and rhabdomyolysis with myoglobinuria from urinary acidification) outweigh the benefits.

Hemodialysis can remove toxins with low molecular weight (<200 daltons), low plasma protein binding, and low tissue binding. Tissue binding often is determined by the volume of distribution. The volume of distribution (Vd) for a drug is calculated as follows:

$$Vd \ (L/kg) = Dose \ absorbed \ (mg/kg)/Plasma \ concentration \ (mg/L)$$

TABLE 71-3
Toxins Removed by Hemodialysis

TOXIN	MEASURED LEVEL SUGGESTIVE OF NEED FOR HEMODIALYSIS*
Acetaminophen	>1000 µg/mL in conjunction with antidote
Arsenic	Only with coexistent renal failure
Bromide	>150 mg/dL and severe symptoms
Chloral hydrate	250 mg/L
Ethanol	500 mg/dL
Ethylene glycol	50 mg/dL
Isopropanol	400 mg/dL
Lithium	4 meq/L in acute overdose as needed for severe symptoms in chronic overdose
Methanol	50 mg/dL
Salicylates	100–120 mg/dL in acute overdose 60–80 mg/dL in chronic overdose

*The decision to perform hemodialysis should be based on physical findings as well as drug levels. Always repeat an elevated level and check units of measurement prior to instituting hemodialysis.

TABLE 71-4
Toxins Removed by Charcoal Hemoperfusion*

TOXIN MEASURED	LEVEL SUGGESTIVE OF NEED FOR CHARCOAL HEMOPERFUSION
Amitriptyline	Based on signs and symptoms
Chloral hydrate	250 mg/dL
Digitoxin	50 ng/mL with antidotal therapy
Digoxin	15 ng/mL with antidotal therapy
Ethchlorvinyl	150 µg/mL
Glutethimide	40 mg/L
Methaqualone	40 µg/mL
Nortriptyline	Based on signs and symptoms
Pentobarbital	50 mg/L
Phenobarbital	100 mg/L
Theophylline	100 µg/mL in acute overdose 60 µg/mL in chronic overdose

*The decision to perform hemoperfusion should be based on physical findings as well as drug levels. Always repeat an elevated level and check units of measurement prior to instituting hemoperfusion.

Hemodialysis is most effective for drugs with a volume of distribution less than 1 L/kg. Toxins that are removed by hemodialysis are listed in Table 71-3. Charcoal hemoperfusion requires diversion of the patient's circulation through a filter in which the toxin is bound to an activated charcoal cartridge. This procedure may allow binding of drugs that are not easily dialyzable because drug removal is less influenced by toxin size and protein binding. Charcoal hemoperfusion is technically more difficult and less available than hemodialysis. Drugs potentially removed by charcoal hemoperfusion are listed in Table 71-4. Less than 1% of pediatric ingestions require extracorporeal methods of elimination enhancement.

Exchange transfusion seeks to replace a significant portion of the blood volume by simultaneous transfusion and removal of red blood cells. In general, blood volume is estimated, and an exchange of two blood volumes is performed to exchange approximately 85% of the blood. Exchange transfusion is indicated for severe methemoglobinemia not responsive to methylene blue or severe carbon monoxide poisoning when hyperbaric oxygen therapy is not available. This modality may be of particular benefit in cases of toxic exposure in neonates and young infants. Exchange transfusion carries the same risk as any high volume blood transfusion including anticoagulation with bleeding, thrombocytopenia, hypocalcemia, hypothermia, and transfusion reaction.

Antidotes help in approximately 3% of poisonings. The most commonly used antidotes and their doses are listed in Table 71-5. It is advisable to involve a medical toxicologist and a regional poison control center prior to administration of antidotes, especially the practitioner if unfamiliar with their use.

Table 71-6 provides the initial management of many commonly ingested agents. The reader is referred to the references for detailed discussion of specific toxins.

SUMMARY

Poisoning remains a common cause of injury in children. All pediatric practitioners should be familiar with the use of the regional poison control center and initial management of common pediatric ingestions. Emergency care of the potentially poisoned child requires stabilization

TABLE 71-5
Common Poisons and Antidotes

POISON	ANTIDOTE
Acetaminophen	N-Acetylcysteine: Loading dose 140 mg/kg, then 17 doses every 4 hrs at 70 mg/kg/dose. Dilute 20% solution to 5%–10% with juice or soda to improve palatability.
Anticholinergics	Physostigmine (*see* Emergency Care of the Poisoned Patient).
Benzodiazepines	Flumazenil (*see* Emergency Care of the Poisoned Patient).
β-Adrenergic antagonists	Glucagon bolus with 50–100 µg/kg, then infuse at 70 µg/kg/hr in 5% dextrose in water. Do not use phenol diluent.
Calcium channel blockers	Glucagon, as above, calcium gluconate 10%, 0.3–0.6 mL/kg (8–16 meq calcium/kg).
Carbon monoxide	Hyperbaric oxygen, consider sodium thiosulfate 25%, for possible concomitant cyanide inhalation if patient suffers from smoke inhalation (*see* below).
Cyanide	Sodium nitrate 3%: dose depends on hemoglobin (*see* cyanide antidote kit package insert). Do not exceed recommended dosage. Do not give to patients suffering from concomitant carbon monoxide exposure. Sodium thiosulfate 25%: dose depends on hemoglobin (*see* cyanide antidote kit package insert).
Digitalis	Digitalis Fab fragments, calculate based on level or dose ingested or 10 vials if acute overdose, 5 vials if chronic overdose.
Ethylene glycol/methanol	Ethanol, 0.6 gm/kg load over 1 hour followed by 100 mg/kg/hr infusion. Pyridoxine and thiamine for ethylene glycol. Folate for methanol. 4-methylpyrazole (investigational).
Iron	Deferoxamine 5–15 mg/kg/hr IV infusion.
Isoniazid	Pyridoxine (*see* Emergency Care of the Poisoned Patient).
Lead	Dependent on level. Lead level 45–69 µg/dL: Dimercaptosuccinic acid 10 mg/kg orally three times a day for 5 days then twice a day for 14 days (may be useful at lower levels) or calcium NaEDTA 50–75 mg/kg/day divided every 6 hrs either IM or slow IV infusion (IV use not FDA approved) Lead level ≥70: Calcium NaEDTA as above and British AntiLewisite (BAL) 3–5 mg/kg IM every 4 hrs for 5 days.
Methemoglobinemia	Methylene blue 1%, 1–2 mg/kg (0.1–0.2 mL/kg).
Narcotics	Naloxone (*see* Emergency Care of the Poisoned Patient).
Organophosphates	Atropine 0.1–0.5 mg/kg initial dose with additional doses as needed to counteract bronchorrhea Pralidoxime 25–50 mg/kg (up to 1 g), for severe cases consider 10–15 mg/kg/hr infusion.
Phenothiazines (dystonia)	Diphenhydramine 1–2 mg/kg IM or IV Benztropine 1–2 mg/kg IM or IV

IM—intramuscularly; IV—intravenously; PO—orally.

TABLE 71-6
Management Guidelines

The following guidelines are designed for children 1 to 5 years of age who are asymptomatic at time of evaluation or phone call and were poisoned within the past 30 minutes. Maximal possible doses less than the amount requiring ipecac do not need treatment. Assume one swallow is approximately 5 mL or 1 tsp.

SUBSTANCE	AMOUNT REQUIRING HOME IPECAC ADMINISTRATION	EMERGENT EVALUATION
Acetaminophen	≥100–140 mg/kg	>140 mg/kg
Antihistamines	≥1–2 times daily dose	>2 times daily dose
Salicylates	≥150–300 mg/kg	>300 mg/kg or any amount of oil of wintergreen: 1 mL = (100%) = 1.4 g salicylate
Azalea	>Three leaves or flowers or nectar of four flowers, evaluate all ingestions of this magnitude	
Camphor	*Never*	>500 mg
Cationic		
Detergents	*Never* if <20% observe	>20% treat as caustic
Clonidine	*Never*	Evaluate all
Codeine	≥1–3 mg/kg	>3 mg/kg
Cyclic antidepressants	*Never*	Evaluate all
Dextromethorphan	≥10–90 mg/kg	≥90 mg/kg
Digoxin	≥50–100 µg/kg	>100 µg/kg
Ethanol	Evaluate if ≥1 mL/kg of 100% ethanol ingested (2.5 mL/kg of liquor/mouthwash, 10 cc/kg of wine, 20 cc/kg of beer)	
Fluoride	≥5–10 mg/kg	>10 mg/kg
Ibuprofen	≥100–200 mg/kg	>200 mg/kg
Iron (elemental)*	≥20–40 mg/kg	>40 mg/kg
Isopropyl alcohol	Evaluate if ≥0.7 mL/kg of 70% rubbing alcohol (approximately two swallows or 10 mL in a 10-kg child)	
Lomotil	*Never*	Evaluate all
Mothballs[†] Naphthalene, or unknown	One bite or half a mothball	>half a mothball or G6PD deficiency
Paradichlorobenzene	≥Three mothballs	Usually not necessary
Mushrooms	One bite	Ask parents to bring a full-sized mushroom for identification
Nicotine	≥One cigarette or ≥three cigarette butts or ≥one cigar butt or ≥8 g chewing tobacco	≥two cigarettes or ≥six cigarette butts or ≥one cigar or two cigar butts or ≥16 g chewing tobacco
Phenylpropanolamine	≥50 mg if regular preparation ≥7 mg/kg if sustained release	
Pseudoephedrine	≥60 mg	
Rodenticide[‡]	≥15–25 mg	>25 mg
Sulfonylurea	*Never*	Evaluate all
L-Thyroxine	≥500–3000 µg	≥3000 µg

*Ferrous sulfate = 20% elemental iron, ferrous fumarate = 33% elemental iron, ferrous gluconate = 12% elemental iron.

†Naphthalene floats in saturated solution of table salt, paradichlorobenzene sinks.

‡Convert to warfarin equivalents: D-Con 0.025% contains 1.25 mg warfarin/5 mL, Talon 0.005% contains 10 mg warfarin equivalents (brodifacoum).

with initial gastric decontamination and administration of substrates and antidotes as indicated; rapid diagnosis of poisoning and toxic agent based on history, physical examination, and ancillary studies; and appropriate management dictated by the identified poison. In the majority of toxic exposures, good supportive care will suffice. In the minority of cases in which elimination enhancement or antidote administration is needed, consultation with a medical toxicologist or regional poison control center is advised for optimal patient care.

BIBLIOGRAPHY

Ellenhorn MJ, Barceloux DG: *Medical toxicology: Diagnosis and treatment of human poisoning.* New York, 1988, Elsevier Science Publishing.

Goldfrank LR, Flomenbaum NE, Lewin NA, Weisman RS, Howland MA: *Goldfrank's toxicologic emergencies,* ed 4, Norwalk, 1990, Appleton & Lange.

Haddad LM, Winchester JF: *Clinical management of poisoning and drug overdose,* ed 2, Philadelphia, 1990, WB Saunders.

Henretig FM, Shannon M: Toxicologic emergencies. In Fleisher GL, Ludwig S, editors: *Textbook of pediatric emergency medicine,* ed 3, Baltimore, 1993, Williams & Wilkins.

Kulig K: Initial management of ingestions of toxic substances, *N Engl J Med* 326:1677–1681, 1992.

Olson KR, Pentel PR, Kelley MT. Physical assessment and differential diagnosis of the poisoned patient, *Med Toxicol* 2:52–81, 1987.

Wiley JF: Drug-related coma in the adolescent, *Adolesc Med State Art Rev* 4:149–166, 1993.

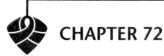

CHAPTER 72

Patient Transport and Primary Care

George A. Woodward

The appearance of a critically ill child in an office setting requires a preconceived plan of action for optimal patient care. Initial intervention and transfer of the patient to a more appropriate facility is required. Anticipation and careful planning can help these situations be managed in the most expedient and beneficial manner for everyone all involved.

Care of a seriously ill child who presents to the office requires appropriate staff and equipment for emergent care or alternative management plans for immediate transfer. It is important for the physician to review procedures, skills, and plans for acute intervention with the office staff on a routine basis because they will most likely not have frequent opportunities to manage acutely ill children. If the office environment is unable to offer advanced life support equipment or skills, plans should be in place for immediate notification of the emergency medical system

(EMS) to transport the patient to the closest facility that can manage and stabilize the patient. Even when initial care capability is excellent, the recognition of need for advanced care and pediatric expertise often will lead to a decision to transfer a child from the office or emergency department to a more appropriate facility. This chapter will serve to review the process involved in deciding to transport a child and will discuss factors that can help lead to improved outcomes.

Identifying the patient who needs transport is not always easy. The job of the primary care physician is to identify those patients who need a different type or level of care than the physician, support staff, or facility can provide. Identification of these types of patients will vary depending on the skill, equipment, and location of the caretakers. For example, the child with a closed head injury might be cared for at a pediatric trauma center, if available, but if the nearest trauma center is 400 miles away, a different approach will need to be followed. A child with second-degree burns covering 25% of the body surface area might be appropriately transported to a local burn center.

When a decision is made to transport a patient, the physician should consider the following:

- How stable is the patient, and is the patient expected to deteriorate?
- What level of medical care is the patient currently receiving?
- What is the appropriate destination for the patient?
- What level of medical expertise is required during the transport?
- What is the appropriate mode of transfer?

PREPARATION AND PLANNING

Prior to the actual need for transport of an ill child, the physician should explore the referral options for his/her area. Community hospital capability for stabilization and diagnosis of an ill or injured child should be evaluated. Names and numbers of contact facilities and personnel should be easily accessible. A plan of action should be reviewed with office staff prior to the actual need of transport. Contact should be made with the local ambulance companies, transport services, and local and specialty hospitals to explore all transport options. Evaluating these services before they are actually needed will lead to a smoother transition of care when used.

Pediatric transport can take place from an office or clinic, but usually an ill patient in those locations places undue stress on personnel and time, even if the proper equipment, medication, and physician expertise are present. Most often these patients should be cared for in an emergency department at a local hospital. If the local hospital does not have adequate pediatric staffing, the skilled primary care physician should consider accompanying the patient in an ambulance to the emergency department and assist in the management of the patient in a more controlled environment. Transport to a more definitive care facility can be arranged simultaneously and the patient then transferred from the emergency department setting. Obviously, these plans depend greatly on the available level of care in the office and the community.

MODE AND LEVEL OF TRANSPORT

Options available for patient transport include a private car, taxi, prehospital (EMS) ambulance with basic or advanced life support capability, generic transport service (one that transports all patients regardless of age or disease process), and specialty transport service such as a pediatric or neonatal team. In many areas, these services are competitive, so many options may be available.

Transport by private car is a valid option for the patient who is being referred for routine medical evaluation or does not have the likelihood of becoming acutely ill in the immediate future. Many physicians will choose the private car option to take a patient to the hospital because they feel it is the most direct, expedient, and inexpensive method for the patient to be transferred to the advanced care center. Although it is possible that a patient could arrive at the referral center quickly and in reasonable condition, one must consider that the patient may not go directly to the referral center and may arrive in a worse state than when they left the office. Not infrequently, a parent will stop at home to wait for another parent to arrive, for other children to come home from school, to pack a bag, or clean the house and may even stop for a meal on the way to the hospital. This situation can happen even with stern direction from the physician that they need to go directly to the hospital. The referring physician needs to understand that he/she is totally responsible for that patient until arrival at the receiving hospital. If a patient decides to go home prior to going to the hospital and has an untoward event or becomes sicker, the physician may be liable for choosing an inappropriate mode of transport. If a patient is ill, the private car option clearly represents a decrease in the level of provided care and allows the physician to be liable under the COBRA/OBRA laws.

Often physicians opt to accompany the patient in a private car in case there is a problem with the patient. Although this option is a noble effort, lack of a medical environment and equipment to intervene as needed may not allow for appropriate care of the patient in case of deterioration. If the patient is stable and the physician believes that a nonmedical transport could be arranged, a taxi may be a viable option. Although there are inherent risks in using a taxi for transportation, such as a lack of seat belts and inability to judge the adequacy and safety of the driver, the physician can be assured that, barring mishaps enroute, the patient will be delivered directly to the referral facility. Again, however, this mode of transport should not be a consideration for a patient who has the potential to become unstable.

The next level of care involves prehospital (EMS) providers. This level of care routinely is used for initial transport to a medical facility. When the physician decides to transport an ill child who is stable, EMS transport is a viable option. A child who needs advanced life support or monitoring, however, may be out of the scope of the prehospital provider. Prehospital care providers may be emergency medical technicians, paramedics, or volunteers with minimal medical experience; therefore, the physician should explore the types and staffing of prehospital care services in the area. Even those ambulances that are staffed and equipped for advanced life support intervention may not be adequate for continuous monitoring of a critically ill child. Prehospital care providers are trained for initial intervention and stabilization, not for ongoing management of critically ill children. This issue can be important when arranging for patient transport over a long distance or period of time.

The need for an increased level of care should then lead to consideration of advanced care transport teams. Transports of acutely ill patients are most often accomplished by ground ambulance or helicopter. The available modes of transportation will vary depending on location.

Transport team composition is variable, consisting usually of a combination of a nurse, respiratory therapist, paramedic, and/or physician. The experience and training of these teams in pediatrics should be explored prior to use of the transport team. The desire to move a sick patient to the receiving center as quickly as possible must be balanced with involving appropriate personnel and equipment.

An advantage with a generic helicopter transport system is that the response time is usually rapid, and the patient is moved from the initial evaluation site quickly. Most helicopter services also pride themselves on a short on-scene time, which is important when responding to the scene of an accident but is not of primary importance when responding to an interhospital transfer of a medical or surgical patient. The larger questions to consider are whether the transport system is providing the best level of care to the patient during the transport and if they are delivering the patient to the best level of care after the transport. If the patient needs specialty care, a specialty transport team should be able to offer sophisticated advice during the initial notification, offer on-site expert care with the arrival of the transport team, and deliver the patient to the referral center in a stabilized and safe condition. This goal can be most effectively accomplished using a dedicated pediatric transport system, if one is available.

The dedicated pediatric transport system should offer immediate response by transport personnel who have ongoing experience with critically ill children. Most specialty teams will have an identified medical command physician who can offer immediate medical advice and direction as needed. Often team composition is variable and can be easily amended to include extra or specific personnel if the patient's status requires. Most specialty teams will have experience in and capability for various modes of transport (ground, rotor, or fixed-wing aircraft) and should be helpful in making decisions regarding the appropriate mode for a specific patient. In most cases, it is appropriate for the primary care physician to contact the specialty transport service and allow them to help decide the mode of transport rather than attempting to determine a mode of transport and then trying to fit a transport team to the transport vehicle. In areas where there are competitive transport services, the physician should explore these options prior to the notification of a transport service for a particular patient.

INFORMATION REQUIRED FOR TRANSPORT

Once the decision to transport a pediatric patient is made, contact with the transport system should take place. Access numbers to the transport system should be easily available to the physician and his/her staff. If they are not available from an identified transport system, the physician should contact the receiving hospital and assess exactly how contact should be made in the most expedient manner. The case should be discussed succinctly with a medical command physician. The acute medical presentation and pertinent past medical history should be presented, vital signs should be available, and any interventions should be discussed in detail, along with the response to those interventions. The physician should avoid the temptation to offer a prolonged history, because this will effectively slow the transport process and may not benefit the patient's immediate care.

The following information should be available for review with the transport team medical command physician:

- Name, location, and phone number of person making the referral
- Patient's name, age, and weight
- Acute medical history and pertinent past medical history, including allergies and infectious disease exposures
- Suspicion of disease process if not clear
- Current vital signs and pertinent physical examination
- Intervention performed and response to those interventions
- Medications given
- Laboratory values, radiograph results
- Limitations in intervention, personnel, or facility capabilities
- Any preferences for physician or service at receiving hospital
- Verification of parental consent

The medical command physician should be expected to offer advice and direction. If the advice and direction are contradictory to what the referral physician believes is appropriate, this should be discussed, as should the inability or unwillingness to intervene as requested for whatever reason. Recognition of the common goal of an optimal patient outcome should allow appropriate care to be rendered.

PARENTAL CONSENT

Part of the transport process involves obtaining consent from the patient's family to transfer the child. The mode of transport and the hospital to which the child is being referred are important topics to discuss with the family prior to the initiation of the transfer request (if possible) or arrival of the transport team. This policy can avoid the embarrassing and expensive mobilization and arrival of a transport team when the parents are unaware or unwilling to transport the child by the particular mode or to the particular hospital. Pertinent records, radiographs, and laboratory tests should be copied. The transport team should not have to take extra time at the scene of the transport to organize or gather these materials and information. Phone and fax numbers as well as addresses of the referring and private physicians and the facility should be made available to the transport team. This demographic information can help the transport team communicate with the referring and private physicians as well as with the referring facility regarding the patient's condition during transport and facilitate patient follow-up information. The referring physician should expect to receive follow-up information from the transport team as to the child's care during transport and disposition within the hospital.

ARRIVAL OF THE TRANSPORT TEAM

On arrival of the transport team, the following information and personnel should be available:

- Acute and pertinent past medical history, including exposures to or suspicion of communicable diseases (written, if time permits)
- Summary of interventions and responses (written, if time permits)
- Copies of laboratory, radiographic, and medical records and other information pertinent to the patient's care
- Physician available in person or by phone for case review with the transport team
- Parents available for brief discussion with transport team personnel
- Parental consent for transfer
- Contact phone numbers and addresses of referring and private physician

When the transport team arrives, a smooth transition of care should take place. Although diplomacy is important, the referring physician should not be offended if the transport personnel's initial attention appears to be focused on the patient and not him/her. Even though the referring physician may have spent a long, stressful period with the patient and family, the transport team needs to be assured on their arrival that the patient is stable at that moment. Once that has been accomplished, a formal transfer of information can be accomplished in an expedient manner.

POTENTIAL PITFALLS

Difficulties with the transport team should be communicated to the personnel who manage and direct the transport team. Heated disagreement regarding patient care at the patient's bedside is often counterproductive and tends to lead to poor outcomes as well as to a lack of confidence in the entire process by the family.

Disagreement is valid, however, and should be approached in a constructive and courteous manner. If a serious disagreement regarding patient care or intervention occurs, and cannot be resolved to everyone's satisfaction, direct communication between the transport medical command physician and referring physician may help to ease the strain.

The transport team is aware of the referring physician's concern to move the patient to more advanced care quickly, but they also are acutely aware that the transport environment is an often unforgiving one, which can be deleterious to the inadequately prepared patient. Time spent stabilizing the patient's airway or vascular access or other similar interventions is usually well spent. Replacement of a poorly secured intravenous line or endotracheal tube in an ambulance or helicopter is difficult in the best of situations.

BIBLIOGRAPHY

Aoki BY, McCloskey K: *Evaluation, stabilization, and transport of the critically ill child,* St. Louis, 1992, Mosby–Year Book.

Baker MD, Ludwig S: Pediatric emergency transport and the private practitioner, *Pediatrics* 88:691–695, 1991.

Bolte RG: Responsibilities of the referring physician and referring hospital. In McCloskey K, Orr R, editors: *Pediatric transport medicine,* St. Louis, 1995, Mosby–Year Book.

Day S, McCloskey K, Orr R, Bolte R, Notterman D, Hackel A: Pediatric interhospital critical care transport: Consensus of a national leadership conference, *Pediatrics* 88:696–704, 1991.

Hackel A, editor: Critical care transport, *Int Anesthesiol Clin* 25:1–173, 1987.

Hageman JR, Fetcho S, editors: Transport of the critically ill, *Crit Care Clin* 8:465–664, 1992.

Jaimovich DG, Vidyasagar D, editors: Transport medicine, *Pediatr Clin North Am* 40:221–463, 1993.

Lee G: Transport of the critically ill trauma patient, *Nurs Clin North Am* 21:741–749, 1986.

McCloskey K, Hackel A, Notterman D, Orr R, Whitfield J, Dudgeon D (Task Force on Interhospital Transport): *Guidelines for air and ground transport of neonatal and pediatric patients,* Elk Grove Village, 1993, American Academy of Pediatrics.

McCloskey K, Orr R: Pediatric transport issues in emergency medicine, *Emerg Med Clin North Am,* 9:475–489, 1991.

Macnab A: Paediatric interfacility transport: Organization and principles, *Paediatr Anaesth* 4:351–357, 1994.

Ramenofsky ML: Prehospital resuscitation and transport. In Touloukian RJ, editor: *Pediatric trauma,* St. Louis, 1990, Mosby–Year Book.

Woodward GA: Responsibilities of the receiving hospital. In McCloskey K, Orr R, editors: *Pediatric transport medicine,* St. Louis, 1995, Mosby–Year Book.

PART TWO

Abuse

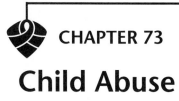

CHAPTER 73

Child Abuse

James E. Crawford

Over the past several decades, the physical abuse of children has become recognized as a problem of epidemic proportions. Society has responded by attempting to improve its ability to identify and assist children at risk. Physicians have become increasingly more involved in recognizing abused children. Kempe's description of "the battered child" in 1962 focused attention on a problem that had not been widely addressed by the medical community. We now recognize that the physical abuse of children results in thousands of cases of significant morbidity and mortality each year. In 1993, there were almost three million cases of child abuse reported to the Departments of Children and Youth in the United States. Approximately 25% of these reports were made in reference to a concern of physical abuse. Because the number of reports to the various hotlines around the country almost surely underrepresents the number of actual assaults that occur, it is clear that abuse is a grave health problem for children in America. Assaults result in the deaths of several thousand children each year. Child homicide is the most frequent cause of injury-related death in children under the age of 1 year and is in the top 10 causes of death for all age groups of children. Many more children face long-term morbidity from trauma suffered as the result of physical abuse. The long-term costs to

children, families, and society as a whole are staggering. For the most part, the perpetrators of these crimes are not strangers on the street, but are typically the child's adult caretakers.

There is no universally agreed upon definition of physical abuse. For example, although some individuals might consider spanking an inappropriate way to discipline children, some state governments not only allow educators to paddle students but protect them from prosecution for having done so. Although some injuries are clearly abusive in nature, such as the neurologic devastation inflicted when an infant is severely shaken, others may be less clear cut. In the broadest sense, physical abuse can be viewed as events or actions that cause a child pain, morbidity, or mortality. The primary care physician must consider a child to be abused when he/she sees evidence of injury that exceeds the reasonable limit of childhood activities.

The physician, in the role as child advocate, must be able to identify those children who are being injured at the hands of their caretakers. Making the medical diagnosis of child abuse is quite easy sometimes and exceedingly difficult at others. Injuries that are observed are usually not pathognomonic for child abuse. Physicians have a unique opportunity to aid children who have been the victims of physical abuse. Whether in the emergency room or a private office, a child's physician may be one of few individuals with whom a child interacts outside of the family unit, particularly for infants and preschool-aged children. Although it may seem like a straightforward concept, children who have been significantly injured usually are taken to a physician for evaluation and treatment; this is true whether the injury is accidental or inflicted. This situation gives the treating physician the opportunity to identify inflicted injuries as being the result of abuse. Making the diagnosis of child abuse is not always easy. A physician rarely hears a parent say, "I just shook my baby, and now she's not moving." There is no serum "child abuse level." Differentiating inflicted injuries from accidental injuries or other medical conditions is sometimes a difficult task.

Making a diagnosis of a nonaccidental injury involves the same steps as any other diagnosis that a physician makes; it should involve the same logical, thoughtful, objective collection of information. The initial aspects of the evaluation involve a complete history with a physical examination. Laboratory studies or radiologic evaluations may be required to define the issues more clearly. The physician needs to observe the interactions between the child and caregiver. To diagnose child abuse, as with any other medical condition, it must be entertained as part of the differential diagnosis. If a physician does not consider that a child's injuries might be the result of abuse, he/she will fail to recognize it as such. It is imperative to recognize that any child could be abused and that any adult could be a potential perpetrator.

THE HISTORY

The history, an integral part in diagnosing abusive injuries, should address the issues listed in Box 73-1. A number of elements to the history may offer clues to the diagnosis of child abuse. A history with any of these characteristics should suggest to the physician that perhaps more has happened to this child than is being revealed. It is important to elicit a history about concerning physical findings, which may be noticed in the context of a visit designated for some other purpose. For example, a physician who notes a burn to the hand of an infant 9 months of age who presented for an evaluation of a suspected otitis

---

BOX 73-1
Pertinent Characteristics of History When Child Abuse is Suspected

Is the mechanism of injury given by the parent or caregiver consistent with the injuries seen in the patient?
Does the child have a "magical" injury, one that no one can explain?
Is the child developmentally able to behave in the manner that the caretaker describes?
Does the caretaker blame someone else for the child's injuries, especially another child?
Is the history consistent over time, or does it change?
Has there been an unexplained delay in seeking medical care?

---

media should elicit a complete history as to how the burn occurred. Precise documentation of the history is very important. Whenever possible, the history should be recorded verbatim, noting who gave the particular history and who was present at the time the history was elicited. If the history were to change over time, this should be documented as well. If the opportunity is available and the child is verbal, both the child and the caretaker should be interviewed separately, in order to assess consistency of the history.

Box 73-2 suggests other important pieces of information that must be obtained from the history.

While trying to determine if child abuse is a concern, it is extremely important for the physician to determine if the history explains the injuries the child has and if it is consistent with the findings of the physical examination. A classic example of a history that is inconsistent with the trauma a child has sustained is the child with significant head injuries and multiple fractures who was reported to have "rolled off the bed." Studies have shown that the vast majority (approximately 80%) of children who fall from a bed or couch sustain no notable injuries. Those that do generally have quite superficial injuries. It is atypical for a child to sustain serious or life-threatening injuries from this particular mechanism. If this mechanism is suggested as the cause of the trauma, the history must be questioned and abuse suspected. This theme is played over and over again in the histories elicited from caretakers who have abused their children.

BOX 73-2

Elements of History That Must Be Elicited When Child Abuse Is Suspected

General
   Identify the child's primary health care provider.
   Determine the frequency of visits to emergency rooms/quick-care centers.
   Obtain a description of the child's general health.
   Obtain a history of previous serious injuries.
   Obtain a history of prior hospitalizations.
Specific
   Obtain a complete history for each injury noted on the physical examination.
   When did each injury occur?
   Determine the location of the child at the time the injury occurred.
   What was the child doing at the time of the injury?
   Who witnessed the event?
   Who else was with the child?
   Who was supervising the child?
   Did the child need medical care at the time of the accident?
   Who took the child to get medical care?
   Was there a delay in seeking medical care?
   How long did any delay last?

In order to recognize histories that misrepresent a child's actions, the physician must be familiar with many aspects of child development. Often the physician obtains a history that states "the baby rolled. . ." If the baby in question is 2 weeks of age, this history is questionable because infants that young are not yet able to roll over. A child's ability to crawl, walk, or manipulate objects is frequently misrepresented. It would not be reasonable, for example, to accept a history as truthful that attributed the scald burns on the hands of a child 13 months of age to the toddler turning on a faucet and trying to wash his/her own hands. Children often are described as being "clumsy" or "accident prone," which is a concerning statement if the injuries sustained fall outside of the realm of what is expected for a child of a particular age and developmental level.

ACCIDENTAL INJURIES

It is critical for the physician to recognize the locations and types of injuries that are an expected part of the life of a young child. Neonates frequently will scratch their faces with their fingernails. These marks are very superficial and are not noted to generate true morbidity. Aside from this injury, young infants do not routinely experience significant bruises or other injuries that are self-generated. Because they neither roll nor crawl, their location is entirely determined by the person who placed them there. A caregiver should be able to explain any significant injury that is noted on examination. Bruises to the face, ears, and head are particularly concerning.

As a child grows and acquires new developmental skills, the pattern of accidental injuries changes. By 4 to 5 months of age, most infants should be able to roll themselves over, which may potentially result in falling from a height if left unsupervised. Injuries sustained while rolling off common surfaces such as couches, beds, and changing tables are usually minor. Although this type of event is in fact a quite common occurrence, it is quite uncommon for an infant to sustain significant or life-threatening injuries from this type of accident. The injuries usually are limited to one area of the body and are not particularly significant. This mechanism would have to be suspect in an infant who has sustained either very significant injury or injuries to more than one area of the body.

Mastering walking is a challenging task for children. It involves a great deal of trial and error. Toddlers are well known for falling. In the course of their normal developmental activities, it is quite expected for toddlers to sustain some degree of bruising, and the bruises occur in predictable locations. The areas most frequently affected by toddlers falling involve bony prominences such as shins, elbows, knees, chin, and forehead. Children tend to sustain accidental injuries to the anterior aspects of their bodies. Frenulum tears, which are not likely to be the result of accidental trauma in a very young infant, are now occasionally seen when toddlers strike their mouths on hard surfaces as the result of falls. Children rarely sustain significant accidental bruises to the buttocks, lower back, genitals, neck, cheeks, earlobes, and inside of the mouth. When bruises occur in atypical areas, the physician must attempt to determine their cause and question their origin.

CUTANEOUS FINDINGS

Cutaneous lesions, especially bruises, are the most common physical manifestation of child abuse. Because children frequently sustain

---

BOX 73-3
Evaluating Cutaneous Injuries When Abuse Is Suspected

More suspicious	Less suspicious
Injuries on the child's	Injuries on the child's
Buttocks	Shin
Cheeks	Elbow
Lower back	Knees
Genitals	Chin
Earlobes	Forehead
Inside mouth	
Multiple bruises	Few bruises
Multiple body planes injured	Bruising limited to one plane
Various stages of healing	Same stages of healing
Clearly identified patterns	Amorphous pattern
History unlikely to produce observed injuries	History consistent with injuries

---

bruising in the course of their everyday activities, attempting to differentiate accidental from inflicted bruising may be challenging. Physicians frequently are asked to determine the age of a bruise. This assessment has been recognized as an inexact science at best. The severity of the bruise, the vascularity of the particular area, and its proximity to the surface are factors that will affect the speed with which the bruise resolves and the color of the surface skin. The general color pattern that occurs during the evolution of a healing bruise is blue/black to blue/green to yellow/brown. The dating of bruises by color can be done as a rough approximation but should not be used as an exact measure of age. A physician can assess whether bruises appear to be the same age. Multiple bruises in various stages of healing suggest that a child has been beaten on more than one occasion. Similarly, a history that suggests a yellowing bruise occurred the evening before is not possible and must be called into question. A child with extensive bruising on his/her body, bruising in unusual locations, and bruises that appear to be in various stages of healing needs to be very carefully evaluated for physical abuse.

The nature of the bruise is important in drawing conclusions about its etiology (Box 73-3). As previously stated, the location of the bruise can make it more or less suspicious. When children experience accidental injuries, the injuries for the most part occur on "one plane." For example, stair falls in children may result in minor bruising to the head or distal extremities, but it is atypical for a child with this history to present with multiple bruises to many body areas. The pattern of the bruise is occasionally suggestive of the object that created the injury. Inflicted bruises are usually due to a child being struck with an object. Perhaps the most common objects with which children are struck are the hands of their caregivers. Slapping, punching, and spanking are the most frequent means of inflicting injury. When an open palm is used, one occasionally can identify a clear outline of fingers in the pattern of the bruise. The pattern of the bruise should be noted. Drawings may be used to delineate the exact location of the injuries, as well as to represent their pattern. When possible, the physician should measure the size of any bruise as exactly as possible. Photographs can be very helpful in documenting the appearance of the bruise.

Bruises that are the result of abuse may have recognizable patterns or bizarre shapes. Patterned loop marks from beatings with electric cords, ropes, or belts usually are easily identified. The object that inflicted these bruises can be inferred by the appearance of the bruise. Because of its flexibility, a cord will wrap itself around the body as a child is struck with it. The resulting bruise will be noted to follow the contours of the child's body. For example, a bruise created when a child is whipped with a cord may be continuous, extending from the child's abdomen, to the side, to the back. This pattern is in contrast to bruises inflicted by other objects such as sticks. These types of objects are less flexible, and the resulting marks will be limited to the area initially struck. The marks will not wrap around a body surface. Other instruments may leave a variety of unusual patterned injuries. Marks left from objects such as hairbrushes or belt buckles may leave patterns that may be difficult to identify. Accidental bruises rarely leave a clearly patterned injury. Significant bruising noted on the hands and forearms may suggest defensive posturing on the part of the child.

Circumferential linear marks are frequently signs of abuse. When these marks are found near the wrist or ankle, it is quite suggestive that the child was bound. Linear marks near the corner of the mouth suggests a gag had been in place. Circumferential neck bruising suggests that the child was choked with a rope or a similar object and that a potentially life-threatening event took place. Ligatures sometimes are applied to the penis of toddler-age boys, frequently in relation to toilet-training issues. This type of assault can result in either bruising or more serious tissue damage, including partial amputation. Bruising to the genitals is an unusual finding.

There are a number of nonabusive conditions that must be considered when presented with a child who appears to have unexplained "bruising" (Box 73-4). These conditions involve both medical illnesses as well as cultural practices that result in marking of the skin. Many of these entities have fairly characteristic presentations or appearances. The distribution of lesions often is suggestive of a particular nonabusive etiology.

As the cultural background of the United States continues to broaden, physicians will progressively see a wider range of health care–related belief systems within the families of their patients. There are a number of cultural practices designed to aid the healing of a sick or injured child with which many American-trained physicians are not familiar. Developing familiarity

with these practices is important so that they are not reported as abusive activity. Cao gio, or *coining*, is the Chinese and Vietnamese practice of rubbing a coin over the skin of a sick child in order to treat fever, headache, and chills. It is not unusual to note bruising and redness. *Cupping* is a practice described among Eastern Europeans used to treat pain. A heated cup is placed against the skin, usually on multiple locations. The resulting marks are usually round, erythematous lesions. These practices are good faith attempts by individuals to alleviate the distress their children are experiencing. It is important to differentiate these acts from those of abuse.

When a child presents with bruises that are concerning, it may be appropriate to undertake a laboratory evaluation to eliminate medical etiologies, although most children with abusive patterned injuries do not require laboratory evaluations. In general, the nontraumatic causes of apparent bruising are the result of a coagulation disorder, a platelet disorder, or a vasculitis. A screening complete blood cell count with hemoglobin/hematocrit and platelet count, prothrombin time, and partial thromboplastin time are usually an appropriate first step. A bleeding time is useful if the physician is concerned about platelet function or von Willebrand's disease. If these screening studies are abnormal, or if the child appears to have a history that is consistent with a bleeding disorder, it would be appropriate to make a referral to a pediatric hematologist. It should be kept in mind that child abuse and bleeding disorders are not mutually exclusive.

BURNS

Inflicted burns represent a serious, and not uncommon, form of child abuse. Approximately 10% to 20% of hospitalizations for abusive injuries are the result of burns. Similarly, 10% to 25% of burns to children are the result of inflicted injuries. Children less than 5 years of age are at the highest risk for both accidental as well as abusive burn injuries. The vast majority (nearly 80%) of burns to young children are minor scald injuries. Flame burns constitute only approximately 13% of burn injuries but, in conjunction with smoke inhalation, cause the highest burn-related mortality. Only a small percentage (2% to 3%) of burns to children are caused by electricity or chemicals.

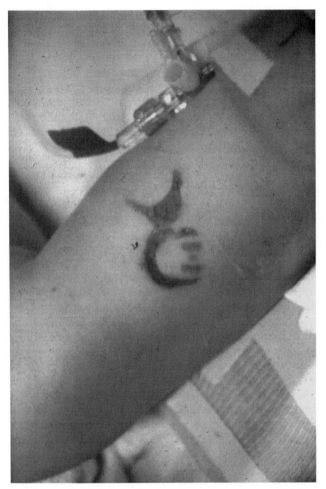

FIG 73-1
Contact burn caused by a disposable cigarette lighter.

The different types of burns tend to have certain age categories associated with them. Scald burns tend to be noted in younger children, primarily infants and toddlers. The most common sources are very hot tap water, hot beverages (tea, coffee), soups, or cooking grease. Scald injuries can be either accidental or inflicted. Many accidental scaldings, especially of young children, are caused when a hot liquid spills from above the child. Burns may be noted to start on or near the head/face and trail or splatter to lower aspects of the trunk or extremities. Flame burns more frequently injure older, school-aged children. Flame burns are an unusual form of inflicted injury, but they do occur. Contact, or branding, burns tend to be noted most frequently in toddlers. These types of injuries occur when a child's skin comes into contact with a heated surface. These types of burns often are caused by irons, curling irons, and hot plates. Inflicted burns are sometimes generated by forcing contact with heating elements from heaters or heated cigarette lighters (Fig. 73-1). Chemical burns may be due to accidental ingestions by toddlers. Electrical burns have a bimodal distribution. They are frequently seen in both toddlers and adolescents due to age-specific behaviors. Physicians are frequently asked to assist in differentiating inflicted from accidental burns. Up to 10% of burns that result in the hospitalization of the child are the result of inflicted injury.

Scald burns are the most common burn injury to children. Burn injuries from spilled liquids are more commonly the result of accidents than abuse. They are usually the result of liquid falling or spilling from a height, onto a child.

The burn is typically more serious around the head and neck. As the liquid flows down the child, it often creates splash patterns to the trunk and lower extremities. The burn will frequently have a nonuniform degree of penetration from top to bottom, with the most severe aspect of the burn being on the superior aspects of the child's body. It is unusual to see children sustaining abusive injuries from having hot liquid thrown on them.

Immersion burns are a very serious form of burn injury. This type of injury involves the child falling or being placed into a hot liquid. When this type of event happens accidentally, a child will attempt as strongly as possible to get out of this very painful situation by kicking, splashing, and struggling. The child will have multiple areas of burned skin, with evidence of splash marks and nonuniformly burned surfaces. This type of pattern is in contrast to what is commonly seen in the injuries sustained by children with forced immersion burns. In this type of injury, the child (or part of the child) is forcibly placed into a hot liquid. If the area of immersion is limited to an extremity, one frequently sees a "glove" or "stocking" distribution to the burn. The burn may be isolated to a single hand and forearm. Frequently there is a very clear line where the burned tissue is separated from the noninjured tissue. This pattern would not be consistent with an accidental event. A "full body" forced immersion burn is the result of a child being held and lowered into a tub of very hot water. One frequently sees involvement of both hands and both feet and buttocks. The central area of the buttocks may be spared if the child is pushed down, forcing contact with the cooler tub surface. Generally, the flexor areas are spared. When the burns occur in this type of pattern they are virtually pathognomonic for abuse. This type of injury is typically associated with toddlers who have soiling and toilet-training accidents.

Contact burns constitute the second leading cause of abusive burns. If a child accidentally comes into contact with a hot surface, he/she will reflexively withdraw from it, resulting in a relatively small burn. The motion of the child often results in relatively indistinct margins to the burn. One edge of the burn may be deeper than the other, due to the unequal pressure being applied while in contact with the hot object. Inflicted burns, in contrast to accidental burns, often have a very distinct pattern imprinted on the skin, akin to a branding. The hot object is applied to the skin with relatively even pressure, resulting in deep imprints with clear margins. Cigarette burns, which are often thought of as "classic" child abuse injuries, are actually fairly unusual.

As with bruises, there are a number of other conditions that might be confused with, and misdiagnosed as, an inflicted burn injury. Accidental burns may be difficult to distinguish from their inflicted counterparts. The patterns, types, extent, and locations will often assist in identifying their accidental origin. Skin infections must be considered as part of the differential of inflicted burns. Impetigo may cause multiple, circular skin lesions about the size that one might expect as being caused by a cigarette burn. Burns caused by cigarettes will be of uniform width; impetiginous lesions will be of varying widths. Similarly, one can see lesions that give the appearance of burned tissue in early staphylococcal scalded skin syndrome and erysipelas. If this condition is suspected, microbiologic tests would be indicated. Epidermolysis bullosa can be confused with burned skin as well. Cao gio, cupping, moxibustion, and other cultural practices also may be confused with abusive burn injuries. Phytophotodermatitis and severe diaper dermatitis also can give the false impression of skin being burned. Severe drug eruptions must also be considered as part of the differential diagnosis.

When a child has been intentionally burned, the physician must consider that he/she may have suffered from other types of physical maltreatment as well, necessitating a complete physical examination of the child to assess the presence of other injuries. In particular, the physician should note the presence of other findings of cutaneous injuries such as bruises or evidence of other burns. The location, measurements, and description of any burn should be clearly documented. Included should be an estimate as to body surface area and degree of burn. Drawings or photographs are useful as adjuncts to the written descriptions. When a child is noted to have multiple burns of different ages, clearly from different events, child abuse must be considered as the most likely etiology. However, it should be remembered that the majority of abusive burn injuries are not associated with other physical injuries. If the child is under

2 years of age, an assessment of the skeleton for evidence of other trauma is appropriate. This should be accomplished with a skeletal survey. If there is any suggestion that the child has suffered some degree of trauma to the head, a computed tomography (CT) scan of the head should be obtained.

SKELETAL TRAUMA

Skeletal trauma is a frequent sequela of inflicted injuries to children. It is the result of either direct trauma to the bone, the bending of bone, traction to an extremity, or a significant rotational force. As with any other injury, the physician must assess the developmental stage of the child and the mechanism offered by the history to determine whether the child may have conceivably injured himself/herself in an accidental manner. A fracture in a child younger than 12 months of age should always be evaluated very carefully. It is uncommon for infants to sustain accidental fractures in the first 12 months of life without a history of significant trauma. An exception to this rule would be birth-related fractures, which most commonly involve the clavicle, humerus, and femur. Skull fractures caused by accidental falls also may occasionally be seen in infants. The characteristics of the skull fracture may be helpful in determining whether it has the appearance of an accidental or an inflicted injury. No isolated fracture is pathognomonic for inflicted injury; however, some are more suspicious than others. Each case needs to be evaluated individually. Rib fractures and metaphyseal fractures are highly specific for inflicted injuries in children under the age of 2 years. It is concerning when bones that are infrequently injured, such as the scapula and vertebrae, are noted to have sustained trauma. Injuries to long bones must be considered on a case-by-case basis to evaluate the circumstances that reportedly caused the injury.

Diagnostic studies are indicated in the evaluation of fractures. A complete skeletal radiographic series is indicated in the evaluation of any child under the age of 2 years as a method of assessing for other bony injuries. The physician may be able to appreciate the presence of occult bone injuries. The presence of multiple healing fractures is indicative of child abuse (Fig. 73-2). In order to assess for the presence of either more subtle or more recent injuries to bone, a radionuclide skeletal scintigraphy study should be utilized. Nuclear studies may pick up trauma that is not detectable by regular radiographs. This study may be able to detect trauma to bone hours after it occurred. Plain films may not detect new fractures, especially in ribs. Follow-up plain films of any suspicious area should be obtained several weeks after the original series was obtained to evaluate the healing process. As bone heals, callus formation becomes apparent, and the sites of previously occult trauma become apparent.

A child with multiple bone fractures may rarely suffer from osteogenesis imperfecta and not be the victim of abuse. A good history, physical examination, and skeletal survey are usually adequate to screen for this rare condition. If a question still remains, referral to a genetic/metabolic specialist may be indicated. A study of cultured fibroblasts obtained from the skin of the child may be used in resolving the question, although this is rarely necessary. Obtaining levels of serum calcium, phosphorus, and alkaline phosphatase are also useful in documenting the absence of other pathology. Rickets, congenital syphilis, leukemia, neuroblastoma, and other oncologic disorders also may cause pathologic fractures or changes in the bone that may mimic abuse.

HEAD TRAUMA

Head trauma, especially to younger children, is a common manifestation of child abuse. Fifty percent to 65% of physical abuse involves trauma to the head, face, and neck. This trauma is caused primarily either by direct blows or shaking. Of the minor injuries, facial contusions are the most common. Frenulum tears, which may be due to accidental trauma in toddlers, are quite concerning when noted on nonambulatory infants. The mechanisms that create this injury generally involve a direct blow to the mouth, which is often associated with contusions, broken teeth and bones, or force feeding with a spoon or bottle, often with no associated injuries. Injuries to the lips most commonly involve contusions, lacerations, and abrasions. Tooth injuries may be due to either accidental or inflicted trauma.

More serious head trauma may result in death or permanent disability. Greater than 90% of all

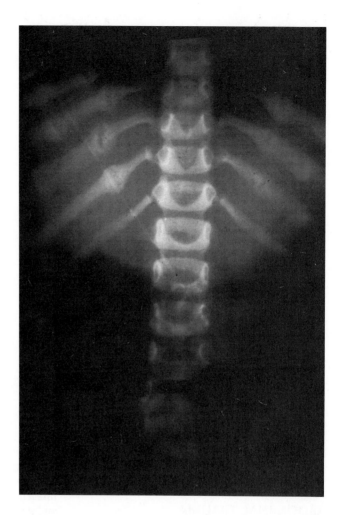

FIG 73-2
Multiple healing posterior rib fractures.

serious head injuries to infants are the result of abusive acts. Injuries sustained from limited falls, such as from a couch or flight of stairs, rarely generate life-threatening injuries. Direct trauma to the head may result in soft-tissue injuries, skull fractures, and intracranial hemorrhages. The typical findings with shaken baby syndrome include subdural hemorrhages, cerebral infarction with brain atrophy over time, retinal hemorrhages (Fig. 73-3), and skeletal injuries. The injury is believed to be generated when an infant is violently shaken with a subsequent impact to some surface. The subdural hemorrhages are believed to occur when bridging veins are shorn by the anterior/posterior movement of the brain within the confines of the skull. The infant may have few, if any, cutaneous signs of abuse. Retinal hemorrhages are commonly seen in the first week of life as a result of birth trauma, however,

they have not been reported to last longer than 5 weeks. When retinal hemorrhages are identified in an infant older than 5 weeks, child abuse must be considered. Infants or children with suspected abusive injuries involving the head should be evaluated with a CT scan. Neurosurgical evaluation should occur as quickly as possible if significant head injury is suspected. If possible, the cervical spine of shaken infants should be evaluated by magnetic resonance imaging, because injuries to this area may occur simultaneously.

Any child or infant with clinically significant head injuries should have an eye examination performed by a pediatric ophthalmologist. Retinal hemorrhages are commonly seen in babies who have experienced violent shaking injuries. When these injuries are noted in an infant without a history of major trauma, the physician

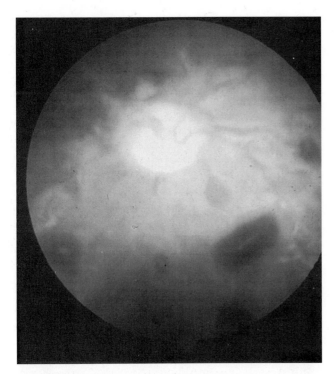

FIG 73-3
Retinal hemorrhages noted in an infant with shaken-baby syndrome.

should be highly suspicious of inflicted injury. Other injuries that may be noted in shaken infants include vitreous hemorrhage and retinal detachment. Ophthalmologic evaluation is important for both diagnosis and management.

ABDOMINAL TRAUMA

Trauma to the abdomen is a common occurrence in abused children. It is the second leading cause of death in child abuse cases, second only to head trauma. It is probably widely underappreciated and underreported. The injuries are generally caused by a blunt force, such as a punch or kick. Penetrating abdominal injuries as a manifestation of child abuse are rare events. Given the relatively weak abdominal musculature and the relatively large size of the organs, a child can sustain significant injuries. The ability of the abdomen to "give" when a blunt force is applied results in less external bruising than might be expected. Only approximately 50% of cases in which a child has sustained serious internal abdominal injuries will have overlying skin bruising. Damage occurs from crushing solid organs, compressing hollow viscera, and shearing of mesentery or hollow viscera. Lacerations of the liver, ruptures of the spleen, intramural intestinal hematomas, pancreatitis, pancreatic pseudocysts, adrenal hemorrhages, and rupture of the stomach can occur from trauma. Children who have sustained injuries that compromise the integrity of the lumen of the bowel may present as an "acute abdomen."

If a child is believed to have sustained a significant injury to the abdomen, it is appropriate to involve a surgeon in the initial evaluation of the child. The earlier a surgical abdomen is recognized, the greater the chance of subsequent survival. An abdominal CT scan is useful in the initial phase of the evaluation. Once a child is stable, studies such as an upper gastrointestinal series with a small bowel follow-through may be useful in documenting the presence of intramural hematomas. The initial evaluation of the child should include a number of laboratory studies, including liver function tests, creatine phosphokinase, amylase, lipase, and urinalysis with microscopy. Any infant or young child who is found to have sustained significant abusive abdominal injury should have a full skeletal series to evaluate for the presence of associated bony injury.

MANDATED REPORTER STATUS

In the event that a physician encounters a child who he/she suspects is being abused, the physician is legally mandated to report those suspicions to the Children and Youth Services that function in his/her state. The responsibility to investigate or prove the abuse falls to the social service and law enforcement agencies. Physicians have been successfully prosecuted for failing to report their suspicions of abuse. In order to identify a child as suffering from abusive injuries, one must acknowledge that any child could be the victim of child abuse and that any adult is potentially capable of being a perpetrator of abuse. The reporting of child abuse is not delegable; the individual who owns the suspicion has the responsibility to report it. All 50 states provide legal protection from lawsuits to physicians who report suspicions of child abuse in good faith. In order to be sensitive and specific in the diagnosis of child abuse, the physician must be both thorough and thoughtful during the evaluation. Many large medical centers and children's hospitals have pediatricians who are specially trained in the medical evaluation of children who are suspected of having been abused. These individuals can be helpful in evaluating difficult cases.

BIBLIOGRAPHY

Cooper A, Floyd TF, Barlow B, et al: Major blunt abdominal trauma due to child abuse, *J Trauma* 28:1483–1486, 1988.

Duhaime AC, Gennarelli TA, Thibault LE, et al: The shaken baby syndrome: A clinical, pathological and biomechanical study, *J Neurosurg* 66:409–415, 1987.

Duhaime AC, et al: Head injury in very young children: Mechanisms, injury types and ophthalmologic findings in 100 hospitalized patients younger than 2 years of age, *Pediatrics* 90:179–185, 1992.

Joffe M, Ludwig S: Stairway injuries in children, *Pediatrics* 82:457–461, 1988.

Johnson CF: Inflicted injury versus accidental injury, *Pediatr Clin North Am* 37:791–814, 1990.

Kempe CH, Silverman FN, Steele BF, et al: The battered child syndrome. *JAMA* 181:17–24, 1962.

Kempe CH, Helfer RE, editors: *The battered child,* ed 4, Chicago, 1987, The University of Chicago Press.

Kleinman PK: *Diagnostic imaging of child abuse,* Baltimore, 1987, Williams & Wilkins.

Lenoski EF, Hunter KA: Specific patterns of inflicted burn injuries, *J Trauma* 17(11):842–846, 1977.

Ludwig S, Kornberg A, editors: *Child abuse and neglect: A medical reference.* New York, 1991, Churchill Livingstone.

Ludwig S, Warman M: Shaken baby syndrome: A review of 20 cases, *Ann Emerg Med* 13:104–107, 1984.

Purdue GF, Hunt JL, Prescott PR: Child abuse by burning—an index of suspicion, *J Trauma* 28(2):221–224, 1988.

Reece R: *Child abuse: Medical diagnosis and management,* Philadelphia, 1994, Lea & Febiger.

Rivara FP, Kamitsuka MD, Quan L: Injuries to children younger than 1 year of age, *Pediatrics* 81:93–97, 1988.

CHAPTER 74

Child Sexual Abuse

Cindy W. Christian

The sexual exploitation of children is not a new phenomenon, although its recognition as a medical problem dates only to the late 1970s. Since that time, a great deal has been learned about the dynamics of child sexual abuse, its varied presentations, and the morbidity related to sexual victimization. Attention to the medical evaluation of sexually abused children has taught us much about normal genital anatomy, genital trauma, and sexually transmitted diseases in young children.

Despite the significant gains made in the past two decades, identifying the sexually abused child remains a challenge for all physicians. The primary care physician has the unique task of identifying young victims of sexual abuse, reporting suspected abuse to the proper agencies for investigation, and maintaining an ongoing, supportive relationship with the child and his/her family. Pediatricians often are asked to provide medical evaluations of children suspected of having been sexually abused. For many children and families, the evaluation is best conducted by the primary care physician, who is a trusted professional and child advocate. The primary care physician who is trained and comfortable with the problem of child sexual abuse can offer continuity of care and ongoing support to both the child and the family. Unfortunately, some pediatricians do not feel they have the experience or training to complete the medical evaluation. Some children will require specialized evaluation or the collection of forensic evidence, which may be best accomplished by physicians with special expertise in evaluating sexually abused children. This chapter will review the approach to the medical evaluation of the sexually abused child and will emphasize the important role the primary care physician plays in these cases.

DEFINITION, DYNAMICS, AND EPIDEMIOLOGY

Like all forms of child abuse, sexual abuse can be defined legally, culturally, and individually. In practice, child sexual abuse can be defined as the involvement of children in sexual activities that they cannot understand, for which they are not developmentally prepared, to which they cannot give informed consent, and that violate societal taboos. Both noncontact activities (eg, pornography; inappropriate observation of the child while dressing, toileting, or bathing; perpetrator exhibitionism directed at the child) and contact activities (eg, sexualized kissing, fondling, masturbation, and oral-genital, oral-anal, genital-genital, and genital-anal contact) are included in the definition. Central to the concept of sexual abuse is the misuse of power and the child's trust by the perpetrator. Child sexual abuse can be an isolated, violent assault, but it is more commonly characterized by ongoing, nonviolent exploitation of the child, in which the child is coerced into sexual compliance. Perpetrators are usually well known to their victims and include parents, other family members, family friends, neighbors, teachers, clergy, and other individuals who have ongoing access to the child. A minority of assaults are stranger related.

The dynamics of ongoing sexual abuse often follow a typical pattern, progressing along stages described by Sgroi in 1982. During *engagement,* the perpetrator establishes a seemingly trusting and affectionate relationship with the child, while coercively introducing the child to nonforcible, but inappropriate, sexual behavior. During the *sexual interaction* phase, the perpetrator manipulates the child into participating in slowly escalating forms of sexual activity. *Secrecy* is essential in order for the perpetrator to have ongoing access to the child and to prevent recognition of the abuse. This secrecy can be accomplished through persuasion, rewards, or real or implied threats. The *disclosure* phase is characterized by accidental or purposeful divulgence of the abuse. The final, *suppression* phase is characterized by the family's desire to "make it all go away." The perpetrator or other family members may exert pressure on the child to retract the disclosure in order to prevent family disruption, financial hardships, or punishment of the perpetrator. Although these five stages represent the classic model of child sexual victimization, cases may not fit neatly into each category. Some children disclose abuse after the first inappropriate encounter; others may not disclose years of abuse. Child victims may care about the perpetrator, may not recognize the abuse as being wrong, or may feel guilty, helpless, trapped, or scared.

The actual incidence of sexual abuse is impossible to determine, because many cases are believed to go unrecognized and unreported. Conservative estimates suggest that between 0.5% to 1% of American children will be victims of some form of sexual abuse each year, with reports of victimized girls far outnumbering boys. This statistic is likely due to both a higher incidence of female victimization and an underrecognition and underreporting of boy victims. Adolescents are also underrepresented in reporting statistics. Homeless, runaway teens, prostitutes, and other adolescents with acting out behaviors may be victims of abuse. Children of all racial, religious, and socioeconomic groups are victims of sexual abuse, therefore the physician needs to consider the diagnosis in all populations of patients.

CLINICAL PRESENTATION

There are very few symptoms that are specific for child sexual abuse, and the more common presenting symptoms are so nonspecific that the diagnosis can only be made if the physician is willing to consider abuse as a possibility. Common symptoms such as school failure, aggressive behavior, phobias, depression, eneuresis, encopresis, abdominal pain, and dysuria are not unique to sexually abused children, although they may be a clue to the diagnosis. Even more suggestive symptoms such as genital infection, hypersexualized behavior, precocious sexual

knowledge, or excessive masturbation are not pathognomonic for abuse and require a thoughtful, comprehensive evaluation.

A child's disclosure of sexual abuse can be purposeful or accidental. The evaluation and management of the child who purposefully discloses abuse is more straightforward and allows for planned intervention. Accidental disclosure of abuse is more problematic, because neither the child nor the perpetrator deliberately revealed the abuse, and the child may be unable or unwilling to discuss the issue. Accidental disclosure may occur in a variety of ways, including a third party discovering the abuse taking place or the child presenting for medical care with unexplained genital injuries, pregnancy, or a sexually transmitted disease. The approach to the evaluation in part reflects the way in which the sexual abuse is discovered.

THE MEDICAL EVALUATION

The primary care pediatrician plays a number of roles in cases of sexual abuse. He/she may be asked to perform a "forensic" examination of a sexually abused child as part of an investigation, he/she may be asked to interview and examine a child who is brought for medical evaluation because of a specific concern of sexual abuse, or, most commonly, he/she may be asked to evaluate a child with nonspecific behavioral or physical complaints that may or may not be related to abuse.

The discovery of child sexual abuse is a family emergency but not usually a medical emergency. Although children are often seen in an emergency department for a medical evaluation, this situation is neither recommended nor desirable. The emergency department is typically a busy, fast-paced environment, staffed with personnel who are not allotted enough time for a proper evaluation. Furthermore, many emergency departments are staffed by physicians who have little training in child sexual abuse. Emergency evaluation of the sexually abused child is recommended for children who are victims of an acute assault (last contact within 72 hours). Children who require the collection of forensic specimens; are involved in an acute stranger assault; have acute genital, anal, or other injuries; may have a sexually transmitted infection; or may be pregnant require immediate medical evaluation and treatment. Children meeting these criteria often can be managed by the primary care pediatrician who has an interest in and knowledge of sexual abuse. The child's best interest is served when the physician involved in the evaluation obtains and documents an objective and complete history and physical examination and makes the appropriate referrals and mandated reports. In all cases, the child's psychological well-being and safety should remain the focus for the physician. The approach to the history, physical examination, and laboratory evaluation of the child will depend on the child's age, history of contact, and symptoms.

HISTORY

The ability to diagnose sexual abuse is usually dependent on the child's ability to provide a history of assault. In a majority of cases, the physical examination fails to identify injuries diagnostic of sexual abuse. Only a minority of abused children incur sexually transmitted diseases. Children who present with possible sexual abuse but have not been questioned about abuse require a comprehensive interview by a professional who is comfortable and knowledgeable about the topic. The primary care physician, although not usually trained in the diagnostic evaluation of child sexual abuse, often is the first professional involved in the evaluation. The child's physician should approach the problem as he/she does others—with a thorough history when indicated, physical examination, and judicious use of laboratory data to determine a working diagnosis and plan. If the evaluation suggests sexual abuse, the physician may need to consult other physicians and professionals with more expertise and training in the evaluation of abuse. If the child has completed investigative interviews before presenting for a medical evaluation, repeated questioning of the child is unwarranted. This does not preclude the physician from discussing the abuse or asking questions relevant to the medical history, including a behavioral and physical review of systems. Children with known sexual abuse need to understand the purpose of the medical visit. The physician might begin by asking the child if he/she knows why he/she was brought for a medical examination and proceed by explaining the purpose and procedures of the examination.

If the child presents with indicators of abuse, but the possibility has never been raised with the child and/or the family, the pediatrician has the opportunity to provide a supportive environment for the disclosure and initial evaluation of the child. The issue of abuse is never easy to raise but can be done in a straightforward, nonaccusatory manner. If the child's symptoms suggest the possibility of abuse, the parents should be told (without the presence of the child, if possible) that there are a number of possible etiologies for the child's symptoms, one of which is sexual abuse. The parents can then be asked if they have had any concerns about possible abuse. This approach provides an opportunity for the parents to disclose any suspicions they may have and brings the topic into the discussion in a nonjudgemental way. Parental denial of abuse cannot be reassurance that the child has not been abused. After talking with the parents, the physician should meet alone with the child.

The initial interview of the child can be both diagnostic and therapeutic for the child. If possible, the interview should be conducted by two professionals, such as a physician and social worker or physician and nurse. It should be tailored to the child's age and development. The interview should begin with the usual introductory conversation and proceed to the topic of abuse in a nonaccusatory fashion. If the child provides a history of abuse, the interviewer should allow the child to give a dialogue of the history. Open-ended questions can be used to help the child with the disclosure. Although leading questions are not to be used, focused and yes/no questions can be used to clarify the history. The interviewer needs to maintain a calm demeanor; it is not helpful when the professional becomes angry, shocked, or upset in front of the child. Some sexually abused children will deny that they have been abused. If the interview fails to uncover abuse that remains highly suspected, the physician should refer the child to a therapist or other professional who is trained in the diagnostic evaluation of abuse. Support should be given to the child during the interview, whether or not the child discloses abuse. If the child discloses abuse for the first time, the physician should acknowledge the difficulty children have in discussing their abuse and let the child know that he/she is interested in the child's well-being and safety.

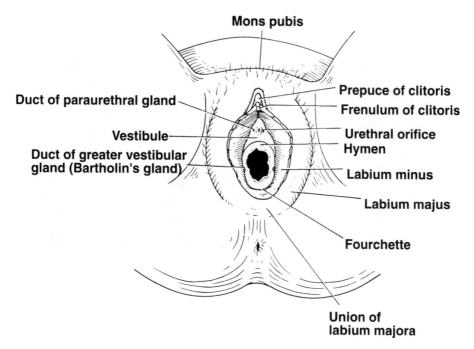

Mons pubis

Duct of paraurethral gland

Prepuce of clitoris

Frenulum of clitoris

Vestibule

Urethral orifice

Hymen

Duct of greater vestibular gland (Bartholin's gland)

Labium minus

Labium majus

Fourchette

Union of labium majora

FIG 74-1
The vulva. [From Snell R, Smith M: Clinical Anatomy for Emergency Medicine, St. Louis, 1993, Mosby–Year Book.]

THE PHYSICAL EXAMINATION

All sexually abused children deserve a physical examination to look for evidence of injury, to assess for the presence of sexually transmitted infections, and, if appropriate, to reassure the patient of his/her physical well-being. The examination of the prepubertal girl is noninvasive and does not involve an internal vaginal/cervical examination. Prepubertal children who require an internal examination for bleeding or a suspicion of a vaginal foreign body are best examined under general anesthesia in the operating room. A pelvic examination is recommended for the sexually abused adolescent. However, not all abused adolescents can tolerate an internal examination, and each case should be individually considered. The child may be given the choice of whether to have a supportive adult in the room for the examination. At no time should physical force be used to complete an examination. The genital and anal examination are done in the context of a complete physical examination.

Since the "discovery" of child sexual abuse as a medical problem, much attention has been focused on describing normal and abnormal prepubertal genital anatomy. The examination of boys is generally straightforward, because most physicians are comfortable examining the penis and scrotum of young boys. The anatomy of young girls is more variable and is often "deferred" during the routine physical examination, making this examination more difficult for many physicians. Both the anatomy and physiology of the female genitalia is largely influenced by hormonal changes throughout childhood, so that individual patients will have enormous variation in the appearance of the genitalia depending on their age.

In the prepubertal girl, the examination focuses on vulvar anatomy, including the labia majora, labia minora, clitoris, urethra, hymen, fossa navicularis, and posterior fourchette (Fig. 74-1).

Some specialists use a colposcope, which is an instrument that provides an excellent light source, magnification, and ability to photograph or videotape the examination. Colposcopic examination is not essential for the completion of the physical examination. The child is usually

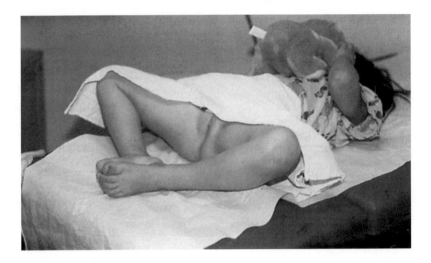

FIG 74-2

Frog-leg position with bottom feet touching. [From Chadwick DL, Berkowitz CD, Kerns D, et al: Color Atlas of Child Sexual Abuse, St. Louis, 1989, Mosby–Year Book.]

examined in the frog-legged position, which involves the child lying in a supine position with the ankles together and the knees abducted (Fig. 74-2). The vulva is best visualized using labial traction, in which the lower portion of the labia majora are gently grabbed between the thumbs and index fingers and the labia are pulled laterally, posteriorly, and toward the examiner. This examination should not hurt the patient.

In the normal prepubertal child, the vulvar mucosa appears slightly erythematous due to the normal appearance of the vasculature in the relatively thin tissue. The labia majora are less prominent, and the labia minora are thin. They meet posteriorly to form the posterior fourchette. There is great variation in the appearance of the hymenal tissue and configuration of the hymenal orifice in young girls. Generally, the hymen is thin and may be translucent, with a lacy vascular pattern. In other children, a normal hymen may appear redundant and more opaque. Hymenal types are generally classified by both the shape of the tissue and the appearance of the opening. Findings are described based on their location in relation to a clock face with 12:00 at the ventral position. Hymens are described as cresentic, annular, septated, cribiform, or microperforate, depending on the location of the tissue and the appearance of the orifice. Unlike the previously

mentioned configurations, an imperforate hymen is abnormal and requires surgical correction. The anal anatomy of infants and young children is the same in both boys and girls. It should appear as a separate opening on the perineum, with symmetric, thin, radiating rugae. Anal tags in the midline position are common and are not necessarily pathologic. The anus should be examined for a brisk wink reflex, lacerations, discharge, bruises, tags out of the midline, or other evidence of trauma. Children with stool in the rectal vault may exhibit anal dilation during examination. This finding should not be considered abnormal.

Only a small minority of children who have been sexually abused have physical findings that are diagnostic of sexual abuse. Even in legally confirmed child sexual abuse cases, a normal examination is common. Many abusive acts do not cause physical injury to the child, and the healing of mucosal injuries is fairly rapid and often quite complete. Subtle changes in hymenal configuration are difficult to interpret if the child's genital anatomy has not been previously documented. Consensus regarding the specificity of findings has not been formalized to date, although certain findings are considered diagnostic of abuse. These findings include the identification of semen, sperm, or acid phosphatase; fresh genital injuries in the absence of an adequate accidental history; the identification of gonorrhea or syphilis other than congenital infection; and transected or absent hymenal tissue without a history of previous known accidental injury or surgery. Although other findings may be suggestive of sexual abuse, caution should be taken in ascribing certainty to the diagnosis based on physical findings alone. A number of medical conditions have been mistaken for sexual abuse, including lichen sclerosus et atrophicus, vulvar hemangiomas and nevi, diaper dermatitis, urethral prolapse, Crohn's disease, straddle injury, and others. Anal injuries are uncommon in sexually abused children. Other than acute injuries that are not otherwise explained, caution is again recommended in interpreting anal findings.

LABORATORY EVALUATION

Universal screening for forensic evidence and/or sexually transmitted diseases is not necessary. Children who are abused within 72 hours of the most recent assault should be considered for forensic studies, although no criteria exist for the completion of "rape kits" in young children. Gonorrhea, syphilis, chlamydia, and other sexually transmitted infections are uncommon in asymptomatic prepubertal children. The decision to test for sexually transmitted infections should be based on the history of contact, characteristics of the alleged perpetrator, patient symptoms, and physical findings. The standard of care for identifying gonorrhea, chlamydia, and herpes simplex virus in prepubertal children is by culture. For children who require sexually transmitted disease testing, gonorrhea cultures should be obtained from the rectum, genitals, and pharynx. Chlamydia cultures are obtained from the rectum and genitals. Universal screening for syphilis, hepatitis, and HIV is not recommended at this time. When done, positive syphilis screens should be confirmed with specific treponemal tests, and HIV testing should be done only after appropriate counseling. For most patients, prophylactic antibiotics are not necessary. Pregnancy prevention is occasionally indicated for adolescents.

DOCUMENTATION AND REPORTING

Proper documentation of the medical evaluation can be essential for the future protection of the child. The patient's history and physical examination should be accurately recorded, because medical records of child abuse cases are often subpoened for either civil or criminal court. Any physician who has been embarrassed by having to review an inadequate medical record in a courtroom recognizes the importance of proper documentation. The history should contain as much detail as possible, using the child's exact words to describe the abusive events. A detailed description of the child's genital anatomy should be recorded. Recording "normal genitals" or "hymen intact" is not appropriate, because these terms are not objective descriptions of anatomy and provide no useful information.

Because the diagnosis of sexual abuse usually is based on the child's history, the conclusion drawn from the medical evaluation needs to be carefully written. Diagnostic injuries or sexually transmitted diseases are not commonly identified, and a normal examination does not exclude the possibility of abuse. Furthermore, the ultimate determination of whether sexual abuse has occurred depends on a multidisciplinary evaluation. The legal determination of abuse is decided in the courts. The child's best interest is served when the physician simply summarizes the historical and physical findings and indicates whether these are suggestive of, consistent with, or unrelated to sexual abuse. In a few instances, the medical findings are diagnostic of sexual abuse. In those cases, it is proper to state this conclusion in the medical record.

The decision to report suspected sexual abuse to child welfare and/or the police is based on a reasonable professional *suspicion* that sexual abuse may have occurred. Reporting laws vary by state, but they generally require a suspicion of abuse for reporting, not proof that abuse has occurred. As mandated reporters, physicians are required to use their education, experience, and good judgement to report reasonable suspicions. All reporting statutes protect mandated reporters from civil liabilities, assuming reports are made in good faith, and not as a malicious attack against an individual. Relatively mild criminal laws, primarily misdemeanors, exist for failing to report suspected abuse cases. Physicians are not exempt from filing reports of suspected abuse based on principles of doctor-patient confidentiality. The family should be informed of the decision to report. Not sharing this information will only serve to foster mistrust and may have negative consequences for the ongoing doctor-patient relationship. In discussing the case with the parents, the physician should remain objective and nonaccusatory. The doctor should not attempt to assign blame or determine guilt or innocence of the parents or other individuals; rather, the focus should be on the need to treat the child and ensure his/her future protection.

Reports regarding child abuse are made to child protective services and/or law enforcement, depending on the circumstances of the case. In general, it is the responsibility of child protective services to investigate abuse that occurs in the child's home or by a caretaker of the child. Child protective service agencies are responsible for ensuring the ongoing safety of the child. Law enforcement's responsibility is in investigating crime. Because all forms of sexual abuse are generally considered crimes, police involvement is common in these cases. Physicians should have an understanding of the reporting laws in their state of practice. Community resources, such as the local child welfare agency or district attorney's office, usually are available to the physician who has questions

related to reporting. Finally, physicians must recognize that involvement in child sexual abuse cases occasionally will result in a subpoena to testify in court. Although few physicians are comfortable in the role of a fact or expert witness, physician testimony is often necessary in either civil or criminal court. Meticulous documentation of the medical evaluation will be of great assistance to the practitioner who is asked to recall details of an examination that was completed in the distant past.

MENTAL HEALTH ISSUES

All sexually abused children require a mental health evaluation, and the majority are believed to benefit from some form of ongoing counseling or therapy. A variety of therapeutic approaches are available for children and families in need of ongoing treatment, including insight-oriented therapy, psychodynamic therapy, behavioral therapy, and individual and group therapy. Unfortunately, empiric data comparing the treatment outcomes of different forms of therapy are lacking. Regardless of the treatment type, the therapist chosen should have training and experience in child sexual abuse, development, and psychology. The physician may serve as a resource for both the child and the family and should maintain a supportive role as the child's advocate after the abuse is recognized and reported.

SUGGESTED READINGS

Adams JA, Harper K, Knudson S, Revilla J: Examination findings in legally confirmed child sexual abuse: It's normal to be normal, *Pediatrics* 94:310–317, 1994.

American Academy of Pediatrics Committee on Adolescence: Rape and the adolescent, *Pediatrics* 81:595–597, 1988.

American Academy of Pediatrics Committee on Child Abuse and Neglect: Guidelines for the evaluation of sexual abuse of children, *Pediatrics* 87:254–260, 1991.

Bays J, Chadwick D: Medical diagnosis of the sexually abused child, *Child Abuse Neglect* 17:91–110, 1993.

Bays J, Jenny C: Genital and anal conditions confused with child sexual abuse trauma, *Am J Dis Child* 144:1319–1322, 1990.

Finkelhor D: *A source book on child sexual abuse,* Beverly Hills, 1986, Sage Publications.

Giardino AP, Finkel MA, Giardino ER, Seidl T, Ludwig S: *A practical guide to the evaluation* of sexual abuse in the prepubertal child, Newbury Park, 1992, Sage Publications.

Guidelines for the clinical evaluation of child and adolescent sexual abuse: Position statement of the American Academy of Child and Adolescent Psychiatry, *J Am Acad Child Adolesc Psychiatry* 27:655–657, 1988.

Krugman RD: Recognition of sexual abuse in children, *Pediatr Rev* 8:25–31, 1986.

Ludwig S: Psychosocial emergencies: Child abuse. In Fleischer GR, Ludwig S, editors: *Textbook of pediatric emergency medicine,* ed 3, Baltimore, 1993, Williams & Wilkins.

Sgroi SM: *Handbook of clinical intervention in child sexual abuse,* Lexington, 1982, Lexington Books.

III

Cardiology

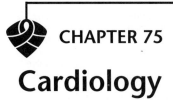

CHAPTER 75

Cardiology

Anthony C. Chang
Bernard J. Clark III

CARDIOLOGY AND THE PRIMARY CARE PHYSICIAN

The primary care physician is often the first medical person to identify a cardiac problem and after referral is responsible for following up the patient in conjunction with the cardiologist. The purpose of this chapter is to present some important, common problems in pediatric cardiology, which will aid the physician in 1) recognizing problems; 2) heightening the awareness of potential problems; and 3) answering some routine office practice questions that arise when dealing with the pediatric patient with heart disease. The following topics are covered: congestive heart failure (CHF), surgical treatments of congenital heart disease; and issues surrounding the handling of fever and preventing bacterial endocarditis, Kawasaki disease, acute rheumatic fever, mitral valve prolapse, hyperlipidemias, and irregular rhythms.

Congestive Heart Failure

Heart failure in infancy and childhood represents a clinical syndrome that reflects the inability of the myocardium to meet the metabolic requirements of the body. Most commonly, failure results from excessive volume overload associated with left-to-right shunts, valvular insufficiency, and iatrogenic causes. Excessive pressure overload (as seen in valvular stenosis, coarctation or interruption of the aorta, systemic hypertension, and pulmonary hypertension) is the next most common cause. Following these conditions are primary myocardial dysfunction from myocarditis, cardiomyopathies, or metabolic and endocrine abnormalities (hypoxemia, sepsis, anemia, hypoglycemia, and electrolyte abnormalities). Finally, rhythm abnormalities from either tachyarrhythmias (supraventricular or ventricular) or severe complete heart block may cause heart failure.

Excessive volume and pressure-loading situations predominate in the infant as causes of CHF. After the child reaches 1 year of age, rheumatic heart disease, bacterial endocarditis, endomyocardial disease, myocarditis, and severe cardiac arrhythmias as well as complications from surgical repair of heart malformations are frequent causes of CHF.

The earliest onset of CHF occurs in the hypoplastic left-heart syndrome, interrupted aortic arch or severe coarctation of the aorta, or severe myocardial disease. Most infants with septal defects or patent ductus arteriosus, endocardial cushion defects, unobstructed anomalous pul-

TABLE 75-1
Causes of Congestive Heart Failure by Age

IN UTERO	
Arrhythmias	Supraventricular tachycardia, atrial flutter, atrial fibrillation, ventricular tachycardia, complete heart block
Volume overload	Atrioventricular valve regurgitation in common atriventricular canal defect or Ebstein anomaly, atriovenous malformations
Primary myocardial disease	Endocardial fibroelastosis, congenital cardiomyopathy, myocarditis, glycogen storage disease
Secondary causes	Rhesus isoimmune disease, feto-maternal and twin-twin transfusion, thalassemia, hypoplastic anemia
NEWBORN AND INFANT	
Volume overload	Large left-to-right shunt: ventricular septal defect, single ventricle physiology without pulmonary stenosis, common atrioventricular canal, pulmonary or tricuspid valve regurgitation, posterior descending artery, aorto-pulmonary window, truncus arteriosus, arterial venous malformation
Pressure overload	Left-sided obstructive lesions (e.g., hypoplastic left heart syndrome, aortic valve stenosis, coarctation of the aorta, interrupted aortic arch), obstructed total anomalous pulmonary venous connection
Arrhythmias	Supraventricular tachycardia, atrial flutter, atrial fibrillation, ventricular tachycardia, complete heart block
Primary myocardial disease	Endocardial fibroelastosis, congenital cardiomyopathy, viral myocarditis, glycogen storage disease
Secondary causes	Asphyxia, sepsis, metabolic (e.g., hypoglycemia, hypocalcemia)
CHILDHOOD	
Residual cardiac defects following surgery	
Volume overload	Residual left-to-right shunts valvar insufficiency, especially aortic and mitral (or left av valve after CCAVC repair)
Pressure overload	Residual RV or LV outflow tract obstruction progressive development of sub-aortic membrane
Myocardial dysfunction	Ventricular dysfunction after atrial switch procedure for TGA or modified Fontan for single ventricle repair (especially if RV is the systemic ventricle)
Acquired heart disease	Viral myocarditis, infective endocarditis, rheumatic fever, Kawasaki syndrome, collagen vascular disease, neuromuscular disease, cardiomyopathy (doxorubicin induced, HIV infection), systemic hypertension, renal disease, thyroid disorders, congenitally acquired syndromes (Marfans, Hurlers, Noonans), pulmonary hypertension, primary or secondary to lung disease

monary venous connections, and less severe coarctation of the aorta usually do not develop CHF until the second week of life or later. Except for newborns with transient myocardial ischemia from perinatal stress causing CHF, patients with anatomic heart disease generally improve only slightly and should be referred immediately for complete evaluation (Table 75-1).

Clinical Manifestations of Congestive Heart Failure

Growth failure may be a sign of CHF in the infant and young child. Feeding difficulties combined with respiratory distress often preclude attainment of adequate nutritional balance. A history of easy fatigability, dyspnea on exertion, or failure to keep up with siblings or peers suggests the presence of CHF. Recurrent pulmonary infec-

tions may be a result of overperfused lungs from large left-to-right shunting defects.

Upon initial examination, the general state of health or illness usually can be readily determined. A baby with reduced oxygen delivery to the tissues, whether from cyanotic heart disease or CHF, will show little spontaneous movement. Dysmorphism of face or body may suggest one of many syndromes associated with congenital heart disease such as Down syndrome (endocardial cushion defect or ventricular septal defect), Turner syndrome (coarctation of the aorta, bicuspid aortic valve), Noonan syndrome (pulmonic valve stenosis), and fetal alcohol syndrome (septal defects and tetralogy of Fallot).

Blood pressure measurements should be obtained in all four extremities for every infant and child evaluated for congenital heart disease to

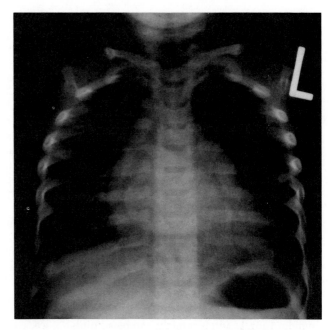

FIG 75-1
Chest radiograph in a patient with heart failure shows enlarged heart and increased pulmonary vascular.

rule in or out the presence of a coarctation of the aorta or other arch abnormality. A heart rate of more than 160 beats per minute in an infant or 100 beats per minute in an older child at rest is suggestive of increased adrenergic tone in response to diminished cardiac output. Tachypnea typically is a part of the clinical picture of CHF. Rapid, shallow respirations with flaring of the alae nasi and retractions with wheezes are characteristic of pulmonary overcirculation. Rales, a late finding in the infant, can be heard in the older child who may also have dyspnea on exertion, orthopnea, and a chronic cough. Hepatomegaly, jugular venous distention, and peripheral edema are all signs of elevated central venous pressure and accompanying CHF.

Examination of the cardiovascular system may reveal specific abnormalities. Palpation of the pulses in upper and lower extremities, an essential part of the examination, can be diagnostic of coarctation of the aorta or one of the various interruption complexes, as well as generalized low-output states in which all pulses are diminished. The heart may be enlarged to palpation or percussion, which will be confirmed with chest radiography (Fig. 75-1). A third heart sound may be present indicating decreased ventricular compliance. Murmurs may suggest an etiology but definitive diagnosis will be made in conjunction with a cardiologist. Auscultation of the rhythm

may suggest an arrhythmia, which can be documented with an electrocardiogram (ECG).

The infant or child with the spectrum of abnormalities previously described requires immediate attention. Such a patient is in a tenuous position and his or her condition may rapidly deteriorate. Therefore, when the diagnosis of possible congenital heart disease with CHF is entertained, the patient is best served by referral to a pediatric cardiologist.

Management of Congestive Heart Failure

Treatment of heart failure includes supplemental oxygen and placement of an intravenous line to aid in drug administration. The patient should be positioned with the head and shoulders elevated to decrease pulmonary blood volume by increasing peripheral pooling. An arterial blood gas analysis should be performed to evaluate acid/base status. If severe metabolic acidosis (pH less than 7.2) is found, bicarbonate therapy should be instituted. Additionally, if respiratory insufficiency or failure is confirmed, positive-pressure mechanical ventilation, which may improve both respiratory and cardiovascular function, should be instituted. It may be difficult in the infant or young child to separate sepsis or pulmonary infection from CHF, and in these circumstances antibiotics may be administered after appropriate cultures have been performed.

TABLE 75-2
Digitalization Schedule for Pediatric Patients (Intramuscular or Oral)*

AGE	WEIGHT (g)	TOTAL DOSE OF DIGITALIS† (µg/kg)
Premature infants	50–1000	20
	1000–1500	25
	1500–2000	30
	2000–2500	30–40
Term to 1 mo		60
1 mo to 2 yr		60–80
2 yr to 10–12 yr		40–60

*The intravenous dose is 75% of oral or intramuscular.
†No dose greater than 1.5 mg.

In most CHF, regardless of the underlying cause, initial pharmacologic therapy will include digoxin and diuretic therapy. Diuretics decrease blood volume and intrapulmonary fluid. Furosemide, 1 mg/kg intravenously, can be administered in the first 24 hours with a dramatic improvement in respiratory status. Because of the kaliuretic effects of the diuretics, serum potassium levels should be monitored during initial therapy and supplemental potassium administered as necessary.

The mainstay of long-term medical management of CHF remains the use of digitalis to improve myocardial function. The digitalization schedule is outlined in Table 75-2. If the patient is in mild or moderate heart failure, the digitalis may be given intramuscularly. In cases of severe CHF, in which absorption of medication from the tissues would be variable and possibly incomplete, the digitalis doses are given intravenously with a 25% reduction in the calculated intramuscular dose. A lower total dose is used in the presence of myocarditis or cardiomyopathy due to an increased predisposition to arrhythmias. A total digitalis dose is given over 24 hours: half initially, one quarter in 8 hours, and the final one quarter in another 8 hours. The patient is monitored for changes in heart rate and rhythm during this period. The daily maintenance dose is one quarter the total digitalis dose divided every 12 hours. The parenteral form of the drug contains 100 µg/mL, whereas the oral preparation contains 50 µg/mL.

The oral bioavailability of digoxin is less than 100% (usually 70%) because it is incompletely absorbed from the gastrointestinal (GI) tract. Disease states or drugs that are characterized by hypermotility may decrease digoxin absorption, whereas drugs that retard GI motility tend to increase absorption. Taking digoxin with meals does not affect the total amount of digoxin absorbed; however, it does retard the rate of absorption. After the administration of digoxin tablets, peak serum levels are reached in 1 to 1½ hours, whereas with intravenous injections, peak levels are obtained almost immediately. After approximately 8 hours, the distribution phase of the drug is completed and the central and peripheral compartments are in equilibrium.

Digitalis Toxicity

A relatively high incidence of toxic manifestations has accompanied the widespread use of digoxin. Intoxication has been reported to be as high as 20% in patients receiving the glycosides. Although the most common and earliest side effects are related to the GI tract (anorexia, nausea, vomiting, abdominal discomfort), disorders of cardiac rhythm are the first manifestation in one third of patients and can be seen in up to 80% of patients with other toxic effects.

Certain ECG abnormalities occur more frequently than others, although none are pathognomonic of digoxin toxicity. The most common abnormalities include bigeminy, multifocal premature ventricular beats, and paroxysmal atrial tachycardia with block. A prolonged PR interval is not a sign of digoxin toxic effect, but it is a sign of digoxin effect. Toxic response may be precipitated by several factors. These include 1) potassium losses (diuretics, adrenocorticosteroids, cathartics); 2) hypercalcemia (usually only with very high serum levels); 3) hypoxemia (accounts for high incidence of toxic effects in patients with cor pulmonale); and 4) renal insufficiency, because digoxin is excreted primarily by this route. A patient with signs or symptoms that can be ascribed to digoxin toxic effects should be referred to a cardiologist.

Although most studies demonstrate elevated digoxin levels (more than 2.0 ng/mL) in patients with digoxin toxic effects, a number of patients with apparent toxic effects have levels in the therapeutic range (1.0 to 2.0 ng/mL). Although the likelihood of toxic effects increases with increasing concentration, there is no precise value that clearly separates toxic from nontoxic levels. Therefore, the serum digoxin level is not, in itself, sufficient for a diagnosis of digoxin toxic

TABLE 75-3
Surgical Procedures for Congenital Heart Defects

LESION	PROCEDURE
Aortic stenosis	Valvulotomy, prosthetic valve insertion (tissue or mechanical)
Pulmonary stenosis	Valvulotomy
Coarctation of aorta	Resection and end-to-end anastomosis, patch angioplasty, subclavian flap angioplasty
VSD	Patch closure through right atrium or ventricle
ASD	Patch or suture closure through right atrium
Endocardial cushion defect	Patch closure of ASD and VSD, division of common AV valve and construction of mitral and tricuspid valves
Tetralogy of Fallot	Various shunt procedures for palliation; patch closure of VSD, relief of right ventricular outflow, obstruction with valvulotomy and outflow patch, with or without resection of infundibular muscle
Transposition of great arteries	Mustard or Senning repairs (atrial baffle and venous return diversion); arterial switch with transplantation of coronary arteries
Tricuspid atresia	Fontan procedure (anastomosis of right atrium to pulmonary artery either directly or via valved or nonvalved conduits)
Pulmonary atresia with associated lesions	Various shunt procedures for palliation; Rastelli procedure (valved or nonvalved conduit from right ventricular outflow tract to pulmonary artery)

response. However, levels may be of value 1) as an adjunct in the diagnosis of toxic effects; 2) in the evaluation of an accidental ingestion; 3) in the assessment of the adequacy of digitalization; and 4) in the management of digitalization of patients with renal insufficiency.

Surgical Treatment of Congenital Heart Disease

The terms *definitive operation, corrective surgery,* and *total repair* are misleading; a definitive repair may be accomplished but residual defects may persist and sequelae or late complications may develop that may jeopardize the well-being of the patient. Therefore lifelong cardiac follow-up should be provided by an experienced cardiologist. Because the events leading to cardiac surgery begin with the primary care physician and because the patient is generally returned to his/her care, it is important for the physician not only to have an understanding of the preoperative anatomy of the defect and knowledge of the types of surgical procedures (Table 75-3), but also of the presence, extent, and likelihood of development of postoperative residua, sequelae, or complications (Table 75-4).

Curative procedures are ones in which no residua or sequelae exist. Today these procedures are confined to division of a patent ductus arteriosus in a patient without pulmonary hypertension and closure of a secundum atrial septal defect (although this may be associated with conduction and rhythm disturbances).

Palliative procedures include shunt operations for tetralogy of Fallot and other lesions associated with inadequate pulmonary blood flow. Valvulotomy for valve stenosis only can be considered palliative surgery, because residual or recurrent stenosis, valvular regurgitation, and continued predisposition for endocarditis remain. Furthermore, prosthetic valves do not grow and if inserted in children will require another operation (possibly more than once) before the patient attains adult size. Both synthetic and tissue valves are at risk for thrombus formation and endocarditis, whereas tissue valves (porcine and pericardial) are associated with calcifications and early degeneration when inserted in children.

Anatomic corrections include closure of ventricular septal defects, correction of endocardial cushion defects, intracardiac repair of tetralogy of Fallot, and arterial switch procedures for complete transposition of the great arteries. Physiologic correction (diversion of blood flow as opposed to anatomic correction) is best represented by the Mustard and Senning procedures (atrial repairs) for complete transposition of the great arteries.

TABLE 75-4
Postoperative Residua, Sequelae, or Late Complications

LESION	RESIDUA, SEQUELAE, COMPLICATIONS
Aortic stenosis	Residual or recurrent stenosis, aortic insufficiency; prosthetic valve dysfunction or stenosis; thrombosis; life-long anticoagulation
VSD	Residual VSD with congestive heart failure; poor ventricular function; AV block; pulmonary vascular disease
Endocardial cushion defect	Mitral, tricuspid regurgitation/stenosis; pulmonary vascular disease; AV block; atrial arrhythmias; residual left-to-right shunt
Tetralogy of Fallot	Residual VSD or pulmonary stenosis; ventricular arrhythmias; AV block; pulmonary tricuspid insufficiency; ventricular dysfunction
Transposition of great arteries	Atrial repair: atrial arrhythmias and conduction disturbances, ventricular dysfunction, caval and/or pulmonary venous obstruction, pulmonary stenosis, tricuspid regurgitation; arterial switch: semilunar valve insufficiency, coronary artery ostia, narrow great vessel stenosis at anastomosis site
Rastelli repair	Conduit stenosis; valve stenosis or insufficiency
Fontan repair	Elevated right atrial pressures at rest and with exercise; abnormal cardiac response to exercise

Despite an initial postoperative success, important residua, sequelae, and late complications have been reported in many of these lesions; the most common of which are presented in Table 75-4. Children, after undergoing repair of coarctation of the aorta, have risks of systemic hypertension as well as of recoarctation. From a recent study of 87 patients seen 5 to 15 years after repair, 14% had recoarctation and 23% had systemic hypertension. In addition to these risks are stenosis and regurgitation of an accompanying bicuspid aortic valve and cerebral complications due to aneurysms of the circle of Willis. Right ventriculotomy used in the repair of several malformations may result in right ventricular dysfunction or conduction disturbances. The conduction defects are the result of peripheral scarring, which may also become a focus of ventricular irritability. Ventricular septal defect closure may result in injury to the proximal conduction system with a late risk of heart block, which may be sudden and life threatening. Intra-atrial repair of transposition of the great arteries, atrial septal defects, and endocardial cushion defects may be associated with sinus node and atrioventricular node dysfunction as well as atrial arrhythmias such as supraventricular tachycardia, atrial flutter, and fibrillation.

Long-Term Postoperative Perspective
Long-term postoperative outlook for children and young adults with congenital heart disease varies. Three groups of patients must be considered: 1) patients who have undergone a definitive operation with no residual disease and no expectation of late complication or future surgery; 2) patients who have had successfully repaired cardiac lesions but in whom significant complications occur with some frequency and in whom further surgery might eventually be necessary; and 3) patients who have had either palliative or limited corrective operations, but who have severe residual disease for which no further palliative or definitive surgical therapy is possible.

Patients in the first group have had lesions such as atrial septal defect (ASD) of the secundum type, ventricular septal defect (VSD), patent ductus arteriosus, coarctation of the aorta, and total correction of tetralogy of Fallot repaired successfully without residua or sequelae. These patients may have normal exercise tolerance, physical examination, ECG, and chest radiographs. Little ambulatory management is required beyond an occasional checkup. No restriction need be placed on regular daily activity, including sports. Prophylaxis for bacterial endocarditis is obligatory in all of these patients except those who have had a patent ductus arteriosus closed. Patients with ASD or VSD closure should be treated prophylactically for 6 months to a year after complete closure to allow for patch endothelialization. Patients who have had a coarctation repair continue to require prophylaxis because of the high incidence (approximately 80%) of an associated bicuspid aortic valve. The low additional risks of having offspring with congenital heart disease as compared with the general population (2 to 4 per 100 vs approximately 1 per 1000, respectively) is the general problem. Although patients with uncomplicated complete repair of tetralogy of Fallot have done well 10 to 15 years after surgery, the long-term status of right and left ventricular function in patients undergoing repair in infancy is unknown.

The patients in the second group have had cardiac malformations corrected but have residua or complications as listed in Table 75-4. Patients with aortic stenosis treated with valvulotomy may develop restenosis or severe aortic insufficiency and require another operation (in as high as 50% of the cases). Some patients with repaired coarctation of the aorta will have systemic hypertension and a number of these will have evidence of recoarctation. Previously competent or minimally regurgitant atrioventricular valves may show progressive insufficiency and require replacement. Although Mustard and Senning repairs of transposition of the great arteries yield physiologic correction, the right ventricle continues to support the systemic circulation and may show progressive dysfunction. The arterial switch procedure theoretically avoids this risk. The operation involves transsecting the great vessels above the semilunar valves and "switching" the arteries so that the pulmonary artery is now anterior, attached to the right ventricle while the aorta is posterior and attached to the left ventricle. The coronary arteries must also be "switched" to the new aorta. However, this procedure is associated with occasional semilunar valve insufficiency and coronary artery ostia narrowing. In patients with conduits, stenosis from pseudointima formation ("peel") or from patient growth requires replacement. Any residua or anomaly may be the site of endocarditis regardless of its functional severity. Periodic evaluation for potential rhythm disturbances, residual lesions, prosthetic valve dysfunction, hypertension, and myocardial dysfunction must be carried out at intervals commensurate with the patient's clinical status and medical or surgical therapy instituted when necessary. Prophylaxis for endocarditis is obligatory in all these patients. These patients may participate in sports activities as long as it is not in a competitive (organized sports) role.

The final group of patients are those with severe residual disease, usually with complex intracardiac anatomy and inadequate pulmonary blood flow. These patients may have had one or more "shunt" procedures for palliation, which may indeed be the only procedures possible. Other patients may have residual pulmonary vascular obstructive disease from previous large systemic-pulmonary anastomoses or despite correction of the basic cardiac defect, such as a large VSD, endocardial cushion defect, or transposition of the great arteries with a VSD. Still others may have chronic progressive myocardial disease and CHF; in such patients no anatomic problem remains that can be corrected surgically. Shunts may be revised or a different anastomosis utilized. A corrective procedure may now be available for certain children previously receiving palliation. If no further surgical procedures are possible or warranted, medical management must be carefully monitored. This includes appropriate treatment of CHF and rhythm disturbances, prophylaxis against bacterial endocarditis, and observation and therapy for progressive polycythemia from persistent hypoxemia (the hematocrit should be measured frequently by venipuncture method and if found to be in excess of 65%, exchange transfusion should be performed).

Fever

Children with congenital heart disease and fever pose challenging problems for the primary physician. In addition to the common viral and bacterial infections that afflict all children, some children with congenital heart disease, particularly those with congestive failure or the small group of patients with heterotaxia syndrome and splenic dysfunction, are at increased risk for serious and even life-threatening bacterial infections. Thus the evaluation of such patients with fever must include an understanding of the underlying heart disease, a willingness to search for a specific cause of the fever, and avoidance of the indiscriminate use of oral antibiotics, which can often confuse and delay diagnosis.

When possible, the treatment of the common respiratory and GI tract infections of childhood should be managed with the same approach taken with children without congenital heart disease: administration of antipyretics and fluids and observation. In small children and infants a search for the specific bacterial source for the fever should be performed. This evaluation should include a chest radiograph if there is tachypnea or abnormal findings on examination of the chest. Often it is difficult to separate evidence of congestive failure from an infectious infiltrate with radiography. In these situations, it is often necessary to admit the patient to the hospital for observation and, if the suspicion of infection is high, for intravenous administration of antibiotics.

If a patient is sick enough to require antibiotic therapy, a blood culture drawn prior to the commencement of antibiotics can be helpful in confirming the presence of a bacterial vs. viral infection and can act as a guide to appropriate antibiotic choice. Because the incidence of endocarditis in young children and infants with congenital heart disease is small, the presence of a positive blood culture should not be taken as evidence of endocarditis. The duration of antibiotics can be limited to treatment of the specific infection. If there is a suspicion of endocarditis, the decision for extended treatment should be made in consultation with the patient's cardiologist.

Subacute Bacterial Endocarditis

Bacterial endocarditis must be ruled out in persistently febrile older children or in patients of any age who have undergone cardiac operations. Often older children will present with only a history of malaise or mild anorexia and weight loss and not have the physical stigmata classically described, such as systemic signs of embolization in the form of splinter hemorrhages or abnormal findings on funduscopic examination. Changes in the character of cardiac murmurs or the appearance of a new murmur should raise suspicion. Laboratory evidence will include an elevated sedimentation rate and, often, evidence of mild anemia and hematuria secondary to an immune complex nephritis. The sine qua non of subacute bacterial endocarditis (SBE) is a positive result of blood culture.

Various regimens have been described to properly gather sufficient blood cultures to rule out SBE. Some guidelines suggest that at least 1% of the patient's blood volume should be cultured over 48 hours, whereas others believe that three properly obtained blood cultures will be sufficient to pick up 97% of cases of SBE. It is now clear that blood cultures can be obtained at any time, because the bacteremia of SBE is continuous.

Sterile surgical gloves should be worn when obtaining blood cultures to rule out SBE and the skin carefully cleansed, because a blood culture result often suggests there was contamination by skin flora. Generally, it is desirable to wait for the identification of an organism prior to commencing antibiotic treatment. In the ill patient, however, therapy with anti-staphylococcal penicillin and an aminoglycoside can be started. Echocardiography has been very helpful in identifying vegetations and should be routinely done in any patient with positive results of blood culture and a suspicion of endocarditis. Once an organism is identified and appropriate antibiotics chosen, the patient should be followed up closely for any sign of embolic phenomena from the breakup of a valvular vegetation.

Duration of treatment is 6 weeks of intravenous antibiotics. Most treatment schedules suggest that an aminoglycoside be added for the first 2 weeks of therapy. The only exception to 6 weeks of antibiotics would be the treatment of *Streptococcus viridans* endocarditis, which has been shown to be adequately treated with 4 weeks of penicillin.

Because the complications of SBE are often not predictable and can occur at any point in the treatment period, most patients should be monitored carefully in concert with a cardiologist skilled in pediatrics or should be referred to a major center for the duration of the antibiotic treatment.

Subacute Bacterial Endocarditis Prophylaxis

Table 75-5 outlines the indications for SBE prophylaxis and type and dose of antibiotic. In general these guidelines are based on the assumption that a surgical procedure that interrupts the epithelial or mucosal surface of an area normally contaminated by microorganisms should be preceded by a sufficiently large dose of antibiotic to provide a level adequate to prevent significant bacteremia. For this reason the antibiotic is guided by the predominant organism in the area to be operated on. The most common situation in which this antibiotic is used is prior to any dental procedure, including routine cleaning and scaling.

Patients who are receiving daily penicillin for either splenic dysfunction or rheumatic fever prophylaxis require a change in antibiotics to erythromycin for dental procedures because of the development of penicillin-resistant oral flora.

TABLE 75-5
American Heart Association Recommendations for Prophylaxis Against Infective Endocarditis*

FOR DENTAL PROCEDURES AND SURGERY OF THE UPPER RESPIRATORY TRACT		FOR GASTROINTESTINAL AND GENITOURINARY TRACT SURGERY AND INSTRUMENTATION	
Oral penicillin for most patients	Children less than 60 lb: 1 g of penicillin V 1 hr before procedure and then 500 mg 6 hr after initial dose.	Ampicillin plus gentamicin for most patients.	Timing of doses is same as for adults. Doses are ampicillin 50 mg/kg and gentamicin 2 mg/kg. Given 30 min before procedure, may repeat once 8 hr later.
Erythromycin for those allergic to penicillin (may also be selected for those receiving oral penicillin as continuous rheumatic fever prophylaxis)	20 mg/kg orally 1 hr before procedure and then 10 mg/kg 6 hr after initial dose.	Vancomycin plus gentamicin for patients allergic to penicillin.	Timing of doses is same as for adults. Doses are vancomycin 20 mg/kg and gentamicin 2 mg/kg.
Ampicillin plus gentamicin for those patients at higher risk of infective endocarditis (especially those with prosthetic heart valves) who are not allergic to penicillin	Doses are ampicillin 50 mg/kg, gentamicin 2 mg/kg, and penicillin V 500 mg (for children uncer 60 lb). Given 30 min before procedure, then penicillin V orally 6 hr after initial dose.	Amoxicillin (oral regimen) for minor or repetitive procedures in low-risk patients.	50 mg/kg 1 hr before procedure and then 25 mg/kg 6 hr after initial dose.
Vancomycin for higher-risk patients (especially those with prosthetic heart valves) who are allergic to penicillin	Vancomycin 20 mg/kg IV over 60 min, begun 60 min before procedure; no repeat dose is necessary.		

*Adapted from Committee on Rheumatic Fever and Infective Endocarditis. Reprinted with permission of the American Heart Association.

Note: In patients with compromised renal function, it may be necessary to modify or omit the second dose of antibiotics. Intramuscular injections may be contraindicated in patients receiving anticoagulants. Children's doses should not exceed adult doses.

Kawasaki Syndrome

Kawasaki syndrome, first described by Tomisaku Kawasaki, MD, of Japan in 1967, is a vasculitis syndrome that involves the medium and large arteries. It is an acute illness characterized by fever for 5 days and at least four of the five following criteria set by the Centers for Disease Control and Prevention: nonexudative, bilateral *conjunctivitis;* nonvesicular, polymorphous *rash; oral mucosal inflammation*—fissuring of lips, pharyngeal erythema, and "strawberry" tongue; *extremity changes*—erythema of palms and soles, desquamation of digits, induration of hands and feet, and transverse nail grooves ("Bow's lines"); and *cervical adenopathy*— usually unilateral and nonsuppurative (at least 1.5 cm or greater in diameter).

Kawasaki syndrome has stirred interest recently because of the potential life-threatening sequelae of coronary artery ectasia, aneurysm formation, and thrombotic occlusion. Coronary aneurysms occur in 15% to 25% of all patients with Kawasaki syndrome with a 1% fatality rate. Risk factors for the development of coronary aneurysms include: age less than 1 year, male sex, fever for more than 16 days, erythrocyte sedimentation rate (ESR) greater than 100, elevated ESR for more than 30 days, hemoglobin level less than 10 g/dL, white blood cell (WBC) count greater than 30,000, arrhythmia, cardiomegaly, and abnormal ECG.

Although epidemiologic data and clinical course seem to support an infectious cause, the exact cause of this disease is still not known. The annual incidence is 0.59 per 100,000 children less than 5 years of age, but there seems to be a seasonal peak in the spring and winter. Although 80% of cases occur in children less than 5 years of age, the peak incidence occurs in children between 12 and 24 months of age. Cases have been reported in patients as young as 2 months of age. In addition, Asians and blacks have higher incidence rates than whites.

Cardiovascular manifestations are not limited to coronary arteritis, and may include myocarditis, pericarditis, pericardial effusion, mitral regurgitation, AV conduction, inflammation, and aneurysm of peripheral arteries (most frequently involving the axillary, iliac, and renal arteries).

Noncardiovascular involvement includes myositis and myalgia, arthritis and arthralgia, urethritis and pyuria, aseptic meningitis, hydrops of the gallbladder, pancreatitis, hepatitis, diarrhea, and pneumonitis.

Diagnosis

Laboratory abnormalities include elevated ESR, elevated WBC count, mild anemia, rise in platelet count (usually in the second week); presence of C-reactive protein (CRP), elevated liver function tests, proteinuria, and cerebrospinal fluid (CSF) pleocytosis. Changes on chest radiographs include cardiomegaly. Changes on ECG include prolonged PR interval, reduced QRS voltages, ST segment changes, and flattened T waves. Findings on echocardiography include pericardial effusion, decreased shortening fraction, and coronary aneurysms.

The differential diagnosis includes Stevens-Johnson syndrome, juvenile rheumatoid arthritis, streptococcal infection, toxic shock syndrome, and other infections (including Epstein-Barr virus, measles, leptospirosis, and Rocky Mountain spotted fever).

The process of the illness starts with an acute phase, which lasts for 1 to 2 weeks, characterized by fever, rash, lethargy, and oral mucosal inflammation. This phase is followed by a subacute phase lasting 3 to 8 weeks. It is during this period that most of the coronary aneurysms occur. The convalescent phase lasts for the next 4 months.

Therapy

Initial therapy for Kawasaki syndrome includes intravenous gamma globulin and aspirin. A variety of gamma globulin regimens have been proposed. The two most common regimens are 2 g/kg intravenous gamma globulin once or 400 mg/kg/day for four doses. Adverse reactions to intravenous gamma globulin can include flushing, diaphoresis, and uncommonly hypotension. Usually infusions should be started at a rate of 0.5 mL/kg/hr for 15 minutes with a gradual increase every 15 minutes to a maximum rate of 4 mL/kg/hr.

Aspirin therapy is begun at the time of diagnosis at 80 to 100 mg/kg/day in divided doses. This can be reduced to low-dose aspirin, 3 to 5 mg/kg/day as a single dose when the patient becomes afebrile. Low-dose aspirin is continued until the sedimentation rate and platelet count return to normal, which may take several weeks.

After the initial period of illness, patients should be followed up with serial echocardiography and ECGs. Cardiac catheterization is used to study the coronary anatomy in detail in selected patients with clinical manifestations of myocardial infarction, ischemic changes on ECG, or echocardiographic evidence of decreased left ventricular function.

The natural course of the coronary aneurysms in Kawasaki syndrome is such that there can be a regression of these lesions in 1 to 2 years. Patients at high risk for coronary aneurysms that persist include those patients who have: fever for more than 21 days, age of onset more than 2 years, aneurysm diameter of more than 8 mm, and aneurysm shape of the saccular type.

The major cause of death appears to be cardiogenic shock caused by acute myocardial infarction. Other causes of death include congestive heart failure, rupture of coronary aneurysm, myocarditis, and arrhythmia.

The characteristic signs and symptoms of Kawasaki syndrome have prompted early recognition and therapeutic intervention by physicians. However, atypical and recurrent cases do occur and may confuse even the most astute clinician.

Children who have had Kawasaki syndrome may be at risk for coronary artery disease in the future, because mural thickening occurs even in the absence of aneurysmal formation. It is important therefore to remember Kawasaki syndrome as a coronary risk factor.

An aggressive approach to Kawasaki syndrome with early diagnosis and treatment is crucial to successful management of this serious illness.

Acute Rheumatic Fever

As recently as the 1920s, rheumatic fever was the leading cause of death in the pediatric population. Furthermore, sequelae from rheumatic fever often resulted in crippling heart disease. However, by the 1970s, rheumatic fever had become extremely rare in the industrialized world, with an incidence of less than one per 100,000 per year.

The recent resurgence of rheumatic fever has younger physicians eager to learn an unfamiliar disease. Outbreaks have occurred in several areas in the United States including Columbus and Akron, Ohio, Pittsburgh, and Salt Lake City. The reason for this recent comeback of rheumatic fever is not certain. Epidemiologic evidence suggests rheumatic fever to be a disease of poverty, because it is more commonly found in overcrowded urban areas and in underdeveloped countries.

It has been known since 1930 that rheumatic fever is caused by an antecedent group A streptococcal upper respiratory tract infection. Although there was a decline in the incidence of rheumatic fever concomitant with the introduction of antibiotics, many authorities do not support the notion that antibiotics were responsible for the disappearance of rheumatic fever.

A set of clinical and laboratory criteria was originally described by T. Duckett Jones in the 1940s and is now revised by the American Heart Association. The diagnosis of rheumatic fever is made if two major criteria or one major and two minor criteria plus evidence of a preceding group A streptococcal infection (e.g., scarlet fever, positive results of culture, elevated or rising streptococcal antibody titer such as ASO or anti-DNAse B) are present.

Major Manifestations

- Carditis (40% to 50%)
- Polyarthritis (60% to 85%): migratory, usually involving large joints
- Sydenham chorea (15%): purposeless, jerking movements occurring in convalescence
- Erythema marginatum (10%): evanescent, nonpruritic rash
- Subcutaneous nodules (2% to 10%): small nontender nodules along tendon sheaths

Minor Manifestations

- Clinical findings: arthralgia, fever, previous rheumatic fever or rheumatic heart disease
- Laboratory data: prolonged PR interval, positive acute phase reactants (ESR, CRP)

Carditis is the most important sequela of rheumatic fever. It can be manifested by a pathologic murmur, pericarditis, or congestive heart failure. Rheumatic heart disease involves the mitral valve in three fourths of the cases and involves the aortic valve in the remaining cases.

The differential diagnosis for rheumatic fever includes systemic lupus erythematosis, juvenile rheumatoid arthritis, infective endocarditis, collagen vascular diseases, infectious arthritis, serum sickness, or viral myopericarditis.

The treatment of acute rheumatic fever involves both eradicating the group A streptococcal infection and reducing the inflammation of arthritis and carditis. The recommendation for *primary eradication* from the Committee on Prevention of Rheumatic Fever of the American Heart Association is intramuscular benzathine penicillin G or oral penicillin V or erythromycin for 10 days. *Secondary prophylaxis,* or prevention of recurrence of disease in a patient who already had rheumatic fever, consists of daily penicillin or sulfadiazine orally or monthly benzathine penicillin G by injection. Children who have rheumatic heart disease and who need *SBE prophylaxis* should receive either erythromycin or vancomycin.

Bed rest and salicylates were and still are the mainstay of therapy for arthritis and carditis in rheumatic fever. Salicylates should not be started, however, until the diagnosis of rheumatic fever is certain. The use of steroids is controversial at present. Some authorities advocate the use of steroids for a short course only in the presence of severe carditis.

The implications of making a diagnosis of rheumatic fever in a patient are not insignificant. Prolonged antibiotic prophylaxis and extended bed rest are more than mere inconveniences. It is vital, however, for primary care physicians to recognize the resurgence of this disease that "licks the joints and bites the heart".

Mitral Valve Prolapse

In 1963 Barlow described a constellation of cardiac findings that has come to be known as mitral valve prolapse (MVP). The hallmarks of MVP on examination include a midsystolic to late systolic click and a systolic murmur. This condition is believed to be caused by redundant mitral valve tissue, which prolapses into the left atrial cavity during ventricular contraction. A great deal of interest has been focused on this problem because of associated symptoms in adults identified with MVP.

Mitral valve prolapse has been found in 1% to 6% of children of all ages. There is a 2:1 female-male ratio. A subset of patients show a familial incidence with approximately 45% of the children of an affected first-degree relative having MVP. The most common auscultatory abnormality in MVP is a midsystolic click and a late systolic murmur. These findings may vary from day to day. In children the murmur may be a honking musical sound, which is loudest just off the left midsternal border. A holosystolic murmur is less common. The diagnosis is confirmed by two-dimensional or M-mode echocardiography. The risk is highest in women in the third and fourth decade of life with a previous syncope or a positive family history of MVP and sudden death. Many of these patients have previous ECGs that show premature ventricular contractions, ventricular fibrillation, or ventricular tachycardia.

Although most children with MVP are asymptomatic, it is very disturbing for parents to find that their child has MVP, especially when they read of the small but significant incidence of lethal arrhythmias in adults with prolapse.

Evaluation of a child suspected of having MVP should include chest radiography, ECG, and echocardiography. In patients with a history of syncope, palpitations, or other symptoms suggesting an arrhythmia, a 24-hour Holter ECG and exercise stress testing may be done. Because of the small risk of SBE, only the patient with a systolic murmur should receive prophylactic antibiotics at the time of surgical procedures.

Chest Pain

One of the most difficult diagnostic dilemmas a pediatrician faces in the office is a patient's complaint of chest pain. Selbst found that 0.59% of all patient visits to the emergency room involved chest pain as a primary or secondary complaint. Patients seen in the office with this complaint tend to have chest pain of a subacute or chronic nature. In all patients with symptoms of chest pain it is important to elicit a thorough history of events surrounding the onset of chest pain as well as aggravating and relieving factors. Studies in emergency rooms and pediatric cardiology offices have shown that the most frequent causes of chest pain are noncardiac. Respiratory or bronchospastic, musculoskeletal, idiopathic, GI, and psychogenic causes are common. Historical and physical findings can lend to distinguishing cardiac from noncardiac chest pain. For example, a recent history of chest wall injury or reproducible chest wall tenderness is most consistent with chest pain of musculoskeletal cause. Patients with associated history of cough and fever are most likely to have a pneumonic or bronchospastic process; those with pain noted after meals have GI disorders.

The differential for cardiac chest pain in children includes inflammation of the myocardium or pericardium, arrhythmia, and structural abnormalities such as aortic stenosis, subaortic stenosis, coronary artery anomalies or coronary arteritis. A normal ECG and chest radiograph can rule out many of these possibilities.

Fyfe and Moodie reviewed patients referred to a pediatric cardiologist for evaluation of chest pain. They found the most common causes of cardiac chest pain to be myocarditis and pericarditis. Myocarditis most commonly follows a viral illness. Patients typically present with shortness of breath, nonspecific chest pain, anorexia, or malaise. Physical examination may reveal the presence of an S3 or gallop rhythm. Chest radiograph typically reveals cardiomegaly, although early in the illness it may reveal normal heart size. ECG reveals changes, most typically ST segment depression and T-wave abnormalities most notably in the inferior leads (II, III, aVF, V6, V7). In these patients, the myocardium is directly affected. Therefore, these patients should have echocardiographic assessment of ventricular function. The inflammation that causes the myocarditis also can directly affect the conduction system, and thus patients with myocarditis may present with arrhythmias. These arrhythmias tend to improve with resolution of the inflammation. In those patients who develop persistent cardiomyopathy, arrhythmias may persist.

In contrast, pericarditis more frequently presents with the acute onset of sharp chest pain, which is lessened by leaning forward. Pericarditis can result from infectious or autoimmune disorders. Physical examination reveals neck vein distention, pulsus paradoxus, and the presence of a friction rub, occasionally with both a systolic and diastolic component. These findings are caused by the presence of pericardial fluid collection resulting from inflammation of the pericardium. In the presence of a large pericardial effusion, ECG often reveals low-voltage QRS complexes. The ECG also can reveal ST-T wave changes, as in myocarditis. When a patient presents with such symptoms, a chest radiograph demonstrating cardiomegaly, or an ECG showing the abnormalities mentioned, referral to a cardiologist is warranted.

Myocarditis and pericarditis result subsequent to an inflammatory process. Most commonly this is a viral process, specifically an echo virus, most often coxsackie B. Viral titers may be helpful in determining specific cause. Other infectious causes include Lyme disease. If myocarditis is suspected in a patient who presents with complaint of chest pain and with a history of tick bite in an endemic area, it is recommended that Lyme titers be obtained. Other inflammatory causes include autoimmune disorders such as lupus erythematosus.

Chest pain in a child with a murmur may suggest left ventricular outflow tract obstruction caused by aortic valve stenosis or stenosis below the aortic valve, as in idiopathic hypertrophic subaortic stenosis. In these patients, chest pain occurs with exercise as a result of a limited ability to increase cardiac output because of a fixed obstruction. This limited response in cardiac output and a fall in systemic vascular resistance during exercise result in coronary underperfusion and subsequent myocardial ischemia. Physical findings in patients with aortic stenosis can include a systolic ejection click, a harsh systolic ejection murmur over the base of a the heart that radiates to the carotid arteries, and frequently a palpable thrill in the suprasternal notch. These patients can have either normal ECGs or ECGs suggestive of left ventricular hypertrophy.

Another variation of left ventricular outflow tract obstruction is hypertrophic cardiomyopathy. IHSS is an autosomal dominant disorder, and a thorough family history is helpful. These patients have a systolic murmur that is enhanced upon standing or subjection to the Valsalva maneuver. These maneuvers decrease left ventricular volume and thus increase the degree of outflow obstruction. Patients with a history of chest pain and a systolic murmur should be referred to a cardiologist.

The diagnosis of anomalies of the coronary arteries such as anomalous left coronary artery or coronary arteritis is uncommon, but when present, the ECG is almost invariably abnormal, with evidence of left ventricular hypertrophy and abnormal ST segments or inverted T waves in the left precordial leads. Most patients with anomalous left coronary artery present in infancy in a shocklike state. It is unusual for this anomaly to present in childhood. When a young child presents with chest pain it is important to inquire about previous Kawasaki syndrome. Fifteen percent of all patients with this diagnosis develop coronary artery aneurysms in the subacute phase of this illness some 3 to 6 weeks after diagnosis. One half of all aneurysms resolve spontaneously.

Chest pain is a common complaint in the pediatric age group, and the incidence of heart disease in this same age group is low. Our approach is to pursue associated signs or symptoms suggestive of cardiac disease. These include: 1) a history suggestive of myocarditis such as a recent viral illness, fever, or malaise; 2) syncope with chest pain as outlined below; 3) suspicion of an arrhythmia as outlined below; 4) ECG abnormalities; 5) cardiomegaly on chest radiograph; or 6) a significant cardiac murmur. If present, these additional findings warrant further investigation and referral to a pediatric cardiologist. In an asymptomatic child with a normal ECG and chest radiograph, observation without referral is prudent.

Cardiac Syncope

The differential diagnosis of cardiac syncope includes left ventricular outflow tract obstruction and arrhythmia. Left ventricular outflow tract anomalies including aortic valve stenosis and subaortic stenosis can cause syncope during exercise for reasons outlined earlier. As previously mentioned, these patients typically present with a systolic murmur. In addition, syncope during exercise may be caused by ventricular arrhythmias. In a patient with syncope during exercise, referral to a cardiologist is indicated.

In patients with a history of syncope and a family history of sudden death, it is essential to rule out long QTc syndrome as the cause of their syncopal episode. Patients with long corrected QT (QTc) syndrome typically have drop attacks associated with life-threatening arrhythmias, including ventricular tachycardia. Patients with syncopal episodes and a family history of sudden death require a 12 lead ECG looking specifically at the QTc interval. This interval is calculated by measuring the QT interval divided by the square root of the R-R interval (QRS-T measured and the previous QRS). The upper limit of normal is 440 msec.

Symptomatic bradycardia caused by sick sinus syndrome or onset of late complete heart block can cause cardiac syncope. This is most commonly seen in children who have undergone cardiac surgery. More specifically, patients with transposition of the great arteries who have undergone correction using an atrial inversion procedure have a high incidence of both automatic atrial tachycardia and sick sinus syndrome. Patients who as part of their repair have had a ventricular septal defect closure may suffer a late complication of intermittent complete heart block. These patients are typically cared for by a cardiologist and have as part of their routine annual follow-up examination 24-hour Holter monitoring to evaluate for these arrhythmias.

Occasionally, a child may present with recurrent episodes of syncope with or without exercise. These patients are frequently referred for cardiac evaluation, which includes 12 lead ECG, echocardiogram and, when indicated, tilt-table evaluation. This relatively new procedure allows more accurate definition of patients with significant recurrent vasodepressor syncope. The patient fasts for 4 hours before the test and is brought to the cardiac catheterization laboratory, where a large-bore intravenous line and an arterial line are put in place. The patient then rests supine for 1 hour. After this period, resting catecholamine levels are drawn by intravenous methods. The patient is tilted upright, and blood pressure and heart rate are continuously monitored. Patients are asked to report any symptoms. Should the patient report dizziness or nausea or should they have alteration in level of consciousness, they are again placed in the supine position for a recovery period. In patients who remain asymptomatic, an infusion of isoproterenol is initiated to further provoke symptoms. Patients with positive tilt-table tests (i.e., those with vasodepressor syncope) are encouraged to increase their intake of fluids. If syncope persists, treatment with Fluronef, a mineralocorticoid, is begun for volume expansion.

To reiterate, the most common cause of syncope in children in noncardiac. Patients with symptoms consistent with vasodepressor syncope need not undergo further evaluation. In patients with recurrent syncope or syncope with associated rhythm disturbances, or in patients with syncope and a positive family history of sudden death, further evaluation by a pediatric cardiologist is warranted.

Hyperlipidemia in Childhood

Because coronary artery disease is the leading cause of death in the western world, many physicians have become increasingly aware of coronary risk factors in the pediatric population. These risk factors are hypertension, diabetes, cigarette smoking, and increased plasma lipids. It is the last of these risk factors that is now most often discussed.

Cholesterol and triglycerides are the two major lipids that are responsible for the genesis of atherosclerosis. These lipids are carried by the four classes of lipoproteins: *chylomicrons* carry fat as triglycerides, *very-low-density lipoproteins (VLDL)* carry triglycerides, *low-density lipoproteins (LDL)* carry cholesterol to the body tissues, and *high-density lipoproteins (HDL)* carry cholesterol back to the liver for removal in the bile.

The Framingham study has shown that increased plasma cholesterol is clearly related to increased risk for developing coronary artery disease. Recent surveys have shown that 5% to 25% of children and teenagers in the United States have serum cholesterol levels above 200 mg/dL. Because of the high percentage of the pediatric population with elevated cholesterol levels, there is a recent emphasis on change in dietary habits as well as on monitoring of plasma cholesterol.

The diagnosis of hyperlipidemia can be made as early as the first or second year of life. A plasma lipid profile, which includes plasma cholesterol, plasma triglycerides, and HDL cholesterol, should be obtained only in pediatric patients who are at high risk; that is, those children from families with hyperlipidemia, sudden death, xanthomas, hypertension, or premature (less than 60 years of age) myocardial infarction, angina, cerebrovascular accident, or peripheral vascular disease.

There are three familial hyperlipidemias that lead to premature atherosclerosis: familial hypercholesterolemia, familial combined hyperlipidemia, and familial hypertriglyceridemia. These genetic disorders affect about 0.5% to 1% of the general population. Causes of secondary hyperlipidemia include: diabetes, hypothyroidism, obstructive liver disease, nephrotic syndrome, excessive dietary intake, and the use of steroids, oral contraceptives, and alcohol.

Therapy for hyperlipidemia includes: dietary modification, weight control, aerobic exercise, and pharmacologic agents. The American Heart Association has recommended that children older than 2 years of age should have decreased amounts of cholesterol and fat in their diets (with cholesterol limited to 100 mg/1000 kcal and with total fat restricted to 30% of caloric intake). This low-fat diet, which restricts total cholesterol and limits saturated fats in the diet, includes five simple modifications: restrict egg intake to three per week, drink low-fat milk, use polyunsaturated fat containing margarine instead of butter, use corn oil in cooking, and limit meat intake and increase intake of fish and fowl. Patients with diagnosed hyperlipidemia should have further restrictions of cholesterol and fat in their diets. In addition, a weight reduction program and an exercise regimen usually is instituted.

Some children may require the use of pharmacologic agents to reduce plasma cholesterol. The drug of choice is a bile acid sequestrant resin such as cholestyramine or colestipol. The main side effects of these agents are constipation, diarrhea, and bloating.

The association of hyperlipidemia and atherosclerotic heart disease is well known in the adult population. Because the process of atherosclerosis probably starts in childhood and adolescence, primary prevention needs to be emphasized by the primary care physician.

Pediatric Dysrhythmias

With the recent further development of sophisticated noninvasive and invasive diagnostic tools such as Holter monitoring, transtelephonic monitoring, electrophysiologic study, esophageal stimulation, and exercise testing, the area of pediatric cardiac dysrhythmias has broadened in scope in the past decade. Dysrhythmias in the younger pediatric patient are often difficult to diagnose. In the newborn infant symptoms of dysrhythmias include such nonspecific findings such as fussiness or poor feeding, whereas preschool children may complain of poorly localized pain or a "funny" feeling in the chest. Syncope can pose an especially difficult differential diagnosis. It is common in school-aged children, has several causes, and the actual incidence of cardiac syncope is small. A complete family history for dysrhythmias, syncope, and sudden death coupled with an ECG to specifically evaluate the corrected QT interval should be part of every evaluation of syncope unless the episode can clearly be ascribed to a noncardiac cause such as a vasovagal attack.

An irregular rhythm is occasionally heard during a routine physical examination. There are several common mechanisms for an irregular rhythm: 1) *Sinus arrhythmia* is an irregular sinus rhythm due to the respiratory cycle (Fig. 75-2). It is benign in children. 2) *Premature atrial contractions* (PACs) are manifested by premature and abnormal P waves. These premature contractions often are seen in the neonate and often disappear in the first few days of life. In infants, although occasional PACs are common, frequent PACs can be associated with supraventricular tachycardia and may require therapy. Although usually benign in children, PACs also occur in the setting of heart diseases such as myocarditis, hyperthyroidism, indwelling lines, or medications. 3) *Premature ventricular contraction (PVC)* (Fig. 75-2) is manifested by a premature widened QRS complex. These premature beats also can be benign, especially if single and uniform and abated with exercise.

Initial workup of PVCs should include: EGG (to rule out prolonged QT syndrome), Holter monitoring, and chest radiography or echocardiography if indicated. Often an exercise stress test is helpful to evaluate PVCs. Predisposing conditions for PVCs include electrolyte abnormalities, drugs, CHF, cardiomyopathy, and after cardiac surgery.

Supraventricular tachycardia (SVT) is the most common symptomatic dysrhythmia in children. An infant with SVT usually presents with poor feeding or lethargy and has a heart rate above 200 beats per minute. The most common cause of SVT in infants less than 4 months of age is idiopathic. Older children with SVT, however, are much less likely to present with CHF because the heart rate is much slower and also because they are capable of verbalizing their symptoms. Older children with SVT are more likely to have a predisposing factor such as congenital heart disease (preoperative or postop-

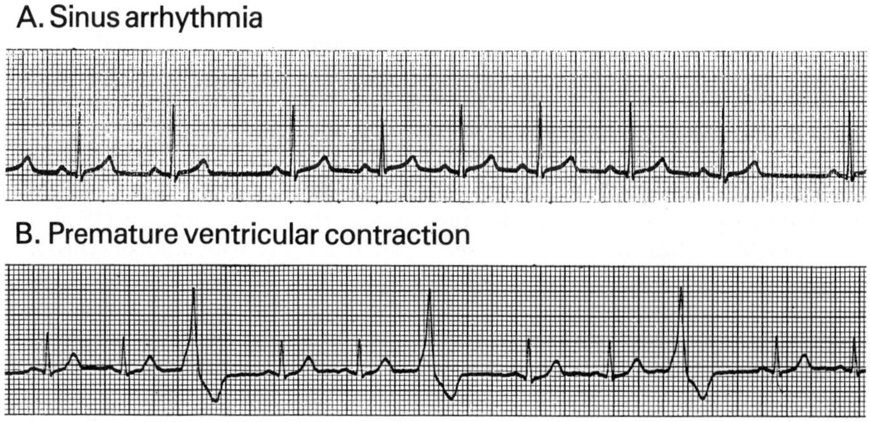

A. Sinus arrhythmia

B. Premature ventricular contraction

FIG 75-2
A, An electrocardiogram of sinus arrhythmia. Note the irregular distance between QRS complexes. **B,** Premature ventricular contractions.

erative), myocarditis, cardiomyopathy, preexcitation syndrome, drugs, or other causes such as hyperthyroidism and usually will undergo an electrophysiologic study as part of their evaluation. Immediate management of SVT includes evaluation of the hemodynamic state. If the patient is unstable, then cardioversion is indicated. If the patient is hemodynamically stable, as are most children who present with SVT, then diagnostic evaluation including a full ECG and the use of vagal maneuvers in children or placing a ice pack over the face of an infant can be tried. Maintenance therapy usually includes digoxin and other drugs, such as propranolol and procainamide as well as newer agents such as flecainide and mexiletene.

BIBLIOGRAPHY

Asai T: Evaluation method for the degree of seriousness in Kawasaki disease. *Acta Paediatr Jpn* 25:170, 1983.

Beerman LB, Neches WH, Patnode RE, et al: Coarctation of the aorta in children: Late results after surgery. *Am J Dis Child* 134:464, 1980.

Bell DM, Morens DH, Holman RC, et al: Kawasaki syndrome in the United States 1976 to 1980. *Am J Dis Child* 137:211–214, 1983.

Bergman AB, Stamm SJ: The morbidity of cardiac nondisease in school children. *N Engl J Med* 276:1008, 1967.

Bland E: Rheumatic fever: The way it was. *Circulation* 76:1190–1195, 1987.

Breslow J: Pediatric aspects of hyperlipidemia. *Pediatrics* 62:510–520, 1978.

Carr RP: Psychological adaption to cardiac surgery. In Kidd BSL, Rowe RD, editors: *The Child With Congenital Heart Disease After Surgery.* Mount Kisco, 1976 Futura Publishing Co.

Dawber T, Kannel W, McNamara P: The prediction of coronary artery disease. *Trans Assoc Life Insur Med Dir Am* 47:70, 1971.

Driscoll D, Glicklich L, Gallen W: Chest pain in children: A prospective study. *Pediatrics* 57:648–651, 1976.

Freedman D, Sriniwasan SR, Cresanta JL, et al: Serum lipids and lipoproteins. *Pediatrics* 80:789–796, 1987.

Furosho K, Kamiya T, Nakano H, et al: High dose intravenous gamma globulin therapy for Kawasaki disease. *Lancet* 2:1055–1058, 1984.

Fyfe D, Moodie D: Chest pain in pediatric patients presenting to a cardiac clinic. *Clin Pediatr* 23:321–324, 1984.

Garson A, Gillette P, McNamara D: Supraventricular tachycardia in children: Clinical features, response to treatment, and long-term follow-up in 217 patients. *Pediatrics* 98:875–882, 1981.

Gilette P: Cardiac dysrhythmias in children. *Pediatr Rev* 3:190–198, 1981.

Kaplan E: The startling comeback of rheumatic fever. *Contemp Pediatr* 4:20–34, 1987.

Kawasaki T: Acute febrile mucocutaneous syndrome with lymphoid involvement with specific desquamation of the fingers and toes in children: Clinical observations of 50 cases (in Japanese). *Jpn J Allergol* 16:178–222, 1967.

Lavie C, et al: Management of lipids in primary and secondary prevention of cardiovascular diseases. *Mayo Clin Proc* 63:605–621, 1988.

McGoon DC: Long term effects of prosthetic materials. *Am J Cardiol* 50:621, 1982.

Newburger JW, Takahashi M, Burns JC, et al: The treatment of Kawasaki syndrome with intravenous gamma globulin. *N Engl J Med* 315:341–347, 1986.

Perloff JK: Adults with surgically treated congenital heart disease: Sequelae and residua. *JAMA* 250:2033, 1983.

Rauch A, Hurwitz E: Centers for Disease Control (CDC) case definition for Kawasaki syndrome. *Pediatr Infect Dis* 4:702–703, 1985.

Rowland TW: The pediatrician and congenital heart disease—1979. *Pediatrics* 64:180, 1979.

Schwartz P: Idiopathic long QT syndrome: Progress and questions. *Am Heart J* 109:399–411, 1985.

Selbst S: Evaluation of chest pain in children. *Pediatr Rev* 8:56–62, 1986.

Talner NS: Heart failure. In Adams FH, Emmanouilides GC, editors: *Moss' Heart Disease in Infants, Children and Adolescents.* Baltimore, 1983, Williams & Wilkins.

Vetter VL, Horowitz LN: Electrophysiologic residua and sequelae of surgery for congenital heart defects. *Am J Cardiol* 50–588, 1982.

III

PART FOUR

Dermatology

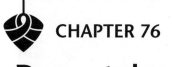

CHAPTER 76

Dermatology

Herbert B. Allen
Paul J. Honig

This chapter covers a number of common dermatologic disorders seen by the primary care provider. Diagnostic characteristics and treatment issues are stressed for each condition.

ATOPIC DERMATITIS

Atopic dermatitis, or eczema, a common skin disease of unknown cause, is found predominantly in children who have a personal history or family history of allergies such as hay fever, allergic rhinitis, or sinusitis. Intense pruritus is the predominant symptom. In fact, atopic dermatitis has been termed "the itch that rashes."

Background

The onset of atopic dermatitis is early in life; 60% of the cases will occur by the age of 1 year. In the early months of life, a severe diaper dermatitis may be the harbinger of future skin trouble. The condition is usually not lifelong, however; 90% of all children recover by adolescence.

In infancy, the rash appears on the cheeks and extensor surfaces of arms and legs as red exudative plaques. Similar lesions may be present in the diaper area. By the age of 2 years, the more characteristic flexural involvement (Fig. 76-1)

has generally evolved, with the common sites being the neck, antecubital, and popliteal spaces (Fig. 76-2). Lesions include erythema, edema, papules, vesicles, papulovesicles, and lichenification. Weeping, oozing, and crusting may be present. The course of the eruption may wax and wane, with chronic relapses being quite common.

In atypical locations the findings are different. If the feet become involved, the soles usually have shiny, peeling skin with painful fissures. Diffuse follicular accentuation, scaling in the scalp (with or without alopecia), hyperlinear palms and soles, pityriasis alba, or fissured or crusted plaques in the auricular folds may variably be present.

Children with atopic dermatitis have poor resistance to superficial viral infections. For example, such children are frequently infected with warts, molluscum contagiosum, and herpes simplex. Eczema herpeticum (Fig. 76-3) can be a serious complication of atopic dermatitis that requires hospitalization and intravenous acyclovir.

The diagnosis of atopic dermatitis is based solely on clinical findings. The laboratory yields no diagnostic assistance. On occasion, elevated IgE, eosinophilia, or positive scratch tests may be found, but these are nonspecific and do not truly confirm the diagnosis.

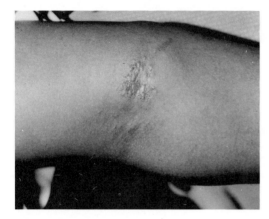

FIG 76-1
Mild atopic dermatitis.

Management

The major therapy for atopic dermatitis is topical corticosteroid application. The potency of the preparation depends on the amount of inflammation, the age of the patient, and the severity of involvement. As the condition improves (generally within 2 to 3 weeks), it is judicious to shift to a moderate or mild topical agent, with 1% hydrocortisone being the mildest of the effective preparations. If there is prominent crusting or erythema, antibiotics such as erythromycin may be employed for 1- to 2-week intervals. These lesions tend to be heavily colonized with *Staphylococcus aureus*. Antihistamines may be helpful in controlling pruritus.

General prevention measures are probably as important as specific treatment and include: 1) decreased bathing; 2) the use of mild soaps—and even these must be used sparingly; 3) the avoidance of irritants, such as quaternary ammonium in perineal wipes; and 4) the generous use of emollients. Soaks (tap water; tea water, especially for feet; Burow's solution; saline solution) are useful if considerable weeping and oozing are present. Lotions, creams, and pastes are also preferable in this instance. For the drier, more lichenified lesions, ointments are generally more effective. Dietary measures may be helpful if the offending food can be identified; however, hyposensitization is not usually indicated in "purely" skin disease. For scalp disease, topical steroid lotions are useful, as is decreased use of shampoos. When the feet are involved, topical steroid ointments and liberal use of petrolatum (whenever the shoes are removed) are helpful.

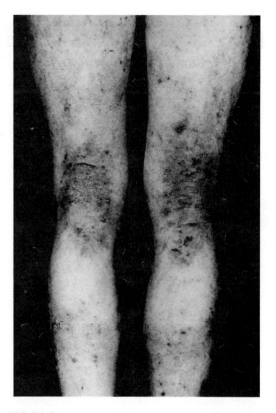

FIG 76-2
Atopic dermatitis. Note the diffuse erythema and excoriated lesions concentrated on the flexor surfaces.

Recently, ultraviolet light and PUVA have both been shown to be beneficial. The use of these modalities may lower the requirement for topical steroid administration.

URTICARIA

Urticaria is a skin condition characterized by hives and itching. It is very common, and many children have had at least one episode in their lives. In the allergic type of hives, a type I immunologic reaction occurs that may be induced by drugs, foods, infections, or other allergens. The classic examples are penicillin for the drug-induced variety, shellfish for foods, and viral hepatitis for infections.

Background

The clinical lesions are widely distributed pink wheals, which may be small or large. Individual lesions usually last less than 24 hours. When

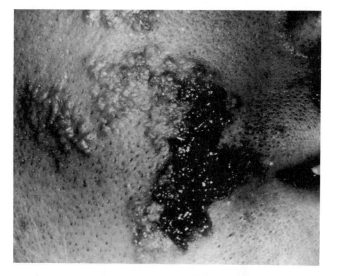

FIG 76-3
Herpes simplex showing grouped vesicles on an erythematous base.

involvement of the respiratory passages occurs, a medical emergency exists.

In general terms, if the hives are of relatively short duration, the offending allergen may be identified. The longer the hives persist and become chronic, the more difficult it is to find the antigenic stimulus. In fact, in chronic urticaria, multiple antigens may be provocative. Subtle antigens such as dyes, salicylates, and preservatives may assume a large role; carefully taken dietary and activity history may be revealing.

Cholinergic urticaria is a condition to be distinguished from allergic hives. In cholinergic urticaria the wheals are tiny at first, then enlarged by coalescing. Adolescents and young adults are more at risk than infants or children. The lesions tend to be distributed on the trunk and are not preceded by an allergen. Dermographism is usually easily demonstrated. Cholinergic urticaria may be provoked by exercise, sweating, rubbing, scratching, emotions, or exposure to either cold or hot temperatures.

Management

If respiratory symptoms are present, treatment with subcutaneous epinephrine, antihistamines, and careful observation should help to alleviate the symptoms. Ordinary treatment involves antihistamines and, possibly, even a short, tapering course of oral corticosteroids. If it does not work, another antihistamine of a different class (ie, cyproheptadine) may be added for concurrent administration. This treatment usually needs to be given for 1 to 2 months, and patients are advised to avoid known precipitating factors and activities.

ERYTHEMA MULTIFORME

Erythema multiforme (EM) is a reaction pattern in the skin somewhat similar to urticaria. It differs in the type of clinical lesion that arises (the iris or "target" lesion [Fig. 76-4] vs the wheal) and in the minimal pruritus present. The skin reaction may be secondary to drugs (such as penicillin, sulfonamides, hydantoin, and barbiturates) or to viral infections. Herpes simplex virus is the most common. Other drugs and other infections also may precipitate the phenomenon.

Background

Lesions generally begin on the distal surfaces of feet and spread centrally; however, they may arise in generalized fashion de novo. The findings may include macules, papules, vesicobullae, and the iris lesion, which has a red or dark center surrounded by pale pink and red rings. When mucous membranes are involved and constitutional symptoms are present, the designation Stevens-Johnson syndrome is used (Fig. 76-5). The lips and oral cavity are most commonly affected. The lips show marked hemorrhagic crusting. Moreover, the conjunctivae, urethra, vagina, perianal area, and even the tracheobronchial and esophageal membranes may be involved.

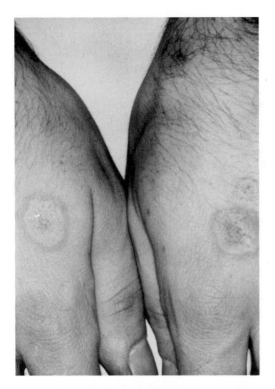

FIG 76-4
Target lesion of erythema multiforme.

Management

The treatment for EM in mild cases is symptomatic. Severe involvement may require corticosteroids to treat systemic effects. Given early (*ie,* in the prodromal phase), a short course (5 to 7 days) of prednisone can even obliterate the development of EM. This response is characteristic in the EM following herpes simplex infection. If eye changes are present, consultation with an ophthalmologist is necessary. For severe crusting of the lips, intermittent warm water compresses should be followed by application of an ointment such as petrolatum. As in urticaria, if a drug is the provoking agent, it should be discontinued. Antihistamines may benefit the patient who is itchy. Chronic acyclovir therapy can be used to prevent recurrent EM secondary to herpes simplex infection.

DRUG ERUPTIONS

In addition to urticaria and EM, drugs may induce maculopapular eruptions, bullous (diffuse or fixed) lesions, vasculitis, nodular lesions, photosensitivity, and toxic epidermal necrolysis. In fact, drugs are an important differential diagnosis in almost all types of skin eruptions.

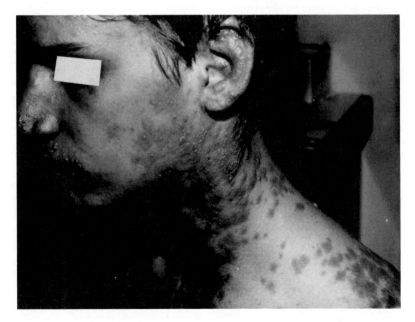

FIG 76-5
Erythema multiforme.

In managing drug eruptions, the offending agent must be discontinued; in cases in which multiple agents are being used, all should be stopped, if possible. When the eruption clears, the least likely agent may be reintroduced followed by the next agent every 3 to 5 days. If the eruption recurs after a drug is taken, that agent is presumed to be the agent producing the rash. Because multiple allergens may be present, a persistent search may be necessary. Subtle allergens may be responsible, such as dyes in liquids, capsule coatings, preservatives, or flavorings. Drug eruptions may be induced by agents patients do not ordinarily term "drugs," for example, nose drops, nose sprays, suppositories, lozenges, and others. A complete review of all such agents is necessary. Frequently, other family members are able to fill in the total picture of ingestants and inhalants.

Other treatments are symptomatic, ranging from antihistamines for control of pruritus to corticosteroids for systemic symptoms. Topical corticosteroids may or may not be useful in drug eruptions because of the diffuse nature of the condition. Soothing baths or compresses (mineral oil or oilated oatmeal) may be used, and, for oozing eruptions, shake lotions (calamine or calamine mixed with equal parts of a moisturizing lotion) may be helpful.

CONTACT DERMATITIS

Allergic contact dermatitis is a form of delayed, cell-mediated hypersensitivity and is less common in children than adults. The incidence below the age of 1 year is rare.

Background
The offending allergen is deposited on the skin, penetrates the stratum corneum, is transcribed or modulated by Langerhans' cells, joins with a carrier protein, and travels to the regional lymph node; after processing by macrophages, it gets recognized by T cells, which then become sensitized. The T cells enter the circulation, migrate to the skin, react with the allergen, and release lymphokines. Six to 24 hours later, dermatitis erupts.

The distribution of the dermatitis may be an important clue to the provoking allergen, for example, contact dermatitis on the neck from perfume or earrings; the mouth, due to dentifrices or

bubble gum; the feet, due to shoes or rubber. The pattern of linear vesicles (Fig. 76-6) in rhus dermatitis (poison ivy) is virtually diagnostic of this form of contact dermatitis.

Clinically, one sees vesicles, bullae, papulovesicles, edema, erythema, crusting, and excoriations. With airborne contactants, there is severe involvement of the eyes. Both upper and lower lids are markedly swollen, and there is generalized facial edema and erythema. Photocontact dermatitis is distinguishable by its presence in areas where sunlight strikes the skin and its absence in nonexposed areas. Nonspecific factors such as trauma, pressure, heat, and sweating may play a role during both the initiation and elicitation phases of contact sensitivity.

Management
Topical steroids are helpful in most cases of contact allergy. In rhus and airborne dermatitis, oral prednisone may be necessary; (a dose of 1 to 2 mg/kg/day for 1 week, with tapering off over 2 to 3 weeks to prevent rebound). Usually the

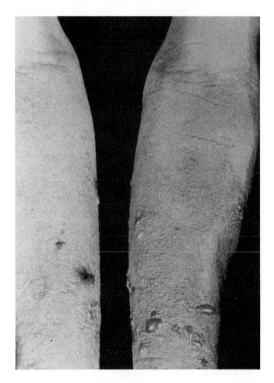

FIG 76-6
Contact dermatitis edematous. Vesicobullous lesions that have sharply demarcated margins.

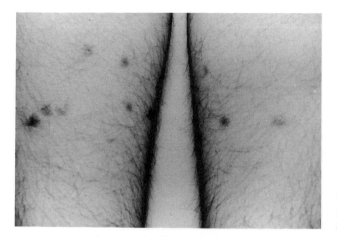

FIG 76-7
Flea bites. Erythematous lesions on exposed surface.

pruritus will disappear 36 hours after the initial dose of prednisone. Then the lesions will flatten, fade, and, ultimately, scale. Soaks, compresses, and shake lotions are useful in the early vesicular, bullous, and weeping eruptions and should be used for 3 to 5 days. Avoid antihistamine-containing lotions because of possible secondary contact sensitization. Ice-water compresses to the eyelids are soothing and beneficial in lessening the edema of airborne reactions and in photocontact sensitivities. Oral antihistamines may be prescribed to reduce pruritus.

Avoidance of the offending allergens is a must or the eruption will recur with repeated exposure. Some "hardening" may occur during the season such that the first case of rhus is ordinarily the worst of the year. Vectors such as pets, clothing, wood, or smoke may carry the allergen to a sensitive person. Secondary contact dermatitis such as sensitivity to the antihistamine in shake lotions or to vitamin E rubbed on the skin may obscure the primary disease. The history and the clinical appearance of the rash are important in recognizing a secondary sensitivity. Patch testing may be useful in all varieties of contact allergy and is especially useful when the specific allergen is unclear.

INSECT BITE REACTION

The common insects that bite children are mosquitoes and fleas. Chiggers, gnats, black flies, "no-see-ums," and others cause bite reactions that are also bothersome but are less common compared with mosquitoes and fleas.

To make the diagnosis, the primary care physician should consider the time of year, the location of the lesions, and the type of lesion. Mosquitoes appear in the warmer months, as do sand fleas. Animal fleas are present year-round on pets or in rugs or furniture.

Exposed surfaces are involved with pink and red papules with a central punctum, papulovesicles, vesicles (Fig. 76-7), and even bullae in highly sensitized patients. Pruritus, intense at times, is the main symptom. Crusting and secondary infection may appear.

Treatment is symptomatic with utilization of ice for acute lesions, antihistamines for pruritus, and shake lotions for soothing. Lotions and creams containing antihistamines may be sensitizing.

The prior use of insect repellents (particularly those that contain N,N-diethylmetatoluamide [DEET]) helps prevent bites but must be applied every 3 to 4 hours because the substance wears off or evaporates. Ingestion of garlic also may help ward off attackers. Avoidance of perfume or perfumed shampoos, rinses, or lotions is also helpful.

DIAPER DERMATITIS

Diaper rash is a common problem in young children. The disorder has many causes, including occlusion, bacterial overgrowth, monilial proliferation, friction, and innate susceptibility (atopic or seborrheic diatheses) having more or less importance in individual cases. Differing types of rashes may be noted when one factor predominates: candidal, atopic, seborrheic, and primary irritant. Mixed types, for example, irritant with monilial overgrowth, are also seen.

Candidal types are recognized by their "beefy red" plaques associated with satellite papules and pustules. Primary irritant eruptions may wax and wane and, when present, have shiny, glazed skin that may become macerated. Atopic and seborrheic eruptions generally are associated with body rashes in typical locations and have appropriate family histories. Bacterial superinfection may occur, and if blistering is present, *S. aureus* infection should be considered.

Treatment of diaper dermatitis consists of allowing the skin to dry as much as possible via air exposure. Candidal infections may be treated with nystatin or the imidazoles such as clotrimazole. Secondary bacterial infections may be treated with triple antibiotic topical agents; inflammation may be reduced by topical corticosteroids. Mixtures of the above may be employed, or an already prepared compound (Mycolog) may be selected. Note that the ointment formula is far less sensitizing than the cream. The use of soap and water should be decreased, and mild soaps should be used. Perineal wipes, especially those containing quaternary ammonium compounds, may be irritating. An alternative to wipes or soap-and-water cleaning for soiled buttocks is the use of a lotion (Keri, Nutraderm, Baby Magic, etc.).

Another useful compound is "triple" paste applied at bedtime. This paste may be removed in the morning by mineral oil, if necessary. The compound itself is soothing, gently drying, and remarkably protective because of its water-impervious nature. A very light dusting of powder may be used to make the substance an even better barrier. Caution must be used with talc-containing powders to prevent inhalation of the substance.

"Id" (diffuse disseminated papules and papulovesicles) reactions generally respond to topical corticosteroids, with 1% hydrocortisone being the safest. Oral nystatin may be necessary to clear an intestinal focus of *Candida albicans*.

TINEA CAPITIS

Tinea capitis is a *dermatophytic* infection of the scalp. It is most common before puberty. The organisms that usually cause tinea capitis are *Microsporum* species and *Trichophyton tonsurans*. There has been a gradual increase in the percentage of cases caused by *T. tonsurans*. Most tinea capitis lesions will not demonstrate fluorescence on Wood's lamp examination due to this changing etiology. Clinically, there are several different forms of tinea capitis. These forms include: 1) patchy, scaling alopecia; 2) boggy, purulent-appearing kerion; 3) diffuse chronic scaling or "dandruff"; and 4) "blackdot," in which the hair is broken off at the scalp, giving the appearance of multiple black dots. These forms vary depending on the infecting organism, the site of infection, the patient's immune response, and state of treatment. The diagnosis of tinea capitis is made by culturing the affected scalp area with dermatophyte test medium.

The management of tinea capitis includes treatment with oral griseofulvin 10 to 20 mg/kg/day in two divided doses for a period of 6 to 8 weeks. It is useful to give the medication with a fatty meal (*eg*, ice cream) to aid absorption. Topical application of selenium sulfide suspension 2.5% (Selsun) in the form of shampoo twice weekly also will decrease the spore count, and thus decrease infectivity. Topical antifungal medications should not be used; they are ineffective. Some dermatologists will treat a painful kerion with steroids, but if the patient requires this therapy, he/she should be referred. The differential diagnosis of tinea capitis includes seborrhea, alopecia areata, trichotillomania, and traction alopecia.

TINEA PEDIS

Tinea pedis is decidedly rare before the age of 11 years but increases in frequency during adolescence. Sweating and occlusion or partial occlusion play large roles in allowing this infection to occur. The ordinary causative organisms are *T. rubrum, T. mentagrophytes,* and *Epidermophyton floccosum*.

The fourth interspace is the most common site of involvement, although other sites may also be troublesome. If the dorsal toes or the ball of the foot is involved at an early age, it is almost never caused by a fungus. Contact or atopic dermatitis are more likely diagnoses. The fungal eruption is characterized by pruritus, which may be intense at times. Scaling maceration and fissuring between toes may be present. Nails are seldom involved early. The diagnosis may be confirmed by potassium hydroxide examination or culture.

Treatment consists of topical antifungals—tolnaftate, miconazole, clotrimazole, econazole, and ciclopirox olamine are all effective. Ordinarily, oral griseofulvin need not be administered. Keeping the foot dry helps prevent recurrences.

ACNE

Acne affects over three fourths of the population during adolescence and early adult life. Although usually mild and self-limited, the disorder can leave many physical and emotional scars. In most instances, these scars can be prevented by control of the disease. Although the pathogenesis of acne is not completely clear, knowledge of current theories makes therapy more understandable.

Background
The target skin appendage is the sebaceous follicle. With initiation of puberty, adrenal androgenic influences cause sebaceous enlargement and secretion. Due to abnormalities in the keratinization process of the follicular lining, epithelial cells are not shed normally, which leads to obstruction within the follicle and retention of sebum. Obstruction then leads to the next step in the cycle, ie, overgrowth of the follicle with *Propionibacterium acnes.* Although most sebaceous follicles are colonized with this organism, acne patients have greater numbers of the bacteria and respond to its presence in an exaggerated fashion. It is this idiosyncratic inflammatory response to *P. acnes* that leads to most inflammatory papules, pustules, and cysts that are seen.

The classic lesions seen in acne are the open and closed comedone (ie, blackhead and whitehead), inflammatory papules and pustules, and cystic lesions (some with connecting sinus tracts). Acne is found wherever sebaceous follicles are present, such as the face, chest, back, upper arms, upper thighs, and buttocks.

On occasion, infants are found to have acne within the first several months of life or later in the first year. Transplacental maternal hormones are the cause. Spontaneous resolution usually occurs with early onset disease.

Management
All treatment is directed toward 1) relieving follicular obstruction, 2) reducing the number of *P. acnes* organisms, and 3) preventing the inflammatory response.

Guidelines for Treatment of Acne
- Put acne in perspective by discussing the problem, the treatment, and usual outcomes.
- Early acne (comedone)
    Retinoic acid: Start with use every other day, then progress to daily treatments
- Mild to moderate acne
    Benzoyl peroxide
- Moderate to severe acne
    Benzoyl peroxide
    Retinoic acid
    Add oral antibiotics (tetracycline, erythromycin)
- Additional options if no improvement:
    Can increase benzoyl peroxide or retinoic acid to twice a day, combine the two treatments, or add topical antibiotics (clindamycin, erythromycin, tetracycline)
- Refer: Problem cystic acne

Therapy begins with the education of patients as to proper skin care. Mild soaps should be used and vigorous scrubbing avoided. The skin should be patted dry and treated gently at all times. Patients should be instructed to avoid squeezing lesions. Certain commonly used cleansers and moisturizers should be avoided because of their comedogenic potential.

Topical retinoic acid is used for open and closed comedones (Table 76-1). This preparation decreases the adhesiveness between cells and relieves obstruction. Topical benzoyl peroxide is used when inflammatory lesions are present as well. Benzoyl peroxide has antibacterial activity as well as acting as an exfoliant and a comedolytic agent. It may cause redness and scaling. With other than mild involvement with inflammatory lesions, systemic antibiotics are required. Severe involvement (ie, diffuse cystic and nodulocystic lesions and sinus tracts) requires the use of 13-*cis*-retinoic acid. Because of the many side effects (including teratogenicity) of this preparation, only physicians experienced with this medication should prescribe it.

When attempts to control acne vulgaris are unsuccessful, referral to a dermatologist is advisable.

TABLE 76-1
Rank Order of Irritancy of Retinoic Acid Preparations*

DEGREE OF IRRITATION	VEHICLE	RETINOIC ACID CONCENTRATION (%)
High	Solution	0.05
	Gel	0.05
	Gel	0.025
	Gel	0.01
	Cream	0.10
	Gel	0.005
Low	Cream	0.05
	Cream	0.025

*From Papa CM: The cutaneous safety of topical tretinoin, *Acta Derm Venereol* [Suppl] (Stockh) 74:128–132, 1975. Used by permission.

LICE

Background

The incidence of pediculosis is gradually increasing in the United States, especially pediculosis capitis. Although crowding and poor hygiene favor infestation, it is now clear that social class is not a factor.

The female louse can lay eggs at a rate of eight to 12 per day, producing large populations of lice within 3 to 4 months. Eggs (nits) are glued to hairs or fibers of clothing. Once hatched, the lice depend on blood meals for survival and therefore cannot exist for more than a few days away from humans.

During feeding periods, toxins released into the skin cause small red or purpuric spots. Continued exposure to these bites results in sensitization, with formation of papules and wheals. Pruritus becomes a major symptom, and secondary eczema occurs due to vigorous scratching.

Three forms of lice infest humans: the head louse, the body louse, and the pubic or crab louse.

Head Louse

The major louse infestation in children involves the scalp. Children are more susceptible to pediculosis capitis than are adults, with girls more often infested than boys. For unknown reasons, blacks are not usually affected. Infestation occurs by direct contact with another individual or indirectly from hats, brushes, or combs.

The female louse attaches her eggs to the hair shaft near the scalp surface. The egg hatches, and the nit is left behind. The numerous nits attached to hair shafts (usually behind the ears or on the occiput) resemble dandruff. Pruritus of the scalp is common. Secondary excoriations and infection with cervical lymphadenopathy frequently occur from vigorous scratching.

Diagnosis is made by differentiation of the nits (which do not easily pull off or move freely along the hair shaft) from dandruff scales or artifacts in the hair (which do). The presence of nits is confirmed by removing a hair and looking for the attached nit under the microscope.

Pubic Louse

Pubic lice infest the hairs and skin of the genital area, the lower abdomen, thighs, and occasionally the axilla. Preadolescents, especially, may have pubic lice in their eyelashes, eyebrows, and scalp lines. Transmission is usually venereal in adolescents and by close contact with infested adults (for example, the mother) in preadolescents. On occasion, indirect transmission occurs from clothing, bedding, and towels.

Excoriations secondary to pruritus frequently occur. With severe infestation, blue macules (maculae caeruleae) can be seen on the thighs, abdomen, or thorax. The exact cause is unknown, but they are thought to result from a substance released by the feeding louse.

Diagnosis is made by identification of nits attached to the hair shaft. Because hair grows slowly in the areas infested by the pubic louse, nits usually are found close to the skin surface.

Usually it is the pubic louse that attaches to eyelashes or eyebrows; on occasion, the head or body louse will. Crusting blepharitis, produced by the infestation, often is misdiagnosed because lice are not considered as a cause.

Body Louse

The body louse lives in clothing or bedding and is found on the body only when feeding. Body lice feed frequently during the day or night when the host is quiet or inactive. They hide in the seams of clothing and attach their eggs to the cloth fibers.

Primary skin lesions are frequently obliterated by scratching. Pruritus is severe. Pressure points beneath collars, belts, and underwear are the usual sites for identifying bites. The face, scalp, hands, and feet are usually spared. Because body lice are not usually found on the body surface, diagnosis is made by searching the seams of clothing for nits or parasites.

Management

Head Lice

Treatment is carried out with 1% permethrin, 1% pyrethrin, 1% lindane, or 10% crotamiton.

1% Permethrin creme rinse (Nix)

1. Shampoo hair and towel dry.
2. Saturate hair with creme rinse.
3. Leave on hair for 10 minutes.
4. Rinse off with water.
5. A single application is sufficient.

1% Pyrethrin (RID, R & C Shampoo, A-200, Cuprex) with piperonyl butoxide

1. Apply to scalp for 10 minutes.
2. Rinse out.
3. Let hair dry naturally.
4. Repeat in 7 to 10 days.
5. Remove nits.

1% Lindane shampoo (Kwell)

1. Protect eyes with towel.
2. Apply enough shampoo to wet hair and scalp.
3. Work thoroughly into hair using water to produce lather and leave in place for 5 minutes.
4. Rinse hair thoroughly and towel dry briskly.
5. Allow hair to dry naturally (do not blow dry).
6. Repeat application of 1% lindane in 7 to 10 days.
7. Remove nits: Soaking hair with 3% to 5% acetic acid solution (NOTE: Regular vinegar is 5% acetic acid; therefore 1 part vinegar plus 2 parts water yields 3% acetic acid.); cover with towel saturated with this solution or apply mineral oil; comb hair with fine-toothed comb (special metal combs available include Medi Comb, Nitex Labs, Boston; Derboc Comb, Johnson Manufacturing, Bonton, NJ; Innomed Comb, Innomed Inc., Greenwich, CT.).

10% Crotamiton (Eurax) cream or lotion

1. Apply to entire scalp.
2. Leave on for 24 hours.
3. Shampoo out.
4. Remove nits.

Pubic Lice

Each of the preparations used to treat head lice also is effective against pubic lice. Contacts must be treated as well. Lice on the eyelashes can be treated with a thick layer of white petrolatum applied two to five times per day for 8 days. Alternatives include 0.25% physostigmine (Eserine) four times a day for 3 consecutive days and 10% fluorescin drops.

Body Lice

Because body lice reside in clothing, patients do not need therapy; however, their clothing must be treated. Clothing and linens should be sterilized by boiling, steaming under pressure, or using a hot iron over seams. The patient should be told to bathe frequently, change clothing frequently, and change bed clothes often. Symptomatic treatment of the skin can be accomplished with antipruritics (antihistamines or topical corticosteroids) and systemic antibiotics for infection.

SCABIES

The major symptom of scabies is pruritus, and the major sign is a nonspecific skin eruption. Frequent misdiagnosis is attributed to the variability and nonspecificity of the skin changes. The astute clinician will consider diagnosis of this disorder when a patient has uncontrolled itching.

Background

The causative organism, *Sarcoptes scabiei,* completes its life cycle in humans. Fertilized female mites burrow into the stratum corneum, laying several eggs per day during a 1- to 2-month life span. Within 2 weeks the ova become adults. It is unusual for pruritus, the major symptom of this disorder, to occur earlier than 1 month after initial infestation. The duration of this latent period seems to indicate that pruritus is a result of sensitization to the organism.

The skin lesions include nonspecific papules, pustules, and vesicles (especially in infants). Linear burrows, rarely longer than 1 cm, occur in only 10% of patients and are frequently distorted by vigorous scratching and eczematization. Therefore, aside from the cardinal symptom of pruritus, the physician must rely on two major clues when making the diagnosis of scabies. Despite diffuse involvement, lesions are concentrated on the skin of the hands and feet (including the palms and soles in infants and young children) and in the folds of the body (axillae, groin, and especially the fingerwebs). Infants are more likely to develop blisters. They also will frequently have involvement of the skin of the face and head, in contrast to adolescents. The second point to elicit is whether family members and caretakers have pruritus and skin lesions.

The primary dermatitis of scabies can become secondarily infected. Persistent reddish brown pruritic nodules may develop. These remain despite adequate treatment and probably represent a reaction to dead mite parts. Norwegian scabies is that form of scabies infestation that produces thick, crusted lesions. It is usually seen in institutionalized, retarded, debilitated, or immunologically deficient individuals.

The diagnosis is made by examination of skin scrapings under the 10× objective for mites, ova, or fecal concretions. Mites are difficult to isolate, but persistence usually yields positive results. The materials required for examination of the skin for scabies includes a glass slide, immersion oil, and a No. 15 scalpel blade. A drop of immersion oil is placed on a glass slide, and the edge of the No. 15 blade is dipped into it (the mite sticks to the oil). The skin is scraped, and the material obtained is placed back into the drop of oil on the glass slide. A cover slip is placed over the oil and the slide examined under the microscope.

Management

Permethrin 5% cream (applied all over in infants and from the neck down in older children and adolescents and then left on overnight) is the treatment of choice for scabies. This treatment may be repeated in 1 week if necessary. Alternative treatments include lindane, crotamiton, or 5% sulfur in petrolatum.

BIBLIOGRAPHY

Atherton DJ, Carabalt F, Glove MT, et al: The role of psoralen photodermotherapy (PUVA) in the treatment of severe atopic dermatitis in adolescents. *Brit J Dermatol* 791–795, 1988.

Caputo RV, Frieden I, Krafchik BR, et al: Diet and atopic dermatitis. *J Am Acad Dermatol* 15: 543–545, 1986.

Jekler J, Larko O: Combined UVA-UVB phototherapy for atopic dermatitis. *J Am Acad Dermatol* 22:49–53, 1990.

Krafchik BR: Atopic dermatitis. *Pediatr Clin North Am* 30:669–685, 1983.

Matthews KP: A current view of urticaria. *Med Clin North Am* 58:185, 1974.

PART FIVE

Endocrinology

CHAPTER 77

Diabetes Mellitus

Marta Satin-Smith
Charles A. Stanley

Diabetes mellitus is one of the most common chronic diseases of childhood. In the United States, one in 350 to 600 children will develop diabetes by the age of 18 years. The most frequent form of diabetes in childhood, by current nomenclature, is called *type I diabetes mellitus* (formerly, juvenile or insulin-dependent diabetes), whereas that seen most frequently in adults is type II diabetes mellitus (formerly, maturity-onset or non–insulin-dependent diabetes). During the past decade, an increasing focus has been placed on efforts to maintain plasma glucose levels close to normal, particularly in adolescents and adults with type I diabetes. This trend derives not only from evidence linking metabolic control to the development of long-term diabetic complications, but also from the development of practical methods to measure blood glucose levels at home and to objectively measure long-term blood glucose control (glycosylated hemoglobin). Efforts to improve glucose control have emphasized the role of the family as primary decision-makers in managing diabetes. The physician's responsibilities are to provide support and supervision for the family as educator, counselor, and medical consultant. This chapter will provide an outline of the approaches to outpatient management and common crises that the primary care physician encounters in children with diabetes.

BACKGROUND

Although type I diabetes can be considered a genetic disease, the inheritance does not follow classic mendelian recessive or dominant patterns. The concordance rate in identical twins is estimated to be approximately 25%; the risk of diabetes in first-degree relatives (siblings, parents, or offspring) is also low, approximately 5%. As is true of other autoimmune diseases, the inheritance of type I diabetes is closely linked to the major histocompatibility loci of chromosome 6, particularly HLA antigens DR_3 and DR_4. The actual gene defect for type I diabetes is not known.

The current model for the development of type I diabetes mellitus involves some inherited predisposing factor that, in association with an environmental insult, leads to autoimmune destruction of the pancreatic β cells. Evidence for an autoimmune process includes the inflammatory round cell infiltrate of the islets of Langerhans seen in children who have died shortly after the onset of disease, and the recent demonstration of circulating antibodies directed against pancreatic β cells. Anti-islet cell antibodies can be demonstrated in most patients with type I diabetes at diagnosis. In a few patients, anti-islet cell antibodies have been found several years prior to diagnosis. This finding suggests that islet-cell destruction may be a chronic process in which clinically apparent diabetes does not occur until late in the disease, when most of the β cells are already destroyed.

There continues to be interest in the nature of the environmental insult responsible for initiating the autoimmune islet cell destruction in the genetically predisposed individual. Circumstantial evidence suggests that viral infections might play such a role. Coxsackie virus, mumps, and rubella have been linked to the incidence of type I diabetes historically and by demonstration of specific autobodies. This is an area of much uncertainty, however, particularly in view of the reports previously noted, that the autoimmune process may begin years before the onset of clinical diabetes.

Long-term complications of type I diabetes include nephropathy, retinopathy and peripheral neuropathy, and accelerated coronary vascular disease. Although few of these problems manifest in the pediatric patient, the more closely one looks for early changes, the more likely one is to see them. The current statistics for complications of type I diabetes are grim: 30% of patients show early changes of retinopathy within 5 years; 50% within 7 years; and 95% within 25 years of disease. Approximately one half of patients with type I diabetes in the United States will develop renal failure caused by nodular or diffuse glomerulosclerosis within 20 years.

Recently published results of the Diabetes Control and Complication Trial (DCCT) have established that better control of blood glucose levels can significantly slow the development of diabetes complications by 35% to 70% in adolescents and young adults. These findings have led to the development of new standards for diabetes management aimed at improving blood glucose control through more intensive therapy. However, because tighter control of blood glucose was associated with a threefold higher risk of severe hypoglycemia, the use of intensive therapy must be approached cautiously, especially in younger children and infants.

DIAGNOSIS

The diagnosis of diabetes in childhood is usually straightforward. The onset of symptoms is most often acute, with a 1- to 2-week history of polydipsia and polyuria. Weight loss of 5% to 10% is common, but the parents may not be aware of it. Although polyphagia is classically part of the triad of symptoms of diabetes, the appetite may decrease as ketosis develops. The majority of patients are now recognized prior to the development of the severe hyperosmolar dehydration and metabolic acidosis that lead to diabetic coma.

The diagnosis of diabetes mellitus should be confirmed quickly to prevent further progression of dehydration and acidosis. A positive urine test for glucose and ketones provides presumptive evidence of diabetes. This evidence can be confirmed by a random or postprandial blood glucose level over 200 mg/dL. Because most children already have markedly elevated blood glucose levels at the time of diagnosis, formal glucose tolerance testing is unnecessary. Stress-induced hyperglycemia may be distinguished from diabetes with serial postprandial blood glucose determinations for several days following presentation. Intravenous glucose tolerance testing should never be used.

MANAGEMENT

In considering strategies for managing type I diabetes, it is helpful to consider "closed-loop" and "open-loop" systems. The normally functioning pancreas provides an example of a close-loop system. Insulin need (due to changes in the levels of plasma glucose, amino acids, hormonal and neural inputs, etc.) is detected by the pancreatic β cell; insulin secretion rate is appropriately altered; and the effect of the change in insulin secretion is continuously monitored to make further adjustments on a minute-to-minute basis. This closed-loop system maintains plasma glucose levels in a narrow range of 80 to 120 mg/dL despite the wide variations in insulin requirements imposed by meals, exercise, and fasting. By contrast, all of the current methods for long-term management of insulin-dependent diabetes are open-loop systems, in which there is no direct connection between insulin require-

TABLE 77-1
Action Profiles of Commonly Used Insulin Preparations

TYPE	TIME (HRS)		
	ONSET OF ACTION	PEAK	DURATION OF EFFECT
Regular	0.5–1	1.5–2	4–6
NPH	1–2	6–12	24–48
Semilente	0.5–1	2–4	10–12
Lente	1–2	6–12	24–48
Ultralente	6	18–24	36+

ment, insulin dose, and insulin effect. This absence of autoregulation explains why type I diabetes has been termed "brittle." To achieve optimal blood glucose control in children with diabetes, it is necessary to focus attention on three areas: 1) insulin administration in a manner that approximates normal β-cell secretion, 2) a diet plan designed to minimize variability in insulin requirements, and 3) methods of monitoring blood sugar responses to provide a basis for making decisions about changes in insulin dose, diet, etc. The patient and his/her family can be viewed as the external decision-makers responsible for working to match insulin dose with insulin requirement in "closing the loop." The sections that follow discuss the three components of the open-loop regulatory system: insulin dose regimens, diet, and monitoring.

Insulin Dose Regimens

Table 77-1 shows the time of peak effect and duration of action of the most commonly used insulin preparations. Familiarity with a short-acting insulin (insulin injection) and an intermediate-acting insulin (isophane insulin suspension or insulin zinc suspension) is usually sufficient, because most insulin regimens now being recommended use a combination of these two preparations. Three forms of insulin preparations are available: human insulin, pure pork insulin, and mixed beef-pork insulin. There is little practical difference between these preparations. Anti-insulin antibody titers tend to be higher with mixed beef-pork insulin, but significant insulin resistance due to such antibodies is rare. Pure pork and human insulins are less antigenic, but cost slightly more than beef-pork insulin.

The goal of insulin therapy is to approximate pancreatic insulin secretion with a low basal level between meals and overnight, and peaks of insulin to coincide with meals. The closest approximation of this pattern is provided with a subcutaneous insulin infusion pump. This device delivers a "background rate" of insulin infusion, and boluses of insulin prior to meals on command of the patient. In combination with close monitoring of blood glucose levels, it is possible to achieve very good diabetic control with insulin-infusion pumps. Insulin-infusion pumps can be used successfully in highly motivated adolescent patients who have demonstrated a commitment to an intensive treatment program. Intensive programs, with three or four injections a day of regular insulin, with intermediate insulin to provide a background level during the night, achieve nearly as good diabetic control.

Most diabetologists recommend two or three daily injections of insulin for children with diabetes. As a rough guide, the total daily insulin requirement equals 1 U/kg (range, 0.5 to 2.0). Two thirds of the total is given 10 to 30 minutes before breakfast in a ratio of one part regular insulin to two parts NPH or lente insulin; the remaining third is given before supper in a ratio of one part regular insulin to one part NPH or lente insulin. In the three-shot regimen, the regular insulin is given before supper, and the NPH or lente insulin is given at bedtime. This distribution must be individualized for each patient, based on experience.

All preparations of insulin now used are 100 units/mL. Premixed insulin (*ie,* 30 U regular/70 U NPH/mL) is available but is not conducive to dose adjustment. Insulin syringes are available in 0.25-mL (25 units), 0.3-mL (30 units), 0.5-mL (50 units), and 1.0-mL (100 units) sizes.

Injection sites should be rotated to avoid lipoatrophy or hypertrophy, using the skin over the triceps brachii, quadriceps, and gluteus medius muscles, and over the abdomen.

Diet

In the context of "open-loop" systems for regulating diabetes, the diet plan can be viewed as an effort to minimize day-to-day differences in insulin requirements. This approach is obviously an approximation, and a consideration of other factors affecting insulin requirements (such as exercise, growth, intercurrent illness, emotional stress, and variable rates of insulin absorption) may be important, particularly in programs designed to achieve "tight" diabetic control. The major elements of any diet plan for type I diabetes are: 1) regularity in the timing of meals and 2) consistency in the amount of carbohydrate eaten at each meal.

The American Diabetes Association (ADA) diet provides a convenient way of teaching patients and their families how to plan meals.

The ADA diet divides foods into three main groups: the carbohydrate group, the meat and meat substitute group (protein), and the fat group. Within these groups, there are exchange lists of foods that are approximately equivalent in carbohydrate, protein, and fat. Meal plans utilizing ADA exchanges should be written with consideration given to the child's usual pattern of intake and food preferences. There is no one diabetic meal plan suitable for all children at a particular calorie level. A registered dietician can provide individualized meal planning and diet instruction. The ADA diet can be used as a guideline for dietary consistency while providing a high degree of flexibility. Current nutrition recommendations are referenced at the end of this chapter.

The diet for children with diabetes should be identical in total calories to that required by nondiabetic children of similar age and size (approximately 1000 calories plus 100 calories per year of age). All diabetic children should have at least four meals a day: breakfast, lunch, supper, and a bedtime snack. The latter is important in avoiding nocturnal hypoglycemia, due to the effects of the evening NPH or lente insulin dose. A midmorning and midafternoon snack may be used in younger children and toddlers or in children who are prone to hypoglycemia in the late morning or afternoon.

It should be emphasized that the diet plan for children with diabetes is not aimed at restricting calories and need not eliminate sugar; with the ADA exchange lists, it is possible to incorporate all types of foods into the diet and plan "treats" of ice cream, cake, etc.

Patients in the intensive treatment group of the DCCT had a tendency to gain more weight than those in the conventional treatment group. Action should be taken to safely decrease calories in patients who are demonstrating excessive weight gain on intensive regimens.

Monitoring

The goal of monitoring is to obtain sufficient data on levels of plasma glucose to permit appropriate decisions about changes in insulin dose. There are a wide variety of home glucose testing devices. Recent technology has eliminated the need to time and wipe blood off of test strips, thus circumventing errors in technique (accidental or deliberate) that result in inaccurate readings. The use of visually read strips (ie, comparison to a color chart) is fraught with errors and should be avoided. Noninvasive glucose testing devices using fiber optic technology are currently being developed. The ADA publishes a buyer's guide to home monitoring equipment in the October issue of *Diabetes Forecast*.

In addition to blood sugar testing, patients with diabetes also should know how to test urine for glucose and ketones. The simplest methods use dipsticks that test both glucose and ketone levels.

The routine times for testing are before breakfast, lunch, dinner, and bedtime snack (ie, when blood glucose levels are likely to be lowest). A useful time to check for possible nocturnal hypoglycemia levels is between 1 AM and 3 AM. Records of test results should be kept to guide adjustments in insulin dose. Implementation of intensive insulin therapy requires close monitoring of blood glucose levels, with a minimum of four tests daily. Urine should be tested for ketones during illness or if blood sugar is above 240 mg/dL.

Goals for Home Management and Guidelines for Dose Adjustment

The primary goals of diabetes management are:

1. Resumption of normal physical and social activities
2. Normal rates of growth and sexual maturation
3. Avoidance of episodes of hypoglycemia
4. Avoidance of symptoms of hyperglycemia
5. Avoidance of ketoacidosis

The secondary goal is to maintain plasma glucose levels as near normal as practical within the limitations imposed by the age of the child, the characteristics of the family, and the intensity of the open-loop system used to manage the diabetes. For example, in infants and children under the age of 10 years, it is necessary to accept higher levels of plasma glucose to avoid hypoglycemia. With blood glucose testing at home and two or three insulin injections, it should be possible to have approximately 50% to 70% of the readings in the range of 80 to 180 mg/dL. To get the majority of blood glucose readings between 80 and 150 mg/dL requires intensive regimens such as the use of multiple daily insulin injections or subcutaneous infusion pumps. In young children, who can not recognize or verbalize symptoms of hypoglycemia, blood glucose levels should fall in the range of 100 to 200 mg/dL.

Adjustments in insulin dose for persistent hyperglycemia should be made gradually to avoid overshooting. Changes equal to approximately 5% of the total daily insulin dose can be made at intervals of 2 to 3 days. Recurrent hypoglycemia should be corrected aggressively by lowering the insulin dose by 20% each day until mild hyperglycemia persists and then readjusting the dose upward in small increments.

CRISIS MANAGEMENT

Hypoglycemia

Hypoglycemia, the most common and most acute medical crisis in home management of diabetes, is the problem that children and parents understandably fear the most.

Hypoglycemia may occur as a result of exercise, a delay in eating, or as a complication of attempts at "tight control." Symptoms of hypoglycemia fall into two groups: those related to central nervous system (CNS) glucose deprivation and those related to adrenergic stimulation. Symptoms related to CNS glucose deprivation include hunger, lethargy, irritability, or confusion and may progress to generalized seizures. Adrenergic symptoms include tachycardia, sweating, pallor, and a feeling of anxiety and tremulousness.

Hypoglycemia must be treated promptly. Mild insulin reactions can be treated orally with the equivalent of 10 to 20 g of glucose. Liquids are preferred, such as 8 oz of fruit juice or soft drink. In emergencies, any source of carbohydrate will suffice, such as candy, bread, fruit, cookies, etc. Patients should be instructed to carry some form of sugar with them at all times. The use of hard candies should be discouraged, because they dissolve too slowly and present the risk of aspiration. Convenient packages of glucose tablets and tubes of glucose-containing gels are now available at drugstores.

Families of children with diabetes should have glucagon available at home for treatment of severe insulin reactions if the child cannot readily eat or drink. Glucagon for injection is available in kits containing 1 mg of glucagon with a vial of diluent. The dose is 1 mg for children of all ages and can be given subcutaneously with an insulin syringe of either the 0.5-mL or 1-mL size. Plasma glucose level will rise within a few minutes and remain elevated for at least 60 to 90 minutes. Clinical improvement is usually rapid but may be slower if the duration of hypoglycemia was prolonged. If the child is not fully alert and oriented within 15 to 30 minutes, the parents should consult with the physician.

Ketoacidosis and Intercurrent Illness

Ketoacidosis is a much less common crisis in home management of children with diabetes than hypoglycemia. The most frequent precipitating event, an intercurrent viral or bacterial infection, leads to an increase in insulin requirements. Less frequent causes include deliberate omission of insulin or emotional stress. Mild ketoacidosis can be corrected with appropriate therapy at home, if recognized early and treated before severe dehydration and acidosis develop.

Patients and parents should be instructed to monitor levels of plasma glucose and urine glucose and ketones more closely during intercurrent illnesses. As a general guide, the specific illness can be treated in the same way as in a nondiabetic child. Medications containing sugar need not be avoided, because the amount of extra sugar consumed is small compared with that already in the diet. Decongestants containing adrenergic drugs may cause mild hyperglycemia; this can be readily managed with small increases in the doses of short-acting insulin (see next paragraph). It is safest not to make increases in the dose of intermediate or long-acting insulin.

For moderate hyperglycemia leading to symptoms of polyuria and for ketonuria, treatment should be started promptly to 1) provide supplemental short-acting insulin and 2) correct any dehydration. In addition to the usual dose of insulin, extra insulin injection should be given every 4 hours until the plasma glucose level falls to 200 mg/dL or less and ketonuria disappears. If ketonuria persists with the plasma glucose level below 200 mg/dL, carbohydrate-containing liquids should be given in addition to supplemental regular insulin until the ketones clear.

The initial dose of supplemental regular insulin should be 10% to 20% of the usual total daily dose; this can be modified upward or downward depending on the degree of hyperglycemia and ketonuria and response to previous doses. Oral fluids should be encouraged to correct deficits and to replace ongoing urine losses (initially, at least 8 to 16 oz hourly). The child's thirst usually provides a good indication of fluid need. Parents should be carefully instructed to seek medical advice if significant improvement is not seen within 4 to 8 hours or if the child is vomiting.

WELL-PATIENT CARE

Regular office visits provide the physician an opportunity to 1) review the diabetes management by the family and the physiologic effects on the patient, 2) determine if there are areas in which the family needs additional education, and 3) assess the psychosocial adaptations of the patient and family. The family should present their blood glucose monitoring records to the physician and discuss adjustments they have made in the home regimen, including diet, activity, and insulin dose. The physical examination includes careful documentation of weight, height, and blood pressure. The funduscopic examination may reveal changes of diabetic retinopathy, although early changes may only be appreciated by an experienced ophthalmologist. The thyroid gland should be palpated routinely, because children with type I diabetes have an increased incidence of Hashimoto thyroiditis. Hepatomegaly may be seen with poor control (Mauriac syndrome). Injection sites should be examined for evidence of lipoatrophy or hypertrophy. Contractures of the interphalangeal joints of the fingers have been described in diabetic patients in poor control. The hands and fingers are placed flat together with the fingers spread. The patient with contractures is unable to bring the palmar surfaces of the fingers into contact along their entire length.

Measurement of glycosylated hemoglobin level is very useful as an objective indicator of glycemic control during the preceding 3 months, a period of time corresponding roughly to red blood cell life span. Normal ranges vary depending on whether total glycosylated or specifically HbA_{1c} is measured and must be obtained from the laboratory. Total glycosylated hemoglobin levels are usually 30% higher than the HbA_{1c} fraction. In the DCCT the intensive treatment group was able to maintain an average HbA_{1c} level of 7%, with normal being less than 6.05%. We recommend that the condition of a child with diabetes be evaluated periodically by a pediatric endocrinologist or diabetologist. There is no substitute for experience in the management of type I diabetes, and the diabetologist may be a valuable resource for the primary care physician both in routine management and crisis care. Current ADA recommendation for monitoring diabetic patients are: 1) total glycosylated hemoglobin or HbA_{1c} fraction on a quarterly basis, 2) urine for microalbumin annually if greater than 12 years of age or disease duration greater than 5 years, 3) ophthalmologic examination annually if greater than 12 years of age or disease duration greater than 5 years, and 4) lipid profile for children greater than 2 years of age. If values are normal this evaluation should be repeated every 5 years.

The psychosocial aspects of diabetes are critical to successful long-term management. Behavioral counseling begins at the time that the diagnosis of diabetes is made. The manner in which the child and family adjust to the diagnosis and education and the resources they are able to mobilize give important indications of potential problem areas. Parenting skills surrounding control vs autonomy issues must be assessed and discussed in terms of the impact that the patient's disorder may have on family dynamics. Strategies for coping with such crises as refusal to test blood glucose level, administer insulin, or follow the meal plan should be worked out by the parents in consultation with the physician.

Behavior problems at home often are attributed to hypoglycemia, and therefore excused by parents. Although we stress that unexplained irritability or lethargy may be a symptom of hypoglycemia, the behavior needs to be addressed in an appropriate manner by the family.

Invariably, there are families whose needs cannot be adequately met with office counseling. Referral to an appropriate psychological or psychiatric therapist should be initiated as quickly as possible. If therapy is to be effective, the primary physician and the therapist must coordinate their efforts to provide the patient and family with unambiguous goals and expectations. The inclusion of the therapist within the health care team emphasizes the importance of the family's involvement in counseling.

Implantable closed-loop pumps and pancreas transplants of β cell may ultimately become the therapy for type I diabetes. Until then, the family's decision-making skills and understanding of diabetes are the key to diabetic management. The family is supported in this by the primary care physician, in the role of educator, counselor, and consultant. The resources of other health care personnel, including dieticians, nurse-educators, and subspecialists such as diabetologists, ophthalmologists, and nephrologists are coordinated by the primary physician. Our goal in this chapter has been to provide a framework for the comprehensive approach to the care of the child with type I diabetes. Managing diabetes is not an easy task. It is time-consuming for the physician and requires an alteration of life-style for the family. With support from the primary care physician and other professionals, the quality of life of the family and child with diabetes can be greatly improved.

BIBLIOGRAPHY

American Diabetes Association Position Statement: Standards of medical care for patients with diabetes mellitus, *Diabetes Care* 17(6): 616–623, 1994.

American Diabetes Association: Nutrition recommendations and principles for people with diabetes mellitus, *Diabetes Care* 17:519–522, 1994.

The Diabetes Control and Complication Trial Research Group: The effect of intensive treatment of diabetes on the development and progression of long-term complications in insulin-dependent diabetes mellitus, *N Engl J Med* 329(14):977–986, 1993.

Travis LB: *An instructional aid on insulin-dependent diabetes mellitus,* ed 10, Austin, 1995, Designer's Ink.

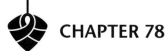

CHAPTER 78

Endocrinology

Stuart Alan Weinzimer
Mary Min-chin Lee
Thomas Moshang, Jr.

Endocrinology involves diagnosis and treatment of chronic endocrine disease as well as differentiation of pathologic patterns of growth and development from variations of normal. The diagnosis of an endocrine disorder often rests on the primary physician's ability to discern subtle abnormalities of growth and development, to recognize clinical manifestations suggestive of disturbances in hormone regulation, and to evaluate commonly available endocrine laboratory tests.

This chapter discusses both the management of some common endocrine problems and the appropriate initial evaluation and subsequent referral of children with more complex endocrine disorders by the primary care physician.

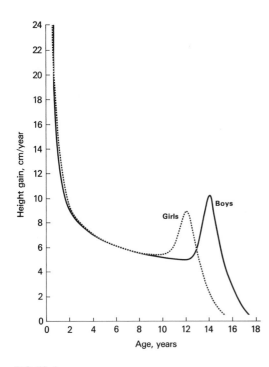

FIG 78-1
Growth velocity chart for children indicates yearly increments of change.

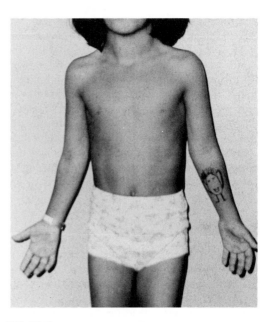

FIG 78-2
Patient with Turner syndrome demonstrates increased carrying angle of elbows.

DISORDERS OF GROWTH

Growth is a dynamic process that reflects genetic potential, nutritional status, and physical and emotional health. Consequently, height and weight measurements are a fundamental and necessary component of all medical examinations. Although clinically useful information can sometimes be derived from isolated heights and weights, normal and abnormal growth patterns can only be recognized through accurate plotting of sequential, consistent measurements on a growth chart. Both the growth rate and the absolute height need to be considered when making a determination of growth failure.

An abnormal growth rate can be defined as a rate of increase in linear height that is consistently below the mean growth velocity for age (Fig. 78-1).

The average full-term newborn measures approximately 20 inches, grows 10 inches within the first year of life, 5 in the second, 3 in the third, and 2 inches a year thereafter until the pubertal growth spurt. A slower than normal growth rate often results in a flattening of the growth curve or a decrease in percentiles on the growth chart. Growth failure is present when the growth rate is subnormal even though the height for age is still normal. The term *short stature* implies a height for age below the 3rd percentile, independent of growth rate. Not all children with short stature have abnormal growth. In variants of normal growth such as familial short stature and constitutional delay of growth and development the absolute height may be below the 3rd percentile, but the growth rate is normal for age.

A patient with an abnormal growth rate signifying growth failure requires further study. The history and physical findings are of major importance in the evaluation. The laboratory evaluation should be directed at confirming the diagnosis suspected by the clinical findings. Screening studies include a complete blood cell (CBC) count, a sedimentation rate, a biochemical profile, a urinalysis, thyroid studies, and a bone age determination. A delayed bone age is compatible with constitutional delay, growth hormone deficiency, or any severe systemic illness and is suggestive of a correctable cause of the growth failure. Because short stature may be the only phenotypic expression of Turner syndrome, a karyotype analysis is a critical screening test in girls (Fig. 78-2).

In some centers, insulinlike growth factor (IGF)-1 (formerly referred to as *somatomedin C*) levels have been used in confirming the clinical impression of lack of illness or in recognizing patients with growth hormone (GH) deficiency. However, low IGF-1 levels are found in normal children in whom physiologic maturation is less than 4 years (as might be found in a child aged 5 or 6 years with a delayed bone age), malnutrition, and systemic illness other than (GH) deficiency. Furthermore, children with (GH) deficiency can have a normal level of IGF-1.

If an intracranial pathologic lesion is suspected, computed tomography (CT) or magnetic resonance imaging (MRI) of the head is indicated. In general, the more common nonendocrine causes of growth failure must be excluded before growth hormone deficiency or other less common disorders are considered.

Constitutional Delay and Familial Short Stature

Constitutional delay of growth and development and familial short stature are two of the most frequently encountered causes of short stature. The hallmark of both constitutional delay and familial short stature is a normal rate of growth and a prominent family history. In constitutional delay, a slowing of the growth rate generally occurs between 1 and 3 years of age with a correspondent delay in physical maturation and bone age. Subsequently, growth is normal, and physical development and bone age progress at a normal rate, although generally 2 or 3 years behind chronologic age. Adolescent development begins 2 to 3 years later than average in these patients, and the ultimate adult height attained is usually within the normal range. Because of the excellent prognosis, an explanation of the disorder and reassurance is the most effective therapy. However, if psychosocial difficulties arise in boys because of their pubertal delay, short-term low-dose testosterone therapy may initiate sexual development in these patients and improve their psychosocial outlook. Testosterone therapy for boys with constitutional delay probably has no effect on ultimate height.

Familial short stature is characterized by short stature, normal rate of growth, normal bone age, and a strong family history of short stature. Therapy is limited to reassurance and general counseling. GH treatment is not indicated in children with constitutional delay or familial short stature. The use of GH in otherwise normal children may result in abusive use of this potent hormone, and related serious side effects may occur (eg, abnormal glucose tolerance, diabetes, tumorigenesis). A questionable increase in the incidence of leukemia has been associated with GH treatment.

Growth Hormone Deficiency

The child with abnormal growth rate can be screened for GH deficiency with measurement of serum growth factors. Because IGF-1 concentrations are low in many chronic diseases as well as in GH deficiency, a low value may not be diagnostic of GH deficiency, but a normal value would indicate probable normal GH production. Measurement of IGF-binding protein 3 (IGF-BP3) may provide a more accurate assessment of the GH axis. IGF-BP3 levels correlate with GH production and exhibit less variation in malnutrition and other systemic disease states. IGF-1 and IGF-BP3 levels correlate with bone age and chronologic age and are lowest during infancy. Consequently, serum levels must be interpreted in light of the patient's bone age and physiologic maturation. The combined use of IGF-1 and IGF-BP3 measurements may allow for the most thorough screening for complete and partial GH deficiency and GH receptor deficiency.

The possible diagnosis of GH deficiency, suggested by clinical findings as well as low IGF-1 and IGF-BP3 levels, needs to be evaluated further with GH provocative tests.

Because GH secretion is pulsatile in nature and basal levels are often low, random GH levels are not diagnostic of GH deficiency. Several tests that stimulate GH secretion are available for the diagnosis of GH deficiency, as shown in Table 78-1. These provocative tests are not free of side effects, and their use is restricted to inpatient or closely monitored outpatient services. It is generally accepted that at least two provocative tests must show subnormal GH response to be diagnostic of GH deficiency.

Human GH usually is given intramuscularly or subcutaneously three times a week. Although hypersensitivity reactions to GH are rare, an occasional patient will complain of minor skin rashes. These rashes will often disappear spontaneously or with small doses of antihistamines. The reconstituted GH is fairly stable and can be conserved for 4 to 6 weeks under refrigeration.

TABLE 78-1
Tests of Growth Hormone Secretory Capacity

TESTS	CONDITIONS	OBSERVATIONS
Physiologic tests		
Exercise	15 min of moderate exercise followed by 5 min of vigorous exercise	Frequent findings of low response in normal subjects
Sleep	Deep sleep (EEG stages 3–4); 60%–70% of normal children will have a response of at least 7 ng/mL of growth hormone during deep sleep	Best utilized in association with sleep EEG
Provocative tests		
Insulin	Regular insulin, 0.05–0.1 U/kg, IV	Severe hypoglycemia
Arginine	0.5 g/kg, IV, over 30 min	Local irritation, numbness, nausea, vomiting, hypoglycemia
Levodopa	0.5 g/m^2, orally	Cardiac and blood pressure changes, nausea and vomiting
Glucagon	0.03 mg/kg, IM, up to 0.5 mg, IM	Nausea and vomiting
Propranolol	1.0 mg/kg up to 40 mg orally; can be used to augment responses to primary stimuli (glucagon, exercise, levodopa or arginine)	Changes in heart rate or blood pressure, hypoglycemia

EEG—electroencephalogram; IM—intramuscularly; IV—intravenously.

Patients should be cautioned that should a precipitate develop on reconstitution, the vial of GH should be discarded.

DISORDERS OF THE THYROID

Thyroid Function Tests

The most common tests utilized to evaluate thyroid function at present include the measurement of total thyroxine (T_4), triiodothyronine resin uptake (T_3RU), and thyroid-stimulating hormone (TSH). Serum T_4 measurement, the most useful indicator of thyroid function, usually correlates well with the clinical disorders. However, the serum T_4 concentration must be interpreted with the knowledge of those factors that may alter the serum T_4 concentration but are not related to alteration of thyroid function. Chronic illness, such as starvation (malnutrition) or hypoxia, may lower serum T_4. Because the determination of serum T_4 measures total hormone, protein bound as well as free (or unbound) hormone, an alteration of the concentration of circulating T_4-binding proteins will result in altered concentrations of serum T_4. Only free T_4 is metabolically active. T_4-binding globulin (TBG), the main binding protein, varies with age, illness, and serum estrogen concentration.

T_3RU is an indirect measurement of TBG and other thyroid hormone–binding proteins. T_4 and T_3RU levels are elevated in hyperthyroidism and low in hypothyroidism. When the T_3RU and the serum T_4 levels are discordant, alterations of thyroid hormone–binding protein concentrations rather than abnormalities of thyroid function should be suspected. The calculated "free T_4 index" (the product of T_3RU and T_4) provides an estimation of free T_4 and correlates closely with measured free T_4. Free T_4 and TBG assays are also available, although they are more expensive.

Because the thyroid gland is under negative feedback control by the pituitary gland, TSH determinations represent a sensitive in vivo measure of the adequacy of thyroid function. Thyroid failure results in elevated TSH levels. With the recent development of a more sensitive TSH assay, the suppressed low levels of TSH seen in hyperthyroidism can now be distinguished from the low basal values seen in the normal euthyroid state.

A number of less common disorders may result in unexpected low TSH findings when the clinical findings suggest hypothyroidism. Low T_4 and low TSH values are found in secondary (pituitary) hypothyroidism, tertiary (hypothalamic) hypothyroidism, and in chronic illnesses ("euthyroid sick syndrome"). The rare syndrome of resistance to T_4 is biochemically characterized

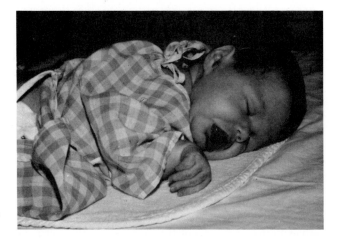

FIG 78-3
Patient with congenital hypothyroidism. Note the large tongue and puffy eyelids.

by high T_4 values, a normal or slightly elevated level of TSH, and a normal TSH surge in response to thyrotropin-releasing hormone (TRH) stimulation.

In general, T_4 concentration and T_3 resin uptake are the most useful tests in confirming the clinical suspicion of hypothyroidism or hyperthyroidism. The measurement of total T_3 should be reserved for the rare occasion when clinical findings indicate hyperthyroidism but the serum T_4 and T_3RU levels are not confirmatory (the syndrome of T_3 thyrotoxicosis). A TSH level should be obtained once hypothyroidism has been established or in the clinical presence of a goiter.

Other useful tests that the endocrinologist might order for delineating the unusual conditions include the TRH stimulation test, radioiodine uptake and scan, ultrasonography, and fine-needle or open biopsies of the thyroid gland.

Congenital Hypothyroidism

Congenital hypothyroidism can be difficult to diagnose clinically. In addition, irreparable neurologic impairment and mental retardation are often established before the clinical findings of hypothyroidism become manifest. Consequently, newborn screening programs have been developed and are now required by law in most states to allow the prompt diagnosis and treatment of hypothyroid infants. With the institution of these programs, the incidence of congenital hypothyroidism has been determined to be approximately one in 4000 newborns (Fig. 78-3).

Thyroid screening tests are designed to identify newborns with T_4 concentrations in the lower 3% of the general population. Most screening programs include determinations of TSH concentrations in patients with low T_4 concentrations. An elevated TSH level in association with a low T_4 concentration is highly suggestive of congenital hypothyroidism. A normal or low TSH level in association with a low T_4 is compatible with congenital TBG deficiency, the "euthyroid sick syndrome" in small or sick newborns or secondary (pituitary) or tertiary (hypothalamic) hypothyroidism. If the screening tests are abnormal, further evaluation with serum concentrations of T_4, TSH, and TBG is necessary for diagnostic confirmation. Radioactive iodine studies, ultrasonography, or serum thyroglobulin determinations may be useful in determining those infants with ectopic thyroid tissue or a hormone synthesis defect.

Treatment is 6 to 8 µg/kg/day of levothyroxine, given as a single daily dose. Serum T_4 and TSH concentrations should be repeated 6 to 8 weeks after treatment is started and every 3 months thereafter to assess the adequacy of therapy. Serum T_4 concentrations are maintained in the upper range of normal. In infants less than 1 year of age, TSH concentrations are very difficult to suppress to normal levels on the usual replacement doses. Consequently, if the T_4 and free T_4 concentrations (as evaluated by the T_3RU or TBG level) are appropriate, slightly elevated TSH levels are acceptable. Using higher than usual doses of levothyroxine in order to suppress the TSH to normal levels in these children may result in complications often associated with hyperthyroidism, such as premature closure of the cranial sutures. The prognosis is usually good if therapy is begun early; however, even appropriately treated infants may have a slight decrease in intelligence when compared with their siblings.

Acquired Hypothyroidism

The causes of acquired hypothyroidism can be classified as primary (thyroid gland dysfunction), secondary (pituitary insufficiency), and tertiary (hypothalamic disease). The most frequent is primary hypothyroidism, often due to chronic lymphocytic thyroiditis (Hashimoto thyroiditis). Other less frequent forms of acquired hypothyroidism include thyroid ectopy, dyshormonogenesis, and pituitary tumors or trauma.

Hypothyroidism usually will present clinically with the slow onset of growth failure; dull, placid expression; myxedema; cold intolerance; constipation; bradycardia; hypotension; brittle hair; and dry, pale skin. Occasionally, the only presenting sign is poor growth and, therefore, a high index of suspicion for thyroid dysfunction is warranted to make the diagnosis. In girls, primary or secondary amenorrhea can be the presenting complaint. An unusual presentation is that of hypothyroidism associated with pseudoprecocious puberty and galactorrhea. The sexual precocity is occasionally complete with breast development, pubic hair, galactorrhea, and vaginal spotting in girls and testicular enlargement in boys. These changes often regress with adequate thyroid replacement. Finally, hypothyroidism can be subclinical or "compensated" when the gland begins to fail but continues secreting adequate amounts of hormone due to increased TSH stimulation.

The diagnosis of hypothyroidism can be easily confirmed by measuring TSH, T_4, and T_3 resin uptake. An elevated TSH level indicates primary gland failure. A low TSH level in the presence of a low T_4 level and low T_3RU is compatible with the diagnosis of pituitary or hypothalamic hypothyroidism or euthyroid hypothyroxinemia secondary to illness.

Once diagnosed, therapy with levothyroxine should be initiated. The usual dose is 3 to 4 µg/kg/day taken as a single oral dose (usually 0.1 to 0.15 mg/day). Adequacy of thyroid hormone replacement should be evaluated clinically and by T_4 and TSH determinations 6 to 8 weeks after starting therapy and every 6 to 12 months thereafter.

Parents should be cautioned that once their child begins thyroid hormone replacement the child will appear livelier and less docile. The child's school work will occasionally deteriorate because of relative hyperactivity and decreased attention span. Most patients will lose their excess myxedematous water weight, and their coarse, dry hair will be lost and slowly replaced by hair of normal texture. Stomach ache (due to increased peristalsis) and headache are occasionally encountered. These complaints are generally transient and do not require specific therapy.

Once the child is euthyroid on levothyroxine therapy, there is no contraindication to full physical activity. There is no increased risk for surgical procedures. In addition, there are no problems with the use of other medications, including those drugs containing iodides.

The prognosis in acquired hypothyroidism is excellent. Normal physical and neurologic development and function can be expected if the patient is receiving adequate replacement therapy. In addition, treatment is easy, inexpensive, and well-tolerated.

Hyperthyroidism

Graves disease, the most common cause of thyrotoxicosis in children, is an autoimmune disorder characterized by the presence of antithyroid immunoglobulins that bind to the TSH receptor of the thyroid gland and stimulate excessive thyroid hormone secretion. In the presence of these thyroid-stimulating immunoglobulins (TSI), the gland, independent of pituitary control, hypertrophies and secretes large amounts of hormone. The older patient often has gradual onset of goiter and complaints of nervousness, palpitations, heat intolerance, increased appetite, and amenorrhea. Younger children often exhibit hyperactivity and behavior problems.

The measurement of serum T_4 and T_3RU level will usually confirm the clinical diagnosis. The syndrome of T_3 thyrotoxicosis is unusual in childhood except during treatment with thionamide drugs. Determinations of serum T_3 levels are generally not necessary until after the initiation of medical therapy. Measurements of antithyroid receptor antibodies or TSI are useful, not only for confirming autoimmune hyperthyroidism but also as an indicator for discontinuing antithyroid medication.

At the Children's Hospital of Philadelphia, the thionamide drugs are the treatment of choice for juvenile thyrotoxicosis. These drugs block the organification of iodide by the thyroid gland and thus decrease the amount of thyroid hormone synthesized. Propylthiouracil and methimazole are the most often used thionamides. The dose of propylthiouracil is 8 mg/kg/day, given three times a day. The dose of methimazole is one tenth that of propylthiouracil. Clinical improvement occurs in several weeks with the thionamides alone. If the patient is very symptomatic or the cardiovascular findings of hyperthyroidism very pronounced, propranolol can be used in conjunction with the thionamides. The dose of propranolol is 1 to 2 mg/kg/day. The dose of the thionamides should be adjusted to maintain the T_4 and T_3 levels within the normal range.

Methimazole and propylthiouracil are both associated with side effects that can complicate medical therapy. Minor side effects include vomiting, stomach upset, leukopenia, arthralgia, arthritis, and urticarial rashes. In general, these are not an indication for discontinuing therapy unless they are very severe. The major complication of thionamide therapy is agranulocytosis. Although rare, it can be life threatening and must be recognized early. Routine blood cell counts are ineffective in predicting this complication because agranulocytosis can appear in a previously healthy patient. However, blood cell counts should be obtained if a patient receiving thionamides develops fever. If agranulocytosis is present, blood cultures should be obtained and antibiotic therapy started immediately. The thionamides should be discontinued and alternate forms of therapy used.

Hyperthyroid patients should be evaluated clinically and with thyroid function tests every 4 to 6 months. At The Children's Hospital of Philadelphia, therapy is discontinued once the patient has been euthyroid for at least 2 years. The patient must be followed-up closely, and if hyperthyroidism recurs, therapy reinstituted.

Failure of medical therapy is due to lack of drug compliance, complications of drug therapy, and unresponsiveness to thionamide drugs. In these cases, thyroid ablation through radioiodine or surgical therapy is indicated. Although the advantages of one form of therapy over the other are a matter of great debate, both are effective forms of therapy. In general, the choice depends on the availability of an experienced surgeon and the patient's personal inclinations.

Thyroid Hormone Resistance

Generalized resistance to thyroid hormone (GRTH), first described in 1967, is defined by the clinical triad of elevated T_4 and T_3 levels, inappropriately normal or elevated TSH level, and peripheral euthyroidism or hypothyroidism. Abnormalities in the thyroid hormone receptors located in the pituitary lead to the continued secretion of TSH in the face of elevated levels of circulating thyroid hormones. These patients are clinically euthyroid or even hypothyroid due to the reduced thyroid hormone receptor activity at the tissue level (pituitary and peripheral resistance). In a variant of GRTH known as *selective pituitary resistance,* inappropriately normal TSH levels in the setting of elevated circulating thyroid hormone levels accompany the clinical features of hyperthyroidism, such as nervousness and tachycardia.

Attention-deficit hyperactivity disorder (ADHD) has been found in up to 70% of children with GRTH. The converse, however, is not true; thyroid hormone resistance itself is a very rare cause of ADHD.

Thyroid Goiters and Nodules

Thyroid goiters are a common occurrence in childhood and can be accompanied by signs of hypothyroidism, hyperthyroidism, or euthyroidism (Fig. 78-4). The most common cause of thyroid gland enlargement in children is chronic lymphocytic thyroiditis, which accounts for 40% to 60% of simple, nontoxic goiters. Chronic lymphocytic thyroiditis is a pathologic diagnosis characterized by interfollicular lymphocytic infiltration of the thyroid gland with formation of germinal follicles and destruction of functioning thyroid tissue. Antimicrosomal or antithyroglobulin antibodies are present in 80% to 85% of patients. Other causes of simple goiters include inborn errors of T_4 synthesis, adolescence in girls, and drugs.

Drug-induced goiters occur more commonly than expected. Drugs implicated in thyroid gland enlargement include iodine (and other halogens), lithium, para-amino salicylic acid, phenylbutazone, thionamides, and the white turnip plants. Breast milk from mothers receiving antithyroid therapy may induce thyroid gland enlargement in their newborn infants.

Thyroid nodules are not uncommon in childhood. Thyroid nodules in children are more often malignant than nodules in adults. The malignant nodule is often "stony hard" and associated with lymphadenopathy. The child with a thyroid nodule should be referred for evaluation and therapy. The evaluation will include radioactive scanning as well as ultra-sonography (Fig. 78-5). A nodule that does not take up the radioiodine, ie, a "cold" nodule, should be surgically removed if ultrasound shows a mixed solid/cystic lesion. A needle biopsy can be performed on a completely cystic lesion before deciding further therapy.

DISORDERS OF THE ADRENAL GLANDS

Adrenal Insufficiency

Adrenal insufficiency may be due to primary failure of the adrenal gland or may be secondary to pituitary or hypothalamic disorders. In childhood, primary adrenal failure due to autoimmune processes, infectious disorders such as tuberculosis or histoplasmosis, and malignancies is relatively uncommon. Primary acute adrenal insufficiency during childhood is more likely to be due to congenital adrenal hyperplasia or meningococcal infections with resulting acute adrenal crisis. Chronic adrenal insufficiency during childhood is more likely to be secondary to either pituitary or hypothalamic disease.

The clinical findings of chronic adrenal failure include weakness, lethargy, exercise intolerance, poor weight gain, anorexia, nausea, vomiting,

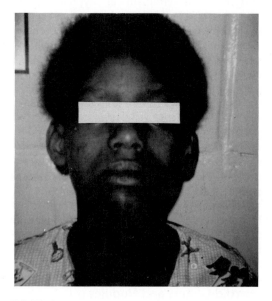

FIG 78-4
Patient with hyperthyroidism with goiter.

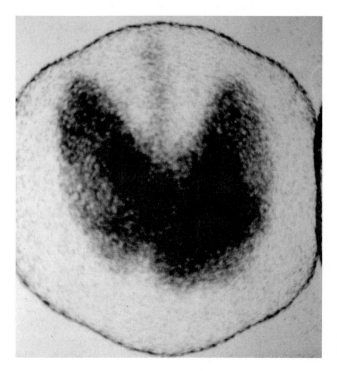

FIG 78-5
^{123}I uptake scan shows goiter and nodule.

headaches, salt craving, polyuria, and dehydration. In primary gland failure, hyperpigmentation may be present and is best noted in the areolae, mucous membranes, extensor surfaces of joints (knees, elbows, and fingers), and surgical scars. Routine laboratory tests may reveal hyponatremia, hyperkalemia, acidosis, and eosinophilia. A morning cortisol level may be low, but a normal level does not rule out the possibility of adrenal insufficiency.

The diagnosis of adrenal insufficiency requires adrenocorticotropic hormone (ACTH) stimulation testing and demonstration of the lack of response in primary adrenal failure or inadequate response of the adrenal in secondary adrenal failure. Once adrenal insufficiency has been diagnosed, appropriate tests should be performed in an effort to elucidate the cause.

Adrenal insufficiency requires chronic replacement therapy with glucocorticoids and, usually, mineralocorticoids. Although a number of glucocorticoids can be prescribed, hydrocortisone is the most frequently used corticosteroid because it is the naturally occurring hormone. Physiologic replacement is achieved with 15 to 25 mg/m^2/day of hydrocortisone taken orally in three divided doses. Mineralocorticoid deficiency requires replacement with a steroid such as fludrocortisone (Florinef) in doses of 0.05 to 0.1 mg once a day.

Patients on corticosteroid replacement will require an increase in their steroid dose during times of severe illness, trauma, or stress. Under these circumstances, patients can be instructed to increase their usual daily dose threefold. They should receive at least 75 mg/m^2/day of hydrocortisone. If vomiting should occur, the oral dose should be repeated in 10 to 15 minutes. If vomiting persists, intramuscular cortisone acetate, at three or four times the usual daily dose, is indicated. This dose can be repeated every 24 hours if necessary for several days. If severe vomiting, prostration, or acute adrenal failure develop, intravenous fluid therapy is required immediately. All patients should be instructed to continue the increased dose of steroids during the acute phase of the illness and to then return to their maintenance dosages within several days.

Patients with secondary (pituitary) adrenal insufficiency are very sensitive to steroid therapy and may not need maintenance treatment or may require only one third to one half the usual physiologic replacement dose. Most of these patients, however, will require increased or pharmacologic doses (75 mg/m^2/day of hydrocortisone) during times of illness or stress. Mineralocorticoid production in these patients is usually normal, and replacement with salt-retaining steroids is not indicated.

Careful follow-up of children on glucocorticoid therapy is essential to ensure that they do not develop signs of steroid excess. Determinations of height and weight are helpful because poor growth and excessive weight gain are often the first signs of corticosteroid excess. Weight loss, nausea, and hypotension may be indicative of insufficient glucocorticoid treatment.

Acute Adrenal Insufficiency (Adrenal Crisis)

Acute adrenal failure is a life-threatening condition that must be treated early and aggressively to ensure survival. Adrenal crisis may be the first manifestation of Addison disease (chronic adrenal insufficiency) or of congenital adrenal hyperplasia. Adrenal crisis also may occur with acute decompensation in a patient known to have these disorders. The patient in adrenal crisis may present in an acutely dehydrated state and be moribund and cachectic. Routine laboratory studies may demonstrate hyponatremia, hyperkalemia, and, occasionally, hypoglycemia.

The most important facet of therapy of adrenal crisis is aggressive fluid and electrolyte management. Most patients present with severe water and salt loss. Cardiovascular collapse is the principal cause of death. To treat hypotension, normal saline containing 5% dextrose should be given as a 20- to 30-mL/kg bolus over 10 to 20 minutes or faster, if necessary. Blood pressure should be monitored closely, and normal saline should be continued until a normal blood pressure is attained. After acute resuscitation, normal saline containing 5% dextrose is infused at a rate to provide maintenance requirements and correct any fluid and electrolyte deficits. If hyponatremia becomes symptomatic (usually less than 120 mEq/dL), it should be corrected immediately and vigorously with 3% saline solution. The dose (in milliliters) of 3% saline solution to be infused over 15 minutes can be calculated by the formula

$$[120 - \text{Na level (mEq/L)}] \times 0.6 \times \text{weight (kg)} \times 2$$

While the resuscitative phase is under way, hydrocortisone in the hemisuccinate form should be given initially as an intravenous bolus in a dose of 2 to 4 mg/kg followed by 200 to 400 mg by constant intravenous infusion over the next 24 hours. If available, desoxycorticosterone acetate at a dose of 2 to 3 mg intramuscularly should be given to provide mineralocorticoid activity. Glucocorticoids can be subsequently supplied by giving cortisone acetate in a dose of 50 to 100 mg intramuscularly every 24 hours. Desoxycorticosterone acetate and cortisone acetate should be continued intramuscularly until the patient is well enough to return to his/her usual therapeutic regimen.

Tapering of Glucocorticoid Administration

Chronic, large-dose steroid therapy is often necessary in children with certain diseases, such as bronchial asthma, nephrosis, nephritis, and leukemia. Consequently, steroid withdrawal often becomes a problem that must be handled with extreme caution. Acute, life-threatening adrenal insufficiency may occur when the adrenal-pituitary axis has not had time to recover following suppressive corticoid therapy. If the patient has not previously received steroid therapy and has received acute, intensive therapy for less than 3 days, it is not necessary to taper the medication, and the steroids can be suspended abruptly. If therapy has persisted for 3 to 10 days, the dose can be tapered quickly, changed to a single morning dose, then to an alternate-day dose, and finally discontinued. If chronic, high-dose therapy has been used, gradual tapering of glucocorticoid dosage is necessary to avoid the possible exacerbation of the primary disease process or the precipitation of acute adrenal failure. Several protocols have been developed for this purpose. In general, if the primary disease permits, the steroid dose can be decreased by 50% each week until maintenance levels are reached. Subsequently, the dose may be decreased by 20% every 3 days until the glucocorticoids are finally discontinued. It is advisable that steroids be given at three times the maintenance doses if the patient is stressed either medically or surgically up to 1 year after cessation of therapy. If signs of adrenal insufficiency develop while corticosteroids are being tapered, the dose should be increased again to previous levels. Symptoms of impending adrenal failure include anorexia, nausea, vomiting, lethargy, headache, and hypotension.

DISORDERS OF THE REPRODUCTIVE SYSTEM

Hirsutism

Hirsutism refers to the increase in short, thick, terminal hair that is usually associated with signs of masculinization. An increase in terminal hair over the upper lips, beard area, upper back, and chest in girls is consistent with hirsutism, especially if accompanied by other signs of virilization, such as clitoromegaly or amenorrhea.

The most common cause of hirsutism is excessive androgen production in late-onset congenital adrenal hyperplasia or in polycystic ovary syndrome. The differential diagnosis of hyperandrogenism must include ovarian and adrenal tumors. Hirsutism can also be familial, a side effect of diazoxide or diphenytoin use, or secondary to hypothyroidism, malnutrition, or central nervous system injury.

In evaluating a patient complaining of hirsutism, it is important to determine if there has been a change in the amount or location of the body hair and if it has been accompanied by a change in weight, voice pitch, or menstrual irregularities. A history of drug intake and a family history of hirsutism should be sought. On physical examination, the location of the body hair, the presence of acanthosis nigricans, and signs of virilization (change in body fat or muscle, clitoral enlargement) should be noted. Patients with true hirsutism, menstrual irregularities, or signs of virilization should be formally evaluated.

The laboratory studies include serum levels of testosterone, free testosterone, dihydroepiandrosterone (DHEA), 17-hydroxyprogesterone, androstenedione, follicle-stimulating hormone (FSH), luteinizing hormone (LH), and prolactin. A karyotype analysis might be necessary. In women, serum testosterone concentrations greater than 200 ng/dL that are not suppressible by dexamethasone suggest the possibility of an adrenal or ovarian tumor. The patient should undergo further evaluation, which would include ultrasound and CT of the abdomen and pelvis.

A mild increase in the serum androgen levels suggests the possibility of an androgen excess syndrome. The serum androgen most often elevated is free (unbound) testosterone. The androgen excess syndromes include late-onset congenital adrenal hyperplasia, polycystic ovary syndrome, and mixed gonadal dysgenesis. To differentiate the various androgen disorders, ACTH stimulation and dexamethasone suppression tests are necessary. The measurement of various steroidal precursors along the cortisol biosynthetic pathway, including 17-hydroxypregnenolone, 17-hydroxyprogesterone, and 11-deoxycortisol, should be determined during ACTH testing. The patient with elevated androgen levels should be referred to an endocrinologist, because the interpretation of the results of the various stimulation or suppression tests is often difficult.

Therapy is to be directed at the underlying pathologic disorder. Surgery is indicated for adrenal or ovarian tumors, whereas glucocorticoids are used for congenital adrenal hyperplasia. Birth control pills containing progesterone have been found to be effective in the polycystic ovary syndrome because they interrupt the constant estrous cycle and lead to normal ovarian function. Because glucocorticoids have been shown to decrease ovarian steroid production, they have also been used as therapy for polycystic ovary syndrome with mixed success. Other medications that have been beneficial include clomiphene citrate, cyproterone acetate, and spironolactone. Cosmetic improvement occasionally can be obtained with electrolysis, although some degree of facial hair usually remains.

Precocious Puberty

Sexual precocity is the appearance of secondary sexual characteristics before 8 years of age in girls and 9 years of age in boys. True precocious puberty refers to sexual precocity produced by an elevation of FSH or LH levels. Pseudoprecocious puberty refers to sexual precocity induced by an increase in sex steroids that occurs independently of gonadotropin stimulation. True precocious puberty is generally complete, with a normal rate of progression of the secondary sexual characteristics. Pseudoprecocious puberty is usually incomplete; not all of the secondary sexual characteristics appear.

The most common problems of premature sexual development in children are premature thelarche and premature pubarche (adrenarche). Both conditions are benign but require separation from true sexual precocity or pseudosexual precocity. Premature thelarche often presents in

the young female infant. The breast development may be present from birth or appear several months after birth and progress slowly from several months to years. The bone age may be slightly advanced, and the vaginal smear may reveal some more mature cells. The general neurologic examination is normal. Levels of LH, FSH, and estradiol are normal. Most often, the breast development progresses very slowly for several months and then stabilizes. Breast tissue in a significant percentage of patients will decrease in size in several years, although a smaller number will persist or continue to increase in size.

Premature pubarche occurs in both boys and girls. There is often a strong family history of premature pubarche. The development of hair in this condition may be as early as 4 years of age, although the most common age for premature pubarche is 6 and 7 years. The bone age is normal to slightly advanced in premature pubarche. Unfortunately, mild forms of the adrenogenital syndrome also may present with premature hair development without attendant bone age advancement. A rapidly developing tumor with marked elevations of androgens might cause pubic hair development with only a slight advancement in bone age. When appropriate, the possibility of androgen excess should be evaluated by determination of serum concentrations of testosterone and androstenedione.

In girls, more than 80% of cases of true precocious puberty are idiopathic, whereas in boys more than 80% have an organic basis. Sexual precocity can be produced by disorders of the hypothalamic-pituitary axis, excessive steroid production by the adrenal gland or gonads, increased sensitivity of the peripheral tissues to circulating sex steroids, and exogenous hormone. Idiopathic precocious puberty is relatively common in girls. In boys, most cases are produced by organic lesions of the central nervous system. Adrenal or gonadal causes and idiopathic sexual precocity is much less common in boys. The aim of the clinical and laboratory evaluation is to separate those boys and girls with an organic cause of precocious puberty from those with idiopathic true precocity. Central precocious puberty, which is suppressible with long-acting gonadotropin-releasing hormone (GnRH) needs to be confirmed by GnRH testing prior to therapy. Central precocious puberty must be distinguished from gonadotropin-independent precocious puberty (McCune-Albright syndrome or familial male precocious puberty). Other than premature thelarche or pubarche, the child with precocious puberty should be referred for evaluation of possible organic causes of sexual precocity and for appropriate treatment.

Therapy is directed at the underlying pathologic disorder. Glucocorticoids are indicated for congenital adrenal hyperplasia and surgery, if possible, for tumors of the adrenal, ovary, or central nervous system. In idiopathic precocious puberty, treatment is directed at suppressing gonadotropin secretion to prevent premature epiphyseal fusion and consequent short stature. The treatment of idiopathic sexual precocity has been unsatisfactory in the past. The drugs used included medroxyprogesterone, cyproterone acetate, and bromocriptine. Although medroxyprogesterone decreased breast size and caused cessation of menses, bone age advancement often progressed, resulting in short stature.

Newly developed synthetic analogs of GnRH with the property of sustained duration of action have been used with great success to suppress FSH and LH secretion by the pituitary. The GnRH analogs leuprorelin, histrelin, and nafarelin are given as a daily subcutaneous injection or long-acting depot intramuscular preparations.

At adequate doses, sexual maturation is halted and may even regress. The increased growth rate and rapid advancement in bone age will also improve. On discontinuation of therapy, pubertal changes will resume and can progress rapidly.

Sexual Infantilism

Sexual infantilism is defined as the lack of secondary sexual characteristics by 13 years of age in girls and 14 years of age in boys. In addition, an age-appropriate onset of puberty but a lack of progression of secondary sexual maturation also may indicate a sexual infantilizing organic disorder. Sexual infantilism can be due to lack of hypothalamic or pituitary stimulation of gonadal maturation (hypogonadotropic hypogonadism) or primary gonadal failure (hypergonadotropic hypogonadism).

Determination of the bone age and measurements of FSH, LH, and testosterone or extradiol levels should be made.

Primary gonadal failure is readily diagnosed by the findings of elevated FSH and LH levels. Because Klinefelter syndrome occurs in one of

every 600 boys and Turner syndrome occurs in one of every 2000 girls, a karyotype analysis should be performed if the gonadotropins are elevated or clinical phenotypic findings of these syndromes are present.

Distinguishing the child with hypogonadotropic hypogonadism from the child with constitutional delay of growth and development can be difficult, because neither sex steroid nor gonadotropin levels will separate the two conditions, and responses to GnRH stimulation are similar. Recently, however, new immunochemiluminetric assays (ICMA) for FSH and LH have been developed with exquisite sensitivity, even in the low prepubertal ranges. These new assays have shown that children with hypogonadotropic hypogonadism do not demonstrate nocturnal augmentation of LH secretion, whereas even prepubertal boys and girls show significant elevation of LH concentrations with sleep. With the ultrasensitive ICMA, clinicians may be able to differentiate these two previously overlapping conditions.

Therapy of sexual infantilism consists of placement of sex steroids. Treatment is generally begun when the bone age is 13 or 14 years or when the patient has reached an appropriate height. In boys, Depo-Testosterone (enanthate or cypionate) is the treatment of choice. For development of secondary sexual characteristics, the usual starting dose is 50 mg intramuscularly once a month. This dose is progressively increased over the next 2 to 3 years until a final adult replacement dose of 300 mg every 3 weeks is attained. The patient also must be referred to a urologist for testicular prosthetic implants, when appropriate.

While receiving testosterone therapy, boys often will complain of breast tenderness, increase in body hair, spontaneous erections, increased libido, and the pain of intramuscular injections. If these symptoms are exceptionally bothersome, a smaller dose of testosterone may be tried until "tolerance" develops. Most patients will be pleased at the secondary sexual development and tolerate the intramuscular injections without major objections.

In girls, estrogens are used to induce pubertal development. Oral ethinyl estradiol in a daily dose of 5 to 10 µg is the preferred therapy. Once secondary sexual characteristics have progressed to a Tanner stage III or IV level, ethinyl estradiol is only administered on the first 21 days of the month. When menstrual bleeding occurs regularly, medroxyprogesterone acetate is given with the estradiol on days 15 to 21 of the month. A monthly cycle is thus established, simulating normal menstrual cycles. If breakthrough bleeding occurs before an appropriate level of sexual and mental maturity is obtained, a smaller dose of ethinyl estradiol should be used. On the other hand, if poor sexual development is observed on 5 to 10 µg of ethinyl estradiol, the dose should be increased to 10 to 20 µg per day.

Ambiguous Genitalia

A newborn infant with genital ambiguity requires urgent attention and expedient referral to a tertiary center for thorough examination. The decision on gender assignment needs to be postponed until results of the initial diagnostic studies are available and should be a joint decision involving the patient's primary care physician, an endocrinologist, a pediatric urologist or surgeon, and a psychologist who is conversant with the parents' concerns. Gender assignment is based primarily on the patient's potential for normal sexual functioning. Future fertility and the feasibility of reconstructive surgery are secondary issues. The chromosomal sex is not critical to the decision.

Vital aspects of the physical examination include the absence or presence of palpable gonads, the location of the urethral meatus, the length and width of the phallus, and the presence of other anomalies. Karyotype analysis is helpful diagnostically in distinguishing an undervirilized boy from a virilized girl, or an infant with chromosome mosaicism. Other useful tests include baseline serum 17-hydroxyprogesterone, testosterone, and gonadotropin concentrations, pelvic ultrasound, and genitourethrography. hCG and cosyntropin (Cortrosyn) stimulation tests, and fibroblast studies for 5_α-reductase activity and androgen receptor disorders may help establish the diagnosis.

Treatment of the patient depends on the cause of the disorder and on the gender assignment and often includes reconstructive surgery and parental counseling. The recent advances in prenatal diagnosis and treatment of congenital adrenal hyperplasia due to 21-hydroxylase deficiency and the institution of newborn screening for 21-hydroxylase deficiency may simplify the diagnosis and treatment of this disorder in the near future.

BIBLIOGRAPHY

Burke CW: Adrenocortical insufficiency, *Clin Endocrinol Metab* 14:947, 1985.

Fisher DA: Hypothyroidism in childhood, *Pediatr Rev* 2:67, 1980.

Foster CM, Kelch RP: New hope for youngsters with precocious puberty, *Contemp Pediatr* 105, 1986.

Frasier SD: Short stature in children, *Pediatr Rev* 3:171, 1981.

Glorieux J, Desjardins M, Letarte J, et al: Useful parameters to predict the eventual mental outcome of hypothyroid children, *Pediatr Res* 24:6, 1988.

Lippe BM, Landaw EM, Kaplan SA: Hyperthyroidism in children treated with long term medical therapy; Twenty-five percent remission every two years, *Pediatr Res* 64:1241, 1987.

Miller WL, Levine LS: Molecular and clinical advances in congenital adrenal hyperplasia, *J Pediatr* 111:1, 1987.

Milner RDG: Which children should have growth hormone therapy? *Lancet* 483, 1986.

New M, Temeck J, Grimm R, et al: An overview of disorders of sexual differentiation, *Res Staff Phys* 31:21, 1985.

Rimoin DL, Horton WA: Short stature, *J Pediatr* 92:523, 1978.

Rimoin DL, Horton WA: Short stature, *J Pediatr* 92:697, 1978.

Root AW: Endocrinology of puberty, II: Aberrations of sexual maturation, *J Pediatr* 83:187, 1973.

Rosenfield RL: Androgen disorders in children: Too much, too early, too little, or too late, *Pediatr Rev* 5:141, 1983.

Saxena KM, Crawford JD, Talbot NB: Childhood thyrotoxicosis: A long-term perspective, *Br Med J* 2:1153, 1964.

White PC, New MI, Dupont B: Congenital adrenal hyperplasia (first of two parts), *N Engl J Med* 316:1519, 1987.

White PC, New MI, Dupont B: Congenital adrenal hyperplasia (second of two parts), *N Engl J Med* 316:1580, 1987.

PART SIX

Gastroenterology

CHAPTER 79

Inflammatory Bowel Disease

Robert N. Baldassano
John T. Boyle

Once considered rare in pediatric practice, chronic inflammatory bowel disease (IBD) is now being recognized with increasing frequency in children of all ages, with greater than 5% of pediatric IBD occurring before the age of 5 years. IBD is a general term used to denote two specific entities: ulcerative colitis and Crohn disease. Ulcerative colitis is characterized by inflammation limited to the colonic mucosa and is continuous along the length of the bowel starting at the rectum. Crohn disease is a transmural inflammatory process that may affect any part of the alimentary tract from the mouth to the anus in a discontinuous fashion. Approximately half of all cases involve the terminal ileum and colon (ileocolitis).

BACKGROUND

Forty percent of all IBD cases occur in the pediatric age group, and 50% to 60% of all cases in this age group are Crohn's disease.

The primary care physician's early diagnosis of IBD and recognition of potential complications makes therapeutic choices more rational. Because there are no specific markers of disease activity, the condition of each patient must be managed according to his/her own specific needs. Thus, experience in dealing with many patients with IBD is essential in deciding on the best medical therapy. Accordingly, these patients should be referred to a pediatric gastroenterologist. The primary care physician, by continuing to administer general pediatric care, develops a unique role as patient advocate and, as such, can collaborate with the subspecialist to provide necessary input in making important management decisions in this chronic illness.

PATHOPHYSIOLOGY

The precise nature of the initiating events involved in IBD are not known; however, considering the increased incidence of IBD seen in the past 50 years, along with the increase in prevalence among first-degree relatives, one must consider both environmental and genetic factors. Environmental factors that are statistically significant in pediatrics include lack of breastfeeding and increased use of antibiotics. Also, there is no simple mendelian genetic mechanism at work in the transmission of IBD, yet multiple familial occurrences are well documented in 15% to 20% of patients. The mechanisms for the spontaneous exacerbations and remissions characteristic of IBD also remain unclear. One hypothesis states

---

BOX 79-1
Clinical Presentations Associated
With Inflammatory Bowel Disease

Nocturnal diarrhea or abdominal pain
Weight loss in excess of 10% of weight when well
Perianal fistula
Fever of unknown origin (rare)
Growth retardation
Delayed puberty, primary amenorrhea
Ankylosing spondylitis and sacroiliitis
Migrating polyarthritis involving large joints
Erythema nodosum and/or pyoderma gangrenosum
Chronic active hepatitis and/or pericholangitis

---

that the bacterial products normally found in the gastrointestinal tract leak through the mucosal barrier during times of transient intestinal injury. In the normal host, this inflammation resolves, but in the genetically susceptible host, a more intense inflammatory response occurs, leading to greater uptake of luminal bacterial products and thus producing the chronic inflammation seen in IBD.

DATA GATHERING

The usual presenting symptoms of crampy pain in the lower quadrant of the abdomen, diarrhea with or without rectal bleeding, weakness, fatigability, and weight loss are common to ulcerative colitis and Crohn disease. The onset of Crohn disease is usually more insidious. A careful history will evoke a positive history of some blood in the bowel movements in both diseases when colonic involvement is present. IBD is always a likely diagnosis in any patient with bloody diarrhea of greater than 3 weeks' duration. Often, however, extraintestinal manifestations or complications of IBD may be the major initial complaint and overshadow the gastrointestinal manifestations. Box 79-1 lists the common clinical presentations associated with IBD. It is important to remember that in ulcerative colitis extraintestinal symptoms are almost always seen concurrently with gastrointestinal symptoms, whereas in Crohn disease extraintestinal symptoms are more likely to overshadow or actually antedate gastrointestinal symptoms.

Severe growth failure occurs in 30% to 40% of patients under the age of 21 years with Crohn disease and in 10% of patients with ulcerative colitis. Typically, children with growth failure have cessation of linear growth associated with poor weight gain, loss of subcutaneous fat, and marked delay in sexual maturation. Most physicians use standard linear growth curves to assess the growing child. Under normal circumstances, the growth of a child is a very regular process. Serial measurements of stature when taken by the same observer show a remarkably smooth, consistent progression from year to year. It is important not to define growth retardation as a height less than the 3rd percentile. In fact, growth retardation is a deceleration in height gain, which is usually manifested by crossing height percentiles. Thus, a patient whose normal growth channel is the 90th percentile for age and whose growth decelerates, crossing percentiles to the 50th percentile, has growth retardation.

A growth velocity curve is the most sensitive indicator of growth deceleration because significant changes may be appreciated before crossing of major percentile lines is observed on standard linear growth curves. In IBD, it is not uncommon to find growth failure preceding the clinical onset of bowel disease, often by years. Growth failure does not correlate with severity of symptoms. Although the etiology of growth failure appears to be multifactorial, dietary insufficiency is the primary factor in most cases. Often despite denying gastrointestinal symptoms, these patients have low caloric intake even for their height age (age at which their actual height would be 50% on a standard growth chart).

DIAGNOSIS

Preliminary workup of suspected IBD should be performed by the primary physician. The importance of the history cannot be overemphasized. History of recent antibiotic intake and family history are important and often overlooked. Abdominal examination is often nonspecific, although a fullness or mass in the right lower quadrant may indicate Crohn disease. Rectal examination is important in detecting perianal disease such as fissures or fistulas as well as appraising stool guaiac (Hemoccult). Laboratory data are also nonspecific. The complete blood cell count may reveal evidence of hypochromic, microcytic anemia. The sedimentation rate is elevated in 90% of patients with Crohn disease. Certainly a normal sedimentation rate should not

---

BOX 79-2
Possible Infective Organisms or Diseases That Mimic Inflammatory Bowel Disease

---

Salmonella species
Shigella species
Campylobacter species
Yersinia enterocolitica
Aeromonas hydrophila
Neisseria gonorrhoeae
Clostridium difficile
Tuberculosis
Entamoeba histolytica
Escherichia coli; enteroinvasive
Chlamydia
?? *Staphylococcus aureus*
?? Cytomegalovirus
Lymphogranuloma venereum
Radiation enteritis
Ischemic enterocolitis
Hirschsprung enterocolitis
Graft-versus-host disease
Vasculitis

---

deter further workup in a suspicious case. The differential diagnosis of infectious disease of the gastrointestinal tract mimicking IBD is described in Box 79-2.

Because IBD is primarily a diagnosis of exclusion, the primary care physician should rule out known infectious causes before referring the patient to a pediatric gastroenterologist. Most microbiology laboratories have the special techniques available to culture *Campylobacter, Yersinia,* and *Aeromonas. Clostridium difficile* is an anaerobe that is the causative agent of pseudomembranous enterocolitis, a complication of antibiotic therapy. Indeed, pseudomembranous enterocolitis has now been described following treatment with almost all routine antibiotics used in pediatric practice, including penicillin, ampicillin, amoxicillin, erythromycin, and trimethoprim-sulfamethoxazole. Rectal cultures for gonorrhea should be obtained, particularly for adolescent girls. This organism extends to the rectum in 20% to 50% of girls with gonorrhea, although development of symptomatic acute colitis is rare (2% to 5%). Practically speaking, amebiasis is the only parasitic infection in the United States that may mimic IBD. This organism is best diagnosed with specific serologic tests that are positive at the time of acute colitis in 90% of patients. Lymphogranuloma venereum is another sexually transmitted

disorder that should be ruled out by appropriate serologic testing if inguinal adenopathy is a finding on physical examination.

Once infectious causes have been ruled out, it is best for the primary care physician to refer the patient to the pediatric gastroenterologist for further diagnostic evaluation. The next diagnostic study should be flexible colonoscopy with colonic and terminal ileal biopsies. A single-contrast upper gastrointestinal tract radiologic series with small bowel follow-up studies is then performed to complete the diagnostic workup. In older children, double contrast radiography (enteroclysis) is the state-of-the-art technique for determining fine mucosal details to detect early ulceration in the small bowel.

It is not necessary to admit most patients with presumed IBD to the hospital for diagnostic workup. Educating the patient and family regarding the disorder and evaluating nutritional parameters are very important issues that must be addressed soon after diagnosis.

MANAGEMENT

Although the primary care physician should not assume direct care of this disorder, for reasons stated previously, he/she should have some understanding of the philosophy of treatment. The general goals of treatment are 1) to attain the best possible clinical and laboratory control of the inflammatory disease with the least possible side effects from medication, 2) to promote growth through adequate nutrition, and 3) to permit the patient to function as normally as possible (*eg,* school attendance, participation in sports). Not all of these goals are always attainable.

The treatment of IBD has changed greatly over the past few years with the development of new agents that can target specific locations within the gastrointestinal tract. Also, nutritional therapies and immunosuppressive therapies have been useful in managing the patient with severe IBD. With our improved understanding of the immune system, many new agents that block specific immune pathways are in clinical trials. It is important to determine the type and location of the disease in order to utilize these therapies (Table 79-1).

Chronic ulcerative colitis usually responds to sulfasalazine, but other 5-aminosalicylic acid

TABLE 79-1
Pharmacologic Therapy for Inflammatory Bowel Disease

	ULCERATIVE COLITIS	CROHN DISEASE
Mild disease and remission	*Sulfasalazine* Azulfidine *Olsalazine* Dipentum *Mesalamine* Asacol Pentasa *5-aminosalicylic acid* Enemas Suppository *Hydrocortisone* Enemas	*Mesalamine* Asacol Pentasa
Moderate disease		Metronidazole Ciprofloxacin Nutritional therapy
	Continue the above therapies with the addition of prednisone, to be tapered to every other day schedule over a 4- to 6-week period, depending on clinical remission.	
Refractory disease	Azathioprine 6-Mercaptopurine Cyclosporin	Azathioprine 6-Mercaptopurine Cyclosporin

(5-ASA) preparations are also successful (Asacol, Dipentum, etc.). At times, steroid therapy is necessary, and indications include poor response to 5-ASA therapy and severe colitis. The fact remains that many gastroenterologists are willing to tolerate mild to moderate active disease or treat with only 5-ASA and symptomatic medication if they believe that the dose of steroids required for complete disease suppression will result in undesirable side effects, especially growth suppression.

Other therapies that have been successful include 6-mercaptopurine (6-MP) and cyclosporin. The toxicity of these drugs must be considered when ulcerative colitis can be cured with a total proctocolectomy. Also, the absolute risk of colorectal cancer 35 years after diagnosis is 40% for those given the diagnosis at less than 15 years of age. The development of several endorectal pull-through procedures, similar to those performed to treat Hirschsprung disease or imperforate anus, have been used to treat ulcerative colitis. Not only are such procedures sphincter-saving, therefore allowing continuity, but the complication of impotence is avoided.

Crohn's disease is often more difficult to man-age because surgery does not cure the disease. It only considered for uncontrollable bleeding, stenotic bowel, or fistulas unresponsive to medical therapy. Strictureplasty is helpful to open up stenotic areas without removing large segments of small intestine. Some success in decreasing recurrence rates after surgery with the use of 5-ASA products (Pentasa, Asacol) have recently been reported. However, until a treatment that prevents recurrence in the majority of cases is developed, medical and nutritional therapy is necessary in treating Crohn disease. The new 5-ASA preparations that work within the small intestine have been shown to have a greater rate of maintaining remission in Crohn disease than placebo. These preparations include Asacol, which dissolves in the ileum and cecum, and pentasa, which is composed of microspheres that release 5-ASA throughout the small intestine.

Recent studies also have shown the usefulness of antibiotic therapy in the treatment of Crohn disease. Metronidazole as well as the combination of metronidazole and ciprofloxacin are helpful in both the management of perianal disease and small bowel and colonic disease.

If there is poor response to the these therapies, steroids may be necessary during an acute exacerbation, but they usually are not helpful in maintaining long-term remission in Crohn disease. New steroid preparations with fewer side effects presently are being studied for effectiveness for long-term use (Budesonide). Multiple immunosuppressive therapies have been successful in controlling Crohn disease, including mercaptopurine, azathioprine, cyclosporin and methotrexate. Nutritional therapy is another important modality for the treatment of disease activity and growth failure seen in Crohn disease.

A dramatic reversal of malnutrition and a change in growth velocity can be expected in all children treated with adequate nutrition in conjunction with medical therapy to adequately control symptoms of IBD. Improvement in nutritional status may be accomplished by a variety of methods. Occasionally, with heightened awareness of the nutritional needs, patients will be compliant for oral supplemental alimentation with any one of a number of high-caloric formulas. When oral supplementation fails, other means of providing nutritional support include overnight continuous nasogastric feeding, intravenous parenteral alimentation in the hospital, or, in select patients, intravenous parenteral alimentation in the home.

In summary, IBD is a chronic disease requiring treatment by a team of experts consisting of a pediatrician, pediatric gastroenterologist, psychologist, nutritionist, and nurse. A critical factor in successful management of this disease is the willingness of the patient to participate and cooperate with the team.

BIBLIOGRAPHY

Baldassano RN, Schreiber S, Johnston RB Jr, et al: Crohn's disease monocytes are primed for accentuated release of toxic oxygen metabolities, *Gastroenterology* 105:60, 1993.

Brown R, Tedesco FJ: Differential diagnosis of infectious disease of the gastrointestinal tract mimicking inflammatory bowel disease, *Intern Med Spec* 5:140, 1984.

Caprilli R, Andreoli A, Capurso L: Oral mesalazine for the prevention of post-operative recurrence of Crohn's disease, *Aliment Pharmacol Ther* 8:35, 1994.

Demling L: Is Crohn's disease caused by antibiotics? *Hepatogastroenterology* 41:549, 1994.

Ekbom A, Helmick C, Zack M: Ulcerative colitis and colorectal cancer, *N Engl J Med* 323:1228, 1990.

Kelts DG, Grand RJ, Shen G, et al: Nutritional basis of growth failure in children and adolescents with Crohn's disease, *Gastroenterology* 76:720, 1979.

Kirschner BS, Klick JR, Kalman SS, et al: Reversal of growth retardation in Crohn's disease with therapy emphasizing oral restitution, *Gastroenterology* 80:10, 1981.

Lichtenstein GR: Medical therapies for inflammatory bowel disease, *Curr Opin Gastroenterol* 10:390, 1994.

Markowitz JF: Inflammatory bowel disease in the child and adolescent, *Pract Gastroenterol* 18:30A, 1994.

Rombeau JL, Gincherman Y: Surgical and nutritional treatment of inflammatory bowel disease, *Curr Opin Gastroenterol* 10:409, 1994.

CHAPTER 80

Viral Hepatitis

Jonathan E. Teitelbaum
John T. Boyle

Inflammation of the liver is not a new disease. Documentation of jaundice dates back to ancient times and in the Ebers papyrus (1552 BC) and the Babylonian Talmud (Fifth century BC). The hepatic diseases resulting from viruses present similar histologic inflammation and necrosis. This chapter will mainly focus on those hepatotrophic viruses (hepatitis A, B, C, D, E, F, and G) with their specific affinity for the liver, rather than systemic viruses that affect multiple organ systems. Knowledge and understanding of viral hepatitis has grown tremendously in the past two decades as an impressive array of sophisticated immunologic, biochemical, and biophysical techniques have been applied to further identify and characterize the disorder. For the primary physician, this knowledge has resulted in improved ability to diagnose hepatitis, to differentiate between acute and chronic infection, to provide treatment, to monitor for short-term and long-term sequelae, and, most importantly, to institute measures to prevent spread of the infection. Prevention demands 1) accurate diagnosis that depends on a high index of clinical suspicion because it is estimated that only 25% of cases are clinically apparent, 2) knowledge of serologic markers that allow specific etiologic identification, and 3) administration of the available vaccines, immunoprophylaxis, and treatments in a timely manner.

BACKGROUND

Hepatitis A

Hepatitis A virus (HAV), a member of the Picornavirus family with single stranded RNA, accounts for approximately one third of the acute viral hepatitis in the United States and the majority of cases in the pediatric population. Because there is no known carrier state in humans, natural perpetuation of the virus is believed to occur outside the human host, most likely in fauna of contaminated water. This theory is supported by an increase in incidence in those areas with poor sanitation. Although human infection can occur from ingestion of contaminated shellfish, particularly clams and oysters, in the majority of cases transmission is human to human, with the most common mode being the fecal-to-oral route through contaminated food and water. The incidence of common-source outbreaks has decreased in the past 5 to 10 years. The previous fall-winter prevalence for school children is no longer observed. Ten percent to 15% of cases in the United States can be seen in daycare centers (especially those that allow non–toilet trained children and infants) and facilities for the mentally retarded. The decrease in incidence of clinical HAV may reflect better sanitation or improved immunoprophylactic measures. Indeed epidemiologic studies suggest that 25% to 50% of the general population have antibody to HAV by 30 to 40 years of age, whereas only 3% to 5% of such individuals report an illness consistent with hepatitis.

The exact method by which HAV travels from the intestine of infected individuals to the liver where it replicates and has its cytotoxic effects is unclear. The incubation period for HAV is 15 to 50 days (with an average of 25 to 30 days). Fecal shedding of the virus (derived from bile rather than replication within the intestine) antedates even prodromal symptoms, although peak shedding occurs during the clinical presentation.

The viral burden is seen mainly within the stool (10^9 virions/mL) and is 10,000 times that seen within the blood during the transient viremic phase. The infectivity of saliva, urine, and semen with their low viral burdens (10^3, 10^2, and 10^2 virions/mL, respectively) remains uncertain. The severity of illness and the ensuing cellular destruction seem to depend on the intensity of viral replication. Most infections are anicteric and self-limited. Fecal viral shedding may continue for up to 14 days after appearance of jaundice, dark urine (brown), or light stool. There is no chronic fecal shedding.

Hepatitis B

Hepatitis B virus (HBV) is a complex double-strand DNA virus, a member of the Hepadnavirus family, which accounts for approximately 43% of the acute viral hepatitis in the United States. HBV has two antigenic components: a core component designated HBcAg and an outer surface component designated HBsAg. The component HBsAg is actually an outer protein envelope manufactured in excess to the core in the cytoplasm of infected hepatocytes. This unique virus contains a third antigenic component, HBeAg, which is the result of proteolytic self cleavage of the core antigen, whose presence indicates ongoing viral replication. Unlike HAV, HBV has an enormous human reservoir because acute infection may lead to a chronic viral carrier state in 5% to 10% of cases. Epidemiologic studies in the United States put the carrier rate in the general population at 0.1% to 0.9%.

Person-to-person spread, including neonatal infections that occur during labor and delivery, is the most common from the blood of carriers. Whereas evidence of HBV virus has been found in all body secretions except feces and urine, a number of studies have shown that the virus is not infectious by the oral, nasal, or respiratory route. Most pediatric cases are acquired through close, intimate contact with an infectious individual by so-called inapparent parenteral spread, involving passage of virus through slight or insignificant breaks in the skin or mucous membrane barrier.

The incubation period for HBV may be as short as 3 weeks or as long as 6 months depending on the inoculum and the route of infection. Unlike HAV, replication and synthetic activity of HBV takes place with minimal or no cytopathogenic impact on the hepatocytes. The hepatocellular injury is dependent on the nature and extent of the host's cell-mediated immune response to the HBV infection. In addition, evidence of immune complex disease with extrahepatic manifestations indistinguishable from serum sickness may be part of the prodrome in 5% to 10% of symptomatic HBV infections. Yet, as with HAV, the most frequent response to HBV exposure is an anicteric, asymptomatic, or self-limited infection. Development of a carrier state does not seem to be related to disease severity. For unknown reasons, infection seems to be ineffectively eliminated and persists either without hepatocyte damage or with histologic evidence of chronic persistent or chronic aggressive hepatitis.

Hepatitis C

Hepatitis C virus (HCV) is a Flavivirus (single-stranded RNA) that accounts for approximately 20% of the viral hepatitis in the United States. Percutaneous spread is the major mode of transmission, and it represents the predominant transfusion acquired hepatitis. The presence of HCV is highly variable within the US population with the highest rates found among intravenous (IV) drug users and hemophiliacs (60% to 90%), moderate rates in hemodyalysis patients (20%), and lower rates in those with high-risk sexual behavior or contacts with HCV carriers (1% to 10%). Despite our increased knowledge of this virus over recent years, 40% to 50% of documented cases are classified as idiopathic with no known risk factors for acquisition.

The incubation period for hepatitis C following transfusion or accidental needle stick has been reported to average 6 to 7 weeks. The resulting viremia is thought to be in significantly lower titers than with HBV. The HCV antibody can appear from 4 to 52 weeks (mean, 21 weeks) after transfusion. In cases of chronic infection (occurring in 50% of those patients with HCV) the HCV antibody persists. Those individuals with HCV antibodies are still thought to be infectious because viral-specific RNA can be found in the serum via reverse transcriptase polymerase chain reaction.

Signs and symptoms of the acute or chronic infectious state are usually absent but may include fatigue and mildly elevated aminotransferases. It is common to have wide episodic fluctuations in alanine aminotransferase (ALT) and aspartate aminotransferase (AST) giving the appearance of quiescence and reactivation.

Eventual outcome appears to be unrelated to disease severity.

Hepatitis D

Hepatitis D virus (HDV) (formally called *delta hepatitis virus* or the *delta agent*) is a defective RNA virus that utilizes the outer coat of HBV with its HBsAg to encapsulate an outer core with HDVAg and a single-stranded circular RNA. This subviral agent replicates only with the assistance of the helper virus, HBV. With this helper, HDV can replicate efficiently within hepatocytes to increase the severity of liver damage caused by HBV infection. The mode of transmission of HDV is similar to that of HBV, with percutaneous being the most efficient and sexual transmission being less so. The incubation period is probably several weeks long. Acquisition of the disease is obtained either as a coinfection, being introduced simultaneously with HBV, or as a superinfection on chronic HBV carriers. People with HBV-HDV coinfection have more severe acute disease and a higher risk of fulmanent hepatitis (2% to 20%) as compared with those with HBV alone.

Once infected the hepatocyte releases both HDV and HBV into the bloodstream with as many as 10^{12} infectious particles/mL of blood. Current serologic studies have shown a high prevalence in certain US populations with rates approaching 50% in (IV) drug users and hemophiliacs and 20% in dialysis patients, prisoners, and some homosexual populations. A person who is a chronic HBV carrier and acquires an HDV superinfection is likely to become a chronic carrier of HDV.

Hepatitis E

Hepatitis E virus (HEV) is an RNA virus and a member of the Calcivirus family. Although the virus is endemic mainly in the Mediterranean basin, the Balkan peninsula, the European Soviet Union, parts of Africa, the Middle East, and the South American Amazon basin, the only cases seen in the United States to date have been "imported." Outbreaks occur most frequently during the rainy seasons or after flooding and are typically associated with poor hygiene and inadequate sanitation. Transmission is through fecally contaminated drinking water, leading to fecal-oral spread and a secondary attack rate among household members as high as 20%.

The virus causes significant mortality among pregnant women, specifically in the second and third trimester with fatality rates averaging 20%. The incidence of fulminant hepatic failure among pregnant women approaches 32%. The typical incubation period for HEV ranges from 2 to 9 weeks (average, 40 days). Subclinical infection occurs in children and adults. The clinical manifestations are similar to hepatitis A in that it is mild, is self-limited, and has no tendency toward chronicity.

Hepatitis F

Hepatitis F virus (HFV) recently has been found to be caused by a silent hepatitis B mutant. Transmission is bloodborne and is similar to hepatitis B. Manifestations of HFV infection include an acute or fulminant hepatitis, as well as chronic hepatitis that can lead to cirrhosis and hepatocellular carcinoma. Research efforts in further characterizing this virus are currently underway with hopes of leading to earlier detection and eventual prophylaxis.

Hepatitis G and Other Hepatotrophic Viruses

Hepatitis G is the name of a recently identified parenterally transmitted Flavivirus linked to acute and chronic hepatitis. Current research efforts will undoubtedly further classify this virus as well as other currently unidentified hepatotrophic viruses.

DATA GATHERING

Symptoms

Most childhood cases of acute hepatitis produce minimal symptoms, are anicteric, and are usually confused with a gastrointestinal flulike illness, particularly in the young child less than 10 years of age. Symptoms of the various viruses overlap and are nonspecific. The frequency of asymptomatic disease decreases with age; for HAV the percentage of asymptomatic infections is 85% for those children 1 to 2 years of age, 50% in children 3 to 4 years of age, and 20% in those greater than 5 years of age. Classically, clinical hepatitis consists of a prodrome of constitutional symptoms, followed by the acute onset of an icteric phase and then recovery. The prodrome consists of low-grade fever (less than 39° C), malaise, easy fatigability, anorexia (greatest with dinnertime meals), nausea, vomiting (rarely prolonged), epigastric or right upper quadrant abdominal pain, headache (seen more with HAV), rhinorrhea, chills, cough, odynophagia, myalgias, photophobia, and arthralgias. Pruritus and diarrhea are rare. Physical examination at this time may reveal tender hepatomegaly and occasional splenomegaly. Ascites and edema are not typical features of hepatitis. The HBV may present with an atypical prodrome consisting of extrahepatic manifestations associated with immune complex disease such as rash, hematuria, proteinuria, arthralgia, and an acute migratory polyarthritis involving the distal joints such as the proximal interphalangeals, symmetrically (seen in approximately 3% to 10% of cases).

The rash is usually a papular acrodermatitis on the face, buttocks, and extensor surfaces of the arms and legs. When such a rash is associated with lymphadenitis and fever, it is termed the *Gianotti-Crosti syndrome.* The syndrome's association with HAV or HBV typically is seen in Japan and Italy, and is unusual in the United States where this papuloacrodermatitis of childhood is secondary to viruses like Epstein-Barr virus (EBV) or cytomegalovirus (CMV). Neurologic involvement without fulminant hepatitis is rare, but Guillane-Barré has been seen with the prodrome of HBV and icteric phase of HAV. Neurologic changes seen on occasions in HAV and HBV include a mononeuritis of either cranial or peripheral nerves.

The icteric phase of viral hepatitis is characterized by the sudden onset of scleral icterus, jaundice, and passage of dark urine and light stools. In this stage, one finds hepatomegaly with a rounded liver edge and mild tenderness in all patients and splenomegaly with posterior cervical lymph nodes in 10% to 15%. Although jaundice and laboratory parameters may increase for several days, the patient feels better. This divergence is classic for acute hepatitis and most often infers a good prognosis. The jaundice disappears gradually over 2 to 6 weeks, with a faster resolution in HAV and in children (typically resolution in 85% by 2 weeks).

Differential Diagnosis

Agents capable of producing a viral hepatitis-like illness include EBV (infectious mononucleosis), CMV, herpesvirus, adenovirus, coxsackievirus, rheovirus, echovirus, rubella, arbovirus, varicella, enterovirus, HIV, mumps, yellow fever, Marburg, Lassa fever, Riff Valley fever virus, leptospirosis, toxoplasmosis, and tuberculosis. Characteristically, these agents produce a predominantly systemic illness with multiorgan involvement. The illnesses caused by EBV and CMV most commonly mimic viral hepatitis. Both rarely produce jaundice, and high fever and diffuse adenopathy are more characteristic.

In teenage girls, *Neisseria gonorrhoeae* or *Chlamydia trachomatosis* perihepatitis (Fitz-Hugh-Curtis syndrome) may occur as an extension of pelvic inflammatory disease. Symptoms and signs include fever, right upper quadrant abdominal pain, jaundice, and elevated levels of transaminases. Pelvic findings of acute salpingitis are present in most cases as well as a history of dysmenorrhea, menorrhagia, or vaginal discharge. Cervical culture may be negative in 15% to 20% of cases.

Wilson disease is a treatable metabolic disorder of copper metabolism that may present with signs and symptoms indistinguishable from acute hepatitis.

Autoimmune hepatitis (formally known as Lupoid hepatitis) typically can be seen in the chronic state with clinical and laboratory evidence of hepatic inflammation for greater than 10 weeks. Major features include female predominance, polyclonal hyperglobulinemia (especially IgG), association with other "autoimmune" disorders, a plethora of circulating autoantibodies, and an often dramatic response to steroid therapy.

All patients with suspected acute hepatitis should be questioned regarding recent medications ingested and environmental toxin exposure.

Diagnosis of Acute Hepatitis

Because most cases of acute hepatitis are mild, presenting only with nonspecific symptoms, it is important to perform a careful abdominal examination in all patients with viral prodromes, because tender hepatomegaly is often the only sign that suggests the correct diagnosis. A history of exposure to hepatitis is uncommon in the young child, more common in the adolescent. Obviously, knowledge of a recent outbreak of hepatitis in a patient's environment is most helpful.

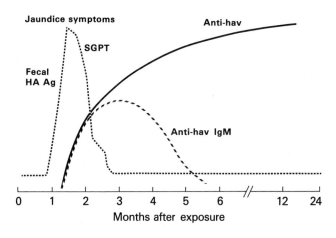

FIG 80-1
Time course of clinical, biomechanical, and serologic events in a typical case of acute hepatitis A.

General Laboratory Tests to Diagnose Acute Hepatitis

Biochemical laboratory tests in cases of suspected acute viral hepatitis include determination of serum transaminase values (AST and ALT); alkaline phosphatase; bilirubin, direct and indirect; complete blood cell (CBC) count; prothrombin time (PT); total protein, albumin, globulin; electrolytes, blood urea nitrogen (BUN), glucose; and ceruloplasmin (if no exposure to hepatitis).

In practice, this testing involves obtaining an automated CBC count and SMA-12 or Chemzyme screen analysis. The most sensitive indicators of ongoing hepatocellular injury are the serum transaminases, AST and ALT. At best, only a rough correlation exists between the structural alterations associated with hepatitis and the corresponding increase in values for transaminases, which arise from hepatocyte destruction and the "leaking out" of its intracellular enzymes. Transaminases may be elevated 10 to 100 times the normal limit, because they rise late in the prodrome and peak after the onset of jaundice. The absolute levels are not important, except when they exceed 3000 U/L. These levels initially fall quickly after they peak; this rate of decline then is not maintained so that minor elevation may persist for a few months. Alkaline phosphatase level is usually normal or slightly increased. If levels are greater than two times the upper limit of normal for age, one should suspect either biliary tract disease, or EBV or CMV hepa-

titis. Direct-reacting or conjugated hyperbilirubinemia (direct fraction greater than 15% of total or absolute value greater than 2) generally peaks 5 to 7 days after onset of jaundice, which coincides with 1 to 8 days after the transaminases peak.

Hyperbilirubinemia may be present in the absence of scleral icterus or jaundice, because these signs usually cannot be appreciated until levels exceed 3 to 4 mg/dL. Absorption of medications and nutrients requiring bile flow should be assumed to be significantly impaired at conjugated bilirubin levels equal to or greater than 7. The bilirubin level then falls rapidly in the convalescent phase, becoming normal in 4 to 6 weeks. Hemoglobin level is usually normal. If hemoglobin is decreased, consider glucose-6-phosphate dehydrogenase deficiency, Wilson disease, or Coombs-positive anemia associated with chronic liver disease. The white blood cell (WBC) count is also usually normal or slightly decreased, such that leukocytosis with WBC count greater than $25,000/mm^3$ is considered a poor prognostic sign. An increased number of atypical lymphocytes may be noted in viral hepatitis as well as in infectious hepatitis. PT is also normal in 95% of cases. Elevation of PT does correlate with disease severity and poor prognosis, especially if level does not correct following intramuscular injection of vitamin K. Total protein, albumin, and globulin levels are normal in acute hepatitis. Decreased albumin or increased globulin levels should suggest an acute flare of chronic liver

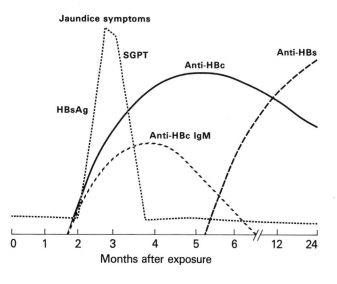

FIG 80-2

Time course of clinical, biomechanical, and serologic events in a typical case of acute hepatitis B.

disease. Baseline electrolytes and BUN are important because dehydration is one of the more common complications of anorexia and vomiting. Hypoglycemia is a major complication of severe hepatitis. Even in mild cases, levels of blood glucose in the range of 60 mg/dL are not uncommon and should not be cause for concern without other abnormal prognostic indicators.

Serologic Diagnosis of Acute Hepatitis

Figures 80-1 and 80-2 contrast the sequence of clinical, serum biochemical, and serologic events in typical HAV and HBV infection. The serodiagnosis of acute hepatitis is best approached by testing first for anti-HAV IgM, anti-HBcAg, HBsAg recombinant immunoblot assay (RIBA) to HCV, and a Mono-spot or EBV serologic analysis. All these tests are now commercially available. A finding of IgM anti-HAV is diagnostic of HAV infection having occurred within the past 2 to 3 weeks to months ago. It appears during the acute phase of illness, peaks within a few weeks, then declines to an undetectable level in 3 to 4 months. A more precise timing of actual infection can be accomplished by measuring total immunoglobulin (both IgM and IgG) anti-HAV because IgG arises after 3 to 4 weeks and then persists indefinitely as the source of ongoing immunity against repeat infection.

HBsAg is the first serologic marker of HBV infection to appear and predates prodromal symptoms, increase in transaminases, or jaundice. A positive finding of HBsAg suggests the diagnosis of HBV in a symptomatic patient, but a negative finding does not rule it out, because HBsAg may rapidly be cleared from the serum within 1 week of onset of symptoms in 5% to 15% of the cases. If there is a strong suspicion, testing for anti-HBc (anti-HBcAg) is indicated to further exclude HBV, particularly if the disease is detected late. Anti-HBcAg rises after the HBsAg and peaks in weeks, persisting long after HBsAg disappears. This allows for diagnosis of acute HBV infection during that "window" of time when the HBsAg is undetectable and its antibody has yet to rise. Indicators of ongoing viremia or viral replication include HBeAg (seen within a few days to weeks of the appearance of HBsAg and disappearing prior to HBsAg when the HBe antibody appears), and HBV DNA, which is seen in the early phase and typically gone in 6 to 8 weeks.

The diagnosis of HCV infection is best made by a positive reverse transcriptase polymerase chain reaction detecting HCV RNA in the patient's blood. Antibody tests such as enzyme-linked immunosorbent assay or RIBA have resulted in false negatives because the immune response does not make detectable antibody to HCV early in the acute disease state.

In acute HDV infection the HDVAg is the first marker to appear; however, it is short-lived, and serologic testing for the antigen is not commercially available. The antibody response is somewhat slow in its appearance with only 40% of patients having antibody by the second week of illness. The IgM anti-HDV is transient in patients with self-limited disease, but persistent in chronic infection.

Currently there are no commercial tests available for the diagnosis of HEV, HFV, or HGV; however, in cases in which there is a high index of suspicion, many tertiary care centers can perform these tests.

Management

Management of Acute Viral Hepatitis

There is no specific treatment for acute viral hepatitis. γ-Globulin has no influence on the course of the disease once symptoms occur. Steroids also have no role in the treatment of infectious hepatitis because they may result in a "rebound crisis" after what may appear to be an initial improvement in the acute symptomatology. Today, the vast majority of patients can be treated with supportive care and symptomatic therapy. Traditionally, a low-fat, high-carbohydrate diet and bed rest have been recommended. Both are probably unnecessary, because neither influences the duration of the disease. Parents should be told to expect that their child's appetite will be poor. Small frequent feedings of a balanced diet may be helpful. Ambulation and activity around the home should be allowed as tolerated. Drugs should be strictly avoided. The key for both the patient and household contacts is personal hygiene. Infants and small children should avoid contact with the infected child even after they have received immunoprophylaxis. Because shedding of virus may occur for up to 2 weeks after onset of jaundice, patients should be kept home and out of school for this time. After this time, they may resume normal activity as tolerated, even if low-grade jaundice persists. Education of school authorities regarding such patients as well as notification of local public health authorities are important functions of the primary care physician.

The indications for hospitalization of the patient with acute hepatitis are as follows:

1. Dehydration secondary to anorexia and vomiting
2. Abnormal prothrombin time persisting after administration of parenteral vitamin K
3. Level of transaminases >3000 U/L

Basically, hospitalization is required for dehydration, the most common complication of hepatitis, or for observation because of the presence of one or more of the factors considered to imply increased risk for fulminant hepatitis. The physician should also consider hospitalization for any patient for whom there is concern regarding poor home environment. Although patients with acute hepatitis who are hospitalized should be isolated, it is not necessary for health care personnel to wear gowns, gloves, and masks when caring for these patients. Personal hygiene is essential.

Management of Fulminant Hepatitis

Fulminant hepatitis is characterized by massive hepatic necrosis, a rare, catastrophic complication of viral hepatitis, and occurs in less than 1% of the cases. Hepatitis B (especially with superinfection with HDV), hepatitis C, and more recently in England, hepatitis E are well-established causes of fulmanent hepatitis. The cause remains unknown in many instances, despite our increasing knowledge. Fulminant hepatitis is extremely rare following HAV. Two modes of presentation are seen. In the first mode, the child develops clinical hepatitis, but instead of improving, jaundice deepens, the level of transaminases starts to fall while the liver begins to shrink, the PT elongates, and progressive neurologic symptoms including impaired mentition, drowsiness, insomnia, and asterixis become apparent. In the second mode, a child manifesting a typical benign course of hepatitis suddenly relapses at a time when jaundice is decreasing. A course similar to the first mode of presentation then occurs. Fever, abdominal pain, and vomiting most often recur during the relapse.

At best, there is only a 20% survival from fulminant hepatitis. Prognosis is definitely related to level of intensive care management. These patients often develop significant cerebral edema and require intracranial pressure monitoring, mechanical ventilation, and mannitol. Additional morbidity stems from the resultant coagulopathy, an insulin-resistant nonketotic hypoglycemia, and hepatorenal syndrome. Patients who have poor prognostic biochemical indicators and whose conditions continue to deteriorate clinically should be transferred to a pediatric tertiary care center equipped to provide the level of intensive care they require. Blood glucose level must be carefully monitored in such patients during transport. Medical management including acid blockers, steroids, and exchange transfusions have not been successful in decreasing mortality.

Course and Follow-up of Acute Hepatitis

The jaundice of viral hepatitis gradually clears over 2 to 4 weeks. It may be 1 to 3 months before levels of transaminases return to normal in hepatitis A. It is not unusual for a mild, short-lived relapse of both clinical symptoms and slight jaundice to occur in 10% to 15% of patients 8 to 12 weeks after the acute illness. This phenomenon has been called *relapsing hepatitis* and usually resolves in 2 to 3 weeks. Rarely, some patients develop a significant cholestatic form of acute hepatitis associated with high levels of direct-reacting hyperbilirubinemia and increased levels of alkaline phosphatase and cholesterol. Such patients usually complain of pruritus. Because of the concern of an extrahepatic biliary tract disorder in such patients, it is wise to perform an ultrasound to examine the gallbladder and bile ducts.

Because HAV infection does not lead to a chronic carrier state or chronic hepatitis, a patient who is positive for anti-HAV IgM can just be followed-up clinically without biochemical studies. Patients with HBV or hepatitis C should have biweekly physical examination, as well as a check of serum bilirubin and ALT until these parameters either return to normal or by continued abnormality greater than 6 months fit the time criteria for a diagnosis of chronic hepatitis. Because HBV and HCV are sexually transmitted, one should consider screening for other sexually transmitted diseases in affected adolescents and adults.

Chronic Type B Hepatitis

In patients with HBV, HBsAg should also be checked monthly. Persistence of HBsAg for 8 to 10 weeks indicates that the patient will probably not resolve the viral infection rapidly but will become a chronic carrier. Approximately 5% to 10% of adults with acute HBV become chronic carriers. This statistic yields an overall US carrier state of 0.1% to 0.9% with the rate among Asian-Americans being 5 to 10 times that of the general population and that of Alaskan-Eskimos 25%.

The number is considerably greater in neonates infected by transmission from their mothers; such that 80% to 90% of infants born to HBV carriers will themselves become carriers (with an increased prevalence among children born to HBeAg-positive mothers). Most chronic carriers are asymptomatic or have symptoms of mild fatigability or right upper quadrant pressure tenderness that can last 3 to 10 years. In the majority of individuals, levels of transaminases gradually fall to normal or near normal. Low-grade inflammation may lead to cirrhosis in some patients, and a small percentage will die from liver failure. HBV carriers are at significantly greater risk for developing hepatocellular carcinoma. For this reason some experts recommend that a baseline ultrasound and yearly alpha-fetal-protein level be checked. All chronic carriers should be followed up on a quarterly basis to determine infectivity status (positive HBeAg) and possible seroconversion to anti-HBe. In the latter case these individuals most likely will not develop severe chronic liver disease. Ten percent to 40% of chronic patients have HBsAg and antibody concurrently, but the antibody is in lower titer with low affinity to HBsAg.

One of the major dilemmas for the primary care physician is the infectivity of HBsAg carriers. One study demonstrated that classroom contact may at times be sufficient to allow for so-called inapparent parenteral spread of HBV. Chronic HBeAg-positive infants could be considered for placement in daycare or nursery schools if they are "non-biters," and universal precautions should be exercised with respect to their secretions and diapers. School attendance in grade school should be allowed with precautions to maximize personal hygiene as best as possible. The dilemma of infectivity of HBV underscores the need to prevent this infection.

Chronic Hepatitis C

Chronically infected persons with HCV should be followed with serial anti-HCVAg until resolution. Of those patients with HCV-related chronic liver disease, chronic active hepatitis or cirrhosis has been found in 29% to 76% within several years of onset. Factors believed to influence the rate of progression to cirrhosis include age of exposure, duration of infection, and degree of damage at the initial biopsy. One study of patients with posttransfusion HCV revealed 20% of patients with evidence of cirrhosis after 10 years and 66% to 71% with cirrhosis after 25 years. Nineteen percent of the infected patients went on to develop hepatocellular carcinoma.

Chronic Hepatitis

Chronic hepatitis should be suspected in a patient who presents with 1) signs and symptoms of acute hepatitis but has markers of chronic illness such as decreased level of albumin or increased level of globulin or 2) a patient with acute hepatitis who continues to have persistent hyperbilirubinemia or elevated transaminases with or without clinical symptoms for 6 to 8 weeks following initial presentation. The etiology is unknown but probably involves the host's immune response to hepatocellular injury. Clinical features include persistent jaundice, relapsing jaundice, extrahepatic complaints such as fever, arthritis, rash (particularly erythema nodosum), colitis, and, rarely, advanced features of liver failure including ascites and encephalopathy. Evidence of autoantibodies, particularly antinuclear antibodies and antismooth muscle antibodies, is found in 60% of patients. Patients who fulfill the two criteria given above should be referred to a pediatric gastroenterologist for further evaluation. A diagnosis of chronic active hepatitis requires liver biopsy.

Although treatment of the chronic hepatitis state is in its infancy, it holds great promise.

Prevention of Viral Hepatitis By Immunoprophylaxis

Prevention of the spread of viral hepatitis should be one of the primary goals of the primary care physician.

Hepatitis A

Conventional immune serum globulin (ISG) with its anti-HAV IgG confers passive protection against clinical HAV infection if given during the incubation period up until 6 days before onset of disease. In fact, 75% of those individuals receiving a dose of 0.02 mL/kg intramuscularly develop evidence of passive-active immunity with anti-HAV IgM with abortion of HAV infection and suppression of clinical manifestations of hepatitis. Fifteen percent to 20% of those receiving HAV immunoglobulin will have a subclinical infection, and thus a proportion of patients develop active immunity with endogenous anti-HAV.

Postexposure immunoprophylaxis is suggested for 1) household contacts and close personal contacts, 2) institutionalized contacts, and 3) contacts within a daycare center. Contacts of an isolated case within a grade school classroom and routine play contacts do not require ISG. However, a second case within a class warrants immunoprophylaxis of the rest of the class. Immune serum globulin is protective for as long as 6 months. One potential method of determining who should receive ISG is to test susceptible contacts for anti-HAV IgG and to give ISG only to those who are negative. Preexposure prophylaxis is required for individuals traveling to areas where HAV is endemic (including North Africa, the Middle East, Central and South America, South Africa, and India). The dose is 0.02 mL/kg intramuscularly. If the stay is to be longer than 3 months, 0.06 mL/kg should be given every 5 months. Vaccines using inactivated strains of HAV have been licensed in countries outside the United States to provide active immunity.

Hepatitis B

IgG against HBsAg is protective, thus preventive care focuses on the immunization of persons using HBV vaccine (a recombinant product with trademarks of Recombivax B or Energix-B) to promote active immunity. Neonates respond superbly with 100% developing anti-HBsAg after three doses, and adults respond somewhat less frequently (approximately 90% to 95%). A three-dose regimen is necessary with intramuscular shots (1 cc if greater than 10 years of age and 0.5 cc if less than 10 years of age) at time zero, 1 month, and 6 months, with the third dose causing peak antibody levels at 7 to 10 months after the first shot. The vaccine has been found to be extremely safe, with no contraindication for pregnant or lactating women. The major side effect is soreness at the injection site. Earlier questions surrounding a possible link to Guillan-Barré is limited only to plasma-derived vaccine (Heptavax B), which is no longer used in the United States. There has been no reported cases of HIV transmission via the vaccine. No antibodies are detected 10 years after vaccination in 13% to 60% of patients; however, in immunocompetent hosts no booster is recommended. Currently the recommendation calls for all newborns and adolescence to be vaccinated.

In newborns born to HBsAg- or HBeAg- positive mothers a vaccination and 0.5 cc of hepatitis B immunoglobulin (HBIG) given at different sites within 12 hours of birth and routine completion of the vaccine schedule results in a protective efficacy of 85% to 95%. Needle sticks to personnel who were previously unimmunized from a known carrier should similarly receive HBIG and the routine vaccination schedule.

Sexual contacts of people with acute HBV should receive 0.6 cc/kg HBIG within 14 days. Intimate contacts with those people who are chronic HBV carriers should receive immunizations without immunoprophylaxis.

Hepatitis C

To date there is no role for immunoglobulin treatment in those individuals who have been exposed to HCV, nor is there an approved vaccine. Prevention rests mainly in limiting exposure to blood products and transfusions.

Hepatitis D

Prevention of HDV infection currently is obtained through prevention of hepatic infection with HBV.

Hepatitis E, F, or G

No current vaccine is available, and the use of immunoprophylaxis is under investigation.

Neonatal Hepatitis B

Infants born to mothers who have had acute HBV infection during the third trimester or chronic carriers of HBV (particularly HBeAg-positive carriers) are at risk to develop neonatal hepatitis B. In the United States where the carrier rate is less than 1%, neonatal acquisition of HBV from carrier mothers is said to be 5% to 10%. In contrast, in the Far East, where 40% to 50% of mothers are carriers, neonatal acqui-

sition is close to 95%. Thus, it seems that the causes of acquisition are multifactorial. Infection seems to occur at birth by ingestion of virus from amniotic fluid, vaginal secretions, or placental or uterine blood, or through postpartum exposure by close contact, or via breastfeeding. Transplacental spread, if it occurs, is rare. The component HBsAg usually is first noted when the infant is 6 to 8 weeks of age. Neonatal HBV is usually an asymptomatic illness. However, a high percentage of the infants, particularly boys, become chronic carriers because of an ineffective immune response. The length of the carrier state is unknown. However, because of the dilemma of infectivity of such infants and children, prevention of neonatal HBV is essential. Current recommendations, therefore, are that all pregnant women in the United States should be routinely tested for HbsAg because testing of only high-risk mothers resulted in 50% of affected mothers going undiagnosed. The expected yield of one to five cases per 1000 tests is higher than that seen in serologic monitoring for syphilis; however, HBsAg testing is much more expensive. The children of infected parents should receive HBIG and HBV vaccine as outlined in the previous section.

No special nursery precautions are indicated because at this point, the infant is not infective, although the carrier mother is infective. Mothers who are HBeAg-positive probably should avoid breastfeeding. Because these infants with carrier mothers will have continued exposure, serologic evaluation when they are 1 year of age should include anti-HBc and anti-HBs. If both tests are positive, passive-active immunity has occurred, and the infant probably has lifelong immunity. If anti-HBs titer alone is positive, it is probably the result of vaccination. Hepatitis C also has been demonstrated to be transmitted vertically to neonates, although with less frequency than hepatitis B.

BIBLIOGRAPHY

Alter M, Mast E: The epidemiology of viral hepatitis in the United States, *Gastroenterol Clin North Am* 23(3):437–456, 1994.

Committee on Infectious Disease: *The red book* 1994, 221–241.

Maddrey WC: Viral hepatitis: A 1994 interim

report, *Gastroenterol Clin North Am* 23(3):
429–436, 1994.

Perrillo RP, Mason AL: Therapy for hepatitis B
virus infection, *Gastroenterol Clin North Am*
23(3):581–602, 1994.

Piccoli D: Viral and infectious hepatitis, unpublished data, 1993.

Purdy M, Krawczynski K: Hepatitis E, *Gastroenterol Clin North Am* 23(3):537–546, 1994.

Taylor JM: The structure and replication of hepatitis delta virus, *Annu Rev Microbiol* 46:253–276, 1992.

Uchida T, Shimojima S, Gotoh K, Shikata T,
Mima S: Pathology of livers infected with
"silent" hepatitis B virus mutant, *Liver* 14:251–256, 1994.

Walker WA, Durie PR, Hamilton JR, Walker-Smith JA, Watkins JB: Viral hepatitis. In *Pediatric gastrointestinal disease, pathophysiology, diagnosis, management,* Philadelphia,
1991, BC Decker.

PART SEVEN

Genitourinary

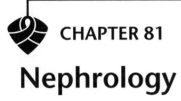

CHAPTER 81

Nephrology

John W. Foreman

Although chronic renal failure occurs in only eight children per 1 million, the primary care physician may be called to see such children for acute illnesses and general pediatric care. Because of this, it is helpful for the general pediatrician to understand certain aspects of this problem, although major renal decisions lie in the realm of the nephrologist. This chapter will describe the major problems associated with chronic renal failure, aspects of chronic dialysis, transplantation, and general indications for a renal biopsy.

PROBLEMS OF CHRONIC RENAL FAILURE

Chronic renal failure is usually without signs or symptoms until significant renal function is lost. Biochemical abnormalities are often not evident until the glomerular filtration rate is reduced to less than 30% of normal. Symptoms suggestive of renal failure, such as fatigue, poor school performance, anorexia, nausea and vomiting, and edema, are usually not noticed until the glomerular filtration rate falls below 25% of normal and often not until it falls to 15% of normal. Because of the marked redundancy of renal function, patients with renal insufficiency are able to survive

without dialysis until the glomerular filtration rate falls below 10% and often 5% of normal. However, with specific disease processes, certain manifestations and symptoms may be evident with only minimal reductions in glomerular function.

The following are specific problems associated with chronic renal failure:

Problems of Chronic Renal Failure
- Growth retardation
- Renal osteodystrophy
- Hypocalcemia
- Hyperphosphatemia
- Acidosis
- Hyperkalemia
- Hypertension
- Edema
- Anemia
- Uremia

Growth impairment, one of the earliest signs of chronic renal failure, may be evident when the glomerular filtration rate is reduced to only 50% of normal. The etiology of the growth failure in renal insufficiency is multifactorial, including acidosis, disturbances in vitamin D metabolism, problems with calcium and phosphate regulation, and disturbances in the growth hormone (GH)–insulin-like growth factor (IGF) axis.

Growth impairment is probably not due to a lack of GH because GH levels in children with renal insufficiency are usually normal to elevated because the kidney is the major site of GH degradation. The growth promoting actions of GH are mediated through IGF. Circulating IGF is made principally in the liver, but many tissues, including epiphyseal cartilage cells, make IGF, and this local production of IGF may be more important in tissue growth. Circulating IGF levels in renal failure are relatively normal, but there also appears to be an increase in IGF-binding proteins that leads to a decrease in unbound IGF levels and its growth-promoting activity. However, therapy with recombinant GH in children with renal failure has led to significant increases in growth velocity and height with few problems.

Disturbances in vitamin D metabolism and calcium-phosphate regulation are also important problems and causes of growth failure in chronic renal insufficiency. The final step in the activation of vitamin D, the formation of calcitriol, occurs in the kidney and is decreased in renal insufficiency. This leads to poor calcium absorption by the gut and decreased mineralization of growing bone. Decreased calcium absorption also leads to hyperparathyroidism, which also interferes with normal bone formation. In addition, the failing kidney is unable to excrete the normal dietary load of phosphate, further increasing parathyroid secretion and bone disease. With severe renal failure the combination of decreased calcitriol and increased serum phosphate levels lead to hypocalcemia and eventually tetany. Treatment of these disorders consists of supplemental vitamin D, usually as calcitriol, and restriction of dietary phosphate. Calcium carbonate is often given, as well, to bind ingested phosphate and prevent its absorption and to provide a source of calcium.

Acidosis is another common feature of chronic renal failure, especially when the glomerular filtration rate falls below a third to a quarter of normal. It may be evident earlier if the renal disease predominantly involves the tubules, such as cystinosis and obstructive uropathy. Acidosis occurs because there are not enough nephrons to excrete the normal dietary load of acid, although individual nephrons excrete supranormal amounts of acid. In the forms of renal failure characterized by tubular disease, acidosis is enhanced by bicarbonate loss from the kidney. In spite of the acidosis, the blood pH rarely falls below 7.2 because the acid that is not secreted by the kidney is buffered by bone. However, the price paid for this buffering is further bone demineralization.

Because the acid production of the average child is 2 to 4 mEq/kg of body weight per day, the treatment of the acidosis of chronic renal failure typically requires a similar amount of alkali given as either sodium bicarbonate or as the sodium or potassium salt of citrate. Citrate is metabolized by the liver to bicarbonate and is easily given to children. When correcting the acidosis of renal failure, especially in severe renal failure, hypocalcemia must be corrected concomitantly to prevent tetany.

The renal handling of sodium and potassium is also often disturbed in chronic renal failure. Sodium problems range from an absolute need for sodium seen in some children with marked tubular or interstitial disease to children who require very restricted intakes of sodium, especially those children with glomerulonephritis. In contrast, many infants with renal dysplasia require supplemental sodium for optimal growth. All children with renal failure tolerate extremes of sodium intake poorly.

Potassium also needs to be followed carefully. Most children with renal insufficiency do not have hyperkalemia until their renal failure is quite advanced; however, hyperkalemia is a common cause of death in such patients. When hyperkalemia is evident, dietary potassium should be restricted. If this is not sufficient, then resins such as sodium polystyrene sulfonate, which bind potassium secreted into the gut, can be employed. Failure of these agents to control the serum potassium level necessitates the institution of dialysis. Some children with renal insufficiency require supplemental potassium, especially those with tubular disorders such as renal tubular acidosis or the Fanconi syndrome.

Hypertension is a very common problem in chronic renal failure, especially that secondary to glomerulonephritis. Hypertension in glomerulonephritis often is evident before there is any impairment of the glomerular filtration rate. Increased blood pressure arises for a number of reasons, including impaired sodium and water excretion leading to volume expansion, and the liberation of vasoactive hormones, especially those of the renin-angiotensin system. (For treatment of this problem, *see* the section on Hypertension.)

Edema, another problem of renal failure, is usually present early in glomerulonephritis, but appears, if at all, late in tubular or interstitial diseases. Edema is present either because of impaired sodium and water excretion leading to expansion of the intravascular space or because of proteinuria with the development of the nephrotic syndrome. In both situations, sodium restriction and often diuretics are helpful in controlling the edema. With severe impairment of renal function and decreased urine output, fluid intake may also need to be limited.

Anemia is a major and predictable consequence of chronic renal failure. It may even be the presenting sign, especially in medullary cystic disease. The anemia, characterized by normal indices and a low reticulocyte count, is caused primarily by decreased production of erythropoietin by the diseased kidney. With the advent of recombinant erythropoietin, this situation usually can be corrected without the need for blood transfusions. Although the rise in red cell mass may cause hypertension or worsen existing hypertension, it usually can be managed by starting or increasing antihypertensive medication.

The diet is very important in children with renal failure. Typically, it must be high in calcium and low in phosphorus, with attention to the amount of sodium. As mentioned before, some children tolerate a normal amount of sodium or even require extra sodium, whereas others need sodium restriction. The diet also must contain an adequate number of calories. This requirement presents a difficult challenge because of the anorexia associated with worsening renal failure. Undernutrition is an especially important problem in infants with renal failure and correction of this problem, often with tube feedings, can significantly improve growth. Protein restriction to 2 g/kg body weight per day in infants and 1 to 1.5 g/kg in older children should be considered when the blood urea nitrogen (BUN) level rises over 70 mg/dL. The protein offered should be of high biologic value, such as egg protein. Obviously, designing a restricted diet that is both nutritious and palatable is quite difficult.

Uremic symptoms usually begin to appear when the BUN level rises above 75 mg/dL and especially when it rises above 150 mg/dL. Early symptoms of uremia are lethargy, increased fatigability, shortened attention span, and poor school performance. Later, persistent nausea and vomiting occur. More serious signs and symptoms of uremia are coma, seizures, pericarditis, and bleeding, especially gastrointestinal, from a platelet dysfunction.

Another important consideration to bear in mind when treating children with renal failure is the adjustment of medication dosages. The kidney is an important excretory organ for many drugs, eg, gentamicin. With renal insufficiency, dangerous levels can develop if adjustments are not made. Recommendations for specific medications are beyond the scope of this chapter, and such questions should be referred to a pediatric nephrologist or nephrology text.

Children with renal failure should receive their routine immunizations, a task that usually falls to the general pediatrician. However, children on dialysis, especially peritoneal dialysis, have low levels of immunoglobulins and impaired responses to vaccines. Therefore, an antibody titer should be checked sometime after an immunization to ensure a protective level.

DIALYSIS

Because there are no precise indications for when to institute chronic dialysis, this decision must be individualized for each child. Usually, chronic dialysis is begun when the serum creatinine rises to 8 to 10 mg/dL or glomerular filtration rate falls to less than 5 to 10 mL/min per 1.73 m^2. In younger children and infants, chronic dialysis may need to be undertaken with much lower levels of serum creatinine reflecting the smaller muscle mass and creatinine production by such individuals. Irrespective of the serum creatinine, dialysis should be considered if other biochemical abnormalities, such as acidosis, hyperkalemia, hyponatremia, hypocalcemia, hyperphosphatemia, and marked azotemia cannot be managed with more conservative means. However, more important than biochemical criteria in making this decision is the presence of progressive fatigue, weakness, lassitude, anorexia, nausea, and vomiting. Furthermore, clinical problems related to volume overload that are unresponsive to sodium restriction, fluid restriction, and diuretics such as anasarca, hypertension, and congestive heart failure will require dialysis, again irrespective of the biochemical status of the patient.

Having made the decision to put a child on

chronic dialysis, the next question to answer is which mode of dialysis is best suited to the patient and his/her family. The choices available are hemodialysis, continuous ambulatory peritoneal dialysis (CAPD), and automated peritoneal dialysis (APD). Each method has advantages and disadvantages, and it is not known which method is most effective in terms of the long-term goals of growth and survival. Therefore, the decision of which modality to use is based on a number of factors including availability of facilities, educability of the family and patient, and the interest and time the family and patient have in performing home dialysis.

The traditional mode of chronic dialysis is hemodialysis. Hemodialysis is accomplished by passing arterial blood along one side of a semipermeable membrane while a balanced salt solution, called the *bath,* is pumped along the other. Because the bath solution does not contain urea, creatinine, or other nitrogenous waste products, these compounds diffuse from the blood into the bath and are removed. Because the blood is pumped along this membrane under pressure, a filtrate of the plasma, composed of water, salts, and waste products, is also forced into the bath, further cleansing the blood and allowing the removal of excess sodium and water.

Vascular access that allows a large blood flow rate (100 to 300 mL/min) is required for hemodialysis. Such access can be achieved by connecting an artery to a vein either directly or via synthetic graft. In small children, proximal vessel grafts, such as the bronchial artery to cephalic vein or femoral artery to saphenous vein, are necessary. The synthetic graft may be used more quickly after surgery than a natural arteriovenous fistula but carries a greater risk of infection or aneurysm formation. Rapid vascular access can be achieved by the percutaneous insertion of a catheter in a large vessel, such as the femoral, subclavian, or jugular veins. Tunnelling the catheter subcutaneously prior to entry into the vein prolongs the usefulness of the catheter and reduces the incidence of infection.

A major problem common to all modes of vascular access is thrombosis. This problem often can be recognized by the loss of the palpable thrill associated with a well-functioning shunt. If detected early enough, it is sometimes possible to remove or dissolve the clot without changing the access site.

Because of the expense and family disruption

that hemodialysis causes, chronic home peritoneal dialysis has become the choice of most families. A peritoneal dialysis catheter designed by Tenckhoff and his colleagues has made this possible by reducing the incidence of infection through the use of a long subcutaneous tunnel prior to the catheter's entry into the peritoneum. In spite of this tunnel, infection remains the major problem associated with chronic peritoneal dialysis. However, it affords the most normal lifestyle for a child with end-stage renal failure.

The two major methods of performing home peritoneal dialysis are CAPD and APD.

In CAPD, dialysate is allowed to remain in the abdomen for 4 to 6 hours and then replaced with fresh dialysate approximately four to six times a day. Extra fluid is removed by this technique by using a concentrated glucose solution in the dialysate. This has been a very effective method of dialysis but does require that either the child or a caretaker constantly change the dialysis solution. With APD, the dialysate exchanges are done every other hour for 8 to 12 hours a night, 5 to 7 days a week. A simple machine can perform this task while the child is asleep, minimizing the disruption that chronic renal failure can wreak on family life. With both modes of peritoneal dialysis, meticulous care of the catheter is necessary to prevent infection of either the subcutaneous tunnel or the peritoneum. Diagnosis and treatment, usually with antibiotics delivered via the dialysis solution, should be undertaken at the first sign of infection. Unfortunately, tunnel infections often require removal of the catheter to eradicate the infection. Also in both forms of peritoneal dialysis, there are constant protein losses into the dialysate, necessitating a more liberal intake of protein than is usually possible with hemodialysis.

TRANSPLANTATION

Because chronic dialysis imposes significant dietary and social restrictions on children, the ultimate goal of most pediatric end-stage renal programs has been successful renal transplantation. Over the past 15 years, renal transplantation in children has become an established procedure. The two potential sources of kidneys that are available to patients with end-stage renal disease are from compatible, healthy, immediate relatives (live related donor) or from a brain-dead but otherwise healthy patient (cadaveric donor).

Transplants from living relatives have longer graft survival and can be performed more quickly once the disease reaches end stage. For these reasons, these transplants are the choice of many pediatric centers.

Life-long immunosuppression is necessary in transplant patients to prevent rejection, usually consisting of steroids, azathioprine, and cyclosporine. Rejections are treated with high doses of steroids and often anti–T-cell immunoglobulin.

A number of problems continue to plague renal transplant patients. Rejection remains the major cause of graft loss, and for this reason continual monitoring of renal function is necessary. All too often, poor compliance with the medical regimen, especially in the adolescent, leads to rejection and graft failure. Infection, especially with viral agents, presents a constant problem because of the immunosuppression. As a consequence, any symptom suggestive of an infection should be evaluated promptly, a task that the primary care physician is often asked to perform in consultation with the transplant center. These patients should avoid routine immunizations, especially with live vaccines, and other individuals who have been recently immunized with live vaccines, such as the poliomyelitis and measles vaccine because of the immunosuppression. Hypertension is very common in renal transplant recipients, often because of the prednisone and cyclosporine. The management is similar to that in other patients. Avascular necrosis, especially of the femoral head, is an uncommon, but disabling, problem of transplant patients and is usually related to the steroids. Finally, poor growth in spite of a functioning renal transplant is still a significant problem in children. Reduction of the steroid dose and the use of an alternate day administration is helpful. Recombinant GH can improve growth in such children, but it is unclear at this time whether GH does or does not adversely affect the graft.

RENAL BIOPSY INDICATIONS

There are few absolute indications for a renal biopsy, therefore the reasons for biopsy vary between nephrologists. A renal biopsy can provide information on both diagnosis and prognosis and occasionally on therapy. Complications arising from the procedure, mainly related to bleeding, are quite low when done by individuals experienced in performing it in children. Recent studies have shown that it need not be performed in prepubertal children in the initial presentation of nephrosis who respond to steroids, because the overwhelming majority have minimal disease change. Because adolescents presenting with nephrosis have less than a 50% response rate to steroids, a renal biopsy is a useful procedure for guiding therapy in these patients. A renal biopsy is not necessary in a healthy child with microscopic hematuria in the absence of proteinuria, urinary casts, and hypertension. Persistent proteinuria, after excluding orthostatic proteinuria, is an indication for a biopsy because there is a high probability for significant renal disease.

BIBLIOGRAPHY

Alexander SR, Honda M: Continuous peritoneal dialysis for children: A decade of worldwide growth and development, *Kidney Int Suppl* 40:S65–S74, 1993.

Campos A, Garin EH: Therapy of renal anemia in children and adolescents with recombinant human erythropoietin (rHuEPO), *Clin Pediatr* 31:94–99, 1992.

Hanna JD, Foreman JW, Chan JCM: Chronic renal insufficiency in infants and children, *Clin Pediatr* 30:365–384, 1991.

Mehls O, Tonshoff B, Haffner D, Wuhl E, Schaefer F: The use of human recombinant growth hormone in short children with chronic renal failure, *J Pediatr Endocrinol* 7:107–113, 1994.

Salusky IB, Ramirez JA, Goodman WG: Recent advances in the management of renal osteodystrophy, *Curr Opin Nephrol Hypertens* 2: 580–587, 1993.

Sanger S, Ettinger RB: Kidney transplantation in children, *Semin Pediatr Surg* 2:235–247, 1993.

CHAPTER 82

Nephrosis

Thomas L. Kennedy III

As every physician in training learns, nephrotic syndrome consists of heavy proteinuria, hypoalbuminemia, edema, and hyperlipidemia. To the nephrologist, the nephrotic syndrome is defined by proteinuria in excess of 40 mg/m^2/hr (approximately 50 mg/kg/day), because the other components are all the consequences of this primary abnormality. To the child and his/her family, however, the nephrotic syndrome is the severe, generalized edema, which can be both frightening and debilitating.

BACKGROUND

Etiology and Epidemiology

The nephrotic syndrome is an uncommon condition in childhood. The exact incidence is unknown, but several studies suggest a yearly incidence of two to seven cases per 100,000 children less than 15 years of age. Although the nephrotic syndrome has occurred in families and some immunogenetic markers are more common in patients with nephrotic syndrome, there is no recognizable genetic pattern, and the vast majority of cases are sporadic. Male patients predominate, with a ratio of approximately 2:1.

The nephrotic syndrome is not a single entity, and the heavy proteinuria that characterizes it may occur in association with virtually any glomerular disease. In childhood, however, one form comprises 80% of all cases of nephrotic syndrome. This entity has gone by several names, including lipoid nephrosis, nil disease, minimal lesion nephrotic syndrome, and the idiopathic nephrotic syndrome of childhood, but minimal change nephrotic syndrome (MCNS) is the term with widest current acceptance. The name originates from the observation that histologic examination of the kidney reveals only slight abnormalities. On light and immunofluorescent microscopy, there are usually no pathologic abnormalities. On electron microscopy, there is "fusion" of the foot processes of glomerular epithelial cells.

The etiology of MCNS is unknown. The observation has frequently been made that the onset and relapses occur in temporal relationship to an infection or an allergic episode. However, such a precipitating event is not always present, and cause and effect cannot be proved. Furthermore, speculation and anecdotal evidence implicating diet and food additives in the nephrotic syndrome have no convincing support. Although minimal change disease may occur at any age, it is most common between ages 2 and 5 years and accounts for more than 90% of cases of nephrotic syndrome in this age group.

Pathophysiology

A persuasive body of evidence has developed that strongly implicates an immunopathogenesis in minimal change disease. Some of this evidence includes clinical observations, and some is derived from in vitro experiments using serum and white blood cells (WBCs) from patients with the condition. Observations exist, however, that cause doubt on a primary immunologic dysfunction. It is possible that the immune abnormalities are secondary to the low serum proteins and the hyperlipoproteinemia.

There is further uncertainty regarding the etiologic role of the immunologic dysfunction and the pathophysiology of the nephrotic syndrome as it is currently understood. The renal glomerulus possesses a filtration barrier that retards the loss of certain substances from the blood on the basis of molecular size, configuration, and charge. The barrier normally possesses a net negative charge that prevents the filtration of anionic molecules such as albumin. In the nephrotic syndrome, the glomerular negative charge is lost and albumin—and, to a more variable extent, other serum proteins—becomes filterable. It is not known how or why the negative charge disappears.

As the kidney loses protein, serum levels begin to decline. The body unsuccessfully attempts to compensate by increasing the hepatic synthesis of albumin. The hypoproteinemia that develops causes a concomitant fall in plasma oncotic pressure and plasma water begins to move from the intravascular to the interstitial space. The serum protein level at which edema develops varies among children but generally is less than 2.4 g/dL.

The elevated levels of cholesterol and lipids are not totally understood but are due, in part, to the nonspecific increase in hepatic synthetic pathways. Also contributing to the hyperlipidemia is the urinary loss of lipoprotein lipases that are important in the metabolism of lipoproteins.

DATA GATHERING

Clinical Manifestations

The child with nephrotic syndrome almost invariably presents with edema. The onset may be dramatic or insidious, but it is usually rapid enough that discovery of heavy proteinuria on a routine screening urinalysis is uncommon. Generally, the swelling is first recognized in the periorbital area, is intermittent, and frequently is attributed to allergic symptoms. As the edema becomes generalized, renal disease is suspected and proteinuria is documented.

The child with nephrotic syndrome should be evaluated for the possibility of associated renal disease. In addition, detailed information and education should be provided to the family. This latter aspect cannot be overemphasized because it is extremely important that the family appreciates the recurrent nature of what is usually a chronic condition and the stress such an illness can place on them. They should understand the pathophysiology of the edema so they see the value of restricting salt intake, but not fluids, during relapses. They must know how to detect proteinuria and be committed to routine urine testing and to keeping a diary. They should appreciate the role of infection in precipitating relapses, the danger of infection in the child on

high-dose steroids, and the expected and untoward effects of prednisone. Hospitalization may be necessary in children with severe anasarca, abdominal symptoms, or infection.

History

In evaluating the child with nephrotic syndrome, important history includes questions that would suggest the presence of preexisting renal disease including previous episodes of nephritis, abnormalities on screening urinalyses, and a history of hypertension or urinary tract infections. Also important is an inquiry regarding a family history of renal disease. Questions must be asked regarding possible infections, because infections not only frequently precede the onset of nephrotic syndrome, but also occur more often in the hypoproteinemic, edematous child and may be life-threatening. A history of oliguria is usually obtained and may be misleading to the extent that it may suggest acute renal failure. Renal failure, however, occurs only rarely in MCNS. More frequently, the oliguria is appropriate and reflects the kidney's response to intravascular volume depletion caused by the hypoproteinemia.

Physical Examination

The physical examination can help document intravascular volume depletion when significant postural changes in blood pressure exist. A fall in systolic blood pressure of 10 mm Hg or more when the patient changes from the supine to the erect position is of concern. Hypertension should make one suspect significant renal disease. After obtaining the patient's height and weight, it is important to determine the ideal weight for height to estimate the amount of edema and to calculate medication doses on the basis of "dry" weight or surface area. Great care must be taken on physical examination to exclude the presence of infection, including those that may not be obvious (eg, sinusitis, perianal abscess, or urinary tract infection) or those that may appear trivial (eg, paronychia, dental or gingival infection). The edema, which tends to be pitting and dependent, may be obvious or may occur as mild ascites and/or pleural effusion. Scrotal and labial edema are of concern not only because of the discomfort they cause but also because an overlying cellulitis may develop. The presence of abdominal discomfort associated with anorexia and diarrhea is often attributable to bowel wall edema, but this discomfort makes careful abdominal and rectal examination essential to assess the possibility of peritonitis. An interesting but clinically insignificant and unexplained finding in the child with nephrotic syndrome is softening of the cartilage in the ear.

Laboratory

Laboratory tests are directed at confirming the presence of nephrotic syndrome, determining whether it is MCNS or part of some other renal disease and excluding the possibility of infection. Laboratory evaluation of the child with nephrotic syndrome is summarized in the following listing.

Laboratory Evaluation
Confirm the diagnosis of nephrotic syndrome
- Urine dipstick for protein (usually 3+ to 4+) or urine protein/creatinine >1.0
- 24-hour urine protein (>40 mg/m^2/hr)
- Determination of serum total protein and protein electrophoresis
- Determination of serum cholesterol and triglyceride levels (not essential)

Rule out other renal disease (not all tests are necessary in every child)
- Determination of blood urea nitrogen (BUN) creatinine
- Glomerular filtration rate (creatinine clearance)
- Urinalysis (sediment examination for cellular casts)
- C3, CH$_{50}$ determinations
- Other serologic tests: antinuclear antibody, antistreptolysin O titers, hepatitis B surface antigen, circulating immune complexes
- Renal ultrasound

Rule out infection
- Complete blood cell (CBC) count
- Cultures (as indicated, including paracentesis for abdominal tenderness)
- Radiographic films (as indicated, including chest, abdomen, sinus)
- Tuberculin skin test (before starting steroids)

The CBC count is helpful in several respects. An elevated hematocrit level may indicate intravascular volume depletion. On the other hand, anemia may occur in long-standing nephrotic syndrome secondary to loss of transferrin in the urine or may indicate the presence of renal insufficiency. The WBC count is a useful guide to the presence of possible infection until steroids are begun. Because of increased levels of fibrino-

gen, cholesterol, and α-globulins, the sedimentation rate is elevated and, therefore, not a reliable indicator of infection in the child with nephrotic syndrome.

Serum protein concentrations show marked reduction in albumin concentrations (frequently in the range of 1.0 g/dL), increases in α$_2$-globulin fraction, and variable changes in the γ-fraction.

Although a 24-hour urine is helpful to quantitate the protein loss, the urine protein-creatinine ratio on random specimens recently has been shown to accurately reflect the nephrotic state.

The use of urine protein electrophoresis and comparison of the renal clearance of different-sized proteins, the so-called protein selectivity index, is not specific enough to be of help in evaluating the condition of an individual with nephrotic syndrome.

The BUN and creatinine levels will indicate or exclude renal insufficiency. The level of BUN may be elevated disproportionately to that of creatinine (prerenal azotemia) as a manifestation of the intravascular volume depletion and decreased urea clearance. A creatinine clearance should be obtained, with the urine collected for protein quantitation for more precise determination of glomerular filtration rate. Although the creatinine clearance is generally normal in MCNS, a reduction at the time of diagnosis usually reflects decreased renal blood flow rather than glomerular disease.

The urinalysis may be helpful in differentiating MCNS from other causes of nephrotic syndrome. Microscopic hematuria may be present in up to one quarter of children with MCNS, but the presence of an "active" sediment, which is the presence of mixed cell types and cellular casts, suggests other renal disease.

Complement proteins are rarely reduced in the child with MCNS and suggest other renal lesions, including acute poststreptococcal, membranoproliferative, or lupus glomerulonephritis.

Other laboratory studies are not routinely indicated for every child. Rather, they should be considered in the child with signs and symptoms of other diseases or with atypical presentation of the nephrotic syndrome.

The renal biopsy remains the definitive diagnostic test, but may be reserved for certain circumstances. These include 1) the child older than 12 years at diagnosis, 2) the child whose presentation and prior evaluation strongly suggest renal disease other than minimal-change disease, 3) the child who is steroid resistant, and

4) the child who is a candidate for immunosuppressive therapy. Most children with nephrotic syndrome do not require a biopsy, and the diagnosis of MCNS is generally presumed rather than documented anatomically.

Differential Diagnosis

The differential diagnosis of nephrotic syndrome is lengthy and may be considered as broad groupings that include the nephrotic syndrome that occurs as the primary manifestation of a glomerulopathy and the one that occurs secondary to a systemic disease or toxic injury. The following classification of the nephrotic syndrome is not exhaustive. Only a very few of the conditions listed occur frequently enough in the pediatric age range to deserve mention in this discussion.

Differential Diagnosis of Nephrotic Syndrome

Primary renal disease
* Without glomerulonephritis
  Minimal change nephrotic syndrome
  Focal segmental glomerulosclerosis
  Congenital nephrotic syndrome
* Associated with glomerulonephritis
  Mesangial proliferative
  Membranoproliferative
  Membranous

Occurrence with systemic disease
* Infections
  Viral (hepatitis B, HIV, Epstein-Barr virus, cytomegalovirus, etc.)
  Bacterial (acute poststreptococcal glomerulonephritis, subacute bacterial endocarditis, shunt nephritis, etc.)
  Parasitic (malaria, schistosomiasis, etc.)
  Congenital syphilis
* Malignant disease
  Lymphoma (eg, MCNS in Hodgkin disease) and leukemia
  Solid tumors (Wilms tumor, carcinomas)
* Metabolic disease
  Diabetic nephropathy
  Hypothyroidism
* Inflammatory disease
  Systemic lupus erythematosus
  Henoch-Schönlein purpura
  Systemic vasculitides (eg, polyarteritis)
* Miscellaneous diseases
  Sickle cell disease
  Hemolytic-uremic syndrome
  Renal venous thrombosis

Associated with exogenous agents
* Allergens
  Pollens, inhalants
  Venoms (eg, bee, snake)
* Immunizations
* Toxins
  Heavy metals
  Heroin
* Medications
  Captopril
  Penicillamine
  Nonsteroidal anti-inflammatory agents

Focal segmental glomerulosclerosis (FGS) comprises approximately 5% to 10% of cases of childhood nephrotic syndrome. It may mimic minimal change disease in its presentation, although a more insidious onset, hematuria, hypertension, and azotemia are all more common. It is generally unresponsive to steroid and immunosuppressive therapy and leads to slowly progressive renal insufficiency. Focal segmental glomerulosclerosis has been reported with increased frequency in children with vesicoureteral reflux, in children with one kidney, and in some families. There are some nephrologists who believe that it may be a transition form of minimal change disease, although this is controversial.

Mesangial proliferative glomerulonephritis also accounts for approximately 5% to 10% of cases of childhood nephrotic syndrome. Its presentation is much like MCNS. Initially, it often responds to steroid therapy, although children with this condition have more frequent relapses and more commonly become steroid resistant. The outlook for this condition is more uncertain than that for MCNS or FGS. As with the other forms of nephrotic syndrome, definitive diagnosis depends on tissue histologic studies obtained by renal biopsy.

Membranoproliferative glomerulonephritis (MPGN; formerly called mesangiocapillary glomerulonephritis) comprises approximately 5% of cases of childhood nephrotic syndrome. Membranoproliferative glomerulonephritis may be divided into three types and is frequently characterized by persistent hypocomplementemia. Although the outlook for patients with MPGN has traditionally been considered unfavorable, chronic drug therapy with prednisone given on alternate days and most recently antiplatelet therapy with aspirin has improved the prognosis.

Membranous nephropathy is noted because it is so infrequent in children while it is the most common form of nephrotic syndrome in adults. There is no adequate therapy, although the course in children may be marked by spontaneous remissions.

The congenital nephrotic syndrome (also called Finnish-type or microcystic disease) is inherited as an autosomal recessive disorder presenting at birth or shortly thereafter and characterized by resistance to any form of therapy. The massive protein loss leads to growth failure, malnutrition, and fatal infection unless aggressive management, such as parenteral alimentation, nephrectomy with dialysis, and eventual renal transplantation, is instituted.

MANAGEMENT

It is important to realize that of all the laboratory tests that may help to diagnose MCNS, the best predictor of MCNS short of a renal biopsy is the response to steroid therapy.

Of children with MCNS, 90% respond to glucocorticoids with complete, albeit usually temporary, resolution of proteinuria. The drug with the widest use is prednisone, begun at a dose of 60 mg/m^2/day (or 2 mg/kg/day, maximum 80 mg) in two to three divided doses. The drug should be given in this manner for a maximum of 1 month or at least 2 weeks after the urine has been protein free. The average time from the onset of therapy until onset of remission is approximately 10 to 14 days. During this interval, it is frequently very difficult for both parents and physicians to stand by and watch the child become more edematous. Measures such as aggressive diuretic therapy are generally ill-advised and potentially dangerous (see supportive therapy). Patience is the most important attribute during this period. Depending on the amount of edema, remission may be associated with a dramatic and marked diuresis that can lead to electrolyte disturbances, including hyponatremia and hypokalemia. After the diuresis, the child frequently will feel fatigued and appear tired with dark discoloration around his/her eyes.

When remission is attained, the prednisone is given on alternate days as a single morning dose with breakfast. The initial alternate-day dose and tapering schedule may vary somewhat among nephrologists, but the majority favor a slow decrease over a 2- to 3-month period. The alternate-day schedule is effective and minimizes steroid toxicity.

Children who have persistent proteinuria after receiving 4 weeks of daily steroids require special treatment or a renal biopsy and therefore require consultation with a pediatric nephrologist.

MCNS can be classified as follows:

1. Steroid sensitive: Patients respond to steroids and can stay protein-free without treatment for various lengths of time.
2. Steroid dependent: Patients respond to steroids but require continuous treatment with low-dose steroids.
3. Steroid resistant: Patients do not respond to steroid treatment.

The child with MCNS who responds to prednisone may follow several patterns. First, the nephrotic syndrome may resolve and never recur. This ideal outcome accounts for only approximately 20% of cases. Second, there may be infrequent relapses (eg, less than two per year) occurring for several years, responding each time to steroids and eventually resolving. This category accounts for approximately 30% of cases. Third, 40% of children have frequent relapses of heavy proteinuria, requiring repeated and often prolonged courses of steroids. These children are at risk of developing steroid toxicity. When such toxicity becomes intolerable, the child should be considered to receive immunosuppressive drugs capable of inducing long-term remissions in both steroid-dependent and steroid-resistant MCNS. The difficulty is deciding when the myriad of steroid side effects becomes intolerable, because the potential toxicities of the alternative alkylating agents are significant.

Steroid side effects such as growth failure, hypertension, aseptic necrosis of bone, steroid-induced psychosis, or severe myopathy are clearly unacceptable. Of these, problems with growth are most common and growth rates must be followed closely.

The impact of other side effects are more variable. For example, the cushingoid changes, acne, and hirsutism may be totally unacceptable and lead to noncompliance in an adolescent woman, so the decision to use alternatives to prednisone must be individualized.

Immunosuppressive Therapy

Only approximately 10% of children with MCNS require immunosuppressive therapy. The drugs that are effective are cyclophosphamide (Cytoxan) and chlorambucil (Leukeran). Each has its proponents, but neither has been shown to be superior to the other. The drugs are given at a lower dose and for a shorter period of time than when used to treat malignant disease (for cyclophosphamide, 2 mg/kg for 8 to 12 weeks; for chlorambucil, 0.2 mg/kg/day for a total dose of 12 mg/kg). For this reason, their potential toxicities are less common when used in children with MCNS. By convention, they are given in conjunction with prednisone (generally 2 mg/kg/day in divided doses for 14 days, then every other day), even when the child is steroid resistant. Short-term side effects of both are leukopenia, and weekly WBC counts should be obtained. Administration is temporarily interrupted for total WBC counts less than $4000/mm^3$ or for total granulocyte counts less than $1500/mm^3$. Other potential short-term effects include anorexia, mild hair loss, hemorrhagic cystitis with cyclophosphamide (good oral hydration must be emphasized), and focal seizures with chlorambucil. All of these are uncommon. Long-term effects include infertility, the possibility of sustained immunologic dysfunction, and the occurrence of malignant disease. Unfortunately, the exact risk is unknown, but it appears to be small. The remissions obtained are frequently prolonged or permanent, but, if not, will sometimes appear to decrease the frequency of relapses. Cases of children who convert from a state of steroid resistance to steroid responsiveness following immunosuppressive therapy are well documented. Other drugs with limited experience and usefulness in the treatment of MCNS include levamisole and cyclosporine.

Long-Term Follow-Up

Relapses

Recurrence of proteinuria may develop at any time in the child with nephrotic syndrome. The most common triggering event is infection, although many times transient proteinuria may occur in association with an infection and disappear when the illness resolves. For this reason, it is wise not to start steroids or increase the dose in a child who develops infection-associated proteinuria until it is clear the protein loss is persistent after the child is well. Likewise, once the decision is made to use steroids, they should be given in full doses (ie, 2 mg/kg/day) and not reinstituted in half-doses or other nonsystematic fashion that can lead to prolonged courses and steroid toxicity. Remission is defined as 5 consecutive days of protein-free urine (dipstick reading negative or trace), and the transition to alternate-day therapy can be made at that time.

Patterns may become apparent for the occurrence of relapse in certain children and, if recognized, the timetable for decreasing steroids can be tailored for that individual. For example, some children may require a more gradual transition from daily to alternate-day steroids, whereas others appear to relapse only when their dose is reduced below some critical level. At any rate, it is good practice to pay close attention to the child on a tapering dose of prednisone and to avoid reducing the dose at the time of an intercurrent illness.

The use of chronic, low-dose, daily (2.5 mg of prednisone) or alternate-day steroid therapy has been advocated to prevent proteinuria in children with frequent relapses. The efficacy of such therapy remains to be fully established.

Supportive Therapy

Dietary measures may be used to aid in the management of MCNS. The diet should include optimal amounts (1.5 to 2.0 g/kg/day) of high biologic value protein, but there is no reason to increase intake above this level because the body will not utilize the excess protein ingested. Moderate salt restriction will help reduce the rate of edema formation but should not be so severe that it will affect the palatability of the diet. Fluid restriction should not be instituted, because thirst in the child with nephrosis frequently indicates intravascular volume depletion.

For the same reason, diuretic therapy should be undertaken with caution. In a child with MCNS who is incapacitated by anasarca, who has respiratory distress because of pleural effusions, or who has abdominal discomfort and anorexia because of ascites, the use of intravenous infusions of 25% albumin (1 g/kg/dose given over 60 to 90 minutes and followed by 1 mg/kg of furosemide) may be used. These infusions may provide significant, temporary relief through the diuresis they evoke. However, this therapy is expensive and not totally without risk. Because the hyperoncotic albumin temporarily increases the intravascular volume through movement of edema from the interstitium, hypertension may develop and the blood pressure must be monitored closely. Routine oral diuretic therapy becomes very useful in chronic forms of nephrotic syndrome, in which the blood volume is not contracted and edema can be minimized.

Other supportive measures include attention to the prevention and prompt treatment of infectious disease. In the child who has had a relapse of MCNS, peritonitis remains a threat. The most common organism is *Streptococcus pneumoniae,* but *Hemophilus influenzae* and *Escherichia coli* also have been reported and antibiotic therapy must be chosen appropriately.

It is important to remember that the nephrotic syndrome is a hypercoagulable state, and venipuncture in deep veins (*eg,* the femoral vein) should be avoided.

Although its efficacy in children with MCNS is unknown, the pneumococcal vaccine should be considered. If the vaccine is administered, it should be given preferably when the child is in remission and off steroids. The same is true for the varicella vaccine, which should be given to any child with MCNS who is not immune.

Despite reports of immunizations precipitating relapses in children with MCNS, such cases are uncommon and the routine schedule of immunizations may be followed at the physician's discretion.

Outcome

The "statistically average" child with MCNS will have approximately five relapses over a 5-year period and then permanently go into remission. However, such prognostication is unreliable for any individual, because some children have no relapses and some children have many relapses extending well into adulthood.

The ultimate outlook for permanent remission and preservation of normal renal function is good for steroid-sensitive patients with MCNS. Of greatest concern is therapy-related morbidity that includes steroid-induced growth retardation and obesity and the long-term dangers of the alkylating agents. The morbidity, if any, related to the hyperlipidemia of MCNS is unknown.

The risk of MCNS transforming into another glomerulopathy such as focal glomerulosclerosis or mesangial proliferative glomerulonephritis is also unknown and, as mentioned earlier, is controversial. If such transformation occurs, however, it is quite uncommon. The physician, therefore, may remain very optimistic when counseling the family of a child with MCNS regarding outcome.

Use of Consultants

The pediatric nephrologist need not provide total care for the child with MCNS. Consultation at the time of diagnosis may provide useful suggestions with regard to the evaluation and initial therapy. The nephrologist can also provide the necessary information the family will need to know to adequately care for their child and realistically deal with the future course. Later, the nephrologist can be helpful in the management of children with frequent relapses who may require many changes in their steroid regimen. The nephrologist must assume responsibility for the child who requires a renal biopsy or the use of immunosuppressive medication and should play an active role in the care of children with nephrotic syndrome other than MCNS.

BIBLIOGRAPHY

Berns JS, Gaudio KM, Krassner LS, et al: Steroid-responsive nephrotic syndrome in childhood: A long-term study of clinical course, histopathology, efficacy of cyclosphosphamide therapy and effects on growth, *Am J Kidney Dis* 9:108, 1987.

Tarshish P, Tobin JN, Bernstein J, Edelman CM: Cyclophosphamide does not benefit patients with focal segmental glomerulosclerosis. A report of the International Study of Kidney Disease in Children Pediatric Nephrology 1996, 10:590–593 #5.

McVicar M, Chandra M: Pathogenic mechanisms in the nephrotic syndrome of childhood, *Adv Pediatr* 32:269, 1985.

Strauss J, Zilleruelo G, Freundlich M, et al: Less commonly recognized features of childhood nephrotic syndrome, *Pediatr Clin North Am* 34:591, 1987.

CHAPTER 83

Urology

William Tarry

Management of urologic problems changes as concepts are modified and evaluations are undertaken. The purpose of this chapter is to discuss the present understanding of common urologic problems that are encountered by a primary care physician. These problems include ureteral reflux, use of the cystoscope, circumcision, cryptorchidism, meatal stenosis, and dysfunctional voiding. These topics are presented so that the physician will be aware of the potential treatments and have a better understanding of the approach taken by the urologist when caring for these patients.

VESICOURETERAL REFLUX

Urinary tract infection (UTI) is one of the most common bacterial infections of childhood. The treatment of UTI in children is discussed in Chapter 96. Every child with a UTI should undergo voiding cystourethrography (VCU) and intravenous pyelography or renal ultrasound after the urine has been sterilized.

Because of the frequency of vesicoureteral reflux, many urologists and nephrologists recommend a VCU after the first infection. The initial VCU assesses the status of the bladder and urethra, ruling out obstructing lesions such as posterior urethral valves, diaphragms, and strictures. It documents the presence and severity of vesicoureteral reflux and demonstrates trabeculation and diverticula that suggest outlet obstruction. To ensure the most accurate assessment of the degree of reflux, the cystogram should be obtained while the child is awake, and the radiographs should be taken at the time of peak flow of the voiding phase. The VCU may not give reliable information about bladder size or postvoid re-

sidual urine. Many children do not empty completely on each voiding, and many will experience a reflex bladder contraction prior to reaching full capacity.

A renal ultrasound will screen the upper urinary tract for obstruction evidenced by hydronephrosis and give reliable information about renal size and growth. Patients in whom reflux is demonstrated should have their kidneys imaged by dimercaptosuccinic acid (DMSA) or glucoheptonate renal scan for the most accurate assessment of renal scars. Ureteral duplications and other upper tract abnormalities coexisting with vesicoureteral reflux represent complex cases, which are managed on an individual basis by a urologist.

Reflux is the most common abnormality discovered in the radiographic evaluation of a child with an infection and one of the most significant congenital anomalies in children in terms of morbidity and long-term disability. In the first year of life, 50% of infants with UTI will have vesicoureteral reflux. Between ages 1 and 16 years, reflux occurs in 15% to 35% of children presenting with UTI. The remainder of this section will consider vesicoureteral reflux and infection in the absence of other anatomic or neurologic lesions.

Vesicoureteral reflux occurs secondary to an abnormality of the ureterovesical junction. The more severe the abnormality, the greater the degree of reflux. Because the ureterovesical junction changes with growth of the child until the age of puberty, the children may "grow out" of reflux.

Grading the severity of reflux helps to predict the likelihood of spontaneous resolution. The international grading system for reflux and the rates of spontaneous resolution by grade are shown in Figure 83-1 and in the chart on page 572:

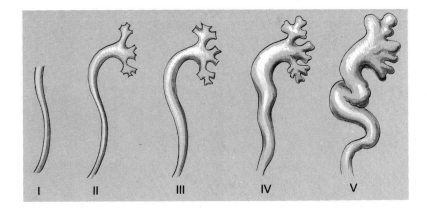

FIG 83-1

International classification of vesicoureteral reflux. Grade I, ureter only. Grade II, ureter, pelvic, and calyces; no dilatation of renal pelvis; no or slight blunting of the fornices. Grade IV, moderate dilatation or tortuosity of ureter and moderate dilatation of renal pelvis and calyces; complete obliteration of sharp angle of fornices. Grade V, gross dilatation of tortuosity of ureter; gross dilatation of renal pelvis and calyces; papillary impressions no longer visible in majority of calyces.

GRADE OF REFLUX	RATE OF SPONTANEOUS RESOLUTION, %
I	85
II	63
III	53
IV	34
V	0

The grading system reflects a combination of aspects of two older systems derived by Perlmutter and Parkkulainen. The system helps the clinician predict the natural history of reflux in a general way; the spontaneous resolution rates observed enable one to pursue the conservative or medical management of reflux with some confidence.

Medical management of reflux consists of 1) prevention of infection by continuous antibiotic prophylaxis and 2) evaluation of progress by periodic radiologic imaging. Efforts should be made to optimize bowel and bladder habits with particular attention to chronic constipation. Some physicians recommend quarterly surveillance urine cultures for the first year. Prophylactic treatment consists of bedtime administration of one fourth to one half of the therapeutic dose of nitrofurantoin or trimethoprim-sulfamethoxazole, and cephalexin, 2 to 4 mg/kg/day, also can be used. These regimens usually do not alter gastrointestinal tract flora or lead to monilial infections. Urine cultures should be obtained any time the child exhibits unexplained fever, abdominal pain, or voiding symptoms. Fortunately, "breakthrough" infections in children on antibiotic suppression occur in less than 10% of children. The addition of anticholinergic drugs such as oxybutynin (Ditropan) to the regimen in children with reflux and "wetting" problems or other symptoms of an unstable bladder may enhance spontaneous resolution of reflux but will aggravate the chronic constipation seen in two thirds of children with recurrent UTI.

Resolution or progression of reflux may be documented by yearly conventional cystography or nuclear voiding cystography, which is more costly but has the advantage of providing less radiation exposure. Renal growth and progression of scarring may be monitored by intravenous pyelogram, renal scanning, or ultrasound. Nuclear and ultrasound studies reduce the radiation dose but may be more subject to errors of interpretation unless carried out by radiologists familiar with such studies in children.

The surgical alternative is ureteral reimplantation (Fig. 83-2). The advancement technique (Cohen reimplant) used in most centers today produces excellent success in correcting reflux with minimal complications. Intravenous pyelogram and VCU are usually performed 3 months after surgery, and, if the findings appear satisfactory, administration of the suppressive antibiotics is stopped. Although in most cases the

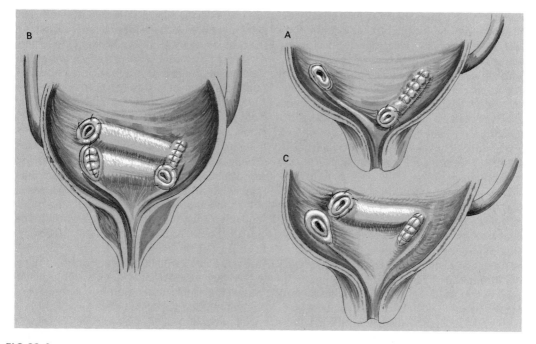

FIG 83-2

Reimplantation procedures. **A,** Anderson advancement. Left ureter is moved distally to prevent reflux. **B,** Cohen procedure. Bilateral transverse tunnel created by moving left ureter through mucosa to right side and right ureter to left. **C,** Cohen procedure. Unilateral reimplantation.

3-month studies will demonstrate a good result, reflux will occasionally persist for up to 1 year after surgery, probably secondary to edema of the trigone area. By 1 year, the success rate should be greater than 95%. Obstruction is exceedingly rare with ureteral advancement techniques; persistent reflux may occur in 2% to 4% of cases. It may eventually resolve if bladder function is normal or may be corrected by a second reimplantation. The patient with normal upper tracts, like one whose reflux resolved spontaneously, probably needs no follow-up beyond a year after surgery. Those patients with scars or poor renal growth are at risk for hypertension and deterioration of renal function and should be followed-up into adulthood. By the time they reach their late twenties, the incidence of hypertension is 23%; the mean age at onset is 19 years and mean interval since surgery 12 years. The risk of end-stage renal disease is approximately 4% for all scarred kidneys.

Several factors influence the choice of surgical therapy. In general, increasing grade, progressive scarring, poor growth or compliance, and breakthrough infections lead one toward surgery either at the onset or after a trial of medical treatment. The relative cost of an operation vs several years of radiographs and medications must be considered, as well as the preference of the family and their level of understanding and reliability. Reimplantation is preferable to loss of renal function due to the patient's being lost to follow-up. The question of the prepubertal girl with persistent reflux remains unresolved. Most urologists think that a girl with persistent reflux and a history of infections should undergo reimplantation before child-bearing age, especially if renal scarring is present. The pregnant woman is at risk for scarring from infected reflux, and reimplantation may prevent some episodes of pyelonephritis; it does not appear to prevent irreversible deterioration of renal function that is rarely observed in pregnant women with scarred kidneys.

ROLE OF CYSTOSCOPY IN CHILDREN

The advent of smaller, more versatile endoscopes has greatly enhanced the ability of the urologist to perform therapeutic maneuvers in even the smallest infants in those rare instances it becomes necessary. Valve ablation is easier and safer. Stricture incision at any level of the urinary tract, antegrade percutaneous endopyelotomy, endoscopic lithotripsy, and short-term internal stenting are readily performed at any age. However, the rarity of stones in children renders most of these procedures infrequent. The availability of constantly improving radiographic techniques obviates cystoscopy and retrograde pyelography, with their requirement for general anesthesia, as diagnostic maneuvers.

In the past, one of the most common indications for cystoscopy was UTI, with or without vesicoureteral reflux. At present, vesicoureteral reflux can be diagnosed and graded with careful VCU, and a reliable prediction can be made on that basis as to the likelihood of spontaneous resolution of the reflux. The endoscopic observation of the bladder and ureteric orifices rarely adds any useful information. Data from the Mayo Clinic and Children's Hospital of Philadelphia indicate that in intermediate grades of reflux, the endoscopic judgment of position and shape of the orifice and ureteral tunnel length was only 50% accurate in predicting resolution of reflux. Associated findings such as cystitis cystica, trigonitis, and urethritis do not alter the management in these cases. Urethral stenosis in women is no longer thought to be a cause of infection or reflux, so that cystoscopy in combination with urethral dilation for recurrent UTI is no longer warranted.

Endoscopy is not helpful in evaluating most hematuria. Episodic asymptomatic hematuria most commonly occurs secondary to benign urethritis (urethrorrhagia) or a lacuna magna (congenital diverticulum of the fossa navicularis), hypercalcemia, or medical renal disease. These conditions are diagnosed by other tests and procedures (*see* Chapter 44).

At present, cystoscopy is useful primarily to confirm a diagnosis made on the basis of a radiograph at the same time that intervention is applied, particularly in cases in which the intervention can be carried out by endoscopic means. Lesions requiring cystoscopy after radiographic diagnosis are urethral valves, strictures, diaphragms, ureteroceles, bladder tumors, and fibroepithelial polyps. Cystoscopy also is useful in completing the evaluation of intersex states and anorectal malformations. It is sometimes used postoperatively to evaluate a reconstructed ure-

thra or bladder neck. Retrograde pyelography is no longer often required, because the ureter can be evaluated both anatomically and functionally by means of careful application of intravenous pyelogram, antegrade pyelography, ultrasound, and renal nuclear scanning techniques.

CIRCUMCISION

The first description of circumcision is found in Egyptian tombs around 3000 BCE. The practice spread from the Egyptians around the eastern Mediterranean, and it has also appeared spontaneously in widely separated geographic areas including the Amazon, central Africa, and Fiji. The practice of circumcision is spotty rather than universal even within those areas, with adjacent tribes in central Africa differing in this custom. The reasons given for circumcision generally are: 1) it is the custom, 2) it confers beauty, and 3) it promotes health. As a custom, neonatal circumcision began to be advocated in the United States in the 1870s and by the mid-20th century had become standard throughout North America. Seventy-five percent to 80% of newborn boys were circumcised as late as the 1980s despite many years of opposition by pediatricians. It is interesting to note that in Britain, with the introduction of the National Health Service in 1948, the doctors no longer received fees per item of service, and the custom of circumcision of babies largely died out. Beauty, of course, is in the eye of the beholder. A circumcised penis, like a pierced ear, is appealing to some and not to others.

Promotion of health has been cited as a reason for circumcision in the United States and recently has received further support by studies showing that boys with circumcised penises have fewer infections than those with uncircumcised penises. Some experts have argued for neonatal circumcision as a preventive measure for balanitis, phimosis, or dyspareunia. In the countries where circumcision is not widespread, these problems are generally treated nonsurgically. Recent epidemiologic studies in the pediatric literature have supported the contention that the presence of the foreskin promotes pyelonephritis in male infants. Statistical and methodological problems with these studies preclude their acceptance as definitive. Even if these conclusions are correct, a positive impact on the cost-benefit ratio for prophylactic circumcision remains to be demonstrated. It should be noted that circumcision does not confer complete protection against urinary tract or other infections. Furthermore, Wettergren showed that the initially high incidence of neonatal urinary and foreskin colonization has declined by 9 months of age. In 1988 Fink published all the available evidence that could possibly support neonatal circumcision, none of which proved that it is better to remove the prepuce rather than merely keep it clean. Only a careful prospective trial would answer the question as to whether rendering the irretractable prepuce retractable under anesthesia in the office would be as effective as removing it in preventing disease and promoting hygiene. As a general rule it seems wise to counsel parents that no proven medical benefit results from routine neonatal circumcision. On the other hand, it is unreasonable to be so dogmatic as to refuse to perform the procedure, remembering that the physician's purpose is to inform rather than argue.

No special care is required by the uncircumcised boy during the first year of life. The normal foreskin is adherent to the glans and gradually separates during the first years of life. The foreskin is nonretractable in 80% of boys at 6 months of age, 50% at 1 year, 20% at 2 years, and 10% at 3 years. In some normal boys, it is not retractable until school age. Forcibly retracting the foreskin is painful to the child and may lead to a true phimosis from traumatic rupture of glans-foreskin adhesions. There are no harmful effects from failure to clean under the foreskin in childhood. By the time a child is old enough to bathe himself, the adhesions usually will have spontaneously separated, and he can be taught normal penile hygiene.

UNDESCENDED TESTIS

The primary care physician's task is to differentiate a retractile testis, which requires no surgical correction, from a truly undescended testis. Retractile testis occurs secondary to the pull of the cremaster muscle on the small prepubertal gonad. Occasionally this distinction is difficult, and in some cases, it can only be made with the patient under general anesthesia. If the testis can be manipulated into a dependent portion of the scrotum without tension on the spermatic cord, it is a retractile testis even though it spends most of its time in the inguinal canal. No harm comes to the gonad. Such testes eventually will reside in the scrotum as the child grows older. Gentle pressure by the fingers on the inguinal region usually will push the testis low enough that it can be grasped by the fingers of the opposite hand and gently drawn into the scrotum. This maneuver requires a relaxed patient and careful manipulation on the part of the examiner. Examining an obese boy in a squatting or "catcher's" position may push the testis down to where it may be grasped and drawn into the scrotum. If it reaches no farther than the pubic bone or upper scrotum or if it cannot be palpated at all, surgical exploration is warranted. If it reaches the scrotum but pops up into the canal as soon as it is released, the testis is undescended and surgery is required.

The cause of testicular maldescent remains unclear. One plausible theory is that decreased local testosterone production produces failure of descent. Mechanical factors have been implicated as well, and the role of the gubernaculum remains to be defined. Maldescent can occur as part of the several syndromes including chromosomal anomalies, endocrine deficiencies, and midline cranial developmental defects. Although undescended gonads are frequent in intersex states, most of these children come to medical attention because of their ambiguous genitalia. One should be aware that a child who appears to be a normal boy but who has no palpable gonads must be assumed to be a girl until proved otherwise, because the adrenogenital syndrome can rarely produce this degree of virilization. A karyotype analysis will clarify this issue. Because approximately one fourth of boys with hypospadias and an undescended testis are found to have an abnormal chromosomal analysis, a karyotype is indicated. Most frequently, a genetic mosaicism is found, requiring only hypospadias repair and orchiopexy. These patients are likely to be sterile.

Treatment of undescended testes by administration of human chronic gonadotropin (HCG) has been popular in Europe, but American urologists have found it unrewarding. Recently, intranasally administered gonadotropin-releasing hormone (GnRH), not yet available in the United

States, has achieved better results. When GnRH is followed by a course of HCG, an overall success rate of 74% has been reported. Such a success rate is seen only with unilateral, prescrotal testes; bilateral and inguinal or abdominal cryptorchid testes fare less well.

Surgical orchidopexy is still the standard treatment of cryptorchidism. Currently, urologists believe that orchidopexy should be carried out by age 2 years because pediatric anesthesia is now quite safe and the results seem to be improved. Histologic changes can be seen as early as 1 to 2 years of age and are progressive. Fertility is poor in the patient subjected to orchidopexy late in childhood. Logic dictates earlier orchidopexy to improve fertility, although no large group has yet been followed-up sufficiently long enough to prove this hypothesis. Orchidopexy can be done on an outpatient basis even when accompanied by intraperitoneal exploration. If both gonads are intra-abdominal, it is wise to stage the procedures.

Approximately 85% of undescended testes will be found in the inguinal canal and are easily placed in the scrotum by one of several standard procedures. Fewer than 5% of testes will be absent, and the remainder will be found within the abdomen along the course of normal descent, usually adjacent to the internal inguinal ring. These testes may require mobilization on a vas-peritoneal pedicle with ligation of the spermatic vessels (Fowler-Stephens orchidopexy). Gonadal survival in these cases is approximately 70%. The role of laparoscopy is still being defined, but it appears to be useful in identifying the 5% of absent testes with minimal morbidity, and laparoscopic techniques may get some intra-abdominal testes into the scrotum without dividing the spermatic vessels, which results in better gonadal survival.

The major considerations in terms of surgical results are fertility and malignant potential. Oligospermia occurs in 20% to 65% of patients after orchidopexy. The highest sperm counts are seen in patients whose orchidopexy was performed prior to age 4 years. No improvement in fertility can be shown to result from orchidopexy at or beyond puberty; therefore, the pubertal undescended testis is usually removed unless it is solitary.

The risk of gonadal malignancy in a cryptorchid testis is approximately 10 times that for a normally descended testis. Malignant potential is greater in the abdominal testis than in the canalicular or ectopic one. Tumors rarely have developed in testes brought down early (under age 4 years), whereas orchidopexy at puberty does not decrease the risk of malignancy, highlighting another reason that undescended testes after puberty should be removed and earlier orchidopexy emphasized. Even at age 10 years, germ cell hyperplasia or carcinoma in situ may be present in 8% of undescended testes.

Most surgeons will follow-up the patient for some months postoperatively to ensure that the testis remains in good position without atrophy. Beyond that, it becomes the burden of primary care physicians to be alert for the development of malignancy, because 10% of germ cell tumors occur in undescended testes. Regular examination of the testis should be carried out after puberty and can be taught to the patient much as self-examination of the breasts is taught to adult women. Any increase in size or change in consistency after completion of pubertal growth warrants referral to a urologist.

MEATAL STENOSIS

Meatal stenosis is a term that is often applied to any urethral meatus that appears to be narrow or pinhole in nature. Such an appearance seems to result from ammoniac and/or mechanical irritation of the exposed meatus in many circumcised boys. The lesion is almost never seen in the uncircumcised patient. An appearance suggesting significant meatal stenosis can often be misleading because the meatus may in fact be quite pliable and can be shown by calibration to be normal. In such cases, the voided stream is completely normal, and the meatal appearance has no functional significance. In boys with functionally significant meatal stenosis, the urinary stream will spray or be deflected, usually dorsally. Such voiding symptoms as frequency and enuresis should not be blamed on meatal stenosis, which should not be regarded as significant obstructive uropathy. Those patients who have a sprayed or deflected urine stream require a meatotomy, which usually can be carried out as an office procedure under local anesthesia. A distinction should be made between this lesion and the meatal stenosis occurring after urethral surgery which, although it is called by the same name, is a result of scarring and can indeed produce significant bladder outlet obstruction.

DYSFUNCTIONAL VOIDING (HINMAN SYNDROME)

Voiding disorders including enuresis, urinary frequency, and diurnal urge incontinence are all related pathophysiologically. At the worst end of the spectrum are a few patients whose disorder includes UTI and upper urinary tract damage. These patients' conditions can progress to end-stage renal disease if not recognized early and managed aggressively. Because bladder dysfunction occurs as a spectrum of disorders, the distinction between true dysfunctional voiding or Hinman syndrome and the more common pediatric uninhibited bladder may initially be difficult.

In infancy, coordinated voiding occurs by reflex; detrusor contraction automatically follows striated external sphincter relaxation, which seems to occur in response to stretch receptor stimulation. Voiding to completion is usual. At the age of toilet training, the child becomes aware of bladder filling and emptying and initially attempts to gain control over a bladder contraction by "holding on" with the striated urethral sphincter. Tightening the sphincter during a bladder contraction raises intravesical pressure, but most children eventually gain the ability to inhibit detrusor contractions by a poorly understood central mechanism that is largely subconscious in nature. During the transition to central control over the bladder, uninhibited detrusor contractions can lead to incontinence either during the day or the night. Attempts to control this wetting by contracting the external sphincter engender the squatting or cross-legged stance that such children exhibit, as well as the sensation of urgency that leads some children to run to the bathroom many times in succession while producing only small amounts of urine. Once central control of the detrusor develops, sustained relaxation of the sphincter during voiding ensues in most cases. In that event, the enuresis or urge incontinence resolves without sequelae. Most of these children do not exhibit abnormalities on radiographs or have significant problems with UTI.

In some instances, for reasons that remain unclear, a transitional pattern persists, and the child fails to relax the external sphincter to initiate voiding. Elevated intravesical pressure during voiding and incomplete bladder emptying results, leading to infection, incontinence, and, in severe cases, hydroureteronephrosis. None of these children has any underlying neurologic or muscular disease, and careful electromyography will demonstrate normal action potentials and conduction velocities in the involved musculature. The role of urodynamic investigation in the care of children with dysfunctional voiding is therefore unclear. The information provided by such investigations usually does not alter the management. The diagnosis may be suspected on the basis of the following historical, physical, and radiographic findings: older child (>7 years), wetting and infection, chronic constipation and encopresis, infrequent voiding and intermittent stream, elevated residual urine volume, increase in anal sphincter tone, trabeculated bladder, and hydronephrosis and reflux. Only the progress of the condition over time will establish the severity of this disorder.

Children with radiographically normal upper urinary tracts may be managed with an anticholinergic, with or without antibiotics; timed voiding; focus on relaxation and sustained stream; relief of chronic constipation; and careful follow-up. Many of these patients ultimately will be shown to have simple, uninhibited bladder or persistent transition-phase voiding. These measures can be applied to patients falling all along the spectrum of voiding dysfunctions up to the point at which upper tract dilation has occurred. Constipation often accompanies these voiding dysfunctions and usually can be resolved with dietary maneuvers that provide more bulk. Follow-up includes urine cultures, and ultrasound or radiographic assessment of bladder emptying and upper urinary tract drainage in patients in whom infections develop or whose conditions fail to improve with this regimen. Any change in the upper tracts dictates referral to a urologist for further treatment. In many cases, clean intermittent self-catheterization has been most successful.

BIBLIOGRAPHY

Bartholomew TH: Neurogenic voiding: Function and dysfunction, *Urol Clin North Am* 12:67–74, 1985.

Fink AJ: *Circumcision: A Parent's decision for life,* Kavanagh, CA, 1988.

Johnston JH, editor: Management of vesicoureteric reflux, vol 10, *International perspectives in urology,* Baltimore, 1984, Williams & Wilkins.

Kaplan GW: Complications of circumcision, *Urol Clin North Am* 10:543, 1983.

Metcalf TJ, Osborn LM, Mariani EM: Circumcision: A study of current practices, *Clin Pediatr* 22:575, 1983.

Proceedings of the 6th International Workshop on Reflux in Children, *J Urol* 148:1639–1760, 1992.

Raifer J, editor: Symposium on cryptorchidism, *Urol Clin North Am* 9:3, 1982.

Snyder HM, Duckett JW: Endoscopic evaluation problems in refluxing orifices, *Dialogues Pediatr Urol* 6:12, 1983.

Walther PC, Kaplan GW: Cystoscopy in children: Indications for its use in common urologic problems, *J Urol* 122:717, 1979.

Wettergren B, Jodal U, Jonasson G: Epidemiology of bacteriuria during the first year of life, *Acta Pediatr Scand* 74:925, 1985.

Wiswell TE, Roscelli JD: Corroborative evidence for the decreased incidence of urinary tract infections in circumcised male infants, *Pediatrics* 78:96, 1986.

Wiswell TE, Cohen ML, Ozere L, *et al.:* Corroborative evidence for the decreased incidence of urinary tract infections in circumcised male infants (letters to the editor), *Pediatrics* 78:951, 1986; 79:649, 1986; 80:303, 763, 1987.

PART EIGHT

Hematology

CHAPTER 84

Common Problems in Hematology

Steven E. McKenzie

The primary care physician will often be the first to see and evaluate patients with hematologic conditions, ranging from mild anemias to easy bruisability to neutropenia. The purpose of this section is to provide a framework for evaluating common office problems and for identification of those patients that might benefit from the advice of a pediatric hematologist. The primary care physician may also choose to share in the long-term care of children with known hematologic disorders. This section will cover some common issues for these children that arise during primary care.

The conditions that primary care physicians may face include: 1) neutropenia, 2) possible bleeding disorders, 3) leukocytosis, 4) questions about inheritance patterns and screening tests, and 5) managing infection in the asplenic child.

NEUTROPENIA

The definition of neutropenia, the most common white blood cell (WBC) abnormality a primary care physician will encounter, depends on the age and ethnic origin of the patient. In patients greater than 1 year of age, the lower limit of normal for the neutrophil count is 1500/mm³. (The absolute neutrophil count is the percentage of band forms plus mature segmented neutrophils times the total WBC count.) Infants will normally have greater than 2500 neutrophils/mm³. Up to 30% of black infants may have neutrophil counts between 500 and 1500/mm³ without adverse consequences. The concern with neutropenia is the risk of life-threatening infection. Although the risk of infection depends on the specific cause of the neutropenia, in general, only severe neutropenia (<500/mm³) that lasts for more than several days confers a substantial risk of life-threatening infection.

Differential Diagnosis

Common Causes of Neutropenia
Congenital
- Benign chronic neutropenia
- Cyclic neutropenia
- Severe congenital neutropenia (Kostmann syndrome)
- Reticular dysgenesis
- Decreased marrow storage pool

Malignant
- Leukemia, lymphoma, solid tumor (*eg*, neuroblastoma)

Toxic
- Drugs
- Radiation

- Heavy metals
- Organic compounds

Infectious
- Viral
- Bacterial
- Rickettsial

Idiopathic
- Aplastic anemia

Immune
- Isoimmune neonatal neutropenia
- Autoimmune neutropenia
- Drug-induced neutropenia
- Complement-mediated
- Collagen-vascular disease

Miscellaneous syndromes
- Shwachman-Diamond (neutropenia and exocrine pancreatic insufficiency)
- Fanconi's anemia
- Chediak-Higashi

In an ill-appearing neutropenic child with a fever or history of fever, prompt evaluation is needed. The hemoglobin level, platelet count, and other elements of the blood smear must be carefully assessed. Even if these elements are normal, diagnosis and treatment may depend on a bone marrow examination coupled with expeditious consultation with the hematologist. In a child with a history of good health without frequent infections, isolated neutropenia is rarely a major problem. Furthermore, rarely is neutropenia found to be the culprit in a child with recurrent infection.

In a healthy child, neutropenia will usually be discovered because a concurrent viral syndrome or focal bacterial infection such as otitis media has led to a complete blood cell (CBC) count. Occasionally neutropenia is discovered when a routine CBC count has been done. This condition is most often a transient neutropenia, associated with either viral infection itself (as in varicella, rubella, influenza, mononucleosis, and hepatitis) or with frequently prescribed antibiotics (such as penicillins, cephalosporins, and sulfa agents). All drugs that can be safely stopped should be stopped, and serial neutrophil counts obtained at least weekly. In 3 to 6 weeks, a normal count should return.

Neutropenia in the newborn may be associated with serious underlying infection, such as bacterial sepsis, meningitis, or congenital viral infection with an agent like cytomegalovirus. Transient neutropenia has been reported with maternal hypertension and birth asphyxia and in preterm infants in association with copper deficiency. After these causes, congenital or familial neutropenia should be considered.

The patient with congenital neutropenia will benefit from evaluation by a pediatric hematologist. The current prognosis in these individuals ranges from excellent (isoimmune neonatal neutropenia and benign chronic neutropenia) to good with supportive care (cyclic neutropenia) to grim (Kostmann syndrome and reticular dysgenesis). For severe congenital neutropenia, including Kostmann syndrome, and cyclic neutropenia associated with infections, daily subcutaneous injections of granulocyte colony-stimulating factor (G-CSF) have been shown to be effective in increasing the neutrophil count and preventing serious infection.

Screening Tests

Evaluation of a neutropenic patient begins with a thorough history including recent viral illnesses, drug exposures, and family history. One reassuring, useful, and inexpensive step is to check the results of any prior CBC counts the child had. The physical examination starts by considering if this is a well child: is he/she growing well, is he/she febrile? In performing the physical examination, extra attention should be devoted to the skin and mucosal surfaces, especially the mouth, and the lymph nodes, liver, and spleen. The primary laboratory test is the CBC count with differential and platelet count. The blood smear should be examined carefully for several reasons. Sometimes the neutrophils clump together and are missed, giving a falsely low neutrophil count. Bizarre neutrophil appearances may provide a clue to a specific syndrome. Finally, even with relatively normal hemoglobin and platelet counts, leukemic blasts might be seen. The diagnosis of leukemia is rarely made when neutropenia is present alone.

Because most primary care physicians will see transient neutropenia in a healthy child, serial CBC counts twice weekly at first and then weekly for 6 to 8 weeks will establish the pattern. If the neutrophil count returns to and remains normal, no further tests are needed. If drug exposure is implicated and there are adequate alternatives, that drug should be avoided in the future.

Anticipated Complications

Neutropenic patients commonly have infections of the skin, oral mucosa, nasopharynx, gingiva, and perianal areas. Often the classic signs of inflammation are diminished or absent. More severe infections include pneumonia; sepsis; meningitis; and septic arthritis caused by *Staphylococcus* species, the gram-negative enteric organisms, especially *Escherichia coli* and *Pseudomonas,* and fungi, especially *Candida* species. These infections may present without fever but with mild redness, tenderness, or fluctuance or they may present with fever only in an ill-appearing child.

Primary Care Treatments

Regardless of the cause of neutropenia, infection must be approached carefully. The use of prophylactic oral antibiotics has not been established. There is no role for prophylactic granulocyte transfusions. The afebrile child with focal infection, such as otitis or pharyngitis, should be treated with broad-spectrum oral antibiotics with mandatory close follow-up for resolution. The febrile, neutropenic child should be admitted to the hospital for at least 48 to 72 hours of broad-spectrum intravenous antibiotics pending clinical resolution and negative results on cultures. At the Children's Hospital of Philadelphia we use an antistaphylococcal penicillin, an antipseudomonal cephalosporin, and an aminoglycoside. Cultures of blood, throat, urine, and any lesion sites for bacteria and fungus are needed. If a positive result on a culture is found, specific intravenous antibiotic therapy continues for an acceptable duration, for example, 7 days after the first negative result on a blood culture in a clinically improved child who had bacteremia. These guidelines are essential to the care of children with a known neutropenic disorder. As mentioned previously, G-CSF is useful for children with severe congenital neutropenia. The effective dose varies among affected children, with a range from 2.5 to 30 µg/kg/day. During viral and bacterial infections, the neutrophil count for these children may fall below 500/mm^3 despite the G-CSF therapy, and the dose may need to be increased temporarily. A generally well child with a viral syndrome or on oral antibiotics for otitis media can be watched closely, with serial physical examinations and CBC counts as outlined previously.

Indications for Referral or Consultation

Congenital neutropenia, persistent or cyclic neutropenia, severe infection at the time of neutropenia, other cell lines affected, or phenotypic abnormalities of the child or his/her neutrophils are indications for referral or consultation. If a self-limited process is not evident, further evaluation begins with a bone marrow aspirate and biopsy coupled with serologic and culture screening for infection. Further useful tests include a Coombs' test, serum folate levels, and serum B$_{12}$ levels. CBC counts in other family members are sometimes revealing. To make a specific diagnosis and prognosis, the hematologist might also consider the antineutrophil antibody assay, antinuclear antibody assay, quantitative immunoglobulins, in vitro neutrophil colony forming assays, a hydrocortisone stimulation test, or tests of exocrine pancreas function, which are abnormal in Shwachman-Diamond syndrome.

POSSIBLE BLEEDING DISORDERS

The question of a bleeding disorder usually arises because of frequent nosebleeds, easy bruising, excessive bleeding after minor trauma, or before elective surgery. The approach to the child with acute onset of clinical bruising and/or bleeding is covered elsewhere in an earlier section. Briefly, those children will be ill and will have one or more abnormalities of the platelet count, prothrombin time (PT), or partial thromboplastin time (PTT). Important diagnostic categories include idiopathic thrombocytopenic purpura, leukemia, and disseminated intravascular coagulation. Likewise, the presentation of the common hemophilias (factor VIII and factor IX deficiency) is discussed in an earlier section. There the predominance of affected men and manifestations that may include bleeding with circumcision and into deep muscles and joints are distinctive.

The differential diagnosis of possible bleeding disorders in a generally well child is listed below, by area of the circulation primarily involved. Severe bleeding under stressful circumstances can certainly occur in these conditions.

Differential Diagnosis

Common Causes of Bleeding Disorders
Plasma
- von Willebrand disease
- Acquired inhibitors of coagulation
- Drug use (coumarins, heparin notably in flush solutions)

- Other factor deficiencies

Platelets (qualitative or functional abnormalities)

- Drug use (aspirin, indomethacin, nonsteroidal agents, occasionally penicillins)
- Storage pool disease
- Glanzmann thrombasthenia
- Other platelet defects

Vascular

- Vasculitis (with or without systemic collagen vascular disease)
- Ehlers-Danlos syndrome
- Other connective tissue abnormalities (*eg,* scurvy)

Screening Tests

A good personal and family history helps screen for the possibility of a bleeding disorder. Scoring systems and forms that incorporate the major historical questions have been devised. A list of relevant questions includes the following:

1. Does anyone in the family have a known bleeding disorder?
2. What skin manifestations of bleeding does the patient have: petechiae, spontaneous bruising, easy traumatic bruising, or prolonged (>1 hour) bleeding from lacerations?
3. Does the patient have nosebleeds lasting more than 30 minutes? Has he/she ever sought emergency care for these or required packing?
4. Is there mouth bleeding: spontaneous, with tooth brushing, after minor trauma, after loss of baby teeth, or after dental work?
5. Is there any deep muscle bruising, spontaneous or with immunization injections?
6. Is there joint bleeding, spontaneous or with minor injury?
7. What operations has the patient had, and was there excessive bleeding or need for transfusion (include circumcision, tonsilectomy, tooth extraction)?
8. Is there excessive vaginal bleeding, with menses, between menses, during pregnancy, or with childbirth?
9. Was there excessive bleeding or delayed separation (after 18 days) with the umbilical cord?
10. Is there any hemoptysis, hematemesis, melena, or hematuria without an identified anatomic abnormality?

A positive family history has one or more relatives (including parents, siblings, grandparents, aunts, uncles, and first cousins) with the same bleeding manifestations sought in the personal history. An epistaxis scoring system has recently been proposed and tested to identify which children with nosebleeds will benefit from further laboratory tests.

An algorithm for evaluating a possible bleeding disorder is presented in Figure 84-1. All individuals with a suspected bleeding disorder should have a CBC count with differential and platelet count, a PT, and a PTT. Screening for disseminated intravascular coagulation is not necessary in an essentially well child. If the CBC count, PT, and/or PTT are reproducibly abnormal, the advice of a hematologist should be sought. If the CBC count, PT, and PTT are normal and the personal and family histories are not highly suspicious, no further testing is needed, with the exception of before major surgery. If the CBC count, PT, and PTT are normal but the personal or family history is highly suspicious or major surgery is planned, a bleeding time test should be done. Other tests, such as clotting time, do not add to the evaluation.

The bleeding time test examines how long it takes a stable clot to form at the site of a small puncture or linear wound. It is done usually on the undersurface of the forearm with a blood pressure cuff inflated to 40 mm Hg on the upper arm, and it may leave a small scar. The result of the test depends on the skill of the technician. Therefore the test is best done by experienced personnel. Normal ranges are established by the specific method and the testing laboratory. To have a normal bleeding time means that virtually all aspects of clotting are functional: plasma factors important to platelet adhesion and aggregation, platelet function, and vascular integrity. This feature makes the bleeding time a quite sensitive, though not specific, test. More importantly, the chances of significant bleeding with a properly performed normal bleeding time are very small.

The evaluation of a prolonged bleeding time begins by ruling out recent drug ingestion. As little as 80 mg of aspirin within as many as 7 days of the test may prolong the bleeding time. Many over-the-counter medications include aspirin. The test should be repeated when no medications have been ingested for a week. If no medications are implicated in a prolonged bleeding time, the hematologist will perform further testing directed initially at detecting von Willebrand disease or a platelet function abnormality.

von Willebrand disease is the most common identifiable disease with a prolonged bleeding

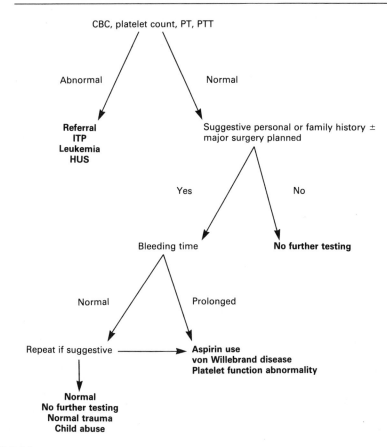

ALGORITHM FOR EVALUATING POSSIBLE BLEEDING DISORDERS

Personal and family history obtained first
Normal physical examination

CBC, platelet count, PT, PTT

Abnormal

Normal

Referral
ITP
Leukemia
HUS

Suggestive personal or family history ±
major surgery planned

Yes

No

Bleeding time

No further testing

Normal

Prolonged

Repeat if suggestive ⟶ **Aspirin use**
von Willebrand disease
Platelet function abnormality

Normal
No further testing
Normal trauma
Child abuse

FIG 84-1

Decision tree for differential diagnosis of possible bleeding disorders.

time. Its incidence is probably close to that of hemophilia A (approximately one in 10,000 individuals in the general population), but its variable clinical manifestations have made precise calculations difficult. Men and women are affected equally. The defect is in the plasma factors needed for platelet adhesion to damaged endothelial surfaces and for platelet aggregation. These factors circulate with the factor VIII molecular complex. They are distinct molecules from the portion that is deficient in hemophilia A. As a result, in von Willebrand disease, the PTT is most often normal. There are several subtypes of von Willebrand disease, which vary in genetics and severity. The predominant subtype, type I, has autosomal dominant inheritance and mild-to-moderate severity. Patients may have mucosal and gastrointestinal bleeding, nosebleeds, bleeding after surgery and dental extractions, and menorrhagia in women. Other less common subtypes have autosomal recessive or dominant inheritance and may be more severe, with similar bleeding as type I but also bleeding into muscles and joints. The diagnosis of von Willebrand disease is made by measuring factor VIII coagulant activity, factor VIII antigen levels, and ristocetin cofactor activity. In the most common type of von Willebrand disease, these are low. The von Willebrand multimer distribution identifies other subtypes. These levels vary over time in the same individual, because some behave as so-called acute phase reactants. Hence when the

TABLE 84-1
Normal Leukocyte Counts*

	TOTAL LEUKOCYTES		NEUTROPHILS			LYMPHOCYTES			MONOCYTES		EOSINOPHILS	
AGE	MEAN	RANGE	MEAN	RANGE	%	MEAN	RANGE	%	MEAN	%	MEAN	%
Birth	18.1	9.0–30.0	11.0	6.0–26.0	61	5.5	2.0–11.0	31	1.1	6	0.4	2
12 hr	22.8	13.0–38.0	15.5	6.0–28.0	68	5.5	2.0–11.0	24	1.2	5	0.5	2
24 hr	18.9	9.4–34.0	11.5	5.0–21.0	61	5.8	2.0–11.5	31	1.1	6	0.5	2
1 wk	12.2	5.0–21.0	5.5	1.5–10.0	45	5.0	2.0–17.0	41	1.1	9	0.5	4
2 wk	11.4	5.0–20.0	4.5	1.0–9.5	40	5.5	2.0–17.0	48	1.0	9	0.4	3
1 mo	10.8	5.0–19.5	3.8	1.0–9.0	35	6.0	2.5–16.5	56	0.7	7	0.3	3
6 mo	11.9	6.0–17.5	3.8	1.0–8.5	32	7.3	4.0–13.5	61	0.6	5	0.3	3
1 yr	11.4	6.0–17.5	3.5	1.5–8.5	31	7.0	4.0–10.5	61	0.6	5	0.3	3
2 yr	10.6	6.0–17.0	3.5	1.5–8.5	33	6.3	3.0–9.5	59	0.5	5	0.3	3
4 yr	9.1	5.5–15.5	3.8	1.5–8.5	42	4.5	2.0–8.0	50	0.5	5	0.3	3
6 yr	8.5	5.0–14.5	4.3	1.5–8.0	51	3.5	1.5–7.0	42	0.4	5	0.2	3
8 yr	8.3	4.5–13.5	4.4	1.5–8.0	53	3.3	1.5–6.8	39	0.4	4	0.2	2
10 yr	8.1	4.5–13.5	4.4	1.8–8.0	54	3.1	1.5–6.5	38	0.4	4	0.2	2
16 yr	7.8	4.5–13.0	4.4	1.8–8.0	57	2.8	1.2–5.2	35	0.4	5	0.2	3
21 yr	7.4	4.5–11.0	4.4	1.8–7.7	59	2.5	1.0–4.8	34	0.3	4	0.2	3

*Numbers of leukocytes are in thousands per mm^3, ranges are estimates of 95% confidence limits, and percentages refer to differential counts. Neutrophils include band cells at all ages and a small number of metamyelocytes and myelocytes in the first few days of life. (From Dallman PR: In Rudolph AM, editor: *Pediatrics,* ed 16, New York, 1977, Appleton-Century-Crofts, p 1178. Used by permission.)

clinical or family history is suspicious, repeat testing is needed. Testing the bleeding time in other family members can be helpful.

Anticipated Complications

The problems with the various bleeding disorders include spontaneous bleeding and bleeding during procedures and trauma. Should inexplicable significant bleeding occur with a procedure or trauma, consultation with a hematologist is recommended. There are cogent reasons for this recommendation. First, advances have made the use of blood products unnecessary in some bleeding disorders. For instance, the drug epsilon-aminocaproic acid (Amicar) can be of great use in oral bleeding and DDAVP (1-deamino-8-D-arginine vasopressin) in type I von Willebrand disease. There are major limitations to the use of DDAVP that make initial use by the primary care physician inadvisable. The recent availability of intranasal DDAVP of appropriate strength and formulation for patients with von Willebrand disease and mild factor VIII deficiency provides a convenient way to treat bleeding episodes and to provide prophylaxis for minor procedures, once the hematologist has approved this therapy for a particular patient. Second, the choice of the optimal blood product requires either a specific diagnosis or recognition of a pattern of clinical bleeding.

Primary Care Treatments

In those patients with an identified bleeding disorder, treatment can be provided by primary care physicians in concert with a hematologist. Topical care is indicated for superficial bleeding, such as packing or cautery for nosebleeds in conjunction with the otolaryngologist. Finally, appropriate family counseling and avoidance of high-risk situations can be offered to those families with heritable bleeding disorders.

Indications for Referral or Consultation

The algorithm serves as a guide for referral based on an office evaluation. In general, treatment decisions for bleeding patients benefit from the advice of a hematologist.

LEUKOCYTOSIS

The primary care physician may find an elevated WBC count during routine screening, a febrile episode, or the newborn period. The elevation may be exaggerated in one specific element, hence the concern will be neutrophilia, lymphocytosis or atypical lymphocytosis, monocytosis, or eosinophilia. The definition of leukocytosis requires knowledge of the upper limits of normal, which depend on the patient's age (Table 84-1).

TABLE 84-2
Differential Diagnosis of Leukocytosis

ETIOLOGY	NEUTROPHILIA	LYMPHOCYTOSIS	MONOCYTOSIS	EOSINOPHILIA
Infection				
Bacteria	x	x(A)		x(D)
Virus		x(B)	x	x(E)
Parasite				x(F)
Mycobacteria	x	x	x	
Other		x(C)		
Systemic illness				
Allergy/asthma				x
Atopic skin disease				x
Collagen vascular			x	
Ulcerative colitis			x	
Hyperthyroidism		x		
Drug reaction				
Steroid	x			
Antibiotic				x
Idiosyncratic				x
Postsplenectomy	x		x	
Malignancy				
Hodgkin disease			x	x
Leukemia	x	x		x
Leukemoid reaction	x			
Down syndrome	x			
Congenital syndromes				
Lofflers				x

A = pertussis, parapertussis; B = Epstein-Barr virus, cytomegalovirus, many others; C = toxoplasmosis; D = scarlet fever; E = *Chlamydia*; F = helminths.

Once true leukocytosis is identified, an orderly evaluation can proceed.

Screening Tests

The history and physical examination are paramount to this workup, because the broad range of diagnoses precludes testing all possibilities. Infection of all types, drug reactions, and systemic diseases outnumbers hematologic entities. Table 84-2 summarizes the differential diagnosis of each type of elevated WBC count, noting some shared and some distinct causes.

The primary distinguishing features of leukemia and leukemoid reactions are the appearance of the cells and the presence or absence of changes in other cell lines. Increased leukocyte alkaline phosphatase has been reported as a marker for the leukemoid reaction. However, definitive distinction may require bone marrow aspirate and biopsy. This is particularly true for children with Down syndrome in whom the risks of leukemoid reactions and leukemia are greatly increased over the general population.

Anticipated Complications and Primary Care Treatments

The breadth of diagnoses precludes any generalizations here, except that treatment of the underlying disorder is the most appropriate approach. Individual references are devoted to specific abnormalities, such as eosinophilia.

Indications for Referral or Consultation

Those causes of leukocytosis beyond identifiable infection, drug reaction, or systemic illness may benefit from the advice of a hematologist.

QUESTIONS ABOUT INHERITANCE PATTERNS AND SCREENING TESTS

The primary care physician may be asked about inherited hematologic disorders. Prospective parents may inquire before pregnancy or during pregnancy, or their questions may arise in the newborn period. An important related question is the availability of prenatal and newborn

TABLE 84-3
Hematologic Disorders: Inheritance Patterns and Screening Tests

DISORDER	POPULATION	DISEASE FREQUENCY	INHERITANCE	SCREENING
Red blood cell				
Sickle cell anemia	A	1 in 600 (blacks)	Autosomal recessive	Newborn (a), prenatal
Thalassemia				
alpha	A⁺	b	Autosomal recessive	Newborn, prenatal
beta	A	1 in 20,000 (c)	Autosomal recessive	Newborn, prenatal
Glucose-6-phosphate dehydrogenase deficiency	A⁺	1 in 5000	X-linked recessive	Newborn
Hereditary spherocytosis	White primarily	1 in 5000	Autosomal dominant (some recessive)	Newborn
Coagulation factor				
VIII (hemophilia A)	All	1 in 10,000–12,000	X-linked recessive	Newborn, prenatal
IX (hemophilia B)	All	1 in 40,000–50,000	X-linked recessive	Newborn, prenatal
von Willebrand disease	All	Unknown (of order 1 in 10,000)	Autosomal dominant (>90%)	Newborn

A = the "malaria belt" populations: Africa, Mediterranean, Middle East, Indian subcontinent, and Southeast Asia; A⁺ = genotypes differ in black and oriental forms with significant consequences; a = this screening is strongly encouraged and legally mandated in increasing numbers of states; b = because there are two genes for alpha globin on each chromosome 16, the inheritance is complex; however, 3% of the American black population lacks two of the four genes and has microcytosis and mild anemia, absence of four genes causes hydrops fetalis and is lethal; c = the incidence varies widely with ethnic group and location, up to one in 10 in some Greek and Oriental locales.

screening for these disorders. In obtaining the family history, the presence of the disorder or trait for that disorder if such exists can be sought in parents, siblings, and other relatives. This reason may well be why inheritance information is sought, although public education has progressed to the point that members of certain ethnic groups are aware of risks for common genetic diseases.

Table 84-3 lists the common red blood cell (RBC) and coagulation factor inherited disorders, the most likely populations at risk, their inheritance and frequency, and the availability of prenatal and newborn screening. Although high-risk populations are defined, these disorders are not limited exclusively to the populations listed. For example, β-thalassemia has been identified in virtually every known ethnic group. WBC and platelet inherited disorders are uncommon enough that interested primary care physicians are referred to primary hematology sources. This information is not provided to act as replacement for formal genetic counseling, an essential service to families at risk that works best when

primary care physicians, hematologists, obstetricians, and human geneticists work together. Rather, the intent is to indicate to the practitioner how disorders are inherited and for which disorders screening can and should be done.

Screening Tests, Anticipated Complications, and Primary Care Treatments

The value of newborn screening for sickle cell disease has been amply demonstrated—it saves lives. The risk of death from sepsis is high, up to 5% of unidentified patients. The risk is greatly decreased by enrollment before the age of 4 months at the sickle cell center with its use of prophylactic antibiotics, immunization, and probably most importantly education about the illness and febrile episodes. Many states have made newborn screening for sickle cell disease mandatory; hopefully, other states will follow. These tests have the additional benefit of identifying essentially all clinically relevant inherited hemoglobin disorders. Electrophoresis with agar gel at an acid pH (6.0) is the method of choice at

Children's Hospital of Philadelphia because of the ability to distinguish abundant fetal hemoglobin from normal and sickle hemoglobin. The test can be performed with 1 mL of anticoagulated blood (purple top tube).

Indications for Referral or Consultation

Any individual whose family history places them at risk for an inherited hematologic disorder may benefit from consultation with a hematologist. All individuals found through screening to have a RBC or coagulation factor inherited disorder will need referral to a hematologist. For the much larger numbers of individuals who are identified with traits for these disorders, ie, heterozygotes for recessive disorders, appropriate counseling can be coordinated by the primary care physician with input as needed by the hematologist and geneticist.

THE ASPLENIC CHILD

The primary care physician may encounter a child who is without spleen function for one of three reasons: the spleen was removed surgically, the spleen is in place but not working, or the child was born without a spleen. The most common reasons for surgical removal include traumatic rupture and certain hematologic processes. This latter group includes splenectomy for idiopathic thrombocytopenic purpura, hereditary spherocytosis, homozygous β-thalassemia, and Hodgkin disease. Functional asplenia occurs in sickle cell disease, after splenic radiation, and with immunodeficiencies. Syndromes with congenital absence of the spleen exist but are very rare.

The danger with reduced or absent splenic function is overwhelming bacterial infection. The spleen serves as a principal filter for bacteria that reach the blood and as a site of antibody synthesis. The risk of fulminant sepsis depends on the cause of diminished function and the age of the child, but the relative risk of death from sudden onset of sepsis ranges from 50 to 1000 times that of the general population. Before the age of 5 years, the risk appears to be the highest, regardless of the cause. Much of our current knowledge about treating asplenic children comes from the natural history after surgical removal and the efforts of the

National Collaborative Study of Sickle Cell Disease.

Screening Tests

In almost all cases the functional or anatomic asplenia of the individual is known. Specialized tests can often identify individuals with impaired spleen function, including the search for Howell-Jolly bodies on the peripheral blood smear and microscopic examination with Nomarsky optics for pitted RBCs.

Anticipated Complications and Primary Care Treatments

Sepsis in the asplenic individual is characterized by the rapid onset of fever and malaise followed by deterioration that can be fatal in hours. The encapsulated organisms are the major offenders, with pneumococcus as the most common offender. Other major pathogens include *Haemophilus influenzae* b and meningococcus. The febrile asplenic child is an emergency case, and evaluation and treatment must be prompt, regardless of oral antibiotic prophylaxis or immunization status. When the temperature exceeds 38.5° C, a careful examination, CBC count, and cultures of the blood, urine, and throat should be followed-up with intravenous antibiotics effective against the likely organisms. There is no need to wait for any test results before treating; in fact, this would be dangerous. Intravenous antibiotics should continue for 48 to 72 hours until the culture results are negative and the patient is improved. Viral syndromes will occur in these children, but all fevers must be evaluated and those above 38.5° C treated as noted previously. Fever of 38.0° to 38.4° C warrants increased oral antibiotic prophylaxis to four times a day for 5 to 7 days and close observation. However, if the child is ill-appearing, intravenous antibiotics are indicated.

Elective splenectomy should be deferred until the age of 5 years or above. It should be preceded by immunization against pneumococcus and *H. influenzae* b. Because the potential benefits outweigh the minor risks, lifelong penicillin prophylaxis is recommended. A program of immunization and penicillin prophylaxis is standard care for the sickle cell patient. If in an emergency the spleen is removed without vaccination against pneumococcus, the vaccination should be given as soon as possible after splenectomy.

BIBLIOGRAPHY

Dickerman JD: Splenectomy and sepsis: A warning, *Pediatrics* 63:938–941, 1979.

Gaston MH, *et al.:* Prophylaxis with oral penicillin in children with sickle cell anemia, *N Engl J Med* 314:1593–1599, 1986.

Katsanis E, Luke KH, Hsu E, Li M, Lillicrap D: Prevalence and significance of mild bleeding disorders in children with recurrent epistaxis, *J Pediatr* 113:73–76, 1988.

Lukens JN: Eosinophilia in children. *Pediatr Clin North Am* 19:969–981, 1972.

Manroe BL, Weinberg AG, Rosenfeld CR, Browne R: The neonatal blood count in health and disease. I. Reference values for neutrophilic cells, *J Pediatr* 95:89–98, 1979.

Montgomery RR, Scott JP: Hemostasis: Diseases of the fluid phase. In Nathan DG, Oski FA, editors: *Hematology of infancy and childhood,* ed 4, Philadelphia, 1993, WB Saunders.

Petersdorf SH, Dale DC: The biology and clinical applications of erythropoietin and the colony-stimulating factors. *Adv Intern Med* 40:395–428, 1995.

Stockman JA, Ezekowitz RAB: Hematologic manifestations of systemic diseases. In Nathan DG, Oski FA, editors: *Hematology of infancy and childhood,* ed 4, Philadelphia, 1993, WB Saunders.

Vichinsky E, Hurst D, Earles A, *et al.:* Newborn screening for sickle cell disease: Effect on mortality, *Pediatrics* 81:749–755, 1988.

Weetman RM, Boxer LA: Childhood neutropenia. *Pediatr Clin North Am* 27:361–375, 1980.

Zarkowsky HS, Gallagher D, Gill F, et al: Bacteremia in sickle hemoglobinopathies, *J Pediatr* 109:579–585, 1986.

CHAPTER 85

Anemia

Mortimer Poncz

The differential diagnosis of anemia in children has already been described under "Pallor" in Chapter 55. In this chapter, four common causes of anemia in childhood are discussed in detail: iron deficiency anemia, the thalassemias, hereditary spherocytosis, and glucose-6-phosphate dehydrogenase (G-6-PD) deficiency. Sickle cell anemia is discussed in the Chapter 88.

IRON DEFICIENCY ANEMIA

Background

Prevalence and Etiology

The most common cause of childhood anemia is iron deficiency. Historically in the United States, approximately 3% of white children and 15% of black children 1 year of age have iron deficiency anemia, whereas another 20% are iron deficient but without anemia. Two major factors account for the high rate of anemia due to iron deficiency in childhood: the rapid increase in body size (and blood volume) and the relative insufficiency of iron in the diet. The two periods of greatest body growth are the first 2 years of life, in which a child more than triples his/her birth weight, and the adolescent years; both periods are also associated with poor dietary iron intake. In infancy, if the formula is not iron-fortified or if whole cow's milk is introduced too early, total dietary iron intake may be inadequate. Poor iron intake may again occur in adolescence because of erratic eating habits or fads that do not include a food source rich in iron.

Blood loss during these two time periods can further stress the limited iron reserve and lead to iron deficiency anemia. For example, a term infant who had significant perinatal blood loss due to transplacental bleeding will be more likely to develop iron deficiency anemia and should receive earlier iron supplementation than a child without a similar perinatal history. After menarche, the adolescent girl will have a greater risk of developing iron deficiency and should receive adequate iron supplementation to her diet. The development of iron deficiency in a child whose age is outside the two major risk ages should lead to a vigorous search for a source of blood loss as body growth is slow, and the diet should be sufficiently varied to contain adequate sources of iron. The blood loss often occurs from an obvious source such as menorrhagia or recurrent epistaxis or rectal bleeding as might be seen in a child with Meckel diverticulum or polyp.

Data Gathering

Most commonly, iron deficiency anemia is diagnosed either from a routine complete blood cell (CBC) count or from a patient's pale appearance. Iron deficiency may result in neurologic dysfunction with increased irritability, shorter attention span, and poor scholastic performance. Well-controlled clinical studies have shown behavioral and scholastic improvements when iron-deficient children are appropriately treated. Whether transient iron deficiency can result in permanent long-term neurologic impairment is unknown.

Other unusual manifestations of iron deficiency include the presence of pica, a persistent or purposeful ingestion of material with no nutritive value. Often the pica disappears with adequate iron replacement. It is presently uncertain whether severely iron-deficient children have an increased incidence of infections reflecting a decrease in the bactericidal activity of polymorphonuclear cells in iron deficiency.

Results of physical examination are often normal although signs of pallor may be present. The child may be irritable and restless, although often this aspect of the child's iron deficiency is only noticed in retrospect after treatment. Physical examination rarely reveals tachycardia and congestive heart failure, because the anemia develops slowly, allowing sufficient time for compensation. Examination of the hands in severe iron deficiency may reveal spooning of the nails (koilonychia). In children with iron deficiency, atrophic glossitis is not seen.

Iron deficiency anemia is a microcytic hypochromic anemia with a low reticulocyte count (Fig. 85-1). The most sensitive and reliable way of confirming the diagnosis of iron deficiency anemia is by measuring the serum ferritin level. An elevated free erythrocyte protoporphyrin (FEP) level can be rapidly detected on 20 μL of blood. Although the test is sensitive and rapid, it is not specific for iron deficiency because the FEP may be elevated in the case of lead poisoning.

Management

In a child with a history and physical examination consistent with iron deficiency anemia and in whom laboratory data reveal a hypochromic microcytic anemia and low serum ferritin level, it is proper to administer a trial of iron supplementation and observe the patient carefully for a therapeutic response under the assumption that the patient has iron deficiency anemia.

Because treatment can be accomplished by the oral supplementation of iron, blood transfusion or intramuscular iron-dextran can be avoided in virtually all cases. The most common iron salt used is ferrous sulfate that is 15% by weight elemental iron. In treating iron deficiency anemia, 6 mg/kg/day of elemental iron should be given, divided into three doses. Larger doses will have increased side effects (mainly constipation) without improved speed of therapeutic recovery. Changes in behavior often are noted by the second day of treatment. At the end of 1 week of therapy, a reticulocytosis occurs that is followed by a rise in the hematocrit level of approximately

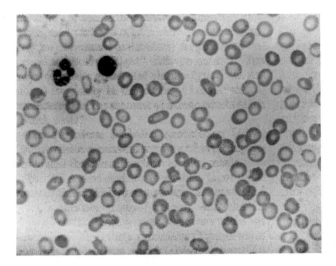

FIG 85-1
A blood smear from a patient with iron deficiency anemia that shows microcytic hypochromic cells with some misshapen red cell forms.

1% per day. A normal hematocrit value for age is achieved during the first month of treatment. Full-dose iron supplementation should be continued for a total of 2 months to ensure adequate iron stores. In addition, therapy should include appropriate dietary counseling and analysis for potential sources of iron loss to avoid a recurrence of the iron deficiency.

Failure to respond to oral iron supplementation is often due to poor compliance or inadequate dosage. This condition often can be verified by finding that the child's stools are not black (as would occur if the iron was properly administered). If on-going blood loss is present, the child may only partly respond to the iron treatment. The presence of a concurrent chronic illness also may interfere with the body's ability to respond to the iron supplementation. Rarely, impaired gastrointestinal absorption may underlie a poor response. Finally, the diagnosis of iron deficiency anemia may have been incorrect. Often children with thalassemia trait are misdiagnosed as having iron deficiency anemia and receive prolonged courses of unnecessary iron therapy. Any child treated for iron deficiency based on a CBC count and an elevated level of FEP should be followed-up to ensure that there is an appropriate response. If there is not an adequate response, part of a further evaluation should be a more extensive evaluation of the child's iron status, including determination of a serum iron level and iron-binding capacity.

THALASSEMIA

Background
Hemoglobin is a tetramer of 2 α-like and 2 β-like globin chains, each of which is bound to a heme moiety. Thalassemia refers to a decreased production of a globin chain (eg, β-thalassemia refers to an underproduction of β-globin chains and α-thalassemia refers to an underproduction of α-globin chains).

The incidence of both α-thalassemia and β-thalassemia are highest in ethnic groups originating from the world's malarial belt. This includes people from the Mediterranean region, Africa, the Near East, India, and Southeast Asia. In some groups, the incidence of the thalassemias can be surprisingly high. In blacks, the α-thalassemia gene can be found in 30% of the population; whereas in Cypriots, the incidence of the β-thalassemia gene is approximately 10%.

Data Gathering
Depending on the exact thalassemia syndrome inherited, the hematologic consequence can vary from an inapparent carrier state, to a mild hypochromic microcytic anemia, to a severe life-threatening anemia, and even to hydrops fetalis and stillbirth. The following discussion will first describe the β-thalassemias and then the α-thalassemias, the two most common thalassemia syndromes. Their pattern of inheritance, clinical manifestations, ethnic groups affected,

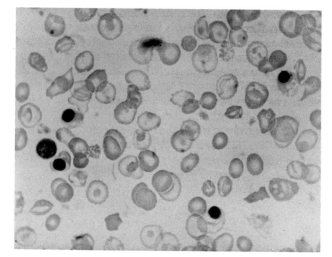

FIG 85-2

A blood smear from a splenectomized patient with thalassemia major that shows severe hypochromia, microcytosis target cells, and nucleated red blood cells.

and laboratory diagnosis are sufficiently different to warrant separate discussions.

There are two β-globin genes in every person, one on each chromosome 11. There are, therefore, three possible patterns of inheritance: 1) completely normal, having inherited two functional β-globin genes; 2) β-thalassemia trait in which one of the two β-globin genes is dysfunctional; and 3) homozygous β-thalassemia in which both of the β-globin genes are dysfunctional. The child with β-thalassemia trait is often of Mediterranean origin (although he/she may belong to any of the other ethnic groups mentioned previously). The anemia is mild (eg, the hemoglobin level is usually 9 to 11 g/100 mL), with a significant degree of hypochromia and microcytosis. There is a greater degree of microcytosis in thalassemia trait compared with that in a child with iron deficiency and a similar degree of anemia. Laboratory evaluation for iron deficiency anemia should be normal. A CBC count of the parents should reveal that at least one of them has hypochromic microcytic red blood cell (RBC) indices, although the parent may not be anemic, because adults with β-thalassemia trait can have a normal hemoglobin level. A quantitative analysis of the hemoglobins present in the child's blood will confirm the diagnosis of β-thalassemia trait revealing an increased level of hemoglobin A_2 (a minor adult hemoglobin). This quantitation cannot be reliably done by photometric scanning of a hemoglobin electrophoresis gel as performed in many hospitals but must be quan-

titated in a laboratory with an appropriate technique such as column chromatography.

Homozygous β-thalassemia (thalassemia major) is very often a severe life-threatening anemia that becomes clinically apparent after approximately 6 months of age when the fetal blood is replaced by adult blood. Usually the child has a severe hypochromic microcytic anemia (Fig. 85-2), often with hepatosplenomegaly that in part is secondary to extramedullary hematopoiesis. Hemoglobin electrophoresis will reveal a predominance of hemoglobin F (fetal hemoglobin) with little or no adult hemoglobin A. The proper management of such a child's condition should be done by a pediatric hematologist trained in the management of such cases.

Every person inherits four α-globin genes, two on each chromosome 16. There are, therefore, five potential clinical states as shown in Table 85-1. In blacks, virtually all the α-thalassemia chromosomes involve a single α gene deletion (α–) and therefore only the silent carrier (α–/αα) or α-thalassemia trait (α–/α–) are seen. In contrast, both the single gene deletion chromosome (α–) and the double deletion (– –) are seen in Southeast Asians. This is the reason that in Southeast Asians, hemoglobin H disease (α–/– –) and hydrops fetalis (– –/– –) are seen as well as the silent carrier and α-thalassemia trait.

The diagnosis of the silent carrier and α-thalassemia trait cannot be made by hemoglobin electrophoresis except in the newborn period in which hemoglobin Bart (consisting of tetra-

TABLE 85-1
Thalassemia Syndromes, Clinical State, and Diagnosis

DIAGNOSIS	ARRANGEMENT OF α GENES*	HEMATOLOGIC STATUS AND LABORATORY DIAGNOSIS
Normal	αα/αα	Normal
Silent carrier	α–/αα	Clinically normal. Less than 2% hemoglobin Bart (γ_4) in the newborn period.
α-Thalassemia trait	α–/α– or αα/– –	Mild hypochromic microcytic anemia. 2% to 10% hemoglobin Bart in the newborn period.
Hemoglobin H	α–/– –	Moderately severe anemia, significant α/β globin chains synthesis imbalance.
Hydrops fetalis	– –/– –	Often stillborn. Incompatible with long-term survival except with a chronic red blood cell transfusion program.

*In the table "α" refers to a functional α gene, whereas "–" refers to a nonfunctional gene. The "/" separates the maternal and paternal chromosomal pattern.

mers of the fetal β-like globin chain called γ) can be detected. The most reliable method at present to detect the majority of α-thalassemia syndromes involves DNA analysis. These studies are done in referral centers and should only be necessary in those cases in which an actual or potential risk exists of having a severely affected child. In a well black child with a mild hypochromic microcytic anemia not due to iron deficiency or lead poisoning (as screened by an FEP determination) or to β-thalassemia trait (shown by a normal hemoglobin A_2 level), the diagnosis of α-thalassemia trait is made by exclusion and no further testing need be done, whereas in an Asian patient, the risk of having more affected children should lead to a more complete genetic evaluation of the family.

Management

Genetic Counseling

The importance of establishing the diagnosis of thalassemia trait in a child is multifold. By confirming the proper diagnosis, unnecessary and potentially harmful administration of iron therapy can be avoided. In addition, proper genetic counseling can be done. In β-thalassemia, the parents of a child with the trait should be tested to be sure that both are not carriers of the thalassemia trait. If both parents are carriers, then there is a one in four risk of having a child with severe homozygous β-thalassemia. The potential risks of the child with the trait marrying another person with the trait should also be discussed. Prenatal diag-

nosis for the thalassemias is now available and should be offered to the parents if a child severely affected with thalassemia is a potential outcome.

In blacks with α-thalassemia, there is virtually no risk of having a severely affected child. Genetic counseling should emphasize this point. However, in Asian families with α-thalassemia the risk of having a severely affected child exists, and the pediatric hematologist who confirms the α-thalassemia diagnosis should also provide genetic counseling.

HEREDITARY SPHEROCYTOSIS

Background

Hereditary spherocytosis, the most common intrinsic RBC membrane defect known, is an autosomal dominant disorder. It results in a hemolytic anemia with spherocytosis. Approximately 15% of cases are sporadic, with neither parent affected. In the United States, the incidence is one in 5000, occurring most commonly in people of Northern European descent.

Recent studies have shown that hereditary spherocytosis is a defect in the RBC membrane's skeleton. The membrane's skeleton contains four proteins: spectrin, actin, protein 4.1, and ankyrin. At least several cases of hereditary spherocytosis are due to a defective spectrin molecule. The membrane abnormality results in an increased influx of sodium ion into cells and in a greater utilization of energy by the RBC to maintain its electrolyte balance. The cells are more susceptible to destruction inside the spleen, resulting in a shortened RBC life span.

Data Gathering

Hereditary spherocytosis can present at any age. In the neonatal period, early and severe hyperbilirubinemia should raise the possibility of hereditary spherocytosis. A palpable spleen is often present. However, in the newborn period, spherocytes also can be seen in other common disorders such as ABO incompatibility. Examination of the peripheral blood smears of the parents can assist in the proper diagnosis.

In older children, the diagnosis is made while evaluating a mild normochromic, normocytic anemia. Occasionally, the patients' initial presentation is due to an acute severe anemia. The etiology of this severe anemia can be either an aplastic crisis with no RBC production or a hemolytic crisis with increased RBC destruction. Both can follow a viral illness. The child has a rapid and significant drop in hemoglobin level, sometimes resulting in heart failure. Deficiency of G-6-PD and autoimmune hemolytic anemia also can present in a similar fashion, and enzyme quantitation studies and Coombs test, respectively, should help in the differential analysis. Again, family studies, with the physician looking at the peripheral blood smears for spherocytes and performing osmotic fragilities on family members, can be of value during the child's acute episode.

Very often the diagnosis of hereditary spherocytosis is suggested by the child's peripheral blood smear on which numerous spherocytes are seen. Spherocytes are small round erythrocytes that lack central pallor. The size of the average cell as measured by the Coulter counter is often normocytic as a result of the balancing influence of the large reticulocytes, although often the mean corpuscular hemoglobin concentration is elevated to over 35 g/dL. The red cell distribution width on the Coulter counter will be very high as a result of the double population of small spherocytes and large reticulocytes.

Bone marrow examination is rarely indicated but shows erythroid hyperplasia unless the patient is in the midst of an aplastic crisis.

In hereditary spherocytosis, the RBCs have an increased osmotic fragility. RBCs from patients with hereditary spherocytosis hemolyze at a higher osmotic concentration than normal RBCs.

This test is the cornerstone on which the diagnosis of hereditary spherocytosis is made. In addition, RBCs from a patient with hereditary spherocytosis have a higher rate of autohemolysis when incubated for 48 hours at 37° C. This problem is secondary to the greater energy depletion caused by the membrane's increased permeability to sodium ion influx. The addition of glucose to the incubating RBCs corrects the degree of autohemolysis.

Management

Splenectomy prolongs the half-life of RBCs in hereditary spherocytosis to 80% of normal, resulting in a disappearance of the anemia and the reticulocytosis. Splenectomy should be considered in all severely anemic patients. Asymptomatic patients also may benefit from a laparoscopic splenectomy, because they have an increased risk of bilirubin stones and biliary colic. The decision to perform a splenectomy should be made in conjunction with a pediatric hematologist.

If possible, splenectomy should be postponed until the child is more than 5 years of age. The risk of life-threatening bacterial infections is much higher in children under 5 years of age who have had their spleen removed. At least 1 month prior to splenectomy, the child should receive a pneumococcal vaccine and *Haemophilus influenzae* vaccine. Also, the child should receive prophylactic penicillin, 250 mg twice a day. After splenectomy, febrile episodes should be vigorously treated. A splenectomized child with a fever over 101.5° F without an obvious source should be hospitalized and treated with intravenous antibiotics until blood cultures prove to be negative.

In addition, until splenectomy, the child with hereditary spherocytosis should receive 1 mg of folic acid daily. The increased hemolysis results in an increased need for folic acid. In some cases of aplastic crisis, folate deficiency may be a contributory factor.

GLUCOSE-6-PHOSPHATE DEHYDROGENASE DEFICIENCY

Background

The most common intraerythrocyte enzymatic defect is G-6-PD deficiency. It is a recessive sex-linked disorder; thus the vast majority of patients are men. The exact clinical picture seen depends on the enzyme mutation present and on the oxidizing stress to which the RBC is exposed.

G-6-PD is the first enzyme in the hexose monophosphate shunt and plays a major role in preventing oxidation of the hemoglobin and membrane components of the RBC. In G-6-PD deficiency, when a RBC is exposed to an oxidizing agent, denatured hemoglobin precipitates in the cell as Heinz bodies, resulting in a shortened RBC life span.

G-6-PD deficiency occurs in the malarial belt of the world, where gene frequency for the disorder can be greater than 20%. In blacks, the most common form of G-6-PD deficiency has a level of enzyme activity that is 10% to 20% of normal. The G-6-PD level is higher in young RBCs. The common Mediterranean form of G-6-PD deficiency has 0% to 5% of the normal activity and is not found at a higher level in reticulocytes. The end result is that given a continued oxidizing stress, a black child with G-6-PD deficiency has a more limited fall in hemoglobin level, with the younger RBCs being protected from further hemolysis, whereas the child with the Mediterranean form of G-6-PD deficiency has a greater fall in hemoglobin level and is not protected from recurrent hemolysis with continued exposures.

Data Gathering

Unless exposed to an oxidizing stress, most patients with G-6-PD deficiency have a normal hemoglobin level. A G-6-PD deficiency may, however, lead to a severe neonatal hyperbilirubinemic state. In Thailand, for example, 65% of infants with a bilirubin level above 15 mg/dL have G-6-PD deficiency. In the United States, the G-6-PD deficiency seen in the black population is associated with an increased incidence of hyperbilirubinemia only in premature infants.

Another common presentation of G-6-PD deficiency is acute hemolytic anemia secondary to ingestion of an oxidizing agent. In the United States, ingestion of moth balls made from naphthalene is the most common ingestion leading to a hemolytic anemia in G-6-PD–deficient children. Other oxidizing agents include several antipyretics and analgesics (but not aspirin or acetaminophen), antimalarials, sulfa drugs, sulfones, fava beans, nalidixic acid, toluidine blue, phenylhydrazine, and methylene blue. After ingesting an oxidizing agent, the G-6-PD–deficient patient has a precipitous drop in hemoglobin level, often associated with jaundice. Congestive heart failure could develop if the fall in hemoglobin level is sufficiently acute and severe.

Rarely, a G-6-PD deficiency can cause a chronic hemolytic anemia. Virtually all such cases are in men, and in 80% of the cases, steady-state hemoglobin values are greater than 10 g/dL. Infections and exposure to oxidant drugs exacerbate the hemolysis. Like other hemolytic anemias, aplastic crisis can occur.

During an acute hemolytic episode, the G-6-PD–deficient patient will have spherocytes, polychromasia, and sometimes eccentrocytes with a clear "blister" area under the cell membrane in the peripheral smear. Special stains such as methyl violet stain are needed to show the presence of precipitated hemoglobin (Heinz bodies) in the peripheral blood. A Coombs test to rule out autoimmune hemolytic anemia and an osmotic fragility test to rule out hereditary spherocytosis may be necessary.

The definitive test is a quantitative measurement of G-6-PD level. In severe deficiency, the level should be low or absent in spite of the resultant reticulocytosis. However, in black children with G-6-PD deficiency, after an oxidizing stress the presence of reticulocytes with their higher level of G-6-PD could result in a borderline or even normal level. Therefore, the degree of reticulocytosis should be taken into account when deciding whether a child has G-6-PD deficiency. A low normal G-6-PD level with an elevated reticulocyte count should be considered suspicious, and the quantitative G-6-PD level should be repeated when the reticulocytosis has resolved.

Management

Other than avoidance of oxidizing stresses and supportive measures during acute hemolysis, there is no specific treatment for G-6-PD deficiency. Severe neonatal jaundice exacerbated by G-6-PD deficiency may require phototherapy or exchange transfusion.

BIBLIOGRAPHY

Bessmar JD, McClure S: Detection of iron deficiency anemia, *JAMA* 266:1649, 1991.

Beutler E: Study of glucose-6-phosphate dehydrogenase: History and molecular biology, *Am J Hematol* 42:53, 1993.

Delgiudice EM, Iolascon A, Pinto L, Nobili B, Perrotta S: Erythrocyte-membrane protein alterations underlying clinical heterogeneity in hereditary spherocytosis, *Br J Hematol* 88:52, 1994.

Poncz M, Cohen A, Schwartz E: Thalassemia, *Adv Pediatr* 31:43, 1984.

Sadowitz PD, Oski FA: Iron status and infant feeding in an urban ambulatory center, *Pediatrics* 72:33, 1983.

Walter T, Kovalsky J, Staked A: Effect of mild iron deficiency on infant mental development scores, *J Pediatr* 102:519, 1983.

Walter T: Infancy: Mental and motor development, *Am J Clin Nutr* 50(suppl):655, 1989.

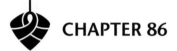

CHAPTER 86

Hemophilia

Catherine Manno

The term *hemophilia* usually refers to the inherited deficiency of factor VIII (hemophilia A) or factor IX (hemophilia B). Because the genes for factors VIII and IX are sex-linked and recessive, hemophilia primarily affects men, but women may rarely be affected. Hemophilia occurs in all races. Approximately one in 10,000 men in the United States is affected with hemophilia A; hemophilia A is four times more common that hemophilia B.

The other factor deficiencies are much rarer. Because they are autosomally inherited, they occur in men and women with equal frequency. von Willebrand disease, the most common inborn coagulation disorder, is inherited autosomally, usually in a dominant fashion. Many variants of von Willebrand disease exist. In the most common form, type 1, levels of factor VIII activity (F.VIII:C), von Willebrand factor antigen (vWF:Ag), and von Willebrand factor activity (ristocetin cofactor activity) are all low. Because von Willebrand factor is necessary for the normal adhesion and aggregation of platelets, the bleeding time is prolonged.

The clinical classification of severity is given in Table 86-1.

Recurrent joint bleeding can lead to crippling joint deformities and chronic arthritis. Appropriate on-demand replacement therapy helps decrease the severity and frequency of joint deformity and can slow the development of arthritis. Prevention of joint disease may be possible in certain patients through adherence to prophylaxis regimens.

Factor concentrates are either plasma derived or produced by recombinant DNA technology. Currently available products have been refined for enhanced purity and therefore contain fewer extraneous plasma proteins than previously available products. Virucidal techniques for

TABLE 86-1
Severity of Hemophilia A or B

SEVERITY	FACTOR LEVEL (%)	CLINICAL MANIFESTATIONS
Severe	< 1	Frequent, spontaneous hemorrhages; hemarthroses common
Moderate	1–5	Occasional hemorrhages; hemarthroses uncommon
Mild	5–20	Spontaneous hemorrhages rare; hemarthroses only after trauma

improving the safety of plasma-derived products include wet heat and solvent detergent treatments. Many patients treated with plasma-derived concentrates that were not virally inactivated became infected with hepatitis and HIV in the 1970s and 80s. AIDS has developed in many hemophilia patients, and the clinical picture is that seen in other patients who received HIV from blood transfusions. The risk for developing such viral infections using today's products is very low.

DATA GATHERING

The diagnosis of hemophilia may be made before birth or in the newborn period, if there is a family history. In many families, prenatal diagnosis of factor VIII deficiency is possible by DNA analysis. In these families, chorionic villous sampling or amniocentesis provides the material necessary for the diagnostic studies. A hemophilia or genetic center can provide the latest information on prenatal diagnosis of factor VIII or IX deficiency. Because neither factor VIII nor factor IX crosses the placenta, a citrated blood sample of cord blood may be used to measure the factor level. Factor VIII is present at normal levels (greater than 50%) in premature and term infants; therefore, the diagnosis of any degree of deficiency may be made at birth. The level of factor IX, a vitamin K–dependent coagulation factor, is lower than normal at birth in normal infants. Although severe factor IX deficiency can be diagnosed, it may be necessary to repeat measurements over a period of several months if the initial value is low and the family history suggests mild or moderate disease. The degree of factor deficiency is consistent throughout affected family members, although the clinical severity may vary somewhat.

In the absence of a positive family history, the diagnosis of severe hemophilia usually is made when there is prolonged bleeding from circumcision or when the family or physician notices unusual bruising or bleeding. Excessive bleeding from a laceration, particularly in the mouth; multiple, elevated bruises; or large ecchymoses following trauma should suggest the presence of a bleeding disorder. In mildly affected patients, the diagnosis may not be suspected until excessive bleeding occurs after dental extractions or surgery.

The studies necessary for diagnosis depend on the deficiency suspected, *eg,* a partial thromboplastin time and factor VIII assay or factor IX assay if hemophilia is suspected. Prolongation of the prothrombin time is not seen in hemophilia A or B. With an isolated prolongation of the prothrombin time, the diagnosis of factor VII deficiency should be considered. Diagnosis of any congenital bleeding disorder should be confirmed at a hemophilia treatment center. Choice of the proper replacement product depends on the precise identification of the deficient factor.

MANAGEMENT

General Care

Ideally, all patients with hemophilia should be enrolled in a hemophilia treatment center where periodic comprehensive evaluations can be made by a hematologist, nurse, orthopedist, dentist, and social worker. Family education and, when appropriate, home care training are offered. Genetic counseling and referral of the mother for carrier testing and prenatal diagnosis, if desired, can be arranged.

The pediatrician or family doctor is central to the care of the hemophilia patient, providing well-child care and treating all nonbleeding-related problems. If the patient lives a long distance from the hemophilia treatment center, the willing primary care physician can guide in the treatment of minor bleeding episodes and in the initial treatment of major bleeding. Patients should be referred to the center for life-threatening bleeding and surgical procedures.

Regular well-child care is important for the child with hemophilia. Immunizations are important but should be given subcutaneously rather than intramuscularly. A 26-gauge needle should be used, and firm pressure exerted at the injection site for several minutes. Immunization for hepatitis B is especially important for the child with hemophilia and may be given subcutaneously. The initial immunization is followed with booster doses 1 and 6 months later. Some pediatricians prefer to give immunizations intramuscularly after a patient has received an infusion of factor concentrate for another reason.

Young children with severe bleeding disorders often require iron therapy in the dose of 6 mg of elemental iron/kg/day to replace the iron lost as a result of external bleeding.

Aspirin should never be used for the child with a bleeding disorder. Its interference with platelet function can markedly increase bleeding. Other drugs that can interfere with coagulation should be used with caution.

Pediatric patients with severe and moderate hemophilia may participate in outdoor activities and in physical education classes. Contact sports (such as football and lacrosse) and activities with a high risk of trauma (such as motor-biking) should be avoided. Many sports, including swimming, golf, and tennis, can be safely pursued.

Hemophilia should not interfere with the child's placement in a regular school. The school nurse should be aware of the patient's diagnosis and the basics of emergency care. Homebound tutoring is only rarely needed. The child should be encouraged to participate fully in those activities that are not specifically prohibited.

Recent advances in the care of hemophilia patients can be attributed to the development of safer factor replacement products and the use of prophylactic therapy in selected patients. Rather than treating bleeding episodes on demand, prophylaxis involves factor concentrates given on a routine basis to prevent bleeding episodes. "Primary" prophylaxis begins soon after a child is diagnosed with severe hemophilia; F.VIII replacement is given every other day, and F.IX is given twice a week. Regular infusions in a young child may necessitate placement of an indwelling catheter. "Secondary" prophylaxis is initiated in a patient only after several bleeding episodes. Prophylaxis is supervised by personnel at hemophilia treatment centers where comprehensive care is offered by multiple specialists. Home therapy for on-demand or prophylaxis therapy allow patients to treat themselves at home, thus eliminating the need for frequent visits to a treatment site for minor bleeding episodes and reducing the financial cost of treatment.

Evaluation of Acute Problems

In the following discussion of problems, the minor bleeding episodes that can be readily managed in the office or emergency room or at home by families on home treatment programs are discussed. Those problems requiring hospitalization will be mentioned briefly. The discussion of treatment in more detail is beyond the scope of this chapter but can be found in the suggested references. The physician who is willing to provide care for minor bleeding episodes should discuss the case of the patient in detail with hemophilia treatment center personnel.

Some bleeding problems may mimic other disorders. The primary care physician must keep in mind at all times that the child has hemophilia and must question whether any acute problem, particularly pain or anemia, can be due to bleeding. In case of doubt, treatment for the bleeding disorder should be given while other diagnostic possibilities are still considered. For example, the young hemophilia patient with abdominal pain should receive factor replacement therapy. The physician must be alert, however, to the possibility that the child has a nonbleeding problem, such as appendicitis or urinary tract infection.

Bleeding episodes can be divided for purposes of management into those episodes that are minor and nonlife-threatening and those that do threaten life or function.

Bleeding can be prevented or stopped by replacement of the missing factor. The levels required to treat bleeding depend on the extent and location of the injury. Most minor injuries can be treated by raising the factor level to 30% for a brief period. Life-threatening bleeding or surgical wounds require higher levels of factor for more prolonged periods and hospitalization. The common bleeding episodes are listed below according to severity.

Common Hemorrhages
Minor
- Joint hemorrhages
- Muscle hemorrhages

- Skin lacerations
- Subcutaneous bruises
- Mouth bleeding
- Epistaxis
- Nontraumatic hematuria

Major

- Intracranial hemorrhage
- Retroperitoneal hemorrhage
     Iliopsoas muscle hemorrhage
     Uncontained bleeding
- Hemorrhage threatening the airway
- Muscle hemorrhage with nerve compression
- Traumatic hematuria
- Gastrointestinal tract hemorrhage
- Surgical procedures

Concentrates of F.VIII are preferred for the treatment of bleeding episodes in hemophilia A. Although cryoprecipitate contains F.VIII, vWF, and fibrinogen, the single donor plasma-derived product has not undergone viral inactivation procedures and is not preferred in treatment of hemophilia. Certain patients with von Willebrand disease and congenital fibrinogen deficiency may be treated with cryoprecipitate, although for von Willebrand patients, F.VIII concentrates that retain vWF activity are currently available. For hemophilia B, prothrombin complex concentrates containing F.II, F.VII, F.IX, and F.X are still available but have been supplanted by coagulation F.IX containing only F.IX as the treatment of choice. Fresh frozen plasma, which contains all the coagulation factors, can be used to treat the other coagulation disorders.

Physicians treating hemophilia patients should keep abreast of the current recommendations of the National Hemophilia Foundation and the Centers for Disease Control and Prevention.

In some patients it is possible to avoid the use of blood products by using desmopressin (an analog of vasopressin), which raises the plasma level of F.VIII:VWF three- to sixfold. Because desmopressin works by causing the release of vWF from endothelial cells it is not effective in patients with severe or moderate hemophilia who have very low factor VIII levels or in patients with those types of von Willebrand disease in which von Willebrand factor is absent or defective. It should be used to treat most bleeding episodes in patients with mild factor VIII deficiency or with the most common form, type 1 von Willebrand disease. Determination of the effectiveness of desmopressin therapy and safe testing

to determine which type of von Willebrand disease a patient has can be done at specialized coagulation laboratories.

Most skin lacerations require no treatment. Firm pressure will generally stop the bleeding. If the cut is larger and particularly if it requires sutures, treatment should be given. Occasionally treatment is needed when sutures are removed.

Subcutaneous bruising is the most common bleeding manifestation. Application of a cold pack, if the child will tolerate it, may decrease the bleeding. If, however, the bruise continues to enlarge or is in a tight area such as the buttock, one treatment may be needed.

Muscle bleeding responds in most cases to one infusion of the factor to raise the level to 30%. Immobilization with a posterior splint is sometimes necessary to prevent reinjury and rebleeding. Cold applications may help limit the hemorrhage.

Bleeding in some muscles requires special precautions. Hemorrhage in the gastrocnemius muscle usually requires several treatments. Exercises, and even physical therapy, may be necessary after the acute bleeding has stopped to prevent tightening of the heel cord. Iliopsoas muscle hemorrhage is treated in the hospital because rebleeding is frequent unless the patient receives multiple infusions. Because bleeding into the thigh can be massive, often resulting in a drop in hemoglobin level of 3 to 4 g/dL, the patient needs repeated treatment in the hospital. Bleeding into muscle compartments such as the forearm or gastrocnemius may cause nerve compression. If there is appreciable swelling in these areas, the patient should be hospitalized for aggressive treatment.

Joint hemorrhages are the most common form of bleeding requiring treatment. Because chronic damage can occur, rapid treatment of all hemarthroses is recommended. Knees, elbows, and ankles are most commonly involved. Even slight bleeding causes pain. As the amount of blood in the joint increases, swelling, warmth, and decreased range of motion follow. One treatment to raise the factor level to 30% is sufficient for treatment of most hemarthroses. If the patient has recurrent bleeding into one specific joint, a more aggressive treatment program including joint aspiration or the initiation of prophylaxis may be designed in conjunction with the hemophilia center. Other measures that are helpful are application of cold to the joint and immobilization of painful joints. Pain usually will cease within several hours of treatment. Continued pain or progression of swelling is indication for repeat factor therapy. Patients with hip bleeding should be admitted for bed rest and repeated treatment.

Mouth bleeding from a cut or a torn frenulum is very common in the young child. With the use of an antifibrinolytic agent such as epsilon-amino-caprioc acid (EACA) as adjunct therapy to prevent lysis of the clot that forms, one treatment with factor to raise the level to 30% is usually sufficient. EACA is given orally in the dose of 100 mg/kg every 6 hours (400 mg/kg every 24 hours) with a maximum dose of 24 g/day. Treatment must be continued for several days until the wound is well healed. EACA must not be given in the presence of hematuria or concurrently with prothrombin complex concentrates. One treatment dose of factor is usually sufficient, but more should be given if the clot is poor or oozing persists. Dry topical thrombin applied with an applicator to the bleeding site is also helpful.

Epistaxis is usually mild and readily controlled by pressure. Prolonged bleeding warrants factor replacement. An occasional patient will have recurrent, severe epistaxis with significant blood loss.

Hematuria unrelated to trauma is very common. Although most episodes probably result from tears in small vessels, other causes such as infection, tumor, and kidney stones should be considered, particularly if the hematuria persists for more than a few days. Most episodes can be managed by bed rest alone. One treatment with factor may help resolve the bleeding. Blood loss is rarely significant, even if the bleeding lasts for days. In hemophilia patients, EACA should not be used for hematuria because extensive clotting with renal compromise has been reported. If there is a history of trauma, costovertebral angle tenderness, or passage of large clots, the patient should be hospitalized for close observation, diagnostic studies, and frequent factor replacement.

Major bleeding episodes are still an important cause of death in those patients who have developed an inhibitor to factor VIII or IX. Patients with inhibitors in high titers do not respond to usual factor replacement. These patients should be treated through the hemophilia center.

Intracranial hemorrhage accounts for most of the hemorrhagic deaths in all age groups of hemophilia patients. Other serious hemorrhages include retroperitoneal hemorrhage (signaled by the presence of abdominal pain and often by the development of guarding and an ileus); hemorrhage in the mouth or throat area that may threaten the patency of the airway; bleeding into muscles in tight compartments that can produce permanent nerve damage; hematuria following trauma; and gastrointestinal tract hemorrhage that can result in massive blood loss.

All major hemorrhages require hospitalization for close observation and repeated treatment. If the patient lives a distance from the hemophilia center, the primary physician may give the first treatment dose calculated to raise the factor to 100% and then arrange for local hospitalization or transfer to the center.

Because intracranial hemorrhage is so serious a threat, injuries to the head should be treated as soon as possible to prevent bleeding. Any injury in which significant force is exerted on the head should be treated, including minor trauma such as occurs from falls or blows from hard, thrown objects, as well as the more traumatic injuries sustained in automobile or other accidents. In the young child, frequent falls may result in many prophylactic treatments. Any blow that the patient or family feels is significant enough to report to the physician should be treated even if there is no external sign of injury and even if there are no neurologic signs. Treatment should not be withheld while waiting for symptoms to appear. Tears in small vessels can be sealed immediately if factor replacement is given. If it is not given, continuing oozing can occur until the hemorrhage is large enough to cause symptoms. By this time, loss of function and death may be imminent.

Only very minor head injuries should be managed in the outpatient setting. In such minor injuries a single dose of factor is given to raise the factor level 100%. Although a 70% level is probably adequate, the higher dose is given to allow for extravascular extravasation. The family should be instructed to observe the patient closely. Further doses are not given if the patient remains well, and repeat examination by the physician is usually not necessary unless symptoms develop.

If the injury is more severe, *eg,* from an automobile accident or a fall down stairs, the patient should receive the initial dose to raise the factor level to 100% and should be admitted for repeated replacement therapy, imaging, computed tomographic (CT) scan or magnetic resonance imaging (MRI) of the head, and close observation.

Intracranial hemorrhage can occur in the absence of trauma. The development of neurologic symptoms such as headache or signs including drowsiness and repeated vomiting must be assumed to be due to intracranial hemorrhage in the hemophilia patient. Careful evaluation by a neurologist or neurosurgeon and diagnostic studies, such as CT scan or MRI, are necessary to exclude the presence of central nervous system or epidural cord bleeding. Patients with neurologic findings should be treated immediately to raise the factor level to 100% and then hospitalized for evaluation of their condition and further treatment.

CONSULTATIONS

The child with hemophilia should receive regular dental care and fluoride administration. Although it is possible to do even extensive dental surgery under factor coverage and with the use of EACA, it is much preferable to prevent dental caries and gum disease. No factor coverage is necessary for cleaning or for placement fillings if anesthesia is not needed. If local infiltrations are to be used, one treatment to raise the factor level to 30% is given prior to the dental appointment. Regional block anesthesia should not be used because hemorrhage in the loose tissue can extend to obstruct the airway. Extensive gum surgery, dental extractions, and any procedure involving the bone require careful planning, factor replacement, and close observation and are best done at the hemophilia center.

The orthopedist is an essential partner in the evaluation and treatment of the severely affected patient. Frequent evaluations may be necessary for the child with frequent hemarthroses and chronically affected joints. For those joints that have developed chronic synovitis due to repeated bleeding episodes, the affected synovium can be removed using either arthroscopic or radionuclide synovectomy. These procedures should be performed by experienced operators. Physical therapists and physiatrists also make important contributions to the preservation of joint function, the rehabilitation of joints affected by acute and chronic bleeding, and the postsynovectomy recovery process.

BIBLIOGRAPHY

Furie B, Limentani SA, Rosenfield CG: A practical guide to the evaluation and treatment of hemophilia, *Blood* 84:3, 1994.

Gill FM: Treatment of hemophilia and von Willebrand's disease, *Med Clin North Am* 68:601, 1984.

Hilgartner MW, editor: *Hemophilia in the child and adult,* New York, 1982, Masson Publishing.

Hoyer LW: Hemophilia A, *N Engl J Med* 330:38, 1994.

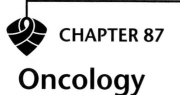

CHAPTER 87

Oncology

Michael N. Needle
Beverly Lange

Each year in the United States approximately 7000 children and adolescents develop cancer. Approximately one third of pediatric malignancies are leukemia, one quarter are brain tumors, and the remainder are solid tumors including sarcomas, lymphomas, Wilms tumor, neuroblastoma, hepatomas, and retinoblastoma. The four common tumors of adults—lung, breast, colon, and prostate—almost never occur in children. Figure 87-1 illustrates the progressive improvement in 5-year survival for children and adolescents with pediatric cancers. Even with the substantial success of the past 25 years, cancer remains the number one cause of nonaccidental death in children over 1 year of age.

No screening tests exist for tumors in children that are comparable to those for adult cancers. Thus, to recognize the child with cancer, the primary care physician must rely on a probing history, a meticulous physical examination, and a prepared mind. Childhood cancer presents in many ways. Some presentations, such as an abdominal mass, are obvious. Others are vague, insidious, and nonspecific such as low-grade anemia, fatigue, and failure to thrive. Finally there are extraordinary presentations such as myoclonus opsiclonus ("dancing eyes, dancing feet") of neuroblastoma or the diencephalic syndrome of an infant with a hypothalamic glioma. Table 87-1 lists the "classic" presentations for many childhood neoplasms. Because the presentation is variable and may be subtle, physicians need some guidelines to help distinguish the child with cancer from the child who has a less serious illness or a functional complaint. For example, pain is often a symptom of cancer. Box 87-1 describes characteristics of cancer pain that are often not present in other kinds of pain, particularly functional pain.

Table 87-2 lists common and not-so common signs and symptoms of pediatric patients that demand a diagnosis. Virtually all of these signs and symptoms require some laboratory test to give them a name and to direct the investigation toward or away from cancer or other serious illness. Obviously cancer is only one of many conditions that can cause these signs and symptoms. Generating both a broad differential diagnosis and a systematic approach to data gathering will help the practicioner recognize the few cases of cancer he/she will encounter.

Occasionally cancer presents as a true emergency. These emergencies occur when a tumor compresses or obstructs a vital organ or causes dangerous endocrine or metabolic derangements or when blood count abnormalities cause life-threatening bleeding, thrombosis, or infection. Emergencies that occur at the time of presentation are listed in Table 87-3. When any of these oncologic emergencies is discovered, it is best to telephone a regional referral center to discuss the immediate management of the child and arrange for safe transport.

Although cancer is often not an emergency, it is almost always an urgency. There is medical urgency to obtain a diagnosis as soon as possible to prevent extension of the tumor. There is a psychologic urgency to relieve both parents and the primary care physician of feelings that there was unnecessary delay and to begin the process of helping families to cope with what is probably the most terrifying experience of their lives.

Standard practice involves referring the child with possible or certain cancer to a surgeon, oncologist, or cancer center. However, in most cases the primary care physician is the one who is faced with telling the parents and patient that cancer is a consideration. At this time the physician needs to be honest, to communicate only the information that is known, and to offer hope. This news often causes shock, grief, and anger.

This chapter reviews the common childhood malignancies. It emphasizes their presenting signs and symptoms and suggests simple diagnostic evaluations that the primary care physician can obtain while contacting the referral center. Finally it discusses treatment complications that a primary care physician may encounter in a patient who is receiving cancer chemotherapy or radiation therapy.

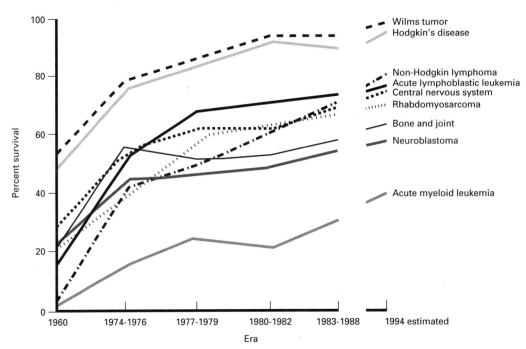

Five-year survival rates for selected pediatric cancers: 1960 to 1994

FIG 87-1

Trends in 5-year survival for the common childhood malignancies based on life-table analysis of cases diagnosed in living patients from birth to 14 years of age. [From Hankey BF, Gloekler-Ries LA, Miller BA, Kosary CL, Edwadrs BK, editors: *Cancer Statistics Review, 1973–1989*, United States Department of Health and Human Services, NIH Publication 92-2789, Bethesda; Robison LL: General Principles of Epidemiology and Childhood Cancer. In Poplack DG, Pizzo A, editor: *Principles and Practice of Pediatric Oncology*, ed 2, Philadelphia, 1993, JB Lippincott.]

TABLE 87-1
"Classic" Presentations of Some Childhood Cancers

MALIGNANCY	PRESENTATION
Acute leukemia	The "dwindles" (fatigue, pallor lingering after minor illness)
	Excessive bruising
Infant acute myeloid leukemia	Skin nodules; hepatosplenomegaly; adenopathy
Chronic myeloid leukemia	Massive splenomegaly in well patient
Wilms tumor	Parent notes an abdominal mass while bathing child
Medulloblastoma	Child with morning vomiting, headache, ataxia
Hodgkin disease	Teenager notes neck mass in mirror
Osteosarcoma	Pain, swelling around knee (sometimes after trauma)
Sarcoma botrioides	Grapelike mass protruding from infant vagina
Retinoblastoma	Cat's eye (white pupil) often noted in photograph

ACUTE LEUKEMIA

Leukemia is the most common malignancy of childhood, occurring in nearly four of 100,000 children under the age of 14 years. Acute lymphoblastic leukemia (ALL) is the predominant leukemia of childhood. Acute myoblastic leukemia (AML) occurs in the remaining 15% to 20% of children with leukemia. Less than a generation ago, there was no effective therapy for ALL. Today, remission can be induced in more than 95% of patients, and cure can be expected in at least 70%.

BOX 87-1

Some Features of Cancer Pain in the Pediatric Patient

Wakens from sleep
Permits daily activities, at least initially
Evolves to unremitting, severe pain
Age/location discordance
  Headache in an infant
  Back pain in an infant or child
  "Lumbago" (sciatica) in any young person
  Limp in an older child or adolescent
  Abdominal pain in the older adolescent (particularly boys)

Data Gathering

Table 87-4 summarizes the most common presenting complaints among children along with their frequency. Signs and symptoms often reflect bone marrow failure, destruction of bone, or distention of periosteum. The physician should question parents about fever, infections that persist, and pains in the chest, bones, joints, and back. This pain may not be severe and can take many forms. The physician should determine if there has been an increase in the frequency of nosebleeds or easy bruising and should ask about lumps or masses. On physical examination, the child with acute leukemia may have a fever. Mucosa and nailbeds may be pale, and there may be boggy or bleeding gums. Cervical, inguinal, and axillary lymph nodes may be enlarged and visible, and splenomegaly and hepatomegaly may be present. The testes should be palpated for enlargement or change in consistency due to infiltration with leukemic cells.

A complete blood cell (CBC) count, with differential cell count, and a serum chemistry profile including urea nitrogen, creatinine, uric acid, calcium, and liver function studies are usually sufficient. Table 87-5 summarizes the presenting characteristics of leukemia in one large pediatric

---

TABLE 87-2

Signs and Symptoms That Demand Diagnosis

AGE	POSSIBLE MALIGNANCY
Birth to 2–3 years of age	
Subcutaneous nodules (<1 year of age)	Leukemia, neuroblastoma
Enlarging head	Brain tumor
Abdominal mass	Wilms tumor; neuroblastoma, hepatoblastoma; teratoma
Extremity mass	Sarcoma
Loss of milestones	Brain tumor; neuroblastoma
Can't bear weight	Neuroblastoma
Failure to thrive	Brain tumor, neuroblastoma, leukemia
Cat's eye (white pupil)	Retinoblastoma
Persistent or recurrent headache	Brain tumor
Any age	
Abdominal mass	Wilms tumor; neuroblastoma; hepatocellular carcinoma; sarcoma; germ cell tumor
Chest wall mass	Sarcoma; lymphoma
Extremity mass	Sarcoma
Hepatosplenomegaly	Leukemia; lymphoma
Lymphadenopathy (Boxes 87-2 and 87-3)	Lymphoma (Hodgkin disease, non-Hodgkin lymphoma), neuroblastoma
Severe pain (Box 87-1)	Leukemia, sarcoma, lymphoma, brain tumor
Increased intracranial pressure (Box 87-4)	Brain tumor
Abnormal bleeding or bruising	Leukemia
Fever of unknown origin	Leukemia, lymphoma, Ewing tumor, neuroblastoma
Periorbital swelling	Rhabdomyosarcoma, Ewing tumor neuroblastoma, acute myeloid leukemia (chloroma)

III

TABLE 87-3
Oncologic Emergencies That May Be the Presenting Feature of Cancer

EMERGENCY	MALIGNANCY	COMPLICATION

Hyperleukocytosis:
  WBC >200,000 in acute myeloid
  leukemia
  WBC >400,000 in acute lympho-
  blastic leukemia
  WBC >600,000 in chronic myeloid
  leukemia
	Leukemia	Cerebrovascular accident
		Pulmonary stasis
		Thrombosis
		Brain herniation

Superior vena cava syndrome/
  superior mediastinal syndrome
	Lymphoma
	Sarcoma
	Neuroblastoma
		Cardiorespiratory arrest with
		  flexion or prone position with
		  sedation or anesthesia

Spinal cord compression	Neuroblastoma Sarcoma Leukemia Central nervous system tumor	Paraplegia
Increased intracranial pressure	Central nervous system tumor	Herniation
Hemorrhagic diathesis	Acute myeloid leukemia; acute pro- myelocytic leukemia	Cerebrovascular accident

Tumor lysis syndrome
  high K^+ and PO_4^-, low Ca^{++}
  high blood urea nitrogen, creati-
  nine, uric acid
	Burkitt lymphoma
	T-cell acute lymphoblastic leukemia
		Renal failure
		Cardiac arrest

Hypercalcemia	Alveolar Rhabdo. Non-Hodgkin's lymphoma; leukemia	Dehydration Renal failure Coma; death

TABLE 87-4
Frequency of the More Common Presenting Complaints Among Children

FINDING	PERCENT
Fever	61
Pallor	55
Hemorrhage	52
Anorexia	33
Fatigue	30
Bone pain	23
Abdominal pain	19
Joint pain	15
Lymphadenopathy	15
Weight loss	13

From Sutow WW, Vietti TJ, Fernbach DC: *Clinical pediatric oncology,* ed 3, St Louis, 1980, CV Mosby. Used by permission.

cancer study group. Further classification as to cell type, morphologic characteristics, leukemia cell surface markers, and karyotype should be performed at the facility where treatment is to be started. With careful guidance by the primary care physician, this transition to the referral center can be accomplished with expediency and with appropriate emotional support of the family.

NON-HODGKIN'S LYMPHOMA

Non-Hodgkin's lymphomas (NHLs) are malignant tumors that originate in lymphatic tissues (eg, lymph nodes, thymus, mesentery, Peyer patches, appendix, and, rarely, spleen). Extralymphatic sites of origin include bone, ovaries, and skin. In contrast to the adult forms in which the disease can remain indolent and localized for years, childhood NHL proliferates rapidly and spreads outside the primary site in weeks to months. Metastasis occurs to the bone marrow and central nervous system (CNS). If extensive marrow involvement occurs, the distinction between NHL and acute leukemia may be extremely difficult. The types of lymphomas seen in children are almost always poorly differentiated and diffuse, and they entirely efface the architecture of the tissue of origin.

Non-Hodgkin lymphomas usually occur before puberty or in early adolescence. The childhood incidence is 0.5 cases/100,000 children under 15 years of age. Patients with any form of immunodeficiency state, either inherited or acquired, have an exceptionally high incidence of

TABLE 87-5
Presenting Characteristics of 1024 Patients With Acute Leukemia as Reported by The Southwest Oncology Group

CHARACTERISTIC	PERCENT
Age (yr)	
<2	14
2–5	47
6–10	24
>11	15
White blood cell count (1000/mm³)	
<10	34
10–24	25
25–49	22
>50	19
Hemoglobin (g/100 mL)	
<7	44
7–11	43
>11	14
Sex (male)	57
Race (white)	85
Hemorrhage (yes)	48
Blasts (%)	
<65	25
65–84	22
85–94	28
≥95	25
Platelets (1000/mm³)	
20	29
20–49	23
50–99	20
≥100	29
Liver enlarged	79
Spleen enlarged	69
Cervical nodes enlarged	62
Inguinal nodes enlarged	54
Axillary nodes enlarged	47

From Sutow WW, Vietti TJ, Fernbach DC: *Clinical pediatric oncology,* ed 3, St Louis, 1980, CV Mosby. Used by permission.

NHL. Those patients having undergone renal or cardiac transplant, patients receiving chronic immunosuppressive therapy, and patients with Hodgkin disease treated with radiation therapy and chemotherapy have an unusually high incidence of NHL.

Classification of NHL is controversial. Histologic, cytologic, and immunologic studies are readily employed. The tumors are also classified according to stage that reflects the degree of tumor burden. The common types of NHL are Burkitt's lymphoma (small noncleaved cell lymphoma), lymphoblastic lymphoma, and large cell lymphoma.

BOX 87-2
Common Presentations of Pediatric Non-Hodgkin Lymphoma

Localized NHL
Large lymph node or group of matted nodes
Unilateral tonsilar enlargement
Nasopharyngeal mass
Acute appendicitis (appendiceal mass)
Jaw swelling (African Burkitt NHL)
Brain tumor in immunocompromised host

Disseminated NHL
Mediastinal mass, ± effusion, ± marrow (lymphoblastic NHL)
Abdominal mass, ± ascites, ± tumor lysis syndrome (Burkitt NHL also called small non-cleaved cell lymphoma)
Generalized adenopathy ± fever, bone pain, weight loss

NHL—non-Hodgkin lymphoma.

Data Gathering

Approximately 25% of NHLs in childhood present as isolated lymph nodes or a group of nodes. The rest are widely disseminated. The common presentations are listed in Box 87-2.

Burkitt lymphoma usually causes generalized abdominal enlargement, pain, nausea, vomiting, constipation, and, in half of the cases, malignant ascites. These symptoms also may suggest a primary tumor arising in the ovaries or in retroperitoneal lymph nodes, but kidney and bowel are sometimes involved. Burkitt tumor cells proliferate exceedingly rapidly, which allows the tumor to extend locally over a period of days to weeks. This condition usually leads to ascites, pleural effusion, and renal failure. Extension of the disease to the meninges and bone marrow is common. If untreated, the tumor is rapidly fatal, usually due to renal failure. Even when treated, the disease sometimes recurs within a few months either in the abdomen or as leukemia.

Mediastinal NHL occurs commonly in boys during late childhood or early adolescence. If untreated, metastasis to bone marrow, CNS, and testes is quite common. Presenting signs and symptoms include the presence of a bulky thoracic tumor in the anterior mediastinum, which may be associated with cardiovascular or circulatory (superior vena cava syndrome) compromise.

Management

When localized NHL is suspected, a biopsy of the lymph node or mass should be obtained promptly. Prior to this, chest radiographs and

BOX 87-3
When a Lymph Node Should Undergo Biopsy

Immediately
>3 cm in diameter, matted, adherent, and/or not
  obviously infectious
Unusual location, not obviously infectious
  Supraclavicular (almost always)
  Low cervical (often)
  Femoral (often)
  Axillary (sometimes)
Associated with mediastinal mass
Associated with fever of unknown origin, anorexia,
  generalized adenopathy, and no definable infec-
  tion

Soon (up to 6 wks)
>3 cm in diameter, possibly infected but unre-
  sponsive to antibiotics
Enlarging under observation or treatment

Later (up to 12 weeks)
>3 cm in diameter, unusual location, or firm, rub-
  bery, or fixed

CBC counts are essential to ensure that there is neither a mediastinal mass nor any evident leukemic process.

Adenopathy is common in children. Box 87-3 lists those features of a node that alert the physician to the need for a biopsy. If a node is suspected to be malignant, the biopsy specimen should be sent to pathology in a sterile container so that immunophenotyping and cytogenetics can be obtained as well as routine histology.

Once the primary care physician has ascertained a suggestion of the type of process involved, expedient referral for definitive therapy should be accomplished. More than 70% of patients with either localized or disseminated NHL are cured with chemotherapy.

HODGKIN DISEASE

Like NHL, Hodgkin disease is a malignancy of the lymph nodes. Usually it begins in a cervical lymph node and spreads in a predictable and orderly sequence from one lymph node region to the next. If left untreated, it progresses to involve organs outside the lymph nodes. In contrast to NHL, spread to the bone marrow and CNS is rare. The malignant cell in Hodgkin disease is the Reed-Sternberg cell, which is thought to originate from either a B-lymphocyte or a histiocyte precursor. Hodgkin disease is classified according to the extent of disease at presentation and the histologic composition of the involved lymph node.

The incidence of Hodgkin disease is similar to that of NHL: 0.6 cases per 100,000 children under 15 years of age. Although Hodgkin disease has been reported in infants, it is rare in children under 5 years of age. In the United States Hodgkin disease tends to occur in the higher socioeconomic classes. Its cause is unknown.

Data Gathering

Hodgkin disease most often manifests as a mass in the neck; approximately 4% of the cases present as masses in the groin. The mass may have been present for days, months, or years. Some patients initially complain of adenopathy localized to a few lymph node regions; others notice generalized adenopathy. Anterior mediastinal masses occur in one half of the patients. Nonetheless, large mediastinal Hodgkin tumors can present with the same cardiovascular or respiratory symptoms as mediastinal NHL. Most patients with Hodgkin disease are well, but 30% will present with fever and involuntary weight loss. At the time of diagnosis, the fever may be low grade or high grade. The typical Pel-Ebstein fever, a high, debilitating fever followed by a drenching sweat, is usually a sign of very advanced disease.

The workup of a patient with Hodgkin disease should include a chest radiograph and a computed tomographic (CT) scan of the chest to define the lower limit of cervical disease and the extent of mediastinal disease. Patients require both an abdominal and CT scan.

Management

Hodgkin disease can be successfully managed using a number of approaches. It is best to involve the referral center early in the diagnostic workup. There are a number of factors to consider. Young children are particularly predisposed to abnormalities of growth from radiation therapy. Postpubertal boys are prone to sterility from high-dose chemotherapy. All patients are at risk for second tumors from radiation therapy and chemotherapy. Most importantly, many patients whose disease recurs after the first treatment for Hodgkin's lymphoma can be retreated and cured.

The traditional model, still practiced by most oncologists, is to treat the patient with limited-disease adult with radiation therapy only. This treatment is possible for patients with disease on one side of the diaphragm and with a mediastinal mass that is less than one third the diameter of the chest. Patients treated with radiation alone should have a staging laparotomy and splenectomy to confirm the limited stage of the disease. Splenectomy is not to be taken lightly; it carries a life-long risk of susceptibility to encapsulated bacteria. In many pediatric centers, children with limited-stage disease will receive chemotherapy both to avoid splenectomy and to permit reduced-dose or elimination of radiation therapy. Patients with advanced disease will all receive chemotherapy, and radiation therapy is reserved for residual disease at the end of chemotherapy.

LANGERHANS CELL HISTIOCYTOSIS

Langerhans cell histiocytosis (LCH), which until recently was called *histiocytosis X* (or eosinophilic granuloma, Hand-Schüller-Christian disease, Letterer-Siwe disease), is a disease characterized by varied presentation and varied progression. Although there are other benign and malignant forms of histiocytoses, they are rare and will not be discussed here.

Data Gathering
The prognosis for a patient with LCH is dependent on the stage of the disease, particularly on the number of organ systems involved. On discovery of a patient with LCH, workup will include a radiographic skeletal survey, as well as a CBC and differential, coagulation profile, liver function, and water deprivation tests. Abnormalities in these tests often will lead to biopsy of the involved organs.

Management
Presentation can be isolated to a skin rash consisting of red to brown papules that are scaly, erythematous, or seborrhea-like, often in the intertriginous regions or on the scalp. The initial manifestation of a bony lesion is a painful swelling. The skull is the most common site, followed by the long bones of the upper extremities and the flat bones. The child with disease limited to one of these lesions will most often have spontaneous resolution or resolve after biopsy and curettage. Involvement of the bone marrow, liver, spleen, lungs, gastrointestinal tract, or brain signify more threatening disease that will require chemother-

apeutic intervention. The most common endocrinopathy is diabetes insipidus. This condition often accompanies skull lesions and abnormalities can be demonstrated on gadolinium-enhanced magnetic resonance imaging (MRI). Patients with advanced disease have a poor prognosis and require transfer to a referral center without delay.

BRAIN TUMORS

A number of advances have improved the treatment options of the child with a brain tumor. Improved noninvasive imaging, such as CT and MRI, have led to earlier diagnosis. The operating microscope has given the pediatric neurosurgeon improved capability to distinguish tumor from surrounding brain. Postoperative MRI with gadolinium enhancement has improved the ability to assess the extent of resection prior to initiation of adjuvant therapy.

Children with brain tumors frequently present with subtle symptoms that are not localizing in nature. Macrocephaly may be the first sign of an infant with a brain tumor. Headache is the most common symptom (Box 87-4). Unfortunately, the classic headache that awakens the patient from sleep and improves throughout the day is uncommon. More commonly, patients present with chronic intermittent headache or a persistent headache. Patients who have intermittent headaches for more than 1 month or persistent headache for more than 1 week need to be evaluated carefully. Other constitutional findings for which a brain tumor needs to be considered, especially if more common etiologies cannot be confirmed, include failure to thrive, loss of development milestones, and deterioration in school performance. Occasionally these symptoms are attributed to psychologic illness before a structural lesion is considered.

Specific neurologic deficits can be helpful in localizing a lesion (Table 87-6).

Most childhood brain tumors are in the posterior fossa (Table 87-7). They can block the 4th ventricle and cause signs and symptoms of increased intracranial pressure secondary to hydrocephalus. New onset ataxia, which in a toddler can manifest as refusal to walk, suggest a cerebellar lesion. Cranial nerve palsies often are the first signs of a brainstem tumor. New onset of focal seizures require that a supratentorial tumor

BOX 87-4
Conditions Associated With Headaches That Warrant a CT or MRI

Age <3 years
Regular morning vomiting*
   Vomiting without nausea
   Relief after vomiting
   Vomiting episodes last more than 2 weeks
Sleep disruption*
Cushing's triad*
   High blood pressure
   Low heart rate
   Slow respirations
Neurologic abnormality
   Ataxia
   Hemiparesis
   Bell's palsy
   Visual changes (diplopia, loss of acuity, squint, field cut)
Associated focal seizure or protracted seizure
Associated metabolic or endocrine abnormality
   Diabetes insipidus
   Precocious puberty
   Growth hormone deficiency or growth deceleration
Associated constitutional disorder
   Neurofibromatosis types I and II
   Tuberous sclerosis
   von Hippel Lindau
History of cranial irradiation for other tumor

*These findings are nonspecific signs of increased intracranial pressure and/or hydrocephalus.

TABLE 87-6
Common Presenting Symptoms of Brain Tumors*

SYMPTOM	PERCENT
Raised intracranial pressure	85
Headache	70
Vomiting	75
Episodic blindness	10
Disturbance of gait	40
Mental symptoms	35
Diplopia	25
Vertigo	25
Hemiparesis	15
Seizures	10
Head tilt	10

*From Gjerris F: Clinical aspects and long-term prognosis of intracranial tumors in infancy and childhood, *Dev Med Child Neurol* 18:145–159, 1976. Used by permission.

TABLE 87-7
Location of Pediatric Brain Tumors*

LOCATION	PERCENT
Posterior fossa	60
Supratentorial	40
Midline region	15
Cerebral hemispheres	25

*From Walker RW, Allen JC: Pediatric brain tumors, *Pediatr Ann* 12:383, 1983.

or not, neurologic consultation and MRI with gadolinium enhancement is indicated.

Once a tumor has been diagnosed, the first step is biopsy and, if possible, surgical excision. This procedure is possible in most cases, excepting tumors intrinsic to the brainstem (pons) or in the deep midline structures such as the optic chiasm, hypothalamus, or thalamus. Because surgery is an invaluable diagnostic and therapeutic intervention, consultation with an experienced pediatric neurosurgeon is critical. This consultation may require referral outside the usual regional center, to an established pediatric brain tumor center.

Surgery is potentially curative in patients with low-grade glioma of the cerebellum or the cerebral cortex. Higher-grade gliomas, such as anaplastic astrocytoma and glioblastoma multiforme, are much more aggressive and require adjuvant radiation therapy and usually chemotherapy. Prognosis remains poor in patients with malignant glioma, with less than 25% cured.

Table 87-8 lists the incidence of brain tumors by histology. Medulloblastoma is the single most common entity.

Medulloblastoma, and the related primitive neuroectodermal tumor of the cerebral cortex, has a high propensity to spread throughout the CNS. Therefore, after surgery, patients will require an MRI of the spine to evaluate for the presence of metastatic deposits. Radiation therapy must include the entire brain and spine. Most patients will require chemotherapy, except perhaps those with posterior fossa tumors that have been completely excised and have no evidence of metastatic spread. These tumors are responsive to adjuvant therapy, and cure is possible in 70% of cases.

Ependymoma is a slow-growing tumor with a propensity for late recurrence. Surgery and radiation therapy are the mainstays of treatment. These tumors spread along the periventricular spaces.

be considered. Visual disturbance, including bumping into things as a sign of loss of peripheral vision, can be the presenting sign of a tumor of the optic nerves or chiasm. In virtually all of these situations, whether the presentation is localizing

TABLE 87-8
Incidence of Brain Tumors by Tumor Histology*

TYPE OF TUMOR	PERCENT
Medulloblastoma	20
Astrocytoma (cerebellar)	17
Astrocytoma (other)	16
Glioblastoma	5
Ependymoma	9
Craniopharyngioma	8
Optic nerve glioma	5
Meningioma	2
Pineal (germinoma)	2
Other[†]	16

*From Bell WE, McCormick WF: *Increased intracranial pressure in children,* Philadelphia, 1978, WB Saunders.
[†]These include sarcomas, pituitary adenomas, oligodendrogliomas, and primitive neuroectodermal tumors.

TABLE 87-9
Tumors in Upper Abdomen*

BENIGN	MALIGNANT
Renal	
Hydronephrosis	Wilms' tumor
Polycystic kidney	Adenocarcinoma
Benign neoplasms	
Renal hypertrophy	
Adrenal	
Adrenal hyperplasia	Neuroblastoma
Benign neoplasms	Ganglioneuroblastoma
	Adenocarcinoma
	Pheochromocytoma
Liver	
Hepatosplenomegaly	Hepatoblastoma
Benign neoplasms	Hepatocellular carcinoma
Benign hyperplasia	Metastatic tumor

*From Jones PG, Campbell PE: *Tumors of infancy and childhood,* Oxford, England, 1976, Blackwell Scientific Publications. Used by permission.

Brainstem glioma is the most difficult tumor to treat. Most tumors are intrinsic to the pons and cannot be safely excised. Radiation therapy is usually administered without histologic confirmation. Survival for most patients is less than 2 years. In contrast, brainstem tumors that are discreet and have an exophytic component are amenable to surgery and have at least a 50% chance of cure after radiation therapy.

Infants with brain tumors present a particular challenge. The developing nervous system is exquisitely sensitive to radiation therapy, virtually precluding its use prior to the third birthday. Infants treated with high-dose radiation have significant cognitive and growth disturbance. Multiple trials using chemotherapy alone have been successful in preserving neurologic development in patients treated without irradiation. Unfortunately, cure is achieved in roughly one in three patients.

ABDOMINAL, GENITOURINARY, AND RETROPERITONEAL TUMORS

The discovery of an abdominal mass requires an immediate orderly investigation to determine its precise nature. As is the case with many signs and symptoms in pediatrics, the etiology of the masses differs among infants and children of various ages. The spectrum of intra-abdominal and pelvic tumors is summarized in Tables 87-9 and 87-10.

Data Gathering

Wilms tumor and neuroblastoma are the most common intra-abdominal neoplasms of young children. Wilms tumor presents as a large flank mass in a well child; abdominal neuroblastoma, outside of infancy, presents as a midline or flank mass in an ill child. Hepatic tumors are sometimes associated with systemic illness. Tumors arising in the pelvis, regardless of cause, may first cause neurologic deficits or abdominal pain.

For most of these tumors, staging usually depends on the amount of tumor that has been removed surgically. Stage I tumors are usually those that are completely removed. If there is microscopic or gross residual or if there is spread to regional lymph nodes, the tumor is considered stage II or III. Tumors presenting with widespread distant metastasis to other organ systems are considered stage IV. Histologic classification is apparent for each tumor category and has gained in significance only recently as survival has improved.

WILMS TUMOR

Wilms' tumor (nephroblastoma), the most common intrarenal neoplasm of childhood, is an embryonal neoplasm of mixed histologic composition. Approximately 5% of all Wilms' tumor occurs bilaterally. Wilms tumor occurs in approximately eight in 1,000,000 children under 15 years of age; 65% of children presenting with

TABLE 87-10
Tumors of Lower Abdomen and Genitalia*

BENIGN	MALIGNANT
Retroperitoneum	
Presacral teratoma	Soft-tissue sarcoma
Anterior meningomyelocele	Bone sarcoma
	Lymphoma
Ganglioneuroma	Neuroblastoma
Lipoma	Teratoma
Bladder and urethra	
Abscess	Rhabdomyosarcoma
Ureterocele	Leiomyosarcoma
Polyp	
Neurogenic bladder	
Bowel	
Appendicitis	Lymphoma
Feces	Adenocarcinoma
Duplication cyst	Carcinoid
Carcinoid	
Female genitalia	
Vagina	
Cysts	Rhabdomyosarcoma
Hydrocolpos	Clear-cell sarcoma
Hematocolpos	Endodermal sinus
Adenoma	
Neurofibroma	
Uterus and fallopian tubes	
Abscess	Rhabdomyosarcoma
Papilloma	Adenocarcinoma
	Embryonal carcinoma
Ovary	
Teratoma	Teratoma
Cyst	Dysgerminoma
Granulosa theca cell	Arrhenoblastoma
Fibroma	Adenocarcinoma
Hemangioma	Choriocarcinoma
	Metastatic tumor
Male genitalia	
Prostate gland	
Abscess	Rhabdomyosarcoma
Testis	
Hydrocele	Rhabdomyosarcoma
Testicular torsion	Embryonal carcinoma
Orchitis	Seminoma
Teratoma	Leukemia
Leydig or Sertoli cell	
tumor	
Spermatic cord	
Hydrocele	Rhabdomyosarcoma
Hernia	Leukemia
Inflammation	
Adrenal rest	
Benign tumors of	
connective tissue	

*From Jones PG, Campbell PE: *Tumors of infancy and childhood,* Oxford, England, 1976, Blackwell Scientific Publications. Used by permission.

Wilms tumor are under 5 years of age. There is a significant association between Wilms tumor and congenital anomalies, including aniridia, hemihypertrophy, genitourinary anomalies, hemangiomas, hamartomas, and cardiac anomalies. There are several case reports of familial Wilms tumor as well as reports of families in which some of the members had the congenital anomalies listed above, whereas other members had Wilms tumor.

Data Gathering

The majority of children with Wilms tumor have an abdominal mass discovered accidentally by their parents while bathing or clothing the child or by the physician on routine physical examination. The mass is solitary and deep in the flank and can be either firm or soft. Abdominal pain, fever, anorexia, malaise, vomiting, and weight loss are rare presenting complaints. Gross hematuria occurs in less than 25% of the cases and usually indicates invasion of the renal pelvis with tumor. Hypertension, seen in a small number of patients, is thought to be the result of excessive renin secretion secondary to renal artery compression. By a related mechanism, polycythemia occasionally occurs. More often, anemia results from bleeding into the tumor.

In performing the physical examination, the physician should note the size of the liver and spleen, the site and size of the mass, blood pressure, and the presence of any of the congenital abnormalities listed previously. Laboratory evaluation should include determination of CBC count, blood urea nitrogen, and creatinine. Renal ultrasound is the most expedient way to evaluate a patient with a suspected renal mass.

At this point, children with a presumed Wilms tumor should be referred to a (pediatric) surgeon experienced in the diagnosis and treatment of this tumor. Wilms tumor exemplifies the advances of multimodal therapy in the pediatric oncology center; disease-free survival rates now approach 90%. Even patients with metastatic disease or bilateral tumors can be treated successfully.

NEUROBLASTOMA

Neuroblastoma is a malignant tumor arising from sympathetic tissue in the adrenal medulla, or in the sympathetic chain along the craniospinal axis in the neck, posterior mediastinum, the

TABLE 87-11
The Many Presentations of Neuroblastoma

PRESENTATION	USUAL AGE
Abdominal mass on physical examination	Newborn
Skin nodules, hepatic failure, ill infant	Neonate
Skin nodules, hepatomegaly, well infant	2–12 mos
Irritability, bone pain, abdominal mass, ±racoon eyes, ±skull nodules	1–4 yrs
Paraplegia	<5 yrs
Refusal to bear weight	<1–5 yrs
Opsiclonus/myoclonus	>1–5 yrs
Intractable diarrhea	<1–>5 yrs
Horner syndrome	<1–>5 yrs
Hypertension	<1–>5 yrs
Posterior mediastinal mass on incidental radiograph	2 yrs to teenage

pelvis, or intra-abdominally. This tumor commonly metastasizes to bone, bone marrow, skin, liver, and lymph nodes. The protean presentations of neuroblastoma are listed in Table 87-11.

After CNS tumors, neuroblastoma is the most common solid tumor of childhood. Approximately 50% occur in children before the age of 2 years, and 80% are found in children under 5 years. Neuroblastoma occurs in approximately one of 100,000 children under 16 years of age.

Data Gathering

Approximately two thirds of patients present with widespread metastases. Signs and symptoms include irritability, anorexia, weight loss, pallor, and subcutaneous lumps. Adrenal neuroblastoma, as well as nonadrenal intra-abdominal tumors, can cause a palpable abdominal mass. When the cervical sympathetic ganglia are involved, Horner syndrome (ptosis, miosis, anhidrosis) can be seen on the affected side, or hoarseness arising from recurrent laryngeal nerve compression can occur. Spinal cord compression syndrome can occur when neuroblastoma arising in sympathetic ganglia extend into and out of the intervertebral foramina. This condition is often referred to as a "dumbbell tumor." Thus, rapidly occurring paraplegia in a child under 5 years of age should be considered neuroblastoma unless another cause has been proved. Skeletal lesions lead to bone pain or pathologic fractures. When periorbital metastasis occurs, proptosis and periorbital ecchymosis or "black eyes" are noted. The physician should not confuse these black eyes for those associated

with battered children. Rarer presentations include opsomyoclonus ("dancing eyes-dancing feet"), hypertension, tachycardia, skin flushing, and chronic diarrhea all manifested as a result of excessive catecholamine secretion from the tumor itself.

Infants with a rare characteristic of neuroblastoma (noted as stage IV-S) demonstrate the ability of the tumor to undergo spontaneous regression or mature to a more benign lesion. These children present in the first few months of life with gross hepatomegaly or skin nodules. The primary tumor may not be obvious. When the primary physician encounters massive hepatomegaly in an otherwise healthy-appearing child, the diagnosis of stage IV-S neuroblastoma should be considered.

Once neuroblastoma is suspected, the evaluation should include a CBC count, abdominal ultrasound or CT scan, chest radiograph, skeletal survey, bone scan, and bone marrow aspiration and biopsy. The latter two procedures are best performed by those physicians prepared to treat the tumor. Patients should have quantitative evaluation of urinary catecholamine levels, including vanillylmandelic acid and homovanillic acid, along with other serologic markers, such as ferritin, which can be obtained at the regional center just prior to surgery.

Management

Surgery cures most tumors totally or near totally resected. Chemotherapy may shrink some unrectable tumors, making them resectable. Chemotherapy and autotherapy marrow transplant are used to treat disseminated neuroblastoma.

Even though the majority of the disseminated tumors respond initially to therapy, most will become refractory to treatment and the disease is often fatal.

RHABDOMYOSARCOMA

Rhabdomyosarcoma arises from striated muscle and is the most common soft-tissue sarcoma of children under 15 years of age, accounting for 6% of all pediatric malignancies. The annual incidence of this tumor is 8.4 in 1,000,000 white children and 3.9 in 1,000,000 black children. Approximately 70% of cases present before the child is 10 years of age. The peak incidence is between 2 to 6 years of age (median age, 5 years), but there is also a considerable number of adolescents with retroperitoneal, chest wall, or extremity rhabdomyosarcoma or other related soft-tissue sarcoma.

Data Gathering

Sarcomas usually occur as a lump in soft tissues. This lump may be painless or painful, and specific symptoms may depend on the location of the tumor. Orbital tumors cause rapidly developing unilateral proptosis. Nasopharyngeal tumors can present with recurrent epistaxis, chronic sinusitis, chronic nasal obstruction, or dysphagia. Middle ear rhabdomyosarcoma can cause chronic otitis media, ear pain, and cranial nerve palsies. Neck tumors can cause dysphagia, hoarseness, or simply a painless lump in the posterior cervical triangle. Urinary tract obstruction or constipation usually is produced when rhabdomyosarcoma arises in the bladder or the prostate. In girls, sarcoma botryoides of the vagina or uterus may present as protrusion of hemorrhagic polyps from the introitus. In a paratesticular region, the tumor presents as an expanding nontender mass in the scrotum, usually located above and separate from the testis; this mass may be confused with a hernia and may be associated with a hydrocele. In the extremities or trunk, a painless mass is the most frequent presentation. Metastasis commonly occurs to the lungs, CNS, bones, liver, bone marrow, and regional lymph nodes. Head and neck tumors usually extend to the base of the skull.

All children with this histologic diagnosis proven with biopsy should have a CBC count and bone marrow evaluation. Radiography of the primary tumor site and the lungs and bone scans should be obtained. All patients with head and neck tumors should undergo tomography of the base of the skull and/or whole-brain CT or MRI. Other tests, such as examination of cerebrospinal fluid, bone radiographs intravenous pyelography, MR imaging, cystography, lymphangiography, and gallium scanning may be indicated depending on the primary site of the tumor.

The primary care physician, when confronted with a soft-tissue mass in a child, should consider cancer in the differential diagnosis and promptly begin the evaluation and biopsy of the mass, or refer the child to a physician or surgeon trained in the care and treatment of the disease. No therapy should be instituted until the final outcome of the staging procedures listed previously are available.

Bone Tumors

Malignant tumors of bone are sarcomas that arise from the cells of cortical or cancellous bone (osteosarcoma) or reticuloendothelial cells of the marrow (Ewing tumor).

Osteosarcoma and Ewing tumor are most common during adolescence, with 50% of the cases diagnosed in the second decade. Approximately 300 cases are diagnosed in the United States each year, giving an incidence of approximately three in 1,000,000 children under the age of 15 years. Sixty percent of all osteosarcomas occur just above or below the knee. Although osteosarcoma shows no racial predilection, Ewing's tumor is an exceedingly rare tumor in blacks.

Data Gathering

Patients with malignant bone tumors complain of pain or a painful lump that frequently is realized after a notable episode of trauma. This lump occasionally may be associated with hemorrhage into the tumor. The pain is usually at night and may awaken the patient. Although most patients with osteosarcoma are well, approximately one third of those with Ewing tumor will have some constitutional symptoms such as fever, weight loss, anorexia, and malaise.

When the tumor occurs in an extremity, examination may reveal a hard, tender swelling. Larger tumors may feel warm, owing to increased vascularity. Trunk lesions, especially those arising in the pelvis, are difficult to diagnose. Because the mass is buried deep in gluteal tissue, neither radiography nor physical examination may offer any clues. These tumors often are massive in size when finally revealed by CT scan, MRI, or pelvic ultrasound.

Bone tumors usually require radiographs and a biopsy of the lesion for confirmation. Plain radiographs may reveal changes associated with a destructive process in bone: "Codman triangle" created from periosteal elevation and the typical "sunburst" appearance produced by tumor blood vessels growing perpendicularly into extracortical tumor tissue. Later, one may see an "onion skin" periosteal reaction caused by repetitive episodes of the lesion pushing out the periosteum and the periosteum responding by producing calcium.

A bone scan or MRI will be especially useful in diagnosing Ewing's tumor if the history and physical examination suggest that trauma alone cannot account for the pain. Other studies including determinations of CBC count, sedimentation rate, and serum alkaline phosphatase in osteogenic sarcoma are often useful. A chest radiograph should be obtained to determine whether there are obvious metastases. This should be correlated further with chest CT.

Once any infectious process has been ruled out, a biopsy is indicated. This procedure should be performed by an orthopedic surgeon who has expertise in the total management of neoplastic bone lesions. The biopsy also must be performed with regard for future attempts at limb preservation at the time of definitive surgery. The clinical course of osteosarcoma is that of a highly malignant neoplasm. The tumor rapidly disseminates hematogenously, with pulmonary metastases generally being the first site of recurrent disease. Prior to recent advances in therapy, metastatic disease occurred within 6 to 9 months from the time of diagnosis, with death ensuing 6 months later. Following the development of pulmonary metastases, dissemination to other bones and visceral organs frequently occurs. With the use of chemotherapy and surgery for osteosarcoma and chemotherapy, surgery, and radiation therapy for Ewing tumor, the incidence of metastases has decreased and those patients who still do develop pulmonary metastases tend to have fewer with a later onset. Today, approximately 60% of patients with osteosarcoma or Ewing tumors are cured.

PRINCIPLES AND COMPLICATIONS OF CANCER THERAPY

Over the past three decades, combinations of surgery, chemotherapy, and radiation therapy have brought about long-term survival and possible cure to as many as two of three children with cancer (Fig. 87-1). The first step for patients with solid tumors is usually surgery to remove as much tumor as possible and to provide tissue for diagnosis. Surgery is rarely curative. Radiation therapy provided to the surgical bed and, perhaps, to areas of local extension can prove curative when added to surgery in children with brain tumors. Most often, tumors require chemotherapy. Chemotherapy treats not only the local area of tumor extension but also treats distant sites of disease. Children with leukemia are treated primarily with chemotherapy. Most children are treated using either

national collaborative protocols or institutional pilot protocols, which are the primary tool used in advancing the state of the art while at the same time providing national standard treatment protocols.

Virtually all malignancies are treated with more than one chemotherapy agent. The use of several drugs reduces the likelihood of the development and growth of resistant tumor populations. If unchecked, these resistant cells eventually will manifest themselves as recurrent or metastatic disease. In many circumstances, chemotherapy or radiation therapy will be used in a prophylactic or adjuvant way; that is, even though the tumor has been completely removed with surgery, therapy is given to prevent the development of metastases rather than treat residual tumor. For example, children with ALL receive intrathecal chemotherapy or intrathecal chemotherapy plus cranial irradiation before the development of leukemic meningitis. This type of prophylactic therapy has made the development of leukemic meningitis, once a common source of treatment failure, a rare event.

Extremely high doses of chemotherapy, once considered too toxic to be used safely, are currently used during bone marrow transplantation. In this procedure, the patient is treated with ablative doses of chemotherapy followed by reinfusion of either their own previously stored bone marrow or bone marrow from a matched donor. Although this procedure is highly toxic, it has added significantly to the cure rate for acute myeloid leukemia and is the only curative therapy for chronic myeloid leukemia. The role of bone marrow transplantation in ALL and solid tumors is investigational.

Most cancer chemotherapy acts by disturbing the normal biochemistry of DNA, RNA, or protein synthesis of proliferating cells. Unfortunately, there is little distinction between the effects on malignant proliferating cells and normal proliferating cells. It is the effect on normal tissue that results in the substantial toxicity from chemotherapy. The toxic effect of chemotherapy includes bone marrow suppression with leukopenia causing immune suppression, anemia, and thrombocytopenia, which can predispose a patient to bruising and bleeding. Nonhematologic toxicity includes an ulcerative mucositis to the gastrointestinal tract and renal insufficiency. It is important to make the point that the most common cause of death in children with cancer, other than the malignancy itself, is infection.

The care and cure of children with cancer has been greatly facilitated by substantial improvements in the supportive care of children receiving treatment.

INFECTION IN THE COMPROMISED HOST

Three infectious conditions occur in the immunocompromised cancer patient: 1) fever and neutropenia, 2) interstitial pneumonitis, and 3) serious viral illness from viruses generally not dangerous in the general population. Most other infections can be managed as in an otherwise healthy child.

Fever and Neutropenia

Neutropenia requiring emergent intervention is defined as an absolute neutrophil count of less than 500/µL and falling. Fever is defined as three temperature readings above 38° C in 24 hours or a single temperature over 38.5° C. Fever, a highly reliable sign of infection, may often be the only sign. However, in patients who have received steroid therapy for months even fever may be suppressed, and clinical deterioration may be the only sign of sepsis. Most ill-appearing children on chemotherapy should be considered septic until proven otherwise. Only 25% of febrile neutropenic patients have microbiologically documented infection. Most bacterial infections are caused by endogenous flora, *Escherichia coli, Staphylococcus aureus,* or *Pseudomonas* species, which have become invasive because of altered host defenses. Although it is recommended that blood and urine cultures be obtained, routine lumbar punctures are not indicated unless the child has clinical symptoms of meningitis. A chest radiograph is warranted in any child with pulmonary symptoms. The child should be treated promptly with broad-spectrum antibiotics, which cover the most common pathogens. Combinations of an antistaphylococcal penicillin or cephalosporin plus an aminoglycoside plus an anti–*Pseudomonas* penicillin are recommended. Some hospitals are able to provide adequate empiric coverage with a single agent, usually a third-generation cephalosporin with antipseudomonal activity, depending on the prevalent pathogens in that community. Specific agents are best discussed with the subspecialist. Shock must be corrected promptly.

Fungal disease is also a cause of fever in neutropenic patients. Candidial esophagitis occurs in some patients receiving steroids and presents as dysphagia and substernal pain or unexplained vomiting. Other invasive fungal diseases occur such as aspergillosis in hospitalized patients receiving antibacterial antibiotics and having prolonged neutropenia. The treatment of choice for invasive fungal disease in most cases is amphotericin B. Most oncologists now add amphotericin B empirically to treat persistent (beyond 6 days) or recurrent fever in the neutropenic patient. Simple thrush can be treated with nystatin, clotrimazole, or fluconazole.

Interstitial Pneumonitis

Twenty years ago, *Pneumocystis carinii* pneumonitis was the leading cause of death in children with lymphoblastic leukemia in remission. Now most children who are at risk for this pneumonia receive prophylactic therapy with oral trimethoprim-sulfamethoxazole. Nonetheless, children not receiving or not complying with prophylaxis are still at risk: *Pneumocystis* pneumonia presents as cough, fever, progressive tachypnea, and cyanosis. Hypoxemia in excess of clinical symptoms is highly suggestive. Chest radiographs show interstitial pneumonitis with prominent hilar infiltrates. Bronchoalveolar layers or open lung biopsy for diagnostic confirmation is most helpful. If a diagnostic procedure is not possible, susceptible children are admitted, given trimethoprim-sulfamethoxazole, observed, and reevaluated. Other causes of interstitial pneumonia include: cytomegalovirus, common respiratory viruses, *Mycoplasma* pneumonia, and, rarely, legionnaires' disease or fungal disease, as well as radiation- or chemotherapy-induced pneumonitis.

Varicella and Rubeola

Although varicella and rubeola do not usually cause life-threatening infections in healthy children, they can be fatal in children with leukemia or lymphoma or in children who have had extensive irradiation and immunosuppressive therapy with agents such as steroids or cyclophosphamide. Varicella can cause pneumonitis, encephalitis, hepatitis, and a hemorrhagic diathesis with disseminated intravascular coagulation. Varicella should be treated promptly with intravenous acyclovir. All chemotherapy, except long-term steroid administration, should be stopped.

More importantly, fatal varicella can be prevented. Protection and prevention are achieved by the parents advising the child's school and friends about the risk of varicella and asking them to acknowledge exposures promptly. Administration of varicella-immune globulin (VZIG) within 72 hours of exposure will attenuate or abort the disease. The child's oncologist should be contacted to discuss interruption of chemotherapy and administration of steroids tapered to replacement levels. Children should receive VZIG if they have a household contact or if they have been playing closely with a child who develops varicella. The disease is contagious 24 hours before the rash and until all lesions have become scabs. Varicella vaccine recently has been licensed, but a consensus regarding the appropriate indications is lacking.

Zoster, or shingles, is common in children with Hodgkin disease or leukemia or in marrow transplant recipients. Zoster also should be treated with intravenous acyclovir.

Children who have received adequate immunization with measles, mumps, and rubella (MMR) vaccine should be immune to rubeola. Those inadequately or unimmunized should receive 0.05 mL/kg of immune serum globulin immediately on exposure and, usually, chemotherapy should be stopped.

Common Childhood Illnesses

If a child does not have neutropenia, is not seriously ill, is not receiving prolonged steroid therapy, is not at risk for *Pneumocystis* pneumonia, and does not have varicella or rubeola, then it is likely that most illnesses can be treated according to the principles of good pediatric practice. Otitis, mild bronchopneumonia, streptococcal pharyngitis, and urinary tract infection can be treated with specific appropriate antibiotics. Bactericidal antibiotics rather than bacteriostatic antibiotics should be used. Rubella, mumps, infectious mononucleosis, enteroviruses, and influenza do not require special care or precautions. Hepatitis B infection is becoming less common because of screening of blood products, but children with leukemia who are hepatitis B surface antigen (HBsAg)-positive shed

extraordinarily high quantities of virus in saliva and stool.

NONINFECTIOUS SIDE EFFECTS OF CANCER AND CANCER THERAPY

In addition to predisposing to leukopenia and opportunistic infection, cancer therapy also causes anemia and thrombocytopenia. Anemia is well tolerated, but packed red blood cell transfusions are used to maintain a hemoglobin level of approximately 8 g/dL in patients who are unlikely to be able to make their own erythrocytes and who are ill or symptomatic. Spontaneous bruising and bleeding occur with platelet counts of under 10,000/μL. Platelets are not given routinely for prophylaxis because they increase the risk of platelet resistance. However, 0.1 U/kg or 4 U/m^2 (maximum of 6 U) are given for bleeding or in patients with falling platelet counts who repeatedly bleed at counts under 20,000/μL. Children with thrombocytopenia should avoid contact sports and should receive platelets for trauma. Blood products should be irradiated to avoid graft-vs-host disease in leukopenic patients and, if possible, cytomegalovirus-negative or leukocyte-depleted blood products should be used in children who are candidates for bone marrow transplant.

Like the marrow, the intestinal tract is susceptible to transient damage from therapy. This condition most often manifests itself as oral ulcers and denuded mucosa. Local and systemic analgesics, good oral hygiene (brushing with a soft toothbrush), a diet with cool bland foods, and, sometimes antibiotics are helpful. Patients should be seen by the dentist for prophylactic care, and dental problems should be treated as soon as possible to avoid abscesses as sources of infection.

Specific drugs have some unusual side effects that should be recognized. These effects are in Table 87-12. It should be noted that temporary hair loss, nausea and vomiting, and hematopoietic toxic effects are almost universal.

IMMUNIZATIONS

Although children may receive diphtheria-pertussis-tetanus (DPT) and influenza immunizations, it is usually best to postpone immuniza-

TABLE 87-12
Acute and Delayed Toxic Effects of Commonly Used Chemotherapeutic Agents

DRUG	ACUTE TOXIC EFFECTS*	DELAYED TOXIC EFFECTS*
Bleomycin	2,7,8	E[†]
Cisplatin	1,2,3,6,13,15	D[†],F[†]
Carboplatin	1,2,3,6,8,12	F[†]
Corticosteroids	See Chapter 78	
Cyclophosphamide	1,2,3,4,6,14,15	A[†],E[†],I[†]
Cytarabine	1,2,3,4,6,7,12	
Dacarbazine	1,2,3,7	
Dactinomycin	1,2,3,5,6,12	B,E[†]
Daunorubicin	1,2,3,5,6,8	B,C[†],E[†]
Doxorubicin	1,2,3,5,6,8	B,C[†],E[†]
Ifosfamide	1,2,3,4,6,14	A,I
L-Asparaginase	7,8,9,10,12	
Melphalan	1,2,3,4,5,6,7	A,I[†]
Mercaptopurine	3,4,6,10	
Methotrexate	1,2,3,4,6,7,10,12	E[†],H
Nitrogen mustard	1,2,3,4,6	A[†],I[†]
Nitrosoureas (lomustine, carmustine)	1,2,3,4,6,7,13	A,D,E,I
Procarbazine	1,3,4,12	I
Thioguanine	3,4,6,10,12	H
Vincristine	2,5,7,11,13,15	
Vinblastine	2,3,5,11	
VM-26 (teniposide), VP-16 (etoposide)	1,2,3,8,11	I

*Explanation of codes: 1, indicates nausea and vomiting; 2, alopecia; 3, myelosuppression; 4, immunosuppression; 5, tissue necrosis with extravasation; 6, mucosal ulceration; 7, fever; 8, urticaria; 9, pancreatitis; 10, chemical hepatitis; 11, neuromuscular pain; 12, rash; 13, renal tubular damage; 14, hemorrhagic cystitis; and 15, syndrome of inappropriate antidiuretic hormone. A, indicates sterility; B, radiation recall; C, cardiac failure; D, renal failure; E, pulmonary fibrosis; F, hearing loss; H, hepatic fibrosis; and I, secondary leukemia.
[†]Effect enhanced by radiation therapy.

tion until 3 to 6 months after chemotherapy is completed. Inactivated (Salk) poliomyelitis vaccine and influenza vaccine may be given. Live poliomyelitis vaccine should not be given to children receiving chemotherapy or their siblings. Inactivated vaccine can be given to siblings. If a sibling receives live poliomyelitis vaccine, the children should be separated. Current recommendations are for 4 to 6 weeks of separation, but these recommendations apply more to recent marrow transplant recipients or for children with severe combined immune deficiency. In children with leukemia it is practical for siblings to avoid any form of fecal-oral contact so that dishes, clothing, towels, and so forth should be kept separate and physical contact and close play avoided. Likewise MMR vaccine should not be given, because measles vaccine may lead to fatal rubeola. γ-Globulin is indicated for protection after exposure to measles or hepatitis A. Haemophilus influenzae B vaccine has been recommended for compromised hosts, and there are data to show that children receiving chemotherapy can respond to H. influenzae–diphtheria conjugate vaccine.

GROWTH AND DEVELOPMENT

Growth is retarded during chemotherapy and radiation therapy. At the time of cessation of therapy, there is usually substantial catch-up growth, although ultimately there may be a reduction in predicted stature. If high doses (>3,000 rad) and large-field irradiation have been used, particularly to the brain, chest, or spine, major growth disturbances occur; skeletal and soft-tissue abnormalities appear months and years later. Late-onset damage to heart and lung are also of great concern. Radiation therapists who specialize in the care of children attempt to minimize these sequelae by limiting the dose and field of irradiation as much as possible.

Children and pubertal or postpubertal patients who have received alkylating agents (cyclophosphamide, melphalan, nitrogen mustard, lomustine, carmustine, busulfan, chlorambucil) or irradiation to the gonads are likely to suffer gonadal failure. This condition may present as delay to develop secondary sex characteristics or more likely infertility. Boys are more susceptible than girls. These problems should have been or should be discussed by the subspecialist who has obtained informed consent for therapy. Thyroid function and pituitary function may be damaged by irradiation to these glands.

Most children are able to resume normal activities and to return to school within weeks or months of diagnosis. However, some therapies may interfere with cognitive development. High doses of irradiation to the brains of infants and young children with primary brain tumors may cause major learning disabilities. In the young child with leukemia, the combinations of moderate doses of irradiation and methotrexate and overt CNS leukemia may cause learning disabilities. Children should be tested and placed in appropriate classes if learning disabilities occur. More importantly, there is much ongoing research about therapeutic alternatives to avoid these problems.

NUTRITION

Parents have many questions regarding nutrition and receive spurious unsolicited advice about nourishing their children. Few guidelines exist, and cancer and some cancer therapy cause wasting and malnutrition. There is no firm evidence that maintenance of an absolutely normal nutritional status favorably or unfavorably influences the outcome of disease. Parenteral hyperalimentation is used for malnourished children without a properly functioning intestine; nighttime nasogastric feeding may be used in the anorectic wasted child who has a normal intestinal tract. General dietary recommendations are the same as for a healthy child, except that when mucosal ulceration is severe, bland, cold foods are soothing. Megadose vitamins are contraindicated. Children may take vitamin supplements that provide the minimal daily requirements of essential vitamins; however, folic acid folinic acid should not be given routinely to children receiving methotrexate. Supplemental iron is usually not necessary because the anemia of cancer comes from arrested production of erythrocytes or low-grade hemolysis, and not from iron deficiency.

DISEASE RECURRENCE AND SECOND TUMORS

Most recurrences occur within the first 2 years after diagnosis. Brain tumors tend to recur with symptoms of headache, vomiting, seizures, and weakness or cranial nerve abnormalities; rarely, they metastasize to the spinal cord or outside the CNS to bone or marrow. Other solid tumors metastasize most commonly to lung, which is frequently detected on routine surveillance radiographs. The tumors occasionally recur at their original site. Leukemia may recur in marrow and often shows itself by reproducing the symptoms that occurred at diagnosis. In approximately 5% of patients, leukemia recurs in the nervous system as leukemic meningitis. This condition may be silent or may cause meningeal signs and symptoms. In boys, leukemia may appear in the testis as painless, hard testicular enlargement.

In most cancers recurrence is a sinister event in that it often means that cure is unlikely. However, in some tumors, such as Wilms tumor, Hodgkins disease, and, rarely, in osteosarcoma and acute leukemia, major changes in treatment strategy appear to be allowing increasing numbers of patients who have had a relapse to achieve long-term survival and possible cure. Patients who do recur can benefit with prolongation of life by a participating in trials of investigational chemotherapy.

COMMUNICATION

Because of the complexity and cost of care of children with cancer, it is necessary for most families to have access to a number of physicians. Currently, many primary care physicians are helping to care for these children by administering chemotherapy or blood products as prescribed by the subspecialist, monitoring blood counts, evaluating and treating intercurrent infections, coordinating activities with the school and other organizations, and caring for the handicapped or dying child. The participation of the primary care physician is essential to help relieve the financial and emotional strain that cancer brings on a family. For the physician the work is gratifying and challenging. However, for shared care to be safe and efficacious, mutual trust and written and verbal communication between the community physician and the cancer center are essential.

Finally, the Leukemia Society, the American Cancer Society, the Candlelighters (a national organization that provides an accurate, incisive newsletter for parents and physicians), and many local charitable and paramedical organizations are invaluable resources in the care of the child with cancer. Local hospice organizations may provide assistance to the family of a child dying at home.

THE CONCEPT OF CURE

Defining "cure" for a child with cancer is not simple. Terms such as "long-term disease-free survival" or "no evident disease" are more likely expressions of our own clinical inadequacies. An equally important problem is that the disease and its treatment frequently are associated with sequelae that prevent complete restoration to normal health or that alter subsequent growth and development.

The primary care clinician should realize that the diagnosis and treatment of cancer, albeit far superior to any prior science and technology thus seen in modern medicine, must still resolve several difficult issues. The construction of medical treatment regimens that minimize acute and late effects and the design of intervention strategies to reduce the psychologic and social impact of the disease on children and families must be further researched.

Society must also undergo some degree of modification of attitudes so that as the number of survivors increase, more acceptance in the community is realized.

BIBLIOGRAPHY

Cline MJ: The molecular basis of leukemia, *N Engl J Med* 330:328–336, 1994.

Constine LS, Woolf PD, Cann D, et al: Hypothalamic-pituitary dysfunction after radiation for brain tumors, *N Engl J Med* 328:87–94, 1993.

Crist WM, Kun LE: Common solid tumors of childhood, *N Engl J Med* 324:461–471, 1991.

Curtis RE, Boice JD Jr, Stovall M: Risk of leukemia after chemotherapy and radiation treatment for breast cancer, *N Engl J Med* 326:1745–1751, 1992.

Davis AM, Bell RS, Goodwin PJ: Prognostic factors in osteosarcoma: A critical review, *J Clin Oncol* 12:423–431, 1994.

Duffner PK, Horowitz ME, Krischer JP, et al: Postoperative chemotherapy and delayed radiation in children less than three years of age with malignant brain tumors, *N Engl J Med* 328:1725–1731, 1993.

Egeler RM, D'Angio GJ: Langerhans cell histiocytosis, *J Pediatr* 127:1–11, 1995.

Lipshultz SE, Colan SD: Late cardiac effects of doxorubicin therapy for acute lymphoblastic leukemia in childhood, *N Engl J Med* 324:808–815, 1991.

Neglia JP, Meadows AT, Robison LL, et al: Second neoplasms after acute lymphoblastic leukemia in childhood, *N Engl J Med* 325:1330–1336, 1991.

Pappo AS, Shapiro DN, Crist WM, Maurer HM: Biology and therapy of pediatric rhabdomyosarcoma, *J Clin Oncol* 13:2123–2139, 1995.

Pollack IF: Brain tumors in children, *N Engl J Med* 331:1500–1507, 1994.

Pizzo PA: Management of fever in patients with cancer and treatment-induced neutropenia, *N Engl J Med* 328:1323–1332, 1993.

Pizzo PA, Poplack DG: *Principles and practice of pediatric oncology,* ed 2, Philadelphia, 1993, JB Lippincott.

Pui CH: Childhood leukemias, *N Engl J Med* 332:1618–1630, 1995.

Rivera GK, Pinkel D: Treatment of acute lymphoblastic leukemia: 30 years' experience at St. Jude Children's Research Hospital, *N Engl J Med* 329:1289–1295, 1993.

Willman CL, Busque L: Langerhans'-cell histiocytosis (histiocytosis X)—A clonal proliferative disease, *N Engl J Med* 331:154–160, 1994.

CHAPTER 88

Sickle Cell Disease

Kim Smith-Whitley
Kwaku Chene-Frempong

BACKGROUND

The term *sickle cell disease* refers to all disorders in which the presence of sickle hemoglobin (Hb S) in the red blood cells (RBCs) leads to a chronic hemolytic disease characterized by vasoocclusive complications. Hb S is produced as a result of the inheritance of the β^S-globin gene, a variant of the normal β^A-globin gene. An A → T mutation in the 6th codon of the β-globin gene alters the normal GAG (codon for glutamic acid) to GTG (codon for valine). The substitution of valine for glutamic acid is the only difference between Hb A $(\alpha^A_2\beta^A_2)$ and Hb S $(\alpha^A_2\beta^S_2)$. The globin genes are autosomal codominant so that individuals inheriting β^A-globin gene from one parent and β^S-globin gene from the other, produce both Hb A and Hb S in their RBCs. These individuals are said to have sickle cell trait.

Other globin gene abnormalities that interact with the B^S-gene to form common variants of sickle cell disease are B^C and $(\beta^{6:\ Glu\ \rightarrow\ Lys})$ and the β thalassemia syndromes. The β^S gene is found predominantly in people of African descent including those of the Mediterranean and Middle Eastern regions and in those of Indian origin. In the United States, 8.5% of blacks have sickle cell trait compared with 15% to 20% in West and Central Africa. The β^C gene is found most commonly in people of West African origin where the prevalence is of the order of 5% to 15%. Approximately 3% of blacks are heterozygous for the β^C gene.

There are four common types of sickle cell disease: SS, SC, Sβ⁺ thalassemia, and Sβ° thalassemia. SS is the most common and often the most severe type. SC is generally less severe, whereas Sβ° thalassemia is as severe as SS. Sβ⁺ thalassemia is the least severe of the common types

of sickle cell disease. Both types of Sβ thalassemia comprise approximately 8%, SC approximately 28%, and SS approximately 63% of sickle cell disease patients in the United States. Combinations of Hb S and other β hemoglobinopathies comprise less than 1%.

The pathophysiology of sickling disorders may be thought of in terms of three interacting processes: 1) chronic hemolytic anemia and its consequences, 2) acute and chronic vasoocclusive tissue damage, and 3) organ failure as a result of the combined effects of processes 1 and 2. Most of the complications of sickle cell disease can be explained on the basis of these processes.

The amino acid substitution in Hb S results in a hemoglobin that is insoluble and polymerizes when deoxygenated. Sickling of RBCs results from the physical distortion and membrane damage caused by the Hb S polymers (fibers). Sickle cells hemolyze easily and have a shortened life span. The usual hemoglobin level is between 6 and 9 g/dL in patients with SS or Sβ° thalassemia and between 10 and 13 g/dL in those with SC and Sβ⁺ thalassemia.

Sickle cells are rigid and not pliable enough to pass through capillaries and precapillary arterioles. They also cause damage to the endothelial lining of large vessels. The damaged vessels develop intimal hyperplasia and thickened walls and become severely stenosed or completely occluded. It is likely that the acute vasoocclusive events such as painful episodes, stroke, and acute chest syndrome involve primarily the occlusion of large vessels, whereas occlusion of capillaries is a constant feature of the disease and contributes to chronic organ damage.

The high level of hemoglobin F present in the RBCs in the newborn protects the cells from sickling in the first few months of life. By approximately 6 months of age, however, the child is susceptible to most of the acute problems encountered in older patients. The most important effect on the young child is the increased susceptibility to serious infection, particularly sepsis and meningitis.

Although many defects in the immune defenses of the sickle cell patient have been found, the most important seems to be the loss of the reticuloendothelial function of the spleen, termed *functional hyposplenia.* Splenic function can be lost even while the organ is enlarged. The spleen's filtering function is most important for encapsulated organisms, such as *Streptococcus pneumoniae* and *Haemophilus influenzae.* The young patient who has not developed many antibodies is most susceptible, particularly to sepsis and meningitis, but the increased risk of infection persists throughout life.

TESTING FOR SICKLING CONDITIONS

Testing for sickle cell disease is recommended for all newborns in the United States. The diagnosis can be made in newborns with several methods including isoelectric focusing, high-pressure liquid chromatography, and citrate agar gel electrophoresis. Rapid sickling and solubility tests are not suitable for use in infants because their high levels of hemoglobin F may cause these tests to be falsely negative. They should not be used to confirm results from newborn screening. In addition, a positive sickling test must always be followed by definitive tests to distinguish between sickle cell trait (AS) and the various types of sickle cell disease. Family studies help delineate the exact form of sickle cell disease.

Early diagnosis is essential, particularly now that penicillin prophylaxis is begun by 2 months of age.

The early months are an important period for family education and formation of a strong family-physician bond. The family should receive genetic counseling about the risk of having another affected child and about the availability of prenatal diagnosis with amniotic fluid fibroblasts or chorionic villi samples.

The value of screening older children for sickle cell disease or sickle cell trait has not been established.

MANAGEMENT

General Care

Well-child care of the infant or child with sickle cell disease does not differ greatly from that of other children. By 4 to 5 months of age, most infants with SS and S-β°-thalassemia have a mild anemia and reticulocytosis. Some have even lost the reticuloendothelial function of the spleen. Penicillin prophylaxis must be started by the age of 2 months in all children with SS and S-β°-thalassemia. A double-blinded, randomized study showed a significant reduction in incidence and in mortality rates from pneumococcal infection in young children with SS who received 125 mg of penicillin-V twice daily compared with the rates in those who received placebo. The role of prophylaxis in SC and S-β-thalassemia has not been studied. Prophylaxis should continue at least to 5 years of age. The need for penicillin prophylaxis in patients after 5 years of age was not established in a recently concluded study.

Routine immunizations including hepatitis B, *H. influenza* type b, and varicella should be administered to children with sickle cell disease. In addition, the polyvalent pneumococcal vaccine should be administered at 24 months then a booster 4 years later. The available pneumococcal vaccines are not fully protective against invasive pneumococcal infection because several vaccine failures have been reported. The influenza vaccine should be given yearly particularly to those children with a history of acute chest syndrome. It is important for physicians to teach parents that penicillin prophylaxis and appropriate vaccination are not guarantees against serious infection. The child with ACD, fever, and other signs of infection must be managed promptly and aggressively.

Good pediatric care is important for children with sickle cell disease. Screening for iron deficiency and lead poisoning are done as for normal children. Diet should be appropriate for the patient's age. Folic acid, 1 mg daily, may help maintain adequate RBC production. Baseline determinations of hemoglobin and reticulocyte levels and spleen size are important, because they are helpful in assessing the condition of the ill child. Yearly urinalysis and assessment of hepatic and renal function can reveal early changes of chronic organ damage.

Intelligence is not affected by sickle cell disease unless the patient has developed cerebral damage. Although more severely affected patients may miss some school days because of their disease, they should be expected to attend regular class and to perform well. Rarely does a child require tutoring at home.

The patients are generally well adapted to their lower hemoglobin levels. The children should be able to play active games and take gym classes at school. They should be allowed to rest when tired, however, and should not be pushed to perform when fatigued. Because of the loss of the ability to concentrate urine, the children may need to leave class to drink water or to urinate.

Nocturnal enuresis is common past the age of 5 years because of the development of hyposthenuria. Parents should be counseled that this condition is physiologic and will resolve as the bladder capacity increases and the child learns to wake to urinate. Fluid intake should not be restricted because of this obligate water loss, but other usual methods of managing enuresis may be helpful.

Education of the patient and family is extremely important. The significance of fever or pallor as a danger signal must be emphasized. Older patients need help in understanding the implications of the disease for their life. Genetic counseling is important for parents and for older patients. The education should be provided by personnel from the sickle cell center and by the primary physician.

As in other chronic disease, patients and their families may need specialized support services from social workers, psychologists or psychiatrists, and vocational guidance counselors. These services usually can be provided by the sickle cell center working with the patient's own physician.

Examination of the Ill Child

Certain symptoms or complaints that might be minor in normal children may herald a more difficult problem in children with sickle cell disease. These include fever (which might herald a serious infection), unusual fatigue and loss of appetite (acute anemia due to aplastic crisis or acute splenic sequestration), abdominal pain (vasoocclusive pain, pneumonia, biliary disease), pain in the extremities (vasoocclusive pain), weakness (stroke), or a limp (stroke, aseptic necrosis). Severe headache may be a sign of severe anemia or, rarely, stroke.

A careful history is important in evaluating the condition of the sick child. Does the child have fever? Duration and height of the fever as well as any accompanying symptoms should be noted. It is important to note whether the child receives penicillin prophylactically because this information may influence the choice of antibiotics.

The history of fluid intake should be noted. Vomiting, diarrhea, and increased sweating can lead rapidly to dehydration in the sickle cell patient, because the ability to concentrate urine is lost by 4 or 5 years of age.

A careful examination should be performed on any ill patient with sickle cell disease. A site of infection may be found in the febrile child. The degree of pallor and jaundice should be noted. Particular attention should be paid to the chest and abdominal examinations. The size of the spleen should be noted carefully and compared with the usual size in the patient. Swelling of joints or extremities may be due to vasoocclusion but may also signal infection. Signs of neurologic deficit require further neurologic evaluation.

Laboratory studies helpful in evaluating the ill child's condition are the complete blood cell (CBC) count with differential. In addition, the reticulocyte count should be determined to be sure that the child does not have an aplastic crisis. If the child has any respiratory symptoms or signs or has chest or abdominal pain with the fever, a chest radiograph should be obtained. It is common for an infiltrate to be found on the radiograph of a child who has no rales or wheezing.

Transfusions of RBCs play an important role in the care of the sickle cell patient. Although transfusions are not used routinely in the care of most patients, they are essential for the treatment of some acute and chronic problems. The formation of alloantibodies is high in this group of patients. Prior to the first transfusion an extensive RBC typing should be done. The patient receiving long-term RBC transfusions must be monitored for the development of excessive iron stores.

Acute Problems

The most common acute problems in sickle cell disease are listed below. Those problems that can be managed on an outpatient basis are discussed in more detail. Those requiring hospitalization

TABLE 88-1
Common Infections in Sickle Cell Disease

INFECTION	COMMON ORGANISMS	COMMENTS
Sepsis	Streptococcus pneumoniae Haemophilus influenzae Escherichia coli	More frequent in young children
Meningitis	S. pneumoniae H. influenzae	Almost always in young children
Acute chest/pneumonia	S. pneumoniae H. influenzae Mycoplasma pneumoniae	Often no organism identified
Urinary tract infection	E. coli Klebsiella	Often associated with positive blood culture
Osteomyelitis, pyogenic arthritis	Staphylococcus aureus Salmonella species S. pneumoniae	Multiple sites possible
Malaria	Falciparum malariae	In malaria endemic regions

are outlined only sufficiently so that their importance and differential diagnosis can be understood. Sickle cell patients who develop a major complication are best referred to a sickle cell center.

Acute Problems in Sickle Cell Disease

- Infection
- Acute anemic episode
  Splenic sequestration
  Aplastic crisis
- Painful episodes
- Acute chest syndrome
- Cerebrovascular accident
- Priapism

Infections

Infection is the major cause of death in the child less than 5 years of age. Fever must be recognized as a danger signal in patients of every age but particularly in the young child. The infections that have an increased incidence in sickle cell disease are listed in Table 88-1.

The most common serious infections in children are sepsis and meningitis. The risk is greatest for patients with SS or S-β°-thalassemia but is also increased for the other sickling disorders. The most common cause of sepsis and meningitis is *Streptococcus pneumoniae,* but *H. influenzae* and other gram-negative organisms also cause serious disease. Meningitis occurs predominantly in the young child. Sepsis can occur in older children and adults and is more commonly due to gram-negative organisms.

Because bacterial sepsis often cannot be separated clinically from a viral febrile illness, guidelines for management of children with sickle cell disease with fever have been developed. These are discussed below.

Osteomyelitis may occur at any age and is most commonly due to *Salmonella* organisms or *Staphylococcus aureus,* but other organisms may be responsible.

Patients with osteomyelitis may present like those with bone infarct, with localized swelling and warmth. Persistence of fever and localized signs and symptoms should alert the physician to evaluate the patient for osteomyelitis. The most useful test for the diagnosis of osteomyelitis in patients with sickle cell disease is local aspiration for culture.

Urinary tract infections are common in patients with sickling disorders. Patients with pyelonephritis usually have a high fever, a positive urine culture, and signs of toxicity. Because pyelonephritis is frequently accompanied by sepsis, sickle cell patients with findings of urinary tract infection and fever should be admitted for treatment. Bacteriuria not accompanied by fever may be managed on an outpatient basis, with antibiotic coverage based on the organism's sensitivity. The guidelines for investigative studies and suppressive antibiotic coverage are the same as for patients who do not have sickle cell disease.

Salmonella and *Shigella* dysentery are fairly common in patients with sickling disorders. Hospitalization is not needed if the diarrhea is mild, the patient afebrile, and fluid intake can be maintained. Despite not receiving antibiotic therapy, most children recover without complications. In malaria endemic regions of the world, the leading cause of death in young children with sickle cell disease is infection due to *Falciparum malariae*. The patient with fever and no discernible source is a problem. Although most of these episodes will be due to viral infections, some represent sepsis. In the young child sepsis may progress to irreversible septic shock within a few hours. For this reason young children are frequently hospitalized and treated with antibiotics before culture results are known. The scheme used at our center is outlined below.

Management of the Febrile Patient

The management of the young febrile child with sickle cell disease is changing as the incidence of pneumococcal sepsis is decreasing due to early diagnosis and institution of penicillin prophylaxis. Previously, children less than 5 years of age with temperature of 38.5° C or higher were admitted and treated with broad-spectrum antibiotics intravenously after obtaining cultures.

Blood, throat, urine, and cerebrospinal fluid (if indicated) are obtained for cultures. In recent years, several centers have adopted outpatient management plans. Patients with fever who do not appear toxic are evaluated, cultures are obtained, and the patients are treated with parenteral ceftriaxone and discharged to be followed-up as outpatients. The success of this method of management depends on the judgment of the examining physician and the availability of the child for close outpatient monitoring. A follow-up visit within 24 hours for reevaluation may be an added measure of security. Children who look ill initially or later are hospitalized.

The child over 5 years of age who has low-grade fever may be treated as an outpatient in almost all cases if he/she feels well and is in a stable hematologic state. Evaluation of fever includes a thorough history as outlined previously, a complete and careful examination, a CBC count with differential and reticulocyte count, and appropriate cultures. Even with apparently minor infections it may be necessary to hospitalize the patient if the fever is over 39° C, if vomiting or diarrhea may lead to insufficient oral fluid intake, if the fever is accompanied by a vasoocclusive crisis that cannot be managed at home, or if the CBC count reveals a marked decrease in the hemoglobin level or the reticulocyte count.

Acute Anemic Episode

Increased pallor and/or increased fatigue may be due to a fall in the hemoglobin level. This condition can be caused by an aplastic crisis or by acute splenic sequestration.

Because RBC survival is shortened, and markedly so in SS and S-β°-thalassemia, cessation of bone marrow production of RBCs for even a few days can cause a marked fall in the hemoglobin level. Viral infections, particularly infections with parvovirus B19 can cause an aplastic crisis in a patient of any age.

The fall in hemoglobin level occurs over several days. Initially, the child may be more tired than usual, irritable, and play less. The older child may complain of headache. As the hemoglobin level drops farther, the child may lose interest in eating and may refuse to walk. Eventually, usually at hemoglobin levels of 2 to 3 g/dL, congestive heart failure occurs.

If the parents report any of these changes in activity or if the child appears to be paler, a CBC count with reticulocyte count should be obtained. The hemoglobin level will be lower than normal, and the reticulocyte count will be 0 or extremely low. The white blood cell (WBC) and platelet counts may also be low. If marrow recovery has begun, nucleated RBCs and reticulocytes will be present in the peripheral blood.

Treatment depends on the degree of anemia and the stage of recovery. If the hemoglobin value is more than 2 g below the usual level, the patient should be hospitalized for observation and possible transfusion of packed RBCs. If the hemoglobin level is only mildly reduced and, particularly, if there are signs of marrow recovery, the child may be reexamined and the hemoglobin and reticulocyte values determined every day or two until the marrow recovers. The child should rest during this period. If the hemoglobin level continues to fall, the child should then be admitted. The aplasia is transient and lasts several days. Children hospitalized with suspected aplastic crisis should be isolated to protect pregnant caregivers, children with hemolytic anemias, or immunocompromised patients from parvovirus infection.

In acute splenic sequestration, the spleen enlarges and blood pools within, resulting in hypovolemia that may be severe enough to cause shock and death. This condition is a medical emergency, because shock may occur within a few hours. The parents usually report that the child seems irritable and pale. There may be abdominal pain as the spleen enlarges. On physical examination the spleen will be larger than usual and very firm. To be considered acute splenic sequestration, the enlarging spleen should be associated with at least a 2-g/dL drop in the hemoglobin with reticulocytosis and/or nucleated RBCs. Often there is a left shift in the WBC differential and lower total WBC and platelet counts than at steady state. In recent experience, an enlarged spleen associated with anemia, reticulocytopenia, and other cytopenias has been recognized in some children. Parvovirus infection has been documented in some of these cases.

Half of these children have recurrent or severe episodes and may require splenectomy. Splenic fibrosis often occurs in children with SS by 6 years of age, but individuals on chronic transfusion protocols or those with SC or Sβ+-thalassemia may have sequestration episodes into adulthood.

Painful Episodes

The most common acute event in sickle cell disease is the painful episode attributed to vasoocclusion. Many episodes, even some of the more painful ones, can be managed at home. Increased intake of fluids may be helpful. Analgesics ranging from acetaminophen, aspirin, and other nonsteroidal anti-inflammatory drugs (NSAIDs) to codeine and other oral opioids may be used at home. Warmth to the painful areas gives comfort to some patients.

If these measures do not give adequate relief, if the painful episode is accompanied by significant fever, or if vomiting or diarrhea limits the amount of fluid that can be taken, the patient should be seen by a physician.

Often patients are managed in emergency room or other acute care settings. Parenteral analgesics, such as morphine plus oral or parenteral NSAID, are usually given. Suspected infections should be treated. If relief is obtained and oral fluid intake is adequate, the patient can be discharged to be treated at home with further analgesia. If relief is not obtained, the patient is hospitalized.

Pain usually involves one or more bones, particularly the extremities. Bone infarcts, particularly in young children, may produce localized swelling, erythema, and tenderness, similar to signs of osteomyelitis. The child with these findings should be hospitalized for observation and appropriate testing.

The child may have vasoocclusion in the small bones of the hand and/or feet, producing the hand-foot syndrome. Swelling is usually present in both hands and feet at once but may be unilateral, and fever is usually present. Most of these episodes can be managed at home with increased fluid intake and oral analgesics. If the fever is high or the findings suggest an osteomyelitis, the child should be hospitalized.

Vasoocclusive crises in some areas may mimic more serious problems such as an "acute" abdomen that requires surgery or orbital cellulitis. In such cases the patient must be hospitalized for observation and appropriate consultation and testing.

Pain in the abdomen may result from vasoocclusion, acute chest syndrome, urinary tract infection, intrahepatic sickling, acute or chronic cholecystitis, or biliary tree obstruction by gallstones. Careful physical examination and appropriate laboratory tests will help sort out these causes. Pain in the right upper quadrant is often due to biliary or hepatic disease. Children with such pain, particularly if it is accompanied by fever or vomiting, should be admitted for evaluation of their condition.

Because of the hemolytic anemia, gallstones are very common in patients with sickle cell disease. In many patients the gallstones will not produce symptoms while others may be symptomatic. Children with recurrent abdominal pain and gallstones demonstrated on ultrasonography or plain radiography may need referral to a surgeon for consideration of a cholecystectomy.

Acute Chest Syndrome

The acute chest syndrome is a pneumonia-like illness that is common in individuals with sickle cell disease, particularly children less than 5 years of age. The etiology is unknown but thought to be due to either infection, infarction, or a combination of these two. The classic definition is a new infiltrate on chest radiograph. Clinically fever, chest pain, an elevated WBC count, and hypoxia often accompany this syndrome. The clinical course is variable and ranges from a mild respiratory illness to respiratory failure and death. Treatment includes antibiotics, incentive spirometry, supplemental oxygen, and bronchodilator breathing treatments when appropriate. Intravenous hydration should be one to one and a half maintenance at most because aggressive hydration can exacerbate pulmonary edema. Simple or exchange transfusion is recommended for children with moderate to severe respiratory distress and/or hypoxia. Recently, it has been reported that frequent use of incentive spirometer in patients with chest wall pain can reduce the occurrence of acute chest syndrome.

Cerebrovascular Accident

Cerebrovascular accident (CVA) is a major complication of sickle cell disease. Those CVAs that are due to occlusion of large cerebral vessels are common in patients in the first two decades of life and affect 5% of children with SS. Hemorrhagic CVA is more common in older patients and often is due to rupture of vessels in the circle of Willis but may be intracerebral.

Occlusive CVA is most commonly manifested as hemiparesis, aphasia, and/or facial palsy. Sickle cell disease patients with these findings must be hospitalized for immediate intravenous hydration, transfusion, and imaging studies of the brain. Some completed CVAs are preceded by transient neurologic abnormalities, such as limp or temporary aphasia. The findings may be explained on a vascular basis and correspond to transient ischemic episodes. Such symptoms and findings must be taken seriously, and the child's condition must be evaluated by a neurologist. If the diagnosis is transient ischemic attacks (TIA), the patient should also receive transfusions. Imaging of the brain soon after a patient presents with signs of CVA is essential to rule out intracranial hemorrhage that may require surgical intervention. Magnetic resonance imaging (MRI) or computerized tomography (CT) often shows areas of infarction corresponding to the deficits on neurologic examination.

The occurrence of nonspecific neurologic symptoms such as headache or fainting is much more difficult to evaluate. These are sometimes warning symptoms of cerebral vascular disease but may occur for other, more usual reasons. Referral of the child with recurring neurologic symptoms to the sickle cell center is advised.

Recurrence of CVA, which has been reported to be as high as 60%, essentially can be prevented by a chronic transfusion program in which the hemoglobin S level is kept below 30%. Such a program can be done on an outpatient basis.

Intracranial hemorrhage is more common in the adolescent and adult. Warning symptoms such as a severe headache may occur, although some patients are first seen in coma. CT should demonstrate the hemorrhage. Some patients survive, and immediate diagnostic studies and hospitalization are essential.

Priapism

Painful, prolonged erection is an acute problem in some boys with sickle cell disease. This condition may occur before puberty but seems to be more frequent around the time of puberty. Almost all episodes of persistent priapism require hospitalization for intravenous hydration, analgesia, and urologic care. In a mild episode, increased fluid intake and oral analgesia may be sufficient treatment.

Chronic Problems

Almost any organ system can be damaged by repeated occlusion of small vessels by sickled cells. Regular evaluation by the primary care physician may diagnose chronic complications at an early stage. The following are the most common sites of chronic organ damage; selected chronic problems are discussed below.

Chronic Organ Damage

Eye: Retinal vessel proliferation
Bone: Avascular necrosis
Skin: Leg ulcer
Heart: Congestive heart failure
Liver: Chronic liver disease
Kidney: Nephrotic syndrome, chronic renal failure
Lungs: Chronic lung disease

Although chronic damage occurs in the heart, lungs, liver, and kidneys, there is no specific preventive therapy available for these complications. The patient should receive appropriate care for the specific problem. For example, renal transplantation has been successful in patients with sickle cell disease.

Eye

Proliferative retinopathy may threaten the vision of patients with sickle cell disease. Evaluation by a retinal specialist is necessary to detect the early lesions, which can be treated, if necessary, by laser phototherapy. Significant retinal disease is rare before 10 years of age. Thereafter, it increases in frequency and is particularly common in patients with SC disease. These patients should be seen yearly after 7 years of age by a retinal specialist.

Bone

Avascular necrosis of the heads of femur and the humerus is very common in sickle cell disease. By 20 years of age, almost 30% of SS patients have radiographic evidence of avascular necrosis. Although both the hip and shoulder are equally affected, the hips are the usual source of complaints because they are weight bearing. It is usually discovered when the patient complains of pain or develops a limp. The pain is usually chronic but may be acute if synovitis is present. Examination of the involved joint usually shows limitation of motion and pain. Diagnosis is facilitated with radiography of the bones.

The patient should be referred to an orthopedist for treatment. The acute symptoms of synovitis usually are controlled by bed rest with traction. Many patients are able to resume normal activities after a period of non–weight bearing. In some older patients, total hip replacement has been successful, although later revisions will probably be necessary.

Leg Ulcers

Leg ulcers are rare in the first decade of life but increase in frequency after the age of 15 years. Although they are not a major health threat, ulcers result in much time lost from school or work. The exact cause of the ulcers is unknown, but therapy is similar to that for stasis ulcers. Good local care with soaking, dressing changes, and antibiotic ointment, if indicated, is extremely important. Bed rest and elevation of the affected limb may help. In children, an infected cut often leads to ulcer formation; oral antibiotic therapy combined with vigorous local care usually results in rapid resolution of small ulcers. In older patients recovery is often very slow. For resistant ulcers, RBC transfusions given over a period of months and other measures such as local hyperbaric oxygen therapy may be helpful.

Skin grafting often is necessary in ulcer therapy; however, the outcome is not always good. Once the ulcer has resolved, the area should be protected with support hose or socks. Recurrence is very frequent.

General Growth and Development

Infants with sickle cell disease grow and develop normally in the newborn period. A minority of children will later have height and/or weight gains below the normal limits. The physician should be sure that food intake is adequate and that other causes of poor growth have been excluded. Some patients have delayed onset of the pubertal growth spurt and sexual maturation. Bone age is delayed, and endocrine studies suggest a prepubertal state. It is very important to reassure the teenager that puberty will occur in a few years. Infertility is not a problem in sickle cell disease.

Birth control is important in sexually active women, because pregnancy is associated with higher risks for the mother and fetus. Most gynecologists recommend low-dose estrogen pills or barrier methods for these women.

Because of the problems of pregnancy in sickle cell disease, pregnant women should be under the care of obstetricians who specialize in high-risk pregnancies.

Consultations

If possible, the child with sickle cell disease should be seen at a sickle cell center at least twice yearly. This allows the child to be seen by hematologists experienced in the care of chronic complications and also allows the family to take advantage of the educational and psychosocial services of the center. Personnel in centers recognize the valuable role of the primary physician and are willing to work with him/her by telephone. For certain problems, however, the patient is treated best in the center's hospital. Patients with CVA, severe and frequently recurring vasoocclusive complications, and ocular disease are best followed at the center.

Because sickle cell disease affects so many organ systems, many medical and surgical specialists are essential for the best care of the patients. Routine evaluations by a retinal specialist are needed as described previously. Regular dental examinations are also important.

Referrals to surgeons are often necessary for acute or chronic problems such as abdominal pain, gallbladder problems, and leg ulcers. Surgery is frequently performed successfully for patients with sickle cell disease. All patients with sickle cell disease must receive a blood transfusion prior to prolonged general anesthesia for surgical procedures. Simple transfusion to increase hemoglobin level to 10 g/dL has been found to be as effective as aggressive transfusion to decrease Hb S percentage in SS patients. Patients with high hemoglobin levels may require exchange transfusion.

Social workers and psychologists or psychiatrists are extremely helpful in the long-term care of sickle cell patients. They provide educational and vocational advice, emotional support, and family and patient counseling.

Definitive Treatment

Allogeneic bone marrow transplantation has been curative for a few individuals with sickle cell disease. Due to the risk of serious complications bone marrow transplantation is reserved for individuals with serious complications and a suitable sibling bone marrow donor.

Hydroxyurea (Hydrea), a well-known chemotherapeutic agent, has been found to increase the level of fetal hemoglobin in sickle cell disease patients. In a recent study on adult patients with SS, those receiving hydroxyurea experienced fewer painful episodes and acute chest syndrome events with relatively minor side effects. However the long-term toxicity of this drug in individuals with sickle cell disease is unknown. Hydroxyurea is presently being studied in children in a phase I/II trial.

BIBLIOGRAPHY

Charache S, Lubin B, Reed CD, editors: *Treatment of Sickle Cell Disease.* United States Department of Health, Education, and Welfare, 1984, Publication 84-2117.

Embury SE, Hebbel RP, Mohandas N, Steinberg MH, editors: *Sickle Cell Disease. Basic Principles and Clinical Practice,* New York, 1994, Raven Press.

Gaston MH, Verter JI, Woods G, et al: Prophylaxis with oral penicillin in children with sickle cell anemia. A randomized trial. *N Engl J Med* 314:1593, 1986.

PART NINE

Infectious Disease

CHAPTER 89

Part I: HIV Infection in Children and Adolescents

Richard M. Rutstein

ISSUES FOR PEDIATRIC PRIMARY CARE PROVIDERS

With HIV-infected children now reported from all areas of the country, and the numbers of HIV-exposed neonates on the rise, pediatric health care providers must be able to provide the evaluation, testing, and comanagement of this illness, which should be thought of as a primary care illness, and a prototypic family illness.

Central to providing quality care for HIV-exposed/infected patients and their families is maintaining an understanding, compassionate view, nonjudgemental attitude, and the willingness to learn the intricacies of a "new" disease. A good reference point can be found in Box 89-1, which lists the role of the pediatric primary care provider in caring for HIV-exposed/infected infants, children, and adolescents as delineated in clinical practice guidelines (prepared by an expert panel of the United States Public Health Services/Agency of Health Care Policy and Research).

For pediatric HIV infection, all exposed/infected patients are best managed by a linkage between community primary care health care providers and centers dedicated to the care of HIV-infected individuals. The methods of this working relationship will vary from community to community.

This chapter will hopefully assist pediatric primary care providers in delivering these critical services to their patients and their families.

TRANSMISSION

HIV is transmitted by three well-defined routes: parenteral exposure to infective body fluids (almost always blood), sexual contact, and vertical transmission from mother to child. There is no evidence to support transmission by "alternative" methods (*ie,* by casual contact, by mosquito, etc.).

Vertical Transmission
More than 95% of new pediatric HIV infections are acquired perinatally. Since early in the epidemic, it was apparent that the virus was transmitted to some, but not all, exposed newborns. In the United States, vertical transmission rates have ranged from 18% to 30%.

Prevention of Vertical Transmission

One of the major advances in the field of perinatally acquired HIV was the result of the AIDS Clinical Trials Groups 076 protocol. This multisite, double-blinded, randomized study showed conclusively that it is possible to reduce the risk of vertically transmitted HIV infections by the use of zidovudine (ZDV). It is now the national recommendation that all HIV-infected pregnant women be counseled about the benefits of ZDV therapy as it pertains to the prevention of HIV infection in their newborns.

Exposure to Infected Blood

Transfusions of blood products are responsible for 3% to 5% of AIDS cases. HIV has been transmitted through transfusion of infected whole blood, red blood cells, platelets, and plasma.

Since April 1985, all donated blood has been screened for HIV by enzyme-linked immunosorbent assay (ELISA) antibody tests. It is still possible, although very unlikely, to acquire HIV through transfusion of HIV-infective but antibody-negative blood.

Exposure to infected blood via the use of nonsterile needles with illicit drug use still continues unabated and remains a major risk factor for HIV infection. In many areas over 50% of intravenous drug users are HIV infected.

Sexual Contact

Sexual intercourse is responsible for the vast majority of new HIV infections worldwide. It appears that male-to-female transmission is more efficient than female-to-male and that anal receptive intercourse carries a higher risk of transmission than vaginal intercourse.

DATA GATHERING

History

The initial hospital or office visit with any patient or family should include an assessment of HIV risk factors in the parents or patient and possible HIV-related signs and symptoms (Box 89-2). In addition, in this era of more widespread HIV testing, pediatric primary care providers should always inquire as to whether the parents and patient have been previously tested for HIV.

Pediatric primary care providers should recognize that the risk factor assessment will fail to detect many infected persons. For this reason, and the real possibility of preventing vertical transmission of HIV, in 1995 the Centers for Disease Control and Prevention and American Academy of Pediatrics both recommended the routine counseling and voluntary HIV testing of *all* pregnant women.

Clinical Assessment

In the neonatal period, HIV-infected infants rarely manifest any signs or symptoms referable to the infection. HIV-infected infants are not more likely to be preterm, although in general infected newborns have a slightly lower birth weight compared with uninfected babies.

Physical findings associated with HIV infection generally become detectable after the first 2 to 6 months of life, and by age 2 years 90% will have one or more abnormalities on physical examination.

The most common clinical manifestations suggestive of HIV infection in infancy and childhood are noted in Box 89-3.

In recent years, there has been an increase in the numbers of perinatally infected children diagnosed after 6 years of age. There is now an appreciation that many HIV-infected children have a disease course paralleling that of adults,

---

BOX 89-3
Indications for HIV Testing

Parents with high-risk history
Teenagers with sexually transmitted diseases, especially syphilis
History of transfusions before 1986 in parents
Chronic conditions
    Failure to thrive, adenopathy, hepatosplenomegaly
    Chronic thrush
    Chronic or recurrent diarrhea
    Chronic or recurrent parotitis
Severe or recurrent pneumonia
Recurrent invasive bacterial disease
Lymphocytic interstitial pneumonia (reticulonodular pattern) on chest radiograph
Progressive developmental delay/encephalopathy, acquired microcephaly
Idiopathic thrombocytopenic purpura, especially if presentation is atypical

---

BOX 89-4
HIV Testing

ANTIBODY TESTS
  IgG —ELISA
      Western blot
  IgM—Not available
  IgA —Western blot
VIRAL PRODUCTS
  p24 Antigen assay
  ICD p24 antigen assay
DETENTION OF VIRAL GENETIC MATERIAL
  Polymerase chain reaction DNA or RNA testing
VIRAL BLOOD COCULTURE

---

with an asymptomatic phase that may last 5 to 10 years. In older children, the presentation is often subtle, with recurrent bacterial pneumonia, thrush, slowed growth velocity, or weight loss as the symptoms that led to HIV testing. At our center, fully 25% of HIV-infected children diagnosed after the age of 5 years were tested simply because a parent or sibling was diagnosed as HIV infected. This statistic illustrates the necessity of testing all family members once a diagnosis of HIV infection is made in a parent or child.

Testing for the Diagnosis

The standard HIV antibody tests are the ELISA and Western blot assays. By convention, the ELISA is run first and, if repeatedly positive, the Western blot is preformed on the same sample. Using the two tests together results in a very high sensitivity and specificity for detecting HIV infection in a patient over 18 months of age. Any positive test should be repeated on another serum sample, and, if positive again, a diagnosis of HIV infection can be made. *See* Box 89-4 for indications.

Rarely children with perinatal HIV infection will be HIV-antibody negative. In a child with family risk factors and an illness consistent with HIV infection, such as severe failure to thrive or opportunistic infections, further tests should be considered if an initial ELISA is negative.

Diagnosing HIV infection in infancy is more problematic. The standard ELISA and Western blot assays measure IgG class anti-HIV antibodies. Because IgG antibodies readily cross the placenta, *all* full-term infants of HIV-infected

mothers will be antibody positive themselves by virtue of the presence of these maternally derived antibodies. These maternal antibodies may be detectable in the infant's bloodstream until 15 to 18 months of age, with the median time to loss of maternal antibodies of 9 to 12 months. Thus a positive HIV antibody test, in an infant less than 15 months of age, merely confirms the mother's infection status.

Methods of diagnosis of HIV infection in infancy include non-IgG antibody–based tests, viral product–based tests, polymerase chain reaction (PCR) DNA detection assays, and HIV coculture methods (Box 89-5).

One promising test detects IgA class antibody employing a Western blot technique. This assay is not sufficiently sensitive in the first 3 months of life but is reliable and fairly sensitive for older infants. Its greatest use will be in regions where more sophisticated tests are not available.

Any positive result on PCR, coculture, or p24 antigen assay must be repeated before a definitive diagnosis is made to the family. One negative PCR or culture in an HIV-exposed infant is insufficient to rule out HIV infection, and one positive test is insufficient to definatively diagnose what is still ultimately a fatal infection.

Laboratory Evaluation Of Immunologic Function

It is important to assess immunologic function in exposed or infected infants. CD4 counts are used as one measure of immunologic status. It must be remembered that normal CD4 counts are age dependent. In an infant less than 12 months of age, normal values range from 1500 to 5000/mm^3, with a median around 3000/mm^3. In noninfected children, normal CD4 counts trend downward

BOX 89-5
HIV Infection Laboratory Diagnosis in Infants*

			% INFECTED PATIENTS IDENTIFIED			
			1 DAY–		AGE OF PATIENTS	
COST	EASE OF TEST	TEST	2 WEEKS	1 MONTH	3 MONTHS	6 MONTHS
++++	+	Culture	50%	_90%	95%	_95%
+++	++	PCR	50%	_90%	_95%	_95%
+	++++	p24 Ag	17%	NA	16%	15%–20%
+	+++	ICD p24Ag	85%	NA	83%	_80%
+	++++	IgA Western blot	<10%	8%	60%	85%

*All tests had false-positive results in cord blood.

with age until reaching adult values of 700 to 1500/mm³ (median 1000/mm³) by age 6 years. When assessing an HIV-infected child's CD4 count, the primary physician should always evaluate it based on age-appropriate normal ranges. Generally CD4 counts are obtained at 1- to 3-month intervals in infected children and exposed infants in the first year of life.

Serum levels of IgG, IgA, and IgM are elevated in >95% of infected children by 6 months of age. Postimmunization antibody titers should be assessed in all infected children. Yearly anergy panels with PPD are performed in all infected children.

Follow-up Care of the Exposed Infant
Infants born to HIV-infected women should have an initial HIV PCR or coculture performed at 1 month of age, along with determination of the CD4 count. If the viral tests are negative, the test should be repeated by 6 months of age, along with a repeat CD4 count. If the viral tests are negative twice, it is very unlikely that the child is HIV infected. The child should be followed-up in a setting familiar with HIV testing of exposed infants. Repeat HIV antibody tests should be done at 12, 15, and 18 months of age, until two successive tests are negative. If the initial CD4 count is low, this should be followed at the same intervals.

Once the child has seroreverted to antibody-negative status, has at least two negative viral tests, and is thriving with a normal examination, further HIV antibody testing is not indicated. If, however, the child exhibits signs or symptoms consistent with HIV infection, such as general-ized adenopathy, failure to thrive, or recurrent bacterial infections, or laboratory evidence of dysfunction of the immune system, repeat anti-body tests and PCR and/or coculture would be warranted. Consultation with a HIV care spe-cialty site would be indicated as well.

Prognosis in Perinatally Acquired HIV Infection
Survival for infants with perinatally acquired HIV infection follows a bimodal course (Box 89-5). Although the overall prognosis is for a median survival of 6 to 8 years of age, 25% of perinatally infected patients develop rapidly progressive disease. Typically these infants have the onset of severe symptoms in the first year of life, and present with *Pneumocystis carinii* pneu-monia (PCP), severe failure to thrive, or progres-sive encephalopathy. The average survival in this group of children is less than 5 years of age.

For the remaining perinatally infected pa-tients, the median survival now approaches 10 to 12 years. Children in this cohort generally do not develop significant symptoms or illnesses related to HIV until 5 to 10 years of age. Many in this group will survive until their adolescence.

CLINICAL SYNDROMES ASSOCIATED WITH PEDIATRIC HIV INFECTION

Pneumocystis carinii Pneumonia
PCP in HIV-infected infants is a rapidly progres-sive pneumonia. The majority of patients progress to respiratory failure within 24 to 48

BOX 89-6
Major Illnesses—HIV Infected Children

Pneumocystis carinii pneumonia	13%–47%
Lymphoid interstitial pneumonia	20%–30%
Recurrent bacterial infection	17%–23%
Candida esophagitis	14%–18%
Progressive encephalopathy	9%–20%
Disseminated *Mycobacterium* *avium-intracellulare*	3%–18%
Cytomegalovirus-related disease	5%–10%
HIV-related cancers	<5%

hours of presentation. A smaller number of patients have presented with a more indolent 1- to 2-week course of cough and low-grade fever (Box 89-6). The patients are generally febrile, with tachypnea. Rales may be heard on auscultation, but rarely is wheezing detected.

Chest radiographs most commonly reveal a bilateral diffuse alveolar infiltrate. Most patients will have a A-a gradient at presentation. Elevated serum lactic dehydrogenase is noted in more than 90% of patients at the time of diagnosis.

The diagnosis of PCP is made by demonstration of the organism on histochemical stains of sputum, lung lavage fluid, or lung biopsy. PCP may be recovered from lung fluid days after therapy is started; therefore, it is imperative to start therapy whenever PCP is suspected while arranging for definitive diagnosis. First-line therapy is 21 days of intravenous trimethoprim/sulfamethoxazole (20 mg/kg/day) and the concomitant use of corticosteroids.

PCP should be considered in any infant with severe pneumonia or pneumonia unresponsive to routine antibiotics.

Lymphocytic Interstitial Pneumonia

The second most common pediatric AIDS indicator illness is lymphocytic interstitial pneumonia (LIP), frequently diagnosed incidentally by chest radiograph. The classic radiographic finding of LIP is a distinctive diffuse reticulonodular infiltrate, reminiscent of miliary tuberculosis. It is most often found in an HIV-infected child 2 to 4 years of age with a relatively intact immune system. Children with LIP tend to have enlarged parotids and generalized adenopathy. The average survival following a diagnosis of LIP is 6 to 8 years, much longer than for any other AIDS indicator illness.

A large number of children with LIP develop mild reactive airway disease. A smaller proportion of the children will develop symptoms of chronic lung disease, manifested first by shortness of breath on exertion and then resting tachypnea. In more severe cases, right ventricular hypertrophy with corpulmonale will develop.

In symptomatic children (those with a resting pulse oxygen saturation of less than 95%) a lung biopsy is performed to confirm the diagnosis. Once proven to be LIP, the treatment is a 1- to 3-month course of prednisone. Any child on prednisone for LIP also must be maintained on PCP prophylaxis, because chronic steroid use predisposes to the development of PCP.

Progressive Encephalopathy

Up to 25% of infected children will develop a progressive encephalopathy, manifested by the loss of development milestones and acquired microcephaly. Neuroradiologic studies reveal cortical atrophy and basal ganglion calcifications. The course is quite variable, with some children having a plateau phase interspersed with periods of deterioration, whereas others have a relentless downhill course.

Recurrent Invasive Bacterial Infection

Up to 25% of infected patients will have recurrent invasive bacterial infection (defined as two or more episodes of pneumonia/invasive disease within 24 months). The most common organism isolated from the blood is *Streptococcus pneumoniae,* with *Salmonella* species also frequently found. Other organisms include *Haemophilus influenzae* type b, and, when indwelling catheters are present, *Staphylococcus aureus* and *Pseudomonas aeruginosa.*

Although patients with more severe CD4 depletion appear at increased risk, the incidence of serious bacterial infection is as high as 10% per year for all patients.

Disseminated *Mycobacterium Avium-Intracellularae* Complex

Disseminated *Mycobacterium avium-intracellularae* complex (dMAC) is a disease of older HIV-infected children with severe immunodeficiency (mean age, >5 years; mean CD4, <100/mm³). The disease presents with prolonged fevers, abdominal pain, anorexia, and diarrhea. The organism can be recovered from blood cultures, bone marrow aspirates, and liver or node biopsies. Treatment is lifelong with three to four drugs active against the organism.

THERAPY OF PEDIATRIC HIV INFECTION

Family Education and Support
Above all else, HIV is a disease that affects families. Infected children and their families most frequently reside in communities afflicted with crime, poverty, substance abuse, and family violence. These families must be cared for by a team cognizant of their daily difficulties. Pediatric primary care providers will need to develop linkages with services available in their community and work within a multidisciplinary team to ensure optimal care for affected families.

Nutrition
Monitoring growth velocity is an important issue when caring for HIV-infected children. Anorexia, chronic diarrhea from formula intolerance, HIV enteropathy, and secondary gastrointestinal infections are very common among HIV-infected infants and children and contribute to the poor growth observed in so many of these patients.

Immunizations
Routine childhood immunizations are an integral part of pediatric care for HIV-infected children. The schedule is the same as for uninfected children with the exception that the inactivated poliovirus vaccine is always substituted for the oral poliovirus vaccine in HIV-infected or -exposed infants, children, and their siblings. However, a live vaccine, measles, mumps, and rubella (MMR), is administered to HIV-infected children at 12 to 15 months of age. This vaccine is based on the fact that measles can be fatal in this population, and there are no reports of untoward side effects from MMR immunization in infected children.

Pneumococcal vaccine is given at age 2 years, and infected children should receive yearly influenzae A/B vaccine.

Intravenous Gammaglobulin
The benefits of IVgg appear to be a slightly lower rate of hospitalizations for febrile episodes, prevention of pneumococcal infections, and prevention of less serious bacterial and viral illness.

BOX 89-7
Pediatric HIV Infection PCP Prophylaxis

Indications
　All infected infants 1–12 mos of age
　All exposed infants pending polymerase chain reaction/culture results
　Infected children >12–24 mos—CD4 <750, or
　　　　　　　　　　　　 <20%
　　　　　　　　 24–72 mos—CD4 <500, or <20%
　　　　　　　　 >6 yrs—CD4 <200, or <20%
　All children with previous episode of *Pneumocystis carinii* pneumonia

---

IVgg is expensive and requires a 4-hour infusion on a monthly basis.

Prophylaxis
One of the major advances in HIV-related medical care has been the ability to prevent or delay many of the opportunistic infections common in late-stage HIV infection. We now have the ability to identify the patients most at risk and can offer effective prophylactic regimens. First and most important is prophylaxis against PCP.

PCP usually can be prevented with trimethoprim-sulfamethoxazole (TMP-SMX) 3 days a week. Alternative therapies include dapsone, aerosolized pentamidine, or intravenous pentamidine.

It appears that all infants with HIV are at risk in the first year of life, although the risk is greatest for infants with CD4 counts less than $2000/mm^3$ (Box 89-7). Because of the high morbidity and significant mortality associated with PCP and the effectiveness, safety, and low cost of TMP-SMX, it is now recommended that all infected infants receive PCP prophylaxis for the first 12 months of life. In addition, all HIV-exposed infants should receive prophylaxis while undergoing evaluation until HIV infection is ruled out.

Prophylaxis against dMAC is now recommended in adolescents and adults with CD4 counts less than $50/mm^3$. In children, it is reasonable to offer prophylaxis once the CD4 count falls below $100/mm^3$. Once daily rifabutin or twice daily clarithromycin are effective in adults in delaying the onset of dMAC.

Future Directions
We must remember that adolescent and adult HIV is a preventable disease. Because a cure still eludes us, we must all redouble our efforts at education and prevention in our offices, schools,

places of worship, and homes. We must demystify the illness, stop demonizing those infected, and not be afraid of openly discussing sexual practices and risk-reduction behaviors. Only then will we have any hope of stemming the tide of this relentless silent killer.

BIBLIOGRAPHY

Annunziato PW, Frenkel LM: The epidemiology of pediatric HIV-1 infection, *Pediatr Ann* 22: 401–405, 1993.

Boyer PJ, Dillon M, Navaie M, et al: Factors predictive of maternal-fetal transmission of HIV-1, *JAMA* 271:1925–1930, 1994.

Church JA: Clinical aspects of HIV infection in children, *Pediatr Ann* 22:417–427, 1993.

Coonor EM, Sperling RS, Gelber R, et al: Reduction of material: Infant transmission of human immunodeficiency virus type 1 with zidovudine treatment, *N Engl J Med* 331:1173–1180, 1994.

Pizzo PA, Wilfert CM: Antiretroviral therapy and medical management of the human immunodeficiency virus-infected child, *Pediatr Infect Dis J* 12:513–520, 1993.

Part II: HIV and Adolescents

Bret Rudy

INTRODUCTION

Infection with HIV is a significant risk for sexually active and intravenous drug–using youth. Normal adolescent development, especially during midadolescence, entails risk-taking and a sense of invulnerability with very little future perspective. Perceived risk of HIV in these adolescents may be very low, although their risk behaviors are very significant. Due to the latency of approximately 10 years from the time of infection to the time of HIV-related symptoms, most adolescents who acquire HIV infection during the teen years are not identified until they are young adults. In those HIV-infected adolescents who are identified during their adolescence, many basic biologic issues have not been investigated in this population. Thus, because adolescents biologically resemble adults more closely than young children, the standards for following and treating adults is most often followed.

TESTING AND COUNSELING YOUTH

Many conflicting opinions exist on which adolescents should be approached concerning HIV counseling and testing. Risk-factor assessment through interviewing youth is ineffective at identifying those youth infected with HIV. One study from Washington, DC, found that risk-factor assessment of youth will only identify 38% of infected youth. In a study from Houston, 49% of youth testing positive for infection with HIV did not acknowledge a significant risk factor. Thus, it may be difficult to determine which youth should be tested for HIV. Many adolescent HIV specialists now recommend HIV counseling and testing for all youth who are sexually active or who report intravenous drug use, especially those who live in areas with a high seroprevalence.

Adolescents have two options for HIV testing: confidential or anonymous. Confidential testing provides the advantage of providing information that may help those health care workers testing the youth to track them should they not return for their test results. However, this system always places the confidentiality of the adolescent at risk with possible disclosure of information that the youth may choose not to share. Anonymous testing maintains the confidentiality of the adolescent; however, there is no way to track the adolescent should he/she not return for the test results. Although up to 50% of youth may not return for test results, this may be independent of the type of testing but rather more dependent on the quality of the pretest counseling. No matter which type of counseling and testing is offered, youth-sensitive protocols should be followed in a youth-friendly environment. The counseling should be done in terms understood and used by teens. More than one counseling session may be required to be certain the adolescent understands the material and can give true informed consent. It is also helpful to have the adolescent identify one support person who can return with him/her to receive test results and act as the teen's primary support. Pretest counseling should include the following: a review of HIV and AIDS and the distinction between the two; an explanation of the test covering both the ELISA and Western blot; the meaning of a positive, negative, and indeterminant test result; mechanisms for linking the youth into care if the test result is positive; and a discussion of how the youth will deal with each test result. Good posttest counseling should include the test results, a review of the limitations of a negative test result in terms of recent infection, and recommendations for future testing should the result be negative or indeterminant. In addition, it is very important to explain to adolescents that a negative test result does not mean that he/she is immune to the infection but rather that they have not yet been exposed or that they were exposed recently enough (in the past 6 months) so that they have not had sufficient time to mount an antibody response. Discussion of the need for retesting in those cases in which the original test results were indeterminant or in which high-risk activity has transpired in the preceding 6 months is essential. Retesting is generally advised 3 to 6 months following the initial test.

BOX 89-8
Laboratory Evaluation of the HIV-Infected Adolescent

Initial Screening Tests
Complete blood cell count with differential
Blood chemistries to include liver function tests, blood urea nitrogen, creatinine
Syphilis screening with rapid plasma reagin
Toxoplasmosis titers
Varicella titers
Quantitative immunoglobulins
CD4 cell count with both total and percentage and CD8 with a CD4/CD8 ratio

Other Screening Tests
PPD with anergy panel
Chest radiograph
Urine analysis
Girls who are sexually active:
  Papanicolaou smear
  Cultures for GC and *Chlamydia*
  Wet preparation for trichomonas
Boys who are sexually active:
  Urethral swabs for GC and *Chlamydia*
  Oral and anal swabs for GC and anal swab for *Chlamydia,* where indicated

---

EVALUATION OF THE HIV-INFECTED ADOLESCENT

A complete medical history is an important first step in caring for the HIV-infected adolescent. First, a general medical history covering previous medical care, major illnesses, hospitalizations, allergies, and immunizations is important. Second, a comprehensive psychosocial history is important to understand risk-taking behavior in the adolescent and support systems. Because much of this information is very sensitive, it may take the adolescent several visits to feel safe in the medical environment. Substance use and abuse must be explored including use of alcohol and other disinhibiting drugs, with discussion of their use around sexual activity.

The sexual history provides the key to effective ongoing risk reduction. All questions should be addressed using gender-neutral terms for sexual partners until a discussion of the gender of the partners is addressed. The number of sexual partners; types of sexual experiences, specifying oral, vaginal, and anal intercourse; pregnancy history; history of sexual abuse; history of previous sexually transmitted diseases; and condom use are important elements in a complete sexual history. The questions surrounding gender of the partners can be tricky because sexual orientation may be very different from sexual behaviors. Asking the question in terms such as "When you have sex, do you have sex with men, women, or both" is effective because it lets the adolescent know that the health care professional is open to a frank dialogue and is not applying labels to him/her. Discussion of sexual behaviors is important to provide good counseling and to completely evaluate for sexually transmitted diseases. In adolescent girls as well as boys who have had same-sex contacts, a discussion of anal intercourse should be included in a complete history. Anal intercourse is by far the most risky sexual behavior in terms of HIV transmission and one that many practitioners find difficult to discuss.

The initial medical evaluation should be very detailed. First, a complete physical examination with special attention to screen for thrush, oral hairy leukoplakia, adenopathy, hepatosplenomegaly, retinitis, and skin manifestations such as petechiae, Kaposi sarcoma, and molluscum. The laboratory evaluation can be fairly extensive and can be completed over two to three visits. First, if the adolescent has not had a second HIV ELISA and Western blot, one should be performed to confirm the original positive test. Other elements of the laboratory evaluation are listed in Box 89-8. All adolescent girls who are sexually active should have a complete gynecological examination because of the increased risk for cervical dysplasia and neoplasia. In addition, screening and treating other sexually transmitted diseases should be completed as part of comprehensive adolescent health care. The Papanicolaou smear should be performed every 6 months. For those with abnormal Papanicolaou smears, colposcopy should be performed. In sexually active male adolescents, a urethral swab should be obtained for detection of *Neisseria gonorrhoeae* and *Chlamydia*. Perianal inspection and cultures for GC should be obtained from those adolescents reporting anal intercourse.

PREVENTION

Presently no prevention programs exist that are 100% effective against transmission of HIV in adolescents. As noted previously, the difficulties encountered in prevention endeavors are encountered primarily due to normal adolescent developmental characteristics. Ongoing prevention efforts with evaluation of effectiveness are essential. The use of peer educators to speak with the adolescents about safer sex practices and facts surrounding HIV transmission has been shown to be effective, especially with adolescent girls. It is also important to address the other stressors in the adolescent's life as well as discussing HIV. To a teenager out on the street with no shelter or regular meals, concern over infection with HIV may be very low on the priorities in his/her life.

BIBLIOGRAPHY

Centers for Disease Control and Prevention: Recommendations on prophylaxis and therapy for disseminated *Mycobacterium avium* complex for adults and adolescents infected with Human Immunodeficiency Virus, *MMWR* 42:17–20, 1993.

Conway GA, Epstein MR, Hayman CR, et al: Trends in HIV prevalence among disadvantaged youth: Survey results from a national job training program, 1988 through 1992, *JAMA* 269:2887–2889, 1993.

D'Angelo LJ, Getson PR, Luban NL, Gayle HD: Human Immunodeficiency Virus in urban adolescents: Can we predict who is at risk? *Pediatrics* 88:982–985, 1991.

Futterman D, Hein K: Medical care of HIV-infected adolescents, *AIDS Clin Care* 4:95–98, 1992.

Hein K, Futterman D: Medical management in HIV-infected adolescents, *J Pediatr* 119:s18–s20, 1991.

Ilegbodu AE, Frank ML, Poindexter AN, Johnson D: Characteristics of teens tested for HIV in a metropolitan area, *J Adol Health Care,* 15:479–484, 1994.

Jabs DA: Treatment of cytomegalovirus retinitis—1992 (editorial), *Arch Ophthalmol* 110:185–187, 1992.

Vermund SV, Hein K, Gayle H, et al: AIDS among adolescents in NYC: Case surveillance profiles compared with the rest of the US, *Am J Dis Child* 143:1220–1225, 1989.

CHAPTER 90

Infectious Diseases of Childhood

Louis M. Bell

The infant, toddler, and child are faced with a vast array of infectious diseases. The child's maturing immune system must control the spread of primary infections, as well as provide the amnestic response needed to attenuate or prevent repeated infections from causative agents.

Despite the development of vaccines that prevent many of the once "common childhood diseases," the physician who cares for children must still be able to recognize a variety of different infections that are unique to this age group.

This chapter describes some of the infectious diseases seen in children beginning with the six childhood exanthems that were known by numbers in the late 19th century. Measles, scarlet fever, and rubella were the first three. The "fourth disease" is no longer recognized. Erythema infectiosum was named the fifth disease, and roseola infantum has been referred to as the sixth disease.

MEASLES

Measles, a highly contagious disease, is spread by the airborne route and has an incubation period of 8 to 12 days. Vaccination with killed measles vaccines from 1963 to 1968 and then attenuated live measles virus vaccine since 1968 has made this a rare infection in the United States, with on average 3000 cases of measles reported each year since 1981. However, the number of cases doubled in 1986 and continues to increase. In 1989 the Centers for Disease Control and Prevention (CDC) received reports of 56 outbreaks of measles, which accounted for an increase of more than 300% in cases over the number reported in 1988. In 1990, 27,672 cases of measles were reported, with 89 deaths. Large outbreaks occurred in Los Angeles, Dallas, New York, Chicago, and Philadelphia. Analysis of these outbreaks revealed the cause to be a failure to adequately vaccinate preschool-aged children against measles. In addition, measles is still prevalent in developing countries and therefore can be seen in the immigrant population of the United States, especially in children under 5 years of age.

Data Gathering

The prodrome of measles lasts approximately 2 to 4 days and begins with symptoms of an upper respiratory infection and fever up to 104° F. General malaise, conjunctivitis with photophobia, and cough increase in severity over this period. It is during this time that Koplik spots (white spots on the buccal mucosa) appear.

Appearance of rash on the face and abdomen occurs classically 14 days following exposure. The rash is erythematous and maculopapular and spreads from the head to the feet. After 3 to 4 days, the rash begins to clear, leaving a brownish discoloration and fine scaling. Fever is usually absent 3 days after the rash appears. Pharyngitis, cervical lymphadenopathy, and splenomegaly may accompany the rash. Diarrhea and vomiting may be seen in the young.

Modified and Atypical Measles

Classic measles as described previously is relatively rare. One is more likely to see either modified measles (occurring in a partially immune individual) or atypical measles (primarily in individuals vaccinated with killed vaccine between 1963 to 1967).

Modified measles occurs naturally in infants less than 9 months of age because of the presence of transplacental acquired maternal antibody or as a result of the administration of immune globulin to an exposed susceptible child. The illness follows the progression outlined previously but is generally mild. Conversely, individuals (young adults) with atypical measles are quite ill with a sudden onset of fever to 103° to 105° F associated with headache. Unlike typical measles, Koplik spots are rare, and the rash appears first on the distal extremities progressing in a cephalad direction. In addition, virtually all patients have respiratory distress with clinical and radiographic signs of pneumonia, often associated with pleural effusion.

Diagnosis depends on recognition of the progression of the clinical illness and on results of acute and convalescent measles antibody serologies, collected 1 to 3 weeks apart.

Complications
Dehydration, pneumonia, myocarditis, pericarditis, encephalitis, and disseminated intravascular coagulation (Black measles) have been associated with measles virus infection.

Subacute sclerosis panencephalitis occurs in one per 100,000 children with naturally occurring measles. After an incubation period of several years, a progressive encephalopathy develops among vaccinated children. The incubation period is shortened and occurs in one in 1,000,000 vaccinees.

Management
Supportive measures are antipyretics, plenty of oral fluids, and room humidification to help reduce cough.

New interest has been aroused in the use of vitamin A to reduce the morbidity and mortality of children admitted to the hospital because of pneumonia, diarrhea, or croup. In April 1993, the American Academy of Pediatrics issued a policy statement concerning vitamin A. In general, the use of vitamin A should be considered for children 6 months to 2 years of age who are hospitalized with measles or its complications and patients over 6 months of age who have an immunodeficiency, ophthalmologic evidence of vitamin A deficiency, impaired intestinal absorption, or moderate to severe malnutrition or who are recent immigrants for areas of high mortality from measles. The recommended dosage for children over 1 year of age is a single dose of 200,000 IU of water-miscible vitamin A on admission, a second dose the following day, and, for children with ophthalmologic evidence of vita-

min A deficiency, a third dose at 4 weeks. Children 6 months to 1 year of age should receive 100,000 IU. The higher dose may be associated with vomiting and headache for a few hours. Vitamin A is available in a 50,000-UL/mL solution and may be given orally.

In an attempt to control the measles outbreaks in the United States, new recommendations for measles immunization have recently been published by the American Academy of Pediatrics. These recommendations include routine vaccination against measles, mumps, and rubella (MMR) at 12 to 15 months and a second MMR vaccination at entrance to middle school or junior high school. In outbreak situations, monovalent measles vaccine may be given to infants as young as 6 months.

If aggressive vaccination programs around the world are pursued, elimination of measles as a cause of human disease is possible. There is no specific antiviral therapy available.

SCARLET FEVER

Scarlet fever is caused by group A β-hemolytic streptococci. The disease is spread by close contact of primarily school-aged children and is rare in infants. Because immunity is short-lived, it may recur every 3 to 5 years during childhood. The rash is a result of hypersensitization to the erythrogenic toxins produced by the organism, which has established a focus of infection. The most likely site of invasion by the organism is the pharynx or tonsils, but other sites such as the skin (impetigo) or perianal area also can be infected.

Data Gathering
The typical course of scarlet fever begins with complaints of sore throat after an incubation period of 1 to 4 days. The pharynx may appear reddened with petechiae on the soft palate, with a swollen uvula and reddened tonsils, often with a whitish exudate. However, the pharyngitis may be subclinical. The tongue also may have swollen papillae giving the appearance of a strawberry.

The rash is typically erythematous with closely grouped fine papules, giving a sandpaper feel to the skin. The rash starts on the face and trunk and is most prominent in the folds of the skin. The rash blanches with pressure. The skin usually will peel after the rash fades in 4 to 7 days. Just as the skin peels, the tongue will typically peel to a smooth surface.

Positive results of a throat culture or from other suspicious skin lesions helps to confirm the diagnosis of scarlet fever. An alternative to cultures are the numerous rapid diagnostic tests that detect the group A carbohydrate antigen. Although the specificity of the tests is usually good, they lack sensitivity, so all negative results should be confirmed with traditional culture methods. One should confirm a group A streptococcus infection because a scarlatiniform rash is sometimes associated with enteroviral infections.

Management

Treatment prevents the suppurative and nonsuppurative complications of group A streptococci infections.

Complications of Group A β-Hemolytic Streptococci Pharyngitis

- **Suppurative**
    Peritonsillar abscess
    Otitis media
    Mastoiditis
    Osteomyelitis of the skull
- **Nonsuppurative**
    Acute rheumatic fever
    Glomerulonephritis

Treatment consists of Benzathine penicillin G or penicillin VK in appropriate doses. Penicillin prevents rheumatic fever, even if therapy is started 7 to 9 days after the onset of acute illness, so even delayed therapy is indicated.

RUBELLA (GERMAN MEASLES)

Rubella is usually a mild erythematous infection spread by infectious droplet with minimal morbidity. However, infection during pregnancy may have devastating effects on the fetus. Vaccination programs, which started in 1969, are aimed at reducing the rubella activity in women of child-bearing age.

Data Gathering

Symptoms of malaise, a sore throat, and low-grade fevers may precede the rash. The rash may start in the malar region of the face, then spread to the trunk and limbs. The rash, which blanches with pressure, clears after 3 to 4 days. The spleen

also may be palpable. Enlarged occipital and postauricular lymph nodes in association with a morbilliform rash should raise the suspicion of rubella. Rubella can be confirmed by the presence of anti-rubella IgM antibodies in the serum.

Complications of rubella include polyarthritis, especially in older girls; encephalitis in one of 5000 cases; and congenital deformities in infants born to mothers with the disease. Commonly described anomalies associated with congenital rubella include cataracts, microophthalmia, chorioretinitis, sensorineural deafness, microcephaly, and mental retardation.

Management

If rubella infection occurs, treatment consists of supportive measures only.

ERYTHEMA INFECTIOSUM (FIFTH DISEASE)

Erythema infectiosum, or fifth disease, is caused by parvovirus B19, a virus first discovered in asymptomatic blood donors in 1975. The infection is probably spread by respiratory secretions. Secondary spread among susceptible family members is common and occurs in 23% to 62% of children and 14% to 38% of adults. The incubation period is 6 to 16 days.

Data Gathering

Erythema infectiosum is a mild childhood illness characterized by prodromal symptoms of low-grade fevers, malaise, and occasionally a sore throat. This prodrome may last 1 to 4 days, followed by a facial rash ("slapped cheeks") over the malar areas of the face. This rash is followed by a diffuse macular or maculopapular rash on the extremities and trunk, which is sometimes described as reticulated or lacelike. Rubella-like, vesicular and purpuric rashes also have been associated with parvovirus B19 infection. The rash may last for up to 10 days and is pruritic in 30% to 50% of cases. The rash may fade but reappear after sun exposure or exercise.

Other common associated symptoms include arthralgias and arthritis. Arthritis is rare in children but can occur in up to 90% of symptomatic adults. The most common joints affected are the knees and hands. There may be only mild swelling of the painful joint. Serologic tests for detecting a specific IgM antibody response to parvovirus are available only in research laboratories. The CDC will make these tests available on a limited basis.

Complications

In children, erythema infectiosum is a mild, self-limited illness during which the child usually remains alert and playful. Adults may have prolonged complaints of joint symptoms. In addition, parvovirus B19 infections have been associated with aplastic crisis in patients with chronic hemolytic anemia, hydrops fetalis, and chronic bone marrow suppression in immunocompromised individuals.

Management

Treatment is supportive. Parents of the child should be counseled concerning secondary spread of this infection among family members. However, when the rash appears, the child is no longer infectious.

Maternal B19 infection has been associated with hydrops fetalis and fetal death. Among pregnant women of unknown antibody status, the risk of fetal death after exposure to B19 has been estimated to be less than 1.5%. Risk to the fetus appears to be greatest if the infection occurs prior to the 20th week of gestation.

ROSEOLA INFANTUM (SIXTH DISEASE)

Roseola infantum (exanthema subitum) is a common acute illness of young children with a year-round incidence. Ninety percent of those infected are less than 2 years of age. It is rare before the age of 3 months. Roseola-like illnesses have been associated with enteroviruses, adenoviruses, and parvovirus B19. Most recently, human herpes virus 6 (HHV-6) has been identified as a major cause of roseola infantum. Although HHV-6 may be the predominant etiologic agent, roseola is a syndrome caused by a variety of viral agents.

Data Gathering

The basic clinical pattern of the roseola syndrome is the sudden onset of fever (usually above 38.9° C [102° F]), which lasts for 3 to 5 days and may rapidly return to normal. Only after defervescence does a rash appear, predominantly on the trunk. The rash is characterized by discrete erythematous, macular, or maculopapular lesions that blanch with pressure. The rash, which lasts for 24 to 48 hours, is not usually associated with pruritis or desquamation. Although febrile, the child is frequently happy and playful. A number of other signs and symptoms have been occasionally associated with roseola, including inflammation of the pharynx and tonsils, infection of the tympanic membranes, suboccipital and postauricular adenopathy, palpebral edema, and bulging of the anterior fontanelle.

Many patients will have leukopenia (with a relative lymphocytosis), which reaches its nadir on the third to sixth day of illness.

Presumably because of the often rapid onset of fever, febrile seizures are the most common of complications associated with roseola. Roseola rarely produces encephalitis, occasionally with permanent central nervous system (CNS) sequelae.

MUMPS

Mumps, caused by a paramyxovirus, was a common childhood infection prior to the introduction of vaccine. Infection affects primarily preschool and grade-school age children, occurring in late winter and early spring. Spread of the infection is via airborne droplets. The incubation period can be from 12 to 22 days. Asymptomatic infection is common, occurring in 20% to 40% of children.

Data Gathering

Rarely is mumps a severe systemic illness. A prodrome of fever, malaise, and headache may precede the parotid gland swelling. Pain and swelling may occur in one or both parotid glands. In trying to differentiate between parotid gland swelling and lymphadenopathy, the examiner should remember that the parotid gland lies in front of the ear, and the uncinate lobe of the gland wraps itself underneath and in back of the ear. Swelling in this area will result in elevation of the earlobe. After unilateral parotid gland swelling, the second parotid gland may become swollen after 1 to 2 days. At times, the submandibular glands may be involved concomitantly with the parotid gland or alone. Redness and swelling of Stenson or Wharton ducts of the affected glands may occur. Eating or drinking may cause discomfort. The swelling may last for 1 week to 10 days.

In addition, patients with mumps usually are febrile for 3 to 4 days. Headache, photophobia, and other signs of meningeal irritation are more common in older children (>15 years of age). The disease is considered noninfectious 1 week after the onset of parotid gland swelling.

Other infectious causes of parotid swelling should be considered in the differential diagnosis.

Infectious Diseases Associated with Parotid Swelling

• **Viruses**
  Mumps
  Enterovirus (coxsackie A)
  Parainfluenza virus
  Cytomegalovirus
  Epstein-Barr virus
• **Bacterial (suppurative)**
  Staphylococcus aureus
  Streptococcus species
  Tuberculosis
  Histoplasmosis
  Cat scratch disease

Complications

Orchitis is probably the most feared complication of mumps. Up to 35% of postpubertal men with mumps may be affected. A new onset of fever with unilateral pain, swelling, and tenderness of the testicle occurs at the end of the first week of illness with mumps. Bilateral involvement is less common but may lead to sterility. Analgesics, support of the testicle, and the application of ice may help to relieve the discomfort. There is no indication for the use of steroids.

Other complications include aseptic meningitis, epididymitis, oophoritis, pancreatitis, mastitis, thyroiditis, arthritis, and deafness.

Management

Supportive therapy is recommended in the treatment of mumps. Analgesics may be necessary, especially if severe headaches are noted. The physician caring for the child may be asked advice concerning the father who has no history of symptomatic infection who is exposed to mumps. Although administration of the live attenuated mumps vaccine is not protective, it may prevent infection due to future exposure. In many cases, the father may have had a subclinical infection as a child.

INFLUENZA VIRUS

Influenza viruses A, B, and C are responsible for acute respiratory tract infections, which have occurred in epidemics throughout history. Although attack rates are highest in children, the major mortality and morbidity rates associated with this infection occur in the elderly or in those with underlying illness such as heart disease, chronic lung disease, chronic renal disease, and in patients with neoplasm or neuromuscular illnesses. Improvements in living standards and the ability to treat the secondary bacterial infections associated with influenza have led to a gradual decline in mortality rates. Influenza viruses A and B cause the majority of human disease. Occurring in the winter months, the infection is spread by inhalation of aerosolized nasal secretions or by direct contact. The incubation period is 2 to 3 days with viral shedding lasting up to 5 days after the onset of clinical symptoms.

Data Gathering

The symptoms of influenza have a rapid onset characterized by fever up to 104° or 106° C with chills, headache, and myalgias. Cough, nasal congestion, and complaints of photophobia or pain with eye movements are also common. In younger children, symptoms of bronchiolitis or the croupy cough of laryngotracheitis may predominate. Symptoms will last from 3 to 7 days. Gastrointestinal symptoms of nausea, vomiting, or diarrhea have been described for both influenza virus A and B epidemics.

Outbreaks of influenza occurring in the winter months along with the characteristic constellation of symptoms facilitate the diagnosis. Virus can be isolated from respiratory secretions to confirm the diagnosis. Generally, isolation takes 1 to 3 days. Currently, new rapid diagnostic techniques are being tested that will allow sameday results. The sensitivity and specificity of these tests remain to be seen.

Complications

Secondary bacterial infections especially in the elderly, may complicate influenza infections. Myositis with myoglobinemia requiring careful fluid management is seen more commonly in children. Reye syndrome has been associated with influenza virus A infections and aspirin therapy. Other more rare complications include encephalitis, pericarditis, myocarditis, and acute parotitis.

Management

Treatment for influenza is mainly rest, fluids, and temperature control with acetaminophen. Aspirin is not recommended because of its association with the development of Reye syndrome. Amantadine or Rimantadine has been shown to be effective against only influenza A and is most efficacious if used as prophylaxis against infection.

Yearly influenza vaccination is recommended for children over 6 months of age with the following conditions:

- Asthma and other chronic pulmonary diseases
- Hemodynamically significant cardiac disease
- Immunosuppressive therapy
- Sickle cell anemia and other hemoglobinopathies

VARICELLA-ZOSTER INFECTIONS (CHICKENPOX AND ZOSTER)

The primary infection of the varicella-zoster virus results in chickenpox, whereas reactivation of latent virus results in a unilateral vesicular eruption localized to the sensory dermatomes, called zoster or "shingles." Chickenpox occurs in the late winter and early spring. The illness is transmitted by respiratory spread and will infect susceptible persons with an 85% attack rate among household contacts. The incubation period of varicella is 11 to 21 days. Most cases of infection occur in children between 5 and 10 years of age. The children are contagious until the vesicular rash is crusted. Although zoster or shingles are more common in the elderly, it is not uncommon in children and may be seen in infants whose mothers had chickenpox in the third trimester. Susceptible individuals exposed to a patient with zoster may become infected.

Data Gathering

In children, chickenpox is usually a mild illness characterized by a low-grade fever (temperature 38.4° to 38.9° C) and a vesicular rash. The hallmark of the rash is that one can observe lesions in different stages of evolution. Individual lesions progress from macules to papules, then to vesicles, and finally to crusted lesions on an erythematous base. The rash starts on the scalp or trunk and may involve the mucous membranes and sclera. It is often pruritic. Crops of lesions may appear over the first 3 to 5 days spreading to the extremities.

Varicella in immunocompetent children is almost always benign. However, in immunocompromised children or infants born to mothers whose rash appeared within 5 days before delivery or within 48 hours after delivery, the infection may be progressive and severe with a mortality rate of 20%. In addition, chickenpox in adolescents and adults tends to be more severe with systemic symptoms and a confluent rash.

The rash of zoster consists of grouped vesicles on an erythematous base. The vesicles are confined to one to three sensory dermatomes. If the vesicles are seen on the tip of the nose, the ophthalmic branch of the facial nerve is affected, and repeat examinations to rule out ocular involvement are necessary. Prior to eruption, there may be a prodrome of pain or tingling.

Complications

Secondary bacterial skin infections with streptococci or staphylococci are the most common complication.

Central nervous system (CNS) manifestations occur as well. Meningoencephalitis can occur and may be severe, appearing early in the course of chickenpox. An acute cerebellar ataxia, which usually appears after 5 to 10 days of the rash, is the most common CNS complication. The prognosis with this type of isolated cerebellitis is good. Reye syndrome appears to occur more frequently in children with chickenpox or influenza.

Idiopathic thrombocytopenic purpura can be associated with varicella infection, occurring after a week of illness. Purpura fulminans is a rare phenomenon characterized by an inflammatory vasculitis and necrosis of the tissues, predominantly the extremities and buttocks.

Management

Uncomplicated chickenpox or zoster in children requires only supportive therapy. Daily bathing will help decrease secondary skin infections, but soap detergents may be irritating. Some recommend oatmeal baths (1 cup oatmeal with 3 cups cold water in a quart jar and shake well) as a soothing cleansing bath. Pruritus can be controlled with antihistamines. Fingernails should be trimmed to prevent secondary skin infections from scratching.

Acyclovir is indicated for immunocompromised children with chickenpox or zoster. The use of acyclovir in immunocompetent children with zoster is probably not necessary but can be considered in children with involvement of the ophthalmic branch of the facial nerve. Situations in which varicella-zoster immune globulin is indicated are published by the American Academy of Pediatrics. Passive immunization has been shown to prevent or modify illness in normal and high-risk individuals.

The first live attenuated varicella vaccine was licensed by the Food and Drug Administration on March 17, 1995, for use in individuals 12 months of age or older. Discussion and recommendations for the use of the vaccine are published in the May 1995 issue of *Pediatrics* (95:791–795). The vaccine is recommended for all healthy children who lack a reliable history of varicella. From age 12 months to 13 years one dose of vaccine is given. After age 13, healthy adolescents who lack a history of varicella require two doses of vaccine given 4 to 8 weeks apart. A third dose of vaccine is not needed if there is an inadvertent delay longer than 8 weeks between doses; however, the child may not be fully protected during the interim.

HERPES SIMPLEX VIRUS

Herpes simplex virus (HSV, types 1 and 2), a ubiquitous virus, infects a majority of people. The wide spectrum of illness includes cutaneous, mucous membrane, ocular, and nervous system infection. Like other herpes viruses (cytomegalovirus, Epstein-Barr virus, and varicella-zoster virus), HSV is able to induce a state of latency in the infected individual that may lead to recurrences of disease. The mechanism leading to recurrence is unknown. People of all ages are susceptible to HSV infection, which can be symptomatic or asymptomatic. The infection is spread among individuals via close contact and is present without regard to socioeconomic group. The incubation period is not well defined but is related to the size of the inoculum and has been estimated to be 2 to 14 days.

Serologically, there are two types of HSV infection. HSV type 1 infection is found in children and adults, with 90% exhibiting HSV-1 antibodies by adulthood. HSV type 2 accounts for the majority of HSV genital infection in adults. As might be expected, HSV-2 infections are the predominate cause of neonatal disease.

Data Gathering

The clinical manifestation of HSV infection can be primary or recurrent, as a result of reactivation of a latent virus infection.

Mucosal Infection

Acute herpetic gingivostomatitis is one of the most frequent manifestations of a primary HSV infection. Young children are usually affected (10 months to 3 years). The child may develop fever 24 to 48 hours prior to the development of gingivirus or mucous membrane ulcers, which involve the anterior tongue and hard palate. The gingiva will be swollen and red, often with exudate at the gum line that may bleed with gentle pressure from a tongue blade. Vesicles may appear around the mouth and on the chin. In children who suck their fingers, the infection can be transferred to the digit causing herpetic whitlow. Fever may last up to 10 days. Associated cervical and submental lymph nodes are often swollen and tender. The most important complication of this infection is refusal to drink fluids with subsequent dehydration.

HSV gingivostomatitis is differentiated from herpangina (*see* next section) by the placement of the ulcers. The patient with herpangina, a manifestation of enteroviral infection, has ulcers on the posterior palate and anterior tonsillar pillars.

Skin Infection

HSV infections of the skin are common and may develop in apparently unbroken skin. More commonly, minor skin trauma in a child becomes infected with HSV by the common habit of "kissing it better." Grouped vesicles on an erythematous base may appear 24 to 48 hours after inoculation. Herpetic whitlow, sometimes confused with bacterial felon or paronychia, can be secondary to autoinoculation in the child with herpetic stomatitis or may be seen in sexually active patients. Health care workers (dentists, nurses, physicians) are also at risk, because they come in contact with oral secretions during care of their patients. Careful hand washing and gloves will prevent such exposure.

Interestingly, erythema multiforme may occur in some patients with recurrent HSV skin eruptions. Thought to be an allergic response, the typical rash appears 7 to 10 days after the HSV eruption. In addition, sports involving close physical contact have been associated with cutaneous HSV infection. Wrestling (herpes gladiatorum) and rugby (scrum pox) are two examples. These infections must be differentiated from impetigo.

Any child with chronic dermatitis, such as eczema, is at risk for secondary infection with HSV. The infection may spread extensively and is recognized as eczema herpeticum, otherwise known as Kaposi varicelliform eruption. Finally, HSV-2 infection can be manifest in the genitalia of both boys and girls (*see* section on Sexually Transmitted Disease).

Herpes Simplex Infection in Neonates

Neonatal herpes infection occurs in infants after exposure either intrauterine, perinatally, or postnatal spread from the mother, father, or hospital nursery personnel. Intrauterine infection is rare but is associated with chorioretinitis, mental retardation, and microcephaly. Postnatal acquisition is also rare but is well described in the literature. The overwhelming majority of infants became infected perinatally. However, many mothers will not have any prior history of HSV infection.

The risk of HSV infection to the infants born vaginally is much higher in those mothers with primary genital HSV infection. The clinical presentation of HSV infection in neonates occurs in three patterns. The infant, usually in the first week of life, may develop a generalized sepsis involving the liver and CNS. Only one third of these infants will necessarily have HSV skin lesions associated with sepsis. Mortality is high. Some infants may have isolated CNS symptoms, whereas some have localized skin and mucocutaneous infection alone.

Central Nervous System Infections

HSV infections may cause encephalitis. In the majority of cases, the encephalitis is caused by a recurrent infection with HSV-1 and can affect people of all ages. The encephalitis may not be associated with cerebrospinal fluid (CSF) pleocytosis but consistently involves the temporal lobe. HSV encephalitis is an acute illness beginning with fever and irritability, which progresses rapidly to CNS symptoms with focal neurologic or altered mental status, coma, and death in the majority of cases if untreated. HSV-2 causes aseptic meningitis usually associated with a primary genital infection. Signs of meningitis (unlike HSV-I encephalitis) are commonly observed.

Eye Infections

Primary HSV infection of the eye may cause an acute superficial conjunctivitis. This condition may proceed to cause ulceration of the cornea. Deep lesions of the cornea and iris are also possible and may be caused in part by a hypersensitivity to the herpes virus.

Diagnosis

Diagnosis of cutaneous herpes infections can be made by the appearance of grouped vesicles on an erythematous base. Clinical suspicion can be confirmed by isolation of the virus in tissue culture from vesicles, genital lesions, CSF, urine, and blood. Fortunately, HSV grows quickly and can be identified in most cases by 3 days. More rapid diagnostic techniques include the Tzank test with the modified Wright stain. In this test, the base of a vesicle is gently scraped and the stained cells are examined for evidence of multinucleated giant cells. The test is nonspecific and will be positive in 60% to 70% of cases. A more sensitive fluorescent antibody test again depends on obtaining HSV infected cells at the base of the vesicle.

Although the diagnosis of herpes encephalitis can be difficult, contrast-material–enhanced computed tomography will often reveal involvement of the temporal lobe. The electroencephalogram will show a characteristic spike wave pattern in the affected temporal lobe. Brain biopsy and isolation of HSV is the gold standard for diagnosis and is necessary in some cases to confirm the HSV infection or to identify other treatable causes of encephalitis.

Management

In neonates with HSV infection, acyclovir and/or vidarabine have been used to treat both localized mucocutaneous lesions and CNS or systemic infections. Acyclovir has less toxicity and is easier to administer and is preferred. Acyclovir is the drug of choice for encephalitis in older patients.

Patients with HSV ocular involvement should receive a topical ophthalmic drug (1% or 2% trifluridine, 1% iododeoxyuridine, or 3% vidarabine) as well as systemic acyclovir therapy.

Topical steroids are contraindicated in HSV infections of the eye.

ENTEROVIRUS INFECTIONS

The genus enterovirus includes coxsackie viruses, echoviruses, polioviruses, and any newly identified enterovirus, which are now classified only by number and not assigned any particular name or grouping. The nonpolio enteroviruses, which are responsible for a variety of human illness, will be discussed in this section.

In general, the peak time of enteroviral illness in temperate climates is late summer and early fall. In tropical regions, no seasonal pattern is apparent. The spread of enterovirus infections is thought to occur only among people usually by the fecal-oral route. Fecal viral excretion may continue for several weeks after the onset of infection. Insects and animals that come in contact with human excreta may spread the infection, especially among people with poor sanitary systems. The primary illnesses occur in infants and children. Many infections are asymptomatic. The incubation period is 3 to 6 days.

Data Gathering

Coxsackie viruses groups A and B, echoviruses, and enteroviruses are associated with specific illnesses that are outlined below.

Coxsackie Viruses, Group A

These viruses are associated with infections of the mouth and skin and are rarely serious. Herpangina is one such infection often caused by subtypes A4, A5, A6, or A10. This illness is characterized by fever and painful vesicles and ulcers on the soft palate and anterior tonsillar pillas. Sometimes ulceration on the buccal mucosa occurs. The illness lasts 4 to 5 days.

Hand-foot-and-mouth disease often occurs in epidemics, usually in children under 4 years of age. The causative agents are subtypes A16, A5, A7, or A9. Scattered vesicles appear in the mouth that quickly ulcerate. In addition, many children develop vesicular lesions on the palms and soles. Occasionally, scattered vesicles appear on the proximal extremities and buttocks. Rarely, a generalized vesicular or macular papular rash occurs that resembles varicella but occurs in only one crop. Several group A subtypes are associated with a febrile disease in infants and young children characterized by a maculopapular rash that begins on the face and spreads to the trunk. The palms and soles are usually spared.

Coxsackie Viruses, Group B

Illnesses associated with group B infections are, in general, more serious and include pleurodynia, sepsis in the neonate, myocarditis and pericarditis, and CNS infections.

Pleurodynia (Bornholm disease, devil's grip) is characterized by an acute onset of severe paroxysmal pain referred to the lower ribs. The pain is made worse by coughing or motion. In some patients, there is a prodrome of headache, malaise, and myalgia. The severe pleuritic pain may radiate to the neck and scapular region and be accompanied by upper abdominal pain and splinting of abdominal muscles. The patients are usually febrile and may have other symptoms such as headache, diarrhea, and vomiting. The illness lasts approximately 4 days, although recrudescence occurs frequently.

Myocarditis and pericarditis have been associated with subtype B1-5. The patient will present with symptoms of congestive heart failure, and/or pericarditis often approximately 2 weeks after a nonspecific febrile or respiratory tract illness.

CNS infection can occur in any age group and be caused by any of the enteroviruses. Aseptic meningitis is the most common illness, but a poliolike paralysis and encephalitis may occur as well.

Neonates may develop any of the manifestations of enterovirus infection outlined previously. However, the neonate will commonly present with a nonspecific sepsislike illness. Subtype B1-5 has been associated with a fulminating encephalomyocarditis in this age group.

Echoviruses

Echoviruses can cause many of the diseases described previously, but certain specific associations of virus subtype and disease are recognized. A petechial exanthem and aseptic meningitis is seen in epidemics, usually among families and is caused by an echovirus 9 infection. There may be a prodrome of fever, sore throat, anorexia, and vomiting followed by an asymptomatic period. This period is followed by fever, signs of meningitis (headache, stiff neck), and a maculopapular rash. The rash is especially frequent in children under 3 years of age. The rash starts on the face and spreads to the trunk and extremities. The rash may become petechial, which raises the differential diagnosis of meningococcemia. The disease lasts 3 to 5 days.

Neonatal hepatic necrosis has been associated with echovirus 11 infection. Hepatitis can be seen in infections with many different enterovirus infections.

Enteroviruses

These newly isolated viruses can cause illnesses similar to those described previously. However, enterovirus 70 may cause acute hemorrhagic conjunctivitis. Recognized in epidemic form only in the past 20 years, this illness has a sudden onset. Symptoms include severe eye pain, photophobia, blurred vision, lacrimation, and edema of the eyelids. Systemic symptoms are rare. Preauricular lymphadenopathy is often present on examination. Recovery is usually complete without sequelae by 7 to 12 days. This disease must be differentiated from epidemic keratoconjunctivitis due to adenovirus type 8.

Diagnosis

Diagnosis is based on the season of the year and the clinical presentation. The suspicion of enterovirus infection can be confirmed by isolation of the virus in tissue culture from the appropriate body fluid or biopsy. Enterovirus can be excreted for weeks in the feces. For that reason, serum antibody titers may be necessary to prove acute infection.

INFECTIOUS MONONUCLEOSIS

The association between Epstein-Barr virus (EBV) and infectious mononucleosis was made more than 20 years ago. EBV infection is spread among human beings by close personal contact. Infection is common early in life, especially among lower socioeconomic groups, as evidenced by serologic studies. EBV infection in the young child may be asymptomatic or a mild illness resembling an upper respiratory tract infection. However, the development of classic mononucleosis seems to be age-related and is most often described in adolescents and young adults. Infected individuals may excrete virus for many months, and approximately 20% of individuals are asymptomatic carriers. The in-

cubation period is estimated to be from 14 to 50 days.

Data Gathering

Symptoms of malaise and spiking fevers (to 40° or 40.5° C), anorexia, and easy fatigability are usually the first symptoms of mononucleosis. The fevers may be associated with chills and sweats. Generalized lymphadenopathy (especially posterior cervical) appears within the first week. The term *anginose mononucleosis* is used to describe the illness in the patient with exudative pharyngitis, marked tonsillar enlargement, petechiae on the hard palate, and cervical adenopathy as a prominent early feature of the disease. The face and eyelids may appear swollen and the conjunctivae infected. Diffuse erythematous macular skin rashes are occasionally seen, particularly in patients treated with ampicillin. Hepatosplenomegaly is often noted as well. Other causes of a mononucleosis-like illness include cytomegalovirus and toxoplasmosis.

Diagnosis

The suspicion of clinical mononucleosis, as described previously, is strengthened if the white blood cell counts show a lymphocytosis of over 50% with 20% atypical lymphocytes. In addition, there may be abnormalities of liver function tests.

Confirmation of the diagnosis depends on either the measurement of heterophil antibodies (Monospot test) or specific antibodies to the EBV. In children over 4 years of age, the Monospot test will detect approximately 84% of those infected. In children less than 4 years, the sensitivity decreases with age from 50% to 5% in the child less than 1 year of age. In children less than 4 to 5 years or in older patients with clinical mononucleosis, specific antibodies to EBV should be measured if the Monospot test is negative.

There are specific antibodies to various components of EBV that appear in the blood at a predictable sequence during recovery from an acute infection. The pattern of positivity to these antibodies can determine current, recent, or past infection in any given patient (Table 90-1).

Management

Treatment of mononucleosis is supportive only. Rarely, short-term steroid therapy is considered if tonsillar enlargement leads to respiratory embarrassment or if rupture of an enlarged spleen is

TABLE 90-1
Epstein-Barr Virus Infection Status According to Antibody Titer

	NONE	CURRENT	RECENT	PAST
IgM anti-VCA	–	++	–	–
IgG anti-VCA	–	++	++	+
Anti-EA	–	+	– or ±	–
Anti-EBNA	–	–	– or ±	+

VCA = viral capsid antigen; EA = early antigen; EBNA = Epstein-Barr virus nuclear associated antigen; + = positive; – = negative.

possible. Patients receiving steroids for these conditions warrant admission to the hospital for close observation. Others have advocated the use of a tapering dose of steroids over 7 to 10 days for more moderate symptoms of mononucleosis given as outpatient therapy.

ROCKY MOUNTAIN SPOTTED FEVER

The cause of Rocky Mountain spotted fever (RMSF) is *Rickettsia rickettsii,* named after Howard Ricketts, who in 1906 proved that ticks transmit the disease. Although first described in the Rocky Mountain region, the disease is predominant in the eastern coastal and southeastern states. The organism is a natural parasite of the dog tick *(Dermacentor variabilis)* in the eastern region and of the wood tick *(Dermacentor andersoni)* in the west. Humans are infected by the bite of an infected tick. The disease occurs in the spring, and approximately 45% of cases occur in children younger than 14 years of age. The incubation period ranges from 3 to 12 days.

Data Gathering

Initially, the patient develops nonspecific features of malaise, headache, and fever that may be high (40° C). Myalgia and muscle tenderness are common complaints. A maculopapular rash will appear within the first 3 days in 50% to 60% of cases. The rash usually starts on the extremities and later involves the trunk and the palms and soles. The rash may become petechial or hemorrhagic in 50% of cases. Edema in the face or extremities is a late sign, indicating that vascular endothelial damage has begun. The patient may progress to shock with disseminated intravascular coagulation. Severe headache with symptoms of meningoencephalitis (restlessness, irritability,

confusion, and delirium) are common and may progress to coma.

Mortality rates of 3% to 6% persist despite prompt recognition and therapy. Long-term neurologic sequelae of RMSF include behavioral disturbances and learning disabilities. Finally, cardiac involvement with electrocardiogram abnormalities is frequently present.

Hyponatremia (in 88%) and thrombocytopenia (in 76%) is reported in children with RMSF. Therefore, a history of tick bite, fever, and rash with laboratory abnormalities as noted previously should alert the physician to the possibility of RMSF. Unfortunately, serologic confirmation of infection with the nonspecific Weil-Felix test (which depends on the common antigens of rickettsia and two strains of *Proteus* bacteria, OX-19 and OX-2) cannot be used as a rapid diagnostic test. This test becomes positive 10 to 14 days after the onset of the illness. Specific serologic tests available on acute and convalescent serum specimens are now the preferred method of diagnosis, but once again cannot be relied on for rapid early diagnosis. The most commonly used specific tests are the complement fixation or indirect fluorescent antibody tests.

Management

Early recognition and treatment with effective antibiotic therapy will ensure the best possible outcome. For this reason, the decision to treat cannot be based on the results of serologic tests but should be based on clinical suspicion alone. Chloramphenicol or tetracycline (for children over 9 years of age) is the drug of choice. Antibiotics should be continued until the patient is afebrile for 2 to 3 days; a usual course is 5 to 7 days. Management of the hyponatremia, shock, and disseminated intravascular coagulation is also necessary in severe cases.

RABIES PROPHYLAXIS

The number of reported cases of rabies in domestic animals (cattle, cats, and dogs) has dropped over the second half of this century. Conversely, rabies in wild animals began to increase in the 1970s, particularly in the midwestern and mid-Atlantic states. An increase in rabies cases among raccoons and skunks constitute the major reason for this increase.

An estimated 18,000 Americans are treated for exposure to rabies each year. The majority of these occur in children under 15 years of age. The decision to immunize the individual who has been bitten is based on the location in which the bite occurred, the circumstances surrounding the attack (eg, unprovoked), and whether the animal can be observed.

Management

Bites by domestic animals should be handled according to circumstance. An apparently healthy animal should be observed for 10 days. If it remains well, no treatment is needed. If the animal appears sick, it should be killed and its head removed and sent in ice (not frozen) to a qualified laboratory for examination, and immunization procedures should be initiated (see below). If the examination proves negative, the immunization can be discontinued. If the state of the animal is unknown (eg, escaped animals) consultation with the local health department can indicate the risk from data of the presence or absence of rabies in the community.

Bites by wild animals, such as skunk, fox, coyote, raccoon, bat, or other carnivores, should be considered as potentially infected. If the animal can be captured, it should be handled as previously noted for sick animals. If the animal cannot be examined in the laboratory, the individual should be immunized (see below).

If immunization procedures are decided on, both passive and active immunization should be given. Passive immunization consists of human rabies immune globulin (HRIG), with a standardized antibody content of 150 IU/mL. The dose is 20 IU/kg of body weight; one half should be used to infiltrate the wound(s) and the rest administered intramuscularly. Wounds in mucous membranes should not be infiltrated; the entire dose should be administered intramuscularly. Concurrently, active immunization should be started with intramuscular injection of 1 mL of human diploid cell vaccine (HDCV). If the laboratory report is negative, no further vaccine need be given. If positive or if the animal is suspected of being rabid, another 1 mL of HDCV should be given intramuscularly on the 3rd, 7th, 14th, and 28th days.

Prophylaxis is advisable for animal handlers or those living in areas where animal rabies is prevalent. Three intramuscular doses of HDCV are given on days 0, 7, and 21 or 28. In addition, an intradermal preexposure vaccine is available, given on the same time schedule. After exposure, these individuals need no HRIG and only two doses of vaccine on the 1st and 3rd day.

BIBLIOGRAPHY

American Academy of Pediatrics: Influenza. In Peter G, editor: 1994 Redbook: Report of the Committee on Infectious Diseases, ed 23, Elk Grove Village, 1994, American Academy of Pediatrics.

Anderson LJ: Role of parovirus B19 in human disease, Pediatr Infect Dis J 6:711–718, 1987.

Annunziato D, Kaplan MH, Hall WW, et al: A typical measles syndrome: pathologic and serologic findings, Pediatrics 70:203–209, 1982.

Balfaur HH, Bean B, Laskin OL, et al: Acyclovir halts progression of herpes zoster in immunocompromised patients, N Engl J Med 308:1448–1453, 1983.

Bloch AB, Orenstein WA, Ewing WM, et al: Measles outbreak in a pediatric practice: Airborne transmission in an office setting, Pediatrics 75:676–683, 1985.

Cartter ML, Farley TA, Rosengren S, et al: Occupational risk factors for infection with parvovirus B19 among pregnant women, J Infect Dis 163:282–285, 1991.

Cherry JD: Enteroviruses. In Feigin RD, Cherry JD, editors: Textbook of pediatric infectious diseases, ed 2. Philadelphia, 1987, WB Saunders.

Cherry JD: Roseola infantum. In Feigin RD, Cherry JD, editors: Textbook of pediatric infec-

tious diseases, ed 2, Philadelphia, 1987, WB Saunders.

Corey L: Infections with herpes simplex viruses, *N Engl J Med* 314:686–690, 747–756, 1986.

Denny FW: Current problems in managing streptococcal pharyngitis, *J Pediatr* 111:797–806, 1987.

Helmick CG, Bernard KW, D'Angelo LJ: Rocky mountain spotted fever: Clinical, laboratory and epidemiological features of 262 cases, *J Infect Dis* 150:480–488, 1984.

Hull HF, Montes JM, Hays PC, et al: Risk factors for measles vaccine failure among immunized students, *Pediatrics* 76:518–523, 1985.

Jubeliner D: Suppurative parotitis. In Feigin RD, Cherry JD, editors: *Textbook of Pediatric Infectious Diseases,* ed 2, Philadelphia, 1987, WB Saunders.

Krajden S, Middleton PJ: Enterovirus infections in the neonate, *Clin Pediatr* 22:87–92, 1983.

Nahmias AJ, Whitley RJ, Visintine AN, et al: The collaborative antiviral study group, *J Infect Dis* 145:829–836, 1982.

Nelson JD: The effect of penicillin therapy on the symptoms and signs of streptococcal pharyngitis, *Pediatr Infect Dis J* 3:10–13, 1984.

Plummer FA, Hammond GW, Forward K, et al: An erythema infectiosum-like illness caused by human parvovirus infection, *N Engl J Med* 313:74–79, 1985.

Rabies Surveillance, United States, 1987, *MMWR* 37:SS–4, 1988.

Sullivan-Bolyai JZ, Hull HF, Wilson C, et al: Presentation of neonatal herpes simplex virus infections: implicatons for a change in therapeutic strategy, *Pediatr Infect Dis J* 5:309–314, 1986.

Sumaya CV, Ench Y: Epstein-Barr virus infectious mononucleosis in children, *Pediatrics* 75:1003–1019, 1985.

Weller TH: Varicella and herpes zoster, *N Engl J Med* 309:1362–1368, 1434–1440, 1983.

Yeager AS, Ashley RL, Corey L: Transmission of herpes simplex virus from father to neonate, *J Pediatr* 103:905–910, 1983.

CHAPTER 91

Lower Respiratory Tract Infections

Craig D. Lapin
Craig M. Schramm

DISCUSSION

The most common forms of lower respiratory tract infection (LRTI) in pediatrics patients are acute bronchitis, bronchiolitis, and bacterial or nonbacterial (atypical) pneumonia. Acute bronchitis is characterized by the presence of cough, rhonchi, and fever in the absence of hypoxemia and significant systemic toxicity. Bronchiolitis is an acute, often first, episode of wheezing in children less than 2 years of age without pneu-

monia or asthma. It is associated with coryza, cough, and fever. Pneumonia is an infection of the terminal bronchioles and alveoli. Unlike bronchitis or bronchiolitis, pneumonia is a parenchymal disease and is often accompanied by high fever and systemic toxicity.

In general, however, most infections occur secondary to aspiration or inhalation of organisms from the nasopharynx and/or oropharynx into the lower respiratory tract. Hematogenous spread to the lungs also occurs but is far less

BOX 91-1
Etiologic Agents of Common Lower Respiratory Tract Infections

BRONCHIOLITIS
 Respiratory syncytial virus
 Parainfluenza viruses (types I and III)
 Adenovirus
 Influenza
 Mycoplasma pneumoniae
PNEUMONIA-VIRAL
 Respiratory syncytial virus
 Parainfluenza viruses
 Adenovirus
 Influenza
PNEUMONIA-BACTERIAL
 Streptococcus pneumoniae
 Staphylococcus aureus
 Pyogenic streptococcus (groups A, B, and D)
 Haemophilus influenzae B
PNEUMONIA-ATYPICAL
 Mycoplasma pneumoniae
 Chlamydia pneumoniae (TWAR)
 Mycobacterium tuberculosis (primary, tuberculous, and miliary)
 Fungal

acquired pneumonia in children over 3 years of age. Bacteria are responsible for a sizable minority (approximately 20%) of pneumonias in children. Common bacterial organisms responsible for community-acquired pneumonia include *Streptococcus pneumoniae, Streptococcus pyogenes* and other α-hemolytic streptococci, and *Staphylococcus aureus. Escherichia coli* and group B streptococci also may cause pneumonias in infants. *Hemophilus influenzae* type B was a frequent etiologic agent in young children until the advent of vaccination. Typeable and nontypeable *H. influenzae* and *Moraxella catarrhalis* remain common bacterial causes of acute bronchitis, particularly in children with host deficiencies or underlying pulmonary disease. Respiratory syncytial virus (RSV), parainfluenza viruses, and adenovirus which, are more frequent in infants and toddlers, and cause disease in older children less often. Lastly, after decades of decline the incidence of tuberculosis in children is increasing globally, especially in urban settings.

common in the normal host, even for bacterial pathogens. Once in the lower respiratory tract, the virulence of the infection and several factors of the host child (*eg,* immunity, nutrition, anatomy) help determine distal spread. Viruses may facilitate bacterial infection by increasing nasopharyngeal secretions and directly inhibiting mucociliary clearance and/or by interfering with the immune response. Hence, LRTIs may not be pure viral or bacterial infections but may result from both, with a secondary bacterial infection superimposed on an initial viral illness.

The incidence of lower respiratory tract infections varies with age. The incidence declines steadily after the age of 2 years. On average, only 1% of those children with pneumonia and 2% of children with bronchiolitis require hospital admission. The most common causes of LRTI are presented in Box 91-1. There is a great deal of overlap in the presentation of bacterial and nonbacterial pneumonia, bronchiolitis, and acute bronchitis. Nonbacterial agents such as respiratory viruses, *Mycoplasma pneumoniae,* and *Chlamydia pneumoniae* (TWAR) are the most common agents of lower respiratory tract disease. Recent studies indicate that *M. pneumoniae* (27%) and *C. pneumoniae* (28%) together cause approximately half the cases of community-

DATA GATHERING

History
When a patient arrives with a complaint of a "chest infection" a myriad of details may be sorted out quickly by history. The absence of fever or tachypnea practically eliminates LRTI, shifting the diagnosis toward upper respiratory infection or asthma. It is important to note that tachypnea often is not noticed by parents of younger infants, whose baseline respiratory rates are higher than older children. Even the history of a loose or productive cough would not suggest an LRTI if fever or tachypnea were not also present. The quality of the cough is not itself a very sensitive or specific indicator, but may at times be helpful. The dry cough of acute bronchitis is usually harsh, whereas in bronchiolitis it is characteristically hacking. Most bacterial pneumonias have a productive cough, whereas viral, mycoplasmal, and mycobacterial LRTIs are often nonproductive. A paroxysmal cough sometimes followed by stridor or apnea is suggestive of pertussis or, more commonly, pertussis syndrome secondary to a viral etiology.

The degree of illness, *ie,* the amount of fever, malaise, anorexia, respiratory distress, and systemic symptoms, may suggest etiologic agents.

Viral or mycoplasmal pneumonias are usually milder in character, more gradual in onset, and associated with low-grade fever. Bacterial pneumonia is associated with the acute onset of more severe respiratory and systemic symptoms. Nevertheless, certain viruses such as influenza, adenovirus, and hantavirus may mimic typical bacterial symptoms. Lethargy, poor feeding, vomiting, or diarrhea may be the presenting symptoms of pneumonia in young infants, in whom coughing may be mild. The presence of diarrhea, vomiting, and/or poor oral intake greatly increases the infant's risk of dehydration. In addition, apnea may occur in very young infants regardless of their infectious agent, although it is most frequent with RSV bronchiolitis. A 1- or 2-day prodrome of rhinorrhea is common in all types of LRTI except *M. pneumoniae* and *M. tuberculosis,* although it may rarely occur even with these agents. Headaches and malaise are more common in mycoplasma and influenza infections. Chest pain is more common in bacterial pneumonia and in acute bronchitis, the latter causing musculoskeletal pain from coughing. Tuberculosis has been called "the great pretender" and may demonstrate almost any respiratory sign. The classic presentation of chronic cough, weight loss, and night sweats is uncommon in children. The vast majority of confirmed *M. tuberculosis* infections in pediatrics are asymptomatic, having only radiographic findings.

After determining at least the possibility of an LRTI, the physician's knowledge of LRTI epidemiology may narrow the diagnosis and suggest causative organisms. The age of the patient is very important when considering etiologic possibilities (Table 91-1). Bronchiolitis classically describes an illness in children 2 years of age or younger. The main infectious agents responsible for infantile bronchiolitis are RSV, parainfluenza, adenovirus, influenza, and mycoplasma. In older children these agents often cause acute bronchitis, pneumonitis, or pneumonia. With nonbacterial pneumonia and bronchiolitis, there is often a history of exposure to others with similar infections. Parainfluenza type 1 is prevalent in autumn (usually on a biannual schedule), whereas RSV and influenza are seen in midwinter. Parainfluenza type 3 is largely endemic but may have outbreaks in the spring. *M. pneumoniae* is usually endemic as well, but 12- to 30-month urban epidemics have occurred. Bacterial pneumonias develop in all seasons but are most prevalent in the winter and spring months, possibly because of increased transmission due to increased indoor dwelling during these months.

One of the most difficult tasks for the physician is differentiating between a viral-induced exacerbation of asthma versus bronchiolitis, bronchitis, or *M. pneumoniae* infection (Table 91-2). Certain historical characteristics can be more helpful than the physical examination. A previous history of similar episodes strongly suggests asthma. Conversely, the first occurrence of cough and wheezing in an infant during "bronchiolitis season" or in a previously healthy, nonatopic older child is more suggestive of an infectious LRTI. In addition, a response to bronchodilators is less common in bronchiolitis than in asthma, and viral-induced asthma attacks may not be associated with fever.

Physical Examination

A certain degree of tachypnea is present in almost all LRTIs, with the possible exception of acute bronchitis. The respiratory rate should be taken while the child is preferably asleep, or at least quiet and relaxed. Normal values for resting respiratory rate vary with age (Table 91-3). Significant conjunctivitis is usually associated with adenoviral or chlamydial infections, and a mild form may be present in RSV bronchiolitis. Rhinitis and rhinorrhea frequently are present in all types of infection except those due to mycoplasma and mycobacterium. Tonsillitis, pharyngitis, and ulcerative stomatitis occur with viral, mycoplasmal, and chlamydial infections, although they may be less prominent as the disease progresses. Exanthems are seen with *M. pneumoniae* infections. Respiratory viruses, with the exception of adenovirus, are less apt to cause skin rashes than other viruses.

Auscultation of the chest has been shown to be insensitive in diagnosing the type of infection, especially in infants and young children. For example, crackles may be heard in bacterial pneumonia, nonbacterial pneumonia, bronchiolitis, or acute exacerbations of asthma. They may be focal or bilateral in pneumonia and are usually bilateral in bronchiolitis. They are generally absent in acute bronchitis. Wheezing is typically heard in bronchiolitis and asthma but is also a common finding in mycoplasmal, mycobacterial, and chlamydial pneumonias. Retractions are frequent in bronchiolitis and nonbacterial pneu-

TABLE 91-1
Relative Frequency of Organisms Causing Community-Acquired Pneumonia in Otherwise Healthy Children

	NEONATE (<1 MO)	YOUNG INFANTS (1–3 MOS) FEBRILE	YOUNG INFANTS (1–3 MOS) AFEBRILE	INFANTS AND YOUNG CHILDREN	OLDER CHILDREN (>5 YRS) AND ADOLESCENTS
Most frequent	Group B streptococci *Escherichia coli* Respiratory viruses Enteroviruses	Respiratory viruses Enteroviruses	*C. trachomatis*	*S. pneumoniae* Respiratory viruses	*Mycoplasma pneumoniae* *Chlamydia pneumoniae* *S. pneumoniae* Respiratory viruses *S. aureus* Group A streptococci *M. tuberculosis*
Occasional	*Haemophilus influenza*, non type *Streptococcus pneumoniae* *Klebsiella* and other enteric gram- negative rods Group A streptococci *Staphylococcus aureus* Varicella Cytomegalovirus Herpes simplex	Group B streptococci *S. pneumoniae* *S. aureus* Group A streptococci *Bordatella pertussis*	*Ureaplasma pneumoniae* Cytomegalovirus	*S. aureus* *B. pertussis* Group A streptococci *M. pneumoniae* *Chlamydia pneumoniae*	
Rare	*Mycobacterium tuberculosis* *Chlamydia trachomatis*	Varicella Cytomegalovirus *M. tuberculosis* Gram-negative enteric bacilli	*Pneumocystis carinii* (HIV infected)	*H. influenza B* *M. tuberculosis*	

Modified from Gilsdorf J: *Semin Respir Infect,* 2:146–151, 1987.

III

TABLE 91-2
Comparison of Findings in Lower Respiratory Tract Infections and Respiratory Diseases

	UPPER RESPIRATORY INFECTION	ASTHMA	BRONCHITIS	BRONCHIOLITIS	ATYPICAL PNEUMONIA	BACTERIAL PNEUMONIA
History						
Cough	Yes	Frequent	Yes	Yes	Yes	Yes
Sudden onset	Yes	Frequent	Yes	Yes	Occasional	Yes
Upper respiratory infection prodrome	—	Frequent	Yes	Yes	Frequent	Occasional
Toxicity	No	No	No	Yes	Occasional	Yes
Fever	No	Low	Occasional, low	Low	Usually low	High
Sputum	Minimal, post-pharyngeal	Infrequently, modest	Copious, purulent	No	Modest	Copious, purulent
Seasonal	Yes	Often	No	Yes	No	No
Examination						
Tachypnea	No	Frequent	Occasional	Yes	Occasional	Yes
Retractions	No	Frequent	No	Yes	Frequent	Yes
Decreased breath sounds	No	Frequent	No	Frequent	No	Focal
Wheeze	No	Usual	Frequent	Yes	Frequent	No
Rales	No	Infrequent	No	Yes	Yes	Yes
Rhonchi	Upper airway	Frequent	Yes	No	No	No
Laboratory						
Hypoxemia	No	Frequent	No	Frequent	Occasional	Frequent
Leukocytosis	No	Occasional	No	Infrequent	Infrequent	Yes
Hyperinflation	No	Usual	No	Yes	Occasional	No
Atelectasis	No	Frequent	Infrequent	Frequent	Occasional	Infrequent
Infiltrate	No	Infrequent	No	Occasional	Yes	Yes
Effusion	No	No	No	No	Mycoplasma	Occasional

TABLE 91-3
Normal Respiratory Rates for Age

AGE	MEAN	UPPER LIMIT
0–2 mos	45	68
3–4 mos	36	52
5–6 mos	31	44
6–12 mos	28	38
1–2 yrs	26	34
2–4 yrs	24	30
4–7 yrs	22	27
7–10 yrs	20	25
10–13 yrs	19	24
13–16 yrs	18	23
16–17 yrs	17	22

monia, particularly in younger children. Decreased breath sounds secondary to atelectasis or consolidation may be present in bronchiolitis, asthma, or pneumonia. If breath sounds are distant, consideration of a pleural effusion should be made, and, if chest wall percussion is not part of the clinician's normal examination, it should be performed in these cases. Tachycardia is common in bacterial pneumonia and bronchi-

olitis but rare in nonbacterial pneumonias. Palpation of the liver and spleen may be possible in patients with bronchiolitis or asthma because of air trapping, and the abdomen may appear distended because of swallowed air. Gastric distention and ileus also may occur in severe cases of pneumonia, usually bacterial. Abdominal tenderness or pain is common in bacterial pneumonia, and may sometimes be the patient's chief complaint in the presence of a basilar pneumonia or pleural effusion.

Diagnostic Testing
Complete blood cell counts should be performed in all children who appear moderately or severely ill, as well as in any infant less than 6 months of age whose history and physical examination suggest LRTI other than mild epidemic bronchiolitis. Hemoglobin should be assessed, because low values (from severe constitutional anemia, anemia of chronic illness, sickle cell anemia, etc.) affect the oxygen carrying content of the blood. Peripheral white blood cell (WBC) counts are quite variable but tend to be less than $15,000/mm^3$ in viral infections. Although there

may be a slight majority of neutrophils (50% to 70%), high levels of immature forms ("bands") are infrequent in viral LRTIs. Conversely, bacterial infections tend to have higher WBC counts with more immature forms.

Radiographic findings vary according to the clinical diagnosis, infecting agent, and age of the patient. Patients with acute bronchitis usually have a normal chest radiograph. Radiographs in patients with bronchiolitis often reveal hyperexpansion, peribronchial cuffing, atelectasis, and occasionally increased interstitial markings. Bacterial infections typically produce well-defined infiltrates, usually involving one lobe and located in the more peripheral lung field. Also, findings of pleural effusion, abscess, or pneumatocoeles are more characteristic of bacterial agents. Viral pneumonias frequently have perihilar or multilobar, poorly defined infiltrates. Scattered areas of atelectasis are more associated with viral pneumonia. *M. pneumoniae* most often presents with interstitial reticular or noduloreticular patterns, although alveolar and lobar infiltrates can occur as well. In addition, hilar or paratracheal adenopathy (approximately 20%) and pleural effusions (approximately 15%) are seen with mycoplasmal infections. In order of decreasing frequency, radiologic findings of *M. tuberculosis* in children include hilar lymphadenopathy, mediastinal or cervical lymphadenopathy, segmental or lobar infiltrate, consolidated pneumonia, atelectasis, pleural effusion, and miliary tuberculosis.

The ultimate diagnosis depends on identification of the etiologic agent with appropriate specimens and testing. Although this step is commonly omitted, this information is helpful when the patient fails or partially fails to respond to initial therapy. For viruses, the specimen of choice is a nasopharyngeal washing, because the latter yields more airway epithelial cells than expectorated sputum. The best technique entails lavaging the nares via a small feeding tube with 1 mL of viral transport media and aspirating a specimen back into the syringe. The specimen may be sent for culture and/or rapid diagnostic screens. Rapid tests based on enzyme-linked immunosorbent assay and fluorescent antibody techniques are commonly available for RSV, adenovirus, parainfluenza, and influenza. If a bacterial LRTI is suspected, expectorated sputum sent for Gram stain and cultures is the optimal test. Alternately, respiratory cultures may be obtained in patients who are unable to expectorate

by applying a throat swab to the posterior pharynx continuously until the patient coughs at least twice on the swab. More invasive tests such as nasotracheal, transtracheal, or transthoracic aspirate cultures usually are reserved for severely ill patients, often in the intensive care setting.

Diagnosis of *M. tuberculosis* may be made from a positive delayed hypersensitivity skin test (*ie,* purified protein derivative [PPD]; *see* American Academy of Pediatrics Red Book for criteria of a positive test). Tuberculosis skin tests should always be done with a control because of the possibility of anergy. Follow-up of a negative tuberculosis skin test with a negative control would include replacement of the PPD with a full anergy panel (more than one control). If the PPD is negative but the history, physical examination, or radiographs suggest tuberculosis, or if the PPD is positive in an area with a high prevalence of drug-resistant *M. tuberculosis,* then three first-morning gastric aspirates should be obtained and sent for bacteriologic analysis. Because respiratory secretions are concentrated in the stomach overnight, the sensitivity of morning gastric aspirates is greater than that of bronchoalveolar lavage in pediatric patients. In older children who are able to expectorate, nebulization of 3% hypertonic saline may be used to help produce a sputum specimen, which approaches the sensitivity of bronchoalveolar lavage. Polymerase chain reaction techniques have been used in research laboratories to enhance identification of *M. tuberculosis,* as well as *C. pneumoniae.* It is only a matter of time before they will be more commercially applicable.

At present, serologic tests are the only way to diagnose *M. pneumonia* infections. The presence of cold agglutinins is suggestive of mycoplasmal infection but is fairly insensitive and nonspecific. False positive results occur in viral pneumonias (especially adenovirus and parainfluenza) as well as in other illnesses. However, with suggestive clinical symptoms and negative viral cultures, a positive cold agglutinin test becomes much more suggestive for mycoplasma infection.

MANAGEMENT

Acute bronchitis is usually a mild, self-limited illness unless secondary infection occurs. Accordingly, therapy is usually symptomatic (*ie,* antipyretics for fever, antihistamines and decongestants for nasal symptoms, antitussives for cough, and analgesics if chest pain is present). If the patient requires hospitalization and if specific respiratory viruses have been isolated, then ribavirin (RSV or influenza) or amantadine/rimantadine (influenza A) should be considered. If the patient has had more than two episodes of bronchitis, a trial of bronchodilators may help to distinguish cough secondary to infection versus viral-induced bronchospastic coughing. If sputum production becomes more copious and/or purulent, then a secondary bacterial bronchitis may be suspected, particularly in a child with underlying pulmonary disease, and an antibiotic to cover β-lactamase–producing organisms is indicated.

Bronchiolitis in most infants and toddlers is relatively mild. In children who do not require hospitalization, families should be instructed how to watch for increasing respiratory distress by assessing sleeping respiratory rates, retractions, and difficulty feeding. Symptomatic treatment of fever and nasal symptoms should be initiated. In wheezing patients, an outpatient trial of bronchodilators, and possibly corticosteroids, is reasonable in an attempt to ameliorate the illness, although they have not been conclusively shown to change the course of the illness. Children with severe bronchiolitis (eg, those with marked tachypnea, severe retractions, listlessness, decreased oral intake, apnea, and/or hypoxemia) should be hospitalized for observation and supportive management. Infants with bronchopulmonary dysplasia or other pulmonary disease, cardiac disease, or immunodeficiencies are at higher risk for severe disease and admission if they develop bronchiolitis. Once admitted, oximetry should be performed, and arterial blood gases obtained if necessary. If the respiratory rate is greater than 60 breaths per minute, caution should be used before considering oral fluids because of the risk of aspiration. Humidified oxygen should be titrated to keep arterial oxygen percent saturation greater than 95% if possible. In addition to alleviating the hypoxemia, oxygen therapy is useful in decreasing dyspnea, respiratory distress, and irritability. Relief of dyspnea may, in turn, facilitate an infant's oral intake. Intravenous corticosteroids should be considered, especially in patients with previously identified reactive airways disease. Aerosolized β$_2$-adrenergic therapy should be given as needed. It should be noted, however, that β-agonists may worsen the hypoxemia in nonresponding infants.

Recently, nebulized racemic epinephrine has been shown to have therapeutic efficacy in bronchiolitis. If nebulized therapy is required more than every 2 hours for worsening respiratory distress or if apnea occurs, hypoxemia worsens, or more listlessness develops, the patient should be transferred to an intensive care unit. Mechanical ventilation may be necessary for increasing respiratory fatigue or failure, especially in young infants. Once ventilated, most patients with bronchiolitis require this type of support for 7 to 14 days.

Ribavirin is an aerosolized antiviral agent that is active against RSV and influenza types A and B. It is most effective when started early in the course of bronchiolitis. Studies continue to discuss whether the duration of mechanical ventilation or supplemental oxygen requirements are improved with ribavirin. It does decrease the length of viral shedding, however. Data indicate that pulmonary function at 6 months and 1 year follow-up are significantly improved in those infants who had received ribavirin. Ribavirin is suggested for treating infants less than 6 weeks of age, for those with bronchopulmonary dysplasia or other pulmonary problems, congenital heart disease, immunodeficiency, and for those infants with severe respiratory distress. Duration of therapy varies from not less than 3 days to no more than 5 days.

Treatment of pneumonia should be directed at the causative organism. If the clinician strongly suspects a viral agent, antibiotics are not necessary. The patient can be observed, and results of cultures may confirm the viral diagnosis. If a nonviral cause is postulated (eg, bacteria, mycoplasma, or chlamydia), mild to moderate infections may be treated at home. The choice of oral antibiotic to begin treatment should cover the most common organisms, pending results of any cultures. Therefore, co-trimoxazole, erythromycin, or clarithromycin may now be the drugs of choice to consider. If a severe infection warrants admission to hospital, intravenous antibiotics that cover both gram-positive and certain gram-negative organisms should be chosen. Cefuroxime and ceftriaxone have excellent broad-spectrum coverage. In cases in which aspiration pneumonia is suspected, combinations of clindamycin, ticarcillin-clavulanate (Timentin®), or metronidazole, and an aminoglycoside should be effective against the gram-positive, gram-negative, and anaerobic organisms except for resistant staphylococci. Only if cultures indicate the presence of methicillin-resistant staphylococcus is the addition of vancomycin warranted.

Therapy for tuberculosis has undergone many changes in recent years. Currently the American Academy of Pediatrics supports short-course, intensive treatment in children with positive signs or symptoms of tuberculosis, including hilar adenopathy. In the first 2 months, pyrazinamide plus isoniazid and rifampin is given daily, followed by 4 months of the latter two drugs given daily or twice a week under direct medical care provider supervision. The latter regimen greatly enhances compliance, and the overall success rate is greater than 95%. Other alternatives are available. Consideration of resistant organisms must be made, especially when the affected child comes from or has been exposed to areas where drug-resistant *M. tuberculosis* is endemic (*eg,* Asia and South America). Preventive therapy for children with positive PPD but no other findings is 9 months of isoniazid daily or twice weekly under supervision.

All children with pneumonia should be evaluated 2 to 3 weeks after initiation of therapy, or sooner if the LRTI is more severe or slower to resolve. If the child has been asymptomatic, has returned to baseline activity, and has a normal physical examination, follow-up chest radiographs are not indicated. If the child has persistent signs or symptoms; if the pulmonary course was complicated by effusion, abscess, or pneumatocoeles; or if the child has underlying pulmonary disease or a previous pneumonia, a follow-up radiograph should be done. Even in uncomplicated pneumonia, approximately 20% of patients will have abnormalities persisting on radiograph for at least 3 to 4 weeks. Assuming clinical improvement, further intervention at this stage is not indicated, but radiographs should be repeated again in 2 to 4 more weeks. If still abnormal, more aggressive investigation may be indicated as discussed below.

PERSISTENT AND RECURRENT PNEUMONIA

Recurrent pneumonia is defined as a reinfection with signs and symptoms of pneumonia after initial resolution of these features. Persistent pneumonia is pneumonia with a clinical course lasting longer than expected. These entities are often hard to distinguish if clearing of chest

---

BOX 91-2
Differential Diagnosis of Recurrent Pneumonia

FREQUENT CAUSES
    Recurrent exposure in otherwise healthy child
    Asthma
    Gastroesophageal reflux/aspiration
    Foreign body
INFREQUENT CAUSES
    Right middle lobe syndrome
    Immune deficiencies
    Bronchiectasis
    Cystic fibrosis
    Congenital lung lesions
RARE CAUSES
    Hemosiderosis
    Hypersensitivity pneumonitis
    Interstitial lung diseases
    Alveolar proteinosis

---

radiographs as well as the complete resolution of signs or symptoms cannot be documented. Radiographic findings with RSV and parainfluenza infection gradually clear over 2 to 3 weeks, uncomplicated pneumococcal pneumonia may take 6 to 8 weeks, and adenoviral pneumonia may take up to 12 months. These considerations again highlight the importance of the clinician trying to establish an etiologic agent. Even if the cause of pneumonia is unknown, a worsening or unchanged chest radiograph (or clinical signs or symptoms) over 2 weeks or more despite broad-spectrum antibiotic therapy for common bacterial agents is suggestive of an underlying problem rather than a simple LRTI (Box 91-2). A systematic approach, with careful reexamination of the patient's history, scrutiny of physical signs, and more extensive tests should yield a primary diagnosis in every child with persistent or recurrent pneumonia. An algorithmic approach to the child with pneumonia is presented in Figure 91-1.

FREQUENT CAUSES OF PERSISTENT OR RECURRENT DISEASE

The initial decision point in a patient with persistent or unresolving pneumonia is whether the findings are due to an unusual organism, an unusual response to a common infecting organism, or a congenital or acquired pulmonary lesion. A myriad of infectious agents are capable of causing pneumonia, and sometimes the history will provide clues to such etiologies. The cough

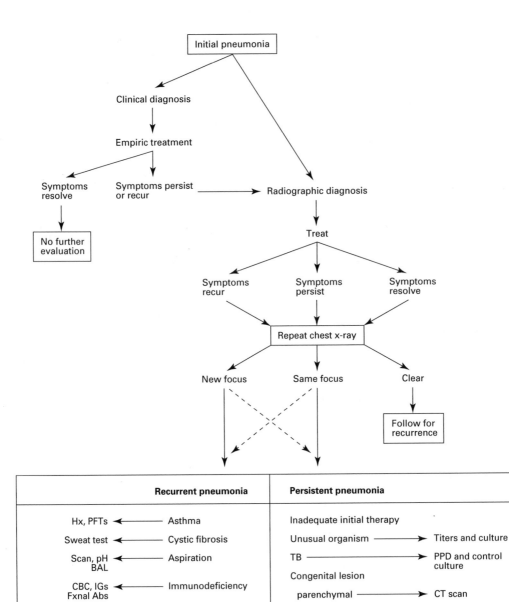

FIG 91-1
Decision tree for differential diagnosis of pneumonia.

TABLE 91-4
Uncommon Infectious Pneumonias in the Nonimmunocompromised Host

PNEUMONIA/DISEASE	INFECTIOUS AGENT	HISTORY	DIAGNOSIS
Bacterial			
Legionnaires' disease	*Legionella* species	Exposure to standing water	Urine fluorescent antibody, rise in titer
Tularemia	*Francisella tularensis*	Exposure to wild animals (especially rabbits, squirrels) or their ticks	Relative bradycardia, rise in titer
Pneumonic plague	*Yersinia pestis*	Southwestern US (exposure to prairie dogs or their fleas)	Rise in titer
Thoracic actinomycosis	*Actinomyces* species	Aspiration	Involvement of chest wall, anaerobic culture
Parasitic			
Eosinophilic pneumonia	*Ascaris lumbricoides*	Endemic areas	Eosinophilia, ova and parasites in stool
Visceral larval migrans	*Toxacara* species	Geophagia (dog or cat exposure)	Marked eosinophilia, high isohemagglutinins
Hydatid disease of the lung	*Echinococcus granulosus* and *E. multilocularis*	Endemic areas	Rise in titer, pathology
Spirochetal			
Leptospirosis	*Leptospira interrogans*	Exposure to animal urine	Meningeal signs, rise in titer
Fungal			
Histoplasmosis	*Histoplasma capsulatum*	Midwestern US	Rise in titer
Coccidioidomycosis	*Coccidiodes immitis*	Southeastern US	Rise in titer
Blastomycosis	*Blastomyces dermatidis*	Southeastern, southwestern, midwestern US	Rise in titer, pathology
Chlamydial			
Psittacosis	*H. capsulatum*	Midwestern US	Rise in titer
Rickettsial			
Q fever	*Coxiella burnetti*	Exposure to cattle, sheep, or goats	Rise in titer
Rocky Mountain spotted fever	*Rickettsia rickettsii*	Endemic area (southeastern US) tick bite	Characteristic rash, rise in titer

Modified with permission from Todd JK: Pneumonia in children, *Postgrad Med* 61:251–258, 1977.

associated with pertussis often persists for up to 6 months after the acute illness, and this diagnosis may be suspected in an incompletely immunized child with the characteristic paroxysmal cough. Infants less than 1 year of age account for nearly 50% of pertussis cases in the United States. Even with full immunizations, there is a 15% failure rate to protect against pertussis. Erythromycin is effective in eradicating the organism from the nasopharynx and can attenuate the development of the paroxysmal cough if administered during the initial catarrhal phase of the disease. It does not, however, shorten the paroxysmal stage of the disease or hasten resolution of the chronic cough. Other rare bacterial and nonbacterial pathogens to consider in certain circumstances are listed in Table 91-4. To the extent that several of these agents require specific

antimicrobials not commonly applied in the empiric treatment of pneumonia, their diagnosis must be pursued vigorously in an ill child who is not responding to conventional therapy.

Asthma is a very common cause of recurrent or persistent radiographic changes. A family history of asthma, atopy, wheezing, and/or cough suggests this diagnosis. Conversely, the presence of clubbing practically eliminates it. Chronic bronchitis is defined in adults as a condition of excessive mucus production and cough present on most days for a minimum of 3 months per year for 2 or more years. However, chronic bronchitis rarely occurs in children. Indeed, it should be emphasized that children with asthma can present with cough only and no audible wheezes ("cough-variant asthma"). Moreover, in addition to the characteristic hyperinflation and peribron-

---

BOX 91-3
Infrequent Causes of Recurrent Pneumonia

Cystic fibrosis
Immune deficiencies
   Immunoglobulin deficiencies
   Complement deficiencies
   HIV
Congenital lesions
   Bronchogenic cyst
   Cystic adenomatoid malformation
   Sequestration

BOX 91-4
Rare Causes of Recurrent Pneumonia

Pulmonary hemosiderosis
Hypersensitivity pneumonias
   Pigeon-breeder's lung
   Farmer's lung
   Humidifier lung—mold
Interstitial pneumonia
   Usual interstitial
   Desquamative
   Giant cell
   Lymphoid
Pulmonary alveolar proteinosis

---

chial cuffing, radiographic changes in asthma frequently involve partial or complete atelectasis of the right middle lobe ("right middle lobe syndrome"), although any lobe may be involved. Thus, asthma may mimic persistent or recurrent pneumonia. Usually, however, asthmatic patients lack fever or other systemic signs of illness despite their radiographic infiltrates. Evaluation of sputum or nasal secretions often reveals eosinophils if allergic triggers are involved. Spirometry and peak expiratory flows, especially with response to bronchodilators, or standardized bronchial challenge tests such as methacholine, histamine, cold air, or exercise, also can help make the diagnosis. Often, an empiric trial of bronchodilators both establishes the diagnosis and resolves the abnormal findings.

In infants, children with neurologic abnormality, and even some normal older children, gastroesophageal reflux (GER), aspiration, and microaspiration can cause recurrent pneumonias. A history of posttussive emesis or dyspepsia may suggest GER. Choking, gagging, coughing, or difficulty feeding may indicate a swallowing dysfunction. Infants who are put to bed with a bottle are at increased risk for aspiration, and, if they have developed caries, they can aspirate purulent material. Once aspiration has occurred, wheezing, crackles, or decreased breath sounds may be auscultated. In infants the right upper lobe often is involved due to the orientation of the bronchus and infants often being supine; however, radiographic and physical findings may be left sided as well. A barium swallow helps to diagnose swallowing problems and anatomic causes of reflux such as tracheoesophageal fistulas and hiatal hernias. Nuclear medicine scans ("milk scans" and "salivagrams") may be useful in studying the patient for aspiration over longer time periods. Unfortunately, the sensitivity of radiologic studies for aspiration is low. Esophageal pH monitoring may demonstrate the presence of GER but, by itself, is not diagnostic of aspiration. Accordingly, given a strong suspicion of aspiration despite negative tests, a flexible bronchoscopy is indicated to rule out a tracheoesophageal fistula and to obtain a bronchoalveolar lavage specimen. The presence of substantial lipid droplets in alveolar macrophages is sometimes the only way to diagnose aspiration in a patient.

A history of sudden choking, violent coughing, wheezing, or brief episodes of cyanosis may suggest aspiration of a foreign body, although up to 20% of children with foreign body aspiration have a negative history. If the foreign body is small and not obstructive, symptoms may be minimal. Focal findings on auscultation would help support this diagnosis, especially decreased breath sounds or wheezing over the affected side. Unilateral change in the shape of the thorax, with overexpansion secondary to air trapping or underexpansion due to atelectasis, may be observed on physical or radiographic examination. Because inspiratory and expiratory films are difficult to get young children to perform, comparison of right and left lateral decubitus films often provide similar information. In selected cases, fluoroscopy or ultrasound of the chest in various projections may be more diagnostic. Removal of the foreign body by rigid bronchoscopy usually is performed by otorhinolaryngologists or general surgeons. If not removed, a late complication of foreign bodies may be hemoptysis. Boxes 91-3 and 91-4 list the less common causes of pneumonia.

COMPLICATIONS OF PNEUMONIA

The majority of pneumonias resolve without consequence. The presence of a pleural effusion strongly suggests a bacterial infection, although many noninfectious causes also exist. A partial list of the organisms that can cause effusions include *S. aureus, S. pneumoniae, S. pyogenes,* anaerobes, *M. tuberculosis, M. pneumoniae,* adenovirus, influenza, coxsackie virus, Epstein-Barr virus, candida, and chlamydia. Laboratory evaluation of pleural fluid for pH, protein, lactic dehydrogenase, glucose, and WBC count establishes the diagnosis of transudate, exudate, or effusion.

Lung abscesses can occur at any age but are quite rare in neonates. Secondary abscesses are more common than primary. Conditions predisposing to secondary lung abscesses in children include severe infections, immunodeficiency or immunosuppression, repeated aspiration, foreign bodies, and cystic fibrosis. *S. aureus* is the most common organism cultured from primary (65%) or secondary (35%) abscesses. A partial list of other agents associated with abscesses includes *Streptococcus viridans, S. pneumoniae, M. pneumoniae,* hemophilus, aspergillus, pseudomonas, and anaerobes. Pneumatocoeles, not to be confused with abscesses, usually occur in the convalescent stages after pneumonia. They are most common with *S. aureus* or measles pneumonia.

Bronchiectasis may be caused by several entities—cystic fibrosis, foreign body aspiration, ciliary dyskinesia, immunodeficiencies, and, most commonly, infections. The most frequent infectious cause of bronchiectasis in developed countries is viral pneumonia, although tuberculosis, pertussis, measles, or histoplasmosis also may be implicated. The typical presentation of bronchiectasis is a persistent streaky radiographic infiltrate, sometimes with characteristic "tram-tracking" of a dilated airway, in a patient with a history of recurrent crackles and infections in that region. The diagnosis can be confirmed in over 95% of cases with a thin-cut computed tomographic scan with contrast enhancement.

Bronchiolitis obliterans is a chronic form of bronchiolitis characterized by the partial or complete obstruction of bronchioles by fibrous tissue following a lower respiratory injury. It differs from classic bronchiolitis in that it can develop at any age, it lacks accompanying upper respiratory infection symptoms, and it typically follows a bronchopneumonia. In children, bronchiolitis obliterans is most commonly preceded by LRTIs caused by adenovirus, influenza, and measles, although it has also been reported following other infections, including parainfluenza and mycoplasma, and in children with chronic aspiration. The clinical and radiographic features wax and wane for several weeks or months, with recurring pneumonia, atelectasis, and wheezing. Radiographic findings include hyperlucency on plain films, a mottled distribution of defects on ventilation/perfusion scan, and a characteristic pruning of distal bronchi on bronchography. Pulmonary functions demonstrate air trapping and fixed airflow obstruction. Some patients can improve gradually over several years, but often the pulmonary dysfunction is permanent.

The adult respiratory distress syndrome (ARDS) is a poorly understood entity attributed to cytokine activation and pulmonary capillary leak. Pulmonary injury from a variety of causes may be complicated by barotrauma and pulmonary oxygen toxicity in a mechanically ventilated patient. For infectious etiologies, ARDS occurs most commonly in the presence of bacterial infection and severe sepsis, but it can develop with a severe pneumonia of any cause, including mycoplasma and viruses. Hantavirus is a newly emerged etiologic agent of ARDS, particularly in the southwest United States and in certain urban areas. The characteristic radiographic presentation is that of low lung volumes and diffuse, progressive alveolar infiltrates. Despite advances in therapy, the mortality rate of ARDS remains as high as 60% to 70%.

SUMMARY

Lower respiratory tract infections are an extremely common problem encountered by all clinicians caring for children. Although the vast majority represent simple, relatively mild illnesses in otherwise healthy patients, the clinician must be alert for the occasional patient who presents atypically, either with unusual findings, an unfavorable response to therapy, or an infrequent complication. The early identification of such patients requires diligent follow-up of children with LRTIs, and the establishment of uncommon etiologies often can challenge the diagnostic and therapeutic acumen of the health care providers. Nevertheless, it is imperative that diagnoses be established for all children with LRTIs, particularly in those with recurrent or persistent "pneumonias," because many of the latter represent other, often progressive, chronic conditions. In many cases, referral of such atypical patients to a pediatric pulmonary sub-specialist may be necessary to establish the diagnosis and assist in the acute and long-term management of the child's pulmonary disease.

BIBLIOGRAPHY

Broughton RA: Infections due to *Mycoplasma pneumoniae* in childhood, *Pediatr Infect Dis J* 5:71–85, 1986.

Gilsdorf JR: Community-acquired pneumonia in children, *Semin Respir Inf* 2:146–151, 1987.

Grayston JT: *Chlamydia pneumoniae* (TWAR) infections in children, *Pediatr Infect Dis J* 13:675–685, 1994.

Jacobs RF, Starke JR: Tuberculosis in children, *Med Clin North Am,* 77:1335–1351, 1993.

Leigh MW: Lower respiratory tract infections in children, *Curr Opin Pediatr* 4:417–425, 1992.

Long SS: Treatment of acute pneumonia in infants and children, *Pediatr Clin North Am* 30:297, 1983.

Panitch HB, Callahan CW Jr, Schidlow DV: Bron-chiolitis in children, *Clin Chest Med* 14:715–731, 1993.

Peter G, editor: *Report of the Committee on Infectious Diseases (The Red Book),* ed 23, 1994, American Academy of Pediatrics.

Regelmann WE: Diagnosing the cause of recurrent and persistent pneumonia in children, *Pediatr Ann* 22:561–568, 1993.

Stark JM: Lung infections in children, *Curr Opin Pediatr* 5:273–280, 1993.

Todd JK: Pneumonia in children, *Postgrad Med* 61:251–258, 1977.

Turner RB, Lande AE, Chase P, et al: Pneumonia in pediatric outpatients: Cause and clinical manifestations, *J Pediatr* 111:194–200, 1987.

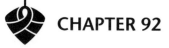

CHAPTER 92

Bacterial Meningitis

Joseph W. St. Geme III

Bacterial meningitis is defined as inflammation of the meninges and evidence of a bacterial pathogen in the cerebrospinal fluid (CSF). Despite the relative rarity of this disease during infancy and childhood, it remains a major cause of morbidity and mortality. Sequelae from men-ingitis occur in 25% to 50% of survivors and include hearing deficits, language disorders, mental retardation, motor impairments, and seizures. Whereas the mortality rate for many infections in children has declined dramatically in recent years, case fatality rates for bacterial meningitis have not substantially changed, remaining at 10% to 20% in the neonate and 5% to 10% in older infants and children.

The attack rate for this infection is highest in newborn infants, with an incidence as high as one per 1000 live births in some nurseries. Most neonatal meningitis occurs during the first week of life (early-onset disease) and results from contact with contaminated amniotic fluid near the time of delivery (ascending amniotic infection syndrome). Susceptible infants either inhale or swallow contaminated amniotic fluid and develop septicemia with bacterial seeding of the meninges. Common neonatal pathogens responsible for early-onset meningitis include group B streptococci, *Escherichia coli, Listeria monocytogenes,* enterococci, and *Klebsiella* and *Enterobacter* species. Late-onset neonatal meningitis occurs between 1 week and 3 months of age and is caused by the same group of pathogens as well as *Streptococcus pneumoniae, Nesseria meningitidis,* and *Haemophilus influenzae.* Late-onset infection may result from colonization at the time of birth (vertical transmission) or via postnatal transmission from nursery personnel, caregivers at home, or community contacts (horizontal transmission). During the past decade, improvements in neonatal intensive care have permitted the survival of a population of very low-birth-weight infants who are hospitalized for many months and are at increased risk for nosocomial infection. Meningitis developing in these infants is caused by a different spectrum of microorganisms, including coagulase-negative staphylococci, *Staphylococcus aureus,* and *Pseudomonas aeruginosa* in addition to the bacteria causing early-onset meningitis.

Among infants over 3 months of age and children, *S. pneumoniae, N. meningitidis,* and *H. influenzae* type b are the agents responsible for approximately 95% of cases of bacterial meningitis. Of these three pathogens, *S. pneumoniae* is probably the most common etiology now in children between 3 months and 5 years of age (*H. influenzae* type b previously was most common in this age group but has waned since the introduction of conjugate *H. influenzae* vaccines). In patients 5 to 19 years of age, *N. meningitidis* is the most frequent bacterial CSF isolate. Infection with all three of these encapsulated bacteria begins with colonization of the nasopharynx followed by invasion of the bloodstream and hematogenous dissemination to the meninges.

Rarely infection may occur from direct extension complicating otitis media, sinusitis, mastoiditis, or fracture through the paranasal sinuses, usually due to *S. pneumoniae* or nontypable *H. influenzae.* Other less common infectious causes of CSF pleocytosis in children include mycobacterial meningitis, Rocky Mountain spotted fever, ehrlichiosis, *Mycoplasma* infection, parameningeal infection, and spirochetal disease such as syphilis, leptospirosis, or Lyme disease. In the immunocompromised child unusual bacteria, certain viruses (especially the herpes viruses), and fungi deserve serious consideration.

In children with bacterial meningitis, several clinical and laboratory findings are predictive of neurologic sequelae. Patients with delayed sterilization of the CSF have significantly more acute complications and a higher incidence of permanent neurologic abnormalities. The presence of focal neurologic deficits at the time of diagnosis and increased bacterial counts in the CSF also correlate with poor outcome. Other factors that may have some bearing on prognosis include seizures for longer than 3 days, CSF protein concentration greater than 1000 mg/dL, CSF white blood cell (WBC) count greater than $10,000/mm^3$, and CSF glucose concentration less than 10 mg/dL.

DATA GATHERING

The presentation of bacterial meningitis is variable. It may be acute and fulminant in association with overwhelming septicemia or insidious, beginning with a nonspecific febrile illness and progressing over a few days. The former mode of presentation is most commonly due to meningococcal infection, whereas the latter is more typical for *H. influenzae* disease, but there is considerable overlap.

History

Common symptoms in children with meningitis include fever, neck stiffness, photophobia, headache, anorexia, and mental status abnormalities such as lethargy, irritability, or confusion. Neonates and young infants generally present with a history of poor feeding, respiratory distress, irritability, and inconsolability; up to one half of them may lack fever, making this finding an unreliable predictor of bacterial meningitis in this population. Approximately 20% to 30% of patients of any age will experience a seizure prior to presentation.

Knowledge about infectious contacts, status of immunization against *H. influenzae* type b, presence of other medical problems, and chronic medications such as immunosuppressing agents may provide clues about the likelihood of specific pathogens. Recent antimicrobial therapy may explain a sterile CSF culture despite CSF cell counts and chemistry values that suggest a bacterial cause. Information about family composition and daycare or nursery school attendance facilitates formulation of a plan for prophylaxis if infection is due to *H. influenzae* type b or *N. meningitidis*. A detailed history of the child's level of development establishes a baseline against which to evaluate recovery.

Physical Examination

In toddlers and older children, classic findings on physical examination reflect meningeal inflammation and include nuchal rigidity and Kernig and Brudzinski signs. Kernig sign is present when pain and resistance are detected on attempted extension of the knee with the hip in 90° flexion. Brudzinski sign is present if passive flexion of the neck induces involuntary hip flexion. These signs can appear late in the young child with meningitis and are generally absent in comatose patients. In the infant signs of meningeal irritation can be minimal, but a bulging fontanelle and diastasis of the sutures (indicators of elevated intracranial pressure) are often observed. Evidence of meningeal inflammation can similarly be subtle in patients with either primary or secondary immunodeficiencies, and suspicion of meningitis in these susceptible children must therefore be high. Despite the frequency of increased intracranial pressure in this disease, papilledema is rarely noted and presence of this sign should raise concern about the possibilities of venous sinus thrombosis, subdural empyema, or brain abscess complicating meningitis. Careful neurologic examination will reveal some alteration of consciousness at the time of hospital admission in the great majority of patients. A variety of focal neurologic abnormalities can also be noted, including deafness, ataxia, limited extraocular movement, asymmetric facial expression, blindness, and motor deficits. Focal neurologic signs occur most commonly in infection due to *S. pneumoniae* and generally result from cortical vein thrombosis or occlusive arterial disease.

In addition to those physical findings directly referable to infection of the central nervous system, a number of other signs can also be present. Hypotension and tachycardia can occur secondary to vomiting and poor oral intake or from septicemia with resultant peripheral vasodilation. The most common skin rash observed is a purpuric or petechial eruption. This rash is observed most frequently with meningococcal infection but can be caused by any of the bacterial pathogens. Occasionally a diffuse maculopapular eruption precedes purpura and petechiae. Other signs can be present as a result of associated focal infection such as otitis media, sinusitis, buccal or periorbital cellulitis, arthritis, epiglottitis, pneumonia, or pericarditis. Recognition of these entities is important because they may influence management.

Laboratory Tests

Collection of CSF for analysis represents the most critical diagnostic step in the child with suspected meningitis. Any child who demonstrates any evidence of meningitis by history or physical examination should undergo lumbar puncture. Although such an approach will lead to a high number of negative lumbar punctures, it will also facilitate early diagnosis and hence allow more expeditious treatment of this serious disease. In the child who has a focal neurologic deficit or signs of elevated intracranial pressure such as papilledema, altered pupillary responses, or increased blood pressure with bradycardia, lumbar puncture should be delayed until a computed tomographic scan has been obtained to avoid the complication of cerebellar or uncal herniation. Other situations in which this procedure should be delayed or withheld include significant cardiorespiratory compromise in a neonate or infection in the area that the needle will traverse to obtain CSF. In all of these circumstances, blood cultures should be obtained and antibiotics should be administered immediately. Lumbar puncture should be performed later when the patient can safely tolerate the procedure. Although short-term antibiotic therapy will reduce the yield of CSF culture and to a lesser extent CSF Gram stain, CSF morphologic and biochemical characteristics will remain unchanged for at least 2 or 3 days.

During lumbar puncture, the opening pressure should be determined whenever possible. This measurement is usually elevated in meningitis, with a mean value of 300 mm H_2O. When the

TABLE 92-1
Normal CSF Values*

PARAMETER	PRETERM NEWBORN	TERM NEWBORN	INFANTS 1–3 MOS	>3 MOS THROUGH CHILDHOOD
White blood cell count (cells/mm^3)				
Mean	9.0	8.2	2.9	
Range	0–29	0–32	0–9	0–7
Polymorphonuclear cells (%)	57	61	0–5	0–4
Glucose (mg/dL)				
Mean	50	52	60	60
Range	24–63	34–119	40–80	40–80
Cerebrospinal fluid/blood	0.74	0.81	0.5–0.65	0.5–0.65
Protein (mg/dL)				
Mean	115	90	40	20
Range	65–150	20–170	20–100	5–40

*Values for preterm and term newborns adapted from Sarff et al: Cerebrospinal fluid evaluation in neonates: comparison of high-risk infants with and without meningitis. *J Pediatr* 1976; 88:473. Other values compiled from Fishman R: *Cerebrospinal fluid in diseases of the nervous system,* Philadelphia, 1980, WB Saunders; Portnoy JM, Olson LC: Normal cerebrospinal fluid values in children: Another look, *Pediatrics,* 75:484–487, 1985; Widell S: Protein content of CSF in normal children. Personal investigations, *Acta Paediatr* 47 (suppl 115):44–57, 1958.

pressure is very high, minimal amounts of fluid should be collected. CSF should be examined immediately, because WBCs begin to disintegrate after approximately 90 minutes. Analysis of CSF should include total WBC count and differential, protein concentration, glucose concentration relative to serum glucose, Gram stain, and culture. Normal values for CSF in newborns, older infants, and children are shown in Table 92-1. In general in bacterial meningitis, the CSF WBC count is greater than 200/mm^3, protein is greater than 100 mg/dL, glucose is less than 40 mg/dL with the ratio of CSF to serum glucose less than 0.5, and Gram stain reveals bacteria. However, patients with meningitis do not always have abnormalities in all of these CSF parameters. Newborn infants can have normal CSF WBC counts as often as 30% of the time and also frequently have normal glucose concentrations and negative Gram stains. In older children with early meningitis, CSF values can also be normal. It is therefore critical to perform a complete evaluation of CSF and await culture results in all cases.

Various immunoassays are available to detect bacterial antigens from group B streptococci, *H. influenzae* type b, *N. meningitidis,* and *S. pneumoniae* in CSF and other body fluids and can be helpful in establishing a causative agent in the child who has received antibiotic therapy prior to lumbar puncture. These techniques include counterimmunoelectrophoresis, latex agglutina-

tion and staphylococcal coagglutination tests, and enzyme immunoassay. Latex agglutination is the preferred test because of its simplicity, rapidity, and high sensitivity and specificity. Occasionally in patients with meningitis, bacterial antigen is detected only in concentrated urine. Therefore, to optimize the yield of this technique, both CSF and concentrated urine should be assayed.

Other laboratory studies that should be obtained at the time of initial evaluation include blood cultures, serum glucose and electrolyte levels, blood urea nitrogen (BUN), serum creatinine, complete blood cell (CBC) count, and possibly coagulation tests. Because most infants and children with bacterial meningitis are initially bacteremic, blood cultures are especially important in the patient in whom lumbar puncture will be delayed until after the initiation of antibiotic treatment. The serum sodium concentration will provide information about the possibility of inappropriate secretion of antidiuretic hormone (ADH) and serve as a baseline level for future measurements. The combination of serum bicarbonate concentration, BUN, and serum creatinine will help in the assessment of the state of hydration and tissue perfusion. A CBC count provides a variety of valuable information. Although peripheral WBC counts are too variable and nonspecific to be useful in confirming or excluding a diagnosis of bacterial meningitis, counts less than 3000/mm^3 suggest severe disease and poor prognosis. Anemia has been described best in association with infection caused by *H. influenzae* type b, resulting from immune hemolysis of red blood cells that are coated with soluble bacterial antigens, but may occur with other pathogens as well. Thrombocytopenia may reflect disseminated intravascular coagulation, and measurement of platelet count in combination with coagulation studies (prothrombin time, partial thromboplastin time, and possibly fibrinogen and fibrin split products) is of particular importance in the child with a petechial or purpuric rash.

MANAGEMENT

Treatment of bacterial meningitis should begin immediately after appropriate cultures are obtained. Initial antimicrobial therapy is based on the likely pathogens.

In newborn infants presenting with meningitis during the first week of life, initial empiric therapy should include a penicillin combined with an aminoglycoside. Ampicillin and gentamicin are generally used because ampicillin has activity against group B streptococci, *L. monocytogenes*, most enterococci, and some gram-negative rods, and gentamicin provides synergism against *Listeria* and enterococci and broader coverage of the Enterobacteriaceae. For infants who present beyond the first week of life but before the age of 3 months, the preferred starting regimen is ampicillin and cefotaxime. This combination is superior to alternative regimens (*eg*, ampicillin plus gentamicin or monotherapy with cefotaxime) because of the excellent coverage it provides against β-lactamase–producing *H. influenzae*, most gram-negative bacilli, *Listeria*, and most penicillin-resistant *S. pneumoniae*, in addition to the other pathogens causing disease in this age group. In infants older than 3 months and children, cefotaxime or ceftriaxone is recommended for empiric therapy. Because cephalosporin-resistant *S. pneumoniae* have been reported in many regions in the United States, the treatment regimen should also include vancomycin, especially if gram-positive cocci are visualized on Gram stain of CSF or the child has received antibiotics during the previous month.

After an organism has been isolated from culture, antibiotic therapy should be tailored according to the results of *in vitro* susceptibility testing. Group B streptococci usually can be treated with either penicillin or ampicillin alone, although some experts advise that gentamicin be included for at least the first few days of treatment. *L. monocytogenes* and susceptible enterococci are generally treated with a full course of both ampicillin and gentamicin. Alternative antibiotics for resistant enterococcal isolates include vancomycin and streptomycin. For neonatal meningitis caused by gram-negative enteric organisms, the synergistic regimen of ampicillin and an aminoglycoside remains the treatment of choice in most cases, but cefotaxime or ceftazidime may be necessary for resistant strains. Isolates of *Enterobacter* species, *Citrobacter* species, *Serratia* species, indole-positive *Proteus* species, and *Providencia* species are optimally treated with an extended spectrum penicillin such as ticarcillin or piperacillin and an appropriate aminoglycoside. For *N. meningitidis* and most strains of *S. pneumoniae,* the preferred regimen is penicillin or ampicillin. Strains of *S. pneumoniae* that are resistant to penicillin (minimal inhibitory concentration [MIC] ≥ 0.1) but sensitive to third-generation cephalosporins (MIC ≤ 0.5) are best treated with cefotaxime or ceftriaxone. Isolates of *S. pneumoniae* that are resistant to broad-spectrum cephalosporins are optimally treated with the combination of cefotaxime or ceftriaxone plus vancomycin. For *H. influenzae,* treatment is with ampicillin if the isolate is sensitive. For ampicillin-resistant strains, cefotaxime, ceftriaxone, or chloramphenicol should be used.

The duration of antimicrobial treatment for bacterial meningitis is determined by the organism causing disease and the clinical response to therapy. For uncomplicated meningitis due to group B streptococci or *L. monocytogenes,* treatment should extend for 14 days following sterilization of CSF. Infants with gram-negative meningitis require a minimum of 3 weeks of therapy, and in cases of delayed sterilization of CSF, 4 to 6 weeks may be necessary. In infants and children with meningitis caused by *N. meningitidis,* 5 to 7 days is considered satisfactory. Uncomplicated infection with *H. influenzae* should be treated for 7 to 10 days, whereas disease due to *S. pneumoniae* should be treated for at least 10 days. The preferred antibiotic(s) and duration of therapy for infection with specific pathogens are summarized in Table 92-2.

TABLE 92-2
Preferred Treatment for Common Causes of Bacterial Meningitis

ORGANISM	ANTIBIOTIC*	DURATION[†] (DAYS)
Group B streptococci	Penicillin or ampicillin (± gentamicin)	Minimum 14
Listeria monocytogenes	Ampicillin and gentamicin	Minimum 14
Enterococci	Ampicillin and gentamicin	Minimum 14
Enterobacteriaceae	Ampicillin and aminoglycoside (cefotaxime or ceftazidime for resistant strains)	Minimum 21
Haemophilus influenzae	Ampicillin (cefotaxime, ceftriaxone, or chloramphenicol for resistant strains)	7–10
Streptococcus pneumoniae	Penicillin (cefotaxime or ceftriaxone ± vancomycin for resistant strains)	10–14
Neisseria meningitidis	Penicillin or cefotaxime or ceftriaxone	5–7

*Ultimate choice of antibiotic must be guided by *in vitro* susceptibility testing.
[†]Duration of treatment is for uncomplicated infection.

During the course of treatment with aminoglycoside antibiotics or vancomycin, one should carefully monitor serum levels, especially in patients with impaired renal function, because of the toxicity of these drugs. Recommended peak serum levels are 4 to 8 µg/mL for gentamicin and tobramycin, 5 to 10 µg/mL for netilmicin, 15 to 25 µg/mL for kanamycin and amikacin, and 20 to 30 µg/mL for vancomycin. Trough serum levels should be less than 2 µg/mL for gentamicin, tobramycin, and netilmicin, less than 10 µg/mL for kanamycin and amikacin, and between 5 and 12 µg/mL for vancomycin. Patients being treated with chloramphenicol also should have levels monitored; monitoring is particularly important in neonates and children with hepatic dysfunction. In addition, one should note that concomitant therapy with phenobarbital, diphenylhydantoin, or rifampin will influence chloramphenicol metabolism and hence serum levels. The recommended peak serum level is 15 to 25 µg/mL.

The inflammatory response plays a critical role in producing the central nervous system pathology and the resultant sequelae of bacterial meningitis. Double-blind, placebo-controlled trials have demonstrated that adjunctive treatment with dexamethasone reduces the incidence of hearing loss and other neurologic sequelae in infants and children with *H. influenzae* type b meningitis. According to these studies, dexamethasone should be initiated before the first dose of antibiotic therapy, or as soon thereafter as possible, and should be administered intravenously in a dose of 0.15 mg/kg. Doses should be repeated every 6 hours to complete 16 doses over 4 days. The role of dexamethasone as adjunctive therapy for meningitis due to other bacterial pathogens is the subject of ongoing study and remains controversial. There is particular concern that dexamethasone may be deleterious in the setting of meningitis due to cephalosporin-resistant *S. pneumoniae,* resulting in delayed sterilization of the CSF. Most authorities agree that dexamethasone should be avoided in infants younger than 2 months of age with bacterial meningitis.

PREVENTION

Vaccination

Primary immunization represents the cornerstone in prevention of meningitis due to *H. influenzae* type b. As shown in Table 92-3, there are currently four vaccines licensed for use against this organism, all containing type b polysaccharide capsular material chemically conjugated to an immunogenic (carrier) protein. The four vaccines differ to some extent with respect to size of the polysaccharide, chemical linkage between the polysaccharide and the carrier protein, or type of carrier protein. In addition, they differ in immunologic characteristics. Based on differences in immunogenicity, three of the four vaccines are licensed for use in infants, and the fourth is approved only for children 15 months of age and older. As a consequence of routine immunization during infancy, the incidence of *H. influenzae* type b meningitis has decreased over 90% compared with the prevaccine era.

For several years a quadrivalent meningococ-

TABLE 92-3
Haemophilus influenzae Type B Conjugate Vaccines Licensed for Use Among Children

VACCINE	TRADE NAME	POLYSACCHARIDE	LINKAGE	PROTEIN CARRIER	LICENSED FOR INFANTS*
PRP–OMP	PedvaxHIB	Medium	Thioether	*Neisseria meningitidis* outer membrane protein complex	Yes
HbOC	HibTITER	Small	None	CRM_{197} nontoxic mutant Diptheria toxin	Yes
PRP-T	ActHIB OmniHIB	Large	6-Carbon	Tetanus toxoid	Yes
PRP-D	ProHIbiT	Medium	6-Carbon	Diphtheria toxoid	No

*Less than 15 months of age.

cal vaccine has been available in the United States that consists of purified bacterial capsular polysaccharide from serogroups A, C, Y, and W135. Most endemic meningococcal disease in this country is caused by serogroup B, for which there is not yet an effective vaccine. As a consequence, routine immunization of children against meningococcal infection is not recommended. However, the quadrivalent vaccine should be administered to children 2 years of age and older who belong to high-risk groups (functional or anatomic asplenia, terminal complement deficiencies). In addition, the vaccine can be used to control outbreaks of disease caused by serogroups A, C, Y, or W135 and may be of benefit to travelers to countries with hyperendemic or epidemic disease.

The 23-valent pneumococcal vaccine contains purified, capsular polysaccharide antigens of 23 pneumococcal serotypes. These serotypes account for more than 95% of cases of childhood meningitis due to *S. pneumoniae.* The existing pneumococcal vaccine has limited immunogenicity in patients younger than 2 years of age but should be administered to children over 2 years of age with sickle cell disease, anatomic asplenia, nephrotic syndrome, HIV infection, or other conditions associated with immunosuppression. Efforts are currently underway to develop a pneumococcal conjugate vaccine that would be immunogenic in young infants.

Chemoprophylaxis

In an effort to reduce the spread of invasive illness (secondary infection) due to *H. influenzae* type b and *N. meningitidis,* antibiotic prophylaxis is recommended under certain circumstances. The intent is to eradicate nasopharyn-geal colonization and thereby interrupt transmission.

The risk of secondary *H. influenzae* disease among unimmunized household contacts less than 4 years of age is substantial, ranging from 2% to 6%. Spread of infection outside the family can also occur, particularly in daycare centers and nursery schools, but the precise frequency remains unclear. When a patient with *H. influenzae* meningitis has a sibling less than 12 months of age, all household contacts should receive rifampin orally once daily for 4 days in a dose of 20 mg/kg (maximum 600 mg/dose). The same applies in households with children younger than 4 years of age who are incompletely vaccinated and in families with a fully vaccinated but immunocompromised child. In addition, when two or more cases of invasive disease occur within a 60-day period among attendees of a child care center, and incompletely vaccinated children attend the facility, rifampin is recommended for all attendees and supervisory personnel. Management after a single case at a child care center is controversial and depends on the age and immunization status of attendees and the duration of daily contact between attendees and the index patient. In all of these circumstances, the primary case also should receive rifampin to eradicate colonization that might persist despite parenteral antibiotics. Therapy should begin during hospitalization. Prophylaxis should be administered to contacts within 7 days of diagnosis of the primary case and sooner if possible.

Secondary infection due to *N. meningitidis* occurs in 1% of family contacts and one per 1000 daycare contacts. Household, daycare center, and nursery school contacts of patients with meningococcal meningitis should receive antibiotic prophylaxis as soon as possible, preferably within 24 hours of presentation of the primary case. In most instances rifampin is the drug of choice in a dose of 10 mg/kg/dose (maximum 600 mg/dose) every 12 hours for 2 days. Some physicians recommend decreasing the dose for infants younger than 1 month of age to 5 mg/kg/dose. Ceftriaxone given as a single intramuscular dose (125 mg for children younger than 12 years, 250 mg for older individuals) is an acceptable alternative and is preferable for pregnant women. Occasionally an isolate will be sensitive to sulfonamides, in which case sulfisoxazole can be used. Patients who are treated with penicillin or ampicillin may still harbor *N. meningitidis* at the end of therapy and thus also should receive rifampin, ceftriaxone, or sulfisoxazole as appropriate before discharge.

Chemoprophylaxis is also a consideration in children at increased risk for pneumococcal meningitis, although the goal is to prevent primary rather than secondary disease. Daily antimicrobial prophylaxis with oral penicillin G or V (125 mg twice daily for children younger than 5 years of age; 250 mg twice daily for children 5 years of age and older) may be particularly useful for children with functional or anatomic asplenia, especially if these children are unlikely to respond to vaccine because of young age or treatment with intensive chemotherapy.

BIBLIOGRAPHY

Baker CJ, Edwards MS: Group B streptococcal infections. In Remington JS, Klein JO, editors: *Infectious diseases of the fetus and newborn infant,* ed 3, Philadelphia, 1990, WB Saunders.

Committee on Infectious Diseases, American Academy of Pediatrics: *Report of the Committee on Infectious Diseases, 1994 Red Book,* Elk Grove Village, 1994, American Academy of Pediatrics.

Feigin RD: Bacterial meningitis beyond the neonatal period. In Feigin RD, Cherry JD, editors: *Textbook of pediatric infectious diseases,* ed 3, Philadelphia, 1992, WB Saunders.

Feigin RD, McCracken GH Jr, Klein JO: Diagnosis and management of meningitis, *Pediatr Infect Dis J* 11:785–814, 1992.

Friedland IR, McCracken GH Jr: Drug therapy: Management of infections caused by antibiotic-resistant *Streptococcus pneumoniae,* *N Engl J Med* 331:377–382, 1994.

Klein JO, Feigin RD, McCracken GH Jr: Report of the task force on diagnosis and management of meningitis, *Pediatrics* 78:959–982, 1986.

Klein JO, Marcy SM: Bacterial sepsis and meningitis. In Remington JS, Klein JO, editors: *Infectious diseases of the fetus and newborn infant,* ed 3, Philadelphia, 1990, WB Saunders.

Nelson JD: Management problems in bacterial meningitis, *Pediatr Infect Dis J* 4:S41–44, 1985.

Schaad UB, Kaplan SK, McCracken GH Jr: Steroid therapy for bacterial meningitis, *Clin Infect Dis* 20:685–690, 1995.

Swartz MN, Dodge PR: Bacterial meningitis—A review of selected aspects, *N Engl J Med* 272: 725–731, 842–848, 898–902, 954–960, 1003–1010, 1965.

III

CHAPTER 93

Otitis Media

Ralph F. Wetmore

BACKGROUND

Acute otitis media is the occurrence of bacterial infection within the middle ear cavity. The presence of nonpurulent fluid within the middle ear cavity is termed *otitis media with effusion.* This fluid may be thin (serous) or thick (mucoid). This condition is alternatively known as serous otitis media, secretory otitis media, or glue ear.

Acute otitis media is the most common cause of bacterial infection in young children. As demonstrated in several studies, one half of children 1 year of age will have at least one episode of acute otitis media. By 3 years of age, one third of children will have had three or more infections, and by age 6 years, 90% will have had at least one infection. Otitis media with effusion is as common as infection in childhood. Increased recognition by the press and improved diagnosis, especially with new technology such as tympanometry, have made otitis media with effusion seem to increase in incidence. Some experts have suggested that there may be an increase in otitis media with effusion due to the treatment of acute otitis media with antibiotics.

The major pathogens of acute otitis media are *Streptococcus pneumoniae, Haemophilus influenzae,* and group A β-streptococcus. Other common organisms include *Branhamella* and *Staphylococcus.* Causative factors responsible for acute otitis media include eustachian tube dysfunction, upper respiratory infection, and allergy. Mechanical or functional obstruction of the eustachian tube allows egress of bacteria into the middle ear cavity. This anatomic problem is the major cause of recurrent acute otitis media in infants. Viral or bacterial upper respiratory infections may result in the spread of infection into the middle ear. Children with allergies are predisposed to upper respiratory illnesses and acute otitis media.

There are multiple factors involved in the pathogenesis of otitis media with effusion. As with acute otitis media, mechanical or functional problems with the eustachian tube is a major element in the development of otitis media with effusion. Tubal obstruction may be due to lymphoid tissue near the orifice of the eustachian tube or edema of the mucosa. In patients with cleft palate, inadequacy of the palatal muscles responsible for opening the eustachian tube leads to frequent problems with otitis media. Adenoid tissue is located in the region of the eustachian tube orifice; chronic adenoid problems including chronic adenoiditis or adenoid hypertrophy have been implicated in the development of otitis media with effusion. The role of allergy in the pathogenesis of otitis media with effusion remains unclear. Symptoms and laboratory evidence of allergy can be found in some patients; however, treatment of allergy has an inconsistent response in the long-term management of otitis media with effusion. Bacteria have been implicated in the pathogenesis of otitis media with effusion in many studies: approximately half of middle ear aspirates in untreated cases have positive results on bacterial cultures. This finding is the major reason for utilizing antibiotics in treatment. In at least one study, the duration of otitis media with effusion appeared to be much shorter in breast-fed infants than in bottle-fed children.

CLINICAL FINDINGS

History

The symptoms of both acute otitis media and otitis media with effusion are often dependent on the patient's age. In neonates and infants (up to 2 years of age), the most reliable symptom of otitis media is a change in behavior such as irritability or lethargy. Fever is an inconstant symptom. Although many infants may tug at their ears, this finding may be seen in the presence of teething or may be just a habit. Decreased appetite, vomiting, or diarrhea may be the result of acute otitis media or its treatment with antibiotics.

Young children (2 to 4 years of age) may be able to verbalize complaints of ear pain. Otalgia may be seen with both acute otitis media and otitis media with effusion, although it is more severe with acute infection. Otalgia secondary to otitis media with effusion is often intermittent and often seems worse at night. Fever may be present with acute otitis media depending on the stage and severity of infection. Fever is typically not a symptom of otitis media with effusion. As with infants, young children frequently show behavioral changes with otitis media. These behaviors may range from lethargy to irritability with acute otitis media and from hyperactivity to indifference with otitis media with effusion. Young children with otitis media frequently complain of noises in their ears. Although specific complaints of hearing loss are not verbalized by them, young children manifest hearing loss by saying "huh" or "what," ignoring directions, mispronouncing words, repeating the wrong words or turning up the television volume. Parents of these children may also complain of speech delay. As with infants, young children may have gastrointestinal symptoms as a result of either infection or treatment.

Children older than 4 years of age usually will complain of ear pain with acute otitis media. This otalgia may be either mild or severe depending on the stage and severity of infection. Fever and change in personality also may be present with acute infection. Children in this age group with otitis media with effusion also may complain of otalgia that is intermittent in nature and seems worse at night. They also may complain of a variety of noises, popping sounds in the ear, or ear fullness. Some children may complain of hearing loss, although hearing loss may be discovered by schoolteachers or through screening audiometry. Indistinct speech frequently will accompany the mild hearing loss seen with otitis media with effusion.

Physical Examination

With acute otitis media, the earliest sign of infection is erythema of the tympanic membrane. This sign should not be confused with hyperemia over the malleus, which is a normal finding.

With many viral syndromes there may be myringitis, which is an inflammation of the tympanic membrane without true infection of the middle ear. This condition is difficult to distinguish from the early stages of acute otitis media and is a cause of misdiagnosis. Hyperemia of the tympanic membrane seen in a crying child frequently may be confused with acute otitis media. This hyperemia may be difficult to eliminate in an infant who cries everytime he/she is restrained or examined. Having the child held in a parent's arms or lap may permit an easier examination of the ears.

As a middle ear infection becomes more intense, physical examination reveals a loss of anatomic landmarks. Normally, the malleus is easily visualized, and in a patient with a translucent tympanic membrane, the incus also can be seen. In acute otitis media, these landmarks disppear as the tympanic membrane becomes opaque and bulges. As the tympanic membrane bulges with purulent fluid, pneumatic otoscopy will demonstrate diminished tympanic membrane mobility. The development of drainage in the external canal during an episode of acute otitis media is indicative of a spontaneous perforation of the tympanic membrane. Usually, these perforations are small and close spontaneously in a few days.

In otitis media with effusion, the color of the tympanic membrane varies according to the color of the fluid in the middle ear cavity. This color may range from clear to amber to gray to blue. In contrast to what is seen in acute otitis media, the malleus, especially the short process, becomes more distinct as the tympanic membrane is retracted. The absence or reduction of tympanic membrane mobility is an essential finding in the diagnosis of otitis media with effusion; thus, pneumatic otoscopy is crucial to its diagnosis. Even in cases in which there is no obvious fluid behind the tympanic membrane, pneumatic otoscopy may indicate reduced compliance consistent with either fluid or severe eustachian tube dysfunction. In cases of prolonged otitis media with effusion there may be either small or large retraction pockets within the tympanic membrane. In severe cases the whole tympanic membrane will become draped over the medial wall of the middle ear.

Audiometric Studies

Middle ear immittance measures (tympanometry and acoustic reflexes) are an important tool in the diagnosis of otitis media. Immittance should not replace good physical examination, but rather should supplement it. The principle behind middle ear immittance measures includes the delivery of an acoustic signal to the tympanic membrane as the air pressure in the external meatus is systematically varied over a range from +200 to –300 mm H_2O pressure. The amount of the acoustic signal reflected from the tympanic membrane is measured under the various conditions of air pressure to derive a tympanometric curve of impedance as a function of pressure. Three general types of tympanometric functions are important to the diagnosis of otitis media which have been labeled types A, B, and C (Fig. 93-1). A normal, or A, curve is seen when the tympanometric function peaks in a range from +50 to –100 mm H_2O. A type C curve is seen in cases of eustachian tube dysfunction in which the peak of the curve occurs anywhere from –150 to –400 mm H_2O. A flat, or type B, curve has no discernible amplitude peak and is seen in cases in which the middle ear system is very stiff, such as that found with otitis media with effusion. A flat curve also will be seen with other stiffening conditions, such as severe thickening of the drum. A perforation of the tympanic membrane also will produce a B curve; however, middle ear volume or static compliance measurements will help to distinguish this condition from otitis media with effusion.

Pure tone audiometry is a procedure that can be performed in the office setting as a screening tool for hearing loss. It has little practical value in the diagnosis of acute otitis media, although it may be abnormal. More importantly, it may confirm a mild hearing loss such as that seen with otitis media with effusion. The typical hearing loss with otitis media with effusion is 20 to 40 dB. A normal hearing test in the office does not rule out otitis media with effusion. Hearing loss greater than 40 dB is suggestive of other conditions, such as an ossicular discontinuity, or a sensorineural or a mixed hearing loss. If office audiometry fails to correlate with either the history or physical findings, a more complete audiometric assessment at a hearing center should be performed.

Tuning fork testing (Weber and Rinne) is important in the diagnosis of hearing loss in adults. Their reliability in children is age-dependent and variable. Normally, the Weber test will lateralize to the ear with a conductive hearing loss. Bone conduction will be greater than air conduction (negative Rinne test) in the presence of a conduc-

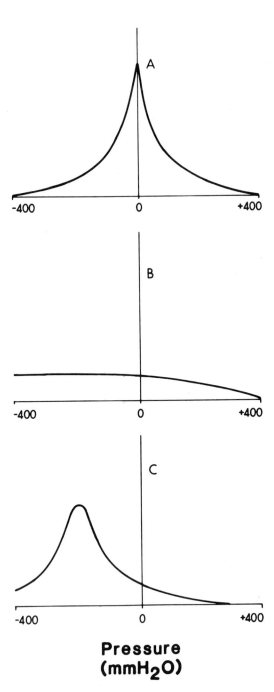

FIG 93-1

Types of tympanograms. **A**, Normal curve. **B**, Curve seen with middle ear effusion. **C**, Curve seen with eustachian tube dysfunction.

tive hearing loss, such as that seen with otitis media with effusion.

Reflectometry is a newly developed screening device that has been used in the office. A signal is transmitted to the tympanic membrane, and the amount of signal reflected can be translated into the degree of middle ear pathologic problems.

EARLY MANAGEMENT OF OTITIS MEDIA

Acute Otitis Media

Although there is evidence that episodes of acute otitis media may be treated expectantly without antibiotics and with minimal sequelae, the current standard of care is oral antibiotic therapy for 10 to 14 days. There are a variety of oral antibiotics that are successful in the management of acute otitis media, and the choice of antibiotic depends on the preference of the physician, the cost, a history of drug allergy, and previous otologic history. Amoxicillin remains the antibiotic of choice in uncomplicated acute otitis media. Other antibiotics such as second- and third-generation cephalosporins (Cefzil, Suprax), erythromycin and sulfisoxazole (Pediazole), trimethoprim/sulfamethoxazole (Bactrim), amoxicillin/clavulanate (Augmentin), and loracarbef (Lorabid) are popular in the treatment of otitis media, especially when resistant organisms are suspected. Antibiotic therapy should continue for 10 to 14 days; treatment courses of shorter duration may allow for the development of resistant organisms. Treatment failure as manifested by a continuation or worsening of pain, fever, irritability, or other symptoms is an indication to switch antibiotic therapy or consider referral to a specialist.

In the past, the use of either decongestants or antihistamine-decongestant preparations was part of the standard care of acute otitis media. Several studies have shown them to have no proven benefit in the management of otitis media.

There are several forms of pain relief available to relieve the otalgia of acute otitis media. Analgesics such as acetaminophen or ibuprofen can be used in infants and young children, whereas codeine can be used in older children. Topical anesthetic drops (Auralgen) and the topical application of heat, such as a hot water bottle, also may provide relief. As noted, the failure of pain to resolve after instituting therapy is an indication to switch antibiotics or refer the patient to a specialist.

In the past, office myringotomy was widely practiced in the early treatment of acute otitis media. This has fallen out of practice today since the advent of successful antibiotic therapy. Injury to the tympanic membrane or the ossicles can occur in inexperienced hands, and emotional trauma related to the myringotomy can make subsequent examinations difficult. There are several conditions in which myringotomy or tympanocentesis should be considered. In neonates less than 1 month of age or hospitalized neonates less than 3 months of age, there may be infection with either gram-negative bacteria or *Staphylococcus*. Tympanocentesis should be part of the septic workup in such neonates when acute otitis media is suspected. Children who are undergoing chemotherapy or who are immunocompromised are often infected with unusual organisms, and tympanocentesis should be considered in these children during episodes of acute otitis media to identify the pathogen. Failure of several oral antibiotics to resolve acute infection or the development of a complication such as acute mastoiditis in an otherwise healthy child is also an indication for tympanocentesis to identify the offending organism and to provide a route of drainage.

Because of the possibility of persistent fluid or failure of complete resolution of infection, a follow-up examination should occur approximately 2 weeks after each episode of acute otitis media. Resolution of symptoms does not guarantee that either all infection or fluid has cleared, and physical examination is necessary to confirm that the ear has returned to normal.

Recurrent bouts of acute otitis media, especially over a short interval of time, are an indication for antibiotic prophylaxis. Although there are no strict criteria for initiating antibiotic prophylaxis, three infections in 3 months or four infections in 6 months are the typical indications for prophylaxis. Although sulfisoxazole (Gantrisin) was initially used for the prophylaxis of recurrent otitis media, amoxicillin in a reduced dosage is also effective.

Otitis Media with Effusion

The major thrust in the early treatment of otitis media with effusion should be antibiotic therapy. Several studies have shown the presence of bacteria in aspirates of middle ear effusions. Other studies also have shown the benefit of antibiotic therapy in the resolution of otitis media with effusion. In many children during the winter months, episodes of acute otitis media may coincide with the presence of otitis media with effusion, and antibiotic therapy is essential in the resolution of both. Antibiotic regimens, utilized in the treatment of otitis media with effusion, may include either therapeutic courses for 10 to 14 days or prophylactic regimens for 4 to 6 weeks. Amoxicillin, cefaclor, trimethoprim/sulfamethoxazole, erythromycin/sulfisoxazole, and amoxicillin/clavulanate are usually utilized for therapeutic regimens, whereas sulfisoxazole and amoxicillin are used for prophylactic treatment. Initial treatment is followed by a repeat evaluation in 4 to 6 weeks.

In the past, decongestants and/or antihistamines were commonly used in the initial therapy of otitis media with effusion. Several studies have shown their ineffectiveness, and their use in otitis media with effusion is no longer essential. A short course of oral steroids has been shown to clear some middle ear effusions; this medication might be tried in children who have had minimal otitis media in the past. Because many children have chronic problems with otitis media with effusion, repeated use of oral steroids is not practical. Nasal steroids have been shown to be ineffective in the treatment of otitis media with effusion.

Older children or adolescents may be taught autoinflation of the eustachian tube. In this procedure, positive pressure is applied to the eustachian tube to attempt to clear negative middle ear pressure or fluid. Although this may prove helpful for some older children, it is not practical in the management of otitis media with effusion in younger children.

Expectant therapy is a reasonable form of management of otitis media with effusion. This is especially true of children who are not having coinciding problems with acute otitis media. During the summer months, the incidence of otitis media with effusion diminishes, and observation of the patient without any medication may result in the resolution of fluid.

COMPLICATIONS OF OTITIS MEDIA

Otologic Complications

Although complications of otitis media are uncommon, they are the major reason why chronic ear infections should be avoided. In the preantibiotic era, acute mastoiditis was a frequent complication of acute otitis media. Today it is seen rarely in infants and young children. These children present with fever, evidence of acute otitis media on physical examination, and postauricular swelling. Mastoid radiographs show fluid in the mastoid air-cell system. Failure to respond to antibiotic therapy may result in coalescent mastoiditis, a destructive infection involving the ear and mastoid. Acute mastoiditis requires prompt and aggressive management including referral to an otologist for possible surgical drainage.

Hearing loss is a frequent symptom of both acute otitis media and otitis media with effusion. During an episode of acute otitis media, there is typically a temporary conductive hearing loss secondary to the purulent material in the middle ear cavity. As long as a middle ear effusion is present, there also will be a persistent hearing loss. In both acute otitis media and otitis media with effusion, the hearing loss will resolve after the purulent fluid or effusion has cleared. The effect of chronic hearing loss in the development of speech and language and in other areas of learning such as reading remains unclear. Significant sensorineural hearing loss clearly affects development; however, with a mild conductive hearing loss, such as that with otitis media, the effects are individual. Some children have no problems with speech development in the presence of chronic fluid, whereas others undergo significant delays with only intermittent fluid. Clearly, the individual needs of each child need to be recognized in the management of otitis media. Sensorineural hearing loss ranging from mild to profound also may be a rare complication of both acute otitis media and otitis media with effusion.

Both acute otitis media and otitis media with effusion can result in chronic perforation of the tympanic membrane. Most perforations with drainage during an episode of acute otitis media close spontaneously, but some may persist. Chronic otitis media with effusion can result in an atelectatic tympanic membrane, which subsequently may form a chronic perforation. Small perforations may close without treatment, but large perforations result in hearing loss and require surgical repair.

Tympanosclerosis is hyalinization of the tympanic membrane, which is frequently the result of otitis media. These white plaques on the tympanic membrane are seen commonly. Typically they do not cause hearing loss, although complete hyalinization of the tympanic membrane may result in a conductive hearing loss.

Cholesteatoma results from keratinizing squamous epithelium being trapped medial to the tympanic membrane. Squamous debris from cholesteatoma continues to enlarge, and subsequent infection results in destruction of normal structures, especially the ossicles and tympanic membrane. Although cholesteatoma may be congenital, most cases are the result of chronic fluid or infection. The characteristic appearance of a cholesteatoma is a white lesion behind the tympanic membrane, although recognition may not always be obvious due to infection. Suspected cases of cholesteatoma should be referred for further evaluation.

Intracranial Complications

Intracranial complications of otitis media include meningitis, brain abscess, subdural empyema, and epidural abscess. In the preantibiotic era, intracranial complications as a result of acute otitis media were a common occurrence. Today these complications are more commonly a result of acute sinusitis.

The intracranial spread of infection from the ear and mastoid may be by one of several pathways: erosion of bone between the mastoid and the intracranial cavity; septic thrombophlebitis with spread of infection into the intracranial cavity; and through preformed pathways between the ear and brain.

The development of an intracranial complication usually follows the onset of acute otitis media by several days. Symptoms of a severe headache or worsening otalgia, a change in sensorium, or the onset of nausea and vomiting signal the development of an intracranial complication. The institution of intravenous antibiotics and further evaluation including computed tomography and lumbar puncture if indicated are the initial therapy. Otolaryngologic and neurosurgical consultations are also necessary.

SPECIALTY REFERRAL

Acute Otitis Media

After initiating antibiotic therapy for acute otitis media, there should be relief of pain within the next 24 to 48 hours. Failure of pain to subside is an indication to switch to a different antibiotic because of the possible presence of a resistant organism. Continued pain also signals the possible development of a complication, and an otologic referral should be made.

Drainage with an episode of acute otitis media indicates perforation of the tympanic membrane. Failure of the drainage to clear with antibiotic therapy is suggestive of an underlying problem such as cholesteatoma. For this reason, an otologic referral should be made if drainage fails to clear with appropriate antibiotic therapy. A culture of the drainage may be helpful in guiding therapy.

The appearance of dizziness or vertigo during an episode of acute otitis media suggests the spread of infection into the cochlea. The resulting labyrinthitis can destroy both the vestibular and cochlear labyrinth, producing a profound sensorineural hearing loss and disturbance of balance. The appearance of this symptom necessitates an immediate referral.

In the management of recurrent acute otitis media, an infection while on a prophylactic regimen constitutes a breakthrough infection. Unless it can be demonstrated that poor patient compliance is the cause of the infection, one must assume that prophylaxis is not effective. A referral should be made for consideration of myringotomy with tube placement.

Some experts believe that a prophylactic regimen for the treatment of recurrent acute otitis media should be used for 3 months. Resumption of infection following this 3-month regimen is an indication for referral to a specialist for consideration of myringtotomy with tube placement.

Otitis Media with Effusion

The persistence of middle ear effusion for approximately 6 to 12 weeks while on appropriate antibiotic therapy should signal referral to an otologist. This referral should be made on an individual basis depending on the time of year, previous otologic history, and current symptoms.

Recurrent bouts of fluid are also a cause for concern. The primary care physician can be misled by the quick resolution of fluid; however, if the child has fluid with each upper respiratory infection that occurs frequently during the winter months, he/she most likely has recurrent otitis media. This produces long-term effects on speech and hearing equivalent to those of persistent fluid, and referral to a specialist should be made to evaluate the child. This is especially true in children who have an underlying sensorineural hearing loss or other developmental delays.

The persistence of a tympanic membrane perforation or the appearance of a white mass behind the tympanic membrane, suggestive of a cholesteatoma, are additional indications for referral to a specialist. A perforated tympanic membrane needs evaluation for damage to the ossicular chain and needs follow-up for possible surgical repair. Cholesteatoma has the potential for continued growth with destruction of the tympanic membrane and ossicles, damage to the cochlea and facial nerve or erosion into the intracranial cavity. For this reason, an expedient referral is necessary for prompt management.

BIBLIOGRAPHY

Bluestone CD, Klein JO: Clinical practice guideline on otitis media with effusion in young children: Strengths and weaknesses, *Otolaryngol Head Neck Surg* 112:507–511, 1995.

Brook I, Yocum P, Shah K, et al: Aerobic and anaerobic bacteriologic features of serous otitis media in children, *Am J Otolaryngol* 4:389–392, 1983.

Cantekin EI, Mandel EM, Bluestone CD, et al: Lack of efficacy of a decongestant-antihistamine combination for otitis media with effusion ("secretory" otitis media) in children, *N Engl J Med* 308:297–301, 1983.

Gates GA, Avery CA, Prihoda TJ, et al: Effectiveness of adenoidectomy and tympanostomy tubes in the treatment of chronic otitis media with effusion, *N Engl J Med* 317:1444–1451, 1987.

Gates GA, Wachtendorf C, Holt GR, et al: Medical treatment of chronic otitis media with effusion (secretory otitis media), *Otolaryngol Head Neck Surg* 94:350–354, 1986.

Healy GB: Antimicrobial therapy of chronic otitis media with effusion, *Int J Pediatr Otorhinolaryngol* 8:13–17, 1984.

Teele DW, Klein JO, Rosner BA: The greater Boston otitis media study group: Epidemiology of otitis media during the first seven years of life in children in greater Boston: A prospective cohort study, *J Infect Dis* 160:83–94, 1989.

Varsano I, Volvitz B, Mimouni F: Sulfisoxazole prophylaxis of middle ear effusion and recurrent acute otitis media, *Am J Dis Child* 139:631–635, 1985.

Wallace IF, Gravel JS, McCarton CM, et al: Otitis media, auditory sensitivity, and language outcomes at one year, *Laryngoscope* 98:64–70, 1988.

CHAPTER 94

Recurrent Infections

Mary Ellen Conley

Every physician who cares for children repeatedly faces the issue of what to do with the child with recurrent infections. Some children seem to be sick all of the time. The parents say they feel as if they live in the doctor's office. The grandparents say something must be wrong. The physician pages through the chart. The child has had many infections, but too many? And, if too many, what can and should be done?

HOW MANY IS TOO MANY?

In a study done of 246 full-term, first-born children, Hoekelman found that although 36% of the children had no infections at all in the first year of life, 13% of the children had four or more infections in the same period. When it is recognized that the children included in this study are in the lowest-risk group and that children who are born prematurely, who have older siblings, or who are in a daycare facility have infection rates that are two to three times greater than these low-risk patients, we estimate that normal children may have up to eight to 10 infections a year in the first few years of life. If these infections are upper respiratory tract infections, otitis, or gastroenteritis; if the child is well between infections; if the screening tests described at the end of the chapter are normal; and particularly if the child is growing normally, there is no need to worry. That is not to say the infections are not a nuisance to the family, but they should not be a cause of worry or considered a harbinger of worse things.

WHEN TO WORRY?

There are certain signs that indicate that a physician should look further into the causes of multiple infections. These signs do not indicate that the patient has an immunodeficiency. Immunodeficiencies are rare, and other causes of recurrent infection are more common. These signs include:

1. Two or more life-threatening infections (requiring hospitalization and intravenous therapy) within 5 years or less.
2. Prolonged infections or infections that are unresponsive to typical therapy.
3. Infections with unusual organisms.
4. Infections interfering with normal growth.
5. Infections in a child with a family history of similar infections, childhood death, or immunodeficiency.

RECURRENT INFECTIONS NOT DUE TO IMMUNODEFICIENCY

The cause of recurrent infections may not be due to a defect in the child at all. Sometimes recurrent infections are caused by a failure to completely eradicate a particularly resistant organism. A child whose otitis media is due to an organism that is resistant to the antibiotic being used may seem to have recurrent ear infections. Another example is the child with recurrent pyoderma. Some staphylococci are unusually virulent. The *Staphylococcus* may be carried by several family members but only one or two are afflicted with the pyoderma. As soon as the patient completes a course of therapy for the pyoderma, he/she becomes reinfected by the asymptomatic carrier. Several circumstances that should increase the physician's suspicion that this is occurring are: 1) recurrent skin infections in an individual who was completely well and without infections for several years prior to the onset of the staphylococcal infections, 2) a chronic skin condition such as eczema or psoriasis in a family member, or 3) employment of a family member in a health care facility or microbiology laboratory.

Recurrent infections may be due to increased environmental exposure to contagious agents. Not only the children who go to daycare centers but the younger siblings of children in daycare centers or kindergarten may have repeated mild infections. Medical students who are doing a rotation in a pediatric walk-in clinic and military recruits who work and sleep in close contact with many individuals are also more subject to infections.

If a child has recurrent infections but only at a single anatomic site, such as the middle ear or the lungs, then a localized defect should be sought. Recurrent pneumonias may be due to cystic fibrosis, α-1-antitrypsin deficiency, foreign body, recurrent aspiration, tracheoesophageal fistula, or other anatomic defects. Asthma with intermittent atelectasis also masquerades as recurrent pneumonia. Asthma and atelectasis should be suspected if the infection is associated with what seems to be a viral upper respiratory tract infection, the "pneumonia" resolves quickly, and the child has a history that suggests an allergic predisposition. Occasionally, a child who has had recurrent meningitis can be found on careful examination to have an abnormal communication between the skin and the cerebrospinal fluid, most often a dural sinus. In these cases, the organisms that cause the meningitis are usually *Staphylococcus* or enteric organisms.

Children with certain systemic defects also have an increased incidence of infection. Worldwide, malnutrition is the most common cause of persistent or recurrent infection. During certain infections (most notably, measles, but also other systemic viral infections), the individual is more susceptible to bacterial infections. Some metabolic diseases, such as diabetes, may be associated with frequent infections. Patients who have had a surgical or a physiologic splenectomy also have a higher incidence of bacterial sepsis.

IMMUNE DEFICIENCIES

In considering the possibility that a child might have an immune deficiency, it is helpful to recognize that defects in each limb of the immune system present with typical clinical findings. The four limbs of the immune system, 1) B cells or antibody production, 2) T cells or cell-mediated immunity, 3) phagocytes, and 4) complement, have overlapping functions to provide maximum protection for the individual, but defects in each limb tend to be associated with particular kinds of infection.

B-Cell Defects
Defects in antibody production are the most common of the immune defects, the easiest to diagnose and often the most amenable to treatment. There are many causes of antibody deficiency including failure of B-cell precursors to mature into B cells, failure of B cells to further differentiate into plasma cells, failure of plasma cells to secrete the immunoglobulin they have synthesized, and loss of immunoglobulin. Some patients have normal serum concentration of immunoglobulins (proteins with certain biochemical properties), but they fail to make specific antibodies (proteins that bind to specific antigens like tetanus toxoid or pneumococcus). Antibody deficiency for any of these reasons tends to result in infections with encapsulated pathogenic bacteria, particularly pneumonococcus and *Haemophilus influenzae*. Congenital agammaglobulinemia usually presents in children between 6 and 18 months of age, after maternally derived antibody has decayed. Presentation is sometimes dramatic, with rapidly progressive sepsis, meningitis, or pneumonia. Otitis, sinusitis, and pneumonia are the most common infections in antibody deficiencies even in children treated with replacement γ-globulin. Children with antibody deficiencies whose conditions are diagnosed early, before they have developed chronic pulmonary scarring or damage at some other site, and who are treated appropriately with γ-globulin replacement and aggressive antibiotic treatment usually do not require repeated hospitalization for acute infections.

T-Cell Defects
T-cell deficiencies, no matter what the cause, tend to present with viral, fungal, or parasitic infections of insidious onset. The infant develops a cold, rhinorrhea, and tachypnea that does not resolve; thrush recurs when therapy is stopped; diarrhea is common and persistent. There may be rashes. Complete congenital T-cell deficiencies usually present as severe combined

immune deficiency because normal antibody production requires T cell help. Babies with severe combined immune deficiency usually come to medical attention between 3 and 6 months of age because of persistent pneumonitis, diarrhea, and failure to thrive. On initial examination they may be found to be infected with as many as four or five different viruses.

The child with DiGeorge syndrome, congenital absence, or hypoplasia of the thymus and parathyroids most often presents not with recurrent infections but with the associated defects of DiGeorge syndrome, cardiac defects, or hypocalcemia. The infections that these children acquire may be as much related to the cardiac defects as to the T-cell immune deficiency.

Phagocytic Defects

For normal phagocytic function to occur, there must be a sufficient number of phagocytes, polymorphonuclear leukocytes, and monocytes in the peripheral circulation. Chemotactic function must be normal; that is, the phagocytes must reach their target. The phagocytes must ingest the foreign particle or substance. Finally, the phagocyte must be able to kill or degrade the invader. If there is a defect anywhere along this pathway, the patient is likely to have infections at the body surfaces, particularly the skin, the oral cavity, the conjunctiva, and the lungs. *Staphylococcus,* enteric bacteria, and fungi, especially *Candida* and *Aspergillus,* are most commonly involved. Some patients also may have intermittent, spontaneously resolving fevers.

Complement Defects

Defects in the complement pathway result in more varied clinical problems than defects in the other limbs of the immune system. Early complement component defects, C1, C2, and C4 deficiencies, may be associated with lupuslike syndromes, or occasionally with recurrent infections due to pathogenic encapsulated bacteria. Defects in the late complement components, C5, C6, C7, and C8, make the patient unusually susceptible to infections with *Neisseria,* both gonococcus and meningococcus. Patients are usually completely well between infections and may not come to medical attention until adolescence or adulthood. Any patient with a systemic neisserial infection who has a past history of severe neisserial infection or a family history of systemic meningococcal or gonococcal disease should be evaluated for a complement defect.

DATA GATHERING

If a child has had recurrent infections, there are several simple laboratory tests that can be done to help evaluate the possibility of an immune deficiency. These include a complete blood count (CBC), quantitative serum immunoglobulins, including serum IgE, functional antibody titers, and a total hemolytic complement (CH_{50}). In a CBC, special attention should be given to the absolute number and appearance of the neutrophils. If a child is neutropenic but does not have an acute bacterial infection and has been previously well, the neutrophil count should be repeated and the child should be followed-up carefully but the physician need not be alarmed. Acute viral suppression is the most common cause of neutropenia in childhood. If the neutropenia persists beyond 3 weeks, the child should be referred to an immunologist or a hematologist. The absolute lymphocyte count also should be noted. Infants with T-cell deficiencies are frequently lymphopenic. Quantitative serum immunoglobulins always should be done rather than a protein electrophoresis or immunoelectrophoresis. The latter two tests are less sensitive and less specific than quantitative serum IgM, IgG, IgA, and IgE. The results of quantitative serum immunoglobulins should always be compared with age-appropriate standards. Children with agammaglobulinemia or hypogammaglobulinemia usually have serum concentrations of IgM, IgG, and IgA that are much less than two standard deviations below the norm. Serum concentrations of IgA do not reach adult levels until the second decade of life. It is not unusual for children to have a delay in production of IgA, so we usually do not make the diagnosis of IgA deficiency before the child is 3 years of age. The quality of antibody production also can be evaluated. Isohemagglutinins or anti–blood group substances are measured in every hospital blood bank and, except in the patient who is blood type AB, can provide good evidence of functional antibody production. In children who have received their measles-mumps-rubella vaccine, an antirubella titer also can be obtained. This test usually is readily available because it is used in obstetrics. The total hemolytic complement assay, or CH_{50}, is a functional assay that gives a normal result only if each of the complement components is present in adequate concentrations.

MANAGEMENT

There are certain management pitfalls that the physician should try to avoid. Sometimes a small child or infant with recurrent upper respiratory tract infections is found to have an IgG concentration at the low range of normal. The physician may be tempted to treat the patient with γ-globulin, but this should be avoided because it can suppress the child's own antibody production and make later diagnostic studies more difficult, and it labels the baby as a fragile, sick child. If the serum IgM level is in the normal range and the child has not had documented systemic bacterial infections, serum immunoglobulin levels should be repeated in 4 to 6 months and the parents should be reassured. Another vexing situation is the child 8 to 18 years of age who has persistent malaise, low-grade temperatures, and headaches or coughs. Findings of all laboratory studies and physical examination are completely normal, and the child is appropriate in height and weight. The parents and the child should be carefully questioned about school attendance under these circumstances. School avoidance frequently presents as persistent undocumented infections. Specific management of school refusal is discussed in Chapter 90.

When a child has had many mild infections, it is sometimes difficult to reassure the parents that the child does not have a significant problem. It can be helpful to point out all the good signs if they are present: normal growth and development, no life-threatening infections, and normal laboratory tests. It is very helpful to point out that each infection has a beginning and an end, rather than it being one prolonged infection. If there is suspicion that the child does have recurrent infection on an immunologic basis, then consultation with an immunologist should be sought.

BIBLIOGRAPHY

Ammann AJ, Wara DW: Evaluation of infants and children with recurrent infections, *Curr Probl Pediatr* 5:11, 1975.

Hoekelman RA: Infectious illness during the first year of life, *Pediatrics* 59:119–121, 1977.

Johnston RB: Recurrent bacterial infections in children, *N Engl J Med* 310:1237–1243, 1984.

Stiehm ER, editor: *Immunologic disorders in infants and children,* Philadelphia, 1989, WB Saunders.

CHAPTER 95

Sexually Transmitted Diseases

Donald F. Schwarz

In addition to the classic sexually transmitted diseases (gonorrhea, syphilis, chancroid, lymphogranuloma venereum, granuloma inguinale), more recently described entities with newly understood frequency include genital papillomas, herpes, candidiasis, nonspecific vaginitis, trichomoniasis, pubic lice, scabies, hepatitis, and HIV-associated disease. These disease entities and their underlying pathogens are becoming increasingly recognized in pediatric practice.

Unlike other infectious diseases, these processes, which are spread through sexual contact, often carry with them both physical and important psychosocial problems. The clinician must be both comfortable with the physical diagnosis and management of the disease entity and sensitive to the associated social issues.

THE PREPUBERTAL CHILD

In the prepubertal child, a sexually transmitted disease must be considered a marker for sexual abuse until proven otherwise. The clinician must remain vigilant for signs and symptoms of child abuse.

In prepubertal girls, vaginitis may occasionally be caused by a sexually transmitted disease. Symptoms of vaginitis include odor, dysuria, frequency, and discomfort. Information from the history, physical examination, and laboratory evaluation help distinguish causes of vaginitis. Common causes of vaginitis that are not related to sexually transmitted diseases include foreign bodies (frequently beads, small toys, or retained tissue; often associated with a particularly foul odor), pinworms, scabies, varicella lesions, streptococcal or staphylococcal disease, and irritative vaginitis (caused by reaction to powders, creams, bubble bath, or poor hygiene). *Gardner-*

ella vaginitis or *Candida* vaginitis may be acquired through venereal or nonvenereal contact. Further investigation is needed in these cases. Papillomas, trichomonal, herpes simplex, gonococcal, or chlamydial disease must carry a high suspicion for sexual transmission. Infectious causes of vaginitis require appropriate antibiotic treatment.

Any pharyngeal or anal infection with a pathogen that is sexually transmitted (including *Gonococcus, Chlamydia,* herpesvirus, or syphilis) must be assumed to be secondary to abuse. In young children with anal symptoms in particular, a directed history and careful physical examination are essential. Diagnostic testing for *Neisseria gonorrhoeae, Chlamydia trachomatis, Treponema pallidum,* and herpes simplex virus should be performed.

Pelvic inflammatory disease (PID), presenting with lower abdominal pain, although reported in young girls, is exceedingly rare. All other causes of abdominal pain must be ruled out before PID is assumed to be present. In cases of lice, scabies, or papillomas of the genital area, the clinician should be careful to inquire about sleeping patterns and shared use of clothing and towels.

For nonvenereal causes of vaginitis, sitz baths and local irrigation with saline solution usually suffice. Occasionally systemic antibiotics are required (for streptococcal infections).

ADOLESCENT WOMEN

Routine screening for sexually transmitted diseases should be performed on all adolescent women who are sexually active; those who are pregnant; those being evaluated for sexual abuse, rape, or incest; and those with a history of sexual activity in the past. In addition, the differential diagnosis for recurrent urinary tract infection should include sexually transmitted disease. Screening tests should be performed at least annually in women who are sexually active; and in women who have multiple sexual partners, an examination should be performed at least every 6 months.

Diagnosis

An evaluation of a patient for a sexually transmitted disease begins with a sexual history. This history should review the age of onset of menses and last menstrual period, pregnancy history, history of previous sexually transmitted diseases, recent use of antibiotics, time of last pelvic examination, symptoms since last examination, number and frequency of partners and their symptoms, and use of contraceptives. Any history of lesions of the genitalia, pain on intercourse, vaginal discharge, pruritis, unexplained rash, joint complaints, urinary discomfort, or infection in a partner should raise the question of a sexually transmitted disease.

After obtaining a history, a complete physical examination is done. Particular attention should be paid to unexplained fever, rash, mucous membrane findings, new murmurs, abdominal symptoms, joint findings, and lesions around the anus. A complete pelvic examination should be performed.

Ulcerating Lesions

The pelvic examination should begin with inspection of the external genitalia. An ulcerating lesion anywhere in the genital area should be considered secondary to syphilis until proven otherwise (*see* below). The classic chancre of syphilis is a nonpainful, indurated, usually single ulcer of several millimeters to slightly over a centimeter in size. It is usually accompanied by firm, nonfluctuant, painless local lymph nodes. It is highly infectious. The chancre of syphilis must be differentiated from the usually multiple and smaller ulcerative lesions of herpes simplex disease. These lesions are frequently clustered and confluent. Herpes may also present with clustered vesicles. These lesions are usually painful, may be pruritic, and progress from vesicle to ulcers to crusted lesions over a number of days. They frequently leave hyper- or hypopigmented areas after the acute lesions have healed (*see* below).

A third cause of an ulcerative lesion is chancroid. Chancroid is the result of infection with *Haemophilus ducreyi* (a gram-negative bacillus). Chancroid is an acute, localized infection that presents with single or multiple papules that progress to painful necrotizing ulcers at the site of infection. Regional adenopathy with painful suppurative lymph nodes is also frequently present. Extragenital lesions do occur. Diagnosis of chancroid is made by culture from the ulcer or from pus from a suppurating lymph node. Chancroid is treated with 1 g of azithromycin orally; ceftriaxone, 250 mg intramuscularly for one dose; or erythromycin base, 500 mg orally four times a day for 7 days.

Granuloma inguinale is caused by *Calymmatobacterium granulomatis,* which causes subcutaneous nodules, vesicles, or papules in the genital area that extend and often ulcerate. The lesions are quite destructive and may be associated with squamous cell carcinoma. Diagnosis is made by punch biopsy or by Giemsa stain of granulation tissue taken directly from lesions. Granuloma inguinale is treated with doxycycline 100 mg twice daily for 21 days.

Rash

External erythematous rash around the genital area, which may be accompanied by discharge, can be caused by candidal infection. Generalized disorders in which genital lesions may occur include erythema multiforme, varicella, aphthous ulcerations of Behçet disease or Crohn's disease, and Kawasaki syndrome. A crusted pruritic rash in the genital area may be caused by scabies. Scabitic lesions of the genital area may or may not resemble those on other parts of the body with a classic linear pattern. Scabies should be treated with lindane or a preparation of pyrethins and piperonyl butoxide. Erythematous, intensely pruritic areas within the pubic hair may be the result of lice infestation *(Pediculosis pubis).* Treatment should be a lindane preparation (Kwell, Scabene) or pyrethins with piperonyl butoxide.

The rash of secondary syphilis may be generalized and accompanied by mild constitutional symptoms. It is described in detail below.

Other Lesions

Inspection of the genital area is not complete without examining the introitus for abscesses of Bartholin glands. Bartholin gland abscesses are caused in the great majority of cases by *N. gon-*

orrhoeae. Treatment is not complete without incision and drainage of the lesions.

Classic wartlike lesions around the genital area are caused by either human papillomavirus (venereal warts) or *T. pallidum* (condyloma lata of syphilis). The two lesions occasionally may be differentiated by the drier, more cornified appearance of common papillomavirus lesions. Condyloma lata are classically moist with a broad base. They are extremely infectious. Definitive diagnosis requires syphilis serologic testing.

Molluscum contagiosum may be transmitted through any intimate contact. Between one and 20 white, translucent, or flesh-colored lesions that are 3 to 7 mm in diameter with central umbilication may be present. They may be accompanied by pruritis or mild irritation. Biopsy is diagnostic.

Adenopathy

After genital inspection, the inguinal lymph nodes are palpated. Diseases that frequently cause regional inguinal adenopathy include syphilis, candida, chancroid, lymphogranuloma venereum, and granuloma inguinale. Lymphogranuloma venereum (LGV) is caused by *Chlamydia trachomatis* types L-1, L-2, or L-3. It is a systemic lymphatic infection beginning often with small, painless, papular or nodular lesions at the portal of entry. This lesion is followed by subacute regional lymphadenitis, usually unilateral. Other symptoms include chills, fever, headache, abdominal and joint pain, and anorexia. Diagnosis is made by culture from lymph node drainage or serum complement fixation tests. LGV is treated with doxycycline 100 mg orally twice daily for 21 days or until lymphadenopathy has resolved.

Internal Examination

After completing inspection and palpation of inguinal lymph nodes, an internal examination is performed with a speculum lubricated only with warm water. On speculum examination, if discharge is present a sample should be taken for wet preparation with saline solution and with 10% solution of potassium hydroxide (KOH). The characteristics of the discharge and the presence or absence of vaginitis, foreign body, and any evidence of vaginal trauma including abrasion and focal vaginitis should be noted. The cervix should be inspected for its transition zone, and any lesions noted. Table 95-1 provides a differential diagnosis of vaginal discharge.

Vaginitis

Herpes simplex vaginitis classically gives a thin, copious, non–foul-smelling discharge. It may be associated with inguinal adenopathy, pruritis, dysuria, labial edema, and pain on intercourse. Diagnosis is made by culture with special viral medium or Tzanck preparation (Wright staining of smears from lesions that reveal multinucleated giant cells and cytoplasmic vacuoles). Serologic tests for herpes simplex virus antibodies are confirmatory but not diagnostic. Treatment is with acyclovir 200 mg orally five times per day for 10 days for initial attacks and for 5 days for recurrence. Suppressive therapy is discussed below.

The discharge associated with *Trichomonas vaginalis* infection is typically thick, frothy, copious, yellow-green, and foul smelling. It is associated with vaginitis and classically causes a strawberry cervix (areas of punctate hemorrhage). Diagnosis of *Trichomonas* is made either by direct visualization of motile organisms on wet preparation with saline (75% sensitive), Papanicolaou smear (80% sensitive), or culture (85% sensitive). Appropriate treatment for *Trichomonas* vaginitis is with metronidazole, either 2 g given once by mouth or 500 mg by mouth twice daily for a week.

Gardnerella vaginalis infection leads to a thick, copious, foul-smelling, white-yellow discharge. It is associated with pruritis and vaginitis and is frequently found in women with *Trichomonas* infection. Diagnosis is made by wet preparation in which clue cells are seen. These cells are large epithelial cells covered with small, hairlike bacteria. The "whiff test" (application of 10% KOH to a sample of vaginal pool discharge yields a fishy smell from amines produced by *Gardnerella* bacteria) is quite specific but not highly sensitive. Culture of the vaginal pool also will lead to diagnosis of *Gardnerella*. *Gardnerella* vaginitis is treated with metronidazole 500 mg orally twice daily for 7 days; clindamycin cream 2%, one applicator intravaginally at bedtime for 7 days; or metronidazole gel 0.75%, one applicator intravaginally, two times a day for 5 days.

Candida albicans (monilial) vaginitis, often associated with intense pruritis, produces a cottage cheese-like discharge. Predisposing factors

TABLE 95-1
Differential Diagnosis of Vaginal Discharge

ORGANISM	DISCHARGE	DIAGNOSIS	TREATMENT
Herpes	Thin, copious, not foul smelling	Culture (special medium)	Acyclovir, oral or topical
Trichomonas	Thick, copious, yellow-green, foul smelling	Wet preparation (75% sensitivity), Papanicolaou smear (80% sensitivity), culture (85% sensitivity)	Metronidazole, 2 g PO × 1 or Metronidazole, 500 mg PO BID for 7 days
Gardnerella	Slightly thick, copious, foul smelling, white-yellow	Wet preparation: clue cells. 10% KOH: whiff test. Culture: send swab	Metronidazole, 500 mg PO BID for 7 days or Clindamycin cream 2%, intravaginally q hr for 7 days or Metronidazole, gel, 0.75%, intravaginally BID for 5 days
Candida	Cottage cheese–like	10% KOH (heat), culture: send swab	Butoconazole, clotrimazole, miconazole, tioconazole, teraconazole intravaginally; fluconazole 200 mg PO × 1
Chlamydia	Any discharge	Culture (special medium) and monoclonal antibodies (rapid-slide). Gram stain (look for 10 or more WBC/hpf).	Doxycycline 100 mg PO BID for 7 days or Azithromycin 1 g PO × 1
Gonococcus	Any discharge	Culture (both Martin-Lewis and chocolate agar).	Ceftriaxone 125 mg IM or Cefixime 400 mg PO or Ciprofloxacin 500 mg PO or Ofloxacin 400 mg PO

REMEMBER: Treat both *Gonococcus* and *Chlamydia* in symptomatic women.

BID—twice a day; KOM—potassium hydroxide; PO—orally; WBC/hpf—white blood cells per high-power field.

to monilial infection include diabetes mellitus, pregnancy, use of broad-spectrum antibiotics, and oral contraceptive use. Diagnosis is made by applying a 10% KOH to a sample of the vaginal pool on a slide and then heating gently. Filamentous hyphae and budding yeast forms may be seen when KOH dissolves cell walls. *Candida* forms are occasionally seen on Gram stain as well. *Candida* can be cultured in laboratories. Simple transport medium is required. Many treatments for Candida vaginitis have been approved for use. Local application of butoconazole, clotrimazole, miconazole, ticonazole, and teraconazole all appear to be equally effective. Fluconazole 200 mg orally as a single dose is also recommended.

Of note, partners of patients with *Trichomonas* vaginitis must be treated to prevent reinfection in women with vaginitis. No treatment is necessary, though, for partners of patients with *Gardnerella-* or *Candida*-induced vaginitis. These are never eradicated from the vaginal pool, and treatment of partners makes no difference to rates of recurrence.

Vaginal discharge in the absence of vaginitis should suggest chlamydial or gonococcal disease. *C. trachomatis* leads to a cervicitis with resulting discharge. Diagnosis is made by culture with special transport medium or with serum antibody testing. Chlamydial infection is treated with doxycycline 100 mg orally twice daily for 7 to 10 days or azithromycin 1 g orally in a single dose.

N. gonorrhoeae also leads to cervicitis without vaginitis. Discharge may be creamy to green-white. Diagnosis is made by culture of endocervical discharge. To maximize the chances of a positive result on culture, pharynx and rectum should also be cultured for *N. gonorrhoeae* in symptomatic individuals. If culture is done, both a restrictive medium such as Martin-Lewis or Thayer-Martin medium and chocolate agar are preferrable, because approximately 10% of *N. gonorrhoeae* will not grow on restrictive media. Plates should be placed in a CO_2-enhanced environment. Transgrow, a modified restrictive medium, contains CO_2 and is suitable for transport for longer than 2 hours. Uncomplicated gonococcal infections should be treated with ceftriaxone, 125 mg intramuscularly; cefixime, 400 mg orally; ciprofloxacin, 500 mg orally or ofloxacin, 400 mg orally, each as a single dose. Alternatively in penicillin-allergic patients, spectinomycin 2 g intramuscularly given once can be used. Ceftriaxone will also eradicate rectal and pharyngeal disease.

To diagnose sexually transmitted diseases appropriately on pelvic examination, the following order should be used for collection of specimens: 1) samples of the vaginal pool for wet preparation and KOH preparation; 2) vaginal culture for *Gardnerella, Candida,* and *Trichomonas* (if appropriate); 3) endocervical specimen for culture for *N. gonorrhoeae,* with a specimen plated on both restrictive and on chocolate agar; 4) a Papanicolaou smear (annually) in all sexually active adolescents; 5) a cervical specimen for *Chlamydia* testing. Chlamydia culture should be the screening test of choice. However, growth of *Chlamydia* in culture is inhibited by the presence of other organisms and pus. As a result, in some centers both *Chlamydia* culture and a rapid diagnostic procedure should be performed.

After completing speculum examination, bimanual examination is performed. Any tenderness on cervical motion, tenderness of the adnexa, or mass should be noted and appropriately handled. In young adolescents, tenderness of the cervix and adnexal structures may be confirmed, after regloving, through a rectal-bimanual examination.

Pelvic Inflammatory Disease

The presenting complaint in patients with PID may range from vague abdominal discomfort to florid signs and symptoms of acute abdomen.

In addition to the classic symptoms of abdominal pain, nausea, vomiting, and fever, the patient may have increased vaginal discharge, menorrhagia, metorrhagia, dysuria, urgency, or urinary frequency. Right upper quadrant pain, pleuritic in quality or referred to the right shoulder and back, suggests Fitz-Hugh–Curtis syndrome, a perihepatitis reported with both gonococcal and chlamydial infections. Physical examination may reveal a mildly to severely ill patient with abdominal or adnexal tenderness; signs of peritoneal inflammation are not uncommon. Adnexal fullness or an adnexal mass suggests tuboovarian abscess; right upper quadrant tenderness or an audible friction rub suggests Fitz-Hugh–Curtis syndrome.

Evaluation should focus primarily on excluding other causes of an acute abdomen that would necessitate prompt surgical intervention. In particular, acute appendicitis and ruptured ectopic pregnancy should be ruled out. Endometriosis or corpus luteum hemorrhage should be distinguished from PID. Fever and laboratory evidence of acute inflammation are not typically a feature of those two disorders.

Toxic shock syndrome, although quite uncommon, should be considered in any severely ill young woman who is menstruating, especially if she uses tampons. Fever, rash, and hypotension are the hallmarks of the disorder, and multisystem involvement is the rule. Abdominal pain, vomiting, and diarrhea are commonly seen.

In patients with symptoms suggestive of urinary tract infection, urinalysis and culture should be performed. In those with abdominal pain and right upper quadrant tenderness, hepatitis secondary to hepatitis virus A, or C, D, or E; cytomegalovirus; and Epstein-Barr virus should be considered. Acute cholecystitis, perforated peptic ulcer, subphrenic or perinephric abscess, acute pyelonephritis, nephrolithiasis, and pneumonia (especially right lower lobe) should be ruled out. Fitz-Hugh–Curtis syndrome is a perihepatitis rather than a parenchymal disease, and for that reason liver function test results are usually normal. On cholecystography, the gallbladder may not be seen early, but subsequent studies will be normal. Like PID, Fitz-Hugh–Curtis syndrome is largely a clinical diagnosis.

In a toxic-appearing patient, particularly a patient in septic shock, the clinician should consider postabortal PID with organisms such as *Clostridium perfringens.*

Several laboratory tests have been used in the initial evaluation of patients suspected of having PID, but none is very sensitive or specific. Less than 25% of patients are estimated to have leukocytosis, and approximately 40% each are estimated to have mild or moderate elevation of erythrocyte sedimentation rate. Organisms isolated from patients with PID include: *N. gonorrhoeae, C. trachomatis,* and mixed anaerobic flora, thus initial therapy while awaiting culture results should include broad-spectrum antibiotics (*see* below). Endocervical, rectal, and pharyngeal cultures for gonococcus isolation should be performed. Cervical cultures or rapid diagnostic testing for *Chlamydia* should be obtained. Pregnancy testing should be performed for all patients with suspected or proved PID. Pelvic ultrasonography may be helpful in the evaluation of patients with adnexal fullness or mass to visualize the occasional tubo-ovarian abscess (TOA), a complication of PID. Gynecologic consultation should be obtained for patients with TOA.

The diagnosis of PID is often clinical and frequently unclear. Because 15% of women have been shown to be infertile after only one episode of PID, the clinician who evaluates a sexually active adolescent woman with abdominal pain must have a high index of suspicion for PID. Treatment should be initiated as early as possible to reduce the risk of complications.

Patients with uncomplicated PID are often adequately treated as outpatients. Outpatient therapy includes doxycycline, 100 mg orally twice a day for 10 days; ceftriaxone, 250 mg intramuscularly; and cefoxitin 2 g intramuscularly with probenecid 1 g orally, or another third-generation cephalosporin. For those patients treated in an ambulatory setting, reevaluation within 72 hours of initiation of therapy is essential. At that time, symptoms should have resolved and fever should have abated.

The Centers for Disease Control and Prevention (CDC) recommend hospitalization for patients with PID in the following situations:

1. If the diagnosis is uncertain.
2. If a surgical emergency, particularly appendicitis and ectopic pregnancy, cannot be excluded.
3. If a pelvic abscess is suspected.
4. If severe illness precludes outpatient management.
5. If the patient is pregnant.
6. If the patient is unable to follow or tolerate an outpatient regimen.
7. If the patient fails to respond to outpatient therapy.

8. If clinical follow-up 48 to 72 hours following the initiation of antibiotic treatment cannot be arranged.

Not mentioned by the CDC, but routinely accepted in many centers, is the policy that all young adolescents (14 years of age and younger) with suspected PID should be hospitalized to ensure adequate treatment and education.

Inpatient therapy for PID may include any of the following:

1. Doxycycline 100 mg intravenously twice a day and cefoxitin 2.0 g intravenously four times a day or cefotetan 2 g intravenously every 12 hours.
2. Clindamycin 600 mg intravenously four times a day and gentamycin (or tobramycin) 2.0 mg/kg intravenously followed by 1.5 mg/kg intravenously four times a day.

ADOLESCENT MEN

All adolescent men who are sexually active, those suspected of being victims of sexual abuse, and those who have a history of previous sexual contact should be considered at risk for sexually transmitted diseases. For sexually active adolescent men, annual screening should be done and should include cultures for gonorrhea and *Chlamydia,* urinalysis, and a serologic test for syphilis.

The visit begins with a sexual history. In boys it is important to determine the time since the last physical examination, the number and frequency of sexual partners, any history of homosexual encounters, any symptoms since the last examination, any history of sexually transmitted diseases, any history of symptoms of disease in partners, recent use of antibiotics, and use of condoms. A complete physical examination should be performed to look for similar systemic symptoms as in adolescent women. The genitalia should be inspected for findings characteristic of syphilis, herpes, *Candida,* scabies, lice, papillomas, lymphogranuloma venereum, chancroid, and granuloma inguinale, as for women. In uncircumcised men, the foreskin must be retracted and inspected for lesions. Any penile discharge should be noted and appropriate cultures obtained.

The physical examination includes palpation of the scrotal contents for tenderness and stripping of the penis for discharge.

Urethritis

Discharge in men should be sent for routine culture for *N. gonorrhoeae,* and either culture or rapid diagnostic testing for *C. trachomatis.* An appropriate sample is obtained with either a swab or wire loop, and samples for *N. gonorrhoeae* should be plated on both restrictive medium and chocolate agar or on an appropriate transport medium. Gram staining of urethral discharge from men, when appropriately done, is 95% sensitive and 97% specific for *N. gonorrhoeae.* Culture is confirmatory. *Chlamydia* culture shows great variability in sensitivity in men. Indications of urethritis can be found with a screening urinalysis. If a spun urine specimen has greater than 10 white blood cells per high-power field, one can be 93% certain that infection is present.

It must be remembered that 45% of men with gonococcal urethritis will also carry *Chlamydia.* The presence of overgrowth of gonococcal organisms and pus inhibit the growth of *Chlamydia* in culture. In men with gonococcal urethritis, the clinician must remember to obtain pharyngeal and rectal cultures. Treatment for gonococcal disease is outlined above for women as is treatment for chlamydial infection. In men with urethritis resistant to these treatments, *Trichomonas* infections should be considered, especially if partners have symptoms of infection. Treatment with metronidazole should be given to men with unresponsive urethral symptoms. Patients who continue to have urethral symptoms after treatment with doxycycline and metroconazole should receive a single 1-week course of erythromycin base, 500 mg four times a day.

Other less frequent causes of urethritis include herpes simplex disease (external lesions are usually present); urethral trauma, such as that caused by accidental insertion or self-insertion of catheters or other instruments (hematuria is frequently present); and Reiter syndrome (usual triad for Reiter syndrome includes urethritis, anterior uveitis or conjunctivitis, and arthritis of lower extremity large joints). In cases of urethritis resistant to antimicrobial therapy, the clinician should consider referral to a urologist for evaluation of urethral stricture, intraurethral ulceration, condyloma acuminatum, or foreign body not readily palpated. Urethrographic or urethroscopic study may be indicated. All men with urethritis should be examined for tenderness and inflammation of the prostate gland.

Epididymo-orchitis

Epididymo-orchitis may be caused by sexually transmitted organisms. It must be differentiated from surgical conditions such as torsion of the testis or appendix testis and incarcerated inguinal hernia. *N. gonorrhoeae, C. trachomatis,* infections, and rarely syphilis cause sexually transmitted epididymitis. Gonococcal infection and chlamydial disease will be diagnosed with cultures, rapid diagnostic, and Gram-stain techniques. Syphilis is diagnosed with serologic testing. Other causes of epididymitis include common pathogenic bacteria such as *Staphylococcus, Streptococcus,* or coliforms extending from a nearby genitourinary focus. Tuberculosis is a rare cause of epididymitis. A positive result of a urine culture in a patient with epididymitis should suggest an underlining genitourinary tract anomaly.

Orchitis is most frequently caused by mumps, coxsackievirus, echovirus, or adenovirus and may be difficult to diagnose. Mumps orchitis is likely in the patient with a history of parotitis 4 to 6 days preceding testicular involvement. Serum amylase values may occasionally be elevated, but often they will have returned to normal by the time testicular swelling has developed.

Scrotum trauma and tortion of the testis, as well as incarcerated inguinal hernia, must always be considered when tenderness is found within the scrotal sac.

SPECIFIC DISEASE ENTITIES

Syphilis

After many years of decreasing frequency, the number of syphilis cases began increasing in the late 1980s. The reported number of cases of congenital syphilis increased by more than 21% in the United States in the second half of 1987.

The natural history of syphilis can be broken down into three stages. Primary syphilis occurs 3 to 4 weeks (range, 10 days to 10 weeks) after initial infection with *T. pallidum.* Primary syphilis is a local infection. Symptoms include large local lymph nodes (draining the portal of entry) and a chancre (nonpainful ulcerating lesion at the portal of entry, which involutes 4 to 6 weeks after initial symptoms). A chancre is more commonly seen in men than in women.

Secondary syphilis, marked by rash and/or condyloma lata, occurs 3 weeks after the onset of

SEROLOGY OF UNTREATED SYPHILIS

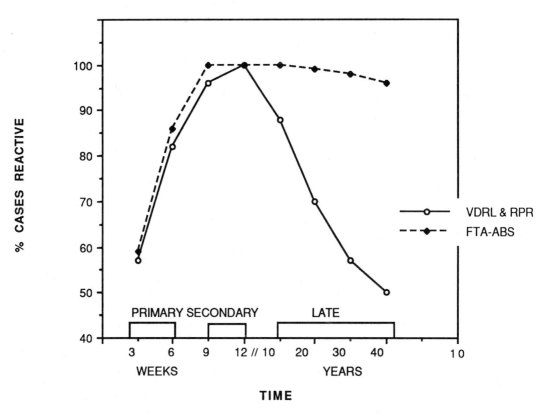

FIG 95-1
The serology of untreated syphilis.

primary symptoms or 6 weeks to 6 months into the course of the disease. Secondary syphilis is a systemic infection and may be accompanied by mild, generalized symptoms. Rash is a common symptom of secondary syphilis. This rash may last weeks to months. It is usually macular, nonpruritic, and located on the extensor surfaces of the extremities and on the chest. It may occur on palms, soles, or mucous membranes. It may be petechial, papular, or even vesicular.

Condyloma lata are moist, warty lesions that usually occur near the portal of entry. They may be found on the vulva, perineum, thighs, or buttocks. Condyloma lata resemble venereal warts caused by human papilloma virus. They can occasionally be differentiated by the wider base and less cornified appearance of lesions due to syphilis. Their surface may be grayish and necrotic.

After symptoms of secondary syphilis abate, a period of latency may occur. This period may happen at any time after primary syphilis. During this time, patients may have recurrent eruptions and lesions on mucosa, skin, eyes, viscera, and bone. One need not progress through primary syphilis to secondary syphilis to latency. It is not unusual to have no primary or no secondary lesions.

Tertiary syphilis, which affects neurologic, cardiovascular, rheumatologic, and integumentary systems should not be seen in pediatric patients because of its long latency period.

Testing for syphilis is done with rapid antibody screening of blood samples. In patients with rapid test results that are positive, a titer is performed. As with other diseases, positive syphilis serology is not diagnostic of current infection in the face of recent treatment with appropriate antibiotics. As shown in Figure 95-1, stages of syphilis, serologic results may be negative at the time of primary lesion. As a result, any suspect lesion in a patient with a history of sexual activity should be appropriately treated at the time of the visit unless follow-up and abstinence can be ensured. In patients with normal serologic results and a primary lesion, a second serologic test should be done 4 to 6 weeks after the initial visit. If serologic test results are positive, treatment should be be initiated. Treatment for early primary syphilis includes either benzathine penicillin, 2.4 MU once; doxycycline, 100 mg orally two times a day for 2 weeks; or tetracycline, 500 mg orally four times a day for 2 weeks. For syphilis of more than 1 year's duration, treatment must include benzathine penicillin G, 2.4 MU weekly for 3 weeks, or tetracycline, 500 mg orally four times a day for a month. All patients with syphilis should be tested for HIV infection. Those patients with HIV infection must be followed closely and are at risk of neurosyphillis, even early in the course of the disease. Cure of syphilis is only suggested when titers begin to decrease.

Human Papillomavirus

Human papillomavirus (HPV) infection leads to condyloma accuminata or venereal warts. One percent to 2% of all Papanicolaou smears in the United States show cytologic signs of HPV. Papillomas may occur in the lower genital tract of women, on the penis, in the urethra of men and women, and on oropharyngeal mucosa. Papillomas may be totally invisible to the naked eye (flat warts). They can be seen only through close inspection with a hand lens or culposcopy after application of 3% acetic acid. Prevalence of HPV infection appears to have been rising since the 1960s when registries began. It is estimated that up to 56% of sexually active women are infected with HPV, and surveys in sexually transmitted disease clinics have found that 90% report having had visible warts. One urban study found a prevalence of 38.2% in sexually active adolescent women.

The virology of papilloma infection is complex. Types 6 and 11 cause exophytic (ie, visible) lesions, which may be associated with itching, burning, and pain. Virotypes 16, 18, 31, and 35 are more likely to cause flat lesions, which are tiny and difficult to see. These lesions may occur on the cervix or external genitalia. They are easier to treat than the more visible lesions but more difficult to diagnose. More than one type of papilloma virus may exist in the same patient at a given time. All serotypes have oncogenic potential. In a 6-year follow-up study of 846 patients with HPV on Papanicolaou smear in 1979, 30 had carcinoma in situ by 1985. Of note, the adolescent cervix is particularly vulnerable to dysplasia because of squamous metaplasia occurring as the squamocolumnar junction migrates outward in adolescence.

External lesions of papillomavirus may have a typical cauliflower-like appearance on the genitalia. These are easily identified. It is important to check the perianal area and the crural folds in patients who have visible lesions on the external genitalia. Cervical condylomas appear as leukoplakia (white spots on the cervix). The presence of HPV is confirmed with Papanicolaou smear; however, the false-negative rate is 20%. In patients with confirmed evidence of HPV on Papanicolaou smear, the smear should be repeated every 3 months. Colposcopy and direct biopsy are usually needed for diagnosis. These should be performed by an experienced gynecologist.

Treatment

Treatments for external lesions include 1) podophyllin, although the long-term cure rate is only 20% and podophyllin is known to be mutagenic and 2) trichloroacetic acid, which is used successfully in many centers in strengths of 25%, 50%, or 85%. Eighty-five percent solutions should be used only by experienced practitioners. If cervical lesions or dysplasia is present, treatment is needed. Treatments include cryocautery, cone biopsy, and laser vaporization of lesions.

Visible HPV lesions of the internal vaginal area in women should be treated with laser vaporization. These treatments are best handled by experienced gynecologists.

In men with HPV lesions, or in partners of women with known papillomavirus infections, diagnosis of flat warts may be made by swathing the genitalia in gauze soaked in 3% acetic acid solution. With a hand lens, lesions will appear as white spots after 5 minutes of soaking. Treatment is generally performed in a urologist's office, because inspection of the distal 1 to 2 cm of the urethra is necessary for complete treatment of HPV lesions in men.

Herpes Simplex

Herpes simplex is a chronic viral infection marked by latency and repeated, recurrent localized lesions. The primary episode of infection is more severe and prolonged than recurrent attacks. The primary attack lasts up to 3 weeks, with initial symptoms beginning 5 to 7 days after infection (range, 1 to 45 days). Lesions are often multiple, bilateral, and coalescent. Lymphadenopathy is commonly found in primary disease. Half of patients will have systemic symptoms with primary disease, including fever, headache, and malaise. Local symptoms include dysuria, pain, itch, and vaginal or urethral discharge. Pain generally lasts 1 to 2 weeks. Ulcers last 4 to 14 days before crusting. All symptoms are more common in women than men. Extragenital lesions occur in as many as one third of patients.

Overall, 60% of patients will have a recurrence. Herpesvirus lives in dorsal root ganglia between attacks. The first recurrence usually occurs within 4 to 6 months of primary symptoms. Recurrent episodes are shorter and milder than primary ones. Only 5% to 10% of patients will have systemic symptoms during recurrent attacks. Lesions in recurrent attacks usually last approximately 10 days. Many patients will have a prodrome 1 to 2 days before an attack. Recurrence is more likely with herpes simplex type 2 infection than with type 1 infection. The average patient will have three to five recurrences per year. Stress, fever, menses, heat, sexual activity, and depression may all bring on a recurrence.

Diagnostic tests for herpes include the Tzanck preparation, in which a scraping is smeared on a slide and Wright stained. The Tzanck preparation is 30% to 50% sensitive for herpesvirus infection. Papanicolaou smears will result in diagnosis in 40% of cases, because of the virus' predilection for the cervix. Available from most large diagnostic centers, herpesvirus culture is between 94% (for vesicular stage) and 27% (for crusting lesions) sensitive. Appropriate diagnostic material from herpes lesions is obtained by unroofing lesions or removing crusts before swabbing for a sample.

Transmission of the virus is through direct contact, although the agent can live on inanimate objects. True asymptomatic shedding does occur in women (from the cervix), though the period of shedding is short (generally 1 to 5 days), and the virus titer is lower than in symptomatic shedding. Virus has been identified in saliva, vaginal fluid, and in semen.

The most feared complications of herpesvirus infection are neonatal acquisition of herpes and cervical carcinoma. Herpesvirus has been isolated from cervical samples obtained from patients with carcinoma in situ of the cervix.

Herpesvirus lesions are treated with acyclovir. Acyclovir inhibits viral DNA polymerase through substitution for a nucleoside base. The drug is available in oral, topical, and intravenous form. Topical acyclovir reduces the duration of viral shedding by 3 to 4 days during a primary outbreak. Ointment is applied four times a day for 7 days. It has little effect on symptoms. In recurrent episodes, ointment may reduce shedding by about 1 day.

Oral acyclovir is more effective than the topical form during primary outbreaks. Dosage for oral acyclovir is 200 mg five times a day for 7 days. Oral acyclovir reduces pain and other symptoms. Oral acyclovir is also effective in treating recurrent infection. To be maximally effective, it must be administered within the first 48 hours of an outbreak.

Oral acyclovir can be used for prophylaxis for recurrent attacks of herpes. Continuous prophylaxis may be helpful in the patient who experiences frequent recurrences, but has no effect on long-term prognosis. Prophylaxis does not prevent asymptomatic shedding.

BIBLIOGRAPHY

Bauwens JE, Clark AM, Loeffelholz MJ, et al: Diagnosis of *Chlamydia trachomatis* urethritis in men by polymerase chain reaction assay of first-catch urine, *J Clin Microbiol* 31:3013–3016, 1933.

Beutner KR, Becker TM, Stone KM: Epidemiol-

ogy of human papillomavirus infections, *Dermatol Clin* 9(2):211–218, 1991.

Brown DR, Fife KH: Human papillomavirus infections of the genital tract, *Med Clin North Am* 74(6):1455, 1990.

Frasier LD: Human papillomavirus infections

in children, *Pediatr Ann* 23(7):354–360, 1994.

Genc M, Ruusuvaara L, Mardh PA: An economic evaluation of screening for *Chlamydia trachomatis* in adolescent males, *JAMA* 270: 2057–2064, 1993.

Gutman LT, St. Claire KK, Everett VD, et al: Cervical-vaginal and intraanal human papillomavirus infection of young girls with external genital warts, *JID* 170:339–344, 1994.

Hammerschlag MR, Golden NH, Oh MK, et al: Single dose of azithromycin for the treatment of genital chlamydia infections in adolescents, *J Pediatr* 122(6):961–965, 1993.

Hook III EW, Spitters C, Reichart MT, et al: Use of cell culture and a rapid diagnostic assay for *Chlamydia trachomatis* screening, *JAMA* 272(11):867–870, 1994.

Ingram DL, Everett VD, Lyna PR, et al: Epidemiology of adult sexually transmitted disease agents in children being evaluated for sexual abuse, *Pediatr Infect Dis J* 11:945–950, 1992.

Martin DH: Chlamydia infections, *Med Clin North Am* 74(6):1367, 1990.

Martinez J, Smith R, Farmer M, et al: High prevalence of genital tract papillomavirus infection in female adolescents, *Pediatrics* 82: 604–608, 1988.

Mertz GJ: Genital herpes simplex virus infections, *Med Clin North Am,* 74(6):1433, 1990.

Remafedi G, Abdalian SE: Clinical predictors of *Chlamydia trachomatis* endocervicitis in adolescent women, Am J Dis Child, 143:1437–1442, 1989.

Rosenfeld D, Vermund H, Wentz S, et al: High prevalence rate of human papillomavirus infection and association with abnormal Papanicolaou smears in sexually active adolescents, *Am J Dis Child* 143:1443–1447, 1989.

Rosenfeld WD, Clark J: Vulvovaginitis and cervicitis, *Pediatr Clin North Am* 36(3):489, 1989.

1993 Sexually transmitted diseases treatment guidelines, *MMWR* 42(RR-14), 1993.

Shafer MA, Schachter J, Moncada J, et al: Evaluation of urine-based screening strategies to detect chlamydia trachomatis among sexually active asymptomatic young males, *JAMA* 270: 2065–2070, 1993.

Shafer MA, Sweet RL: Pelvic inflammatory disease in adolescent females, *Pediatr Clin North Am* 36(3):513, 1989.

Vogel LN: Epidemiology of human papilloma virus infection, *Semin Dermatol* 11(3):226–228, 1992.

CHAPTER 96

Urinary Tract Infection

Mary B. Leonard
Kathy N. Shaw

The high prevalence and significant morbidity of urinary tract infection (UTI) in children make the diagnosis and treatment of UTI an important issue for the practicing clinician. Nuclear scans suggest that a majority of febrile young children with UTI have pyelonephritis, requiring prompt treatment and putting them at risk for scarring and the long-term sequelae of hypertension, preeclampsia, and renal failure. UTI in young children is also the primary indicator of an underlying anomaly such as vesicoureteral reflux (VUR) or obstruction, which have been associated with progression to end-stage renal disease (ESRD). Unfortunately, classic symptoms of UTI often are not present in young children. Fever is the most common presenting complaint. Thus, the practitioner must be aggressive in the evaluation, treatment, and follow-up of children with UTI because a delay in the diagnosis and treatment puts the child at risk for significant long-term sequelae.

TERMINOLOGY

Simply stated, a UTI can be defined as the growth of bacteria in the urine, which ordinarily should be sterile. UTIs can be subdivided based on the level of infection. It is necessary to localize the site of infection because of differences in therapy, prognosis, and follow-up. Cystitis is inflammation of the bladder. Pyelonephritis is inflammation above the ureterovesicular junction, involving the renal parenchyma, calyces, and pelvis. Unfortunately, in children with febrile UTIs, clinical and laboratory findings cannot adequately differentiate upper tract infection. However, imaging studies of the urinary tract anatomy may ascertain the level of infection.

PATHOGENESIS

The general route of infection of the urinary tract is ascending. Although UTI in newborns and young infants commonly is associated with bacteremia, this condition may be a consequence rather than a cause of UTI. Periurethral colonization is facilitated by lack of circumcision and perineal irritation or bacterial soilage. Subsequent transurethral migration of bacteria into the bladder is normally prevented by low urine pH, high urine osmolality, urinary bactericidal substances, and the local immune response. Bacteria also may be introduced into the bladder by instrumentation or indwelling catheters.

Once the bladder has become contaminated, the likelihood of subsequent cystitis depends largely on the patient's voiding habits. School-aged children may void infrequently and incompletely, allowing bacteria prolonged time to multiply in the urine. Children with urinary tract abnormalities that cause obstruction or incomplete bladder emptying (such as neurogenic bladder) are at greater risk for the establishment of UTI. In addition, bladder uroepithelium defense mechanisms may be compromised for several months following an infection. Sexual activity also is associated with bladder contamination.

VUR is a pathologic event in which urine progresses in a retrograde fashion from the bladder to the ureter, and potentially to the kidney. VUR may be due to congenital deficiency of ureter insertion or chronic bladder overdistension and increased intravesicular pressures. VUR is found in 20% to 50% of patients with symptomatic UTI. In infants with UTI, 70% have VUR; this percentage decreases to 25% in children 2 to 8 years of age. Although it is controversial to what degree VUR increases susceptibility to recurrent infection, it is suggested that the combination of reflux and infection, by transporting bacteria to the renal parenchyma, predisposes to scar formation. This result has the potential long-term sequelae of reflux nephropathy and the potential for progression to chronic renal failure and ESRD.

Voiding disturbances also contribute to the pathogenesis of UTI. Dysfunctional voiding occurs in otherwise healthy normal children and may represent delayed maturation. Voluntary obstruction occurs when the child tries to prevent wetting by tightly squeezing the urinary sphincter in response to contractions. The resulting high pressure can lead to VUR and UTI. Constipation is associated with UTI and may exert its pathologic effect by also inducing bladder hyperactivity. Voiding dysfunction does not occur before the age of toilet training.

Most UTIs occur without either obstruction or VUR. It is important to recognize that VUR is only present in a minority of patients with pyelonephritis and subsequent renal scarring.

The establishment of clinical infection and the consequent injury to the urinary tract are due to the complex interplay between the characteristics of the invading bacteria and the characteristics of the host's urinary tract. Given the presence of upper tract infection, the following factors contribute to the development of renal parenchymal scarring: younger age at diagnosis, therapeutic delay, and anatomic or functional abnormalities.

EPIDEMIOLOGY

The first and most important step in preventing UTI-related renal damage is to identify the child with UTI. Because fever is the primary present-

TABLE 96-1
Interpretation of Urine Culture Results by Method of Obtaining Specimen

METHOD	DEFINITE	SUSPICIOUS	INDETERMINANT	CONTAMINANT*	NEGATIVE
Suprapubic	$\geq10^2$ CFU/mL One pathogen	Any growth One pathogen	Any growth Two pathogens or mixed culture[†]	Nonpathogens only	0
Catheterization	$\geq10^4$ CFU/mL One pathogen	$\geq10^3$ CFU/mL One pathogen	$\geq10^3$ CFU/mL of mixed culture[†] ≥500 but <1000 of pure pathogen	≥500 CFU/mL Nonpathogens only or 500–999 of mixed culture	<500 CFU/mL Any organisms
Clean-catch	$\geq10^5$ CFU/mL One pathogen Two cultures	$\geq10^5$ CFU/mL One pathogen One culture	10^4 CFU/mL of mixed culture[†] ≥5000 but <10^5 for pure pathogen	≥5000 CFU/mL Nonpathogens only 5000–9999 of mixed culture	<5000 CFU/mL Any organisms

CFU—colony-forming units.
*Cultures with >two organisms are considered contaminated.
[†]Mixed culture = pathogen + nonpathogen or two pathogens.

ing symptom of most babies and young children for UTI, the practitioner must have a high index of suspicion and a low threshold for screening for UTI in febrile children. Babies without a source of fever, or even a minor source of fever such as an upper respiratory infection or gastroenteritis, may have a UTI. Prevalence of UTI in febrile young children varies depending on age, sex, circumcision status, and prior history of UTI or urinary tract anomaly.

Community studies have shown that the incidence of UTI in girls 1 to 3 years of age is 10 times that in boys of the same age. Febrile UTI or pyelonephritis becomes significantly less common after the first year of life in boys and gradually decreases in girls as they approached school age. Boys who are uncircumcised may have up to a 10-fold increased incidence of UTI compared with circumcised male infants. Thus, uncircumcised boys, boys under 1 year of age, and young girls are at higher risk for UTI and pyelonephritis. Sexually active girls also have a higher incidence of UTI, which is usually lower tract.

Fifteen percent to 30% of cases of ESRD are believed to have been related to urinary infection, especially in infants and younger children. Repeated infections, occurring in 30% to 80% of children with febrile UTIs, may lead to hypertension, ESRD, and toxemia in pregnancy.

The most common pathogen for UTI in children is *Escherichia coli.* Other common pathogens in community-acquired UTI include *Enterococcus, Proteus mirabilis,* and *Klebsiella* species. *Enterobacteria cloacae,* group B β-hemolytic

streptococcus, *Staphylococcus aureus, Citrobacter,* and *Pseudomonas* also can be pathogens in both healthy and immunosuppressed children. Antibiotic usage may select for resistant species, especially in children with urinary tract dysfunction or anomalies. Adolescent girls may have lower tract symptoms from low colony counts of *Staphylococcus saprophyticus.* Nosocomial and catheter-related UTIs are more commonly polymicrobial and are due to organisms such as *Pseudomonas, Citrobacter,* and *Candida.*

CRITERIA FOR DIAGNOSIS

A positive urine culture varies by the method of collection and is not uniform in the literature. Table 96-1 defines UTI as "definite," "suspicious," "indeterminant," "contaminated," or "negative" by method, colony count, and number of pathogens. It is important to distinguish organisms that are commonly pathogens from those that are not. This table must be interpreted in light of the clinical presentation, past history of UTI or urinary tract anomalies, antibiotic usage, and examination of the urine for pyuria and bacteriuria. Most children whose cultures fall into the "definite" or "suspicious" category would be assumed to have UTI. Older children usually will have classic symptoms of UTI and presence of pyuria (≥5 white blood cells [WBCs]/high-power field [HPF]) or bacteriuria (bacteria on Gram stain or by microscopy per HPF). However, lower urine colony counts, more than one pathogen, and absence of pyuria have been reported in babies and children with documented pyelonephritis by nuclear scan or UTI by superpubic aspiration. This result may occur if there is concomitant antibiotic usage, dilute urine from babies that void frequently, or difficulty in obtaining a sterile specimen in a young child. Thus, an "indeterminant" culture may indicate UTI in young babies and children and those patients taking antibiotics. Repeat cultures should be obtained if the clinical suspicion is high for those children with "indeterminant" or "contaminated" urines.

DATA GATHERING

Clinical Features

The clinician must have a high index of suspicion and a low threshold for culturing for UTI in children. In infants and children, there may be considerable overlap between symptoms of upper and lower tract involvement. Acute pyelonephritis is classically characterized by constitutional symptoms of high fever, malaise, abdominal pain, nausea, and vomiting in addition to flank pain and costovertebral angle tenderness. Cystitis is characterized by symptoms of dysuria, urgency, and frequency, usually without fever. As the patient ages, the signs and symptoms become more specific to the urinary tract. Symptoms of UTI in young infants are particularly nonspecific and may include vomiting, irritability, or poor feeding. Fever is the most common symptom in infants less than 1 year of age. Other less common findings of UTI in babies include abdominal pain or distention, jaundice, and failure to thrive. Astute parents will recognize dysuria or malodorous urine. Poor urinary stream may be noted, suggesting the possibility of urinary tract dysfunction and subsequent infection. Unfortunately, the presence of another minor source of fever such as upper respiratory infection, gastroenteritis, or serous otitis media does not preclude a UTI. Thus, babies less than 1 year of age, uncircumcised boys, and preschool-aged girls with fever should be screened for UTI unless there is another documented source of fever on examination.

In older children, the classic symptoms of UTI are more commonly present. However, these signs may not be specific for UTI. Dysuria may indicate urethral irritation from bubble baths or friction. Frequency may be a sign of diabetes, excessive drinking, or masses pressing against the bladder. Urgency, enuresis, and incontinence may occur with normal potty training or relapses from training in normal toddlers and preschoolers. Hematuria actually may be hematachezia or dyes from ingested fluids. Urine may be malodorous when it is concentrated secondary to dehydration.

Abnormal voiding habits such as infrequent urinary voiding, urgency, straining on urination, poor stream, chronic constipation, and enuresis should alert the physician to dysfunctional voiding or underlying structural or neurologic conditions. The patient's past medical history also should be assessed for the recent use of antibiotics, recurrent unexplained fevers, and evaluation of previous UTIs. The family history should be questioned for evidence of UTI, renal disease, or hypertension.

Upper tract infection is difficult to distinguish from lower tract infection on physical examination. Vital signs should be taken including temperature and blood pressure. Fever, flank pain, and nausea or anorexia may not always be present. Some children will present with signs of acute abdominal tenderness suggestive of gastroenteritis or appendicitis. Examination of the external genitalia may reveal local irritation, meatal stenosis, labial fusion, vaginitis, or evidence of sexual abuse. Examination of the lower spine may reveal evidence of occult spinal dysraphism. A pelvic examination should be performed in adolescent girls to distinguish pelvic inflammatory disease from pyelonephritis.

Laboratory Diagnosis

Several urine rapid screening tests are available to aid in the diagnosis and early treatment of UTI in children. These tests include the conventional microscopic urinalysis for pyuria or bacteriuria in urine sediment, urine cell count per mm^3, urine Gram stains of unspun urine, and a rapid filter test for bacteriuria. The urine dipstick for leukocyte esterase or nitrite is equivalent to the conventional urinalysis in detecting UTI in children, is cost-effective, and is easily used in the office setting. Any color change ("trace" or greater) in the dipstick leukocyte esterase is equivalent to ≥5 WBCs/HPF, whereas a positive dipstick for nitrite is very specific for UTI. Although these tests may be useful in indicating the need for a urine culture in older children, they may lack sensitivity in babies. An estimated 10% of young babies who have pyelonephritis documented by nuclear scan lack pyuria. Alternatively, sterile pyuria may occur with trauma, dehydration, febrile illness, viral infection, or chemical irritation. Although rapid testing can be used to make the diagnosis and to begin treatment in the majority of young children, a sterile urine culture always should be sent to confirm infection. Laboratory studies such as serum C-reactive protein, erythrocyte sedimentation rate, leukocyte count, and the presence of antibody-coated bacteria in the urinary sediment have not proven useful in distinguishing upper UTI from lower UTI in children.

The method of obtaining a urine culture in children has major impact on the results. Contaminated cultures are a major problem. Specimens obtained by clean bag technique should not be sent for urine culture because they have contamination rates ranging from 12% to 83%. Often the clinician has only one chance of obtaining a specimen before antibiotics are started. Suprapubic aspiration of the bladder is the most sterile way of obtaining specimens uncontaminated by the perineum's vaginal and fecal flora. However, because of pain and a low success rate, bladder catherization is usually preferred. This method has a contamination rate of approximately 2%. Midstream clean-catch urine, the preferred method for toilet-trained children, has a 0% to 29% contamination rate. Better results occur in older children, uncircumcised boys, and when the girl is positioned backward on the toilet seat (to help spread the labia). Due to the high contamination rate in young preschool-aged children, it is better to obtain two clean-catch specimens or a specimen by catherization before beginning antibiotic therapy.

Urine obtained sterilely should be refrigerated immediately or plated in a microbiology laboratory within 2 hours. Alternatively, it can be plated on a dipslide immediately. The cultures and dipslides should be incubated at 35° C and examined for growth daily for 2 days.

Blood cultures usually are obtained in young babies with high fevers (>39° C) and suspicion of pyelonephritis to detect concurrent bacteremia, which is reported to occur in approximately 10% of babies less than 4 months of age. The WBC count and erythrocyte sedimentation rate (ESR) may be helpful in distinguishing upper versus lower tract infection. Most children with positive dimercaptosuccinic acid (DMSA) scans for pyelonephritis have ESRs greater than 25 mm/hr and WBC counts above 12,000. However, some children with positive nuclear scans have had low ESRs and WBC counts. Nuclear scans appear to be the only reliable indicator of pyelonephritis.

MANAGEMENT

Optimal management of UTI includes early diagnosis, effective antibiotic therapy, and prevention of further infections. Because pyelonephritis in young children may lead to irreversible renal damage and eventually to arterial hypertension or renal insufficiency, early identification and prompt treatment is essential to reduce the incidence of renal scarring. Whereas cystitis can be treated with a short course of orally administered antibiotics, renal parenchymal infection usually requires intravenously administered antibiotics. Therefore, after establishing the diagnosis of UTI, a thorough evaluation is necessary to determine the extent and level of infection and to reveal structural and functional anomalies of the entire urinary tract.

Treatment of the Acute Infection

Once infection is verified, blood urea nitrogen and serum creatinine levels should be checked in patients with suspected upper tract involvement. Antimicrobial therapy depends on the age of the child, severity of illness at clinical presentation, presence of anatomic abnormalities, and the response to initial therapy.

Infants are at risk for serious sequelae and are best treated with intravenous antibiotics in the hospital. Initial therapy generally includes intravenous ampicillin and an aminoglycoside. A repeat urine culture should be obtained after 48 hours of treatment to ensure that the urine is sterile. If the infant has improved clinically and is without fever after 3 to 5 days and the urine has sterilized, oral antibiotics may be given to complete a 10- to 14-day course. For patients with genitourinary abnormalities and patients with evidence of pyelonephritis, at least 7 days of intravenous antibiotics are recommended followed by oral antibiotics to complete a 2- to 3-week course.

Children over 6 to 12 months of age with normal urinary tracts who are able to tolerate oral fluids and medications, are not toxic appearing, and have no evidence of upper tract disease on radiographic evaluation may be treated as outpatients with oral antibiotics. Cultures should be obtained prior to therapy. Because the most likely organisms in uncomplicated lower UTIs is *E. coli* with broad susceptibilities, initial therapy may be ampicillin, amoxicillin, nitrofurantoin, or the combination trimethoprim/sulfamethoxazole, depending on any recent antibiotic exposure. All of these medications are readily absorbed from the gastrointestinal tract and are concentrated in the urine. A repeat urine culture should be obtained after 48 hours of treatment to ensure that the urine is sterile, and sensitivities of the initial cultures should be checked. Antibiotic therapy in such uncomplicated cases of lower tract infection is continued for 7 to 10 days.

Radiographic Evaluation

The subject of imaging the urinary tract in patients with UTIs has been vigorously debated in the pediatric literature for years. Proper evaluation should identify the level of infection; identify and grade VUR; reveal structural anomalies, which may have predisposed to the infection and which require treatment to reduce the risk of further infections and progressive renal damage; and identify evidence of renal scarring and contractures from previous infections. The triad of sonography, radiography, and nuclear medicine provide all the necessary information.

Renal ultrasound is the preferred method of initially evaluating the kidneys. Ultrasound provides information about the size, shape, and location of the kidneys; detects cystic changes; and reveals dilation of the collecting system secondary to obstruction. It is noninvasive and does not expose the patient to radiation. However, it cannot assess renal function and is insensitive in detecting VUR, acute inflammation, and early renal scars.

The voiding cystourethrogram (VCUG) assesses the presence and severity of VUR and provides adequate assessment of the bladder and urethra. Radionuclide cystography is an alternative approach that results in significantly less radiation exposure but grades reflux less precisely and poorly outlines the bladder and urethral structures. Hence, it may be more appropriate for follow-up evaluation rather than primary investigation. The VCUG may be performed during the acute illness or after completing therapy. Although VUR is more likely to be demonstrated when the VCUG is performed during acute inflammation, it is important to know if reflux occurs during infection because that is the time of greatest injury to the kidney. If the VCUG is obtained at a later date, antibiotics should be continued until the VCUG is completed.

Over the past 5 years, renal cortical scans have become an essential part of the standard evaluation of UTI. Renal cortical scans demonstrate a high degree of sensitivity and specificity in identifying pyelonephritis. Two common renal cortical scans are the technetium-labeled DMSA scan and the glucoheptonate scan. A DMSA scan provides high-quality images to assess for acute pyelonephritis and permanent focal scars but does not assess renal function. Glucoheptonate can give an estimate of renal function; however, the images are often of poorer quality. Many cases of tubular dysfunction secondary to infection identified on renal cortical scan have been shown to be reversible with aggressive therapy.

The role of VUR in the pathogenesis of pyelonephritis has been brought into question; the contribution of reflux to scar formation might be less than previously considered. Because the majority of children with pyelonephritis have a normal ultrasound and VCUG, one cannot exclude the diagnosis of pyelonephritis or subsequent renal injury on the basis of normal sonogram and a normal VCUG. Once acute pyelonephritis has occurred, ultimate renal scarring is independent of the presence or absence of VUR.

The younger the patient and the more severe the symptoms, the more aggressive the workup should be. An approach to the evaluation of the first UTI is outlined in Figure 96-1. The first UTI in all boys and in girls less than 3 years of age should be evaluated radiographically with a VCUG, renal ultrasound, and renal cortical scan. The VCUG may be deferred in children less than one year of age who have no history of UTI or unexplained recurrent febrile illnesses, have a normal renal ultrasound and renal DMSA scan, and have no family history of VUR. In girls greater than 3 years of age, if there are clinical signs and symptoms suggestive of infection of the upper tract or there is or a history of unexplained recurrent fevers, the full protocol should be followed. If there are no such indications, an ultrasound should be obtained. If it is abnormal,

Management of the First UTI

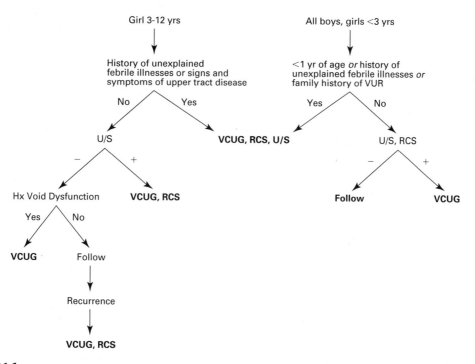

FIG 96-1

Management of the first urinary tract infection.

a VCUG and renal cortical scan should be done. If the ultrasound is normal and there is no history of dysfunctional voiding, the patient can be followed-up. However, should a recurrence occur, the workup should be completed with VCUG and renal cortical scan. If there is a history of dysfunctional voiding, a VCUG should be done. For girls older than 12 years of age, UTI is usually lower tract and does not usually require further investigation. Exceptions would include girls who have a past history of UTIs but no previous workup or a history of recurrent unexplained febrile illnesses.

FOLLOW-UP

A recurrence rate of 30% following the first UTI, with higher recurrence rates following subsequent infections, has been reported. Most recur-

rences occur within 2 years. Better means of identifying, evaluating, and treating patients with UTI may reduce this high rate of recurrence. Figure 96-2 represents an approach to the follow-up management of UTI.

Dysfunctional Voiding

In patients with a normal radiologic evaluation, other etiologic factors for UTI should be considered, including disturbances of bladder and bowel function, which increasingly are recognized as a cause of UTI in children. Symptoms of childhood voiding dysfunction that are seen in the absence of a UTI include urgency and urge incontinence, day and night wetting, daytime frequency, infrequent voiding, and urinary retention. Treatment of dysfunctional voiding or constipation may prevent recurrence of UTI and potentially hasten the resolution rate of associated VUR. Therapeutic protocols employ blad-

**Follow-up Management of Children with
Suspected Upper Urinary Tract Infection**

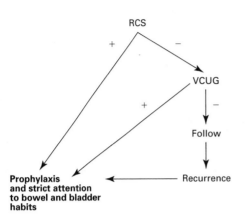

FIG 96-2
Follow-up management of children with suspected upper urinary tract infections.

der retraining with timed voiding regimens or double voiding regimens, biofeedback, urotropic medication, dietary manipulation, stool softeners, and timed defecation programs. Urodynamic testing may be required in patients with daytime irritative symptoms.

Vesicoureteral Reflux
Although the combination of VUR and infected urine may be destructive to the kidneys in young children, the role of VUR in the pathogenesis of pyelonephritis and renal scars is poorly defined. It is now recommended that all patients with UTI and evidence of renal involvement on renal cortical scanning should be treated with long-term prophylaxis, regardless of the presence of VUR. The majority of children with VUR are managed nonoperatively. It is the custom to treat patients with any VUR with prophylactic antibiotics to maintain sterility of the urine, anticipating that the reflux will eventually cease, and the renal parenchyma will be protected in the meanwhile. Spontaneous resolution of VUR as patients get older is seen in 85% of patients with grade I to III VUR, compared with 41% in more severe grades. Medical management also should include careful attention to perineal hygiene and normalization of bladder and bowel habits.

The drugs most commonly used for prophylaxis are trimethoprim/sulfamethoxazole or nitrofurantoin. The exception, in addition to drug allergies, is the newborn infant in whom penicillin or ampicillin is preferred. The prophylactic dose is one half of the therapeutic dose and is given at bedtime so the antibiotic will be in the urine during the longest stasis interval of the day. Should infection occur while on a prophylactic antibiotic, that drug should be stopped and specific treatment with another antibiotic should be instituted based on reculture and sensitivity studies. Once the infection is successfully treated, the same prophylactic antibiotic may be used again. If reinfection occurs multiple times, a different prophylactic antibiotic should be used and noncompliance should be considered. Suppression is continued until reflux has resolved either spontaneously or surgically.

During nonoperative therapy of VUR, the patient must be monitored closely. Monitoring entails interval urine cultures, upper tract imaging every 6 months with ultrasound or renal cortical scan, and yearly assessment for VUR by a nuclear medicine VCUG. Absolute indications for surgical management with ureteral reimplantation include grade V reflux, progressive renal injury, or breakthrough infections despite suppressive management. Relative indications include failure of reflux to resolve following 4 years of successive therapy and entry into adolescence at which time further maturation and spontaneous resolution are unlikely. In addition, if patients cannot or will not comply with long-term prophylaxis, surgery remains an alternative.

These suggestions for the examination and management of a child with a first UTI will certainly undergo modification as more data is accumulated. Cost-effectiveness analysis and outcome research may allow the physician to tailor the evaluation and follow-up for the patients at greatest risk.

Indication for Referral
The physician should consider referral to a pediatric nephrologist for any child with a workup suspicious for upper tract infections, structural abnormality of the urinary tract, or abnormal voiding history. Referral to a pediatric urologist should be considered for children with high-grade reflux, posterior urethral values, or other obstructive lesions.

BIBLIOGRAPHY

Andrich MP, Massoud M: Diagnostic imaging in the evaluation of the first urinary tract infection in infants and young children, *Pediatrics* 90:436–441, 1992.

Benador D, Benador N, Slosman DO, et al: Cortical scintigraphy in the evaluation of renal parenchymal changes in children with pyelonephritis, *J Pediatr* 124:12–20, 1994.

Conway JJ, Cohn RA: Evolving role of nuclear medicine for the diagnosis and management of urinary tract infection, *J Pediatr* 124:87–90, 1994.

Haycock GB: A practical approach to evaluating urinary tract infection in children, *Pediatr Nephrol* 5:401–402, 1991.

Heldrich FJ: UTI diagnosis: Getting it right the first time, *Contemp Pediatr* 12:110–133, 1995.

Hellerstein S: Evolving concepts in the evaluation of the child with a urinary tract infection, *J Pediatr* 124:589–592, 1994.

Hoberman A, Chao HP, Keller DM, et al: Prevalence of urinary tract infection in febrile infants, *J Pediatr* 23(1):17–23, 1993.

Koff SA: A practical approach to evaluating urinary tract infection in children, *Pediatr Nephrol* 5:398–400, 1991.

Landau D, Turner ME, Brennan J, Majd M: The value of urinalysis in differentiating acute pyelonephritis from lower urinary tract infection in febrile infants, *Pediatr Infect Dis J* 13:777–781, 1994.

Lerner GR: Urinary tract infections in children, *Pediatr Ann* 23:463–473, 1994.

Shaw KN, Hexter D, McGowan KL, Schwartz JS: Clinical evaluation of rapid screening test for urinary tract infection in children, *J Pediatr* 118(5):733–736, 1991.

Sheldon CA: Vesicoureteral reflux, *Pediatr Rev* 16:22–27, 1995.

Sherbotie JR, Cornfeld D: Management of urinary tract infections, *Med Clin North Am* 75:327–338, 1991.

Wiswell TE, Roscelli JD: Corroborative evidence for the decreased incidence of urinary tract infections in circumcised male infants, *Pediatrics* 78(1):96–99, 1986.

PART TEN

Neurology

CHAPTER 97

Seizure Disorders

Robert Ryan Clancy

Recurrent epileptic seizures are a common pediatric neurologic disorder affecting approximately 0.5% of children. The majority of affected individuals can have the epilepsy successfully diagnosed, evaluated, and managed by a knowledgeable primary care physician. This chapter will review recent developments in the medical and neurologic approach to children with epilepsy in the setting of an office practice. Neonatal seizures, status epilepticus, and seizures complicating acute medical or neurologic illnesses will not be addressed.

BACKGROUND

The key to the successful management of a seizure disorder is an initial accurate diagnosis of epilepsy and the correct classification of the type of seizure. Children are vulnerable to a wide variety of nonepileptic medical or neurologic disorders that abruptly "seize" them, provoking sudden attacks of disordered consciousness, behavior, involuntary movements, disturbed body tone, posture, or sensation. These nonepileptic abnormal events (eg, migraine, gastroesophageal reflux, and breath-holding attacks) may mimic genuine epilepsy and lead to an initial incorrect

diagnosis and inappropriate or unnecessary evaluation and treatment.

The term *seizure* means literally to "grab hold of." For example, it would be correct to state "a child was *seized* with a fit of laughter" without any connotation of epilepsy. Similarly, the term *convulsion* implies any forceful involuntary contraction of the voluntary muscles. It would, therefore, also be correct to state that "a child coughed *convulsively,*" with no implication of an epileptic mechanism. Epilepsy, however, is a sign of a neurologic disorder characterized by *recurrent* attacks of abnormal brain function (the seizures themselves) arising from abrupt, uncontrolled, repetitive electrical discharges of cortical neurons. Convulsive epileptic seizures (eg, grand mal) display prominent motor signs. Nonconvulsive epileptic seizures (eg, simple petit mal) lack these motor features.

The classification of seizures (Table 97-1) has recently undergone another revision reflecting an increased understanding of the correlation between epileptic clinical and electroencephalogram (EEG) phenomena. The new classification broadly divides all seizures into partial or focal onset (arising from a limited area of cortex of one hemisphere) or generalized onset seizures (arising simultaneously from both cerebral hemispheres).

TABLE 97-1
Revised Classification of Seizures

Partial seizures
Simple: Preserved consciousness   *Complex:* Loss or clouding of consciousness
Simple or complex partial seizures may display motor signs (*eg,* clonic jerking, distorted posture), somatosensory
symptoms (*eg,* simple tingling, warmth), special sensory symptoms (*eg,* simple distortions of smell, taste, vision),
autonomic signs (*eg,* sweating, pallor, piloerection), or psychic symptoms (*eg,* fear, anger, complex hallucinations). Psychic symptoms are far more common with complex partial seizures than with simple partial seizures.

Generalized seizures
Nonconvulsive   *Convulsive*
Typical absence seizure; true petit mal with 3 cps   Tonic (abrupt increase of muscle tone)
  spike wave discharges on EEG   Atonic (abrupt decrease of muscle tone)
Atypical absence seizure: EEG shows "slow" spike   Clonic (repetitive muscle jerking)
  slow wave discharges at 1 to 2 cps: onset and ter- Tonic-clonic (the classic grand mal seizures)
  mination of absence seizure may be gradual rather   Myoclonic (brief, shocklike muscle contractions)
  than abrupt

EEG—electroencephalogram.

Simple partial seizures are focal onset seizures that do not impair consciousness (consciousness implies full awareness of self and the environment and a normal ability to react to external stimuli) but rather manifest as a restricted disturbance in muscle control (eg, isolated twitching of facial muscles), general sensation (eg, warmth or tingling of an extremity), or special sensation (eg, unformed visual hallucinations). Some simple focal seizures may gradually evolve into a complex partial seizure, signified by an altered consciousness. Either may culminate in a grand mal convulsion. Complex partial seizures are focal onset seizures that disturb or impair consciousness. The older terms (temporal lobe, psychomotor, or limbic lobe seizures) have been largely abandoned because partial seizures that disturb consciousness can arise from any lobe of the brain.

Generalized seizures appear simultaneously and symmetrically in both cerebral hemispheres. Consciousness is disturbed immediately, and motor manifestations, if any, are bilateral. The commonly recognized grand mal seizure exemplifies a generalized convulsive seizure composed of a predictable sequence of loss of consciousness, and tonic stiffening of the trunk and limb musculature followed by a series of coarse clonic jerking of the extremities. The familiar petit mal seizure typifies a generalized nonconvulsive seizure producing partial or complete mental arrest or "absence" but lacking forceful muscle contractions.

Clinical observations alone may sometimes be insufficient to correctly discriminate between some of the classified types of seizures, and information gathered from the EEG and other ancillary tests may assist the correct classification of seizures. For example, it is now recognized that automatisms (involuntary, semicoordinated purposeless integrated motor activities that appear during or after the clouded consciousness of a seizure) may accompany petit mal seizures and are not pathognomonic for complex partial seizures. This distinction is more than of academic interest because it provides the basis for selecting the preferred anticonvulsant regimen. Ethosuximide (Zarontin) is highly effective in controlling petit mal absence but has little value in controlling the mental lapses of complex partial seizures. Conversely, carbamazepine (Tegretol) may completely abort attacks of altered consciousness due to complex partial seizures but will not eliminate petit mal attacks.

DATA GATHERING

The initial medical and neurologic examination of the child with suspected seizures seeks to: 1) provide a precisely detailed description of the sequence of events that comprised the attack, including the presence of a warning or aura, loss or preservation of consciousness, presence or absence of unilateral or bilateral motor signs, and postictal signs and symptoms; 2) clarify the medical context in which the seizures arose; 3) define the past and present neurologic health of the patient, including a detailed physical and neurologic examination; and 4) provide specific therapy to remove the cause of the seizures or to treat the seizures themselves with appropriately selected anticonvulsants. The history also should inquire about unusual circumstances of the seizures (*eg,* extreme sleep deprivation) or the possibility of an environmental factor responsible for triggering the attack. The latter might include flickering lights (television, discotheques), reading, tactile stimulation, sound, or musical passages.

The medical and neurologic etiologies of seizures are legion. It is not feasible or desirable to devise a single rigid diagnostic formula that can successfully evaluate all children with seizures. The patient's age, prior medical and neurologic health, type of seizure, and the medical context in which the seizures arose should be thoughtfully integrated to provide a reasonable framework to tailor the patient's evaluation. For example, a thorough toxicology screen is necessary to adequately evaluate the condition of a teenage boy whose first seizure arose during a party. On the other hand, a lumbar puncture is usually performed to fully assess the condition of an ill-appearing infant after the first febrile seizure.

THE ELECTROENCEPHALOGRAM IN EPILEPSY

The EEG remains the most commonly used tool to complement the history and physical examination of patients with suspected epilepsy. The EEG provides unique information to help confirm the diagnosis of epilepsy, classify the type of seizures, assist in discriminating focal onset from generalized seizures, raise the suspicion of an underlying structural central nervous system (CNS) abnormality, suggest the preferred drug treatment, and sometimes formulate a neurologic prognosis.

The EEG cannot substitute for clinical judgment in establishing the diagnosis of epilepsy. A normal interictal EEG does not refute the diagnosis of epilepsy, nor does an "epileptically" abnormal EEG confirm it unless a seizure is clinically recognized. All EEG studies of epileptic patients report a sizable number of patients with normal interictal EEGs. The yield of epileptically abnormal EEGs can be increased by recording the EEG within 1 week of a clinical seizure, obtaining serial tracings, and by enhancing or activating procedures. These activating procedures include recording a portion of the tracing during sleep, prior all-night sleep deprivation, hyperventilation, photic stimulation, and sometimes the use of special recording electrodes such as nasopharyngeal leads. In general, the yield of abnormal EEGs is not materially influenced by the patient's consumption of anticonvulsants except for petit mal epilepsy. The administration of ethosuximide or valproic acid can normalize the EEG in petit mal. Certain historical facts can be ascertained to increase the likelihood of recording an epileptically abnormal EEG. For example, some patients' seizures are clustered in the early morning. Scheduling the tracing for the early morning, therefore, might show an abnormality that may not be present if recorded later in the day.

A small number of healthy, nonepileptic children may display incidental focal or generalized epileptiform abnormalities on their records obtained for evaluating nonepileptic phenomena, such as headaches or learning disabilities. The results of the EEG examination should be carefully correlated with the patient's clinical complaints in all instances. At times, it is necessary to discard the epileptic EEG abnormality as irrelevant to the clinical complaints at hand rather than assuming that epilepsy is the basis for the problem.

Many patients with epilepsy will continue to manifest abnormal EEGs despite good clinical control of their seizures. The often repeated advice of treating the patient rather than the EEG is particularly relevant in this circumstance. Routinely repeating the EEG examination on an arbitrary annual basis contributes little to the patient's neurologic care. It is unnecessary to automatically repeat EEGs at regular intervals if the clinical attacks or seizures are under good control. Repeating the EEG is indicated if there is a poor response to treatment, if a new type of seizure appears, if pseudoepileptic seizures are suspected, and when the physician contemplates discontinuation of treatment after a suitable period of seizure-free existence.

NEURORADIOLOGY FOR THE CHILD WITH EPILEPSY

It is recognized that a variety of structural CNS abnormalities are responsible for provoking seizures in some children with epilepsy. Cerebral hemorrhage, localized infection, contusion, tumor, stroke, calcification, porencephaly, vascular anomalies, and CNS malformations may announce their presence with a focal onset or generalized seizure. The clinician often desires an image of the intracranial contents to exclude a structural cause for epilepsy.

The yield of clinically useful information obtained from routine plain skull radiographic films is surprisingly low in children with chronic epilepsy. Its greatest application presently is to detect linear or depressed skull fractures immediately after head trauma. Computed tomographic (CT) scanning and magnetic resonance imaging (MRI) have largely supplanted the routine skull radiographic film in the evaluation of epilepsy in children.

Several studies have examined the utility of CT scanning in children with epilepsy. The incidence of any CT scan abnormality in children with normal intelligence and neurologic examinations who have generalized seizures is approximately 5%. Children with focal onset seizures have a much higher rate of abnormal CT scans, but most of the findings are nonspecific focal or generalized abnormalities, such as cerebral atrophy, cortical "scars," porencephalic cysts, and other conditions that have no therapeutic import. The yield of therapeutically significant clinical information, such as the demonstration of a resectable tumor or vascular anomaly, is less than 2% in CT scans obtained from children with focal seizures.

One common variety of partial epilepsy does not necessitate routine CT scans: so-called benign focal epilepsy of childhood (rolandic epilepsy, central-temporal epilepsy, sylvian seizures). This inherited form of partial seizures usually begins at 4 or 5 years of age. The clinical seizure may be confined to sleep or may arise diurnally. A witnessed attack is usually heralded by focal twitching of the facial muscles, speech arrest, and salivation and may culminate in a grand mal convulsion. The EEG reveals a characteristic pattern of sharp waves in the central-temporal (sylvian) regions. A family history of similar seizures is present in approximately 30% of cases. This form of epilepsy is considered benign in spite of its focal nature, because it is not associated with any underlying structural CNS abnormality. Furthermore, seizure control is typically achieved easily and the disorder generally remits during later adolescence.

A single CT scan or MRI examination performed during the initial evaluation of the child with epilepsy is generally sufficient in most cases. Repeating the studies annually or on a routine basis is usually not necessary. The appearance of new signs or symptoms, such as headaches or hemiparesis, is a clear indication for repeating a scan, even if the original study was entirely normal. Some low-grade gliomas are not radiologically apparent early in their course, but may appear months or years after the onset of seizures. Children with neurofibromatosis and tuberous sclerosis are especially vulnerable to develop intracranial tumors so a high index of suspicion should be exercised for these individuals.

The introduction of MRI can identify structural abnormalities previously undisclosed by routine CT scans, especially in those with complex partial seizures. The superior resolution of this imaging modality allows small hamartomas, tumors, arteriovenous malformations, and focal scars to be more readily identified. MRI is also useful in detecting mesial temporal sclerosis. However, calcifications may be missed with MRI and are best identified with CT. In some individuals, both CT and MRI examinations will be necessary for the full radiographic evaluation of possible structural abnormalities.

MANAGEMENT

The Single, Unprovoked Seizure

The term *epilepsy* implies the presence of *recurrent seizures*. However, a single, unprovoked seizure may arise as a solitary experience that interrupts the lives of otherwise healthy individuals. The risk of additional seizures and, therefore, epilepsy, following an initial isolated seizure is estimated at between 27% and 43% in adolescents and adults. In young children the risk is higher. Individuals who have suffered a single seizure require the same careful medical and neurologic evaluation as those who have suffered repeated attacks, but neurologists disagree whether all such patients must be treated with anticonvulsants. Many prefer to await the second seizure before embarking on a commitment to chronic use of anticonvulsants.

TABLE 97-2
Simple and Complex Febrile Seizures

CHARACTERISTICS	SIMPLE FEBRILE SEIZURES	COMPLEX FEBRILE SEIZURES
Description of seizure	Generalized tonic, clonic, or tonic-clonic; sometimes atonic (limp)	Focal motor
Duration of seizure	≤15 min	>15 min
Repetition	One seizure within 24 hr	Clusters within 24 hr
Previous health	Normal	Suspected or definite neurologic abnormality
Family history	Negative for epilepsy; may be positive for febrile seizures	Positive for idiopathic or genetic nonfebrile epilepsy
Electroencephalogram	Nonspecific background slowing in the immediate postictal period; usually normal if recorded 7–10 days after the febrile seizure	Frank focal or generalized epileptiform abnormality
Risk for future nonfebrile seizures (epilepsy)	Approximately equal to the general population	≤10%

Febrile Seizures

Approximately 4% of children between the ages of 6 months and 5 years will experience one or more febrile seizures. The clinical characteristics of the seizure, past medical and family histories, physical and neurologic examinations supplemented by the results of the EEG examination will permit most cases to be classified as either simple or complex febrile seizures (Table 97-2).

Children with simple febrile seizures have approximately the same risk of later life (nonfebrile) seizures as their healthy counterparts. This condition is considered an age-dependent CNS response to fever and is distinguished from genuine epilepsy. Although the risk of later nonfebrile seizures is acceptably low, affected children may experience repeated febrile seizures until they have sufficiently matured. The risk of repeated febrile seizures is greatest in infants whose first febrile seizure appeared before 1 year of age. The goal of treatment of simple febrile seizures is, therefore, the prevention of recurrent *febrile* seizures. There is no evidence that treatment reduces the risk of future (nonfebrile) epilepsy. The daily prophylactic administration of phenobarbital to achieve a minimum blood level of 15 µg/mL substantially reduces the risk of recurrent febrile seizures. Phenytoin (Dilantin) is not efficacious as a prophylactic drug. Carbamazepine (Tegretol) is not useful in cases of phenobarbital failure. Divalproex sodium (Depakote®) does protect against recurrences;

however, the risk of serious or fatal adverse side effects in children under 2 years of age precludes its widespread use for this generally benign and self-limited condition. Anticonvulsants usually are administered for at least 2 years and discontinued 1 year after the last febrile seizure.

Children with complicated febrile seizures, preexisting neurologic abnormalities or a family history of idiopathic or genetic nonfebrile seizures face up to a 10% risk of future epilepsy. Prophylactic anticonvulsant treatment is usually prescribed for these children.

Recurrent Nonfebrile Seizures

The goal of treatment of recurrent nonfebrile seizures is the complete elimination of further attacks without exposing the patient to significant systemic, cognitive, or behavioral adverse side effects. The key to the successful management is an accurate initial diagnosis of epilepsy (by carefully considering and excluding nonepileptic events that may mimic true seizures), the identification and removal of the possible cause of the seizures, the correct classification of the type of seizure disorder, and the selection of the appropriate type and dosage of anticonvulsant.

Ideally, the smallest dose of a single anticonvulsant that empirically controls the seizures is the "correct" amount of medication. If low doses of a single drug are unsuccessful, the dosage is gradually increased until seizure control is achieved or dose-related drug side effects appear. When clinical toxicity appears before acceptable seizure control, a second drug is introduced and gradually substituted in place of the initial ineffective drug. After trials of single anticonvulsants have been exhausted, two-drug combinations can be tried.

The selection of the particular anticonvulsant is largely determined by the classified type of seizure. Table 97-3 lists specific anticonvulsants that are considered generally useful for various types of seizures. Maintenance dosages and pharmacokinetic properties are outlined in Table 97-4. For many medications, a lower dose is introduced initially and gradually increased until a maintenance level is achieved.

TABLE 97-3
Anticonvulsants Useful for Different Types of Seizures

Tonic-clonic	Classic petit mal	Atypical petit mal
Carbamazepine	Ethosuximide	Valproate
Divalproex sodium	Divalproex sodium	Clonazepam
Phenytoin	Lamotrigine	Diazepam
Lamotrigine	Clonazepam	Clorazepate
Phenobarbital	Methsuximide	Lamotrigine
Primidone	Trimethadione	Adrenocorticotrophic hormone
Mephenytoin	Acetazolamide	Ketogenic diet
		(Felbamate)
Myoclonic	**Atonic**	**Focal**
Divalproex sodium	Divaiproex sodium	Carbamazepine
Ethosuximide	Clonazepam	Phenytoin
Clonazepam	Ketogenic diet	Gabapentin
Diazepam		Lamotrigine
Clorazepate		Divalproex sodium
Adrenocorticotrophic hormone		Phenobarbital
Primidone		Primidone
Ketogenic diet		Clorazepate
		Methsuximide
		Mephenytoin
		Ethotoin

TABLE 97-4
Dosages, Pharmacokinetics, and Therapeutic Blood Levels of Commonly Prescribed Anticonvulsants

ANTICONVULSANT		APPROXIMATE TOTAL DAILY DOSE (MG/KG [CHILDREN])	DOSAGE INTERVAL (DOSES/DAY)	SERUM ELIMINATION HALF-LIFE (HR)	TIME TO REACH STEADY STATE (DAYS)	THERAPEUTIC BLOOD RANGE	
GENERIC NAME	TRADE NAME						
Phenobarbital	Luminal	3–6	1–2	46–136	14–21	15–40	µg/mL
Phenytoin	Dilantin	3–8	2	10–34	7–8	10–20	µg/mL
Carbamazepine	Tegretol	20–30	3	12–25	3–6	6–12	µg/mL
Primidone	Mysoline	5–20	3	5–16	2–3	5–12	µg/mL
Ethosuximide	Zarontin	20–50	2	20–60	5–11	40–100	µg/mL
Divalproex sodium	Depakote	15–60	3–4	6–15	1–2	50–100	µg/mL
Methsuximide*	Celontin	5–20	1–2	70	15	10–40	µg/mL
Diazepam	Valium	0.1–2.0	3	24–53	5–8	200–600	ng/mL
Clorazepam	Tranxene	0.1–1.0	1–2	48	10	15–40	ng/mL
Clonazepam	Klonopin	0.1–0.35	2–3	18–50	4–9	10–70	ng/mL
Trimethadione	Tridione	20–40	3–4	10	2	20–40	µg/mL

*Methsuximide is rapidly converted to its active metabolite, N-desmethylmethsuximide. Figures reflect the pharmacokinetic properties of this metabolite.

DETERMINATION OF SERUM DRUG LEVELS

Many clinical laboratories offer the clinician direct measurements of serum levels of anticonvulsants that are available for delivery to the nervous system. Therapeutic blood levels of anticonvulsants are usually reported as a range of values. For example, the therapeutic range of phenobarbital is often cited as 15 µg/mL to 40 µg/mL. This range implies that many, but not all, patients will require a minimum blood level of 15 µg/mL to achieve seizure control, and that many, but not all, patients will experience dose-related side effects at blood levels exceeding 40 µg/mL. These therapeutic range values should be regarded as approximate guidelines rather than absolute barriers to be blindly observed. Therefore, it would be allowable to exceed the upper therapeutic range if the patient has experienced a definite, but incomplete, response with a lower dose of medication and remains free from drug-related side effects. Similarly, it would be unwarranted to increase the dose of an anticonvulsant if the patient already experiences side effects despite a blood level that strictly falls within the therapeutic range.

The determination of blood levels of anticonvulsants can only materially benefit the patient if the information is thoughtfully integrated with the entire clinical picture. The routine determination of blood levels without a specific question or goal in mind will probably not benefit the patient. Tables 97-5 and 97-6 outline some practical guidelines to suggest the timing and interpretation of anticonvulsant blood level determinations.

POLYPHARMACY

Some patients with epilepsy do not achieve acceptable seizure control when receiving standard doses of one or two anticonvulsants. It is then tempting for the physician to prescribe a complex regimen of high doses of multiple anticonvulsants in an attempt to completely prevent more seizures. There is little evidence that this

---

TABLE 97-5
Anticonvulsant Serum Levels

TIMING OF SERUM LEVEL DETERMINATIONS
After introducing a new drug and establishing a maintenance dose
After changing the dose of a drug that has been chronically administered
After adding a new medication that affects the metabolism of the first
To adjust the dose in growing children with changing drug requirements
To ensure a maintenance level above the minimum therapeutic range in patients with infrequent seizures in whom treatment response cannot easily be titrated against the administered dose
To determine which of several administered drugs is responsible for clinical toxicity
To adjust the dose in patients with concurrent renal or hepatic disease

---

TABLE 97-6
Anticonvulsant Serum Levels

INTERPRETATION OF SERUM LEVELS	
LOW DRUG LEVELS DESPITE A CORRECTLY PRESCRIBED DOSE	HIGH DRUG LEVELS DESPITE A CORRECLTY PRESCRIBED DOSE
Noncompliance; incorrect dose or wrong drug	Patient accidentally or deliberately taking more than prescribed dose
Determination of blood level before steady-state is achieved (about five elimination half-lives: 5 × half-life)	Reduced metabolism or excretion due to drug interaction
Reduced gastrointestinal absorption	Unique, individual variation in gastrointestinal absorption and/or metabolism
Pregnancy	Hepatic or renal disease
Increased metabolism due to drug interaction	Laboratory error
Increased metabolism due to unique, individual biochemical variations (uncommon)	
Laboratory error	

practice of polypharmacy substantially improves seizure control. Moreover, considerable evidence has suggested that high doses of single or multiple anticonvulsants can produce subtle but measurable disturbances of mental functions including intelligence, mood, perception, short-term memory, attention, concentration, and speed of problem solving.

The effects of anticonvulsants on mental function in children have received abundant attention recently. Most physicians are aware that phenobarbital frequently provokes unwanted behavior (moodiness, hyperactivity, and sleep disturbances) in treated children. However, there is not a similar broad awareness of and sensitivity to the mental side effects of commonly prescribed anticonvulsants. Moreover, the presence of cognitive side effects may not be discernable with the customary clinical observation in the physician's office or via the traditional neurologic examination. Rather, the impairment of cognitive function requires specific, sensitive neuropsychological evaluations.

A few practical conclusions can be drawn on the basis of the investigations presently available: some anticonvulsants expose patients to fewer mental side effects than others. Valproate, phenytoin, and carbamazepine have a more favorable profile of cognitive side effects than agents such as phenobarbital, primidone, and benzodiazepines. For all anticonvulsants, mental side effects are more likely to appear at higher dosages and drug levels than at lower ones. The coadministration of two or more drugs (polytherapy) may have additive mental side effects.

The practice of polypharmacy is often ineffective and may be frankly detrimental to the patient. The clinician must, therefore, carefully weigh the benefits of marginal improvement in seizure control against the risk of impaired mentation due to drug toxicity. For some individuals, total seizure control at the expense of chronic intoxication may be undesirable, and the patient may have to be willing to accept occasional seizures.

MEDICALLY REFRACTORY SEIZURES

Despite the best efforts of the primary care physician, some children's seizures persist with sufficient severity or abundance that they interfere substantially with their intellectual, academic,

personal, and social development. Patients with medically refractory seizures deserve referral to a neurologist who is knowledgeable in epilepsy or to a regional comprehensive epilepsy center. Many programs provide facilities for intensive monitoring of the EEG and anticonvulsant blood levels and expert manipulation of the patients' medications. Patients may enjoy substantial benefits by exposing an incorrect diagnosis or classification of epilepsy, determining the presence of unsuspected pseudoepileptic seizures, or obtaining the safe reduction or elimination of polypharmacy. Some children with intractable epilepsy may be selected as suitable candidates for "seizures surgery." If their habitual focal seizures consistently arise from a single expendable brain region, a sharp reduction or total cessation of seizures can be achieved by excising the offending area. Similarly, children with refractory generalized epilepsy may benefit from surgical transection of the corpus callosum that prevents the free transmission of epileptic discharges between the cerebral hemispheres.

RECTAL ADMINISTRATION OF ANTIEPILEPTIC DRUGS

There are circumstances that arise commonly enough in which the rectal administration of an antiepileptic drug (AED) might be considered and may result in less seizure morbidity and an enhanced quality of life. Hospitalizations and emergency room visits can be reduced if prolonged or recurrent seizures can be reduced by the intermittent use of diazepam. For some children with epilepsy, patterns may emerge with the passage of time in which special circumstances conducive to seizures or status epilepticus are identified. A common observation is the presence of an intercurrent illness, particularly those that produce fever, that frequently precipitates a worsening of seizures. In these cases, the temporary, prophylactic administration of a fast-acting AED such as diazepam can be considered. This drug has the advantage of providing extra protection against seizures when the patient's "seizure threshold" is especially low. Because the administration of diazepam is short-lived, tachyphylaxis is not an issue. It is perfectly acceptable for the child to consume diazepam orally. If the presence of seizures makes oral consumption undesirable or if the child is "NPO" (nothing by mouth) for any reason, diazepam can be given rectally.

When the liquid (injectable) formulation of diazepam is given rectally, it is rapidly absorbed by passive diffusion through the rectal mucosa, and peak blood levels are obtained within 4 to 5 minutes. If seizures do not stop within approximately 15 minutes of administration, a second dose may be given. A typical rectal dose is 0.5 mg/kg, and no more than 20 mg should be given per session. Most children tolerate the rectal administration of diazepam with little consequences except drowsiness. As might be expected, some children experience transient respiratory depression, so this possibility must be managed by informing and educating the family. Rectal diazepam is most effective in the setting of preventing clusters of seizures or status epilepticus.

Many other AEDs can be delivered by the rectal route if necessary due to vomiting or refusal to take the medication orally. Sodium valproate syrup (250 mg/5 mL) can be diluted (1:1 by volume with tap water) and administered as a retention enema. The suspension formulation of carbamazepine and elixir of phenobarbital can be administered rectally as well.

NEW ANTIEPILEPTIC DRUGS

Up until 1993, there had not been a new AED approved by the Food and Drug Administration (FDA) since the introduction of sodium valproate in 1978. At the present time, there are now three novel agents approved but specific indications for pediatric usage are lacking. The issue of AED drug testing and approval for children has received much attention recently, but still the majority of AEDs (and for that matter drugs in general) do not have specific approval for children.

Felbamate

In July 1993, the FDA had approved the general release of felbamate (Felbatol), a meprobamate analog, following clinical testing in the United States. This agent was especially welcome because it demonstrated efficacy in the treatment of the Lennox-Gastaut syndrome, wherein medically refractory seizures are common. As clinical experience accrued, it became apparent that there was an unacceptably high incidence of

serious, sometimes fatal bone marrow depression (aplastic anemia) and acute hepatopathy. As a result, a strong warning has been issued by its manufacturer, but the drug was not withdrawn from production and remains available to those who have responded well to this drug alone. The lesson here is that at the introduction of a new AED, chronic toxicities cannot always be anticipated based on the amount and duration of preclinical testing before FDA approval. Consequently, the physician must always remain alert to the possibility of the patient developing adverse drug reactions.

Lamotrigine

Lamotrigine (Lamictal) is a unique chemical compound that is structurally unrelated to any existing AED. It is believed that it exerts its effects on the CNS by blocking a class of (voltage sensitive) sodium channels, which inhibits the release of the *excitatory* amino acid glutamate from synapses.

Lamotrigine is rapidly absorbed from the gut and results in peak blood levels within approximately 3 hours. It is metabolized in the liver by conjugation with glucuronic acid with a typical half-life of approximately 25 hours. This nominal half-life is shortened considerably by the coadministration of enzyme-inducing AEDs such as carbamazepine, phenytoin, and phenobarbital. Conversely, valproate (a hepatic enzyme inhibitor) substantially prolongs the half-life.

Lamotrigine primarily has been studied as an "add on" or adjunctive treatment of resistant forms of epilepsy such as generalized tonic-clonic seizures, typical and atypical absences, and complex partial seizures. Like all other AEDs, some rare patients report the actual worsening of seizures, especially myoclonic attacks.

The general typical daily target dose of monotherapy is 2 to 10 mg/kg/day divided into two daily doses. Blood levels are not routinely available at the present time, and dosage titration is performed on clinical observations of seizure response and patient tolerance. The target dose of lamotrigine changes if other AEDs are coadministered. Because valproate inhibits its metabolism, the starting dose is much smaller and the increases are more gradual. The most common and potentially serious side effect is skin rash (up to 10% of patients treated with both lamotrigine and valproate). Clinical experience

TABLE 97-7
Schedule for Introducing Lamotrigine

	LAMOTRIGINE MONOTHERAPY (MG/KG/DAY)	LAMOTRIGINE PLUS VALPROATE (MG/KG/DAY)	LAMOTRIGINE PLUS INDUCING ANTIEPILEPTIC DRUGS (MG/KG/DAY)
Weeks 1 & 2	0.5	0.2	2
Weeks 3 & 4	1.0	0.5	5
Maintenance	2–10	1–5	5–15

indicates that this risk is dose dependent and may be reduced by the gradual introduction of lamotrigine at a rate of approximately 0.25 mg/kg/week. The half-life of lamotrigine with valproate can be as high as 44 hours, whereas with enzyme-inducing drugs such as phenobarbital, the half-life falls as low as 7 hours. Table 97-7 summarizes a scheme for introducing lamotrigine as monotherapy or as polytherapy with enzyme-inducing AEDs or valproate.

Lamotrigine is only available as scored tablets (25, 100, 150, and 200 mg), but these can be crushed and mixed with food or beverages.

Gabapentin

Gabapentin (Neurontin) was developed and designed with the specific intention of augmenting the inhibitory influence of its analog, the neurotransmitter GABA. It was FDA approved in December 1993. Curiously, its clinical efficacy as an AED now appears to arise independently of any gabamimetic effects, and its actual mechanism of action is unknown. Based on the results of experiments with animal models of seizures, its spectrum of activity appears broad. Consequently, it is theoretically reasonable to consider its use against a wide assortment of seizure types, although premarketing clinical trials emphasized its use as an add-on for refractory partial seizures.

Gabapentin is rapidly absorbed from the gut after oral administration with peak serum values achieved within 2 to 4 hours. This AED is not metabolized in the body but rather is excreted unchanged in the urine, following first-order kinetics that parallel the patient's creatinine clearance. Gabapentin does not pharmacokinetically interact with other AEDs; consequently, its dosage need not be adjusted during polytherapy. In teenagers and adults, a typical starting dose is

300 mg/day, which can be rapidly titrated upward within a few days to an eventual target dose of 600 to 1800 mg/day. Some individuals tolerate doses ranging from 2400 mg/day to 3600 mg/day. In younger children, the usual target dose is 30 mg/kg/day, administered in divided doses (three or four times a day). The range of daily dosage varies from 20 to 60 mg/kg/day.

Gabapentin is generally well tolerated and has little known toxicity. At the beginning of therapy, transient complaints of excessive drowsiness, headache, or ataxia may be noted.

RESTRICTIONS ON THE CHILD WITH EPILEPSY

Young people with epilepsy must be urged to explore the same activities and aspire to the same goals that challenge all children. They should not be sheltered from the hard work, struggles, discipline, failures, and disappointments that are healthy experiences during normal growth and development. Maturity, performance, independence, and self-confidence will remain dormant if the epileptic child is denied the opportunity to meet a challenge, prove his/her competency, and claim responsibility for both success and failure.

Reasonable limitations are imposed by all parents on their children. Parents of children with epilepsy should be equally expected to exercise their authority and discipline. Either capricious restrictions or overindulgence may harm their children. However, some special restrictions do apply to the child with epilepsy. Water submersion accidents represent a genuine threat to the life of the child with epilepsy. Swimming and boating must be meticulously supervised by an accompanying adult. Scuba diving cannot be sanctioned. Similarly, climbing at high elevations along narrow ledges or bicycling along the edge of a road could prove fatal if a seizure caused the child to lose control.

Society also places restrictions on individuals with epilepsy. Driving privileges are not extended to people with epilepsy unless they have been seizure-free for a predetermined period of time. People with epilepsy may not be inducted into the armed forces, and some employers have public hiring policies excluding individuals with epilepsy. Whether or not these restrictions are fair or necessary, they nevertheless exist.

Part of the clinician's obligation to his/her patients with epilepsy is to advise them regarding these restrictions so that educational and career planning are realistic.

PSYCHOSOCIAL ASPECTS OF EPILEPSY

The majority of children with epilepsy are otherwise intelligent, well-adjusted, healthy individuals. Still it is recognized that educational, behavioral, psychiatric, and socialization disorders are over-represented among the epileptic population. The relative contributions of biologic factors (the epilepsy itself, possible underlying brain injury, AED side effects) and environmental influences vary among individuals. The intrusion of this unwanted, socially embarrassing illness amid the normal turmoil of childhood and adolescence can precipitate unwanted behavior or a frank psychiatric disturbance that can be more disabling than the seizures themselves. In some cases, the anticonvulsant (particularly barbiturates) may incite the untoward behavior, and reduction of dose or substitution with another drug can ameliorate the symptoms. If this simple maneuver fails, the clinician should not resign the child to this unhappy state. Skilled psychological or psychiatric intervention can be and often is effective in helping the child and family cope with this facet of the illness.

BIBLIOGRAPHY

American Academy of Pediatrics Committee on Drugs: Behavioral and cognitive effects of anticonvulsant therapy, *Pediatrics* 76:644–647, 1985.

Camfield CS, Camfield PR, Smith E, Dooley JM: Home use of rectal diazepam to prevent status epilepticus in children with convulsive disorders, *J Child Neurol* 4:125–126, 1989.

Clancy RR: New anticonvulsants in pediatrics: Carbamazepine and valproate, *Curr Prob Pediatr* 17:133–209, 1987.

Commission on Classification and Terminology of the International League Against Epilepsy: Proposal for revised clinical and electroencephalographic classification of epileptic seizures, *Epilepsia,* 22:489–501, 1981.

Dodson WE, Pellock JM, editors: *Pediatric epilepsy: Diagnosis and therapy,* New York, 1993, Demos Publications.

Freeman JM, Vinning PG: Decision making and the child with afebrile seizures, *Pediatr Rev* 13:305–310, 1992.

Graves NM, Kriel RL: Rectal administration of antiepileptic drugs in children, *Pediatr Neurol* 3:321–326, 1987.

Hauser WA, Anderson VE, Lolwensen RB, et al: Seizure recurrence after a first unprovoked seizure, *N Engl J Med* 307:522–528, 1982.

Kriel RL, Cloyd JC, Hadsall RS, et al: Home use of rectal diazepam for cluster and prolonged seizures: Efficacy, adverse reactions, quality of life, and cost analysis, *Pediatr Neurol* 7:13–17, 1991.

McLean MJ: Clinical pharmacokinetics of gabapentin, *Neurology* 44:S17–S22, 1994.

Pedley TA: Differential diagnosis of episodic symptoms, *Epilepsia* 24:S31–S44, 1983.

Schumberger E, Chavez F, Palacios E, et al: Lamotrigine in treatment of 120 children with epilepsy, *Epilepsia* 35:359–367, 1994.

Sheridan PH, Joacobs MP: *The development of antiepileptic drugs for children. Report from the NIH workshop.* Bethesda, 1995, Epilepsy Research (in press).

Shinnar S, Berg AT, Moshe SL, et al: Discontinuing antiepileptic drugs in children with epilepsy: A prospective study, *Ann Neurol* 35:534, 1994.

PART ELEVEN

Ophthalmology

CHAPTER 98

Ophthalmology

III

Richard W. Hertle
Gary Diamond

The primary care physician is an important member of the team concerned with the care of a child's vision. The initial contact and referral, as well as periodic follow-up of the postoperative patient, are usually the role of the primary care physician or pediatrician. This chapter is intended to help the nonophthalmologist to better understand the reasons for and timing of ophthalmologic referrals and postoperative problems of their patients.

In this chapter, the following problems will be discussed: strabismus, cloudy cornea, hemangioma, ptosis, tearing, conjunctivitis and corneal abrasion, cataracts, glaucoma, retinoblastoma, and rhabdomyosarcoma.

STRABISMUS

Strabismus is the condition in which the visual axes of the eyes are nonparallel, *ie,* not directed at the same object. Four percent of the population has some form of the more than 100 different types of strabismus. Comitant strabismus occurs when the deviation of the eyes is the same in all positions of gaze, whereas incomitant strabismus occurs when the deviation between the eyes

changes with changing gaze position. Strabismus appearance also is classified as *esotropia* when the eyes are crossed, *exotropia* when the eyes are divergent, and *hyper/hypotropia* when an eye is up or down. Strabismus is due to either a supranuclear (visual cortex) inability to use the eyes together, which usually results in comitant strabismus, or an infranuclear disorder of the extraocular muscles or their respective cranial nerves, which results in incomitant strabismus. Interruption of visual development in an eye during infancy and childhood (*eg,* retinoblastoma tumor) also can result in strabismus. Most forms of strabismus are comitant and begin either in infancy or early childhood. Adults with strabismus have either decompensated comitant childhood strabismus (approximately two thirds) or acquired incomitant strabismus (approximately one third). Approximately 30% of children with strabismus have family members with strabismus. Inheritance is multifactorial with a parent with strabismus having a 12% to 17% chance of having a child with strabismus (compared with 4% who have no family history). Approximately 50% of children with strabismus under 9 years of age will develop amblyopia (loss of vision) in one eye if the condition is left untreated. Older children and adults develop constant disabling diplopia due to spatial malperception. Longstanding strabismus results in secondary shortening, tightening, and contracture of extraocular muscles, which limits eye excursion and binocular visual fields. Chronic strabismus is disfiguring and results in decreased self-esteem, poor self-image, and aberrant social interaction.

Prompt diagnosis and treatment offers the best results, although no therapy will "cure" most forms of childhood strabismus because we cannot yet reverse the synaptic problem serving binocular function in the visual cortex. Successful treatment includes promoting use of a more primitive cortical form of binocular cooperation. This use prevents amblyopia and is characterized by intermittent recurrence of the deviation due to fatigue and sedation or complete recurrence as an older child or adult.

First medical then surgical treatments are used. All strabismus treatment includes improving vision and then correcting alignment. Spectacle correction of significant refractive errors is accomplished as early as 4 to 6 months of age. Penalization of the preferred eye with patching or cycloplegic drops improves vision due to amblyopia. Spectacles with or without bifocals or optical prism alone may be sufficient in some strabismus types (accommodative esotropia, convergence insufficiency, intermittent exotropia). Topical miotic drops (phospholine iodide) can manipulate accommodation and improve ocular alignment in some forms of esotropia. Visual training "exercises" are somewhat useful, but are limited. Extraocular muscle surgery is performed in an attempt to mechanically move the eyes into a more advantageous position for the brain (within 5°). This result is successful with one operation in 75% to 80% of patients, with 20% to 25% requiring a second procedure. This operation is performed as an outpatient procedure and requires only topical postoperative antibiotics and minimal follow-up or interruption of normal activities. With new techniques, instrumentation, and safe anesthesia, the incidence of complications is rare (less than 1%).

CONGENITAL CLOUDY CORNEA

The cornea of newborns may be transiently hazy immediately after birth, especially in premature infants. Within hours it should have a clear, lustrous appearance such that the irides, pupils, and red reflexes are readily visible. An ophthalmic emergency exists if the cornea remains hazy or becomes cloudy during the neonatal period. In this case immediate ophthalmic consultation is required because this sign may herald serious ophthalmic or systemic disease. Untreated congenital corneal opacification also results in irreversible vision loss due to amblyopia. Common causes of corneal cloudiness include:

- Glaucoma
- Trauma
    Forceps
- Developmental abnormalities
    Sclerocornea
    Dermoid cyst
    Anterior segment dysgenesis (Peters anomaly)
- Inflammation
    Corneal infection
      Herpes virus
      Bacterial ulcer
      Syphilis
    Uveitis
- Mucopolysaccharidoses
    Hurler syndrome

In addition, certain instances of cloudy cornea are associated with heritable disorders of metabolism, such as cystinosis, and may represent the first clue to the diagnosis of a systemic disorder.

CONGENITAL EYELID PTOSIS

Congenital eyelid ptosis manifests as a "droopy" upper lid or lids that are positioned lower on the eye. It is caused by a dysfunction of either the levator palpebrae superioris or Mullers sympathetic tarsal muscle. Congenital ptosis is present from birth and is associated with poor lid movement and poor closure of the eyelid voluntarily and during sleep. Congenital ptosis is often familial and is most commonly due to poor development of the levator muscle of the upper lid, although cranial nerve palsies, tumors, orbital anomalies, and neurodegenerative diseases (eg, myasthenia, botulism) must be ruled out. Depending on the degree of ptosis, the patient may lift his/her chin to use both eyes together. In addition to the obvious cosmetic disturbance, ptosis is often associated with significant astigmatism in the ptotic eye. Amblyopia is common in the ptotic eye due to either image degradation or a refractive difference between the eyes.

Treatment is largely surgical, although spectacles and amblyopia treatment (patching) also may be necessary. Surgery is indicated if significant asymmetry exists or if the lid position is interfering with visual acuity or the superior visual field or contributing to amblyopia. The surgery is performed on an outpatient basis with an initial success rate of 80% to 85%. Complications are rare, although inherently poor lid movement sometimes results in corneal and ocular surface inflammation due to excessive exposure.

PERIOCULAR HEMANGIOMA

Capillary hemangiomas frequently involve the periocular tissues and eyelids. At birth they are clinically insignificant, but they can grow rapidly during the first months of life. Superficial hemangiomas are referred to as *strawberry nevi*. Subcutaneous hemangiomas present as soft, blue masses. These lesions can be extensive and include the orbits, facial structures, and central nervous system. Many of these lesions need ophthalmic treatment due to their propensity to cause amblyopia. This result is usually caused by a combination of image degradation and high unilateral astigmatism in the involved eye. Treatment of these vascular tumors begins most commonly in infancy and involves corticosteroids either orally or by local injection. Periocular hemangiomas regress naturally by 7 to 10 years of age leaving variable combinations of skin abnormalities and structural deformities.

TEARING

The primary care physician should refer a child with tearing at age 3 months because the condition may represent a blocked nasolacrimal system or increased intraocular pressure. The age for referral requires communication with the ophthalmologist because opinions vary. Occasionally, tearing is indicative of structural eyelid abnormalities that cause the lashes to encroach on the cornea. A mass at the medial canthus should prompt immediate referral because it may represent dacryocystitis secondary to obstruction of the nasolacrimal system, or, more rarely, a malignancy.

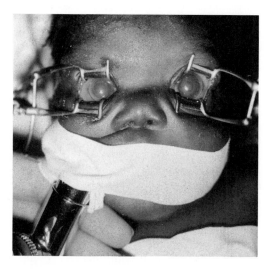

FIG 98-1
A patient with congenital glaucoma prior to surgery. [Courtesy of David Schaffer, MD.]

CONGENITAL CATARACT

The mainstay of modern therapy for congenital cataract is early diagnosis and surgery (Fig. 98-1). If the cataracts are bilateral and complete, it is essential that surgery be performed on both eyes before 3 to 4 months of age. If the cataract is unilateral and the decision is made to operate, the surgery should be performed before 6 to 8 weeks of age, the earlier the better.

The current practice involves outpatient surgery if the child is over 3 months of age or an overnight stay the day of surgery if the child is younger. Using a microscope for visualization, with the patient under general anesthesia, a small incision is made in the eye to remove the lens by a mechanized vitreous cutting device. Some ophthalmologists leave the posterior capsule of the lens and perform a discussion of this capsule at the time of surgery or shortly thereafter; other surgeons remove the posterior capsule and perform an anterior vitrectomy. After discharge, the patient is fitted with an eye patch and plastic shield. Therapy with topical cycloplegic eyedrops, steroid eyedrops, and broad-spectrum antibiotics follows. The patient should have daily outpatient examinations for 1 week and, when possible, be fitted with a contact lens 1 or 2 weeks postoperatively. The ophthalmologist will perform visual acuity examinations and refraction every week or two, depending on the age of the child.

In considering a diagnosis of congenital cataract, the primary care physician should be alerted to the following possible associations:

- Inherited mendelian disorder
  Autosomal dominant
  Autosomal recessive (rare)
  X-borne recessive (rare)
- Associated with chromosomal abnormalities
  Trisomy 21
  Turner syndrome (XO)
  Trisomy 13
  Trisomy 18
- Associated with head and face abnormalities
  Oxycephaly
  Crouzon disease
  Apert syndrome
  Hallermann-Streiff syndrome
  Pierre Robin syndrome
- Associated with skeletal disease
  Conradi syndrome
  Stippled epiphyses
- Associated with central nervous system syndromes
  Sjögren-Larsson syndrome
  Marinesco-Sjögren syndrome
- Associated with renal disease
  Lowe syndrome
  Renal insufficiency and renal dialysis
  Congenital hemolytic icterus
- Associated with metabolic disturbances
  Galactosemia
  Galactokinase deficiency
  Hypocalcemia
  Hypoglycemia
  Diabetes mellitus
  Wilson disease
  Fabry disease
  Refsum syndrome
  Mannosidosis
- Associated with muscular disease
  Myotonic dystrophy
- Associated with embryopathies
  Rubella
  TORCH association (toxoplasmosis, rubella, cytomegalovirus, herpes virus, and syphilis)
- Associated with drug therapy
  Corticosteroid

The primary care physician is in an ideal position to work with the ophthalmologist in the workup of systemic associations of cataracts such as galactosemia, Lowe syndrome, TORCH asso-

ciation, and others. In addition, the primary care practitioner provides valuable support for parents through the period of patching and contact lens manipulation, recognizing that this is a very difficult time for many parents who expected to be bonding with their child in an entirely different manner.

On discharge from the hospital, the physician should be alert for a cloudy cornea (which may indicate a secondary glaucoma), hemorrhage in the eye, or red eye with a discharge. If any of these conditions is noted, the operating ophthalmologist should be contacted immediately.

CONGENITAL GLAUCOMA

The primary care physician should suspect congenital glaucoma in a child with photophobia, tearing and enlarged corneas, a red eye, a cloudy cornea, breaks in the cornea (Haab striae) (Fig. 98-2), and with a positive family history.

As with congenital cataract, the mainstay of therapy demands early diagnosis and early therapy. Present surgical techniques involve creating a channel between the anterior chamber and Schlemm canal by incision of the trabecular meshwork. It is uncertain whether children with congenital glaucoma have an imperforate membrane blocking aqueous outflow or whether faulty attachments of the muscle of the ciliary body are to blame.

Surgery precedes an overnight stay in the hospital if the child is younger than 3 months of age. If the patient is older, the procedure usually is performed on an outpatient basis. A patch and shield are placed on the eye postoperatively; often, a topical steroid and antibiotic eyedrops are prescribed. The ophthalmologist usually examines the child each day for 1 week following surgery, then approximately every 3 months thereafter. Examination under anesthesia will be performed until evaluation of the optic nerve and intraocular pressure can be accurately ascertained with the child awake. It should be noted that in approximately 50% of cases of congenital glaucoma, it is necessary to repeat the surgery.

Because the management of congenital glaucoma in a child is lifelong (a significant percentage of these children will develop secondary glaucoma as teenagers or young adults), the primary care physician's role is crucial in participating with the ophthalmologist in the care of the

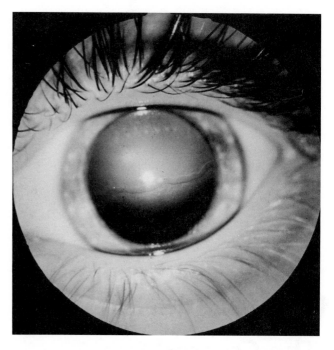

FIG 98-2
Haab striae (breaks in the cornea) in a patient with congenital glaucoma. [Courtesy of David Schaffer, MD.]

patient and providing support to the family. In addition, preoperative control of pressure with osmotic agents or acetazolamide (Diamox) may be necessary. As in the case of congenital cataract, the primary care practitioner is in a position to collaborate on the workup of systemic associations of glaucoma, such as Lowe syndrome, aniridia, Sturge-Weber syndrome, and neurofibromatosis.

The primary care physician should examine the postoperative patient for red eye with discharge, return of presenting signs and symptoms of congenital glaucoma, and increased irritability in the child. If any of these conditions appears, the ophthalmologist should be consulted without delay.

RETINOBLASTOMA AND RHABDOMYOSARCOMA

The two ophthalmic conditions presenting to the primary care practitioner that have potentially life-threatening consequences are retinoblastoma and rhabdomyosarcoma. A patient with a retinoblastoma often presents with leukokoria (white pupil) and should be referred for ophthalmologic examination. Other causes of leukokoria are as follows: congenital cataract, choroidal

coloboma, retinoblastoma, persistent hypertrophic primary vitreous, Norrie syndrome, Coats disease, *Toxocara,* cloudy cornea, retinopathy of prematurity, and toxoplasmosis.

Any child with a poor red reflex or in whom fundus details cannot be examined should be considered to have a retinoblastoma until proved otherwise. The majority of patients present at 5 years of age or less, although there are cases that have been described at later age. Retinoblastoma can present as strabismus in a young child if the visual axis is compromised by tumor.

If this tumor is left untreated it is almost uniformly fatal, but, with modern methods of treatment, the survival rate is over 90%. It occurs in approximately one in 20,000 live births. The tumor arises from primitive retinal cells, thus its clinical presence usually occurs prior to 4 years of age. Retinoblastoma is seen in both hereditary and nonhereditary forms. The genetic basis of retinoblastoma—etiology, inheritance, and pathophysiology—has been a model for the study of other malignancies. Treatment modalities include enucleation (advanced intraocular tumors), radiation, and chemotherapy (for metastatic disease).

Rhabdomyosarcoma is an orbital tumor that presents in older children, commonly between the ages of 6 and 10 years. It is often a rapidly progressive lesion causing proptosis and signals immediate referral. With increasingly effective radiation therapy and chemotherapy available, the prognosis for saving of life is much improved, so timely referral may have a significant effect on outcome.

BIBLIOGRAPHY

Beller R, Hoyt CS, Marg E, et al: Good visual function after neonatal surgery for congenital monocular cataract, *Am J Ophthalmol* 91:559, 1981.

de Luise V, Anderson D: Congenital glaucoma, *Surv Ophthalmol* 28:1, 1983.

Taylor D: *Pediatric ophthalmology,* Cambridge, 1990, Blackwell Scientific Publications.

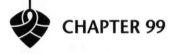

CHAPTER 99

The Crossed Eye

Graham E. Quinn

Strabismus, a general term for describing eyes that are not parallel, is apparent in approximately 2% of children, and twice that number of children may have latent eye muscle imbalances. The recognition of eye muscle problems is often the responsibility of the primary care physician, whereas classification and treatment depends on the ophthalmologist. This chapter will deal with the basic types of strabismus seen in the pediatric age groups and how to screen for these problems in the outpatient office.

If there is a question of strabismus, the primary care physician can examine the child initially in the office to determine if a referral should be made. Depending on the interest and expertise in using the tests described below, the examiner can make an informed judgment concerning the presence or absence of strabismus. Further evaluation and treatment of the condition should be carried out by the ophthalmologist who has the necessary equipment to conduct a full eye examination and the experience in treating these problems in children.

BACKGROUND

Essential to a discussion of strabismus is an assessment of the visual acuity in each eye and the presence or absence of amblyopia. Amblyopia or poorer vision in one eye when compared with that of the fellow eye has many causes, including strabismus, anisometropia (difference in refractive error between the two eyes), and structural ocular abnormalities such as macular scars and cataracts. Because many children aged 2 to 3 years are able to read a simple chart like the HOTV or E-game with a little review and encouragement, it is frequently possible to document vision acuity objectively in this age group. In the examination of the preverbal (or more likely precooperative) child, one may simply have to observe the child's reaction to occlusion with the examiner's thumb or an eye patch to see if there is objection or a marked change in behavior when each eye is covered individually. Be suspicious of ambylopia of the uncovered eye if different behavior is noted with occlusion.

TYPES OF STRABISMUS

Disturbances of fine sensory and motor forces may cause strabismus to be either manifest or latent. The manifest deviation is always present and observable. There is no need for the observer to bring the deviation out with manipulation or by altering the use of two eyes together. Such deviation is called *heterotropia*. The prefix *hetero-* may be deleted in favor of a prefix that has directional value and more accurately describes the deviation, *eg, eso*tropia (in-turning), *exo*tropia (out-turning), or *hyper*tropia (one eye higher).

Phoria, on the other hand, is noted only when fusional mechanisms have been disrupted. This deviation usually remains latent in normal visual functioning, but may cause symptoms of eye fatigue or blurring when the patient "breaks down" from a latent to manifest deviation.

In-turning of the eyes is called *esotropia* if it is constant and *esophoria* if fusion must be broken to demonstrate it. Exotropia and exophoria refer to out-drifting of one eye with respect to the other eye in a similar manner. The prefixes, *hypo-* and *hyper-* refer to one eye being on a different vertical plane from the other; *eg,* left hypertropia means that the vertical alignment of the left eye is higher than that of the right eye.

One last set of terms is necessary to define strabismus accurately: comitant and noncomitant. A deviation is comitant when the amount of the deviation is the same in all directions of gaze. For example, a patient who has sixth nerve palsy cannot have comitant strabismus, because he/she is unable to fully abduct the affected eye and therefore has noncomitant strabismus.

Strabismus may be constant or intermittent, congenital or acquired, and an effort should be made to determine which category the condition fits, because therapy, prognosis, and outcome depend on these variables.

DATA GATHERING

Several basic tests for screening for suspected strabismus are available. In all of these tests, the examiner must be confident that the child is fixating on the target and has useful vision in each eye.

To understand if a patient has "straight" eyes, it is essential to know what the child is focusing on at any given moment. One must use an object of sufficient interest to the child to be able to control where he/she is looking and how much accommodation (or focusing power) the child is using. For this reason, the best circumstance for screening strabismus is to have the child focus on a letter or target some distance away (preferably infinity). Realistically in the young age group, controlling near-fixation with a small puppet or toy that is sufficiently interesting is adequate for most purposes.

The Hirschberg test or corneal light reflex test is done by holding a small light source approximately 33 cm directly in front of the patient. By noting where the light reflex is on each cornea, one may get a rough measurement of the degree of strabismus. The light reflex is normally in mirror-image position from one eye to the other (Fig. 99-1), and each millimeter of horizontal or vertical disparity corresponds to 7° of squint. An in-turned (esotropic) eye usually will have a light reflex that is displaced temporally from the center of the pupil, and the out-turned eye (exotropic) will have a nasally displaced light reflex.

A more accurate way of assessing alignment is the cover-uncover test (Fig. 99-2), which demonstrates the presence or absence of tropia of any type. The child with heterotropia has one eye that is not aligned with the object of interest, and, when one covers the fixating eye, the deviating eye will move to take up fixation. Each eye must be covered in turn because the examiner may not know which is the fixing eye initially.

First, the examiner covers the right eye and observes for a fixation movement in the left eye. Then he/she removes the cover and after a few seconds moves to cover the left eye and observes the right. If no movement occurs, there is no tropia; if movement is noted, the direction of the movement should be noted and the diagnosis of heterotropia made (Fig. 99-2). Outward movement of the eye as it takes up fixation suggests esotropia; inward movement, exotropia; and upward movement, hypotropia.

The alternate cover test demonstrates phorias and tropias. As in the cover-uncover test, each eye must be tested in turn, but here the cover is quickly moved to occlude the other eye. Fusional mechanisms (coordinated binocular function) are thereby disrupted. The examiner covers one eye and then rapidly moves the cover to the other eye. If no movement is noted, then no tropia or phoria has been demonstrated. If movement is

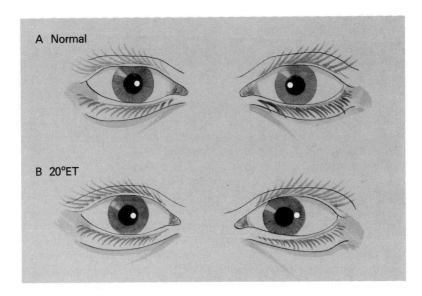

FIG 99-1
Hirschberg or corneal light reflex test. **A,** Normal light reflex. **B,** Light reflex demonstrating 20° esotropia.

noted, then a phoria, tropia, or both have been elicited. Based on the outcome of the cover-uncover test, the examiner knows the presence of tropia and then can interpret the results of the alternate cover test.

The ophthalmologist will quantitate the degree of misalignment by using the same tests while introducing prisms of increasing strength to change the angle of incident light to one eye.

A funduscopic examination is an integral part of any evaluation for strabismus. Cataracts, corneal clouding, and chorioretinal abnormalities from trauma, infection, or congenital malformation, as well as life-threatening conditions such as retinoblastoma and papilledema, may present as strabismus and may be observed first with a careful funduscopic examination by a primary care physician.

MANAGEMENT

Pseudostrabismus

Pseudostrabismus, or false impression of esotropia related to facial configuration of the infant, is sometimes very difficult to distinguish from true esotropia. A broad, flattened bridge of the nose and prominent epicanthal folds can make the most experienced examiner hesitate on examination, and many of these families can be reassured

by demonstration of the Hirschberg corneal light reflex test. When there remains a question, the child should be referred to an ophthalmologist for examination and care.

Esotropia

Esotropia in infants or older children is abnormal. Constant esotropia in early infancy must be differentiated from bilateral sixth nerve palsy or extraocular muscle abnormalities. Once other ocular and systemic pathologic conditions are ruled out, the child may be said to have an infantile esotropia, and unless the child has proper visual alignment prior to 2 years of age, he/she has little chance of ever acquiring binocular capabilities. Because more than one surgical procedure or other therapy may be necessary to align the eyes, the child should be referred as early as possible to allow for properly paced therapy. Most ophthalmologists suggest performing surgery as early as the angle of the strabismus is reproducible and the infant can safely tolerate a surgical procedure, usually at approximately 6 months of age.

Esotropia in the child from 1 to 7 years of age can be quite different in presentation from infantile esotropia and is usually related to a focusing imbalance caused by either farsightedness or abnormal accommodative powers. Regardless of the cause, the fusional mechanisms that allow

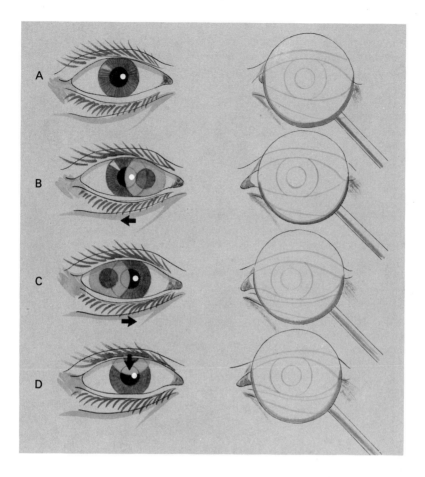

FIG 99-2

Cover-uncover test. **A,** Left eye covered elicits no movement of right eye. **B,** Left eye covered elicits outward movement of right eye, suggesting esotropia. **C,** Left eye covered elicits inward movement of right eye, demonstrating an exotropia. **D,** Left eye covered causes downward motion of the right eye; right hypertropia is present.

the child to keep straight eyes have been overcome, and the child turns the eyes in too much for the object distance. The amount of the in-turning is variable. After referral, the child most likely will receive some sort of antiaccommodative therapy, such as glasses for farsightedness or certain drugs that help control accommodation. The child with esotropia is at significant risk for developing amblyopia. If the isotropia is left untreated, the child usually will develop an unvarying component to the esotropia that does not respond to antiaccommodative therapy.

Exotropia

Exotropia may be constant, latent, or most commonly, intermittent. The intermittent type usually is seen in a child between 1 and 4 years of age and is noticeable when the child is daydreaming, recently ill, or very fatigued. It is most noted at distance fixation at first and can be very difficult to diagnose in the office because obtaining distance fixation in a young child is difficult. Suspect intermittent exotropia when the child constantly closes one eye in sunlight or the parent gives a vague history of poor eye contact and eye muscle problems.

Constant exotropia is relatively uncommon in childhood. In general, the ophthalmologist seeing a child with congenital exotropia will approach the problem in a manner similar to that used for the patient with infantile esotropia. In older children, constant exotropia usually is acquired or a sequel to untreated intermittent exotropia. Treatment belongs in the hands of an ophthalmologist.

Other Types of Strabismus

Vertical deviations often present with an abnormal head posture, and a child with a consistent head tilt or chin position without obvious skeletal or neck muscle abnormalities should be examined for a vertical eye muscle problem. The most common problem is a fourth nerve palsy, which manifests as a head tilt to the opposite side from the affected muscle. Other noncomitant strabismus problems that may present in the office include A and V patterns, oblique muscle problems, muscle palsies, and certain developmental defects such as Duane syndrome and Möbius' syndrome. These problems require a complete ophthalmologic examination for documentation and should be referred for evaluation and treatment.

BIBLIOGRAPHY

Archer SM, Helveston EM: Strabismus and eye movement disorders. In Isenberg SJ, editor: *The eye in infancy,* St. Louis, 1994, Mosby–Year Book.

Ehrlick MI, Reinecke RD, Simons K: Preschool vision screening for amblyopia and strabismus: Programs, methods, guidelines, 1983, *Surv Ophthalmol* 3:145–163, 1983.

Friendly DS: Preschool visual acuity screening tests, *Trans Am Ophthalmol Soc* 76:383–480, 1978.

Ing MR: Early surgical alignment for congenital esotropia, *Ophthalmol* 90:132–135, 1983.

Moody E, Gibson G: Ophthalmic examination of infants and children. In Harley RD, editor: *Pediatric Ophthalmology,* Philadelphia, 1975, WB Saunders.

Parks MM: *Ocular motility and strabismus,* New York, 1975, Harper & Row.

von Norden GK, Maumenee AE: *Atlas of strabismus,* ed 2, St Louis, 1973, CV Mosby.

PART TWELVE

Otolaryngology

CHAPTER 100

Otolaryngology

Ralph F. Wetmore

Frequently, primary care physicians share responsibility for their patient's care with an otolaryngologist. The primary care physician with a better understanding of the management of an otolaryngologic problem is better able to coordinate the patient's overall treatment and communicate more effectively with the patient and his/her family. In this section, the following topics will be discussed: 1) diagnostic evaluation of hearing loss, 2) management of ear ventilation tubes, 3) current indications for tonsillectomy and adenoidectomy, 4) management of a foreign body of the upper aerodigestive tract, and 5) management of a chronic tracheostomy.

DIAGNOSTIC EVALUATION OF THE CHILD WITH HEARING LOSS

The three major categories of hearing loss include 1) conductive, 2) sensorineural, and 3) mixed. An accurate determination of the type of hearing loss has important implications for prognosis and management.

A conductive hearing loss can result when sound is impeded at any point from the external auditory meatus to the footplate of the stapes. This may include a cerumen impaction of the external canal, a perforation of the tympanic membrane, or a disruption of the ossicular chain. Conductive hearing losses are often reversible by medical or surgical therapy.

Damage to the cochlea, the cochlear nerve, or the brain stem may result in sensorineural hearing loss. This type of loss may be secondary to infection, metabolic abnormality, or genetic transmission. With rare exceptions, most cases of sensorineural hearing loss are not reversible. A mixed hearing loss has both conductive and sensorineural components. Each component can be evaluated and treated separately.

An audiogram, including both pure-tone and speech thresholds, remains the keystone in the evaluation of hearing loss (Fig. 100-1). In children, the skill of the audiologist and the age and cooperation of the subject determine the accuracy of the test. Hearing loss greater than 20 dB is abnormal, and the patient should be referred to an otologist for further evaluation.

The evaluation of a child with conductive hearing loss begins with a detailed history, including its duration, previous occurrence, and presence of a recent ear or upper respiratory tract infection. Physical examination of both ears should be made with attention to possible occlusion of the external canal with either cerumen or a foreign body. A tympanic membrane perforation or evidence of infection such as purulent

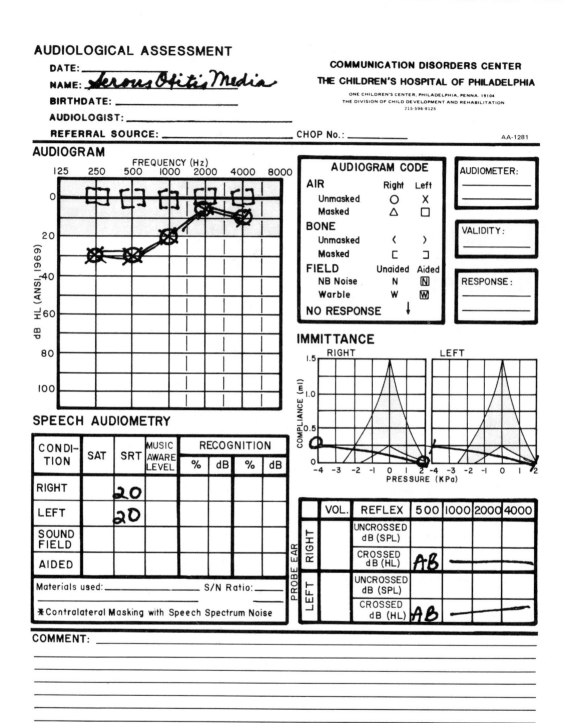

FIG 100-1

Hearing test. Decreased air conduction in 250 to 1500 Hz range. Tympanogram on both sides shows a flat curve, indicating minimal tympanic membrane motility.

drainage also may result in a conductive hearing loss. Assessment of tympanic membrane mobility by pneumatic otoscopy is crucial in the evaluation of a conductive hearing loss. Tuning-fork testing (Weber and Rinne) can be used to confirm a unilateral conductive hearing loss. In the Weber test, the sound produced by the tuning fork will lateralize to the ear with the conductive hearing loss. By demonstrating that bone conduction is louder than air conduction in the Rinne test, one can verify a conductive, as opposed to a sensorineural, hearing loss.

In addition to an audiogram, which should confirm the amount of the conductive hearing loss, additional information can be obtained by impedance audiometry (tympanometry), an additional method of quantitating tympanic membrane mobility (see Fig. 93-1). Normal mobility is indicated by a type A curve, with the peak at O. An A_D curve has an extremely high peak, characteristic of hypermobility of the tympanic membrane. This finding may occur in the presence of an ossicular discontinuity or with a very atrophic tympanic membrane. An A_S curve has a shallow peak, indicative of stiffness of the tympanic membrane. This may be seen in conditions such as otosclerosis or tympanosclerosis. B (or flat) curves demonstrate little or no tympanic membrane mobility, such as seen in otitis media with effusion. C curves peak in the negative-pressure range, indicating varying degrees of eustachian tube dysfunction.

Occasionally, additional confirmation of conductive hearing loss in a young or difficult-to-test child may require brain-stem evoked response audiometry. Brain-stem audiometry does not require subjective responses from a patient to determine the level of auditory acuity. Objective data obtained by this procedure can support routine audiometry.

Evaluation of sensorineural hearing loss also includes a complete medical history with special attention to episodes of meningitis, major neurologic insults, or family history of hearing loss. Otologic examination in most cases of sensorineural hearing loss is normal. Routine audiometry confirms and quantitates the degree of hearing loss. In infants, brain-stem audiometry can supplement behavioral testing. Brain-stem audiometry is also useful in the difficult-to-test or malingering patient. Tympanometry is usually normal in a purely sensorineural hearing loss

although the stapedial reflex may be absent if a substantial loss is present.

Sensorineural hearing losses follow one of several audiometric patterns. With flat losses, all frequencies are affected equally. A sloping high-frequency loss consists of a progressive increase in hearing loss with an increase in testing frequency. The development of high-powered audio and stereo equipment has increased the susceptibility of adolescents to noise-induced hearing loss. Depending on the intensity and duration of exposure, this type of loss may be temporary or permanent. Noise-induced hearing loss produces a characteristic sloping pattern, with the greatest loss at 6000 Hz.

In most children with a sensorineural hearing loss, the etiology cannot be determined. Metabolic abnormalities affecting hearing may be discovered by a series of tests including: complete blood cell count, urinalysis, serologic analysis, serum lipids determination, thyroid function studies, and serum glucose determination. A mastoid radiologic series may pinpoint genetic abnormalities of the cochlea.

MANAGEMENT OF THE CHILD WITH EAR VENTILATION TUBES

The child with tympanostomy tubes need not have any restrictions of activity other than avoidance of water in the ears. Because tympanostomy tubes provide ventilation of the middle ear cavity, children with functioning tubes should have no difficulty adjusting to changes in pressure, such as that experienced on airplane flights.

Because cerumen tends to collect lateral to the tympanic membrane, it rarely blocks the tympanostomy tube. Blockage of tubes occurs when attempts at cleaning force cerumen deeper into the canal and obstruct the tube. Superficial amounts of cerumen may be carefully debrided in most children with a cerumen curet. The pinna can be pulled in a posterior-superior direction, exposing the external meatus. The lateral portion of the canal may then be inspected and cleaned. With large or deep impactions, use of eardrops, such as those normally used for infection in the patient with tubes (eg, Cortisporin Otic Suspension, a polymixin B-neomycin-hydrocortisone suspension), may prove helpful. *Use of hydrogen peroxide drops or irrigation with water should be avoided.*

The participation of children with ventilation tubes in water activities remains controversial. Some otologists recommend complete avoidance of such exposure to water, although most tend to allow such participation if care is taken to prevent infection of the tubes. The use of earplugs or molds provides an excellent method of excluding water from the ear canal. The other option is to place an antibiotic eardrop in the ear canal after exposure to water.

The management of ear drainage in the child with tubes usually includes either oral antibiotics, antibiotic eardrops, or both. Strict avoidance of water exposure should be practiced until the drainage has stopped. Failure of the ear to clear within 2 weeks on such a regimen should signal the need for an otologic referral. On occasion, a tympanostomy tube will become blocked with dried secretions. Antibiotic eardrops may prove useful in such situations to restore patency of the tube.

CURRENT INDICATIONS FOR TONSILLECTOMY AND ADENOIDECTOMY

Although tonsillectomy and adenoidectomy have been widely practiced for more than a century, no definite criteria have ever been established as absolute indications for surgery. Recurrent infection remains one of the major indications for tonsillectomy and adenoidectomy, including recurrent episodes of either tonsillitis, adenoiditis, or adenotonsillitis. Because it may be difficult to obtain cultures prior to beginning antibiotic therapy, documentation of recurrent bacterial infections with positive throat cultures is often lacking. In some patients, cultures remain negative even in the presence of a bacterial infection. Infection deep within the tonsillar crypts is often difficult to culture and completely eradicate with antibiotics. This failure to clear the infection may account for complaints of chronic sore throats in the absence of clinical signs of infection.

Prior to the development of ear ventilation tubes, adenoidectomy or tonsillectomy and adenoidectomy were widely practiced in the treatment of recurrent acute otitis media and otitis media with effusion. Whereas tympanostomy tubes remain the standard surgical treatment for otitis media, several studies have demonstrated the efficacy of adenoidectomy in the management of chronic otitis media with effusion.

Chronic upper airway obstruction provides another major indication for tonsillectomy and adenoidectomy. Obstruction may be due to adenoid, tonsillar, or adenotonsillar hypertrophy. Symptoms of upper airway obstruction are often more prominent during sleep. Loud snoring is indicative of partial obstruction, whereas complete obstruction may result in apnea. Sleep disturbances including abnormal positions and enuresis are not uncommon. Chronic mouth-breathing, hypersomnolence, complaints or dysphagia, and failure to thrive are the major daytime symptoms of chronic airway obstruction. Because many children have minor obstructive problems with large tonsils and adenoids, the point at which these problems become serious enough for surgery is subjective and judgmental. Most patients with severe obstruction have relief after surgery; the majority of patients with mild-to-moderate symptoms improve with no treatment.

Formerly, tonsillectomy was recommended in all patients with peritonsillar abscess, several weeks after the infection cleared. This recommendation was based on a presumed significant recurrence of abscess formation. More recent studies have shown this recurrence rate to be lower than suspected. Tonsillectomy should be considered when peritonsillar abscess fails to respond to aggressive antibiotic therapy or if the patient has a history of recurrent tonsillitis.

In rare situations, significant tonsillar asymmetry or other symptoms suggestive of a tumor within a tonsil are also indications for tonsillectomy. Although some tonsillar asymmetry may be present as a result of infection, sudden enlargement of one tonsil in the absence of infection is highly suggestive of neoplasm. In children, the occurrence of a tonsillar neoplasm is rare.

Occasionally, a child may have large tonsils without symptoms of chronic upper airway obstruction or recurrent infection. In these cases, tonsillectomy is usually not indicated, because the lymphoid tissue will decrease as the child ages.

MANAGEMENT OF FOREIGN BODY IN THE UPPER AERODIGESTIVE TRACT

The child who has aspirated a foreign body that has lodged in the larynx or upper trachea, producing partial airway obstruction, typically presents with dyspnea and stridor. There may or may not be a witness to the aspiration or a history consistent with such an event, eg, choking, gagging, or acute paroxysms of coughing. No attempts to dislodge the foreign body should be made, because this may result in complete obstruction of the airway. If the situation permits, a radiologic evaluation, including lateral neck and chest radiographs, may prove helpful; however, the child should be accompanied by a physician at all times during these studies. At the same time, a referral should be made to a physician skilled in airway management.

If a partial obstruction is converted to a complete obstruction, a potentially fatal situation develops. Management of complete obstruction remains controversial at present; some physicians favor a Heimlich maneuver, whereas others suggest the use of a physical slap to the midportion of the back. During such a critical event, both should probably be used to try to convert a complete obstruction to a partial one.

The child with a foreign body of the lower trachea or bronchus also will have a history of choking, gagging, or coughing. Nuts, raw vegetables, and popcorn are commonly aspirated materials. Physical examination of the chest frequently reveals diminished breath sounds and wheezing over the affected lung areas. A chest radiograph may demonstrate a radiopaque object. The presence of a radiolucent foreign body may be more difficult to confirm. A hyperlucent lung field distal to a radiolucent foreign body may be demonstrated by fluoroscopy, comparison of inspiratory and expiratory radiographs, or failure of the mediastinum to shift on a decubitus film. A child with a suspected upper respiratory tract foreign body should be referred to an endoscopist skilled in its removal.

The child with a foreign body lodged in the esophagus also may present with a history of gagging and choking. There also may be an inability to swallow secretions. An object located high in the esophagus may press on the larynx from a posterior position, causing stridor. Some children may point to the area of the neck in which they feel the sensation of the foreign body; however, this is not a valid indication of where the foreign body is located.

The initial evaluation should include lateral neck and chest radiographs. These tests may confirm the presence of a radiopaque object. Air in the upper esophagus may provide a clue to a radiolucent foreign body in that region. A barium swallow also may help to pinpoint radiolucent objects, but a negative study does not always exclude a foreign body. As with foreign

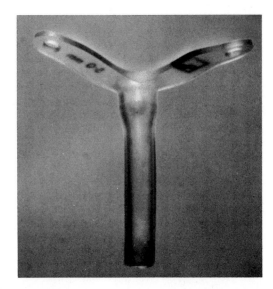

FIG 100-2
A plastic tracheostomy tube.

bodies of the airway, suspicion of an ingested foreign body can only be excluded definitely by an endoscopic evaluation of the esophagus.

MANAGEMENT OF THE CHILD WITH A CHRONIC TRACHEOSTOMY

Although many parents and even some physicians fear caring for the child with a tracheostomy, anxiety may be reduced by good training and adherence to a few basic principles of chronic care.

Although plastic tracheostomy tubes have replaced those made of metal, there are still physicians who favor tubes made of stainless steel or silver. Metal tubes have the advantage of possessing an inner cannula, which can be removed periodically for cleaning without replacing the entire tube. Today, most pediatric tracheostomy tubes in use are made of plastic, which can be either disposed of when soiled or cleaned and resterilized (Fig. 100-2). To prevent stomal infection, tracheitis, or occlusion with secretions, tracheostomy tubes should be changed on a regular basis.

Cloth tapes with foam rubber lining are the best material for securing the tracheostomy tube. In small children who are prone to decannulation, a harness can be fashioned with cloth tapes under the axillae to secure the tube more adequately.

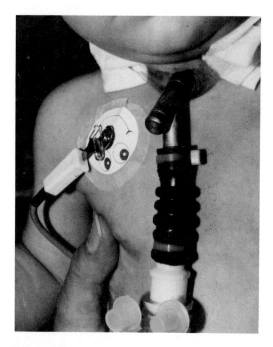

FIG 100-3
Swivel attachment connects tracheostomy tube to humidifier.

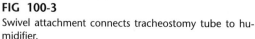

airway occlusion and tracheostomy-related mortality. Most problems with accidental decannulation occur soon after the tracheostomy has been performed, before the stoma has matured. Even in a child with a mature tracheostomy site, decannulation of the tube may result in severe hypoxia or death. To avoid such a calamity, a family member or friend skilled in tracheostomy care, including tube replacement, should always be near a child who has a chronic tracheostomy. Use of a pulse oximeter or cardiorespiratory monitor at night or when the child cannot be closely observed may provide an early warning of airway problems.

Plugging of the tracheostomy tube may occur if secretions are allowed to collect and crust within the tube. Dyspnea and noisy breathing are early signs of occlusion and indicate a need for tube replacement. Routine tracheostomy care, including humidification, suctioning, and periodic changing of the tube, and treatment of infection tend to prevent acute plugging.

Infection of the tracheostomy stoma usually is indicated by erythema and crusting of purulent secretions around the tube. Mild infections can be treated with antibiotic ointment, whereas more serious involvement requires a systemic antibiotic. Because the pathogen is frequently *Staphylococcus aureus,* antibiotic therapy should include coverage for this organism. Skin lacerations caused by the tracheostomy tapes can be managed best with a dressing, to prevent further irritation and to keep the area dry.

Tracheitis, an acute bacterial infection of the trachea, occurs in patients with a chronic tracheostomy. Diagnosis is made by the development of purulent tracheal secretions. Fever and radiographic evidence of infection may or may not be present. A Gram stain of secretions will show the presence of both bacteria and polymorphonuclear leukocytes. A culture of secretions often will indicate a predominant organism. Humidification and appropriate systemic antibiotics are the keystones of management.

Routine tracheostomy care usually consists of daily cleaning of the tracheostomy stoma with either water or half-strength hydrogen peroxide. Soiled tracheostomy strings can be changed as necessary. Suctioning need not be done at regular time intervals, but rather as needed if the patient is having difficulty clearing secretions. Because the tracheostomy bypasses the nose and pharynx, which normally warm and humidify the inspired air, use of a humidifier is recommended to help thin secretions and prevent excessive drying of the tracheal mucosa (Fig. 100-3).

The major problems with a chronic tracheostomy include maintaining the patency of the airway and managing infection. Accidental decannulation and plugging of the tracheostomy tube with secretions are the usual causes of

BIBLIOGRAPHY

Gates GA, Avery CA, Prihoda TJ, et al: Effectiveness of adenoidectomy and tympanostomy tubes in the treatment of chronic otitis media with effusion, *N Engl J Med* 317:1444–1451, 1987.

Gates GA, Avery C, Prihoda TJ, et al: Delayed

onset post-tympanotomy otorrhea, *Otolaryngol Head Neck Surg* 98:111–115, 1988.

Jackson C: Foreign bodies in the air and food passages, *Otolaryngology* 5:1–94, 1983.

Kennedy AH, Johnson WG, Studevant EW: An educational program for families of children with tracheostomies, *Maternal-Child Nurs* 7:42–49, 1982.

Laks Y, Barzilay Z: Foreign body aspiration in childhood, *Pediatr Emerg Care* 4:102–106, 1988.

Line WS, Hawkins DB, Kahlstrom EJ, et al: Tracheostomy in infants and young children: The changing perspective 1970–1985, *Laryngoscope* 96:510–515, 1986.

Luxford WM, Sheehy JL: Myringotomy and ventilation tubes: A report of 1,568 ears, *Laryngoscope* 92:1293–1297, 1982.

Meyerhoff WL: Symposium on hearing loss—The otolaryngologist's responsibility. Medical management of hearing loss, *Laryngoscope* 88:960–973, 1978.

Paradise JL: Tonsillectomy and adenoidectomy. In Bluestone CD, Stool SE, editors: *Pediatric Otolaryngology,* ed 2, Philadelphia, 1990, WB Saunders.

PART THIRTEEN

Respiratory

CHAPTER 101

Asthma and Other Allergic Disorders

Robert Anolik

Asthma, allergic rhinitis/conjunctivitis, and urticaria are among the more common diseases seen in the primary care physician's office. All are a cause of significant morbidity. Recently the mortality rate of asthma has been rising. Among chronic illnesses, asthma is the number one cause of school absenteeism. This chapter presents the more common allergic problems seen by the primary care physician in an attempt to facilitate diagnosis and subsequent treatment.

DIAGNOSIS OF ALLERGY

As is the case in most areas of medicine, a thorough history and complete physical examination are prerequisite to the diagnosis of atopy. Atopic diseases are IgE mediated, resulting in an immediate hypersensitivity reaction. This sensitivity develops in an individual who has a genetic predisposition to IgE antibody formation directed against allergens or antigens. Then there must be repeated exposure to the allergen, resulting in sensitization, with the formation of antigen-specific IgE. Numerous IgE antibodies bind to mast cells. Subsequently, when the individual is exposed again to the allergen, a bridging reaction occurs at the surface of the mast cell and results in the release of various chemical

mediators, such as histamine and leukotrienes. These mediators in turn affect various target organs.

When pursuing a diagnosis of allergy by history, clues should be sought to help differentiate allergic from other causes of the child's problems. One needs to know the kind of illness, its duration, and factors that affect its course. It is particularly important to link clinical symptoms and signs in time with events or exposure to potential allergens. Particular attention should be placed on examining the home and especially the child's bedroom. Exposure outside of the home such as in school, in a babysitter's home, or at a job also may play a significant role. The presence of a familial history of atopy also lends support to the diagnosis of allergy.

A number of features can be found on the physical examination that lend support to the diagnosis of atopy. The examination of the face should include evidence of "allergic shiners" (dark circles below the eyes), eyelid edema, conjunctival injection, and cobblestoning from lymphatic hyperplasia. Examination of the nose should consist of checking for allergic creases on the anterior surface. The interior of the nose can be examined easily in most children by bending the tip of the nose upward with one's finger and illuminating the interior surfaces with an otoscope. In most children it is not necessary to actually insert the otoscope head in the nose. The presence of pale, boggy, enlarged nasal turbinates supports the presence of an allergic diathesis. Associated eustachian tube dysfunction contributes to the production of fluid in the middle ears. In examining the oropharynx, one should look for enlarged tonsils and a cobble-stoned appearance to the posterior pharyngeal wall. The presence of a gaping habitus, high-arched palate, and maxillary overbite (allergic facies) supports the diagnosis of atopy. Examination of the chest should include a check for a barrel-chest deformity due to chronic airway obstruction. During auscultation, one should pay attention to the inspiratory-expiratory ratio. With subtle airway obstruction, there often is a prolonged expiratory phase. The presence of wheezing, rhonchi, or end-expiratory wheezing also should be sought. The skin examination should include a search for eczematoid changes and the presence of dermatographism.

A number of techniques both in vivo and in vitro have been developed to aid in the diagnosis of allergy. An elevated total eosinophil count is helpful but it is not diagnostic of allergy. In addition, many children with severe atopic problems do not have an elevated peripheral eosinophil count. Likewise, the presence of eosinophils in nasal secretions can provide evidence of allergy, but in children the specimens are difficult to obtain and eosinophils are not always found when allergic rhinitis is present. In addition, in the entity, non-allergic rhinitis with eosinophilia, eosinophils are found in the nasal smear even though a link with specific allergens cannot be found. Elevated IgE levels can provide support for the diagnosis of allergy, but other illnesses can elevate the total IgE level. In addition, a child might have a high level of allergen-specific IgE with a normal total serum IgE level.

The major in vitro test for diagnosis of allergy is the radioallergosorbent test (RAST), or modifications of it. The RAST is generally more expensive and less sensitive than properly performed skin tests. In children with severe dermatitis, RAST can offer an advantage. The RAST, unlike skin tests, is not altered by prior use of an antihistamine.

There are two major types of in vivo skin testing. Epicutaneous testing includes the prick, the scratch, and the Multitest methods, in which only the epidermis of the skin is stimulated.

Intradermal testing involves the injection of allergen into the dermis.

Epicutaneous testing can be accomplished either on the back or on the forearm. The back is preferable because it is less accessible to the child and is a more sensitive skin test site. In the prick test, the allergen or antigen is placed on the skin, and the skin is subsequently pricked by a sterile needle. This prick is done so superficially that blood is not drawn. The scratch test is similar but involves abrading the skin after the antigen is applied. The scratch test is less sensitive, and consistency is more difficult to attain. The Multitest technique involves the use of a disposable sterile device that has eight test heads so multiple antigens are applied simultaneously in a uniform fashion. Studies have shown that the sensitivity of this technique correlates well with intradermal testing and the presence of clinical disease. The technique has advantages that include speed of application and consistent application of allergen to the skin.

Intradermal testing involves the use of a more dilute form of allergen in a larger dose. The intradermal technique is more sensitive than the epicutaneous technique, but there is a greater likelihood of false-positive results.

Skin testing should be done with appropriate positive and negative controls. Histamine is normally used as a positive control and the diluent that is used in preparing the testing material is used as a negative control. This helps rule out reactions that might be due to an irritant effect. When scoring skin tests, one is primarily interested in the wheal or the amount of edema that develops. The skin test response can be altered by antihistamines, and therefore the patient should not be given antihistamines for several days before the testing is performed. If nonsedating antihistamines are being used, these drugs must be withheld for a longer period of time. Steroids and all asthma medications presently available do not interfere with the skin test response.

Allergy testing by one of the skin test methods or by RAST is most sensitive and specific for inhalant and stinging insect sensitivities. Food testing materials are not very pure, and false-positive results occur more frequently. Therefore, all positive food test results must be correlated with clinical history and should be confirmed by two or three challenges (unless there is a history of anaphylaxis).

A number of other testing techniques being used have not been proved valid by controlled studies. These tests include the Rinkel skin test titration technique, provocative testing by sublingual and subcutaneous techniques, and leukocytotoxic testing. The American Academy of Allergy and Immunology in a position statement has recommended that these techniques be abandoned until proper studies are done.

ASTHMA

Background
Prevalence figures for asthma are difficult to obtain, but estimates range from 5% to 10% of school-age children. Prior to puberty, asthma in boys outnumbers asthma in girls by a ratio of 2:1. After puberty, this ratio evens out and in adults is actually reversed. This section will emphasize the new understanding of the pathophysiology of asthma and changes in treatment modalities. A comprehensive discussion of emergent treatment, and the treatment of hospitalized patients is beyond the scope of this section.

Pathophysiology
Asthma can be classified in a number of ways with the most recent approach being based on disease severity.

- Mild asthma
    Infrequent short episodes of coughing and/or wheezing
    Good exercise tolerance
    Good school attendance
    Peak expiratory flow rate (PEFR) >80% of predicted
    1-second forced expiratory volume (FEV$_1$) >80% of predicted
- Moderate asthma
    Coughing/wheezing more often than two times per week
      Urgent care required several times per year
    Decreased exercise tolerance
    School attendance affected
    PEFR 60% to 80% of predicted
    FEV$_1$ 60% to 80% of predicted
- Severe asthma
    Daily coughing/wheezing
      Urgent care and hospitalizations necessary

Poor exercise tolerance
Poor school attendance
PEFR <60% of predicted
FEV$_1$ <60% of predicted

Asthma has been characterized by hyperresponsiveness of the airways, due to underlying inflammation, and reversible airway obstruction. A number of pathophysiologic changes have been found in asthma, including smooth muscle contraction, submucosal edema, and increased mucus production. These changes all lead to various degrees of airway obstruction. Most recently, asthma has been viewed as a disease of diffuse airway inflammation characterized by an inflammatory cell infiltrate resulting in mediator release. The early asthmatic reaction or acute phase reaction occurs within minutes or several hours of exposure to a trigger. The late asthmatic reaction or late-phase reaction can occur 6 to 8 hours after exposure to an inciting agent. A late asthmatic reaction can occur whether or not there has been an early asthmatic reaction. Unlike the early-phase reaction, which is quite transient and normally easily reversed, the late-phase reaction tends to persist for a longer period of time and requires anti-inflammatory therapy. Because it does not occur with an obvious temporal relationship to the inciting agent, triggers are often missed.

Management
Drug therapy for asthma should include consideration of the late-phase reaction as well as airway inflammation. Table 101-1 summarizes the actions of a number of asthma medications on the airway.

The goals of asthma therapy should include:

1. Normal exercise tolerance
2. Normal or nearly normal PEFR and FEV$_1$
3. Prevention of daily asthma symptoms and signs
4. Prevention of acute flares
5. Avoidance of medication side effects

Pharmacologic therapy of asthma should be based on asthma severity classification. Treatment can be increased in a stepwise fashion.

- Mild asthma
    Pretreat with β_2-agonist, cromolyn sodium, nedocromil sodium
    Inhaled or oral β_2-agonist prn

TABLE 101-1
Pharmacotherapy of Asthma

DRUG	BRONCHODILATOR	↓ NONSPECIFIC REACTIVITY	BLOCK EARLY–PHASE REACTION	BLOCK LATE–PHASE REACTION
Theophylline	Yes	No	Yes	No
β-agonists	Yes	No	Yes	No
Anticholinergics	Yes	No	Yes	No
Cromolyn sodium	No	Yes	Yes	Yes
Corticosteroids	No	Yes	No	Yes
Nedocromil sodium	No	Yes	Yes	Yes

- Moderate asthma
  Inhaled anti-inflammatory agent(s)
    Cromolyn sodium, nedocromil sodium, corticosteroid
    (Alternate therapy: sustained release theophylline)
  Inhaled β$_2$-agonist
    Prn: short acting only
    Routine therapy: short or long acting
- Severe asthma
  Inhaled anti-inflammatory agent(s)
    Increased doses of inhaled corticosteroids required
  Inhaled β$_2$-agonist
    Routine therapy likely needed
  Sustained release theophylline
    Use as additional therapy, not alternate therapy to anti-inflammatory agent(s)

Theophylline, a methylxanthine, has been available for more than 50 years for the treatment of asthma. It is now viewed as alternative therapy to an anti-inflammatory agent in the child with moderate asthma. Even though controversy exists as to how theophylline acts at cellular and metabolic levels, it induces smooth muscle relaxation and inhibits submucosal edema formation. Concerns have been raised about the effect of theophylline on cognitive behavior and its subsequent effect on school performance.

β-Agonists also have been available for a number of years for the treatment of asthma. They are available in oral (both syrup and tablet), inhaler, and nebulizer forms. The more commonly used β-agonists include albuterol, terbutaline, pirbuterol, and salmeterol. Oral β-agonists have the advantage of ease of administration, but concerns have been raised about drug tolerance with long-term use. Several long-acting oral forms are available. Tolerance is much less likely to occur with an inhaled form. Albuterol, terbutaline, and pirbuterol are short-acting β-agonists that are used for acute relief of asthma symptoms and as pretreatment agents. Salmeterol is a long-acting β-agonist that is used for maintenance asthma therapy. It should *not* be used as a pretreatment agent or as a drug for relief of acute asthma symptoms.

Anticholinergic agents such as ipratromium bromide have been found to have a limited role in the treatment of childhood asthma. They are bronchodilators, but both theophyllines and β-agonists are more potent bronchodilators. Anticholinergic agents are more useful in the treatment of chronic bronchitis and chronic obstructive pulmonary disease.

Cromolyn sodium and nedocromil sodium are nonsteroidal anti-inflammatory agents for first-line drug therapy. Cromolyn is available in several forms including nebulizer solution and metered-dose inhaler. Nedocromil is available only as a metered-dose inhaler. Peak therapeutic benefit for cromolyn usually is apparent within 4 weeks, whereas nedocromil has a faster onset of action. Both medications are very safe but are not as potent anti-inflammatory agents as are the inhaled corticosteroids. Given their well-established safety profiles, however, they may be considered for preferential use in infants and young children.

Corticosteroids are the most potent (approved) anti-inflammatory agents for the treatment of asthma and are appropriate for moderate and severe asthma therapy. All inhaled corticosteroids (beclomethasone, triamcinolone, flunisolide fluticasone) are available as metered-dose inhalers. To decrease oropharyngeal deposition and associated side effects (dysphonia, candidiasis) they should be used with a spacer or holding chamber. In addition, all patients should be instructed to rinse their mouth or brush their teeth. All available inhaled preparations do have some, albeit small, systemic absorption, and therefore the potential exists for side effects, especially in the growing child. The risk of side effects is directly related to the total number of puffs used.

Oral corticosteroids, when administered daily or on alternate days or when given frequently for short periods of time, pose a much greater risk for side effects. Optimal asthma therapy should necessitate infrequent oral steroid use.

Corticosteroid Side Effects
- Growth suppression
- Increase in appetite
- Cushingoid facies
- Acne
- Hirsutism
- Electrolyte abnormalities
- Myopathy
- Cataracts
- Increase in susceptibility to infection
- Peptic ulcers
- Delay in sexual development
- Menstrual changes
- Adrenal suppression
- Mood/behavioral changes
- Hypertension
- Osteoporosis
- Diabetes mellitus

In addition to the pharmacologic treatment of asthma, precipitating and aggravating factors must be considered. Among those factors listed, sinusitis and gastroesophageal reflux are common precipitating triggers. If asthma becomes difficult to control, allergic bronchopulmonary aspergillosis (ABPA) in addition to reflux and sinusitis must be considered.

Asthma Precipitating and Aggravating Factors
- Infections
  - Viral
  - Mycoplasma
- Allergy
  - Inhalants
  - Foods
- Irritants (including tobacco smoke)
- Weather changes
- Emotions
- Sinusitis
- Gastroesophageal reflux
- ABPA
- Aspiration
- Immune compromise

The recognition of subclinical or cough variant asthma is important. Children with low-grade airway inflammation can present with chronic cough without evidence of bronchospasm. Pulmonary function tests at rest sometimes show evidence of airway obstruction, and most children show evidence of airway obstruction after exercise. The cough, often precipitated by crying, laughter, and sports activity, is frequently intense in the early morning hours. If spirometry is not available, measurement of peak expiratory flow rates before and after exercise can be helpful. In children who have been coughing for more than several weeks, a trial with an inhaled β-agonist in combination with an anti-inflammatory agent can be helpful diagnostically.

Sinusitis can result in asthma that appears resistant to normal medical therapy. Suggested mechanisms for this condition include direct soiling of the tracheobronchial tree, heightening of airway hyperirritability, stimulation of irritant or cholinergic receptors, and enhancement of underlying β-adrenergic blockade. Prolonged antibiotic therapy often is needed for control of sinusitis.

Gastroesophageal reflux also can trigger asthma through direct soiling of the tracheobronchial tree if gastric contents are refluxed into the pharynx and subsequently aspirated. A number of studies also suggest that reflux without aspiration that results in esophageal inflammation also can trigger acute and chronic bronchospasm. This event occurs through stimulation of irritant or cholinergic receptors and subsequent reflex bronchospasm and airway inflammation.

As will subsequently be discussed, immunotherapy does play a role in the treatment of asthma in a very specific patient population.

Children with asthma should lead normal lives. They should be able to participate in sports both casually and competitively. Children with asthma should not be routinely restricted from normal activities. In addition, the parents of a child with asthma should not live with the constant fear that wheezing might develop.

The fact that a child wheezes should not be used as an excuse for lack of discipline or school absence.

ALLERGIC RHINITIS/CONJUNCTIVITIS

Background
The terms *hay fever* and *rose fever* are misnomers that describe fall and spring upper airway allergy symptoms, respectively. In temperate zones, fall allergies typically are due to weed sensitivities, and in the spring, seasonal allergies are caused by tree and grass sensitivities. Flowering plants are usually not significant aeroallergens because their pollens are heavy and are spread by insects rather than by air currents.

Data Gathering
Allergic rhinitis/conjunctivitis can be grouped into perennial and seasonal types. It is not uncommon for many children to have both varieties. Perennial allergic rhinitis-conjunctivitis is caused by allergens that are present year-round. The most commonly identified allergens are as follows:

Inhalant Allergens
• Perennial
  House dust mite
  Animal dander and hair
  Mold spores
  Cockroach
  Latex
  Kapok
  Pollens: trees, grasses, weeds (tropics, subtropics)
• Seasonal
  Pollens: trees, grasses, weeds (temperate regions)
  Mold spores (temperate regions)

The pollens, including trees, grasses, and weeds, are the most important seasonal allergens. In temperate zones, molds also can contribute to seasonal difficulties. Pollen counts are usually highest in the morning and can therefore affect the way in which upper airway allergies present.

Common features of allergic rhinitis include allergic shiners (dark circles below the eyes), Dennie's lines (creases below the lower eyelids), gaping habitus or adenoid faces (long drawn-out face with open mouth), allergic salute (upward rubbing of the nose), and allergic creases (transverse lines on the nose). In the examination of the nose, white, pink, or pale blue boggy enlarged nasal turbinates are often seen. Presentations of allergic rhinitis include sneezing, sniffing, throat clearing, nose rubbing, congestion, and clear rhinorrhea. Signs and symptoms of allergic conjunctivitis include eye rubbing, pruritis, edema of the conjunctival tissues, erythema of the conjunctiva and sometimes the sclera, and a pebbly appearance of the conjunctival sac known as cobblestoning.

Vasomotor rhinitis, uncommonly seen in children, is clinically similar to perennial allergic rhinitis. It is caused by irritants such as tobacco fumes, perfumes, deodorants, as well as changes in temperature. Some individuals have allergic rhinitis and vasomotor rhinitis.

Chronic allergic rhinitis/conjunctivitis is not without consequence. Chronic nasal congestion combined with eustachian tube dysfunction can result in serous otitis media and sinusitis. The chronic mouth breathing associated with allergic rhinitis also can result in maxillofacial abnormalities including maxillary overbite and associated malocclusion. Nasal obstruction leading to mouth breathing also can complicate asthma and exercise-induced asthma because the air is not warmed, humidified, or cleaned.

Treatment
A number of treatment modalities are available for allergic rhinitis and allergic conjunctivitis. First and foremost is avoidance of environmental triggers. Efforts should be undertaken to remove the offending allergens from the home. This task is more easily accomplished with horse hair in an old couch than with a dog or a cat that has been with the family for a long period of time. Avoidance of outdoor allergens is more difficult, but the closing of windows and the use of air conditioning during periods of high pollen counts in the spring and fall, and during periods of high mold spore counts during humid weather can be quite helpful.

H_1 antihistamines usually in combination with a decongestant have been the hallmark of treatment for years. Most patients find that oral antihistamines or decongestants will afford them with some relief but usually will not eliminate all symptoms. Several nonsedating antihistamines including loratadine, terfanadine, fexofenadine, cetirizine and astemizole are available. Therefore, side effects can be minimized. In the more severe cases, adequate relief often is not attained.

Antihistamines are most effective when given prior to allergen exposure. If oral antihistamines do not effectively relieve allergic conjunctivitis symptoms, several opthalmic preparations are available.

Antihistamine-decongestant ophthalmic combinations are available by both prescription and over the counter. They provide prompt symptomatic relief. Levocabastine is a new effective antihistamine preparation approved for use in patients over the age of 12 years. Cromolyn sodium and lodoxamide are effective prophylactic agents that decrease mediator release. Ketorolac is a novel nonsteroidal anti-inflammatory agent useful for short-term therapy in individuals over the age of 12 years.

A more potent and effective means of treatment of allergic rhinitis are the topical steroid nasal sprays. They are available both as powders propelled by an inert gas as well as aqueous preparations. Nasal corticosteroids currently available include beclomethasone, triamcinolone, flunisolide, budesonide, and fluticasone. Some have been approved by the Food and Drug Administration for children as young as 6 years of age. Systemic absorption is limited, and the drug undergoes first-pass liver deactivation. Therefore, risk of side effects at the recommended doses is minimal. Peak benefit will usually occur after 3 to 5 days of consistent treatment. The smallest possible dose that alleviates the child's symptoms should be used.

Immunotherapy does play a role in the treatment of allergic rhinitis and allergic conjunctivitis. Studies support the use of desensitization primarily for pollen and dust mite sensitivities. Therefore, children with a strong seasonal pattern in temperate zones or significant dust mite sensitivity who have a perennial pattern are those who would benefit most from this course of treatment.

Long-term studies in children have demonstrated that immunotherapy has an excellent safety profile. In the warmer climates such as the tropics and subtropics, pollen sensitivities occur in all seasons. Treatment decisions, therefore, cannot be based on the presence of a seasonal pattern alone.

Treatment of allergic rhinitis and allergic conjunctivitis should not be trivialized. In addition to the previously described sequelae of nasal obstruction, individuals with significant upper airway allergic reactions do not feel well. Severe congestion can result in mood and behavioral changes and can affect a child's performance in school. School performance also can be affected by the sedative or stimulatory side effects seen with antihistamines and decongestants. Given the wide array of treatment modalities available, children should not have to suffer.

URTICARIA AND ANGIOEDEMA

Background

Urticaria (hives) and angioedema (swelling) are similar lesions caused by mediator release from mast cells. Urticaria is manifest as a wheal and flare reaction of the upper portion of the dermis, whereas angioedema involves changes in the deeper subcutaneous tissues. In the prevention and/or treatment of urticaria and angioedema, an attempt must first be made to classify the type of lesion and determine its cause.

Urticaria and angioedema can be induced by three distinct mechanisms. In an IgE-mediated or true allergic reaction, allergen binds to mast cells inducing a change in the membrane of the cells and mediator release follows. Immune complex reactions such as those seen in acute serum sickness also can induce formation of hives and angioedema. Lastly, mast cells can be induced to release chemical mediators by the direct effect of a number of agents that are not IgE mediated. Examples include foods (strawberries, tomatoes), drugs (opiates, antibiotics), and radiographic dyes.

Data Gathering

Urticaria can be divided into three major categories. The first is acute urticaria in which hives occur transiently. By definition, they cannot last more than 6 weeks. Although in most cases the cause for acute urticaria is not determined, the common known causes include viral illnesses, drugs, and foods.

Chronic urticaria persists for longer than 6 weeks. It is an entity that occurs much more commonly in adolescents and adults than in younger children. Most studies have shown that in more than 80% of the cases, the cause for chronic urticaria remains elusive. Because chronic urticaria can be the first manifestation of an underlying illness such as occult infection, cancer, or collagen vascular disease, these problems should be considered in the assessment of the patient. The first and probably most important part of the evaluation process is a thorough history and complete physical examination. Suggested laboratory tests include complete blood cell count, differential, erythrocyte sedimentation rate, liver function tests, antinuclear antibody, antithyroid antibodies, urinalysis, and urine culture. If these tests are unremarkable, the focus of attention then turns to the treatment of the lesions. In most situations, allergy testing by either an in vivo or in vitro technique will not be helpful.

Physical urticarias are those in which the hives are induced by physical stimuli. The most common manifestation is dermatographism in which stroking of the skin, particularly the back, will induce a wheal and flare reaction. Less commonly, exposure to cold water or cold air will induce hives in an individual with cold urticaria, and, in cholinergic urticaria, heat and/or exercise can precipitate very small pruritic hives. Less commonly seen physical urticarias include solar urticaria, aquagenic urticaria, vibratory angioedema, and delayed pressure urticaria.

Treatment

Acute urticaria should be treated with an H_1 antihistamine such as diphenhydramine or hydroxyzine. In most children, the drug can be used on an as-needed basis. In persistent cases, routine use of the medication until the lesions resolve is often helpful. In refractory cases, the combination of an H_1 antihistamine with an H_2 antihistamine, or a short course of corticosteroids can be used.

Chronic urticaria is somewhat more difficult to treat. Often a single antihistamine is not effective. Treatment options include the use of the above combinations as well as doxepin hydrochloride. Doxepin is a tricyclic antidepressant medication that has been shown to be helpful in refractory cases. Doxepin exerts both H_1 and H_2 antihistamine effects. In most instances, salicylate- and tartrazine-free diets or other dietary changes have not been consistently demonstrated to be beneficial.

The treatment of physical urticaria is determined by the specific type. Dermatographism usually does not warrant treatment. Terfenadine and brompheniramine have both been shown to be effective. Cholinergic urticaria is more difficult to treat, but hydroxyzine has been shown to be the drug of choice. Often high doses are needed, and the dose has to be titrated to the individual patient's need. Cyproheptadine, on the other hand, has been shown to be the most effective antihistamine for the treatment of cold urticaria. Individuals with cold urticaria are at risk for acute anaphylaxis with intense cold exposure such as occurs when jumping into cold water. Pretreatment is necessary and the child or family should be educated so that acute changes in temperature are avoided. Some individuals with cholinergic urticaria also are at risk for systemic anaphylaxis. In these instances, there is an exaggeration of the cholinergic response, which has been termed *exercise-induced anaphylaxis*. Again, caution must be exercised and pretreatment is helpful.

STINGING INSECT ALLERGY

Background

The stinging insects, honeybees, bumblebees, wasps, hornets, yellow jackets, and imported fire ants, tend to invoke fear in patients and physicians alike. Fortunately, true anaphylactic sensitivity to the stinging insects is uncommon. Nonetheless, stinging insect allergy accounts for approximately 75 to 100 deaths in the United States per year.

In most cases of stinging insect anaphylaxis the responsible insect is not identified by history. In addition, some children present with acute anaphylaxis without a history or skin lesion to suggest an insect sting as the triggering factor.

Data Gathering

The order Hymenoptera contains the insects responsible for anaphylaxis. The honeybee and bumblebee are members of the superfamily Apoidea. Despite its impressive size, the bumblebee is a rare cause of insect sting and in turn anaphylactic reaction. Honeybees are also mild-mannered insects but will sting to protect themselves or the hive. The superfamily Vespoidea includes wasps, white-faced and yellow hornets, and yellow jackets, which are much more common causes of anaphylactic reactions. Wasps tend to build their nests in the overhangs of buildings or under other sheltered areas and will sting when they are disturbed. Hornets build dome-shaped nests that hang from trees and shrubs and occasionally from buildings and will also sting when bothered. Yellow jackets build their hives at ground level, usually under logs, branches, or in the ground itself. They are more commonly disturbed, therefore, and are the number one cause of insect sting reactions. Recently, a member of the superfamily Formicidae, the imported fire ant, has been recognized as a cause of anaphylactic reactions due to both its bite and sting. The imported fire ant has been identified primarily in southeastern and south central states.

Reactions to the stinging insects can be classified as follows:

Stinging Insect Reactions
- Local: Erythema and edema at sting site
- Large local: Extensive swelling contiguous with sting site
- Dermal anaphylaxis: Urticaria or angioedema anywhere on body
- Systemic anaphylaxis: Respiratory, gastrointestinal, or vascular compromise

Local reactions occur within minutes or several hours of the insect sting and are characterized by pain, pruritis, swelling, and erythema. Large local reactions are characterized by extensive swelling, but the erythema and edema are always contiguous with the insect sting site. If the sting occurs on the foot and the leg is swollen to the knee this would be classified as a large local reaction. If, on the other hand, the sting occurred on the foot and there was swelling of the face, the reaction would be classified as dermal anaphylaxis. Systemic or anaphylactic reactions can be divided into two categories. The first, as suggested by the previous example, is anaphylaxis involving only the skin. Urticaria or angioedema anywhere on the body following an insect sting would be included in this category. An anaphylactic reaction that results in respiratory compromise, such as laryngeal edema or bronchospasm; gastrointestinal reactions including vomiting, cramps, or diarrhea; or a change in sensorium due to vascular instability needs to be considered separately. Children in this latter category have true life-threatening anaphylactic sensitivity.

Management
Local, large local, and dermal anaphylactic reactions can be managed with antihistamines, especially diphenhydramine, ice to the insect sting site, and if necessary a short course of corticosteroids. Children in all of these categories are not at significant risk for life-threatening reactions with subsequent stings. Despite the ominous appearance of diffuse urticaria and angioedema, subse-

quent sting risks do not warrant insect testing or consideration of immunotherapy in children.

Children who have a history consistent with life-threatening anaphylaxis should undergo venom insect testing as potential candidates for venom immunotherapy. All five insects (six if the child lives in an area endemic for the imported fire ant) need to be tested for, because cross-reactivity does occur. Sensitivity to each insect is tested with a series of prick and intradermal tests. Several companies have marketed kits for this purpose. A child who has a positive skin test reaction to one or more of the stinging insects and a history that correlates with it should receive venom immunotherapy. Venom immunotherapy has been shown to be extremely protective through deliberate and inadvertent sting challenges. The risks for both local and systemic reactions from venom immunotherapy are greater than those with inhalant immunotherapy, and therefore the shots should be given in an office with personnel experienced in administering insect venom and treatment of potential reactions. At present the optimal duration of venom immunotherapy has not been determined; consensus is that it be continued for a minimum of 5 years. If at the end of a 5-year period an individual's skin test reaction has become negative or has decreased, then venom immunotherapy might be discontinued. If there is no decline in skin-test reactivity, immunotherapy should be continued, particularly if the initial anaphylactic episode was very severe.

The imported fire ant causes sensitivity both by biting and stinging. Like other members of the order Hymenoptera, it can cause large local, dermal anaphylactic, and systemic anaphylactic reactions. For children who have had previous life-threatening reactions to the imported fire ant bite or sting, immunotherapy with a whole-body extract has been effective.

Despite the efficacy of venom immunotherapy, the potential for anaphylaxis must still be realized. Children should wear an identification bracelet that indicates their sensitivity. In addition, epinephrine and an H_1 antihistamine should be available at all times.

The treatment of stinging insect allergy also includes avoidance. Children who are allergic to insects should not be allowed outdoors barefoot and should avoid wearing brightly colored clothing as well as scented toilet-ries. Caution should also be exercised in doing yardwork, because this often disturbs the yellow jacket. Many stinging insects are attracted to food, and precautions should be taken in orchards, at picnics, and around trash containers.

ATOPIC DERMATITIS

Background
Atopic dermatitis, an intensely pruritic form of eczema, is often associated with other allergic conditions, especially asthma, allergic rhinitis-conjunctivitis, and urticaria. Even though the pathophysiologic mechanisms involved in atopic dermatitis have not been well defined, most cases are amenable to treatment.

Data Gathering
Atopic dermatitis can be characterized by the age at which it presents and the areas of the skin that are affected. In the infantile type of atopic dermatitis, the rash presents by 4 to 6 months of age and often involves the cheeks. The lesions can spread to other parts of the face, neck, upper trunk, and sometimes onto extensor surfaces. Even though the lesions result in discomfort, especially intense pruritis, many children improve by 2 to 3 years of age. Childhood atopic dermatitis generally presents between 2 and 4 years of age. In contrast to the areas involved in the infantile stage, flexor surfaces are most intensely affected. Unlike the infantile type of atopic dermatitis, this eczema often persists for many years. In the adult phase of atopic dermatitis, flexor surfaces are also involved. In addition, discrete areas such as the neck, wrists, hands, ankles, and feet also might be affected. Investigations that have attempted to define the pathophysiology of atopic dermatitis have found abnormalities of the immune system, cellular biochemical defects, and abnormal skin physiologic responses. Despite these studies, a thorough understanding of the disease process is lacking. Nonetheless, in all children with atopic dermatitis, dry skin, intense pruritis, and a tendency for secondary infection are seen. Studies have shown that 30% to 60% of children with atopic dermatitis have a food allergy, the most common of which is egg. In addition, airborne allergens, such as the dust mite and mold, also can trigger the disease process.

Management
Basic management principles are important to emphasize although details are discussed elsewhere (Chapter 56). Irritants and allergens should be kept away from the skin because they can serve as triggers for the vicious cycle in which irritants (or allergens) stimulate pruritis and subsequent scratching followed by more pruritis. The skin must also be well hydrated by avoiding baths or by applying emollients to the skin immediately after bathing. Soaps, even those with a neutral pH, tend to dry the skin and should be used sparingly. Topical corticosteroid preparations as well as oral corticosteroid preparations play a role in management depending on the severity of the lesions. Any sign of secondary infection should be treated aggressively, because acute flares often will not resolve without systemic antibiotics.

In the more difficult-to-control cases, allergy testing for possible food and/or inhalant sensitivities is appropriate. In some children, skin testing is more problematic than in those without atopic dermatitis, given the hyperirritable state of the skin. In most instances, however, it can be accomplished. If necessary, the RAST can be used as a substitute, although it is not as sensitive.

To date, immunotherapy has not been shown to be effective for atopic dermatitis. In a child with severe respiratory allergies as well as atopic dermatitis, treatment with immunotherapy is reasonable for the former problem. However, immunotherapy as the sole treatment of atopic dermatitis is not appropriate given our present knowledge.

FOOD ALLERGY AND INTOLERANCE

Background
Reactions to foods can be characterized as either immunologic or nonimmunologic. The immunologic reactions are true IgE-mediated phenomena. Nonimmunologic food reactions or food intolerances can be classified as pharmacologic, toxic, metabolic, or idiosyncratic.

Data Gathering
Food allergy is less common than one would expect, given reactions that are coincidental or nonimmune mediated. Food reactions are most likely to occur with early introduction of cow's

milk or solid foods. The most common food allergies are milk, egg, peanut, wheat, and soy. The majority of children allergic to milk, egg, wheat, and soy lose their sensitivity by 2 to 3 years of age. Once a diagnosis of food allergy has been established, the offending allergen should be strictly avoided. Because allergic reactions result from proteins in the food, heating or cooking the food decreases its allergenicity. For example, peanut oil is usually not allergenic in peanut-sensitive individuals. After 2 years of age, it is reasonable to periodically challenge the child with the offending food(s) to see if the sensitivity has dissipated. If a child has a history of an anaphylactic reaction to a food, then challenges should be done in a physician's office where resuscitative equipment is available. It is better that challenges be done in a controlled setting as opposed to a school lunchroom where sandwiches are traded.

The nonimmune reactions or food intolerances are often mistaken for allergic reactions. Pharmacologic reactions are those due to chemicals inherent in the food such as caffeine in cola, theobromine in chocolate, and tyramine in cheese. Toxic reactions are characterized by food-induced release of histamine, or by histamine already present in a contaminated food. In both instances, a true allergic or immediate hypersensitivity reaction does not occur. There is an abnormality in the normal breakdown and processing of a food in metabolic reactions. Examples of this include lactose intolerance and phenylketonuria. Idiosyncratic reactions are unexpected, non–dose-related reactions that occur from very small amounts of the food. Adverse reactions to food dyes and preservatives fall in this category.

Food allergies can result in respiratory, dermatologic, gastrointestinal, occasionally neurologic, and systemic anaphylactic reactions. Claims that occult food allergy are the cause of hyperactivity, developmental delay, enuresis, and seizures are unsubstantiated in controlled, blinded studies.

Management
Most children with food allergy will outgrow their sensitivity by 2 to 3 years of age. Therefore, avoidance of the offending food(s) is the treatment of choice. Foods are classified on the basis of plant families, and cross-reactivity can occur within families. If reactions to a member of a specific family have been severe, caution should

be exercised in eating all foods in that particular family. Clearly, the fewer allergens an infant's immature gastrointestinal tract is exposed to, the less likely the child is to develop food allergy. The introduction of cow's milk should be delayed to 12 months of age, and the introduction of solid food should be delayed to at least 4 to 6 months of age. Breastfeeding should be advocated as a means for preventing food allergy, especially in highly atopic families.

Desensitization (orally, sublingually, or parenterally) plays no legitimate role in the treatment of food allergy. Prophylactic administration of oral ketotifen and cromolyn sodium have been studied. At present, the value of this modality of treatment has not been established.

Most food intolerances can be treated by avoidance of the offending foods and associated agents. Unlike food allergy, however, many of these reactions will persist throughout childhood and into adult years.

ADVERSE REACTIONS TO DRUGS

Background
Adverse reactions to drugs occur commonly in children, but true IgE-mediated allergic reactions are rare. Reactions ascribed to a medication are often a result of the underlying illnesses, because many viruses can cause an exanthem. It is important to be able to differentiate true allergic from nonallergic reactions so that appropriate medications can be administered. Penicillin allergy has been the best studied drug reaction. Given the availability of alternate antibiotics, the need for penicillin testing and desensitization has decreased.

Data Gathering
Drug reactions can be classified as allergic, toxic, intolerance, and idiosyncratic. Toxic reactions are those due to an overdose of the medication and are therefore dose related. The side effects are predictable. Drug intolerances result in predictable side effects, but only a very small dose of the drug is needed to precipitate the reaction, which is the result of an individual's susceptibility to the side effects and is not an allergic reaction. Idiosyncratic reactions are unpredictable, non–dose-related side effects. Again, an IgE-mediated mechanism for this kind of reaction has not been shown. Anaphylactoid reactions

TABLE 101-2
Indications for Immunotherapy

ALLERGENS	DISEASE	PROVED
House dust mite	Allergic rhinitis/conjunctivitis	Yes
	Asthma	Yes
Pollens: trees, grasses, weeds	Allergic rhinitis/conjunctivitis	Yes
	Asthma	Yes
Standardized cat extract	Allergic rhinitis/conjunctivitis	Yes
	Asthma	Yes
Stinging insect venom	Systemic anaphylaxis	Yes
Molds	Allergic rhinitis/conjunctivitis	Controversial
	Asthma	Controversial
Foods	Allergic rhinitis/conjunctivitis	No
	Asthma	No
	Behavioral changes	No

mimic a true allergic reaction without an immediate hypersensitivity reaction occurring. A prototypic reaction in this category is one induced by radiologic contrast material.

Management

Penicillin allergy occurs infrequently in children, although rashes often lead to an inappropriate label. Allergy to penicillin can be confirmed by testing and challenge. Several protocols have been developed for penicillin testing, although the testing material used is not optimal. Desensitization protocols by both the oral and parenteral routes have been well established and can be undertaken in an intensive care unit when necessary.

Reactions to radiologic contrast material occur much more commonly in adults than children. Recent developments in the field of radiology have produced contrast media with fewer side effects. If there is a history of reactions to contrast material, then pretreatment with corticosteroids and diphenhydramine will prevent subsequent reactions in most instances.

Insulin allergy also is more commonly seen in adults than children. With the availability of synthetic human insulin, the incidence of both local and systemic reactions has decreased. Nonetheless, in incidences of true allergy, desensitization can be accomplished with a subcutaneous protocol.

IMMUNOTHERAPY

Immunotherapy, hyposensitization, or desensitization is only part of the total treatment of the child with allergies. Immunotherapy should not be viewed as a substitute for the pharmacologic management of allergies or for allergen avoidance. Immunotherapy has been used since 1911 with various degrees of success. The immunologic mechanisms involved have now been defined, and a true science is evolving. Immunotherapy induces a decrease in clinical sensitivity or tolerance to the allergen for which treatment is being given. This goal is accomplished by a number of mechanisms including an increase in IgG blocking antibody levels, a reduction in white blood cell sensitivity to allergens, and suppression of the seasonal rise in IgE antibody levels.

Controlled studies have shown efficacy for immunotherapy in specific disease states for specific allergens as indicated in Table 101-2. The efficacy of immunotherapy in allergic rhinitis-conjunctivitis has been shown for pollens (trees, grasses, weeds), house dust mites, and recently, a standardized cat dander extract. Immunotherapy also has been shown to have a role in the treatment of asthma that is exacerbated by dust mites, pollens, and cats. Immunotherapy blunts the late-phase reaction as well as the early-phase reaction. Immunotherapy also may play a role in the child with upper respiratory tract allergies as a means of decreasing the child's chance of developing asthma.

Mold immunotherapy in some studies has been shown to have benefit in the treatment of allergic rhinitis-conjunctivitis but not as consistently and not to the degree that has been shown for other allergens. Immunotherapy at the present time does not play a role in the treatment of food allergy, urticaria-angioedema, atopic dermatitis, or vasomotor rhinitis. Immunotherapy has also been shown to be effective in the management of stinging insect allergy.

Immunotherapy or allergy shots should be given deep subcutaneously, preferably over the triceps brachii muscle. The closer the shot is to the muscle, the more local discomfort will be experienced. Small local reactions that resolve within 24 hours are not of concern, and the child's immunotherapy schedule can be followed. Reactions that are large, do not resolve within 24 hours, or induce systemic side effects should not be repeated without consultation with the prescribing physician. Even though the risks of immunotherapy for inhalant sensitivities are small, immunotherapy should always be given with physician supervision and with oxygen, a tourniquet, epinephrine, and diphenhydramine readily available.

Over a period of several months, immunotherapy injections are advanced from initial concentrations diluted to as low as 1:100,000 of the offending allergen to concentrations at maintenance of approximately 1:100 to 1:50. Improvement in the child's symptoms should be seen after the maintenance dose of immunotherapy has been attained. This improvement normally takes a period of several months with injections being given weekly. After the maintenance dose of immunotherapy has been attained, injections can be normally given on a monthly schedule.

Severe reactions to immunotherapy are uncommon. The most commonly experienced reaction is local swelling, erythema, and pruritis. Systemic reactions are infrequently seen. At present, there are no well-documented cases of long-term, adverse effects from immunotherapy in children. Allergy shots are usually given for a 3- to 5-year period and then discontinued. Most children will show prolonged benefit from allergy shots after they are stopped. If within 1 or 2 years of initiation of immunotherapy improvement is not apparent, the treatment should be discontinued and the situation reassessed. Treatment for more than 5 years does not offer any documented advantages.

BIBLIOGRAPHY

Anderson TA, Sogn DD, editors: Adverse reactions to foods, Rockville, MD, American Academy of Allergy and Immunology Committee on Adverse Reactions to Foods and the National Institute of Health and Human Services, NIH Publication No 84–2442, 1984.

Blumenthal MN, Selcow J, Spector S, et al: A multicenter evaluation of the clinical benefits of cromolyn sodium aerosol by metered-dose inhaler in the treatment of asthma, *J Allergy Clin Immunol* 81:681–687, 1988.

Bock SA: A prospective appraisal of complaints of adverse reactions to foods in children during the first 3 years of life, *Pediatrics* 79:683–688, 1987.

Casimir GJA, Duchateau J, Gossant B, et al: Atopic dermatitis: Role of food and house dust mite allergens, *Pediatrics* 92:252–256, 1993.

Eggleston PA: Immunotherapy for asthma: Don't count it out, *J Respir Dis* 9:13–21, 1988.

Furukawa CT, Shapiro GG, Bierman CW, et al: A double blind study comparing the effectiveness of cromolyn sodium and sustained-release theophylline in childhood asthma, *Pediatrics* 74:453–459, 1984.

Larsen GL: The pulmonary late-phase response, *Hosp Pract* 22:155–169, 1987.

Lieberman P: Rhinitis. Allergic and nonallergic, *Hosp Pract* 23:117–145, 1988.

Maguire JF, O'Rourke PR, Colan SD, et al: Cardiotoxicity during treatment of severe childhood asthma, *Pediatrics* 88:1180–1186, 1991.

Marks MB: Physical signs of allergy of the respiratory tract in children, *Ann Allergy* 25:310, 1967.

Matthews KP. Management of urticaria and angioedema, *J Allergy Clin Immunol* 72:1, 1983.

National Institutes of Health: National Heart, Lung, and Blood Institute: Global Initiative for Asthma, Publication No. 95–3659, January 1995.

National Asthma Education Program: National Institutes of Health, National Heart, Lung, and Blood Institute. Guidelines for the diagnosis and management of asthma, Publication No. 91–3042, August 1991.

Ormerod AD, Greaves MW; Physical urticaria and angioedema. In Lichenstein LM, Fauci AS, editors: Current therapy in allergy, immunology, and rheumatology, ed 3, Toronto, 1988, BC Dekker.

Rachelefsky GS, Katz RM, Siegel SC: Chronic sinus disease with associated reactive airway disease in children, *Pediatrics* 73:526–529, 1984.

Rachelefsky GS, Wo J, Adelson MA, et al: Behavior abnormalities and poor school performance due to oral theophylline use, *Pediatrics* 78:1133–1138, 1986.

Rasmussen JE: Recent developments in the management of patient with atopic dermatitis, *J Allergy Clin Immunol* 74:771, 1984.

Reisman RE: Insect sting allergy in children. In Lichenstein LM, Fauci AS, editors: Current therapy in allergy, immunology,and rheumatology, ed 3, Toronto, 1988, BC Dekker.

Scarfone RJ, Fuchs SM, Nager AL, Shane SA: Controlled trial of oral prednisone in the emergency department treatment of children with acute asthma, *Pediatrics* 92:513–518, 1993.

Shapiro G: Childhood asthma, *PIR* 13(11):403, 1992.

Sheffer AL, Rachelefsky GS, editors: Asthma '84: Pharmacologic update, *J Allergy Clin Immunol* 76:249, 1985.

Spitzer WO, Suissa S, Ernst P, et al: The use of β-agonists and the risk of death and near death from asthma, *N Engl J Med* 326:501–506, 1992.

CHAPTER 102

Cystic Fibrosis

Thomas F. Scanlin

Cystic fibrosis (CF), the most common lethal inherited disease in white populations, has an incidence of one in 3300 live births. One in 29 persons is a carrier of the CF gene. CF does occur in blacks, although the incidence is approximately one in 15,300. Most homozygotes for the disease have the "classic triad" of clinical findings: 1) chronic pulmonary disease, 2) malabsorption secondary to pancreatic insufficiency, and 3) elevated concentration of sweat electrolytes. Although there is a great variability in the severity and the clinical course of the disease, the course of CF is generally a chronic progression of the pulmonary disease.

Since the gene responsible for CF was first identified in 1989, there have been more than 500 mutations described in this gene. Prenatal diagnosis in families with known CF mutations is now highly accurate, but positive carrier identi-

fication in individuals without a family history is prohibited by the high number of mutations. The discovery of the gene has raised the hope for a more specific therapy such as gene therapy, but this will require further development before this hope becomes a reality.

Many more patients with CF are now surviving to adulthood; the mean age of survival in the United States is now approximately 30 years. More effective antibiotics, earlier diagnosis, comprehensive care in CF centers, and aggressive treatment of complications contribute to this improved survival. The goal of this chapter is to provide guidelines for the practitioner in the treatment of patients with CF. The discussion of this treatment will necessarily be rather brief; however, the reader is referred to several excellent and comprehensive reviews for further details. The primary care practitioner is also en-

TABLE 102-1
Electrolyte Abnormalities in Two Infants with Cystic Fibrosis*

PATIENT	AGE (MO)	ELECTROLYTES				SERUM pH
		Na	K	Cl	CO$_2$	
1	9	123	2.2	49	48	7.60
2	6	125	2.4	55	41	7.63

*From Scanlin TF: Cystic fibrosis. In Fleisher G, Ludwig S, editors: *Textbook of pediatric emergency medicine,* Baltimore, 1988, Williams & Wilkins. Used with permission.

couraged to form a close working relationship with a CF center and to freely use the CF center for consultation on the management of this complicated chronic disease.

DIAGNOSIS

The diagnosis should be considered in children who present with a variety of acute and chronic problems listed below:

Common Signs and Symptoms of Cystic Fibrosis
- **Neonates**
  Meconium ileus
  Prolonged obstructive jaundice
- **Infants and children**
  Persistent cough
  Recurrent pneumonia, bronchitis, or
    wheezing
  Failure to thrive
  Frequent, bulky stools
  Rectal prolapse
  Intussusception
  Edema, anemia, and hypoprothrombinemia
  Hepatomegaly
  Nasal polyps
  Heat intolerance
  Metabolic alkalosis

Failure to thrive and a history of chronic respiratory or gastrointestinal symptoms is a fairly typical presentation of CF. The respiratory symptoms may vary from a mild but persistent cough to recurrent pneumonia and atelectasis. Expiratory rhonchi and low-pitched wheezes are sometimes found on auscultation of the chest in CF patients. The atypical patient with asthma who has digital clubbing, bronchiectasis, or a cough productive of purulent sputum may also have CF.

Frequent passage of pale, bulky, loose, and excessively foul-smelling stools is characteristic of CF. Patients with this presentation often are misdiagnosed as having chronic diarrhea or milk allergy and are treated with repeated formula changes. Other intestinal problems include rectal prolapse and intussusception or volvulus.

CF should also be considered in cases of dehydration in warm weather, especially if diarrhea alone cannot account for the dehydration or if a metabolic alkalosis occurs. In a typical case, anorexia followed by lethargy are the predominant symptoms. The electrolytes usually show a slight hyponatremia with a profound hypochloremia. Examples of the electrolyte abnormalities that were seen in two infants are shown in Table 102-1.

The cornerstone of the diagnosis of CF is a carefully performed sweat test. The sweat test should be done by the quantitative pilocarpine iontophoresis method. If there is not an accredited CF center nearby where the sweat test can be done, then the patient should be sent to the laboratory that has the most experience with this quantitative method. Sweat tests done by other methods are not reliable because they produce too many false-positive and false-negative results. All siblings of CF patients should have a sweat test performed. First cousins of CF patients should have sweat tests if they have any symptoms that could possibly be due to CF. Genotyping of newly diagnosed patients is useful because it can confirm the diagnosis, facilitate the future use of prenatal diagnosis for the parents, and permit the identification of carriers in the family.

CF is a complex and varied disease, and a number of presentations that are less common than those listed earlier have been described. These presentations are described in the general references and will not be discussed. The symptoms of CF may remain mild for many years, and the diagnosis of CF should not be excluded because "the child looks too good to have CF."

At the time of diagnosis, each patient should have a thorough evaluation to assess the functions of the lungs, pancreas, and liver as well as a careful assessment of nutritional and developmental status. Often this is best accomplished in the hospital setting. Hospitalization also provides a good opportunity to monitor the response of the patient to each component of the therapeutic regimen and to counsel the entire family on the diagnosis, prognosis, and treatment of CF.

APPROACH TO GENERAL MANAGEMENT

Nutrition

The following aspects of nutritional care will be considered: salt replacement, vitamin supplementation, diet, enzymes, and nutritional supplementation.

Because of the defect in the reabsorption of sodium and chloride by the sweat glands in CF, patients with CF are at risk for the development of salt depletion during febrile episodes and periods of warm weather. For these reasons, patients with CF must have a continuous salt replacement program established. Because of recent changes in guidelines and recommendations, many infant formulas and infant foods have less salt than they did a few years ago; therefore, the salt replacement program must be established in infancy. Because infants may need an extra gram of salt each day, this can be done by adding approximately one quarter teaspoon of salt to the infant formula over the course of the day, usually by adding a pinch to each feeding. When vegetables are introduced to this diet they should be salted. Older children are encouraged to salt their food liberally, and salty snacks are encouraged.

As a minimum, patients with CF should take a double or twice daily dose of a standard multivitamin preparation to ensure an adequate absorption and maintenance of adequate levels of vitamins. During the first year of life, infants should receive a supplement of vitamin K, 1.25 mg twice weekly. After the first year of life, supplementation is usually only necessary for patients with known liver involvement or those receiving continuous antibiotics. The need for vitamin K supplementation is guided by prothrombin time

determination. Because many patients with CF have low serum tocopherol levels despite taking multivitamins, vitamin E supplementation is recommended. However, exact requirements and recommended dosages have not been well established. Currently, we give 50 U per day for infants; 100 U per day for children 1 to 2 years of age; and 200 U for children older than 2 years of age.

The concept has emerged that patients with CF need more than 100% of the recommended daily allowance of calories. The older notion that patients with CF all had voracious appetites has not been borne out by clinical experience. Although some centers have recommended severe fat reduction and/or a special elemental diet, our experience is that good growth can be achieved with an adequate intake of a well-balanced diet and enzyme supplementation for those patients in need of pancreatic enzymes. Many infants with CF will do well on a standard cow's milk formula or breast milk if they receive supplementation with pancreatic enzymes. Soybean formulas are generally not recommended for CF patients because of the increased risk for developing hypoproteinemia and anemia. Some infants who have had an episode of severe failure to thrive or who have had meconium ileus and subsequent surgery will require an elemental formula such as Pregestimil for several months at least. All patients with CF will benefit from frequent evaluation for nutritional assessment by an experienced nutritionist. Newly diagnosed patients with CF and their parents should have a complete nutritional assessment and have a nutritional program outlined that will enable them to achieve the necessary caloric intake in a well-balanced diet to ensure adequate growth and nutrition. Ongoing assessment of patients with CF in many specialized centers now includes measurements of resting energy expenditure.

The development of an enteric-coated pancreatic enzyme preparation was a major advance in the therapy of CF. These specially coated preparations have allowed patients with CF to achieve better absorption and to reduce the symptoms and the complications of malabsorption while taking a much lower total amount of pancreatic extract. Although the improvement in enzyme preparations has been a major advance, the push to concentrate enzymes above 20,000 U of lipase per capsule was associated with colonic strictures, and these products have been recalled.

It has been suggested that 2000 U of lipase/kg/meal is the ideal dosage. However, in our experience many patients will require approximately 5000 U of lipase/kg/meal to achieve optimal results. This amount is still less than the excessive doses that were associated with colonic strictures. It is prudent to manage patients on the minimum dosage required to control symptoms and maintain growth. The use of an H_2 blocker (Zantac) may be helpful in this regard. For infants and children who cannot swallow the whole capsule, the microspheres may be given in a small amount of applesauce immediately before or during the meal. Besides being more effective at a lower dose, the newer preparations have eliminated some of the other problems that occur from using the powder preparations, such as irritated mucosal surfaces and respiratory allergy from inhaling the powder preparations. The goal of therapy should be to ensure adequate absorption for growth while reducing bowel symptoms. Fat restriction is only recommended if a patient is required to take an excessively high dose of enzymes and still has bulky stools.

Although the general nutritional program outlined previously works well for most patients with CF, there may be several categories of patients who will have nutritional problems despite such a program, and these patients may require special supplementation measures. One such patient is the infant with meconium ileus who has undergone a resection of a significant portion of the small or large bowel. Intravenous hyperalimentation for several weeks postoperatively has resulted in a good outcome for many of these patients. A special formula such as Pregestimil and a pancreatic enzyme preparation can be introduced slowly while the patient is receiving intravenous hyperalimentation. Patients who have severe failure to thrive prior to diagnosis may require additional supplementation. Some centers have recorded success with either continuous or intermittent nasal gastric tube feedings at night. An advantage to the nasal gastric tube feedings at night is that the patient can continue to eat regular meals during the day and use a formula such as Vivonex, which does not require enzyme supplementation. Some older patients with moderately severe lung disease also reach a point at which there is either no weight gain or weight loss over a period of many months, despite what appears to be adequate nutritional therapy. If there is no response, even

after treating the pulmonary disease, aggressive nutritional supplementation either by gastrostomy or by nasal gastric tube feedings may be of benefit to these patients.

Pulmonary Therapy and Antibiotics

Most patients with CF have some degree of small airway abnormality, although the degree of severity of the small airway disease may vary greatly from patient to patient. Two factors, mucus viscosity and infection, are most important. The respiratory tract mucus in CF is more viscous because of abnormal physiochemical properties, and this mucus is responsible for the airway obstruction, whether it is complete or partial, focal or diffuse. This thickened mucus results in either hyperinflation or atelectasis of lung segments distal to either a partial or a complete obstruction of the airway (Fig. 102-1). Chronic recurrent pulmonary infection also contributes to airway disease. The respiratory tract in CF is commonly colonized with bacterial pathogens. Early in the course of the disease *Staphylococcus aureus* and later *Pseudomonas aeruginosa* are the most characteristic organisms in CF, but other gram-negative bacteria also may be found, such as *Klebsiella, Haemophilus influenzae,* and *Escherichia coli.* The combination of obstruction with thickened mucus and colonization and infection with bacterial pathogens produces a gradual destruction of airways resulting in both diffuse and focal bronchiectasis.

Therapy for the lung disease in CF is designed to clear the obstructing mucus from the airways and to treat the bacterial infection. An important part of the therapy of CF is chest physiotherapy or percussion and postural drainage, which is aimed at clearing these thickened mucus secretions from the lungs. Although adequate controlled studies to determine the optimum regimen of physiotherapy for either prophylaxis or therapy have not been done, most CF centers use physiotherapy as the cornerstone of their pulmonary therapy, and good documentation exists in a controlled crossover study that there is a decrease in pulmonary function when regular, twice-daily chest physiotherapy is discontinued. This decline is reversed when regular chest physiotherapy is resumed. If it is to be effective, it is important that the parents, caregivers, or other family members are carefully trained in the technique and that they administer it conscientiously and thoroughly. We generally recommend that

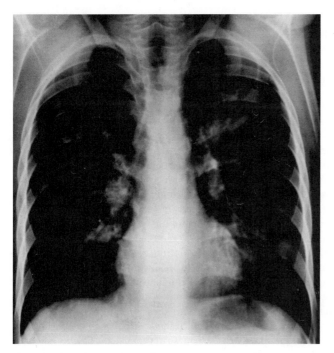

FIG 102-1

Chest radiograph of patient with cystic fibrosis demonstrating hyperaeration, increased bronchial markings and nodular cystic densities.

most patients who are diagnosed as having CF begin a twice-daily chest physiotherapy treatment in early morning and evening. During exacerbations of pulmonary symptoms we usually recommend that an additional treatment be given each day, and often for exacerbations we recommend that an intermittent aerosol be used prior to the percussion and postural drainage, although these are not generally prescribed for regular use. Chest physiotherapy is a difficult and time-consuming treatment. Periodic assessment of technique is helpful because the therapy needs to be modified as the patient grows. Because parents and patients often have difficulty complying with this therapy, the review of procedures serves to reinforce and support the parents in administering this home therapy.

Many CF centers now use an intermittent aerosol therapy as part of their therapy for the pulmonary disease in CF. Whereas some of the intermittent aerosol therapy seems to provide a clear benefit for many patients, controlled studies to provide exact guidelines as to which agent should be used and whether the treatment should be prophylactic or therapeutic, continuous or intermittent, are not available. Although it was a common practice two decades ago, almost no CF centers now prescribe nocturnal mist tent therapy for their CF patients. We recommend that a dilute 5% solution of *N*-acetylcysteine be given by nebulizer prior to percussion and postural drainage in those patients who have copious, thickened pulmonary secretions or only during periods of exacerbation of pulmonary symptoms. Most cases of bronchial irritation occur when a 20% solution is used. We have found very few side effects and reasonable efficacy using a 10% solution diluted 1:1 in saline solution, resulting in a 5% solution. Although many centers routinely use bronchodilators for patients with CF, some patients with CF do not need bronchodilators and some may even have adverse reactions to them. We therefore evaluate the need for bronchodilators on an individual basis, and patients who have reversible bronchospasm are treated with either oral or inhaled bronchodilators using guidelines that are established for the therapy of asthma.

The newest mucolytic agent available is α-dornase (Pulmozyme®). A large multicenter trial demonstrated a 5% improvement in FEV_1 after 6 months of treatment, whereas control groups showed no improvement. The drug has not been tested in patients under 5 years of age. Some patients have a clear and dramatic benefit from the drug, whereas others do not. Our practice is to give a trial of Pulmozyme 2.5 mL inhaled once each morning to patients over 6 years of age who have mild to moderate pulmonary function abnormality and/or significant sputum production. The patients are reevaluated after 1 and 6 months to decide on continued use. Hopefully future studies will clarify the optimal use of this new agent and will determine if there is a role for other dosing strategies or intermittent use of this expensive drug.

Corticosteroids have been used with good results in infants with severe obstructive airway disease that does not respond to antibiotics and bronchodilators and in patients with CF in whom the pulmonary disease is complicated by either severe asthma or allergic bronchopulmonary aspergillosis. Preliminary observations suggested that patients with CF may benefit from the long-term administration of corticosteroids on alternate days. The presumed effect of the corticosteroids is decreased inflammatory response of the airways. However, this treatment regimen was evaluated in a multicenter trial, and it has not been recommended for general use in CF. However, there is a subgroup of patients with CF who may benefit from judicious use of steroids for limited time periods and with close monitoring.

Recently, more attention has been given to the negative impact that chronic airways inflammation has on the course of CF. A controlled study of a small group of patients with CF demonstrated a beneficial effect of 4 years of treatment with a high dose of ibuprofen. However, as in the steroid study, a large multicenter trial should help to clarify the role of this agent in CF. These two studies, taken together, provide hope that the future may bring the development of a selective agent that will control the pulmonary inflammation in CF without having significant side effects.

The development of newer and more effective antibiotics has resulted in a marked improvement in survival of patients with CF and a decrease in pulmonary morbidity. However, once again, controlled studies on the most effective antibiotic regimens, whether continuous or intermittent, have not been established. Our general approach is to treat with antibiotics during exacerbations of pulmonary symptoms, that is, when patients show an increased cough or an increased amount of purulent sputum, when there are new or increased rales on chest auscultation, or when respiratory rate and effort increase. The decision of which antibiotic to use is guided by the results of sputum culture.

Even in young infants, some useful information can be obtained by culture of sputum obtained by a cough swab. In patients who have *S. aureus* colonization and in whom symptoms are not too severe, treatment with an oral antistaphylococcal penicillin and an increase in the chest physiotherapy and intermittent aerosol use at home are usually adequate to treat an exacerbation. Cephalosporins are useful antibiotics for both *Staphylococcus* organisms and some of the gram-negative organisms. Trimethoprim-sulfamethoxazole combination is used if *H. influenzae* is cultured or in combination with cephalosporin (Keflex) if *Staphylococcus* plus a gram-negative organism is present.

The choices are more difficult when *P. aeruginosa* or other species are cultured in the sputum and the patient is having increased symptoms. There are only a few effective oral antibiotics for *Pseudomonas.* For some patients, chloramphenicol may be useful as some percentage of the *Pseudomonas* strains are sensitive to it, and often there is a good clinical response in spite of a lack of *in vitro* sensitivity. Many centers will use trimethoprim/sulfamethoxazole for long-term or suppressive therapy in patients who have *Pseudomonas* in their sputum.

The past few years have seen the introduction of ciprofloxacin, an oral quinolone, that is effective against many strains of *Pseudomonas.* The drug has been very useful in treatment of CF. However, resistance develops relatively quickly after repeated or prolonged courses of treatment. However, patients who are showing an increase in symptoms who are not responsive to oral antibiotics and who are culture-positive for *Pseudomonas* will probably have to be treated with intravenous antibiotics. The preferred regimen is a combination of an aminoglycoside and a semisynthetic penicillin such as tobramycin and ticarcillin given for 14 days. Longer courses of antibiotics (*ie,* 2 to 4 weeks in duration) are occasionally necessary for the patient with CF with severe pulmonary involvement.

The decisions regarding the initiation and duration of intravenous antibiotic therapy are often best guided by pulmonary function testing when serial data on pulmonary performance can be used to document deterioration and improvement in pulmonary function. There have been several limited reports on the benefits of inhaled gentamicin. We use this agent when a patient begins a pattern of requiring admission every few months. Gentamicin 2 to 4 mL of a 40 mg/mL solution inhaled twice daily after chest physiotherapy often will stabilize a patient for a prolonged period after admission.

High-dose inhaled tobramycin given in doses of 600 mg of preservative-free tobramycin in 30 mL of solution four times daily has been shown to have a beneficial effect on pulmonary function. The determination of the precise role of this treatment in the CF regimen and the optimal dose for therapeutic effect will require further study.

Recent reports from several large centers have indicated an increasing incidence and prevalence of infections with *Pseudomonas cepacia* in patients with CF. Most of these organisms are highly resistant. This increase has led to the development of cohorting strategies in most CF centers to prevent prolonged contacts between patients with CF who are colonized with these resistant organisms and those who are not. Synergy studies often will provide useful information for selecting a combination and dose of antibiotics that will be effective against even these multiresistant organisms.

Psychosocial Support

Skilled psychosocial support for the patients and families of those affected by this chronic and ultimately fatal disease is required. Psychosocial support should be started while the diagnosis of CF is being made and should continue throughout the course of the patient's lifetime. At the time of diagnosis, the facts concerning CF should be explained thoroughly to the patient and parents of the newly diagnosed patient. These conferences are best conducted in several long sessions separated by an interval of several days so that the patients and family have time to ask questions concerning what they have previously been told and to clarify any misconceptions they may have. This sequence also provides an initial opportunity for the physician and social worker to assess how the family is beginning to cope with the diagnosis of CF. As soon as the diagnosis of CF is confirmed, it is important that the family be educated in the details, techniques, and rationale of the care regimen for CF. This is best accomplished in individual sessions with skilled health care professionals from medicine, nursing, physical therapy, nutrition, and respiratory therapy departments. Although the seriousness

of the diagnosis of CF cannot be ignored in these educational sessions, it is important to emphasize that the average survival of patients with CF has improved dramatically over the past two to three decades because of the effective care regimen that has been developed during this time. The combination of a thorough educational program along with the facts concerning the improved survival of patients with CF and the ever more realistic hope that basic research may provide better answers for patients with CF provide the patient and the family with a realistically optimistic attitude and a positive approach to living with CF. The identification of the CF gene in 1989, the subsequent increased understanding of the role of the gene product in the pathogenesis of CF, and the initiation of phase I gene therapy trials in patients with CF all provide a more realistic foundation for instilling a sense of optimism in patients, parents, and other family members.

We encourage all patients and families to provide a conscientious home care regimen for the patient with CF but to otherwise encourage the child to live an unrestricted and active life. We encourage the parents to plan for their child to participate in all the activities of his/her peers. A skilled and experienced team of CF care providers can help the family and provide support by anticipating some of the common problems that CF may create as the child progresses through normal developmental stages and moves through the different stages of the educational process. The patient and the family should be given guidance and assistance in answering questions and explaining the diagnosis of CF to friends and family. We recommend that all the relatives be informed of the diagnosis of CF because of its autosomal recessive pattern of inheritance. And we encourage patients and family members to inform close friends and those who need to know, such as teachers and school nurses, of the diagnosis of CF. They should also be informed that the patient is being cared for regularly in a CF center and that, other than providing the opportunity to take the prescribed medications and treatments, no preferential treatment need be given to the child.

During periods of exacerbations of the disease, patients and parents often become anxious and depressed. It is important to provide a skilled assessment of the patient and family as the disease progresses, and should serious emotional or psychiatric symptoms develop, an appropriate referral should be made for psychiatric care. However, by providing support during periods of exacerbation, a physician, social worker, and experienced CF health care professionals usually can provide the necessary support. Often, when the condition of the patient improves in response to medical therapy, the anxiousness and depression abate considerably, and psychiatric intervention will not be required.

As long as is reasonably possible, we encourage patients and families to set goals and work with the medical team to achieve them. However, when it becomes evident that the patient's pulmonary insufficiency is increasing despite an aggressive medical regimen, the patient and family should be prepared for impending death. The possibility of a fatal outcome and the way in which the patient and family would be most comfortable in facing this reality must be discussed. Many patients and families prefer to remain in the hospital, even when medical therapy can no longer improve the increasing respiratory failure. However, this does not mean that extreme or heroic measures must be provided for what is obviously progressive and irreversible respiratory failure. Instead, every effort should be made to make the patient and family comfortable and able to face the patient's death in a dignified and humane fashion. Some families and patients will prefer to have the patient at home if oxygen and other therapies to ensure the patient's comfort can be provided. However, support of the CF center team is not withdrawn when the patient is discharged to home. It is extremely helpful if a physician, nurse, and social worker are able to visit the home; to assess the situation, strengths, and support that the family has; and to provide guidance in what to expect and how to cope with the signs and symptoms of terminal respiratory failure. Guidance in how to comfort and support the patient and each other also should be provided to family members.

The increasing success of lung transplantation has provided an alternative to patients with CF who are approaching the end stage of their disease. Current practice is to refer patients whose FEV_1 is below 30% of predicted for evaluation for lung transplantation. Three-year survival with this procedure is now approaching 60% worldwide. However, the unfortunate fact is that because of a very limited availability of donor organs many patients with CF will die while they are on a waiting list to receive transplanted lungs.

APPROACH TO SPECIFIC SYMPTOMS AND COMPLICATIONS

Rectal Prolapse

Rectal prolapse occurs most commonly in younger children with CF when pancreatic enzyme therapy has been inadequate. Although the appearance of the first prolapse may be quite frightening, it usually can be easily reduced by placing the infant in a comfortable position and using a lubricated glove for manual reduction. It is extremely unusual that an intussusception will be associated with the prolapse or that there will be a danger of bowel strangulation. Surgery rarely will be needed to correct a recurrent rectal prolapse. By adjusting the patient's intake of fat and matching the fat intake with appropriate pancreatic enzyme dosages, the recurrent prolapse usually can be controlled.

Abdominal Pain

Patients with CF frequently give a history of either acute or chronic crampy abdominal pain. If the examination of the abdomen is normal, the pain usually can be treated by adjusting the pancreatic enzyme dosage to meet the intake of fat and protein. A careful history often will uncover the fact that the patient is eating significant amounts of food between meals but is taking pancreatic enzymes only with meals.

If the physical examination reveals a tender fecal mass in the right lower quadrant, more aggressive therapy is necessary. In this instance, we recommend that the patient be given a Fleet enema to clear the rectum. The patient is placed on clear liquids for 24 hours, and N-acetylcysteine (30 mL in 30 mL of cola) followed by mineral oil are given orally. This is usually effective in clearing the inspissated fecal material. If there are signs and symptoms of abdominal obstruction either on physical examination or on a radiograph of the abdomen, a barium enema will be necessary. If a nonreducible volvulus or intussusception is seen, emergency surgery is necessary. If only a fecal mass is present without an associated volvulus or intussusception, medical management using Gastrografin (diatrizoate meglumine) and saline enema usually results in dissolution of the impacted feces. Pressure other than hydrostatic should not be used to instill the Gastrografin. External pressure to the abdomen is also contraindicated. These procedures should be done in consultation with surgeons so that they may be prepared to intervene. Some patients for whom this is a recurring problem will benefit from chronic treatment with lactulose.

Heat Intolerance

Patients with CF have high concentrations of sodium and chloride in their sweat. They are at risk to develop vascular collapse during periods of hot weather when the amount of sweating increases. We recommend that patients salt their food liberally, take salty snacks, and drink liquids such as Coca-Cola, Pepsi Cola, or Gatorade, which contain electrolytes, during periods of warm weather. However, during an intercurrent illness in a period of warm weather, symptoms such as an abrupt decrease in oral intake may be followed by lethargy. In this situation, patients may become dehydrated rapidly and may have serum electrolytes similar to those shown for the two patients in Table 102-1. For such patients, prompt fluid replacement with isotonic saline is critical; 20 to 30 mL/kg should be given within 15 minutes if there are signs of shock or within 1 hour in less severely ill patients. Potassium chloride should be administered as soon as urine output is established. Frequent determinations of serum electrolyte levels will be necessary to guide further therapy until fluid and electrolyte correction has been completed.

Pulmonary Exacerbation

Patients with CF may have an increase in respiratory symptoms such as cough and in the rate and effort of breathing shortly after the onset of a mild upper respiratory tract infection. These patients require careful evaluation. A chest radiograph should be obtained to determine if pneumothorax or local consolidation or atelectasis are present. However, in many cases the radiograph will show only diffuse peribronchial thickening with a varying amount of fluffy infiltrates and hyperinflation. It is most helpful in assessing the degree of acute change in the symptoms and radiograph if comparison can be made in consultation with medical personnel who are familiar with the patient's previous course. Establishment of the network of CF centers by the Cystic Fibrosis Foundation for the comprehensive care of patients with CF has helped to ensure

that such information will be available even on an emergency basis.

If such guidance is not available and if lobar atelectasis, significant respiratory distress, or hypoxia is present, the patient should be treated in a hospital setting with vigorous chest physiotherapy and antibiotics effective against *S. aureus* and *P. aeruginosa* (until the results of sputum culture are available). Oxygen therapy should be guided by arterial blood gas determination.

Pneumothorax

Pneumothorax is being reported with increasing frequency in older patients with CF. It usually presents as the sudden onset of chest pain often referred to the shoulder and sometimes is associated with the acute onset of dyspnea and cyanosis. It is most important to realize that recurrences are very common in patients with CF. Therefore, after the pneumothorax has been treated by tube thoracostomy by an experienced surgeon or chest physician, some attempt should be made to use either chemical sclerosis (eg, with a high concentration of tetracycline) or open thoracostomy and pleural abrasion to prevent further recurrences.

Hemoptysis

For many patients with CF, a small amount of blood streaking in the sputum is a fairly common occurrence. Although the first such episode may be very alarming to the patient and parents, there is no need for a major change in the patient's usual home care regimen other than considering an appropriate course of antibiotic therapy to treat any intercurrent pulmonary infection. Significant hemoptysis (arbitrarily defined as the expectoration of at least 30 to 60 mL of fresh blood) should be treated in the hospital setting. The proposed mechanism is the erosion of an area of local bronchial infection into a bronchial vessel. If the bleeding persists or increases after hospitalization, vitamin K (5 mg initially) and antibiotics should be administered. The patient's blood type should be determined in the event that transfusion is necessary. Some patients with CF occasionally present with an episode of massive hemoptysis with volumes of blood loss ranging from 300 to 2500 mL. Massive hemoptysis is a life-threatening situation and in addition to instituting the measures described previously, the intervention of a skilled team including a bronchoscopist, anesthesiologist, and thoracic surgeon may be necessary to maintain an airway and to locate and ligate the bleeding vessel. When an experienced angiographer is available, bronchial artery embolization has been shown to be an effective procedure to treat recurrent or persistent hemoptysis in patients with CF.

Respiratory Failure

When a patient presents with respiratory failure (ie, hypercarbia, $P_{A_{CO2}}$ greater than or equal to 55 mm Hg), the management decisions are extremely difficult. If the respiratory failure is complicated by cor pulmonale and if this is the first such episode, the patient may respond well to the regimen described for pulmonary exacerbation with the addition of oxygen and diuretics. However, if the patient does not respond to medical therapy, the management decisions become extremely difficult. Patients with CF in general do not respond as well to mechanical ventilation and have more complications from mechanical ventilation when they are compared with patients with other forms of chronic obstructive pulmonary disease.

If an acute episode, such as viral pneumonia or status asthmaticus, precipitates respiratory failure in a patient who has had a history of good pulmonary function prior to the episode, mechanical ventilation should be considered. There are many factors that must be considered in making this decision; however, objective guidelines are not currently available. One large retrospective study found that a history of prior hypercarbia indicated a poor prognosis. It seems reasonable that good pulmonary function prior to the acute episode provides an opportunity for a good result. However, when mechanical ventilation is used for a patient with CF, a skilled intensive care team must be prepared for a potentially difficult course. When respiratory failure with increasing hypercarbia occurs in a patient with CF after a course of progressive pulmonary insufficiency despite adequate medical therapy, mechanical ventilation is not indicated. However, consultation with the physicians providing the chronic care for the patient is important before choosing this course. Some of the factors that must be considered in supporting the family and the patient who is in irreversible respiratory failure are discussed in the previous section on psychosocial support. Members of the family must be educated about signs and symptoms of terminal respiratory failure and also given guidance in how to comfort and support the patient and each other.

SUMMARY

The aggressive treatment of the pulmonary disease and nutritional deficiencies of CF coupled with an interdisciplinary team approach to provide anticipatory guidance and support has improved both the length and the quality of life for patients with CF. Major breakthroughs in elucidating the molecular basis of CF provide realistic hope for a specific therapy that will further improve the outlook for patients with CF.

BIBLIOGRAPHY

Collins FS: Cystic fibrosis: Molecular biology and therapeutic implications, *Science* 256:774–779, 1992.

Davis PB, editor: *Cystic fibrosis,* New York, 1993, Marcel Dekker.

Desmond KJ, Schwenk WF, Thomas E, et al: Immediate and long-term effects of chest physiotherapy in patients with cystic fibrosis, *J Pediatr* 103:538–542, 1983.

Eigen H, Rosenstein BJ, FitzSimmons S, et al: A multicenter study of alternate-day prednisone therapy in patients with cystic fibrosis, *J Pediatr* 126:515–523, 1995.

Fellows K, Khaw KT, Schuster S, et al: Bronchial artery embolization in cystic fibrosis: Technique and long-term results, *J Pediatr* 95:959–963, 1979.

Fuchs HJ, Borowitz DS, Christiansen DH, et al: Effect of aerosolized recombinant human DNase on exacerbations of respiratory symptoms and on pulmonary function in patients with cystic fibrosis, *N Engl J Med* 331:637–673, 1994.

Gibson LE, Cooke RE: A test for concentration of electrolytes in sweat in CF of the pancreas utilizing pilocarpine by iontophoresis, *Pediatrics* 23:545–549, 1959.

Lloyd-Still JD, editor: *Textbook of cystic fibrosis,* Boston, 1983, Wright PSG.

McLaughlin FJ, Matthews WJ, Strieder DJ, et al: Pneumothorax in cystic fibrosis: Management and outcome, *J Pediatr* 100:863–869, 1982.

Ramsey BW, Farrell PM, Pencharz P, et al: Nutritional assessment and management in cystic fibrosis: A consensus report, *Am J Clin Nutr* 55:108–116, 1992.

Redding GJ, Restuccia R, Cotton EK, et al: Serial changes in pulmonary functions in children hospitalized with cystic fibrosis, *Am Rev Respir Dis* 126:31–36, 1982.

Riordan JR, Rommens JM, Kerem BS, et al: Identification of the cystic fibrosis gene: Cloning and characterization of complementary DNA, *Science* 245:1066–1073, 1989.

Ruddy R, Scanlin TF: Abnormal sweat electrolytes in a case of celiac disease and a case of psychosocial failure to thrive: Review of other reported causes, *Clin Pediatr* 26:83–89, 1987.

Ruddy R, Anolik R, Scanlin TF: Hypoelectrolytemia as a presentation and complication of cystic fibrosis, *Clin Pediatr* 21:367–369, 1982.

Saiman L: Treatment of infections in patients with cystic fibrosis, *Infect Med* 10:37–43, 1993.

Scanlin TF: Cystic fibrosis. In Fishman AP, editor: *Pulmonary diseases and disorders,* ed 2. New York, 1988, McGraw-Hill.

Scanlin TF: Cystic fibrosis. In Fleisher G, Ludwig S, editors: *Textbook of pediatric emergency medicine,* ed 3. Baltimore, 1993, Williams & Wilkins.

Stern RC, Borkat G, Hirschfeld SS, et al: Heart failure in cystic fibrosis, *Am J Dis Child* 134: 267–272, 1980.

Taussig LM, editor: *Cystic fibrosis,* New York, 1984, Theime-Stratton.

Welsh MJ, Tsui L-C, Boat TF, Beaudet AL: Cystic fibrosis. In Scriver CR, Beaudet AL, Sly WS, et al, editors: *The metabolic and molecular bases of inherited disease,* ed 7. New York, 1995, McGraw-Hill Book.

PART FOURTEEN

Rheumatology

CHAPTER 103

Rheumatology

Balu H. Athreya

Primary care physicians are likely to encounter various problems related to the diagnosis and management of children with arthritis and other rheumatic disorders. These problems include difficulties with over- and underdiagnosis of rheumatic diseases, follow-up and coordination of care for these children with chronic multisystem diseases, and dealing with the adverse effects of antirheumatic drugs.

DIAGNOSIS OF ARTHRITIS

The primary care physician is the one most likely to see children in the initial phases of arthritis. Initial tasks include the establishment of the diagnosis and a search for the cause of the arthritis. The following criteria must be fulfilled for a diagnosis of arthritis: 1) swelling or effusion of a joint or 2) two or more of the following: limitation of range of motion, tenderness or pain on motion, increased heat.

Swelling of the joint, due to synovial thickening, is felt as a soft, velvety cushioning between the skin and the bony landmarks. Soft, gentle palpation is required to appreciate this finding. Effusion can be elicited by displacement of the fluid in the joint. Even if fluid can be demonstrated inside the joint, it is clinically impossible to say whether it is blood, inflammatory fluid, or noninflammatory fluid without looking at the fluid directly. Therefore, joint fluid aspiration and analysis are essential, particularly in single-joint disease (monarticular arthritis).

Patients with isolated joint pain or stiffness do not have arthritis. In the absence of swollen joints, two or more of the additional criteria mentioned above must be present.

Figure 103-1 summarizes an algorithm developed at the Children's Hospital of Philadelphia as a guideline in the differential diagnosis of arthritis in children. This approach helps the physician to separate acute arthritis from chronic arthritis. Acute arthritis, particularly of a single joint and associated with fever or rash, needs immediate attention. Chronic arthritis, on the other hand, is most often associated with one of the rheumatic disorders.

Causes of Acute Arthritis in Children
Monarticular (single joint)
- Trauma
    Stress fracture
    Child abuse
    Foreign body synovitis
    Acute chondrolysis of the hip
- Sickle cell disease
- Hemophilia

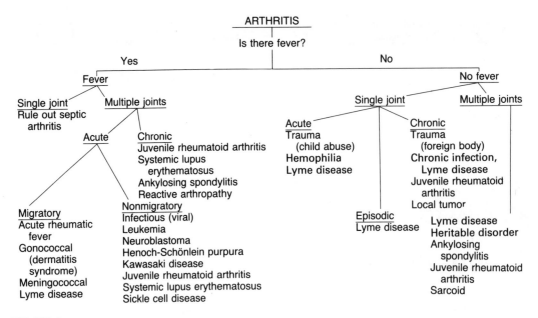

FIG 103-1
Algorithm developed at Children's Hospital of Philadelphia as a guide in the differential diagnosis of arthritis in children.

- Infectious agent (septic) arthritis *(eg, Staphylococcus, Haemophilus influenzae, Gonococcus)*

Polyarticular (many joints)
- Infectious agent arthritis
    Rubella
    Parvovirus
    HIV
    Gonococcal dermatitis-arthritis syndrome
    Enteric pathogens
- Rheumatic disorders
    Acute rheumatic fever
    Henoch-Schönlein purpura
    Serum sickness
    Kawasaki disease
    Juvenile rheumatoid arthritis
- Hematologic
    Sickle cell arthropathy
    Leukemia

Causes of Chronic Arthritis in Children
Monarticular
- Congenital lesions (*eg,* discoid meniscus in the knee)
- Foreign body arthritis (*eg,* plant thorn synovitis)

- Infectious agent arthritis (*eg,* tuberculosis, fungus, Lyme arthritis)
- Juvenile rheumatoid arthritis
- Local tumors: Hemangioma
- Other: Hemophilia, joint hypermobility with recurrent effusions

Polyarticular
- Rheumatic disorders (*eg,* juvenile rheumatoid arthritis, systemic lupus erythematosus, ankylosing spondylitis)
- Chronic inflammation: Sarcoidosis, Lyme arthritis
- Other: Heritable disorders of connective tissue, hypertrophic osteoarthropathy (*eg,* cystic fibrosis)

Common errors in the diagnosis of arthritis are 1) mistaking conditions involving periarticular structures for arthritis, 2) mistaking true arthritis for other conditions, 3) mistaking aches and pains for true arthritis, leading to overdiagnosis of rheumatic disorders, and 4) excessive reliance on laboratory tests, such as rheumatoid factor (RF), antinuclear antibody (ANA), and HLA-B27.

Mistaking Conditions Involving Periarticular Structures for Arthritis

Conditions such as urticaria, cellulitis, tenosynovitis, and osteomyelitis may mimic arthritis. Careful history taking, clinical examination, and proper application of criteria for arthritis mentioned earlier should help differentiate among these conditions.

It is relatively easy to recognize urticaria from the history, characteristic physical appearance of the lesion, and the observation that there is no swelling of the joint all around. There is thickening over only portions of the skin around the joint. The joint also will have full range of movement.

Cellulitis can produce swelling all around the joint. The skin is tender and hot, making it difficult to decide whether there is an associated arthritis. Usually, the child can move the joint through a full range of motion by himself/herself, although he/she may not allow others to do so. Laboratory studies may not be helpful in differentiating cellulitis from septic arthritis, because high white blood cell count, elevated sedimentation rate, and positive blood cultures may be seen in both conditions. Plain radiographs of the area and technetium or gallium scans may be necessary to rule out underlying osteomyelitis or arthritis. Caution should be exercised in aspirating the joint or bone, because passing a needle through an area of cellulitis may carry the infection to deeper structures.

Swelling of the tendons around the joint due to tenosynovitis also may present with pain, swelling, and limitation of motion. The swelling of tenosynovitis is diffuse, extending proximally and distally to the joint, in contrast to localized swelling of the joint. Tenderness along the tendons and inability to extend the fingers are clues to tenosynovitis of the flexor tendons of the hand. In addition to complete blood cell (CBC) count, sedimentation rate, and blood cultures done as routine investigations, aspirations of tendon sheaths for culture may be needed.

Leukemia may present with joint pain and swelling. In children with leukemia, the bone pain is more prominent, and the severity of pain is often out of proportion to the swelling of the joint. A CBC should often give clues to the actual diagnosis, although there are reports of children with a prolonged history of arthritis (up to 6 months) without evidence of leukemia in the peripheral smear. Bone marrow aspiration should be done when the index of suspicion is high. Radiographs may show the characteristic "leukemic" lines. Neuroblastoma also may present with joint pain and swelling.

Mistaking Joint Pains (Arthralgia) for True Arthritis

Confusing arthralgia (joint pains) with true arthritis leads to overdiagnosis of specific rheumatic disorders such as acute rheumatic fever, juvenile rheumatoid arthritis (JRA), and systemic lupus erythematosus (SLE). This in turn leads to unnecessary referrals, laboratory tests, and treatments. The anxiety generated is often disabling.

Of the 110 children referred with a diagnosis of acute rheumatic fever, JRA, or SLE to our pediatric rheumatology center during 1 year, only 60 had a true rheumatic disorder. Criteria for the diagnosis of these common rheumatic disorders have been developed by the American Rheumatism Association and are available in standard textbooks of rheumatology. Strict application of criteria, wise use of laboratory data, and the use of consultants should help to rule out these diagnoses. The following are some of the common reasons for the overdiagnosis of these conditions.

Common Causes of Overdiagnosis of Rheumatic Disorders

- **Overdiagnosis of acute rheumatic fever**
  Interpretation of arthralgia as arthritis
  Interpretation of innocent murmurs or murmurs of congenital valvular lesions as murmurs of acute rheumatic fever in a patient with arthralgia
  Overinterpretation of laboratory results, such as elevated erythrocyte sedimentation rate and antistreptococcal antibody titers
  Overinterpretation of echocardiographic finding
- **Overdiagnosis of JRA**
  Mistaking bone pain and musculoskeletal pain for arthritis
  Diagnosis too early in the course of the disease
  Diagnosis before exclusion of other conditions
  Overreliance on laboratory results, such as RF and ANA

- **Overdiagnosis of SLE**
  Loose application of criteria
  Diagnosis before exclusion of other conditions
  Overreliance on laboratory tests, such as ANA

Overreliance on Laboratory Tests

Rheumatic disorders are difficult to diagnose because they are chronic and, except for acute rheumatic fever, evolve over time. There are no specific laboratory tests, except in the case of SLE, and diagnosis is made on the basis of clinical findings and exclusion of other diseases.

RF is *not* a diagnostic test for JRA. The sensitivity of this test at the Children's Hospital of Philadelphia is less than 5%. Because the prevalence of the disease is less common in the community than at a tertiary center, this test is useless as a screening test for JRA in office practice. However, once a child is known to have JRA (by using standard criteria), an RF test will be of help in defining the subset of JRA and as an aid to prognosis.

ANA also is *not* a diagnostic test for JRA. However, it is a good screening test when a rheumatic disorder is suspected on good clinical grounds. Looking for ANA in children with only joint pain (without true arthritis) or in those with nonspecific symptoms such as fatigue and generalized aches and pains may identify some patients with false-positive ANA leading to unnecessary anxiety and referrals to specialists. Once a diagnosis of JRA is made, the presence of ANA may help define the subset of JRA (pauciarticular arthritis in young girls, and with high risk for iridocyclitis), or may also suggest that the child's disorder may evolve into SLE or scleroderma. In the diagnosis of SLE, however, the ANA is an excellent screening test.

FOLLOW-UP OF CHILDREN WITH JUVENILE RHEUMATOID ARTHRITIS

Rheumatic disorders are chronic disorders with varying courses, indefinite prognosis, exacerbations, and remissions. Management of rheumatic disorders requires the expertise of various specialists, including pediatric rheumatologists, orthopedic surgeons, nephrologists, dermatologists, ophthalmologists, and allied health per-

sonnel such as nurses, physical therapists, occupational therapists, social workers, and child guidance specialists. Therefore, a team leader who can coordinate the activities of these specialists and therapists and who can tailor the therapy to the needs of the child and the family is a necessity. The primary care physician is an ideal candidate for this leadership position. This topic is fully discussed in Chapter 138.

The main goal of therapy in the management of children with JRA is to keep the children active and allow them to lead as normal a life as possible. Therefore, in addition to helping with the treatment of JRA and other acute medical problems, the primary care physicians should take care of the routine medical and developmental needs of these children. Routine immunizations, including rubella vaccination, should be completed *except in those children on steroids and on immunosuppressive drugs,* who should not receive live-virus vaccines. Developmental assessments and counseling should be continued as for normal children.

Some of the specific problems associated with arthritis that may come to the attention of the primary care physician are 1) generalized growth retardation, 2) localized growth abnormalities, 3) eye problems, 4) fever, 5) morning stiffness, 6) anemia, and 7) adverse effects of drugs. In addition, the primary care physician may be called on to answer questions by the physical and occupational therapists.

Growth Retardation

Growth retardation is common in children with systemic and polyarticular-type JRA. The exact cause is not known, although it is probably related to chronic inflammatory disease. In some children, growth retardation is related to steroid therapy with or without vertebral collapse.

General attention to good nutrition is essential, as in any chronic disease, but there is no proven benefit to any of the popular diet therapies. In patients with growth retardation due to steroid therapy, every effort should be made to withdraw the medication. Localized growth disturbances such as leg-length discrepancy and small feet are also common in JRA.

Eye Problems

Iridocyclitis, a major cause of disability in children with JRA, is a particular problem for children with pauciarticular arthritis, who also exhibit ANA in their serum. The onset is insidious and may be asymptomatic. Therefore, all children with JRA should have an initial comprehensive eye evaluation. Guidelines for routine eye examination of children with JRA recommended by the American Academy of Pediatrics are shown in Table 103-1.

Once the disease enters remission, the slit-lamp examination should be repeated every year for at least 4 to 7 years because iridocyclitis can occur even after arthritis has cleared.

Fever

When a child with JRA develops a fever, it is difficult to decide whether the fever is related to JRA or is due to some other cause. Statistical probability favors the possibility of an intercurrent respiratory or urinary tract infection as the most likely explanation for fever. However, there are some specific problems to consider in children with JRA.

First, these children are on aspirin or one of the other nonsteroidal anti-inflammatory drugs. Therefore, when fever occurs, one of the questions is whether to add another drug. Generally, it is not necessary. An occasional dose of acetaminophen (one or two doses per day) should not cause any harm.

Some of the nonsteroidal drugs, specifically indomethacin, may mask localized evidence of inflammation. Therefore, one should perform a thorough physical examination and appropriate laboratory tests to rule out common infections, such as otitis media and urinary tract infection.

Children with systemic JRA who have recurrence of fever always present a diagnostic dilemma. The fever may represent recurrence of JRA or an intercurrent infection. Absence of localizing signs of infection, a fever pattern resembling the earlier course associated with the characteristic rash should suggest exacerbation of the disease. Because leukocytosis may be seen as part of systemic JRA, a white blood cell count may not help in differentiating fever of JRA from that of an infection. Urinalysis and cultures of other body fluids need to be obtained as indicated.

In any child with JRA and fever, there is always a concern that septic arthritis has been added onto the rheumatoid process. The usual findings are increased pain in the affected joint, warmth, and limitation of range of movement. Pain on moving the joint is very intense, and the child

TABLE 103-1
Frequency of Ophthalmologic Visits for Children With JRA and Without Known Iridocyclitis*

	AGE OF ONSET	
JRA SUBTYPE AT ONSET	<7 y[†]	≥7 y[‡]
Pauciarticular		
+ANA	High risk[§]	Medium risk
−ANA	Medium risk	Medium risk
Polyarticular		
+ANA	High risk[§]	Medium risk
−ANA	Medium risk	Medium risk
Systemic	Low risk	Low risk

*High risk indicates ophthalmologic examinations every 3 to 4 months. Medium risk indicates ophthalmologic examinations every 6 months. Low risk indicates ophthalmologic examinations every 12 months.
[†]All patients are considered at low risk 7 years after the onset of their arthritis and should have yearly ophthalmologic examinations indefinitely.
[‡]All patients are considered at low risk 4 years after the onset of their arthritis and should have yearly ophthalmologic examinations indefinitely.
[§]All high-risk patients are considered at medium risk 4 years after the onset of their arthritis.
(Guidelines for ophthalmological examinations in children with juvenile rheumatoid arthritis from the Section on Rheumatology and Section on Ophthalmology of the American Academy of Pediatrics, *Pediatrics* 92(2):295–296, 1993.)
ANA—antinuclear antibody; JRA—juvenile rheumatoid arthritis.

usually does not allow even minimal degrees of motion. Joint fluid aspiration for cell count and culture is absolutely necessary if septic arthritis is suspected.

Morning Stiffness

Morning stiffness can be disabling for some children with JRA. Two of the measures that can ameliorate this symptom are 1) a warm tub bath for 10 to 20 minutes in the morning, and 2) sleeping in a sleeping bag at night.

Anemia

Anemia seen in association with JRA may be due to the chronic inflammatory process, iron deficiency, or both. The anemia is usually of the normocytic normochromic type, but associated iron deficiency may give a microcytic hypochromic picture. Serum iron concentration is low, as in iron deficiency anemia, but iron-binding capacity is normal in anemia of chronic disease. Oral iron therapy may be tried, but is not always successful. The anemia corrects itself when the disease enters remission.

Other causes of anemia in JRA are blood loss through the gastrointestinal tract, hemolysis (either related to the disease or to drugs), and drug-related bone marrow depression.

PHYSICAL THERAPY

The goals of physical therapy measures are 1) relief of pain, 2) maintenance or improvement of range of motion, 3) improvement of muscle strength, and 4) improvement of activities of daily living.

Splinting of an acutely inflamed joint is the best method of achieving pain relief. It is easy to make splints for the knee and the wrist using plaster of paris. The splint should be removed twice daily and the child allowed to move the joint actively. If this is not possible, the child should be taught to do muscle-setting exercises.

Various types of exercises are used to maintain the range of movement of joints and of muscle strength. They vary from passive (therapist moves the limb) to active range (child voluntarily moves the limb), active assistive (child contracts the muscle with help from the therapist), and active resistive (child contracts the muscle against resistance supplied by the therapist).

In children, therapy measures should take into account the child's developmental status and the need for motivation. Play activities that are age-appropriate and that include principles of physical therapy are more likely to be acceptable to children than are drab daily routines. For example, swimming is an excellent exercise for children with arthritis. A tricycle can be used to improve the range of movement of the knee joint.

WORKING WITH LOCAL REHABILITATION CENTERS AND SCHOOL SYSTEMS

JRA is characterized by morning stiffness and arthritis in all cases. Fever, rash, and eye disease are seen in certain subtypes of JRA only. All children with JRA take daily medications, and a dose may have to be administered at school. Although the general philosophy in the manage-

ment of these children is to keep them active and leading as normal a life as possible, there are times when some restrictions are needed. During a flare, a child may not be able to take part in regular physical education activities. All of these disease features create some problems in relation to school attendance and activities.

In the presence of morning stiffness, the child may not be able to arrive in time for the first class period or may be stiff and unable to move rapidly from one classroom to another. Therefore, he/she may have to start earlier than the others at the end of each class. These children may need two sets of books, one for home and one for school, to spare them having to carry heavy books. The physical education teacher may need a note from the physician to excuse the child completely or to arrange a special program for the child. (The latter is ideal, so that the child does not become totally excluded.) If the hands are severely involved, these children may be allowed to do their homework and reports with a tape recorder, rather than having to write.

In the presence of fever and rash, schoolteachers and school nurses often feel nervous and send the child home. This action may be appropriate before the diagnosis is made but unnecessary once the diagnosis is certain and the child is receiving treatment. Children with eye problems may need special seating arrangements.

To aid in the management of all these problems, and many more, the schoolteacher and the school nurse require resources and support. Many specialty clinics in academic centers have special programs to work with the school systems. There are monographs and books that may be of use to the school nurses. However, as a person living in the community who knows its resources, as a leader in the community, and as one who knows the family and the school system, the family practitioner is the ideal resource person for the school system.

ADVERSE EFFECTS OF ANTIRHEUMATIC DRUGS

Most of the drugs used in the management of rheumatic disease have major side effects. Table 103-2 summarizes the drugs used in the management of JRA and their usual side effects.

Aspirin is not used as commonly as it used to be because of the frequency of adverse effects and

TABLE 103-2

Nonsteroidal Anti-inflammatory Drugs Commonly Used in the Treatment of Rheumatic Diseases and Their Side Effects

DRUG	USUAL DOSAGE	SIDE EFFECTS
Acetylsalicyclic acid (aspirin)	80–100 mg/kg/day (in young children); in older, larger children and adolescents, start with approximately 6–8 tablets of 375 mg each in divided doses	Rapid breathing, easy bruising, GI tract irritation, tinnitus, temporary hearing loss, allergy, hepatotoxic effects (elevated aspartate aminotransferase, alanine aminotransferase); rarely Reye syndrome
Tolmetin sodium (Tolectin)	20–30 mg/kg/day; maximum 1800 mg/day	GI tract irritation, hematuria proteinuria, hepatotoxic effects, drop in the hematocrit reading (due to hemodilution)
Indomethacin (Indocin)	1.0–2.0 mg/kg/day; maximum 100 mg/day	Headache, dizziness, GI tract irritation and bleeding, dermatitis, masking of infections
Ibuprofen (Motrin)	Approximately 20–40 mg/kg/day; maximum 2400 mg/day	GI tract irritation, tinnitus, hepatotoxic effects, aseptic meningitis syndrome, allergy
Naproxen (Naprosyn)	15–20 mg/kg/day in two divided doses; maximum 750 mg/day	GI tract irritation, GI tract ulcer, headache, tinnitus, hepatotoxic effects, allergy, pseudoporphyria

GI—gastrointestinal.

a particular concern about its association with Reye syndrome. To avoid this serious potential complication, children with JRA on chronic salicylate therapy are expected to receive yearly doses of influenza vaccine, and aspirin therapy must be discontinued if they exposed to chickenpox. Because of these concerns, children with JRA frequently are started on one of the other nonsteroidal anti-inflammatory drugs (NSAIDs) listed in Table 103-2 such as Tolectin or Naprosyn. Although all NSAIDs are comparable in their efficacy, there are individual differences in response. Therefore, it is best to initiate therapy with one of the NSAIDs and give an adequate trial of 8 to 12 weeks at maximum recommended dose before switching to another NSAID.

Depending on the seriousness of systemic features and arthritis, one may wish to try therapy with two or three NSAIDs before trying one of the second-line agents (Table 103-3). With the introduction of methotrexate in the treatment of JRA, the other drugs on this list are not used as commonly, except for corticosteroids.

Adverse effects of NSAIDs are similar, with skin rashes and gastric irritation being the most common. Most of the rashes are minor, although pseudoporphyria may be a significant problem with some NSAIDs (eg, Naprosyn). Hemodilution with mild drop in hemoglobin is common soon after the NSAID is started. Anemia, leu-

copenia, and thrombocytopenia can occur. Mild abdominal discomfort is common in children and is usually not an indication for withdrawal of the NSAID. Persistent pain, nighttime abdominal pain, fall in hemoglobin, and melena require withholding of NSAID and investigations to rule out gastric or duodenal ulcer. Major problems with kidneys include acute renal failure, interstitial nephritis, papillary necrosis, and nephrotic syndrome. Severe hepatoxicity with diffuse intravascular coagulation can occur with aspirin but not with other NSAIDs.

Major toxicity with D-penicillamine and gold include bone marrow suppression, skin rash, and nephritis/nephrosis. Therefore, a strict protocol of monitoring for these effects must be followed. Six monthly eye examinations including visual fields is required when chloroquine or hydroxychloroquine is used.

Potential adverse effects of methotrexate include bone marrow suppression, abdominal discomfort, oral ulcers, megaloblastic anemia, hepatotoxicity, and an allergic pneumonitis (which can be severe). Some of the hematologic effects may be ameliorated with the use of folic acid supplements. Our practice is to monitor CBC count and liver functions (AST, ALT, serum albumin) every 2 weeks for the first 3 months of therapy and every month for 3 more months. If the child remains longer on methotrexate, liver

TABLE 103-3
Second Line Agents Used in the Treatment of Rheumatic Diseases and Their Side Effects

DRUG	USUAL DOSAGE	SIDE EFFECTS
Hydroxychloroquine (Plaquenil)	5–7 mg/kg/day; maximum 400 mg/day	Dermatitis, keratopathy, retinopathy, GI tract irritation, bone marrow depression, change of hair color, myopathy
Parenteral gold preparations (Myochrysine or Solganal)	Weekly injections; gradual increase in dose; maximum dose of 1 mg/kg for once-weekly injection	Rash, bone marrow depression, renal toxic effects, aphthous ulcers
Oral gold (Ridaura)	0.15–0.2 mg/kg/day in one dose at bedtime; maximum 6–9 mg/day	Diarrhea, rash
D-Penicillamine	5–10 mg/kg/day; maximum 750 mg/day	Same as for gold, plus myasthenia, dermatomyositis and lupuslike syndrome
Corticosteroids	Varies with preparation, eg, prednisone 0.5–2.0 mg/kg/day	Growth retardation, Cushingoid facies, hirsutism, elevated blood pressure, osteoporosis, fractures, aseptic necrosis, collapse of vertebrae, GI tract irritation, peptci ulcer, cataracts, psychosis, myopathy, opportunistic infections, masked infections
Methotrexate	Given orally once a week; dose 10–20 mg/m^2/wk; maximum 15 mg/week in adults	Gastric irritation, stomatitis, hepatotoxicity, bone marrow toxicity, pneumonitis

GI—gastrointestinal.

functions are monitored every 2 months. At present, liver biopsy is not recommended unless therapy is continued for 4 or more years.

Steroids are used only in the presence of fever that is uncontrollable by other drugs, pericarditis, rapidly progressive arthritis with severe pain and limitation, and eye disease. Topical steroids are used for the treatment of iridocyclitis. Intra-articular injections also are used.

Combinations of drugs often are used in the treatment of rheumatic diseases. Many of these drugs are associated with serious side effects, and some are potentially lethal (eg, bone marrow depression due to gold administration). These potentially dangerous drugs should be used by physicians with experience, and it is imperative that there is communication between the specialists who initiate treatment with these drugs and the primary care physician.

ACKNOWLEDGMENT

My thanks to David B. Rosenberg, MD, of Vineland, NJ, who helped formulate the ideas expressed in this chapter.

BIBLIOGRAPHY

Athreya BH: Differential diagnosis of arthritis in children, *Pediatr Digest* 18:12–14, 1976.

Brewer EJ, Giannini EH, Person DA: Juvenile rheumatoid arthritis. In *Major problems in pediatrics*, Philadelphia, 1982, WB Saunders.

Cassidy JT, Petty RE: *Textbook of pediatric rheumatology*, ed 3, Philadelphia, 1994, WB Saunders.

Fithian J, editor: *Understanding the child with a chronic illness in the classroom*, Phoenix, 1984, Onyx Press.

Jacobs J: *Pediatric rheumatology for the practitioner*, ed 2, New York, 1992, Springer-Verlag.

Miller ME, editor: Pediatric rheumatology, *Pediatr Clin North Am* 42(5):999–1318, 1995.

PART FIFTEEN

Trauma

CHAPTER 104

Head Trauma

Frederick W. Tecklenburg

Head injury is one of the most common childhood accidents confronting the primary care physician. Each year approximately 5 million children present to medical attention for evaluation of head trauma. Because the majority of these injuries may be managed on an outpatient basis, the physician's office frequently will be the site of assessment and disposition. Alternatively, roughly 200,000 children will be hospitalized, primarily for careful and serial neurologic observation. At least 30,000 patients suffer more severe craniocerebral trauma requiring prolonged hospitalization and an additional 7000 pediatric patients die. An untold number of children sustain permanent neurologic sequelae. The key to appropriate management of head injuries is early recognition of potential complications, coupled with the rapid and orderly initiation of therapy.

Brain injury due to head trauma has been conceptualized as primary and secondary injuries (Fig. 104-1). Primary injuries are the direct biomechanical damage to the head incurred at the moment of trauma. Fractures, cerebral contusions and lacerations, and the initial neuronal and vascular damage that occur at traumatic impact are examples of primary injuries that unfortunately are seldom amenable to therapy. Secondary brain injuries are the result of reactive central nervous system (CNS) lesions such as brain swelling, intracranial hemorrhages, and seizures, or the result of systemic pathologic conditions, including hypoxia, hypercarbia, hypotension, anemia, hyperthermia, and electrolyte imbalance. If a child deteriorates after the traumatic event, a secondary factor is responsible. These multiple secondary factors are treatable, but if left unchecked, they will ultimately lead to additional brain insults via hypoxemia, ischemia, or increased intracranial pressure. Thus, the goal of the primary care physician is to sort out those patients with minor head trauma and to recognize and refer those patients who may need management of severe primary injuries or secondary head injury factors.

ANATOMIC CONSIDERATIONS

The infant and young child's head occupies proportionately more of the total body mass than the adult. The brain weight and head circumference of the newborn are, respectively, 25% and 60% of adult values; by 2 years of age, these dimensions are 75% and 87% of adult average values. This relative cephalic preponderance, coupled with the child's inquisitive nature and

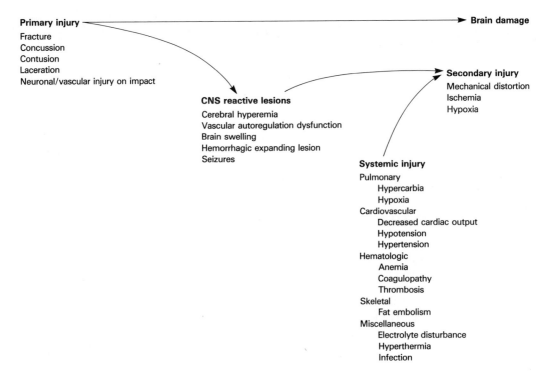

FIG 104-1
Pathophysiology of head trauma. Factors in primary injury and CNS systemic factors that lead to brain damage.

lack of judgment, creates a predisposition to head injury.

Scalp

The scalp consists of several layers, easily remembered by the acronym SCALP: *s*kin, *c*onnective tissue, *a*poneurosis, *l*oose areolar tissue, *p*eriosteum.

The connective tissue is a very vascular subcutaneous layer that anchors the skin to the aponeurosis (galea) via fibrous septa. The minimal adhesiveness of the aponeurosis to the pericranium accounts for the large flaps, "scalping" injuries, and gaping wounds that occur when the galea is lacerated. Underneath this layer is a clinically significant potential space consisting of loose areolar tissue and the emissary veins. A subgaleal hematoma results from hemorrhage into this space, and in the infant it may be sufficiently expansive to induce anemia and, occasionally, shock. The periosteum is the outermost covering of the individual cranial bones.

The Skull

The infant's skull is more flexible than the adult's because of the intrinsic nature of young bone, the flexible sutural ligaments, and the fontanelles. This resiliency has a protective effect by absorbing some of the local traumatic impact forces, but the calvarial elasticity may also allow more detrimental movement of the brain during acceleration and deceleration of the head.

The base of the skull contains the anterior, middle, and posterior cranial fossae. By early childhood these surfaces become more irregular and sharply defined, predisposing the brain to parenchymal damage by sudden accelerative forces. The ridged orbital roofs and cribriform plate of the ethmoid form the floor of the anterior fossa, a potentially injurious surface to the inferior portions of the frontal lobes. The middle cranial fossa's anterior anatomic boundary, the lesser wings of the sphenoid, presents a damaging obstacle to any anterior motion of the temporal lobes. The multiple foramina and air sinuses traversing through bones of the middle cranial fossa make this portion of the base especially prone to fracture. Fractures into these spaces have obvious clinical implications as discussed below.

The Meninges

The meninges envelop the CNS and are integral to the intracranial vascular system. Vessels superficial to the meninges include the middle meningeal arteries that are the most common source of epidural hemorrhages. The dura mater, the outermost meningeal covering, consists of two layers: an endosteal layer tightly adherent to the inner table of the skull and a meningeal layer surrounding the brain parenchyma. The latter separates from the outer layer to penetrate certain crevices of the brain, creating the falx cerebri, tentorium cerebelli, falx cerebelli, and diaphragma sella. These anatomic septa limit the amount of brain rotary movement, and fold upon themselves to form the major venous sinuses. The tentorium cerebelli separates the posterior fossa from the occipital lobes of the cerebrum and is clinically most important. Anteriorly, this membrane opens to form the tentorial incisura, an aperture for the midbrain, posterior cerebral artery, and oculomotor nerves. Pressure differentials at this membrane may lead to brain herniation through the tentorial opening and compression of the structures traversing it.

Interior to the dura is the arachnoid mater, a thin impermeable membrane that contains the cerebrospinal fluid (CSF) in the subarachnoid space. The CSF cushions the brain from trauma and easily exits into the spinal subarachnoid space to dissipate increasing intracranial pressure. The subarachnoid space also contains the cerebral vasculature, which branches from the internal carotid and vertebral arteries. Disruption of these cerebral arteries and veins produces bloody spinal fluid and the clinical stigmata of subarachnoid hemorrhage. The pia mater is the innermost meningeal membrane, closely adhering to the brain surface.

The Brain

Consciousness requires a state of alertness and cognitive function or, on a neuroanatomic basis, an intact ascending reticular activating system and cerebral cortex. Numerous mechanical and/or biochemical factors can affect these anatomic sites and, thus, the level of consciousness.

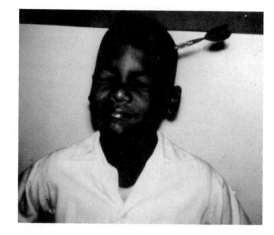

FIG 104-2
Missile injury to the head that fortunately missed injuring the brain.

DATA GATHERING

History

The initial history should include the details of the traumatic event, the patient's neurologic status before and after the accident, the suspected presence of associated injuries, and any care administered prior to the patient's presentation. Questions should address the presence or absence of loss of consciousness, tonic-clonic movements, somnolence, irritability, abnormal behavior or verbalizations, emesis, ataxia, or weakness. Knowledge of the patient's mental status before and after the accident and, more importantly, any progression of neurologic signs or symptoms is crucial to patient management. If the patient is verbally responsive, the examiner should elicit any complaints of head or neck pain, visual changes, paresthesias, or amnesia.

It is important to ascertain the height of fall, the quality of impact surfaces, and the shape and velocity of striking objects (Fig. 104-2). The mechanism of injury will influence the clinician's diagnostic and management plans. For example, a two-story fall necessitates a careful search for associated injuries and a longer period of in-hospital observation. A diving injury immediately dictates that a cervical spine fracture be ruled out.

Finally, the history may reveal discrepancies or unlikely events that could suggest a diagnosis of child abuse. Routine, yet essential, information regarding allergies, chronic illness, and current medications should be known.

Physical Examination

The physical examination of the alert and conscious patient may proceed in a routine, thorough manner, with emphasis placed on the head, neck, and neurologic examinations. Examination of the head includes careful palpation of the calvarium, fontanelles, and facial bones; inspection of scalp wounds for underlying fractures; and the search for signs of any oral or mandibular trauma. If there are no complaints of neck pain or evident neck spasm, cervical range of motion and palpation of the cervical spine should be tested. A complete neurologic examination should include evaluation of mental status, cranial nerves, cerebellar function, sensation, deep-tendon reflexes, and muscular tone and strength. Nonspecific but important signs to recognize in the infant include irritability, pallor, high-pitched crying, "ocular apathy," or poor social interaction. The fundoscopic examination is especially important in infants to rule out retinal hemorrhages, which frequently provide the most diagnostic sign of an abused, shaken baby. Notation of the vital signs, especially pulse and blood pressure, is essential information for a complete neurologic assessment.

The patient with moderate or severe head trauma often requires simultaneous physical examination and therapy, which should always follow the sequence in the acronym ABCD: airway, breathing, circulation, disability. Cervical spine neutrality should be maintained in these patients with altered mental status. After ensuring an adequate airway, ventilation, and circulation, the physician must rapidly assess the neurologic disability. The remainder of the physical examination may then be completed, emphasizing repeated ABCD evaluation to optimize the care of the patient with a head injury.

A neurologic flow sheet facilitates an objective and serial recording of the patient's neurologic status. The descriptive terms of consciousness (alert, lethargic, obtunded, stuporous, comatose) should be replaced with the Glasgow coma scale. This scale is reliable in the hands of multiple observers, and the score itself has management and prognostic implications. The scale consists of scores for three responses: eye opening, verbal, and best upper limb movement (Table 104-1). The eye-opening response to speech does not

TABLE 104-1
Glasgow Coma Scale

Eye opening	
Spontaneous	4
To speech	3
To pain	2
None	1
Verbal response	
Oriented	5
Confused	4
Inappropriate	3
Incomprehensible	2
None	1
Best upper limb response	
Obeys	6
Localizes	5
Withdraws	4
Abnormal flexion	3
Abnormal extension	2
None	1

require a command to open the eyes, and the response to painful stimuli should not include facial stimuli. A note should be made if the eyes are open but not blinking or if they are occluded by periorbital edema. The verbal response score for nonverbal patients (infants and young children) has not been standardized. The painful stimulus for the best upper limb response should be nailbed or supraorbital pressure. Raising the hand above the chin in response to supraorbital pressure is a localizing response. An abnormal flexion and extensor response are decorticate and decerebrate posturing, respectively. The Glasgow coma scale ranges from 3 to 15; morbidity and mortality rise sharply with scores from 7 to 3.

Radiology

Skull series have no place in the evaluation of the unstable patient with closed head trauma. Computed tomography (CT) of the head is the procedure of choice in the patient with a persistently altered or deteriorating level of consciousness, or the patient with focal neurologic findings.

Criteria for skull radiographic films in the stable child with a history of head trauma include the following: 1) clinical signs of basilar or depressed skull fractures, 2) history of loss of consciousness greater than 5 minutes, 3) missile or open injuries, and 4) age less than 12 months, with a history of significant traumatic force, *eg,* a fall greater than 2 ft. The location and extent of fractures are more important variables regarding management. Fractures overlying the middle meningeal groove, deep venous sinuses, or the rim of the foramen magnum have potential intracranial vascular complications and warrant careful patient observation. Skull radiographs should include a stereolateral pair (one upright to rule out a sinus air-fluid level), posteroanterior and Towne views. Alternatively, in the patient who must remain supine and immobile, the lateral views may be obtained with a horizontal beam; the other views, with anteroposterior beams. If facial fractures are suspected, a Waters view may be indicated. Other views can be obtained if a fracture is detected in the initial series.

MANAGEMENT

After the initial assessment of the stable head-injury patient, serial observation is a mainstay of management. Any deterioration must be recognized and addressed promptly to reduce the potential morbidity of craniocerebral trauma. In the alert and responsive child, this continued observation may be carried out by reliable caretakers. The decision for home disposition should meet several criteria: absence of a life-threatening mechanism of injury, no neurologic symptoms other than a resolved momentarily altered consciousness, dependable parents, and a normal neurologic examination. Instructions to parents should include obvious signs and symptoms of deterioration or complications as summarized below.

The physician should be contacted if any of the following exist:

1. A fall greater than the child's height
2. Sleepiness, or difficulty arousing from usual sleep time
3. Vomiting or pallor
4. Severe headache
5. Weakness or dizziness
6. Complaints of visual disturbance
7. Fluid draining from ear or nose
8. Stiff or painful neck

Emergency care should be sought if:

1. The child is unresponsive
2. Seizures develop

The decision to hospitalize a child for observation after minimal head trauma is based on several considerations:

1. History of loss of consciousness
2. Amnesia
3. Vomiting
4. Skull fracture
5. Age of patient; infant or neonate
6. Associated injuries
7. Mechanism of injury
8. Social issues
9. Systemic disease
10. Seizures
11. Change in level of consciousness

Most authorities on head trauma recommend hospitalized observation if a history of loss of consciousness for more than 5 minutes is obtained. This recommendation must be tempered with the parents' ability to estimate time elapsed in an emergency setting. Although retrograde amnesia is common in uncomplicated concussion syndromes, anterograde amnesia is indicative of a more severe injury and warrants further observation until cleared. One or two episodes of emesis within the first couple hours of trauma is often associated with mild head injury, but vomiting associated with somnolence or persistent vomiting requires a longer period of medical surveillance. Frequently, a head CT scan is required to rule out neurologic pathology. The clinical significance of isolated linear fractures that do not cross underlying vasculature is debatable. There is no question, however, that open, basilar, or depressed fractures mandate immediate neurosurgical attention. The physician's threshold for admission should be lowered in the infant or neonate with any symptoms or signs. The mechanism of injury is another consideration in the decision regarding hospitalization. A child who was struck by a moving vehicle or fell a significant distance often requires prolonged observation for head and other associated internal injuries. Social issues include a parent's ability to observe the child and the suspicion of child abuse. Chronic conditions or diseases such as coagulopathies, osteogenesis imperfecta, or ventricular shunts may predispose to intracranial hemorrhages or fractures. A history of a brief seizure on impact or within several hours of head trauma should prompt admission for closer observation, although the stable patient does not require anticonvulsant therapy. Finally, any symptom or sign suggesting a change for the worse in the level of consciousness will necessitate longer periods of observation and neuroimaging studies.

Specific Clinical Situations

Scalp Lacerations

When scalp lacerations are extensive, local hemostasis is a management priority. Under sterile conditions, the wound should be inspected for debris, and the skull palpated for fractures. Evidence of bone fragments or open or depressed fractures dictates neurosurgical evaluation prior to closure. The galea must be sutured first to achieve normal healing, and the more superficial scalp sutures may be ligated slightly tighter than usual to achieve further hemostasis. A pressure dressing also helps stem continued bleeding.

Subgaleal Hematoma

The subgaleal hematoma is a common scalp lesion that presents as a localized or diffuse fluctuant swelling. Bloody fluid accumulates in the potential space between the galea and periosteum, dissecting the two layers. A clinically significant hemorrhage may occur into this space in the young child or infant, but surgical treatment is rarely, if ever, indicated. These lesions do not transilluminate and may require several weeks for resolution. There is an increased incidence of skull fracture associated with subgaleal hematomas.

Subgaleal Hygroma

A subgaleal hygroma is an uncommon scalp accumulation of CSF usually occurring secondary to a laceration of the dura and arachnoid membranes by a skull fracture. Clinically they resemble a subgaleal hematoma, but a positive transillumination and skull fracture suggest the diagnosis. Neurosurgical referral is indicated.

Cephalohematoma

A cephalohematoma is a subperiosteal hematoma of an individual cranial bone. It most commonly affects the parietal bone after parturition and on palpation is firm with a central depression (due to its organized perimeter). It does not cross the suture line and does not transilluminate. Calcification of the elevated periosteal layer not uncommonly occurs, and resolution may require 2 weeks to 3 months. No therapy is required; aspiration is contraindicated.

Skull Fractures

Skull fractures indicate a significant traumatic force occurrence, but the fracture per se does not necessarily correlate with the presence or absence of intracranial pathologic conditions. The linear fracture is the most common fracture and has little serious clinical implication unless it overlies a vascular channel or penetrates an air sinus. On radiographs, the linear fracture usually appears relatively straight and nonbranching; it rarely crosses sutures. Occasionally, a linear fracture is diastatic, in which case the clinician should beware of an underlying contusion or laceration. In addition, diastatic sutural fractures occur with trauma in young children and have significant intracranial hemorrhage potential. The lambdoid suture that overlies the transverse venous sinus is most commonly affected. Increased intracranial pressure at a young age also can lead to generalized split sutures before the sutural ligaments calcify.

A late and rare complication of linear fractures is a "growing" fracture. Growing fractures are thought to arise because the meninges have been lacerated on initial injury and a pulsating arachnoid cyst forms that erodes the fracture margin. The reshaped fracture widens into an irregular bony defect and a leptomeningeal cyst develops. These scalp masses become evident several months to years after the initial fracture and may pulsate and transilluminate. Neurosurgery is usually required.

Depressed fractures often result from significant traumatic forces acting on a small cross-sectional area (eg, a blow from a hammer) and have obvious implications for underlying brain tissue. Unless seen in a tangential view on radiographs, these fractures often appear as an increased sclerotic density because of overlapping bone surfaces. Occasionally, these fractures are open (a compound fracture) or comminuted, and, thus, require neurosurgical debridement and inspection for parenchymal injury. Most neurosurgeons would consider surgical elevation of the bone edges if the depression is either greater than the thickness of the skull or 5 mm.

Basilar skull fractures are in the basal portion of the skull—specifically the frontal, ethmoid, sphenoid, temporal, and occipital bones. Clinical indicators of these fractures include periorbital subcutaneous hemorrhages ("raccoon eyes"), CSF rhinorrhea or otorrhea, cranial nerve palsies, hemotympanum, or postauricular ecchymosis (Battle sign). In the young child, the dura closely adheres to the basilar skull accounting for the associated meningeal tears in basilar fractures. These skull fractures are often difficult to demonstrate on routine radiographs, although sphenoid and frontal sinus air-fluid levels or opacification and pneumocephaly may suggest their presence.

CSF rhinorrhea implies a fracture near the cribriform plate of the ethmoid and may require tomography or CSF radionuclide studies to identify it. Fractures of the temporal bone's petrous ridge causing otorrhea or hemotympanum can be equally hard to demonstrate radiologically. The CSF leaks often increase with coughing or head-down position, and on filter paper the leaks display a "water-ring" if bloody. Infectious complications, primarily pneumococcal or *Haemophilus influenzae* meningitis, are the main reason for clinical concern. There is no clear consensus on the use of prophylactic antibiotics. Fortunately, in many cases the CSF leaks close within a week.

Concussion

Concussion is a mild closed head injury, with an associated brief impairment of consciousness. Although an organic lesion is not consistently demonstrable, the ascending reticular activating system and cerebral cortex are the probable sites of this temporary neuronal dysfunction. Clinically, the child exhibits variable degrees of impaired consciousness, from coma to lethargy, and often has associated anorexia, vomiting, or pallor. Sleepiness, confusion, or abnormal behavior may continue for several hours. The older child or adult often reports amnesia for the events leading to the accident (retrograde amnesia). A posttraumatic or anterograde amnesia reflects a temporary difficulty forming new memories after the injury. The length of the posttraumatic amnesia correlates with the severity of the head injury. There is usually an uneventful recovery in concussions.

An alternate presentation of concussion, especially in infants and younger children, is the pediatric concussion syndrome. A delayed deterioration of consciousness occurs minutes to several hours after seemingly minimal head trauma. The change in mental status usually is heralded by pallor, vomiting, and irritability. The patient may be mildly ataxic and often becomes somnolent. There are no focal findings,

and the syndrome resolves in several hours. The differential diagnosis of delayed deterioration of consciousness also includes posttraumatic seizure manifestations, brain swelling, and intracranial hemorrhage. Neurosurgical consultation and CT scan are warranted in this setting.

Cerebral Contusion or Laceration

Contusions are hemorrhagic bruises of the brain demonstrable on CT scan and are often associated with local swelling. The sites of contusions tend to be in the cerebral cortex adjacent to significant focal skull impacts or in areas of the brain anatomically predisposed to accelerative forces (the anterior and orbital surfaces of the frontal lobes, anterior temporal lobes, and areas adjacent to free falx edges). A cerebral contusion does not necessarily cause unconsciousness, although prolonged impairment of consciousness is common. The neurologic signs depend on the site of the contusion and are often focal.

Lacerations are tears in the brain substance that occur at similar sites. In addition, the unmyelinated state of nerve fibers in young infants predisposes their white matter to tears on rotational accelerative forces. The major morbidity of lacerations is related to the site and extent of the tear itself and secondary vascular complications (*ie,* intracranial hemorrhages).

Intracranial Hemorrhage

Epidural Hemorrhage—Epidural hematomas are relatively rare (less than 10%) in pediatric severe head trauma, but early recognition and prompt treatment will improve outcome. They occur more frequently in older children and have a mortality rate of 10% to 20%. The majority of epidural hematomas originate from a hemorrhaging middle meningeal artery that quickly separates the meningeal dura layer from the inner table of the skull. In children, however, a substantial minority of epidural hematomas are due to meningeal and diploic vein hemorrhage. These hematomas may occasionally occur in the posterior cranial fossa secondary to a bleeding deep venous sinus. Another crucial anatomic difference in young children is the dura mater's tight adherence to the skull. These factors are probably responsible for the variable and occasionally subacute presentation of pediatric patients with epidural hemorrhage.

Patients with an epidural hematoma often present with a rapid and focal neurologic deterioration without regaining consciousness. This type of injury often has an arterial source of bleeding and associated brain lesions. Not unexpectedly mortality is higher with an earlier presentation. Some patients will present with the classic triad of concussion, intervening lucent phase, and then neurologic deterioration. The period of "lucency" is usually not a totally asymptomatic interval but simply an improvement in the level of consciousness. Over a variable period of time, the child progressively develops neurologic signs of increased intracranial pressure and impending transtentorial herniation. In supratentorial epidural hematomas, the CT scan reveals a biconvex increased density with varying amounts of "midline shift." The incidence of cranial fractures is at least 50% in pediatric epidural hemorrhages, and approaches 100% in adults. In the pediatric patient epidural hemorrhage also may occur in the posterior cranial fossa after occipital trauma, and commonly causes nuchal rigidity, cerebellar signs, vomiting, and continued impaired consciousness. An occipital fracture is usually present.

Subdural Hemorrhages—Posttraumatic subdural hemorrhages are an important source of neurologic morbidity in pediatric patients. Subdural hematomas occur more frequently than bleeding in the epidural space and tend to affect infants more often than older children. The subdural hemorrhage is almost exclusively venous in origin, most frequently from cerebral vein disruption at the sagittal sinus. These anastomoses are very sensitive to the shearing forces generated by rotational acceleration.

The young infant occasionally presents subacutely after seemingly minor head injury because of the venous source of bleeding and the increased calvarial compliance. Nonspecific symptoms such as vomiting, irritability, and low-grade temperature may develop. In the subacute phase, the subdural blood organizes into a hemorrhagic cyst over several weeks and expands in size via the osmotic pressure of red blood cell breakdown products. Regardless of time course, the majority of patients with subdural hemorrhage will eventually have a focal or generalized seizure. Physical examination often reveals an irritable or lethargic baby with a bulging fontanelle, "sunsetting" eyes, and hypertonicity. Only a minority of these patients have an associated skull fracture. The CT scan will commonly demonstrate bilateral crescentic-shaped subdural collections. If the subdural hemorrhage is older than 1 week, the collection may appear isodense on CT, necessitating contrast medium to establish the diagnosis. The morbidity seen in patients with subdural hematomas is higher than in patients with epidural hemorrhage, due to underlying brain damage. Older children with subdural bleeding tend to present in a more acute state, with symptoms and signs of increasing intracranial pressure and impending transtentorial herniation.

Subarachnoid Hemorrhage—Although the major cerebral vessels traverse the subarachnoid space, the more fragile and smaller leptomeningeal vessels are often the source of subarachnoid hemorrhage. The clinical course is usually dominated by associated brain injuries, although headache, nuchal rigidity, and low-grade fever may occasionally be attributed to subarachnoid blood. Rarely, a communicating hydrocephalus develops due to hemorrhagic debris blocking the CSF circulation. On CT scan, a linear increased density is commonly seen in the interhemispheric fissure.

Intraparenchymal Hemorrhage—Acute intracranial hemorrhage is a common finding in fatal head injuries. Clinically this lesion is indistinguishable from other severe intracranial mass lesions. The hemorrhages predominate in the frontal and temporal lobes and may have associated focal neurologic findings.

Brain Swelling

Acute brain swelling is a common occurrence in the pediatric patient with severe head trauma. A child with a deteriorating neurologic status after a period of "lucency" is more likely to have generalized cerebral swelling rather than an intracranial hemorrhage. The initial basic pathophysiology is increased cerebral blood volume or cerebral hyperemia. The CT scan reveals a small ventricular system and decreased subarachnoid cisternal spaces. This form of brain edema can dramatically increase the intracranial pressure.

Seizures

Seizures develop in approximately 10% of children hospitalized for head trauma. Posttraumatic seizures can be temporally divided into immediate, early, and late seizures. An "immediate" seizure manifests within seconds of impact and probably represents a traumatic depolarization of the cortex. It may occur with mild trauma, is brief, and probably has no prognostic significance.

"Early" seizures account for about half of the posttraumatic fits and take place within the first week of the traumatic event. They are usually due to focal injury by contusion, laceration, ischemia, or edema. Young children seem more susceptible to development of early posttraumatic seizures. The majority of affected patients present in the first 24 hours after the trauma. Roughly equivalent numbers of patients have generalized or focal seizures, and 10% to 20% will develop status epilepticus. Approximately one fourth of patients with early seizures will continue to have seizures after the first week (*ie,* posttraumatic epilepsy).

Late posttraumatic seizures that occur 1 week or longer after trauma probably reflect cortical scarring. The severity of head injury, dural laceration, and intracranial hemorrhage are all factors in this form of seizure. Close to 5% of hospitalized head trauma patients have late posttraumatic fits. The long-term prognosis is more guarded; as many as three fourths of these patients will develop epilepsy.

BIBLIOGRAPHY

Bijur PE, Haslum M, Golding J: Cognitive and behavioral sequelae of mild head injury in children, *Pediatrics* 86:337, 1990.

Bruce DA, Alavi A, Bilaniuk L, et al: Diffuse cerebral swelling following head injuries in children: The syndrome of "malignant brain edema," *J Neurosurg* 54:170, 1981.

Division of Injury Control, Center for Environmental Health and Injury Control: Childhood injuries in the United States, *Am J Dis Child* 144:627, 1990.

Duhaime AC, Alario AJ, Lewander WJ, et al: Head injury in very young children: Mechanism, injury types, and ophthalmologic findings in 100 hospitalized patients younger than 2 years of age, *Pediatrics* 90:179, 1992.

Kelly JP, Nichols JS, Filley CM, et al: Concussion in sports: Guidelines for the prevention of cataschropic outcome, *JAMA* 266:2867, 1991.

Levin HS, Aldrich EF, Saydjari C, et al: Head injury in children: Experience of the traumatic coma data bank, *Neurosurgery* 31:435, 1992.

Masters SJ, McClean PM, Arcarese JS, et al: Skull x-ray examinations after head trauma, *N Engl J Med* 316:84, 1987.

Snoek JW, Minderhoud JM, Wilmink JT: Delayed deterioration following mild head injury in children, *Brain* 107:15, 1984.

Tecklenburg FW, Wright MS: Minor head trauma in the pediatric patient, *Pediatr Emerg Care* 7:40, 1991.

Ward JD: Pediatric head injury: A further experience, *Pediatr Neurosurg* 30:183, 1994.

CHAPTER 105

Facial Trauma

Dee Hodge III

Almost every child experiences facial trauma several times in his/her life. Some children, due to their level of activity or type of play, experience it several times a day. Most facial trauma is minor and does not require the attention of a physician. In other instances, because the face is the site of the vital sensory organs, facial trauma is more of a concern, and the child is brought to the pediatrician or family practitioner.

In this chapter the more common forms of facial injuries will be discussed in regard to their evaluation, diagnosis, treatment, and conditions for referral.

EYE

In evaluating injuries to the eye, it is important to have a general approach to the examination and a few useful tools. Minimal equipment needed by the physician includes: eye chart for evaluation of visual acuity, adequate light and magnification, topical anesthetic (eg, proparacaine hydrochloride [0.5%]), fluorescein dye, and dilating or cycloplegic drops (eg, tropicamide 1%). Lid retractors and a slit lamp are useful but not essential in the office setting. A good history is most important in determining what happened, when, where, and how the child is doing now. Having a standard approach will aid in the evaluation of the injured eye; for example:

1. Evaluate visual acuity.
2. Check extraocular movement.
3. Check face and periorbital area for asymmetry ecchymosis, eyelid laceration.
4. Examine conjunctiva and fornices including eversion of upper lid.
5. Evaluate cornea including examination with use of fluorescein.
6. Examine anterior chamber and compare with other side.

7. Note pupil size and shape.
8. Examine lens and posterior chamber.
9. Conclude with funduscopic examination.

Chemical burns and occlusion of the central retinal artery are the only true ocular emergencies. They should be referred immediately because minutes count as far as survival of the eye. Medical attention within hours is needed for the other injuries noted here. They are divided into nonpenetrating and penetrating injuries of the eye.

Nonpenetrating Injuries of the Eye

Abrasions
Abrasions of the lid can be treated in the same manner as any abrasion to the skin. Special care should be taken to clean the abrasion of any imbedded foreign material to prevent long-term retention of the foreign body or tattooing.

Corneal abrasions are the most common injuries to the eyes of children. Presenting signs and symptoms include uncomfortable sensation, blurred vision, red eyes, tearing, and photophobia. The examination is facilitated by the use of topical anesthesia followed by fluorescein dye to demarcate the abrasion. Most abrasions can be treated in the office. Antibiotic drops or ointment with follow-up in 24 hours is the treatment of choice. The use of patching is controversial and often is not needed. Follow-up is extremely important at 24- or 36-hour follow-up visit, and any large abrasion that has persisted should be referred to an ophthalmologist.

Contusion
Contusion of the eyelid or "black eye" results from blunt trauma to the orbit and surrounding structures. A careful examination is needed to rule out any associated injury to the globe or bone structures. If the injury is isolated to the eyelid, then cold compresses and analgesics are the only

treatment needed. Often these injuries will look worse on the day after the injury, and parents should be prepared for this progression.

A contusion to the globe usually results in subconjunctival hemorrhage. This type of hemorrhage also may occur spontaneously or in association with nose blowing or forceful vomiting. After complete examination, if there is no suspicion of a bleeding tendency or child abuse, assurance may be given to the parents that it will resolve in a few weeks with no need for further follow-up.

Hyphema

Hyphema is defined as accumulation of free blood in the anterior chamber. The most common cause is blunt trauma resulting in rupture of iris or ciliary body blood vessels. Spontaneous hyphemas are known to occur, most often in diseases that include purpuric skin lesions, sickle cell disease, ocular tumors, and congenital and acquired coagulation factor deficiencies. Most fill less than 30% of the anterior chamber and last from 5 to 7 days. Loss of full visual acuity due to the hyphema may produce drowsiness, but the physician must be careful not to overlook concomitant neurologic trauma.

The diagnosis is made by examining the eye and finding blood in the anterior chamber. This blood is easily seen when a light source is placed lateral to the eye and shone across the anterior chamber. A slit lamp will show even microscopic amounts of blood. Hyphemas have been graded based on the amount of blood occupying the anterior chamber: in grade I, one fourth of the chamber is filled; grade II, one half; grade III, three fourths; grade IV, the entire chamber is filled with blood, or "black ball" hyphema.

Management of hyphema, which is the responsibility of the ophthalmologist, includes hospitalization for daily observation, systemic aminocaproic acid, topical atropine, and bedrest. All patients without history of trauma should have determination of prothrombin time and partial thromboplastin time and a sickle preparation done. Complications include rebleeding that may occur on the fourth to fifth day, elevation in intraocular pressure, and corneal staining.

Corneal and Conjunctival Foreign Body

Foreign bodies are also a common problem in the pediatric patient population. A foreign body may be the cause of a corneal abrasion and, indeed, the signs and symptoms are the same. Visual acuity is normal. The sensation of a foreign body is useful in locating the foreign body, and, therefore, the use of anesthetic drops should be avoided in this situation. Fluorescein also may be useful in locating the offending object. Most of the objects can be removed by lavage or by lifting the object with a cotton swab. More resistant objects may need to be removed with the aid of a slit lamp and magnification by the ophthalmologist.

Penetration of the globe by a foreign body is a true emergency and must be ruled out. If the history and the physical examination are compatible with a high-velocity foreign body or vision is decreased, or if the eye is more inflamed or softer than expected, the patient should be promptly referred to an ophthalmologist.

Chemical Burns

Chemical burns are one of the true ophthalmologic emergencies. Alkali burns are more devastating than acid burns. Acids precipitate tissue protein so the injury is more superficial and slower to penetrate into the tissues of the eye. Alkali, on the other hand, allow rapid deep penetration into the tissues of the eye because of saponification of fat and destruction of cells.

Initial treatment by parents at home is essential and consists of irrigation with water for 20 minutes before transport to the office. There should be continued irrigation in the office with 2 L of fluid or until the pH level of the conjunctival sac is between 7.3 and 7.7. Immediate referral to an ophthalmologist is indicated.

Rupture of Eyeball

Rupture of the eyeball may result from a number of different types of injuries but most commonly is caused by blunt trauma. The most common site is along the limbus, although rupture may occur occasionally around the optic nerve. If rupture is suspected, the primary care physician should not try to force the eye open but should place a hard patch around the orbital rim and refer the patient immediately to an ophthalmologist.

Penetrating Injuries of Eye

Any suspected penetrating injury, as mentioned earlier, needs prompt treatment by an ophthalmologist. Every lacerated eyelid should be considered to have a penetrating wound to the globe. Other signs and symptoms of penetration are decreased vision on physical examination, lacerated cornea or conjunctiva, localized scleral swelling, shallow anterior chamber, distorted or peaked pupil, external presentation of the iris or other intraocular contents, or a white pupil. If penetration of the globe is suspected, vigorous examination should be avoided at all cost because the increased pressure on the globe may cause extrusion of the intraocular contents. If intraocular foreign bodies are suspected, radiographic films of the orbit and ultrasound are useful in locating the foreign body. It is again stressed that all patients with suspected penetrating injury must be referred.

Lid Lacerations

Lacerations to the lid comprise the majority of lid injuries after contusion and abrasions. Lacerations that do not involve the lid margins may be sutured in the usual manner using 5-0 or 6-0 nylon after instilling topical anesthetic without epinephrine. Lacerations near the inner canthus frequently involve the canaliculi and should be evaluated by the ophthalmologist. Any through-and-through laceration should raise the suspicion of injury to the globe and also should be referred for examination by an ophthalmologist.

Periorbital Trauma

Blunt trauma to the orbit causes a sudden increase in intraorbital pressure. The medial wall and orbital floor are the weakest bones of the orbit, thus giving way. Orbital floor fractures may result in entrapment of orbital fat, inferior rectus muscle, inferior oblique muscle, or a combination of the above. Examination may reveal proptosis or an inability of upward gaze. Radiographic film of the orbit may show entrapment of the inferior rectus, the so-called "teardrop sign." If no intraocular injury is found, then conservative treatment is advocated. This treatment includes ice, to reduce swelling during the first 24 hours, followed by heat. Oral antibiotics are considered helpful by some to reduce the chance of infection across the violated sinus. All children with orbital fractures should be referred to an ophthalmologist.

NASAL TRAUMA

Epistaxis

Bleeding from the interior of the nose may be caused by injuries, infections, septal perforations, tumors, and blood dyscrasias; however, most nosebleeds are not associated with any of these conditions. Drying of the mucosa and trauma from nose-picking are the most common cause of bleeding from the area of Kesselbach plexus in the anterior nasal septum.

Bleeding from the anterior septum often stops with simple measures. Pinching the nostrils for a full 10 minutes will stop the bleeding in most instances. If bleeding continues, identifying the exact source of bleeding is necessary. The anterior nasal chamber often can be adequately visualized through a surgical head otoscope fitted with a nasal speculum. If no active bleeding is seen, more equipment is needed including optimal illumination and exposure with a head mirror, nasal speculum, and suction tip. If the bleeding point is identified, dry the area and cauterize it with a silver nitrate stick or touch the area with cotton dampened with 2% tetracaine and 3% ephedrine.

Exact sites of bleeding deep within the nose rarely can be identified. Usual sites include the posterior ethmoid, a branch of the external carotid, or septal branch of the sphenopalatine artery. Posterior nasal hemorrhage usually requires sedation, postnasal packing, and hospitalization. The need for posterior packing used in conjunction with anterior packing is very rare in children.

Without a history of recurrent epistaxis, workup of bleeding disorders is unwarranted. Recurrent epistaxis is defined as greater than 10 nosebleeds per year without history of nasal trauma or nasal allergy (*see* Chapter 54 for more details).

Nasal Fractures and Septal Hematoma

For many children with nasal trauma, medical attention is not sought unless the injury is severe enough to cause swelling, cosmetic deformity, airway obstruction, or epistaxis. The child's nose does not respond in the same way as an adult's because of differences in structure. Because of more cartilage, incomplete fracture is more often seen, and with less likelihood of mobility and crepitus. Nasal fractures fall into four categories: 1) *Greenstick*—an incomplete fracture that is never compounded by tearing of the underlying mucosa. The diagnosis cannot be made with conventional radiography. The diagnosis can be made clinically by the finding of point tenderness, but it is impossible to make the diagnosis in the presence of edema. 2) *Linear fracture*—a simple fracture without displacement or communition. 3) *Lateral fracture*—the most common type of fracture found in children. There is an inward fracture of the traumatized nasal bone and an outward fracture of the opposite nasal bone. Findings of radiographic film are often positive. 4) *Frontal fracture*—caused by a straight-ahead blow to nose.

The primary diagnosis of fracture may be difficult. Signs in order of frequency include: epistaxis, swelling of nasal dorsum, ecchymosis of the eyes, tenderness of the nasal dorsum, obvious nasal deformity, and crepitus of the nasal bones. Any change in appearance of the nose since injury may be helpful. Any deviation is pertinent, but seeming absence of deviation may be misleading because of edema. If edema is present, delay definitive palpation until it subsides in 3 to 4 days. Crepitus, if present, is considered diagnostic. Internal examination of the nose is important. Any deviation of the nasal septum increases likelihood of later abnormality. Radiographic film examination is diagnostic in only 50% of the cases.

A septal hematoma also may result from nasal trauma and occurs more frequently in children because the septal cartilage tends to buckle more easily. Small hematomas must be searched for and treated if present. Evacuation of the hematoma is necessary to prevent the possibility of avascular necrosis of the septal cartilage and septal abscess. Consultation with an otorhinolaryngologist is advised.

Foreign Bodies of the Nose
Many times children will present with the complaint of a foreign body in the nose, but more often than not the complaint is of a unilateral foul-smelling discharge. Foreign bodies are often visible in the anterior antrum with a nasal speculum. Foreign bodies include paper, toys, beads, and so forth; thus, the majority are radiolucent. The physician may try to remove the foreign body if it is in the nasal vestibule and can be grasped easily with forceps. The child must be well restrained. The mucosa may be sprayed with a topical vasoconstrictor such as phenylephrine (Neo-Synephrine) to decrease edema and bleeding. The object should never be pushed posteriorly or irrigated because of the danger of aspiration. Once the object is removed, the patient should be treated with amoxicillin, 25 to 50 mg/kg/day for 10

days. If removal is impossible, referral is indicated.

Maxillary and Mandibular Fractures
Problems in diagnosis and treatment of these fractures are often secondary to difficulty in examination, small size of the structure, and lack of development of paranasal sinus. Fortunately, these injuries are rare. Because a lack of pneumatization, the flexibility of developing bone, and mixed dentition produce more stable structures, and therefore a greater force is needed to cause these fractures. When mandibular or maxillary fractures are present they may be associated with intracranial and cervical spine injuries. Rapid evaluation for other injuries is necessary. Management of the airway and treatment of shock, as always, are of first priority. Facial bones heal rapidly; therefore, stabilization is required within 5 days of injury lest malalignment occur.

Fractures of the maxilla are secondary to excessive force directed at a small area. Fractures to the maxilla are frequently associated with nasal injury, soft-tissue trauma, and involvement of the orbit. Examination of any suspected bone facial injury should follow these sequential steps: First, the supraorbital ridges are palpated. Next, the infraorbital ridges are palpated using the examiner's first three fingers to determine symmetry or fracture. The zygomatic arches are then palpated. The infraorbital rims, zygomatic bodies, and maxilla are inspected from the top of the head and then palpated to determine depressions and/or displaced fractures. Next, the nasal bones and maxilla are examined for stability, and the nose is examined intranasally to determine septal placement. Occlusion is observed to determine dental relations. Finally, the mandible is palpated, then distracted to determine sites of discomfort and possible mandibular fracture. If a fracture is suspected or confirmed by radiographic film, then referral of the patient is in order.

Fractures of the mandible are most often caused by direct blow. Fracture is unusual in children but, when seen, most commonly occurs at the subcondyle. Other fracture sites include the angle of the jaw, symphyseal, and body of the mandible. Diagnosis is based on change in occlusion and pain or difficulty opening the mouth. If a fracture is suspected, the child should be referred to an otorhinolaryngologist or dental surgeon.

EAR

External Trauma

External trauma to the ears includes laceration, blunt injury, and thermal injury. Lacerations are common and may be treated in the same manner as lacerations in other areas of the body. Special care and consultation may be needed if there is extensive damage to the auricular cartilage. Blunt injury is typified by ecchymosis and hematoma. Ecchymosis is treated conservatively, but hematomas must be evacuated immediately because of the likelihood of damage to the cartilage. Treatment of burns and frostbite is described in the Chapter 108, Environmental Trauma.

Foreign Bodies

Foreign bodies in the external canal are extremely common and include stones, beads, paper, erasers, and, frequently, insects. Objects may be rolled out with an ear curet or grasped and removed with forceps. Irrigation of the ear with body temperature water is another useful method of removing these objects, provided that the object, such as a dry pea, will not absorb water and become more impacted. It must be noted that insects must be killed with alcohol or mineral oil before removal is attempted. Once the object is removed, the external canal should be treated with antibacterial otic suspension.

Trauma to Middle Ear

Trauma that results in injury to the tympanic membrane or structures of the middle ear must be referred to the otorhinolaryngologist. Minor abrasions along the external auditory canal may be cleansed by irrigation and treated with antibacterial otic suspension for 3 to 5 days.

BIBLIOGRAPHY

Castalano RA: Eye injuries and prevention, *Pediatr Clin North Am* 40:827–839, 1993.

Crouch ER Jr: Traumatic hyphema, *J Pediatr Ophthalmol Strabismus* 23:95–97, 1986.

Levin AV: Eye emergencies: Acute management in the pediatric ambulatory care setting, *Pediatr Emerg Care* 7:367–377, 1991.

Luyk NH, Ferguson JW: The diagnosis and initial management of the fractured mandible, *Am J Emerg Med* 9:352–359, 1991.

McDonald TJ: Nosebleed in children: Background and techniques to stop the flow, *Postgrad Med* 81:217–224, 1987.

Potsic WP, Handler SD: Otorhinolaryngology emergencies. In Fleisher G, Ludwig S, editors: *Textbook of pediatric emergency medicine,* ed 3, Baltimore, 1993, Williams & Wilkins.

CHAPTER 106

Dental Trauma

Mark L. Helpin
Evaline A. Alessandrini

Physicians, nurses, and other health care providers are often the first to see children with injuries to the teeth or mouth. It is therefore important for them to be able to evaluate these injuries thoroughly and provide emergency care. The objective of this chapter is to describe information to familiarize nondental personnel with the diagnosis and treatment of such injuries. This knowledge becomes even more valuable when health care providers work with their dental colleagues to offer optimal care for injured children.

ANATOMY

Enamel is the outermost layer of the tooth. It is variable in thickness and covers the surface of the tooth crown. It has no innervation from the dental pulp, and, because it has no blood supply or viable cells, it cannot regenerate itself. It is the hardest calcified substance in the body (Fig. 106-1).

Dentin is the second layer of the tooth and comprises the bulk of tooth structure. It is found under the enamel and cementum and covers the pulp. It is innervated and does contain viable cells (odontoblasts), which can form some secondary inner layers of dentin next to the pulp. These cells cannot, however, regenerate outer layers of dentin next to the enamel.

Pulp tissue is the soft tissue contained within the hard body of the tooth. It consists of blood and lymph vessels, nerve fibers, fibroblasts, connective tissue, and defense cells.

Cementum is the hard tissue covering the dentin on the root. Its purpose is to provide a medium for the tooth to attach itself to bone.

EPIDEMIOLOGY

Injuries to primary teeth occur in 30% of children. The prevalence of trauma to primary teeth is approximately equal for boys and girls. Most injuries in primary teeth occur in toddlers, who are learning to walk but are not yet well coordinated. Injury may occur from falls onto the floor, from a chair, or from bumps into furniture. They also occur in motor vehicle collisions. Health care providers also should be aware that 50% of abused children suffer injuries to the head or neck region. Tears of the frenulum may be an important indicator of child abuse in the young patient population because they may be due to forceful pushing of bottles into infants' mouths. The maxillary incisors are the most frequently traumatized primary teeth. Trauma to primary teeth most often causes a displacement type of injury within the alveolar socket rather than tooth fracture. This result is due to the soft, spongy nature of the alveolar bone in which the primary teeth sit.

Injuries to permanent teeth occur in 20% of children, with boys becoming injured twice as often as girls. Most of these injuries occur due to falls during play or contact sports. Peak ages of injuries to permanent teeth are between the ages of 10 to 11 years. In teenagers, motor vehicle collisions are also a cause of injury to the permanent teeth. Because the alveolar bone has matured in older children, injuries to permanent teeth are more often fractures of tooth structure rather than displacement types of injuries. The maxillary incisors are, again, the teeth that are most frequently involved.

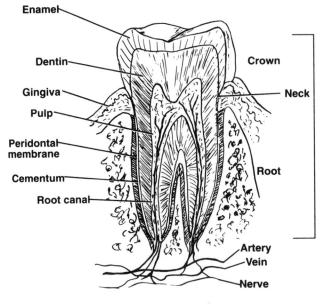

Enamel
Dentin
Gingiva
Pulp
Peridontal membrane
Cementum
Root canal
Crown
Neck
Root
Artery
Vein
Nerve

FIG 106-1
Anatomical structures of the tooth.

EVALUATION OF MEDICAL STATUS

Assessment of the child's general health status must always be addressed first. In the acutely injured child, evaluation of airway, breathing, circulation, and disability must supersede evaluation of dental injuries. A thorough medical history must be elicited, because the child's dental treatment may be influenced by underlying medical conditions. For example, children with cardiac defects or illnesses causing immunosuppression often will require antibiotic therapy or other modifications to routine care. Immunization status, particularly tetanus vaccination, also must be determined.

A complete physical examination of the head and neck must be performed. During the oral examination, the health care provider should make an effort to determine if any tooth or piece of tooth is missing. If the tooth has not been located, then the missing piece should be searched for in the soft tissue of the lips, cheeks, or tongue. The need for radiographic survey of the chest or soft tissue must be considered if missing pieces, or whole teeth, cannot be found.

EVALUATION OF DENTAL STATUS

Lacerations (Intraoral and Extraoral)

When treating intra- and extraoral lacerations, care should be taken to examine lips, tongue, buccal mucosa, and gingiva. Although intraoral lacerations often heal rapidly, especially in the young child, debridement of these wounds and placement of sutures should always be considered. However, placement might be delayed until after necessary dental treatment has been delivered. Recall that if portions of teeth are missing, they may be lodged in the oral tissues. Care also should be taken to ensure that lip and tongue lacerations are not through-and-through, because they will require different treatment than that of a simple laceration. Extraoral facial lacerations should be evaluated and a determination made regarding the need for consultation with a plastic surgeon.

Fracture of Facial Bones

Fractures of the mandible in children usually occur in the neck of the condyle. Falls onto the apex of the chin place the condylar region at great risk for such fractures. They are most often greenstick in nature and rarely require treatment.

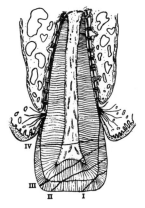

FIG 106-2
Classification of tooth fracture.

The physician should assess the child for pain, asymmetry, or difficulty with mouth opening. Palpation of the condyles themselves, by placing fingers anterior to the tragus or in the external auditory meatus, also might reveal asymmetric movement, pain, or step-off of the mandible. Mandibular fractures also should be suspected if there is malocclusion or a swelling hematoma under the tongue. The ability to move bony segments of the mandible also will help to determine the diagnosis of a fracture.

Facial fractures also are suggested by depression in portions of the face and orbits. If a facial fracture is suspected, the child should be evaluated for numbness of the lips, cheeks, or infraorbital areas. Radiographic examinations of the face, including a dental panographic exposure, may assist greatly in the diagnosis of many facial fractures.

Fractures of the alveolar bone, the bone immediately surrounding and supporting the teeth, can be determined if a segment is noted to be displaced. If force on the dental arch causes movement of a portion of the arch itself or the teeth within the arch, a more subtle fracture may be diagnosed.

Occlusion (Bite)

When the child closes his/her teeth fully, the physician should check to see if the teeth interdigitate maximally and comfortably. He/she also should check if any displaced teeth prevent the jaw from closing normally. If the patient is old enough to understand, the child should be asked if the bite feels the same as before or if it feels different. If the bite feels different, reevaluation of previously examined areas should be performed to determine the cause.

Tooth Mobility

Mobility is evaluated by applying digital pressure alternately on the buccal and lingual (front and back) sides of a tooth. Subluxation injuries are those injuries resulting in tooth loosening without displacement. A child's primary teeth will begin to fall out normally between 5 and 7 years of age, and excessive mobility may not be secondary to trauma.

Tooth Displacement

Evaluation of whether or not a tooth is in its pretrauma position is performed by comparing it with other teeth, and by asking the patient or accompanying family member how the teeth and alignment appear to them. The most serious displacements are those that prevent the child from closing the mandible normally. Tooth displacement within the alveolar socket is also known as a *luxation injury*. There are four common directions of luxation injuries: 1) intrusion (into the alveolar bone); 2) extrusion (partially out of the alveolar bone); 3) lingual (in toward the tongue); and 4) buccal (out toward the lip). Complete removal of the entire tooth root and crown from the alveolar bone is known as *tooth avulsion*.

TOOTH FRACTURES

A simplified classification permits the health care provider to evaluate and describe tooth fractures (Fig. 106-2). A class I fracture involves only enamel. It generally is not very large and is rarely sensitive, because no dentin is involved. Although the fractured tooth structure itself does not have normal form and anatomy (compared with the contralateral tooth), it does have the same color all over its surface. A class II fracture involves both enamel and dentin. This fracture usually involves a greater loss of tooth structure than in a class I fracture. The dentin here appears slightly yellow. With deeper class II fractures there may be an area with a pinkish hue, which is caused by the pulp showing through the thin layer of dentin left over it. A class III fracture involves a small portion of the pulp tissue, observable as a bleeding spot. This fracture is usually quite sensitive. A class IV fracture involves a large part of tooth structure, and a great deal of the clinical crown will be missing. A large exposure of the pulp will be noted. Fractures of the root are often difficult to diagnose and most often require the expertise of a dentist.

MANAGEMENT OF INJURIES

When considering treatment of injuries to primary teeth, the health care provider should be aware that the risk of damage to an associated permanent tooth also must be weighed. Injury to a primary tooth affects not only that tooth but also can cause problems for the permanent tooth that is developing in the nearby alveolar bone.

Subluxation, Luxation, and Avulsion

Dental concussion (injury without loosening or displacement) rarely requires treatment. This injury is diagnosed when percussion of a nonmobile traumatized tooth causes pain. It should be evaluated by a dentist within several days because the trauma can cause pulpal damage and eventual abscess formation.

Treatment for subluxation is based on the degree of mobility the tooth demonstrates. Extremely mobile primary teeth will probably need to be removed to prevent aspiration. A slightly mobile tooth will most likely revert to strong fixation in a short time, however, splinting by a dentist may be necessary. If a child cannot cooperate enough for splint placement, the involved teeth may be carefully observed for a period of time. Permanent teeth that demonstrate severe mobility should be splinted by a dentist. Treatment of concussion and subluxation injuries includes several days of a soft diet and pain medication.

Treatment of intrusion (movement of the tooth into the alveolus) is very different in primary and secondary teeth. Ninety percent of primary teeth reerupt within 6 months without intervention and require only observation during this period. On the other hand, permanent teeth rarely re-erupt on their own. They usually need to be surgically repositioned either immediately or during several weeks of orthodontic therapy. Mature intruded permanent teeth will be strong candidates for endodontic (root canal) therapy.

Treatment of extrusion or lingual and buccal luxation displacement injuries is based on the presence or absence of interference with occlusion and tooth mobility. When there is interference with occlusion and a child cannot close the mouth normally, then treatment by a dentist is necessary. Teeth should be repositioned and splinted when possible. Primary teeth that are severely extruded or luxated are usually extracted in order to minimize risk of harm to the developing permanent tooth.

Treatment for avulsed primary and secondary teeth is, again, quite different. Avulsed primary teeth are not replanted. Permanent teeth should be replanted as quickly as possible. If this cannot be done at the place of injury or in the home, then the tooth should be brought to the physician's office, emergency department, or dentist's office in a transport medium. Hank's balanced salt solution (available in prepackaged kits called Save-a-Tooth), milk, or saliva are preferable transport media. Saline or water are less desirable. Extraoral time is critical to the survival of an avulsed tooth. Prognosis is best when replantation is completed within 30 minutes of the injury. To replant a permanent tooth, the clot should be aspirated, not scraped, out of the alveolar socket and then the tooth replaced using firm pressure. The tooth itself, especially the root, should only be very gently rinsed or cleansed of debris. It should not be rubbed or placed in disinfectant. After the tooth is in its original position, the alveolar bone should be compressed around it. A dentist should then place a splint. Antibiotics, usually penicillin or amoxicillin, and a pain medication such as acetaminophen should be prescribed for 7 to 10 days. The patient should be instructed to eat only a soft diet. Depending on the stage of root development, permanent teeth that have been avulsed may need endodontic therapy.

BOX 106-1
Timing of Dental Referral

Immediate
Class III or IV tooth fractures
Avulsed permanent teeth
Luxation injuries with malocclusion or significant
    tooth mobility
Urgent (within 48 hr)
Class II tooth fractures
Tooth subluxation
Nonurgent (within 1 week)
Class I tooth fractures
Avulsed primary teeth
Tooth concussion

Tooth Fractures

Class I fractures most often require only minimal emergency treatment. Sharp edges should be filed until smooth to prevent soft-tissue injury. Cosmetic restoration of missing enamel can be performed at a later time.

Class II fractures require urgent dental referral so that the sharp edges can be smoothed and the dentin and pulp can be protected. This is most often achieved by the dentist placing a composite "bandage" (covering) and special dental materials over the involved dentin. If the exposed dentin is sensitive to air, then placement of a warm saline or water-soaked gauze over the tooth will help make the child more comfortable until dental referral.

Class III and IV fractures require immediate dental referral (Box 106-1) to minimize contamination of the exposed pulp tissue. Significant crown fractures in primary teeth might require extraction.

Regardless of the depth of the fracture, placement of moist gauze can make the child more comfortable than if the tooth is simply left exposed to the air and to oral fluids.

Soft-Tissue Injury

Lacerations of gingiva and oral mucosa may require suturing, depending on their size and the approximation and stability of the wound edges. Suturing of these tissues is often delayed until definitive treatment of the teeth is completed. Suturing of the lip and tongue after through-and-through laceration is done following thorough debridement of the wound to avoid foreign body contamination and infections. Repair of lip and tongue lacerations may require deep as well as superficial layers of suturing. Again, the necessity for this treatment depends on the size and approximation and stability of wound edges. Oral suturing is usually performed using 3-0 or 4-0 chromic gut suture. Antibiotic coverage with oral penicillin or amoxicillin for 5 to 7 days is recommended.

Bone

If there is a comminuted fracture of the alveolar bone, splinting of the teeth by a dentist can optimize healing. Splinting primary teeth, however, can be very difficult because of dental anatomic considerations and the child's ability to tolerate splint placement. Extractions often are performed for a segmental fracture of the alveolus involving only primary teeth. If segmental alveolar fractures involve permanent teeth, the segment will need to be repositioned and a dental splint placed. Acid-etch resin splints are now preferable to wire and/or arch bar splints because they are so much kinder to the teeth and soft tissues.

Fractures of the maxilla and mandible are not considered simple dental injuries and should be treated in conjunction with an oral and maxillofacial surgeon or other surgical service.

SUMMARY

Prevention of dental injuries should be of importance to all health care providers. Encouraging and endorsing the use of mouth guards and facial protection will do much to prevent oral injuries and improve the general health status of children. Health care providers should remember that initial management of dental injury effects the long-term prognosis for the child. However, treatment of the emergency situation itself is only the first step in care because damage secondary to dental trauma often takes months or years to become evident. Long-term follow-up with a dentist is, therefore, an important component of good comprehensive care for children. Special dental radiographs will be important to diagnose accurately the extent of the dental injuries. Many, but not all, dentists will be comfortable managing patients with traumatic oral injuries.

BIBLIOGRAPHY

Andreasen JO, Andreasen FM: *Essentials of traumatic injuries to the teeth,* Copenhagen, 1990, Munksgaard.

Krasner P, Person P: Preserving avulsed teeth for replantation, *J Am Dent Assoc* 123:80–88, 1992.

Mathewson RJ, Primosch RE: *Fundamentals of pediatric dentistry,* ed 3, Chicago, 1995, Quintessence.

McDonald RE, Avery DR: *Dentistry for the child and adolescent,* ed 6, St. Louis, 1994, CV Mosby.

Pinkham JR: *Pediatric dentistry, infancy through adolescents,* ed 2, Philadelphia, 1994, WB Saunders.

Ravn JJ: Sequelae of acute mechanical traumata in the primary dentition, *J Dent Child* 35:281–289, 1968.

Sicher H: *Orban's oral histology and embryology,* ed 11, St. Louis, 1991, CV Mosby.

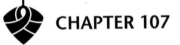

CHAPTER 107

Orthopedic Trauma

Henry H. Sherk
Robert S. Cummings

Children with a complaint of musculoskeletal pain and a history of injury comprise a large group of patients brought to the office of the primary care physician. Because of the frequency with which such patients are seen and the commonness of the diagnoses with which they present, there is a tendency to label such patients as "routine" and proceed rather quickly and automatically along a line of investigation and treatment. However, such children require not only a full awareness of the diagnostic possibilities on the part of the physician but also a careful diagnostic evaluation. Without an organized approach to the assessment of an injured child, one can either miss important injuries or order unnecessary studies, prolong the evaluation, and possibly overtreat.

The child with physical findings that are suggestive of injury and confirmed radiographically requires treatment, not decision-making. If, however, the child has no physical findings, the physician must decide whether the complaint and severity of injury justify radiography, whether symptomatic treatment should be given, and whether additional evaluation is indicated should the symptoms persist. If the patient has positive physical findings and radiographs reveal no musculoskeletal injury, the physician must make similar decisions regarding symptomatic treatment and the need for additional evaluation. A child with musculoskeletal pain and no history of injury requires an assessment that may lead to a wide variety of diagnostic considerations. In such an individual, examination and radiography can very quickly establish the diagnosis of an occult fracture or a dislocation. If, however, there are no abnormal physical findings and if radiographs reveal no musculoskeletal injury,

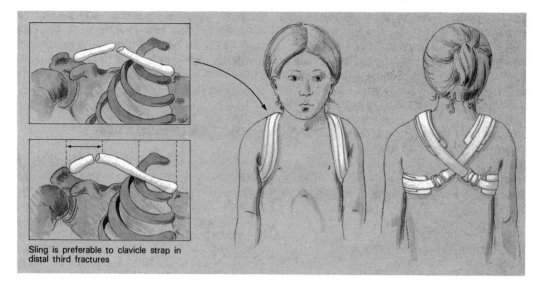

Sling is preferable to clavicle strap in distal third fractures

FIG 107-1
The method for applying a "figure-8" bandage to a fractured clavicle.

one must be alert to the possibility of developmental abnormalities such as the osteochondroses or more serious diseases such as an infection or tumor.

This chapter deals with the common minor fractures, dislocations, sprains, and benign developmental conditions seen in office practice. In each section specific entities (*ie,* upper limb, lower limb) are reviewed with regard to data gathering and management.

FRACTURES OF THE CLAVICLE

One of the most common injuries in children is a fracture of the clavicle. In older children the diagnosis is usually unmistakable on clinical examination, but in infants and very young children it may be less obvious. Overriding of bone fragments, severe swelling, ecchymosis, local tenderness, crepitus, and drooping of the shoulder on the affected side lead the physician to the diagnosis. At times, this symptom complex allows the child and parent to make the diagnosis before the injured patient is brought to the physician for treatment of the "broken collar bone." However, in greenstick fractures the findings are more subtle, because there may be no deformity and very little swelling. The patient may permit passive motion but more often is fretful and has a pseudoparalysis due to pain when mobilization of the shoulder is attempted. Radiographs, of course, establish the diagnosis in doubtful cases and confirm it in more obvious situations.

Treatment is gratifying in almost every case. Children under 6 or 7 years of age require no reduction even if the fracture is displaced. Symptoms resolve quickly over a period of 2 weeks, with a clavicle strap or a posterior figure-of-8 bandage (Fig. 107-1). In infants, even this degree of support may be unnecessary, particularly if there is minimal displacement of the fracture. One can expect rapid union of the fragments and obliteration of the deformity noted on radiography as remodeling and remolding take place with further growth. Older children may require a longer period of support with the bandage until discomfort subsides and union occurs. Reduction is rarely necessary and is difficult to maintain, so that even strikingly comminuted displaced clavicle fractures can be expected to heal well.

Congenital pseudoarthrosis of the clavicle is probably not related to trauma and rarely causes enough deformity, functional impairment, or discomfort to justify surgery. Patients most often request surgery for cosmetic reasons, but the postoperative scarring and frequent recurrence rate make cosmesis an inadequate indication for surgical treatment.

An interesting, though unusual, variant of a clavicle fracture is an epiphyseal separation at the proximal end of the clavicle at the sternoclavicular joint. It is recognizable clinically as swelling and tenderness at the medial end of the clavicle after an injury. Because of the late ossification of the proximal clavicular epiphysis (at the age of 17 years), the diagnosis is difficult to make with radiographs. Treatment should be as conservative as possible with local adhesive strapping and a posterior figure-of-8 bandage for support.

FRACTURES OF THE PROXIMAL HUMERUS

Some dislocations of the shoulder are rare in young children. The patient under 7 years of age with swelling and pain about the shoulder probably has a transverse fracture of the proximal humerus just below the lesser tuberosity. From the age of 7 years to adolescence, shoulder injuries are usually epiphyseal separations, and after adolescence patients usually sustain shoulder dislocations or acromioclavicular separations. Fractures of the proximal humerus in very young children have a propensity to unite quickly, even in the face of bayonet apposition or even a moderate degree of angulation. In an office setting, it is possible to treat such patients with a Velpeau dressing or sugar-tong plaster splints with an excellent chance of satisfactory healing. The bone deformity can be expected to remodel well over a period of several months.

Displaced epiphyseal fractures in older children, on the other hand, probably require more aggressive treatment than can be provided on an outpatient basis. Such patients may require anesthesia for reduction, plaster support in the "salute position," or overhead traction to maintain alignment. Rarely, a patient with this type of injury may need open reduction to disengage the biceps tendon when it is trapped between the fragments. In patients who have minimal deformity, however, the outpatient setting may suffice, and a Velpeau dressing or shoulder spica cast can secure sufficient immobilization to permit uncomplicated healing. Malunion of this type of fracture results in anterior angulation of the humerus just below the humeral head. Patients

with this type of residual deformity have limited shoulder flexion and if outpatient treatment seems suitable for a given individual, adequate follow-up radiographs must be taken frequently in the early stages of treatment to prevent this complication.

SHOULDER DISLOCATIONS

Shoulder dislocations occur infrequently in young children and are uncommon until adolescence. Nevertheless, in an outpatient practice youthful athletes often present with this type of injury and may benefit from prompt treatment by the primary care physician. Recognition of the injury is not difficult. Patients have severe pain with an acute shoulder dislocation, and the appearance of the affected shoulder is obviously different even to the untrained eye. The acromion is very prominent. Often the head of the humerus is visible and palpable beneath the corocoid process, and the shoulder has a square appearance, lacking the normal roundness of the deltoid muscle.

Before undertaking treatment, a radiograph is essential. If the radiograph reveals no fracture, the primary physician often can treat the patient's severe shoulder pain by reducing the dislocation promptly. Some sedation may be necessary in heavy muscular adolescents, but longitudinal traction against the countertraction of a sheet passed under the axilla can very often achieve reduction without resorting to general anesthesia. If manipulation does fail, anesthesia may be necessary to permit the reduction.

Following a first episode of shoulder dislocation, in adolescent patients recurrent dislocation of the shoulder is a frequent complication. Prolonged support in a sling and swath or shoulder immobilizer may minimize the possibility of a recurrence, and young patients with this injury should be restricted in this way for 4 to 6 weeks. The external support should allow the anterior ligaments, capsule, and subscapularis muscle to heal such that these anatomic structures will be competent enough to prevent another episode. Before the external support is withdrawn completely, the patient should carry out a program of range of motion and muscle-strengthening exercises. It should be noted that adult patients do not require prolonged support after an initial shoulder dislocation because the older age groups have a low incidence of recurrence but a high incidence of shoulder stiffness after this type of injury. Older patients can begin the exercise program immediately, using a sling only for comfort for a few days.

FRACTURES OF THE SHAFT OF THE HUMERUS

Fractures of the shaft of the humerus in newborns may be the result of a difficult delivery, but in infants and young children the presence of this type of fracture suggests parental abuse or at least a direct blow to the upper arm. Falls in young patients usually result in fractures of the wrist, forearm, or shoulder, and not the shaft of the humerus.

Fractures of the humeral shaft have an excellent prognosis and heal promptly with the Velpeau wrap-around dressing in infants or with a sugar-tong splint in older children.

INJURIES ABOUT THE ELBOW

The most serious bony injury of the upper limb is a supracondylar fracture of the humerus. This fracture is not generally suitable for office treatment, and, in general, most patients with this injury should be admitted to the hospital. Patients with displaced supracondylar fractures have intense discomfort, severe swelling, and obvious vascular compromise so that there is usually little debate over the need for prompt emergency treatment in a hospital setting.

Other types of elbow injuries, however, also may have major potential for causing long-range impairment but may present less dramatically. Hence, they may receive less attention and possibly go unrecognized and untreated. The most significant injury in this regard is a fracture through the capitellum. It is well known that this fracture fails to unite unless open reduction and pin fixation achieve and maintain a virtually perfect alignment. Even minor degrees of displacement permit the capitellar fragment to migrate and fail to heal. Nonunion of the capitellum causes the distal fragment to migrate proximally and, in turn, the elbow develops a valgus deformity traction neuropathy, with stretching of the ulnar nerve and late degenerative arthritis of the elbow. Patients with fractures through the capi-

tellum, therefore, require recognition by the primary physician and referral for definitive treatment.

Other elbow injuries seen commonly in patients in ambulatory care settings are fractures of the radial head and medial humeral epicondylar fractures. Treatment of these injuries should be as conservative as possible. Radial neck fractures can be permitted up to 30° of angulation before requiring open reduction (never an excision, as in adults), and medial humeral epicondylar fractures need open reduction only if they are displaced into the elbow joint or if they are so displaced as to compromise the ulnar nerve as it passes posteriorly behind the medial humerus. In general, both of these fractures—radial neck and medial humeral epicondyle—can be treated with splinting for 4 weeks before permitting active motion. If in doubt, however, the primary care physician should refer the child for consultation and discussion of the possible need for open reduction.

Elbow dislocation may occur without fracture but before manipulating the injury, radiographs must be obtained to rule out the presence of a complicating bone injury. If one establishes the fact that the patient's pain, deformity, swelling, and ecchymosis are solely related to dislocation of the elbow joint, the primary care physician might consider reduction with traction with the elbow at a right angle. Reduction of a dislocated elbow in a child is usually easily done, and only in older patients might anesthesia be required. After reduction the physician should protect the elbow in a splint for 3 to 4 weeks before removing support and permitting active use of the elbow joint.

Pure dislocations of the elbow, however, are rare in children, and one should be on the lookout for associated fractures of the medial epicondyle, radial neck, capitellum, and olecranon. In general, complex elbow injuries require specialized care and should be referred from the primary care setting.

NURSEMAID'S ELBOW

A common minor elbow injury in children is the pulled elbow, nursemaid's elbow, or radial head subluxation. The lesion is usually present in young children and results from pulling the child vigorously by the wrist or hand. The mechanism of the injury is longitudinal traction applied while the arm is in pronation. This action pulls the radial head part way out of the encircling annular ligament. Part of the annular ligament thus is caught between the radial head and the capitellum. When traction is released, the annular ligament remains in that location and prevents the forearm from returning to a supinated and fully extended position. The child refuses to move the arm and complains of pain in the elbow. Radiographs are normal. One can reduce the subluxation usually by supinating the forearm and extending the elbow slightly. Occasionally one can feel a click or snap as this is done. Young children cry loudly when the elbow is reduced, so that it may be wise to carry out the procedure after warning an apprehensive parent about what will happen. When the reduction is achieved, the pain disappears quickly, and the child will begin moving the arm rather freely. Recurrence of the subluxation is not unusual, but, despite this, support with a sling for a week seems all that is required in the way of postreduction treatment. Most young children will not conform to the sling once the reduction is achieved. After the second or third recurrence, the child may require immobilization in a long arm cast. Nursemaid's elbow is not seen in children over 4 or 5 years of age.

FOREARM AND WRIST INJURIES

The primary care physician can and should be involved in the treatment of forearm and wrist injuries. Because some injuries are more complex, the physician should have a working knowledge of the types of injuries encountered and realize which injuries will need more aggressive treatment than is possible to provide in an office setting.

In a primary care setting minimally displaced fractures often can be treated successfully simply by immobilization. The physician should have adequate skill in applying the cast, remembering to apply plaster smoothly and evenly over adequate padding and making sure it is well molded over bony prominences. Casts should not be circular or tubular but should be contoured to follow the cross-sectional configuration of a limb. Patients should have adequate checks after the cast has been applied for evaluation of neurovascular status, and they should have careful follow-up with serial radiography to rule out late displacement. In general, patients with displaced forearm and wrist fractures should be considered for referral because reduction may require anesthesia.

Classification of Forearm and Wrist Fractures
- Distal third fractures of the radius or ulna
  Greenstick
  Displaced
- Shaft fractures of the radius or ulna
  Greenstick
  Displaced
- Epiphyseal fractures of the distal radius, with or without involvement of the distal ulna
- Fracture dislocations
  Monteggia
  Galeazzi

Fractures of the Distal Third of the Forearm
Angulation of the distal end of a bone readily self-corrects with growth in young children and up to 30° of deformity is acceptable in children under 6 years of age. In these injuries the treating physician would be justified in applying a long arm cast without manipulation. In undisplaced fractures and "buckle fractures" a short arm cast will suffice.

In patients with severely angulated greenstick fractures or displaced fractures of the distal third of the radius and/or ulna, reduction is considered necessary. Remodeling and remolding might eliminate deformity with time in young children, but angulation of 30° or more might result in a permanent deformity and thus should be corrected if possible. A gentle manipulation (with the patient under sedation or with local anesthesia injected into the hematoma) might be attempted in greenstick fractures, but displaced fractures of the distal third of the forearm are more difficult to reduce and often require more vigorous treatment. This type of treatment usually requires general anesthesia. The fracture should be immobilized after manipulation in pronation and slight flexion.

Shaft Fractures of the Forearm
Greenstick fractures develop progressive deformity and angulate rather markedly if not treated correctly. One must break through the intact cortex on the side of the bone away from the

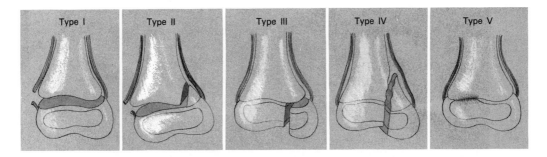

FIG 107-2
Salter Harris classification of epiphyseal fractures.

fracture and then reduce the malalignment prior to casting. It is possible to engage in this type of treatment in a primary care setting but usually results are better and the entire situation less stressful for the patient if the manipulation is done under general anesthesia.

Complete and displaced fractures of the forearm also require suitable analgesia and adequate reduction to avoid permanent deformity and for these reasons are best splinted by the primary care physician and referred for definitive treatment.

Epiphyseal Fractures

Epiphyseal separations to the distal radius can occur above or in conjunction with a fracture of the distal ulna. Minimal displacement requires no reduction, but patients should be immobilized in a long arm cast for 5 or 6 weeks (Fig. 107-2). Patients with displaced epiphyseal separations present more serious problems. Vigorous manipulation or delayed manipulation may so damage the epiphyseal plate that growth arrest occurs and patients may develop a significant radial shortening. Therefore, patients with this type of injury are, in general, not good candidates for treatment in a primary care setting.

Fracture Dislocations

Fracture dislocations of the forearm are complex injuries that usually involve a fracture of a shaft of one bone and dislocation of the radial head or distal ulna. In the Monteggia fracture and its variants, the radial head is dislocated and the ulna fractured. In the Galeazzi fracture the distal radioulnar joint is separated and the distal radius is fractured. In general, these fractures may present more difficulty in treatment than the primary care physician would want to accept. It is essential, however, that one make the diagnosis, a requirement that mandates radiographs with views of the ends of the bones as well as their midshafts. In addition, one should suspect a diagnosis of a dislocation in a fracture of a single bone of the forearm.

HAND INJURIES

Hand injuries in children usually consist of finger fractures and fingertip injuries, although teenagers occasionally present with fractures of the carpal navicular. The severe industrial cases—the cornpicker injuries and crush injuries with clothes wringers—are now much less common in small children. Most minor hand injuries are suitable for care in the primary setting, provided that the physician recognizes several common pitfalls.

For example, fractures of the proximal phalanx at or just distal to the epiphyseal plate occur very frequently and usually are minimally displaced. Such fractures can be treated by "buddy taping" or strapping with adhesive the injured finger to an adjacent digit. The same type of treatment is also suitable for undisplaced fractures of the shaft of a phalanx. In treating fractures of the phalanges, one should remember not to immobilize only one digit and one should avoid rotational malalignment. The physician should ask the patient to flex all four fingers while looking at the hand from the volar direction. All four fingertips should come together to point to the proximal part of the carpal navicular. If rotational malalignment is not corrected, the involved finger will not do this and will overlap an adjacent finger.

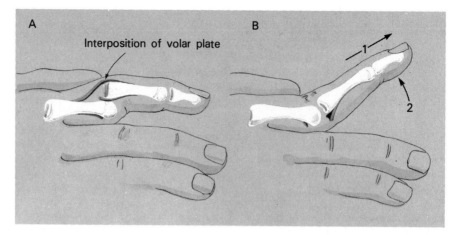

A

Interposition of volar plate

B

1

2

FIG 107-3
Technique for the repositioning of a dislocated finger.

Fractures of the fifth metacarpal usually result from fighting. They merit only very conservative treatment; even if the child or young adolescent maintains a considerable degree of angulation at the fracture site, the functional result will be good. These injuries should be treated with volar splints for 3 or 4 weeks until union is sufficient to permit normal activities.

Fractures of the condylar parts of the phalanges and fractures of the distal phalanx of a digit may not be amenable to treatment in the primary care setting. Displaced condylar fractures can leave the child with permanently angulated fingers unless the fracture is openly reduced and pinned. Fractures of the tendinous insertions of the extensor digitorum communis on the base of the distal phalanx can leave the child with a permanent mallet finger unless splinted in hyperextension. Such fractures may also require pin fixation to prevent deformity but usually splinting in extension is sufficient. In young children a mallet finger deformity is usually caused by an epiphyseal separation. In adolescents the deformity results from a fracture through the epiphysis into the growth plate.

Dislocation of the metacarpal-phalangeal joint may not permit reduction by closed means because the joint capsule and flexor tendon can become interposed between the distal end of the metacarpal and proximal part of the proximal phalanx (Fig. 107-3). If one or two gentle attempts do not achieve reduction of this type of injury, open surgical reduction should be carried out as soon as possible. This reduction is accomplished by splitting the interposed volar plate and retrieving the displaced tendon.

Tendon lacerations and open fractures should be referred from the primary setting for definitive treatment in a hospital.

LOWER LIMB INJURIES

Fractures of the pelvis, hip fractures, femoral shaft fractures, and epiphyseal separations about the knee are all major injuries that probably would not involve the primary care physician. These injuries require hospitalization and prolonged care in a hospital setting. Some undisplaced tibial shaft fractures in young children may be treatable with splinting or cast fixation in the office, but, in general, patients with significant long bone fractures in the lower limb require hospitalization.

AVULSION FRACTURES OF THE PELVIS

Major fractures of the pelvic ring usually result from severe injury, but the primary care physician may be called on to treat avulsion fractures of the pelvis. These occur in immature adolescents who with vigorous muscle contraction avulse a muscle origin. The anterior superior and anterior inferior iliac spines are common sites of injury, with avulsion of the origins of the sartorius and rectus femorus, respectively. The hamstring muscles, in addition, avulse the ischial tuberosity. The patients usually have a good deal of swelling, ecchymosis, and pain, and there is little chance that the physician will not order a radiograph to establish the diagnosis because the patients have such an acute clinical picture. Treatment with bed rest, analgesics, and an ice bag usually suffices. These patients can most often be treated at home after the diagnosis has been made. It usually takes 2 months for the fractures to heal sufficiently to permit a return to regular activities.

KNEE INJURIES

Knee injuries in children are generally different from those seen in adult patients. The torn menisci and ruptured cruciate and collateral ligaments of the adolescent and older athlete are much less common in young patients. The bone-cartilage interface of the epiphyseal plate is the weakest component of the knee in children. In young adults, the epiphyseal plates have closed and the bone is young and very strong. In children, therefore, a major stress on the knee will most likely cause an epiphyseal separation, whereas in a young adult the same step will produce a ligamentous tear. In elderly patients with osteoporosis, the same injury will probably produce a tibial plateau fracture. The implications of the foregoing are that in children internal derangements of the knee are unusual, and a child suspected of having one more likely has an epiphyseal separation. This type of injury may require more aggressive diagnostic measures and treatment than can be provided in the office setting. The injuries that occur in such cases are fractures of the tibial spines, epiphyseal separations of the distal femur or proximal tibia, and intraarticular fractures of the femoral condyles.

Patellar fractures and dislocations, however, may not require more specialized care than is available in the outpatient setting. Acute dislocations of the patella can be reduced and immobilized by the primary care physician. If adequate radiographs including tangential views have established the fact that no osteochondral fracture fragments are loose in the joint, then support in plaster for a few weeks should let the soft tissues heal satisfactorily. Patients should, of course, restore quadriceps and hamstring

strength with an exercise program before resuming athletics. If an osteochondral fragment is loose in the joint, it should be removed.

Recurrent subluxations and dislocations may require surgical correction. Fractures of the patella do not occur very often in children, and it is easy to mistake a bipartite patella (a congenital lesion) for an injury. Fractures of the patella in children may require open reduction and should probably be referred for consideration of that possibility.

TIBIAL STRESS FRACTURES

Stress fractures of the tibia are often not recognized as such, and as a diagnostic problem, they may prove troublesome. They usually cause pain in the lower leg that is associated with a good deal of local tenderness. Patients often have negative findings on radiographs at first. With passing time, a radiograph will reveal hazy callus forming external to the tibia at the level of a transverse radiolucent line. The appearance of the radiograph also may suggest a tumor of bone or an early infection. A bone scan is positive in all three conditions so that the true diagnosis occasionally can only be inferred. Treatment with reduction of activities, weight bearing with crutches, and analgesics usually permits healing to occur with minimal discomfort. An occasional patient may require a long leg cast.

ANKLE FRACTURES

Some ankle fractures can be treated quite successfully by the primary care physician. Undisplaced fractures of the distal fibula, for example, respond well to 3 or 4 weeks of support in plaster and can be treated quite successfully in the office. The caveat here, however, is the recognition of the fact that children—especially young children—do not often "sprain" their ankles, and swelling and pain of the lateral ankle in this age group is probably a minimally displaced fracture of the distal fibula through the epiphyseal plate.

The pitfalls to be avoided in treating ankle injuries in children are related to the Tillaux, triplane, and medial malleolar fractures. The primary care physician's responsibility in the management of this type of case is recognition, because these injuries may require open reduction for the best result. The Tillaux fracture occurs through the lateral part of the distal tibial epiphysis, and the lateral half of the epiphysis is displaced for various degrees from its normal position. If a Tillaux fracture is associated with a complete distal tibial separation with a retained metaphyseal spike (Salter II) (*see* Fig. 107-2), the injury is a triplane fracture. With such severe damage to the epiphyseal cartilage, growth arrest can occur and adequate reduction with internal fixation is necessary to minimize that complication. Medial malleolus fractures in children also have the potential for causing growth arrest, with subsequent varus deformity and shortening. This type of injury also probably requires at least consideration of open reduction and is best referred.

FOOT INJURIES

Injuries of the hindfoot are uncommon except for cases with major crushing injury. In children with a painful swollen ankle and a "normal" radiograph, however, one should be sure to look for an osteochondral fracture of the talus. This lesion is recognizable as a small fragment of bone at the edge of the superior surface of the talus, where it articulates with either the medial or lateral malleolus. Under most circumstances the fracture can be expected to heal with support in a non–weight-bearing short leg cast. Occasionally, however, the fragment may separate itself from the talus and become a loose body in the joint. Under these circumstances, the patient will require an arthrotomy of the joint for its removal.

Fractures of the os calcis in children are very unusual. They require only a compression dressing and elevation under most circumstances. Unless potential skin necrosis complicates the fracture, the primary care physician should be able to treat this patient on an outpatient basis.

Most of the children with foot injuries who present in an office setting have metatarsal fractures or phalangeal injuries. The fracture most often seen is at the base of the fifth metatarsal and is not to be confused with normal ossification of the epiphysis in that location. One can recognize the difference because in younger children the epiphyseal plate is disposed longitudinally. Fractures of the fifth metatarsal, however, are transverse. Metatarsal fractures in children heal promptly with a compression

dressing or short leg cast for 3 or 4 weeks. Older athletic adolescents may fracture the base of the fifth metatarsal repeatedly, however, and eventually develop nonunions. Surgical treatment may be necessary in established nonunions, and one should protect such individuals with casts for longer periods.

Fractures of the phalanges of the toes usually require little formal treatment. When undisplaced or minimally displaced, they can be supported with adhesive strips securing the toe to an adjacent digit. Angulated broken toes should be reduced by passive manipulation before taping the digit.

OSTEOCHONDROSES OF THE LOWER LIMB

The term *osteochondroses* refers to a group of conditions that occur during the juvenile period and are characterized by similar radiologic findings of increased density and fragmentation of an epiphyseal or apophyseal center. The epiphysis, which is located at the metaphyseal ends of long bones, is where bony growth is occurring, and the apophysis is the name given to the location where muscle or tendon attaches to the bone. Historically, the cause of the bone fragmentation has been attributed to avascular necrosis.

However, recent evidence indicates that many of these lesions—especially the apophyseal lesions—are actually due to abnormalities of enchondral ossification, possibly due to mechanical factors related to traction on the bone via the muscular attachment. Therefore, the osteochondroses are a radiologic classification and not an etiologic classification. There are very classic locations where this phenomenon occurs and each is identified by its own eponym. A brief description of each syndrome will follow.

In general, the patient presents with a history of progressive pain in a particular location. There is usually no history of a definite traumatic episode. Some patients may make reference to some minor traumatic event or date the onset of symptoms, but a good etiologic correlation or explanation is usually not confirmed. The pain generally is exacerbated with activities and subsides with rest. The management, which for the most part is always conservative, consists of various forms of immobilization, rest, and anti-inflammatory medications.

Freiberg Infarction (Osteochondrosis of the Metatarsal Head)

This lesion represents true avascular necrosis of a metatarsal head. It usually involves the second metatarsal head but occasionally involves one of the more lateral metatarsals and, rarely, the first metatarsal. On radiographs, there is the appearance of a crushed and fragmented distal metatarsal head. It more commonly occurs in individuals in whom the first metatarsal is shorter than the second, and increased stress from repetitive weight bearing has been implicated as an etiologic factor.

The typical patient is an adolescent who presents with localized pain and swelling of the involved metatarsal head. On physical examination, swelling and limitation of motion of the involved metatarsal phalangeal joint are noted. As stated previously, the findings on radiography are characteristic.

Treatment in the adolescent initially should always be conservative and nonoperative. Initial management should consist of recommending that the patient wear a low-heel shoe with a metatarsal bar or pad to redistribute the weight bearing away from the involved metatarsal and prescribing anti-inflammatory medication depending on the severity of symptoms. If the pain is severe or persists, then a short leg walking cast is used for 3 to 4 weeks. If this fails, a brief period of non–weight bearing with the aid of crutches is instituted until the symptoms resolve. If symptoms were to arise in a patient who is skeletally mature, then the treatment would be resection of the involved metatarsal head.

Köhler Disease (Osteochondrosis of the Tarsal Navicular)

Köhler disease is also a true avascular necrosis of the tarsal navicular. It is believed that repetitive compressive forces lead to fragmentation and loss of blood supply. The navicular bone occupies the apex of the longitudinal arch of the foot and is subjected to constant stress during weight bearing. It is also the last tarsal bone to ossify. The combination of late ossification and constant stress is believed to be the reason why the tarsal navicular is at risk for this particular problem. This theory is supported by the fact that Köhler disease is more common if tarsal navicular ossification is delayed. It is more common in boys because their navicular ossifies later than that of girls.

Typically, the patient presents with a history of progressive pain and swelling around the medial aspect of the midfoot in the region of the tarsal navicular. The average age of onset for this phenomenon is 4 years in girls and 5 years in boys. Physical examination reveals pain and swelling of the tarsal navicular. Two variations on radiography should be noted: the tarsal navicular may either appear as a thin wafer of bone with patchy increased density suggestive of collapse or may appear normal in size and shape with minimal fragmentation but definite uniform increase in density compared with surrounding tarsal bones.

Treatment is again symptomatic. First, treatment with an arch support and restriction of activities is instituted. If the pain persists, a short leg walking cast is applied, and usually the pain subsides within 4 weeks. Refractory cases can be treated with guarded weight bearing with either a pediatric walker or crutches, depending on the age of the child. Short courses of anti-inflammatory medicines such as aspirin are often a good adjuvant. This condition is usually a self-limited problem with normal ossification within 2 years of presentation.

Sever Disease (Calcaneal Apophysitis)

Sever disease is not a true avascular necrosis but merely represents a self-limited traction apophysitis of the calcaneus at the insertion of the Achilles tendon. This condition is more common in boys, possibly reflecting their type of athletic activity. Age of presentation is usually between 6 and 10 years. The typical patient presents with pain and tenderness over the posterior aspect of the calcaneus. The patient complains of an insidious onset of pain that is aggravated by activity (especially running and jumping activities) and is relieved by rest. Physical examination may reveal pain, tenderness, and mild swelling around the insertion of the Achilles tendon. The pain is exacerbated by resisted plantar flexion and passive hyperdorsiflexion of the foot. The appearance on radiographs is classic, showing increased density and fragmentation of the posterior calcaneal apophysis.

The treatment again is conservative and consists of a mild restriction of activities (mainly running and jumping) and a 1-in heel pad to elevate the heel and decrease the tension of the Achilles insertion. In severe cases a short leg walking cast may be required for 3 to 4 weeks.

Aspirin for a short course is helpful. Once the symptoms have resolved heel-cord stretching exercises should be instituted to prevent any recurrence.

Osgood-Schlatter Disease (Traction Apophysitis of Tibial Tubercle)

Osgood-Schlatter disease is quite similar to Sever disease but occurs at the anterior tibial tubercle where the patellar tendon inserts onto the tibial tubercle. It is a traction apophysitis similar to Sever disease, but anatomically the tibial tubercle is located right at the proximal tibial epiphysis and some investigators refer to this entity as traumatic or traction epiphysitis. Regardless of the name, it is basically an inflammation of the tibial tubercle at the insertion of the patellar tendon. The typical patient is an adolescent boy, aged 11 to 15 years, who is active in sports. The patient presents with pain and local swelling around the tibial tubercle. The pain is exacerbated by running activities, stair climbing, bicycling, or any other activity that involves active contraction of the quadriceps mechanism. Physical examination reveals local pain and swelling around the tibial tubercle. In addition, resistive knee extensions and passive hyperflexion cause increased pain around the tibial tubercle.

On radiographs, Osgood-Schlatter disease in younger patients reveals soft-tissue swelling anterior to the tibial tubercle and occasionally thickening of the patellar tendon. Bone changes are usually seen in older adolescents and appear as prominent irregular tibial tuberosities or with fragmentation, often with one large fragment located anterior and superior to the tibial tubercle. This condition is often referred to as an ossicle or unresolved lesion. Osgood-Schlatter disease is usually self-limited and subsides when the tibial tubercle fuses when the patient is about 15 years of age.

Treatment for Osgood-Schlatter disease is symptomatic. If the symptoms are severe enough to interfere with a patient's activities, then a mere decrease in activity level usually suffices. It is most important to cease the aforementioned activities of running, bicycling, and stair climbing. Anti-inflammatory drugs such as aspirin and a knee immobilizer are adjuvants. The knee immobilizer is worn during symptomatic episodes and serves the purpose of keeping the knee in full extension, thereby resting the quadriceps and decreasing the tension on the tibial tubercle. For refractory cases, a plaster cylinder cast can be applied for 4 to 8 weeks. Surgery is reserved for patients with refractory symptoms in whom a definite, separate large fragment or ossicle is identified on a radiograph and could thus be excised surgically. Full return to function without residual impairment is the usual outcome.

BIBLIOGRAPHY

Alpar EK, Thompson K, Owen R, et al: Mid shaft fractures of forearm bones in children, *Injury* 13:153, 1981.

Blount WP: *Fractures in children,* Baltimore, 1955, Williams & Wilkins.

Canale TS: Fractures and dislocations in children. In Crenshaw AH, editor: *Campbell's operative orthopedics,* St Louis, 1987, CV Mosby.

Chapcahal G, editor: *Fractures in children,* New York, 1981, Thieme-Stratton.

Green DP: Hand injuries in children, *Pediatr Clin North Am* 24:903, 1977.

Kennedy JC, editor: *The injured adolescent knee,* Baltimore, 1979, Williams & Wilkins.

Peiro A, Aracil J, Martos F, et al: Triplane distal tibial epiphyseal fractures, *Clin Orthop Related Res* 160:196, 1981.

Pollen AG: *Fractures and dislocations in children,* Edinburgh, 1973, Churchill Livingstone.

Rang M: *Children's fractures,* ed 2, Philadelphia, 1983, JB Lippincott.

Rockwood CA Jr, Wilkins KE, King RE editors: *Fractures in children,* Philadelphia, 1984, JB Lippincott.

Sharrard WJW: *Pediatric orthopaedics and fractures,* ed 3, London, 1993, Blackwell Scientific Publications.

Slater RB, Harris WR: Injuries involving the epiphyseal plate, *J Bone Joint Surg (Am)* 45: 587, 1963.

Tachdjian MO: *Pediatric orthopedics,* ed 2, Philadelphia, 1990, WB Saunders.

Weber BG, Brunner C, Freuler F, editors: *Treatment of fractures in children and adolescents,* New York, 1980, Springer-Verlag.

CHAPTER 108

Environmental Trauma

Dee Hodge III

Environmental trauma refers to those environmental conditions that may injure the child because they are so extreme. These include: 1) heat illness, 2) sunburn, 3) cold exposure, and 4) frostbite.

HEAT ILLNESS

Heat-related illnesses encompass three distinct syndromes: 1) heat cramps or involuntary cramping of muscles; 2) heat exhaustion, which is characterized by hypotension and weakness secondary to acute depletion of the extracellular fluid space by sweating; and 3) heatstroke, which is an acute medical emergency related to the failure of thermoregulatory control. There is a common pathophysiologic mechanism to all of these syndromes.

Heat transfer between the environment and the skin is effected by conduction, convection, radiation, and evaporative cooling. The rate of net heat loss is dependent on the balance of heat production and heat loss. Although each mechanism of heat transfer plays a part, it is evaporative cooling that is the principal avenue of heat loss. When the atmospheric temperature is equal to, or in excess of, that of the skin temperature, sweat loss becomes the principal means of dissipating heat. The higher the humidity, the less sweat evaporates and, therefore, little cooling occurs. High humidity and high ambient temperature are the adverse environmental conditions setting the stage for heat-related illnesses.

Children do not adapt to extremes of temperature as effectively as adults when exposed to high temperature levels. This is true for several reasons including: 1) Children have a greater surface-area-mass ratio than adults, which induces a greater heat transfer between the environment and the body. 2) Children produce more metabolic heat per unit mass with even minimal exercise. 3) Sweating capacity is not as great in children as in adults. 4) The capacity to convey heat by blood from the body core to the skin is reduced in the exercising child. Obesity, febrile state, cystic fibrosis, gastrointestinal tract infection, diabetes insipidus, diabetes mellitus, chronic heart failure, caloric malnutrition, anorexia nervosa, sweating insufficiency syndrome, and mental deficiency all potentiate the risk of heat stress.

Data Gathering

Heat cramps occur acutely during or after intense physical exercise. The physiologic basis for heat cramps is related to the acute loss of sodium through sweating. Water replacement may be sufficient but does not compensate for the electrolyte loss. The ensuing alteration in the sodium-potassium balance in the muscle membrane results in involuntary painful contraction of the muscle.

Heat exhaustion is the most common of the heat stress injuries. There are two identifiable subsyndromes: heat exhaustion due to water depletion and heat exhaustion due to salt depletion. In heat exhaustion due to water loss, the individual is usually sweating. The body temperature may be mildly elevated to 38° C to 39.5° C (100° F to 103° F), but not to the levels encountered in acute heatstroke. Postural or frank hypotension is present. This form of heat exhaustion may progress to heatstroke. In heat exhaustion due to salt depletion, water replacement is adequate, but sodium intake fails to meet sodium losses incurred by intense sweating. Body temperature is normal, thirst is unusual, and muscle cramps may be present, but hypotension and increased heart rate are common.

Heatstroke is classically defined by the triad of hyperpyrexia, neurologic symptoms, and anhydrosis. Temperature is in excess of 41° C (106° F). Multiple organ systems may be involved, resulting in hepatic abnormalities, electrocardiogram (ECG) changes, renal abnormalities as a result of either hypotension, myoglobinuria, or thermal injury, and hematologic abnormalities.

Management

As in any injury, prevention is better than treatment. Intense exercise should be banned under environmental conditions that are conducive to heat stress. The American Academy of Pediatrics Committee on Sports Medicine has outlined criteria for acclimatization and curtailing exercise.

In heat-related illness the following guidelines are suggested for treatment:

Heat Cramps

Oral salt replacement (or occasionally intravenous [IV] salt replacement) is an important measure. Massage of the affected muscles should be carried out.

Heat Exhaustion

Remove the patient to a cool environment to avoid further sweat loss. Obtain blood pressure and rectal temperature. If the patient is hypotensive, IV fluid challenge with 10 to 20 mL/kg of normal saline over 1 hour is recommended. If the patient is normotensive, oral administration of an electrolyte preparation is all that is necessary. Appropriate fluids that contain sodium and potassium include Sportsade, Gatorade, and Pedialyte.

Heatstroke

The most urgent treatment is rapid lowering of the body temperature. Direct cooling with use of ice packs can be accomplished in the office or at the scene, while awaiting ambulance transfer to the hospital. If IV fluids are available, these should be started to support blood volume. The remainder of the treatment should occur in the hospital where continuous hemodynamic monitoring can be accomplished.

SUNBURN

Sunburn is the result of exposure to sunlight in excess of its beneficial aspects. Ultraviolet solar radiation (UVR) in the 290- to 320-nm range is responsible for sunburn and is referred to as the "burn band" (UVB). Factors that increase the exposure and intensity of UVB, and thereby the risk of sunburn, include high altitude, latitudes close to the equator, spring and summer months in the northern hemisphere between 10:00 AM and 2:00 PM, and wide-open spaces of sand or snow that reflect UVR.

There is no single accepted theory for the pathogenesis of sunburn. The minimal erythema dose is defined as the least amount of radiation capable of inducing barely perceptible redness. The erythema is due to vasodilation of blood vessels in the dermis. There is also increased vascular permeability, which results in edema of the dermis. Prostaglandins also seem to play a role in pathogenesis, although it is not understood at this time.

Data Gathering

After the exposure to the minimal erythema dose, there is an immediate erythema that appears and then fades. This erythema is followed by delayed erythema that appears approximately 4 to 6 hours later, becomes maximal at 15 to 24 hours, and lasts up to 3 days. Maximal tanning appears at approximately 3 to 5 days. With sunburn there is erythema and edema of the dermis associated with itching and tenderness. Severe overexposure results in fever, vomiting, delirium, and shock. Severe cases with greater than 70% surface-area burn have a similar clinical picture to that of extensive first- and second-degree thermal burns. Healing occurs with desquamation of the skin.

The condition of the sunburned patient is usually easily assessed by history together with the clinical signs. Marked photosensitivity may be due to drugs or systemic disease. Drugs causing phototoxic reaction include: psoralins, tetracyclines, sulfonamides, thiazides, and retinoic acids. Drugs causing photoallergic reactions include: phenothiazines, sulfonamides, para-aminobenzoic acid esters, and halogenated salicylamides. Systemic disorders associated with photosensitivity include polymorphous light eruption, erythropoietic protoporphyria, and systemic lupus erythematosus.

Management

Prevention is the most effective management. Other than protective clothing, sunscreens offer the best protection for susceptible individuals. There are two types of available sunscreens: chemical screens that filter and reduce the intensity of UVR reaching the cells of the skin, and physical screens that are opaque and reflect and scatter light.

Treatment of mild sunburn includes application of cool tap water or compresses with 1:10 dilution of Burow solution for 15 minutes, four or more times a day. Emollients or plain emulsifying ointments are used to soothe and relieve dryness. Aspirin is effective for pain relief. Local anesthetics do not appear to have a major effect, and topical steroids have been shown to be noneffective in relief of many of the symptoms of sunburn. In moderate-to-severe sunburn, the treatment is the same as in mild sunburn but, in addition, hospitalization and the administration of IV fluids may be indicated (*see* Chapter 49).

COLD EXPOSURE

Hypothermia is defined as a core temperature of less than 35° C (95° F). Although more common in the adult population due to old age, lack of adequate housing, alcohol and drug ingestions, endocrine disorders, and central nervous system disorders, in children the condition may be due to prolonged exposure after automobile accidents, cold water immersion, or becoming wet and exhausted during winter sports activities.

Maintenance of body temperature involves a balance between heat production and heat loss. In response to cold exposure, the thermoregulatory center in the hypothalamus sets in motion a coordinated response including increased thyroid and adrenal output via the pituitary (nonshivering thermogenesis), sympathetic nervous system output leading to peripheral vasoconstriction and increased heart rate, and shivering of skeletal muscles leading to increased heat production. Accidental hypothermia occurs when these mechanisms cannot compensate for exposure to low ambient temperatures.

Data Gathering

The clinical signs of hypothermia are related to the decrease in the core temperature. Mental confusion, impaired gait, lethargy, and combativeness are all early signs. Shivering is a useful sign, but patients whose temperature has fallen below 33.3° C (92° F) may not shiver or even feel cold.

"Paradoxical undressing," described in adults, is believed to be due to the failure of peripheral vasoconstriction at low body temperatures, ap-

parently causing a sensation of heat, leading some confused hypothermic patients to take their clothes off.

Acidosis may be respiratory, secondary to ventilatory failure, or metabolic, secondary to circulatory collapse and increased lactic acid production. Urine flow is increased, resulting in a "cold diuresis." Increased urine output combined with extracellular fluid shifts can lead to significant volume depletion.

Cold insult to the cardiovascular system causes decreased cardiac output and hypotension. Cold-induced myocardial irritability leads to conduction disturbances, with ventricular fibrillation. Other ECG changes include sinus bradycardia, T-wave inversion, prolonged intervals, atrial fibrillation, and the characteristic Osborne "J" wave. A useful staging guide to hypothermia has been developed for adults but has not been correlated for pediatric patients: *Mild hypothermia* (35° C to 32° C) is usually benign. Ataxia, slight clumsiness, slowed response to stimuli, and dysarthria are common. Shivering starts at this stage. In *moderate hypothermia* (32° C to 25° C), shivering stops and is replaced by muscular rigidity. Delirium, stupor, and coma may be present. The patient is often arousable and can be conversant. Temperatures below 30° C are particularly dangerous. Basal metabolic rate is less than 50% of normal. In *severe hypothermia* (less than 25° C) death may ensue if hypothermia is present for more than 2 hours. The patient is unresponsive; purposeful movements and reflexes are absent. The pupils are unreactive. Vigorous cardiopulmonary resuscitation may be required.

Patients who appear dead after prolonged exposure to cold temperatures should not be considered dead until they have a near-normal core temperature and are still unresponsive to cardiopulmonary resuscitation.

Management

Therapy may be divided into two categories: general supportive measures and specific rewarming techniques. Recognition of cold injury is the key. In the field, wet clothing should be removed and further heat loss prevented by blankets, body heat, and, if available, administration of heated humidified oxygen. If possible, warmed IV solutions without potassium should be administered. Hospitalization and intensive monitoring is required by all but the mildly hypothermic patient. Minimal and artful handling is needed because of the ease of precipitation of ventricular fibrillation in the cold heart. Specific rewarming techniques should not be used in the field or in the office situation.

FROSTBITE

Extreme cold injury is uncommon in civilian life, but the number of cases has continued to increase during recent years as the number of participants in outdoor winter sports has increased. The incidence in children is unclear, but those most likely to be injured are those who become wet or exhausted.

The precise mechanism of tissue injury is still unclear, but the extent of injury is determined by the duration of exposure, humidity, wind speed, contact with water or metal, immobility, and dependency of a part. Frostbite is a thermal injury, and the tissue damage is similar to a burn in many respects. High-altitude frostbite is produced by rapid freezing. This type of injury is seen in extremely cold temperatures (−40° C to −52° C), with vasoconstriction and deposition of ice crystals in tissue. Slow freezing is most commonly seen. The initial response is vasoconstriction of the exposed part. With continued exposure, there is decreased blood flow, with stasis and, ultimately, occlusion of the vessels.

Data Gathering

Traditional classification describes four degrees. *First-degree* frostbite is characterized by erythema of the skin and edema of the involved part without blister formation; *second-degree* frostbite, by blister and bleb formation; *third-degree* frostbite, by necrosis of the thick layers of the skin and subcutaneous tissues without loss of a part; and *fourth-degree* frostbite, the most severe, by complete necrosis with gangrene and loss of the affected part. Many experts now advocate a simplified classification: superficial and deep.

Initially the frozen tissue exhibits pallor. As early as 1 hour after freezing, subcutaneous edema becomes manifest as the part thaws. A line of demarcation between frozen and unfrozen tissue, a hyperemic zone owing to reactive vasodilatation, may be seen. Edema becomes maximal approximately 48 to 72 hours after thawing and gradually subsides. It may take as long as 60 to 90 days before a final line of demarcation between viable and nonviable tissue becomes obvious.

Management

Superficial Frostbite

"Frost nip" is the only type of frostbite that can be treated satisfactorily in the field. Adequate rewarming can be accomplished by the removal of clothing from the affected part and placing the part into the axilla or against the torso of a partner or parent. Rubbing the frostbitten part with snow or exercising it in an attempt to hasten rewarming will cause further damage.

Deep Frostbite

Rewarming should not be attempted until adequate facilities are at hand. Once the rewarming process has begun, refreezing or weight-bearing on the affected part will result in additional injury. Rewarming should be accomplished via water bath maintained at 40° C to 42° C (104° F to 108° F). Rewarming should be continued until a flush has returned to the most distal tip of the thawed part, approximately 20 to 30 minutes. After rewarming, thawed parts, like burned tissue, are extremely sensitive to trauma and susceptible to infection. The patient should be kept warm. Dependent position of the affected part should be avoided, and blisters should be left intact. Tetanus toxoid is recommended, and extreme care should be taken to prevent infection and avoid abrasion or other trauma. Ibuprofen should be given for pain at a dose of 5 to 10 mg/kg. The topical application of aloe vera as a thromboxane inhibitor also has been recommended. Whirlpool baths are recommended once or twice daily until healing is complete. Conservative surgical management is recommended.

BIBLIOGRAPHY

Bross MH, Nash BT Jr, Carlton FB Jr: Heat emergencies, *Am Fam Physician* 50:389–398, 1994.

Horowitz BZ: The golden hour in heat stroke: Use of iced peritoneal lavage, *Am J Emerg Med* 7:616–619, 1989.

Tek D, Olshaker JS: Heat illness, *Emerg Med Clin North Am* 10:299–310, 1992.

Simon HB: Hyperthermia, *N Engl J Med* 329:483–487, 1993.

Squire DL: Heat illness: Fluid and electrolyte issues for pediatric and adolescent athletes, *Pediatr Clin North Am* 37:1085–109, 1990.

Potts JF: Sunlight, sunburn, and sunscreens: Preventing and remedying problems from 'too much fun in the sun,' *Postgrad Med* 87:69–63, 1990.

McCauley RL, Heggers JP, Robson MC: Frostbite: Methods to minimize tissue loss, *Postgrad Med* 88:67–77, 1990.

Steele P: Management of frostbite, *Physician and Sports Med* 17:135–144, 1989.

CHAPTER 109

Office Management of Minor Surgical Problems

John M. Templeton, Jr.

Minor surgical problems in children have the following characteristics: 1) the disorder is relatively superficial and can be diagnosed by simple inspection and palpation, and 2) procedures required for treatment can be performed within 15 minutes using local anesthesia. These procedures can be easily handled in an office setting with a relatively low investment in equipment and expense. Performing the procedures in the office is cost-saving for the parent and may be less anxiety provoking for the patient.

The main drawback in performing minor surgical procedures in the office is the limitation in time for the busy primary care physician. Nevertheless, if one takes the time to instruct office staff, the receptionist or office nurse usually will identify which patient needs a procedure and prepare the child in a designated, well-equipped treatment room. The nurse can initiate local cleansing and soaks if indicated. If local anesthesia is required, the primary care physician can instill local anesthesia and then see another patient while waiting 15 minutes for the local anesthetic to take full effect.

The only other drawback to the primary care physician performing minor surgical procedures in his/her office is a medical-legal one. If the procedure is not minor and if a qualified surgical consultant is readily available, the physician may be advised to refer the patient. However, if surgical help is not readily available and the physician feels comfortable in managing the problem, the patients and their families will be grateful for having the procedure done by a physician they know and trust.

ABSCESSES

An abscess is an area of local pyogenic infection that has produced tissue breakdown with the development of pus within this area. An abscess can occur anywhere in the body. When they occur deep to fascial and muscle planes, they are best thought of as complex. Patients with such abscesses often require admission to the hospital for the purposes of general anesthesia to facilitate adequate drainage and the use of intravenous antibiotics. Fortunately in children, most abscesses are superficial. Because of the child's size, such abscesses tend to point earlier and lend themselves to easy incision and drainage. The infective organisms generally reflect the bacteriologic composition of adjacent body compartments. The bacteria grown from a perianal abscess, therefore, are likely to be different from those obtained from a cervical abscess.

In taking a history, one may discover a predisposing basis for the abscess. Examples of this include a puncture wound or insect bite or the presence of a preexisting cystic mass or superficial sinus tract. Most abscesses slowly evolve from an area of apparent cellulitis with erythema, swelling, and tenderness. Over the course of 1 to 3 days, the surrounding erythema becomes brighter red; blanching on palpation becomes more prominent; and the skin begins to take on a shiny quality beneath which there is a somewhat distinct mass that is quite tender. By palpating the mass between one's two index fingers, one often can appreciate fluctuance indicating that frank accumulation of pus has occurred and that incision and drainage is indicated. If these features are not present, one may be dealing with a cellulitis rather than a mature abscess. Because many cases of cellulitis can be treated adequately with frequent warm soaks and antibiotics and never develop an abscess, an incision and drainage in an area of cellulitis is not likely to be helpful. If it is unclear whether a local infection represents cellulitis or an abscess, needle aspiration can be used to help in the assessment. Attaching a 22-gauge needle to a 5-mL syringe that contains 0.5 mL of nonbacteriostatic sterile water, and after thorough prepping of the involved area, one can insert the needle for a distance of 1 to 2 cm while applying back suction. If no purulent material is obtained, the nonbacteriostatic water can be injected into the tissue and then aspirated to provide enough material for culture and sensitivity. If, on the other hand, purulent material is obtained, the needle can be detached from the skin and left in place to serve as a guide for incision and drainage. The purulent material in the syringe can be sent for culture and sensitivity.

Whether or not a needle has been used for

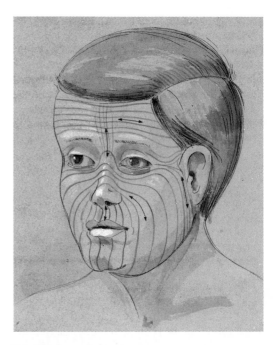

FIG 109-1
Natural skin lines of the face. Incisions of the face as elsewhere should be made in lines parallel to these lines.

initial assessment, the tissue around the suspected abscess site should be thoroughly cleansed and prepared. The final preparation should be with a strong topical antiseptic such as povidone-iodine (Betadine). The field should be draped to isolate the area and to prevent spread of purulent material from beyond the immediate area of drainage. Next, an attempt should be made to identify natural skin lines in the area of the abscess. In most cases, the incision should be planned in a line parallel to natural skin lines to minimize any subsequent scar formation (Fig. 109-1).

The instillation of local anesthesia such as 1% lidocaine (Xylocaine) is often useful because it eliminates the initial pain when the incision is made. The physician must confirm that the patient is not allergic to the anesthetic. At a minimum, an area at least 1.5 cm long should be anesthetized. This step is necessary because an incision for drainage of an abscess that is less than 1 cm may often prove to be inadequate. If an assistant is present, he/she can spray ethyl chloride on the planned site of incision and drainage a second before the incision is made. In using ethyl chloride, it is important to make sure that none of it sprays into the face of the patient. In addition, enough spray is needed to make a prominent white area develop before adequate anesthesia is achieved. Even in the presence of an intense local white reaction, the local anesthetic effect wears off within 5 to 10 seconds. It is difficult, therefore, for a single person both to "freeze" the abscess area and then to perform the incision.

In spite of adequate anesthesia to the skin, the second stage of the procedure is always somewhat painful. Once the incision has penetrated the center of the abscess, a blunt hemostat should be inserted and spread widely in order to break any internal loculations and to ensure adequate drainage. One should have a means of collecting some of the pus for culture. Although most abscesses are due to a coagulase-positive *Staphylococcus,* the organism should be identified in case the patient does not respond properly to treatment.

Once the abscess has been evacuated, it is helpful to place some packing within the center of the abscess. This step is usually best accomplished by lightly inserting 0.25- or 0.5-in width iodoform gauze to the point that a small portion is left protruding from the skin incision. Although there initially appears to be bleeding with the incision and drainage, gentle pressure on the wound margin for 3 to 5 minutes usually will result in complete hemostasis. A bulky sterile dressing should then be applied over the drainage area. In some cases it is advisable to start the patient on a 5-day regimen of oral antibiotics such as cephalexin (Keflex) or dicloxacillin.

Follow-up instructions should include the following: 1) 24 hours after drainage ceases, the dressing and the underlying packing should be removed. Removal of this packing results in some additional debridement effect. Unless the cavity is quite deep or the length of the incision is inadequate, further packing of the wound is not needed. 2) Whether or not further packing is used, the abscess area should receive warm soaks three times a day. These soaks may be done by using local compresses or preferably by immersing the involved area under water. With each soak, the prior dressings and any remaining packing should be removed. At the end of the soak, a sterile dressing should be reapplied. 3) When the wound has closed successfully by secondary intention, soaks and protective dressings may be discontinued. 4) One can arrange to

see the child in 3 to 7 days following the procedure. The family should be instructed to bring the child back sooner should there be progressive inflammation and tenderness in the area surrounding the site or if the child shows persistent fevers or signs of toxic effects.

Contraindications to drainage of an abscess in the office include: 1) A known preexisting medical problem such as a bleeding disorder, an immunologic deficiency, or diabetes mellitus. Complications often occur in such patients, and they should, therefore, be treated in a hospital setting. 2) A child who already has evidence of systemic toxicity, including a high fever and poor appetite. 3) A child who is less than 6 months of age and has a large abscess in the head and neck area.

There are a number of specific types of superficial abscesses that may be encountered in children.

Lymphadenitis

Any area in which there is a concentration of lymph nodes such as the neck, inguinal area, or axillae may develop lymphadenitis and subsequent abscess. If the child has little or no systemic symptoms, and if the child is older than 6 months of age, the majority of these abscesses may be drained in the office. Most children with lymph node abscesses will have them in the cervical area. Although it is possible to treat some of these abscesses with repeated needle aspiration, success in this approach generally requires continuous intravenous antibiotics because of the incomplete drainage obtained from needle aspiration alone. Although incision and drainage may result in residual scar, the child will have more rapid relief of symptoms. From the viewpoint of cost, patient benefit, and time expended, formal incision and drainage is still the standard of care for managing most abscesses.

Perianal Abscess

The origin of perianal abscess, in most cases, is an inflammation in the depth of one of the anal crypts. If this local cryptitis breaks through the epithelium of the anal canal, infection extends through the superficial fibers of the adjacent external sphincter muscle until the skin is reached. The child may have 1 or 2 days of fretfulness and pain on passing stool before the infection becomes obvious. Most abscesses in this area appear in the skin just lateral to the anocutaneous junction. They are rarely larger than 1 cm, are usually bright red, and are tender when palpated locally. When one examines the rectum, but is careful not to touch the abscess, there is usually no other evidence of tenderness or disease around the rectum. The purpose of the rectal examination prior to performing drainage of an apparent perianal abscess is to make sure there is not a larger area of induration and tenderness extending more deeply into the pelvis alongside the rectum. In such cases the infection has broken through the deep portion of the external sphincter mechanism and has now entered easily dissected planes in the ischiorectal space. These deep infections can be quite extensive and life-threatening. When there is any doubt about the possibility of a more deeply extending infection, the patient should be admitted to the hospital and should undergo incision and drainage under general anesthesia so that the physician can adequately break up any loculated pockets of pus within the abscess cavity.

Most children with perianal abscess are less than 1 year of age. Perianal abscess in the neonatal period may indicate immune deficiency. A perianal abscess in an older child should raise the concern of a possible underlying inflammatory bowel condition. In general, the typical perianal abscess is rounded, superficial, and quite discrete. It, therefore, lends itself readily to a localized incision and drainage in the office. It is hard to keep packing inside these superficial abscesses. It is, therefore, better to start the child on frequent sitz baths in the tub, starting 4 to 6 hours after the incision. In most cases the abscess cavity will appear to have healed by secondary intention within 1 week. Parents should be cautioned, however, that one in three children with an episode of perianal abscess will develop recurring local infections. These infections often will drain spontaneously and finally evolve into a fistula in ano. Once a fistula in ano is well established and mature, an elective operative procedure will be required to excise the fistula.

Secondary Abscess in Congenital Cysts

There are a number of cysts or sinus tracts that can be present in children on a congenital basis. In the head and neck area, two of the most common types of superficial congenital malformations are a thyroglossal duct cyst and branchial cleft cysts, with or without a sinus tract. A thyroglossal duct cyst occurs in or quite near to the midline anterior neck in the region of the hyoid bone. It tends to move prominently when the child swallows. Prior to secondary complications such as infection, it is usually smooth, fairly discrete, and slightly mobile. Because these cysts often maintain a sinus tract communication with the foramen cecum, they are susceptible to infection.

The origin of branchial cleft sinus tracts or cysts is the result of failure of complete fusion between each of the branchial arches during fetal development. These cysts or sinus tracts often retain some potential communication with the pharynx or skin, rendering them susceptible to secondary infection. Every child with a preexisting lump or cyst in these areas should be referred to a pediatric surgeon for elective removal because of the increased likelihood of developing secondary infection. When infection does develop, the definitive management of these lesions is complicated. Initially, a formal incision and drainage are required because the preexisting cystic cavity has become an abscess. Then the infection in the congenital cyst will need to heal completely before it is safe to proceed with definitive surgical resection. Some of the branchial cleft sinus tracts, especially those of the second branchial cleft variety, are associated with a small but visible pore entering the skin along the medial margin of the sternocleidomastoid muscle. Patients who are found to have such a skin pore, especially if there is intermittent mucus drainage from the pore, should be referred for evaluation by a pediatric surgeon. The sinus tracts are also susceptible to secondary infection. Their management is, therefore, much easier if they can be handled on an elective basis before an abscess occurs.

One other type of congenital cyst that frequently is associated with a skin pore is a dermoid cyst or sebaceous cyst. The visible pore in the skin in such cases immediately overlies the cyst. Because such lesions have a potential for the entry of bacteria, a secondary abscess often will develop. When an abscess in a dermoid cyst does develop, it requires initial incision and drainage and complete healing before one can proceed with definitive treatment.

Pilonidal Sinus Abscess

Some young children may be noted to have a dimple in the midline in the interbuttocks groove in the region of the coccyx. If the opening of the dimple is wide enough to allow viewing of the base of the dimple, secondary infections are unlikely. On the other hand, some pilonidal sinuses have a very narrow tract. With the onset of puberty, increased growth of hair may occur in this area. Often one or several strands of hair may extend along this small sinus tract, impeding normal drainage and resulting in the development of an abscess. The patient and the family may not be aware of any abnormalities in this area until progressive pain and tenderness is noted overlying the coccyx. Within a few days a frank abscess may present. The usual organisms involved are *Staphylococcus* or *Escherichia coli*. Once an abscess is clearly established, a formal incision and drainage will be required. In addition to evacuation of the purulent material, one should look for and remove any hairs that are seen extending down along the sinus tract. Because the abscess cavities are often fairly large by the time the patient presents for treatment, the family should be instructed in how to provide local hot soaks followed by repacking with new iodoform gauze two to three times a day. These abscess cavities may take 2 to 3 weeks before they close entirely. One to 2 months after infection has fully resolved, the patient should then undergo an elective excision of the still present pilonidal cyst.

MINOR SURGICAL PROBLEMS OF THE HAND

For a number of reasons, the hand is often a site for infections and trauma. Younger children often are unaware of dangers in the environment. When they fall, the hand often takes the brunt of the injury. Likewise fingers may be caught in narrow spaces or crushed in a car door. Many children have the propensity to chew or suck on their fingers, giving rise to infections.

Although many hand problems, if recognized early, can be treated on an outpatient basis, what may appear initially to be a minor problem may within 24 hours turn into a major problem. Because the hand is so important in human development and function, no hand problem should ever be taken lightly. Warning signs and symptoms that a more serious process is involved include generalized swelling of the palm or dorsum of the hand, evidence of dissemination of infection such as lymphangitic streaking, generalized pain on moving the finger joints, or inability to perform simple tasks such as pinching or

curling and uncurling of fingers. The presence of any one of these signs makes it mandatory that the patient be referred for care by a hand specialist in the hospital setting.

Nevertheless, there are a number of localized and early problems involving the hand that are appropriate for care in the office. The following are examples of such localized problems:

Felon

An infection in the pulp of the distal digit is called a *felon*. If the felon occurred as a result of a discernible puncture of the overlying skin, an abscess in the skin at the puncture site may develop. This abscess may be treated with incision and drainage followed by frequent soaks and antibiotic ointment dressings. Often, however, a felon will not show signs of pointing. This undrained infection within the pulp of the fingertip can produce serious complications. Excessive pressure in the pulp's base may lead to ischemic necrosis of soft tissue. Because most felons are the result of infections from coagulase-positive staphylococci, fat between the septa is often destroyed. Dissemination of infection may extend to the underlying phalanx, with extension along the flexor tendon sheath. In this manner the whole finger and even the hand may be jeopardized.

On examination the fingertip is painful, red, and tense. Even slight pressure worsens the pain. Frank fluctuance is rarely present. Early drainage is mandatory. Anesthesia for fingertip problems is best achieved by a digital nerve block. The hand should first be thoroughly cleansed with surgical antiseptic soap and then prepped with antiseptic solution such as povidone-iodine. After the hand has been draped and isolated, 1% lidocaine can be used to infiltrate the proximal digital dorsal and volar nerves on each side. It is important to make sure that there is no epinephrine in the lidocaine solution. Epinephrine instilled around the digital arteries may produce such sustained vascular occlusion that necrosis of a portion of the finger may occur.

As shown in Figure 109-2, the needle can be inserted on the side of the flexor aspect of the finger near the web space and then advanced down to the proximal phalanx. When the periosteum is hit with the needle, the needle can be drawn back 1 or 2 mm. The syringe is aspirated to make sure that blood is not obtained, and then an initial 0.5 to 1.0 mL of anesthetic can be instilled. Next, the needle can be drawn back

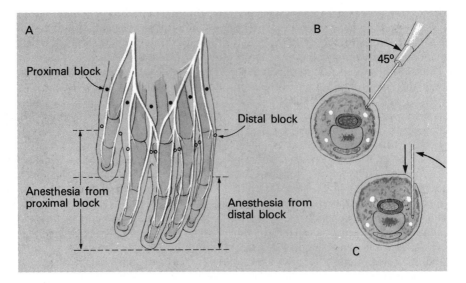

FIG 109-2

A, Nerves supplying the hand with sites for proximal block (black dots) and distal block (white dots) with corresponding areas of anesthesia. For most distal lesions of the digits, a distal block is preferred. **B,** Insert the needle at 45° angle until the periosteum is reached, then retract 1 to 2 mm in, aspirate, and inject 0.5 to 1 mL of anesthesia. **C,** Advance the needle toward the extensor surface, aspirate, and inject 1 to 2 mL of anesthesia.

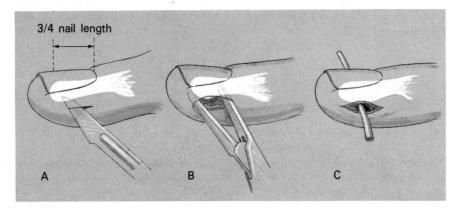

FIG 109-3

Drainage of felon. **A,** Incision of the felon parallel to the edge of nail. **B,** A hemostat advanced along anterior surface of bone. **C,** A small drain is placed.

partway and then advanced toward the extensor surface of the finger, near to the phalanx. Additional anesthetic can be instilled. Usually 1 to 2 mL is sufficient to provide block of the two digital nerves within 10 minutes. The same procedure should be done to block the dorsal and volar digital nerves on the opposite side of the phalanx.

As shown in Figure 109-3, an incision should be made close to and parallel to the edge of the nail. An incision at this point will minimize potential damage to digital nerves and avoid troublesome scar formation. A curved mosquito hemostat can be advanced first to the side of the phalanx, and then further advanced along the anterior surface of the bone. A similar counter-incision on the opposite side can then be made, and the mosquito hemostat tip can be advanced

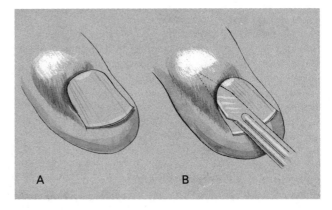

FIG 109-4
A, Paronychia involving the base of the nail.
B, After digital nerve block, a local incision of abscess along the surface of the nail will provide drainage. If the overlying skin is necrotic, it should be debrided as well.

out through this counterincision. A small piece of Penrose drain or sterile rubber band can be pulled through this space and left in place. Dicloxacillin therapy should be started, and the patient should be seen again within 24 hours to make sure that the infection is responding appropriately. If the patient is doing well, the drain may be removed after 48 hours and the patient may start frequent warm soaks.

Paronychia

At the base of the fingernail is a flap of thin epidermis called the *eponychium* (cuticle). This area is vulnerable to trauma, including that which occurs as a result of biting or sucking of the fingers. As a result bacterial invasion may occur, leading to a local cellulitis overlying the base of the nail. When the infection is fairly early and localized, it can be managed by local hygiene and maneuvers to foster spontaneous drainage. Three times a day the entire hand should be washed with warm soap and water for 20 minutes. Then a loose-fitting finger cot that is partially filled with povidone-iodine or polymyxin β-bacitracin-neomycin (Neosporin) ointment can be applied over the finger so that maceration of the inflamed skin occurs. With maceration, spontaneous drainage usually follows. Usually 2 to 3 days with such treatment is sufficient. It is important to make sure that the finger cot is loose enough so that it does not produce a tourniquet effect at the base of the finger.

If the infection is more advanced, the entire base of the nail may be involved. There often will be a collection of pus that is visible under the skin. As shown in Figure 109-4, local incision and occasionally debridement of the skin overlying the abscess is usually necessary. A digital

nerve block should be utilized in such cases before undertaking such drainage.

If the paronychia is far advanced, the proximal base of the fingernail may serve as a foreign body and thereby perpetuate the infection. In such cases one must first excise the overlying eponychium and then excise the involved portion of proximal nail that frequently is surrounded by pus on all sides. When formal drainage of a superficial or deep paronychia is required, therapy should be started with dicloxacillin or cephalexin until the specific culture report is returned. Hot soaks three times a day followed by the application of sterile loose dressing is important until healing is complete.

Subungual Hematoma

A direct blow to the fingernail, as with a hammer, often will cause bleeding between the nail bed and the nail. This bleeding will result in a hematoma that slowly expands over several hours leading to persistent and often throbbing-type pain. At this point one usually will notice a blue-black zone under the nail at the site of the hematoma. Drainage of the hematoma will provide immediate relief of pain and will minimize any potential for secondary pressure effects. If the hematoma extends almost to the tip of the nail, then the nail can be separated from the end of the nail bed resulting in drainage. Usually, however, the hematoma is under the proximal portion of the nail. The easiest maneuver to achieve drainage is to heat a straightened portion of a paper clip with a burning match until it is red-hot and then apply it with slight pressure to the nail over the center of the hematoma. Doing this two or three times will slowly burn a hole through the nail until there is a sudden extrusion

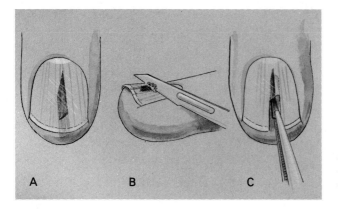

FIG 109-5
Removal of a splinter. **A,** A splinter embedded under the nail, too deep to reach by the distal approach. **B,** Shaving a portion of the overlying nail to expose the splinter. **C,** Removal of the splinter with a hemostat.

of dark watery blood. One can also use a no. 11 scalpel blade to cut through the nail overlying the hematoma (Fig. 109-5). This cutting is done in a rotary fashion until a hole is cut through the nail down to the hematoma. This technique requires a moderate amount of pressure, however, and will add to the patient's pain and discomfort unless one has initially used a digital nerve block. After the blood has been drained, one should soak the finger two to three times a day and then keep a light dressing over the area until the dead space has closed in completely.

Subungual Splinter
While playing, children occasionally catch a splinter under the fingernail. Usually the splinter is wood, but other items such as a sliver of metal or plastic can produce the same injury. Because it is a penetrating injury, bacteria are often present. The presence of bacteria and a foreign body may lead to local infection and complications. Removal of the splinter is, therefore, important for both comfort and treatment. If the splinter is not totally embedded, it is better not to pick at the wooden splinter, because it may cause it to break into fragments making removal of the deeper portion more difficult. Instead the edge of the nail should be trimmed back as closely as possible to the tip of the finger. Then after thorough cleansing of the hand, the object often can be caught against the undersurface of the nail with a needle or a scalpel tip and gently stroked out of its pocket. If the splinter has broken off and is embedded under the nail, direct exposure of the splinter can be obtained by scraping a portion of the overlying nail away as shown in Figure 109-6. Once the splinter is exposed, it can be removed and local cleansing

can be done. The hand should be soaked three times a day, after which an antibacterial ointment dressing should be applied. As with all wounds involving foreign bodies, one should make sure that the patient has adequate protection against tetanus.

Fingertip Amputations
Children are prone to crush injuries or amputation injuries of the tip of the finger. In most cases such injuries involve only the distal half of the distal phalanx. They usually involve part or all of the nail bed. In many cases, the bone of the tip of the phalanx is partially exposed or amputated. In contrast to the treatment for adults, it is very important when treating children to avoid at all costs debriding back bone or the nail bed to obtain a primary closure. After placement of a digital nerve block, any frankly necrotic tissue should be gently debrided. After thorough cleansing with the use of dilute antiseptic surgical soap followed by saline lavage, the fingertip should be dressed with a sterile petrolatum gauze and bulky absorbent gauze to immobilize and protect the finger. Such relatively minor fingertip injuries usually will heal spontaneously in a few weeks with a quite acceptable cosmetic and functional result. In cases of a more severe or proximal injury or the development of secondary infection, the patient should be referred immediately to a hand specialist.

Entrapped Rings
Children have a fascination for rings and often will put more than one on a hand. Sizing of rings for children is often not accurate, especially if one child borrows another child's ring to try it on. This practice can lead to the ring becoming

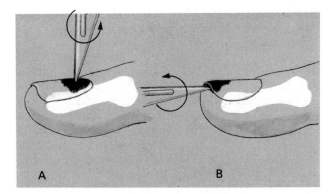

FIG 109-6
Drainage of subungual hematoma. **A,** A proximal hematoma drained through the nail. **B,** A distal hematoma drained directly.

trapped proximal to the proximal interphalangeal (PIP) joint. Very often the parent or child will have attempted to pull off the ring by using soapy water or mineral oil. In such cases prolonged attempts at pulling on the ring may have resulted in edema of the distal portion of the finger, making removal even more difficult.

Commercial ring cutters are available. When the ring is an inexpensive one or is thin, removal of a ring in this fashion is quite easy. A thick ring may take more time and effort. An alternative to using a ring cutter is to attempt to milk the edema and swelling out of the distal finger so that the ring may be slid over the PIP joint. A no. 1 silk suture works well in such cases. One end of the silk is used to wrap the soft tissues of the finger tightly, beginning at the distal end and slowly wrapping the silk more and more proximally, thereby squeezing any edema back toward the hand. The wrapping is continued all the way down to the ring, at which point the proximal portion of the silk is passed underneath the ring. Then this end of the silk is lifted outward at right angles to the axis of the finger and unraveled in the reverse direction. This maneuver thereby coaxes the ring up and over the blockage at the PIP joint. This maneuver is greatly assisted by having the patient's hand and involved finger kept in an elevated position over the head for 10 to 15 minutes before attempting the ring removal.

Hair Strangulation of a Digit
Young children, particularly those in the first year of life, often grab their mother's hair or loose threads. Occasionally a single strand of hair or thread may completely encircle a finger or toe, leading to constriction of the digit. Distal to the constricting band, the digit becomes swollen and

red. One usually can identify a clear line of demarcation between the normal proximal tissue and the edematous distal tissue.

On examination the constricting material may not be immediately discernible because it has cut so deeply into the skin. This is particularly true in the case of a strand of hair if the hair was wet when it became wrapped around the finger. Subsequent drying will lead to further shrinkage and constriction of the digit. Retraction of the skin surrounding the indentation will finally reveal the constricting object. It is imperative to remove this band as soon as it is identified. It is helpful to use a magnifying lens to see and remove all of the material producing the constricting band. In most cases the band can be grasped with the tip of a fine mosquito hemostat. The portion that has been grasped with the hemostat can then be cut with a no. 11 scalpel blade. If one is sure that the constricting band is a hair fiber, one may also use a depilatory agent (*eg,* Nair) to dissolve the hair. After removal of the band, the hand should be placed in an elevated position to allow further resolution of edema in the distal digit. If the digit has not been irreversibly compromised, it should return to normal within 48 to 72 hours.

OTHER MINOR SURGICAL PROBLEMS

Foreign Bodies
Because of their general level of activity and their occasional lack of attention to safety measures, children are prone to soft-tissue injuries that result in the embedding of foreign bodies. Falls in an area where bits of rough gravel or cut glass are present often result in small lacerating inju-

ries that may not suggest the presence of a foreign body. Carrying sharp items or not paying attention to where one steps or sits may result in the embedding of a broken pencil tip or penetration of the foot or buttocks by pins or other sharp objects.

It is very important for the physician to obtain an accurate history as to the location and circumstances in which a child may have incurred a small puncture-type injury. If there is any reason to suspect entry of a foreign body a radiograph should be obtained. Metallic items and glass will be seen on a radiograph, whereas organic material such as wood splinters is usually not radiopaque. If a foreign body is seen on a radiograph, it usually is removed before complications develop. The presence of organic material in the tissue, however, may go unrecognized and is, therefore, more often associated with complications. Moreover, such material is likely to elicit a greater inflammatory response than is a smooth-surfaced object such as glass. Because of the concomitant presence of bacteria, this enhanced inflammatory response results in a purulent reaction that soon evolves into a localized abscess. The abscess is helpful in that it tends to enhance the body's attempt to extrude the foreign material and points the way for the physician who is called on to treat the problem. Such a localized abscess should be prepared and opened as described previously. Exposure of the abscess cavity will usually result in extrusion of the foreign object. Subsequent treatment should be the same as with any abscess.

Foreign objects that are appropriate for removal in an office setting are those that are in the subcutaneous tissue and/or are readily palpable. The end of the needle, for example, may be palpated just under the surface of the skin, although the tip of the needle may extend more deeply. When a foreign body cannot be felt and radiographs show that the foreign body is deep to superficial fascia, the patient should be referred to an appropriate surgical specialist for assessment and probably removal of the object. This is particularly true in the case of penetrating objects in the foot and buttocks because much time and effort can be saved by removal of the foreign body under fluoroscopy. As with all penetrating injuries, it is very important to make sure that the patient is immunized for tetanus.

Fishhook Injuries

Fishhook injuries can occur in almost any part of the body, usually as a result of misadventures with casting. Often, attempts to remove the fishhook at the scene of the injury result in the fishhook becoming more deeply embedded.

Occasionally, when the fishhook has punctured a slender structure such as a finger or an auricle the bared end of the hook will be seen to have partially exited on the side opposite to the point of entry. In such cases the tip of the fishhook may be grasped with a hemostat. Next, the shank of the fishhook is cut flush with the skin at the entry site. Then the distal fragment can be drawn out with little or no discomfort.

In most cases, however, the fishhook is deeply embedded in the patient's soft tissues. Any attempts to remove the fishhook should be designed to neutralize the effect of the barb at the end of the hook. Most techniques involve some manipulation of the fishhook that may be a bit painful and frightening to the child. Therefore, after local cleansing with surgical soap and antiseptic solution, one should instill 1 or 2 mL of local anesthetic around the entry site and around the embedded portion of the fishhook. The most commonly used technique to neutralize or disengage the barb is to place a piece of heavy silk around the exposed curve of the fishhook and to loop this silk two or three times around the index and ring fingers of one hand. With the other hand, one should grasp the straight shank of the fishhook with a thumb and middle finger and use the index finger to press the curve of the shank downward, thereby disengaging the barb from the tissue within. Holding this downward pressure with one hand, one can then use the other hand to pull on the silk suture steadily outward in a line that is parallel to the straight shaft of the fishhook. This will have the effect of straightening the curve of the hook slightly enough to allow extraction of the fishhook.

Insect Bites

There are a number of insects that have the ability to penetrate the skin for sucking, as in the case of mosquitoes, or to puncture the skin, often accompanied by the release of an irritating or toxic material. The more serious forms of insect bites include those of poisonous spiders. Because the effect of their envenomation can lead to serious local and systemic symptoms, children with such bites should be referred to a hospital. Much more common than spider bites are stings from insects of the Hymenoptera order. Honeybees, wasps, yellow jackets, and hornets can live and thrive in environments close to man. For certain susceptible individuals, stings from these insects can be life-threatening. It is estimated that 40 to 50 people die each year in the United States as a result of anaphylactic reactions following a sting from one of these insects. Immediate treatment with subcutaneous epinephrine 1:1000 (0.1 to 0.3 mL) and a tourniquet above the site of the sting may help to lessen the life-threatening effects of an anaphylactic reaction. Even in individuals who are not so sensitive, a systemic toxic reaction can occur when 10 or more stings have occurred. Such systemic symptoms may include vomiting, diarrhea, muscle cramps, headaches, and dizziness. Rarely, convulsions may occur. If such symptoms are pronounced or protracted, the patient should be taken to a hospital. If these symptoms pass quickly, however, one may then proceed with local care and treatment of each sting site. One should first cleanse the area with soap and water. Then, using a knife blade held at a right angle to the surface of the skin, the stinger can be scraped out of the skin. Cold compresses may provide local symptomatic relief. One can then apply a solution of one fourth of a teaspoon of meat tenderizer (chymopapain) and 1 teaspoon of tap water to the sting site. In addition one can give the patient diphenhydramine (Benadryl) 5 mg/kg/24 hr in four divided doses by any route. This medication may particularly help to reduce any associated systemic signs and symptoms.

Zipper Injury to the Penis

On occasion a young boy who is in a hurry to get back to playing after urinating will zip up the fly of his trousers so quickly that the skin of the shaft of the penis is caught in the zipper. If the portion of skin that is caught is small and appears to be caught by only one of the small zipper teeth, one can quickly pull the zipper back, detaching the skin. This action will be painful for a moment, but then the problem will be resolved.

If the skin is tightly entrapped, involving several of the small teeth of the zipper, one should attempt first a relatively nonthreatening approach with the use of mineral oil. The zipper and the entrapped skin are liberally coated with mineral oil. The involved area is then further soaked with mineral oil for 10 minutes. At this point the zipper often can be gently pulled free of the entrapped skin with little difficulty. If this does not succeed, one can then clean the skin and infiltrate the skin around the entrapped area with 1% xylocaine without epinephrine. Because of the partially closed nature of the zipper, one will not be able to see the entire circumference of the shaft. Instead, the anesthesia can be instilled subcutaneously down for a distance of 1 cm beyond where one can see. With effective anesthesia the child can be reassured that he will have no more pain and discomfort. It may then be possible to thrust the zipper handle quickly downward to try and disengage the zipper from the skin. If this is not feasible because of the secondary development of edema, it is better to take a pair of heavy scissors and cut the involved portion of zipper off of the pants. With the patient's pants removed, one can better see the entrapped area. Then the teeth with their attachment to the cloth of the zipper can be individually pulled and cut away until the entrapped skin is released.

After removal of the zipper, the involved area of skin should be thoroughly washed and cleansed and dressed with polymyxin β-bacitracin ointment (Polysporin) and a light, fluffy dressing. It is a good idea for the child to lie down for the rest of the day to help to resolve any local edema. Starting the next day the child should take sitz baths two or three times a day, after which a local polymyxin β-bacitracin ointment dressing should be applied until the area has healed satisfactorily.

BIBLIOGRAPHY

Barkin RM, editor: *Emergency pediatrics,* St Louis, 1984, CV Mosby.

Fleisher GR, Ludwig S, editors: *Textbook of pe-diatric emergency medicine,* ed 3, Baltimore, 1993, Williams & Wilkins.

Kanegaye JT, Schonfeld N: Penile zipper entrapment: A simple and less threatening approach using mineral oil, *Pediatr Emerg Care* 9:90–91, 1993.

Oosterlinck W: Unbloody management of penile zipper injury, *Eur Urol* 7:365–366, 1981.

Pascoe D, Grossman M, editors: *Quick reference to pediatric emergencies,* ed 3, Philadelphia, 1984, JB Lippincott.

Reece, RM, editor: *Manual of emergency pediatrics,* ed 2, Philadelphia, WB Saunders.

Welch KJ, Randolph JG, editors: *Pediatric surgery,* ed 4, Chicago, 1986, Year Book Medical Publishers.

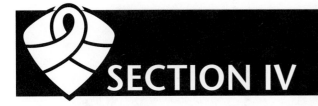

SECTION IV

Developmental Disabilities

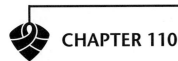

CHAPTER 110

Myelomeningocele

Edward B. Charney
Nathan J. Blum

Spina bifida with myelomeningocele is one of the most significant handicapping conditions of childhood. It is a birth defect that may adversely affect the motor, sensory, psychosocial, emotional, and cognitive development of the child, and may produce tremendous psychological and economic stress on the entire family. By the nature of its multisystem involvement, many children with this disorder receive specialized care from a multidisciplinary team that often consists of a developmental pediatrician, neurosurgeon, orthopedist, urologist, nurse, social worker, and physical or occupational therapist. The primary care physician, however, may be the one to whom both the family and team of specialists turn for day-to-day medical management, assistance in locating community resources, and provision of ongoing emotional support. Famil-

iarity with the nature of the birth defect, its functional implications, and management issues can be valuable in the physician's fulfillment of this role.

NATURE OF THE BIRTH DEFECT

Spina bifida describes the separation or nonfusion of the vertebral spinal arches, whereas myelomeningocele describes the cystic dilatation of the meninges around a malformed neural tube (Fig. 110-1). Neural tube defects including myelomeningocele, meningocele (cystic dilatation of meninges around a normal spinal cord without neurologic deficits), anencephaly, and encephalocele result from incomplete neural tube closure at around 28 days' gestation. It occurs in approxi-

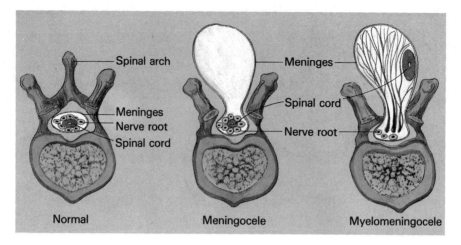

FIG 110-1
Nomenclature of neural tube defects.

mately 0.6 to 1.0 per 1000 live births in the United States.

Although many theories for etiology have been proposed, the cause remains unknown. There is, however, a well-documented higher incidence in affected families with estimated recurrence rates 50 times higher than the general population; increased frequency of other congenital malformations (*ie,* cleft palate/lip, congenital heart disease) among both the affected child and family members; and a higher incidence in Ireland (four per 1000 live births) with lower, but still increased incidence among Irish descendants living elsewhere. On the basis of these observations and other epidemiologic data, it has been suggested that a predisposition with polygenic mode of inheritance exists.

Environmental factors also play a contributory etiologic role. Recent studies suggest that supplementation with folic acid in the periconceptional period can reduce the risk of myelomeningocele by 50% to 70%. Use of valproic acid during pregnancy has been associated with the occurrence of myelomeningocele.

Prenatal diagnosis may be established through amniocentesis at 16 to 18 weeks of pregnancy. Fetuses with open neural tube defects will have an increased amniotic fluid level of α-fetoprotein, an α-globulin synthesized by normal embryonal yolk sac, liver cells, and gastrointestinal tract. Ultrasonography and amniotic fluid levels of acetylcholinesterase can significantly enhance prenatal diagnosis.

The level in the spinal cord at which neural tube closure was incomplete, determines the degree of motor paralysis and sensory loss of the child (Fig. 110-2). Sensation is either totally or partially absent in the skin over the paralyzed muscle groups. Musculoskeletal deformities develop primarily around those joints that are either totally or partially paralyzed. Deformities may develop on a dynamic basis with imbalanced muscle strength about the joint, or on a positional basis where effects of gravity and/or position lead to contractures about a totally paralyzed joint. Spinal deformities of scoliosis or kyphosis may be associated with congenital anomalies of the spine and rib cage, such as hemivertebrae or fused ribs.

Often there is not just an isolated birth defect of the spinal cord and spine, but rather there commonly are associated congenital malformations of the brain. Ninety percent of patients with myelomeningocele have an Arnold-Chiari type II malformation of the hindbrain, in which there is downward displacement of the medulla and posterior cerebellum into the cervical vertebral canal (Fig. 110-3). Hydrocephalus develops in 60% to 95% of patients with myelomeningocele, as cerebrospinal fluid flow and absorption are compromised from the Arnold-Chiari malformation as well as from the frequently accompanying aqueductal stenosis or occlusion. Additional clinical complications of this malformation include cranial nerve palsies with strabismus, vocal cord paralysis with stridor, swallowing diffi-

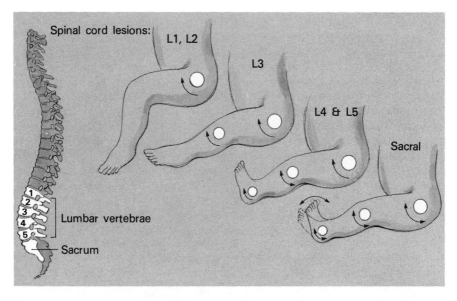

FIG 110-2

Motor activity and level of the spinal cord lesion. Lesions a L-1 and L-2 allow only hip flexion, whereas lesions at L-3 allow extension of the knee. Patients with lesions at L-4 and L-5 dorsiflex flex ankles, and those with sacral lesions also can plantarflex ankles and move toes (*see* Table 110-1).

culties, and apnea. Other less well-defined anatomic lesions in the brain may contribute to seizure disorder in 15% of patients with myelo-meningocele, mental retardation in 35%, and visual perceptual problems in 80%.

FUNCTIONAL IMPLICATION

Infants and children with thoracic lesions have flaccid paralysis of both lower extremities with variable weakness in abdominal and trunk musculature. Those children with high lumbar lesions (L-1, L-2) have voluntary hip flexion and adduction but flaccid paralysis of the knees, ankles, and feet (*see* Fig. 110-2). Ninety percent to 95% of children with thoracic or high lumbar paralysis have associated hydrocephalus. They also are particularly prone to musculoskeletal deformities of the spine, hips, and entire lower extremity. These children may be capable of walking; however, they require extensive bracing and crutches for independence (Table 110-1).

Children with midlumbar (L-3) paralysis have strong hip flexion and adduction and fair knee extension, but paralyzed ankles and toes (*see* Fig. 110-2). Approximately 85% have associated hydrocephalus. Musculoskeletal deformities of the lower extremities may be common and independent ambulation can be accomplished with either extensive, moderate (Fig. 110-4), or minimal bracing.

Children with low lumbar lesions (L-4, L-5) have strong hip flexion and adduction, knee extension, and ankle dorsiflexion with often weak or absent ankle plantar flexion, toe extension/flexion, and hip extension (*see* Fig. 110-2). Seventy percent have associated hydrocephalus. They are particularly prone to deformities of the ankles or feet and often need moderate, minimal, or no bracing for independent ambulation.

Children with sacral lesions usually only have mild weakness of the ankles and/or toes (*see* Fig. 110-2). Approximately 60% have associated hydrocephalus. Musculoskeletal deformities are usually of the feet, and the vast majority will walk independently with only minimal or no bracing.

Bladder and bowel problems are present in at least 90% of these children, irrespective of their degree of lower-extremity paralysis. Motor and sensory innervation of both organs are normally mediated through the S2-4 level of the spinal cord and, therefore, incomplete neural tube clo-

IV

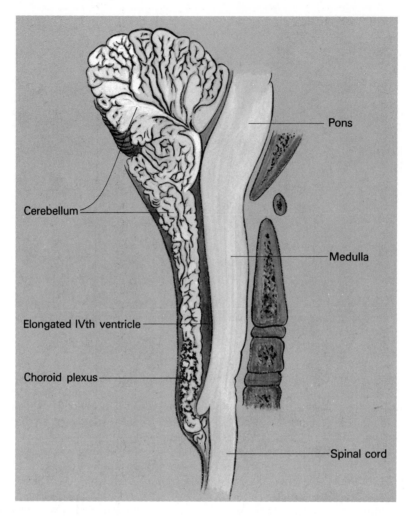

Pons

Cerebellum

Medulla

Elongated IVth ventricle

Choroid plexus

Spinal cord

FIG 110-3
Arnold-Chiari malformation.

TABLE 110-1
Degree of Paralysis and Functional Implications

PARALYSIS	HYDROCEPHALUS (%)	AMBULATION	BOWEL/BLADDER INCONTINENCE (%)
Thoracic or high lumbar (L-1, L-2)	95	"May" walk with extensive braces and crutches	>90
Midlumbar (L-3)	85	"Can" walk with either extensive, moderate, or minimal braces and usually with crutches	>90
Low lumbar (L-4, L-5)	70	"Will" walk with moderate, minimal, or no bracing with or without crutches	>90
Sacral (S-1 to S-4)	60	"Will" walk with minimal or no braces and usually without crutches	>90

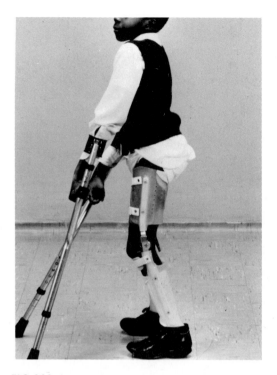

FIG 110-4
Knee-ankle-foot orthosis or long leg bracing with Lofstrand (forearm) crutches.

sure of this area results in a neurogenic bladder and bowel. In general, there are two major types of neurogenic bladder, one that fails to empty adequately or one that fails to store adequately (Fig. 110-5). Failure in emptying usually is associated with paralysis or ineffective bladder detrusor contractility and/or ineffective urethral relaxation. Infants and children with this type of bladder are at risk for urinary tract infections associated with urinary stasis, hydronephrosis (when abnormally increased bladder pressure and vesicoureteral reflux are present) (*see* Fig. 110-5E), and overflow incontinence. Failure to adequately store urine is often a result of either uninhibited bladder detrusor contractility and/or ineffective urethral resistance. Although urinary tract infections and hydronephrosis are relatively uncommon complications of this bladder type, urinary incontinence is usually present.

Problems in bowel control are primarily related to either ineffective involuntary relaxation or contraction of the internal anal sphincter (Fig. 110-6). The inability to establish relaxation results in constipation with a full rectum that is unable to completely empty its fecal contents through a tight sphincter. Unless the rectum is emptied regularly, constipation will produce a hugely dilated colon with "overflow" or "bypass" diarrhea interspaced with infrequent passage of hard stools. Inability to maintain some normal contraction of the internal sphincter, on the other hand, usually results in frequent diarrhea and a tendency for rectal prolapse. Irrespective of the status of the internal sphincter, almost all children with myelomeningocele have no anal or perianal somatic sensation. This lack of sensation, along with an inability to voluntarily control their external sphincter, makes them unable to sense or control stool passage.

MANAGEMENT

Treatment of children with myelomeningocele should be individualized according to the needs of both child and family. There is also considerable variation of these needs with the different developmental stages of the child. When reviewing management issues it is best, therefore, to examine separately the child with myelomeningocele as a newborn, infant, preschooler, school-aged child, and adolescent. Recognition of the importance of developmental stages in management affords the clinician a somewhat easier task when formulating a whole-child total care plan.

Newborn
Controversial issues in the newborn management of myelomeningocele have included both the selection process and optimal time for surgical intervention. During the 1950s and 1960s, early surgical back closure was performed on most infants, irrespective of their clinical severity, as advances in surgical technique were made and the ventricular shunt was improved. The enhanced survival of these infants, however, was observed to be associated with an increased number of more severely disabled children. Retrospective and prospective studies in the 1970s identified a number of "adverse criteria" at birth that were associated with severe disabilities later in life. These "adverse criteria" included: thoracolumbar lesions with paralysis of the legs below the knees, congenital hydrocephalus with head circumference greater than the 95th percentile, congenital kyphoscoliosis, birth anoxia, and other severe birth defects. A selection process

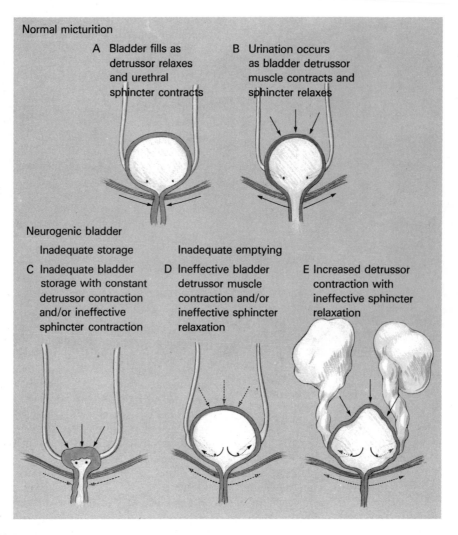

FIG 110-5
Normal functioning bladder (**A** and **B**) vs neurogenic bladder (**C, D,** and **E**).

was then advocated and practiced whereby infants with one or more of these criteria did not receive surgical intervention. Although survival rates diminished, as approximately 90% of those without surgery died during the first year, the number of severely impaired survivors decreased among those selected for surgical intervention.

Consideration of withholding life-prolonging measures for any handicapped newborn is an ethical and moral dilemma for both physician and parents. Resolution of this dilemma often necessitates a decision-making process over a period of time. Until recently it was believed that delay in surgical closure of the myelomeningocele beyond 48 hours was associated with increased morbidity. Current data, however, suggest no increase in morbidity or mortality if surgery is delayed 1 to 2 weeks. This additional time may afford both the physician and parents a period to seek additional consultation and emotional support before establishing a treatment plan for the newborn.

When surgical intervention is decided on, the infant will usually first have surgical closure of the myelomeningocele defect. Evaluation for

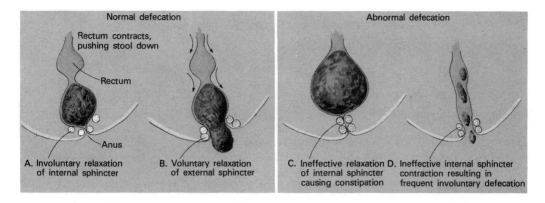

FIG 110-6
Normal functioning bowel (**A** and **B**) vs neurogenic bowel
(**C** and **D**).

development of hydrocephalus may then be done by head circumference measurements and brain ultrasound or computed tomography (CT). Management of the hydrocephalus usually involves a shunting procedure whereby cerebrospinal fluid from the ventricular system is internally diverted to another place in the body for better absorption. A ventriculoperitoneal shunt is commonly utilized; however, a ventriculoatrial shunt may be used when peritoneal absorption is poor (Fig. 110-7). Urologic evaluation also should occur during the initial hospitalization. A renal ultrasound or intravenous pyelography (IVP) and voiding cystography should be obtained to identify hydronephrosis and/or structural abnormalities in the kidney or collecting system. Poor bladder emptying may require a vesicostomy or intermittent catheterization of the bladder. A vesicostomy (Fig. 110-8) usually results in decompression of the bladder and upper tracts by permitting complete emptying. The infant's care is simpler than with intermittent catheterization because only a diaper is required.

Infant

During the infant's first few months at home, most parents will have considerable concern over whether or not their child's shunt is working. Approximately 50% of all infants with shunts will require at least one revision during the first year of life. Mechanical shunt malfunction without infection is far more common than shunt infection alone as a cause of shunt revision. Signs and symptoms of shunt malfunction may be insidious or acute. Often, the earliest sign in the younger infant may be an increased velocity in head growth accompanied by a fullness or bulging in the anterior fontanelle. Lethargy, vomiting, and irritability are particularly common symptoms of the older infant with shunt dysfunction. If these signs and symptoms are reflective of increased intracranial pressure alone, then the clinical signs of common childhood febrile or afebrile illnesses including otitis media, diarrhea, or upper respiratory illness are usually absent. Although shunt infections also may present with lethargy, irritability, and vomiting, they often have an otherwise unexplained fever and commonly occur within a shunting postoperative period of several weeks to months. Other signs of increased intracranial pressure in the infant may include an acute onset of a sixth nerve palsy with abduction paresis or vocal cord paralysis and stridor. A croupy cough and stridor in an infant with myelomeningocele is often more likely associated with shunt malfunction than it is with an infectious respiratory process such as tracheolaryngobronchitis. Diagnostic studies for assessing the functional status of a shunt often include brain CT or ultrasound for ventricular size; plain radiographs of head, neck, chest, and abdomen for continuity of shunt tubing; and sterile collection of ventricular fluid through the shunt system for chemical and bacteriologic analysis.

Motor paralysis or weakness may contribute to both the development of musculoskeletal deformities and delays in gross motor skills during the first year. Parental instruction in proper positioning and passive stretching exercises for the child

IV

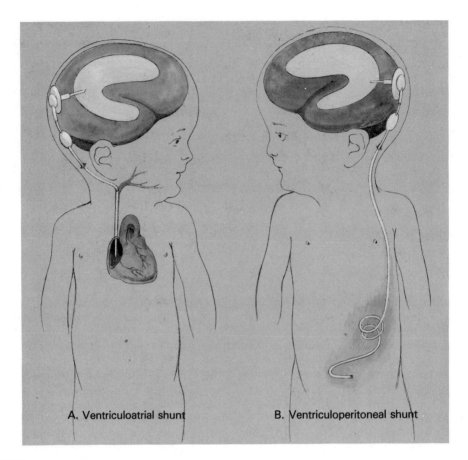

FIG 110-7
Ventricular shunting procedure for hydrocephalus. **A,**
Ventriculoatrial shunt. **B,** Ventriculoperitoneal shunt.

often can minimize the development of these
deformities.   Some infants, however, such as
those with rigid equinovarus deformities (club
feet), will require casting and/or surgical correction during this time. Delays in gross motor skills
including head and trunk control and independent sitting, crawling, and standing are common,
particularly among those with significant motor
paralysis. The valuable developmental experience of independent environmental exploration
may be compromised by these delays. Individualized therapy plans are therefore developed so
as to enhance gross motor as well as other developmental skills in these young children.

Management of the neurogenic bladder during
infancy is directed at ensuring adequate emptying, preserving normal upper tracts, and preventing urinary tract infection. Although the Credé

maneuver with suprapubic pressure has previously been recommended for bladder emptying,
recent evidence has been accumulating that suggests it may often be unnecessary and, at times,
harmful. Surveillance to ensure adequate bladder emptying and prevention of hydronephrosis
therefore utilizes repeat renal ultrasound and/or
IVP, often at 6 months and 1 year of age. The
prevention or control of urinary tract infections
often is dependent on regular collections, either
by midstream or urethral catheterization, of urine
specimens for culture. In general, during infancy
even asymptomatic bacteria is treated with a
course of oral antibiotic therapy. The indication
and efficacy of daily low-dose prophylactic antibiotic therapy remains controversial.

Bowel difficulties generally require no more
intervention than the routine well-baby dietary

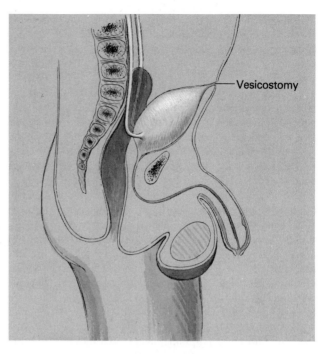

Vesicostomy

FIG 110-8
Vesicostomy with dome of bladder brought out to skin.

counseling. If after such counseling constipation persists, a trial of a daily mild rectal suppository (*ie,* glycerin) may be employed to avoid the complications of a persistent distended rectum. Dietary counseling is also important in avoiding obesity, because many of these infants have decreased caloric requirements on account of decreased motor activity. Obesity later in childhood can significantly compound and complicate an existent motor and/or psychosocial disability.

Anticipatory guidance for parents of these young infants is a critical part of their routine well-baby care. Parents often need repeated explanations of their child's birth defect, including its effect on the infant's overall development, what to expect as potential complications or management interventions, and the emotional effect of such a disability on both parents and siblings. A process of better appreciation and understanding of these issues on the part of parents often affords them a somewhat easier time in coping with a child's problem later in life. The primary care physician has the unique opportunity of seeing these infants and parents on a regular basis and may thereby be instrumental in establishing both the medical and emotional support necessary for this process.

Preschool-age Children

One of several major goals of management during the preschool years is independence in mobility. Sometime between 12 months and 5 years of age a child with myelomeningocele may learn to walk, depending on the level of paralysis, with or without the assistance of braces and/or crutches. Motor strength in the legs alone, however, does not ensure success in walking. Rather, a developmental readiness in both cognitive skills and motivation must be complemented by a therapeutic program before many of these children learn to walk. For some, musculoskeletal deformities of the hips, knees, or feet may interfere with functional standing or walking. Surgical management of these deformities during these years may then become necessary. Postoperative care may include casting of an immobilized joint for several weeks. It is not uncommon for these children to sustain fractures soon after cast removal, because their slender and osteoporotic bones fracture easily with minimal trauma. Painless swelling and redness of the involved leg usually develops within several days. Most lower-extremity fractures will heal with only temporary discontinuation of weight bearing while maintaining the child in braces, rather than casts. Sores to anesthetic skin often become problematic as the child becomes mobile, and anticipatory guidance should be directed at avoiding sunburn, tight-fitting shoes or braces, crawling on rough surfaces, and excessively hot baths.

Another major goal of management at this time is the achievement of fecal and urinary continence. Success in this area may afford the child an enhanced self-esteem while enabling him/her to remain clean and free of soiling and odor. Between 2 and 3 years of age, the family is encouraged to sit the child on the potty for several minutes after every meal. Often with the benefit of the postprandial gastrocolic reflex and gentle abdominal pressure or the Valsalva maneuver, the child may learn to have a regular timed bowel movement, thereby avoiding accidents other times of the day. If by 3 or 4 years of age this method of timed evacuation has not produced continence, then the families are instructed in the use of a nightly rectal suppository (*ie,* glycerin or bisacodyl) to stimulate regular emptying. Constant soiling or frequent loose bowel movements may be a sign of constipation with "bypass" diarrhea. More complete bowel emptying can then be accomplished with intermittent use of an enema. If modification of stool consistency is necessary for continence, then dietary manipulation is generally utilized rather than oral medications.

Attempts at achieving urinary continence are generally introduced after bowel continence has been achieved. This process usually involves a clean intermittent catheterization (CIC) program wherein parents and child are instructed in the clean, but not sterile, insertion of a catheter through the urethra approximately four times a day. If parents and child are compliant and there is complete bladder emptying without uninhibited detrusor contractions or diminished urethral resistance, continence may be achieved. In those children with bladders that cannot store urine adequately, a pharmocologic intervention may be necessary, consisting of either anticholinergic agents (*eg,* propantheline bromide, oxybutynin chloride) to diminish uninhibited detrusor contractions or adrenergic agents (*eg,* imipramine hydrochloride) to increase urethral resistance. Once adequate storage is accomplished, continence may be achieved with regular bladder emptying by CIC. Complications of CIC including epididymitis or urethral injury are rare. Asymptomatic bacteria is common. Courses of oral antibiotic therapy are utilized primarily in those with vesicoureteral reflux, upper tract damage, or symptomatic infections (*ie,* incontinence, fever). Urinary tract surveillance continues during these years with regular renal ultrasound or IVP. Development of vesicoureteral reflux with hydronephrosis may be managed initially with either a trial of CIC or vesicostomy for minimizing bladder pressure and enhancing emptying (*see* Fig. 110-8).

Although shunt malfunctions are most common during the first year of life, they can occur at any age. The older the child is, the more likely he/she will complain of headache as a manifestation of the increased intracranial pressure. Nausea, vomiting, lethargy, and/or strabismus also are frequently associated with malfunctioning shunt systems in the older child.

Assessment of the child's motor, language, and psychosocial development is another important aspect of overall treatment in these young children. Early intervention programs or other community educational resources may be extremely helpful for both the child with developmental delays and his/her family. When the child reaches the age to enter either kindergarten or first grade, psychological evaluation for school readiness may be available through the local community school system. Ideally, decisions regarding appropriate school or classroom setting should be based primarily on the child's cognitive and emotional development, rather than on the degree of physical disability.

School-age Children

Throughout the school-age years, emphasis in management must be directed at establishing and/or maintaining independence in self-care skills and self-respect. The latter is usually dependent on independence in mobility, toilet needs, avoidance of obesity, and success in school. Socialization among both disabled and nondisabled peers also must be developed for all the extensive medical and surgical intervention to be of value in producing a successful long-term functional outcome.

In general, the vast majority of children who can walk both at home and in their local community with braces and crutches will have achieved this skill by 6 years of age. For those children who are unable to walk on the basis of either severe paralysis, mental retardation, obesity, poor motivation, or severe musculoskeletal deformities, independent mobility in a wheelchair is encouraged. Progressive spinal deformities of

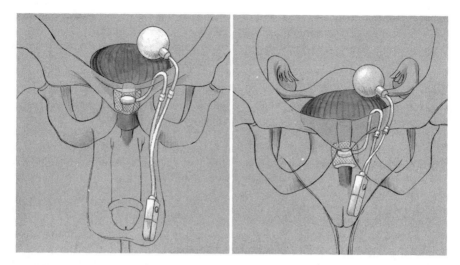

FIG 110-9

Artificial genitourinary sphincter (Scott-American Medical Systems). Pressure in cuff around bladder neck-urethra maintains continence. When pump in scrotum or labia is activated, fluid is transferred from the cuff to the retroperitoneal balloon, permitting bladder emptying. After several minutes, the cuff automatically refills, restoring continence.

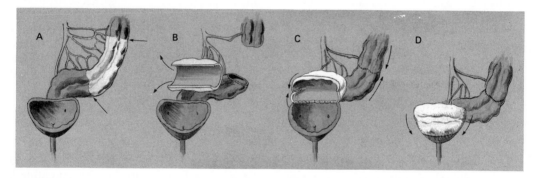

FIG 110-10

Augmentation sigmoid cystoplasty. **A,** A segment of sigmoid to be used for augmentation is outlined, and the bladder has been widely opened. **B,** The sigmoid segment converted into a patch in order to eliminate effective peristaltic contraction. **C,** Bowel continuity restored by intestinal anastomosis. The sigmoid patch being sutured to the bladder. **D,** Augmentation sigmoid cystoplasty completed.

scoliosis or kyphosis may interfere with functional sitting, standing, or walking during this time. In extreme situations, these deformities also may result in restrictive lung disease and cor pulmonale later in life. Although initial management of these deformities might include a plastic body jacket for trunk support, some may progress in severity and necessitate surgical fusion of the spine.

When CIC is successful in establishment of urinary continence, the child is encouraged to be an active participant in his/her toilet needs by performing self-catheterization, being responsible for the care of catheters, and regulating timing of the procedure. When continence has not been achieved, surgical intervention may be considered in a well-motivated youngster with urodynamic study evidence of a dysfunctional bladder that is unresponsive to pharmacologic measures. There are several surgical procedures for incontinence, including insertion of an artificial urinary sphincter (Fig. 110-9) or bladder augmentation with an intestinal patch (Fig. 110-10) that can enhance low-pressure bladder storage capacity and thereby afford the child an opportunity to be continent. Surveillance of the upper tracts is continued throughout these years with renal ultrasound or IVP and routine blood pressure measurement is utilized for identification of the unusual, but still possible, complication of hypertension secondary to renal damage.

The visual perceptual motor deficits that are frequently present in children with hydrocephalus commonly result in poor school performance. Unfortunately, the child's inability to attain the academic level of his/her classmates may be misinterpreted as either laziness, immaturity, or mental retardation, when in fact it may be symptomatic of a specific learning disability. Recognition and appreciation of this potential complication on the part of the school system can lead to early identification of the problem through appropriate psychometric testing. Remedial help may then be arranged with resource room or full-time specialized educational classroom settings. A successful experience in school, both in academic achievement and social acceptance by peers, can then contribute significantly to the establishment of an enhanced self-respect that is critical for a smoother emotional transition into adolescece.

Adolescents

Although a significant part of adolescent treatment is directed toward establishing emotional well-being, appropriate schooling, and realistic planning for the future, there are still some physical problems requiring attention. As some adolescents, particularly those with high paralysis, become more dependent on wheelchairs for mobility, they are prone to development of pressure decubitus ulcers of their anesthetic buttocks. Local wound care and avoidance of additional pressure or trauma is the major mode of therapy. Prevention of these sores may be accomplished by reminding the adolescent of the need for frequent positional changes while in the wheelchair and for maintaining adequate seating adaptations.

Sexual counseling is particularly important during the adolescent years. Abnormal sexual function is associated with a neurogenic bowel and bladder, because organ innervation is similar through the sacral portions of the spinal cord. For men, penile erection may be partial or not sustained, ejaculation may be absent or retrograde, and orgasm may not be precipitated by direct genital stimulation. Surgical management with artificial penile implants may be beneficial, and orgasm can be attained through stimulation of nonanesthetic erotic areas of the body. Women are generally fertile and can undergo normal labor and delivery. Both men and women have a 1 in 10 risk of parenting an infant with a neural tube defect.

It is not surprising that many of these children, by the nature of their disability, have significant problems in adolescent adjustment. Achievement of self-identity and independence is often difficult, and depression with social isolation is not uncommon. Although anticipation of these problems with appropriate intervention plans throughout childhood may be effective, additional support systems are often necessary during the adolescent years. Professional counseling may need to supplement guidance counseling through the school and social groups in the community. Parents of these teenagers and other family members also can benefit from additional emotional support and guidance.

SUMMARY

With recent advances in medical, surgical, and diagnostic technology, the majority of children with myelomeningocele now have the opportunity to live a normal life span. The quality of this life, however, is dependent to a considerable degree on supportive services available to them on both a national and local level. Emphasis must be placed, therefore, on the responsibility that society has to these disabled individuals if they are not only to survive, but also to become functional and productive citizens in the world.

BIBLIOGRAPHY

Brocklehurst G, editor: *Spina bifida for the clinician,* Clinics in Developmental Medicine, no 59. London, 1976, Spastics International Medical Publications.

Charney EB, Weller S, Sutton LN, et al: Myelomeningocele newborn management: Time for a decision making process, *Pediatrics* 75:58–64, 1985.

Charney EB, Weller SC, Sutton LN, et al: Management of Chiari II complications in infants with myelomeningocele, *J Pediatr* 111:364–371, 1987.

Freeman J: *Practical management of meningomyelocele,* Baltimore, 1979, University Park Press.

Liptak GS, Bloss JW, Briskin H, et al: The management of children with spinal dysraphism, *J Child Neurol* 3:3–20, 1988.

Rieder MJ: Prevention of neural tube defects with periconceptional folic acid, *Clin Perinatol* 21:483–503, 1994.

Shurtleff DB: Myelodysplasia: Management and treatment, *Curr Probl Pediatr* 10:1–90, 1980.

Shurtleff DB: *Myelodysplasias and extrophris: Significance, prevention, and treatment,* New York, 1986, Grune & Stratton.

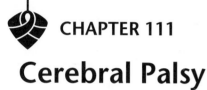

CHAPTER 111

Cerebral Palsy

Louis Pellegrino

Cerebral palsy is defined as a nonprogressive motor impairment. It comprises several syndromes that result from abnormalities in the early development of the brain. These syndromes are grouped together because they result in similar experiences and have similar functional and therapeutic implications.

CLASSIFICATION

Cerebral palsy often is subcategorized according to the type of motor impairment that predominates (Boxes 111-1 and 111-2). Cognitive and sensory impairments frequently accompany motor impairments in cerebral palsy, but they are not invariant features and are not included in the definition or classification of cerebral palsy. In spastic cerebral palsy, the predominant abnormality in muscle tone and motor control results from dysregulation of the stretch reflex. A lowered reflex threshold results in markedly increased deep tendon reflexes and sustained clonus. Although the whole body may be involved, for particular patients specific muscle groups tend to be more affected than others. Spastic cerebral palsy is further classified according to the distribution of limbs affected. In spastic diplegia, the lower extremities are mainly affected. In spastic hemiplegia, one side of the body is most affected. In spastic quadriplegia, all four limbs and usually the trunk and oral motor apparatus are affected. Dyskinetic cerebral palsy is characterized by tonal abnormalities, which by definition involve the whole body. Changing patterns of muscle tone from hour to hour and day to day are typical. These children often will exhibit rigid muscle tone while awake and normal or decreased muscle tone while asleep. Involuntary movements, although sometimes difficult to detect, are the hallmark of this type of cerebral palsy. Choreoform movements and athetosis are seen in athetoid cerebral palsy, a subtype of dyskinetic cerebral palsy. In dystonic cerebral palsy, rigid posturing centered in the trunk and neck is characteristic. Ataxic cerebral palsy is characterized especially by abnormalities of voluntary movement involving balance and position of the trunk and limbs in space. These abnor-

BOX 111-1
Definitions

Cerebral palsy:
A syndrome characterized by motor impairments that result from injury to or dysfunction of the developing brain. It is nonprogressive (*ie,* static encephalopathy).

Spasticity: Velocity-dependent increase in the resistance of a muscle to passive stretch (hypertonia) associated with increased deep tendon reflexes (lowered threshold for eliciting the stretch reflex), sustained clonus, and the clasp-knife response (a sudden decrease in resistance to passive stretch when a spastic muscle is stretched past a certain length).

Rigidity: Type of hypertonia seen in dyskinetic forms of cerebral palsy. It is characterized by fluctuating tonal abnormalities, antagonistic contractions of muscles across joints, "lead-pipe" rigidity (repeated stretching of muscle "works-out" tone), normal or slightly increased deep-tendon reflexes, clonus (if present) not sustained, no clasp-knife response.

Dyskinesia: Abnormal involuntary movements, often seen in dyskinetic cerebral palsy. Includes choreoform movements (rapid, random, jerky movements) and athetosis (slow, writhing movements).

Ataxia: Abnormality of voluntary movement, characterized by disordered amplitude and tempo of movements, associated with unsteady gait, past-pointing, intention tremor, and nystagmus.

BOX 111-2
Cerebral Palsy Classified According to Predominant Motor Impairment

Pyramidal	Spastic cerebral palsy	
	Diplegia	Involving primarily the lower extremities
	Hemiplegia	Involving primarily one side of the body
	Quadriplegia	Involving all four extremities, trunk, and oral motor structures
Extrapyramidal	Dyskinetic cerebral palsy	
	Athetoid	Characterized by choreoform movements or athetosis
	Dystonic	Characterized by dystonic posturing
	Ataxic	Characterizied by signs of cerebellar dysfunction
	Other	Meets the definition of cerebral palsy but cannot be categorized into main cerebral palsy types
	Mixed	Two or more motor impairment types equally predominant

malities may be associated with increased or decreased muscle tone in particular children. Cerebral palsy is classified as mixed when more than one type of motor pattern is present and one pattern does not clearly predominate over another.

The terms *pyramidal* and *extrapyramidal* refer to the presumed mechanisms for the motor abnormalities seen. Pyramidal cerebral palsy is synonymous with spastic cerebral palsy and implies abnormalities in the direct and indirect corticospinal pathways or cerebral gray matter. Extrapyramidal cerebral palsy refers to all other cerebral palsy types and implies pathologic involvement of the basal ganglia or cerebellum. The physiologic mechanisms suggested by these terms are presumptive and in some cases contro-

versial; the clinically descriptive terms *spastic, dyskinetic,* and *ataxic* are therefore preferable.

EPIDEMIOLOGY AND ETIOLOGY

The prevalence of cerebral palsy is approximately two in 1000 and has remained fairly constant despite efforts to remediate the clinical conditions that are presumed to lead to the development of cerebral palsy. Recent epidemiologic evidence strongly favors prenatal factors over perinatal problems in the pathophysiology of cerebral palsy, suggesting that improvements in obstetric care may have only marginal benefits in reducing the prevalence of cerebral palsy. Improved survival of very low birthweight infants, who are at increased risk for the development of cerebral palsy, has resulted in an increased representation of former premature infants in populations of children with cerebral palsy, thus helping to maintain the prevalence rate. In theory, efforts to reduce the rate of prematurely born infants would have the greatest impact toward decreasing the prevalence of cerebral palsy.

Epidemiologic and genetic studies suggest that multiple factors, especially those factors related to conditions during pregnancy, are responsible for predisposing an individual to cerebral palsy. Although a number of statistically significant risk factors have been defined in populations of children with cerebral palsy, none robustly predicts the development of cerebral palsy for the individual child. With regard to pathophysiologic mechanisms, a unique vulnerability of the periventricular white matter probably contributes to the development of spastic cerebral palsy in some former premature infants. An increased incidence of hypoxic-ischemic events (not necessarily perinatal) is suggested for some children with dyskinetic cerebral palsy. Ataxic cerebral palsy has been associated with specific genetic syndromes, such as Angelman syndrome. Given the heterogeneity of the motor impairment syndromes that are encompassed by the term *cerebral palsy,* it should not be surprising that a variety of etiologic factors would apply.

DIAGNOSTIC ISSUES

There are three distinct diagnostic issues that must be addressed when approaching a child with possible cerebral palsy: 1) making the diagnosis of cerebral palsy and determining the subtype; 2) making an effort to find the etiology of cerebral palsy, and 3) diagnosing associated impairments and disabilities.

Making the Diagnosis of Cerebral Palsy

The diagnosis of cerebral palsy rests on the recognition of severely delayed motor development associated with deviancy in muscle tone and motor control. Detailed knowledge of normal patterns of motor development in infancy is a prerequisite to diagnosis. During the first 2 years of life, an orderly sequence of events unfolds that results in the establishment of independent

---

BOX 111-3
Management of Spasticity

Physical modalities
  Range of motion/bracing/casting
  Heat/cold
  Electrical stimulation
Medication
  Diazepam
  Baclofen
  Dantrolene
Chemical neurolysis
  Nerve blocks
  Motor point blocks
Botulinum A exotoxin
Intrathecal baclofen
Selective dorsal rhizotomy

---

dent bipedal ambulation and exquisitely controlled fine motor skills. During the first year of life, primitive "reflex" patterns of motor activity seen at birth are gradually integrated into more complex voluntary patterns of behavior. During the same period, automatic, protective, antigravity reactions develop as an adjunct to voluntary movement. By the time a child reaches preschool age, he/she is no longer hindered by immature motor patterns and has all of the skills and fail-safe mechanisms needed to navigate freely and safely in his/her environment.

In contrast, the child with incipient cerebral palsy has significantly delayed motor milestones. There is a similar delay in the integration of primitive reflexes (which for some never disappear) and the emergence of protective reactions (which for some never appear). The child typically will present to the pediatrician when a concerned parent realizes that the child is not progressing as expected. A number of diagnostic difficulties arise at this juncture. The first difficulty is in recognizing how significant a motor delay is. In general, if a child has not achieved a milestone at an age (corrected for prematurity) when more than 90% of children do, then the delay must be considered significant (*eg,* greater than 7 months of age for sitting without support, greater than 15 months of age for walking independently).

The second difficulty relates to the cause of motor delay. Global developmental delay, not cerebral palsy, is the most common cause of significant motor delay. Delay in motor development alone is not sufficient for the diagnosis of cerebral palsy.

IV

The third difficulty is that the typical pattern of motor deviancy for a particular child does not fully emerge until 2 to 3 years of age. For example, many children who will eventually meet the criteria for spastic quadriplegia will be hypotonic or will have truncal hypotonia and mild hypertonia of the limbs during infancy and will only gradually develop global hypertonia. Children with athetoid cerebral palsy may not exhibit characteristic involuntary movements until 2 to 3 years of age. Ataxia may be difficult to appreciate in a nonambulatory child.

The fourth difficulty relates especially to former premature infants. Some of these children will show mild tonal abnormalities (ie, increased tone in the lower extremities, seen as scissoring and extensor posturing, associated with mild truncal hypotonia), which resolve by 2 years of age; many of these children are prematurely diagnosed with cerebral palsy. Although it is important to recognize abnormal patterns of motor development and begin appropriate monitoring and remediation, it is hazardous in most cases to make a definitive diagnosis of cerebral palsy before a child is 2 years of age.

Etiologic Diagnosis

Given the heterogeneity of neurologic conditions grouped under this condition, it is not possible to create a diagnostic algorithm for the determination of etiology that would apply to every child with cerebral palsy. It is also important to consider the goals in pursuing an etiologic diagnosis. In most cases, an etiologic diagnosis does not result in a change in recommendations for the child's care. It is important that the child's parents understand this before embarking on a course of extensive and expensive testing. A notable exception to this rule relates to the pursuit of inborn errors of metabolism and other neurodegenerative disorders. In some cases a specific treatment may be indicated that could result in improved prognosis or even cure. Sometimes children who are diagnosed as having "cerebral palsy" because of physical findings consistent with upper motor neuron dysfunction also have a history of neurologic deterioration that is chronic or episodic (therefore excluding them from a diagnosis of cerebral palsy by definition). When episodes of deterioration are associated with vomiting, changes in diet, or sudden weight loss, this should increase concerns about possible metabolic disease. The results of brain imaging studies (such as white matter anomalies on magnetic resonance imaging), and ophthalmologic examination (such as retinal abnormalities and inclusions) may point to particular metabolic syndromes. Typical laboratory studies include electrolyte studies to allow the calculation of the anion gap (increased in the presence of a fixed acid), ammonia levels (elevated in urea cycle disorders), lactate and pyruvate (levels and ratios help to distinguish carbohydrate and respiratory chain disorders), and blood amino acid and urine organic acid determinations. An increasing number of metabolic conditions, including storage disorders and leukodystrophies, will not be discovered by routine metabolic testing, however. If a high clinical suspicion remains, further evaluation by a metabolic specialist is indicated.

Another reason to pursue an etiologic diagnosis is for the purposes of family and genetic counseling. A careful history and physical examination are required to raise suspicion about genetic disorders and should guide the selection of further laboratory data. A careful pregnancy history may suggest a specific prenatal etiology such as infection. A family history should include questions about neurologic, developmental, and psychiatric conditions and also should explore any history of recurrent fetal loss or prematurity. An infant who was small for gestational age or who has a number of physical anomalies not attributable to the child's neurologic condition is more likely to have an identifiable genetic syndrome. A child with ataxic cerebral palsy is also more likely to have an identifiable genetic syndrome. In cases in which no specific etiology is suggested by the history and physical examination, an empiric risk of 10% to 20% for cerebral palsy in subsequent children has been suggested.

Diagnosis of Associated Impairments and Disabilities

Other impairments and disabilities frequently found in association with the motor impairment characteristic of cerebral palsy can be classified into three groups: sensory, cognitive, and physiologic.

Sensory impairment in children with cerebral palsy is very common and can be easily overlooked in the clinician's zeal to address motor abnormalities. There is a high incidence of visual impairments, including myopia, amblyopia, visual fields defects (especially in children with hemiplegia), and cortical blindness. Oculomotor disturbances such as strabismus are also common and predispose to the development of amblyopia. There is an increased incidence of hearing loss, especially among former premature infants. Many children have somatosensory deficits (eg, abnormalities of proprioception), but these are difficult to test for and quantify, and the benefits of intervention strategies for these deficits are unclear. It is therefore recommended that all children with cerebral palsy have early and regular examinations by a pediatric ophthalmologist, and hearing should be tested by a licensed audiologist with experience in the evaluation of children with developmental disabilities.

For many individuals with cerebral palsy, cognitive disabilities pose a greater obstacle to fuller functioning in society than do limitations in mobility. It is estimated that approximately one half of children with cerebral palsy have mental retardation as a second developmental diagnosis. This figure may be an overestimate: most centers that collect such statistics see a sample of children that is biased toward more severe impairment and disability. Although children with more severe motor disability tend to have higher rates of mental retardation (eg, mental retardation is more common among children with spastic quadriplegia than among children with spastic diplegia), this is not invariably true, and normal intelligence may be found in individuals with very severe motor impairments. Among those with normal intelligence, there is an increased incidence of learning disabilities, developmental languages disorders, and probably attention deficit/hyperactivity disorder.

For the medical professional, the physiologic impairments associated with cerebral palsy are of particular concern. Conceptually these may be divided into impairments that are a direct manifestation of the central nervous system dysfunction that gave rise to the cerebral palsy and impairments that are a secondary consequence of the primary disturbance in neuromotor function. For example, spasticity may be seen as a primary manifestation of cerebral palsy in a particular child, whereas musculotendonous contracture is the long-term consequence of persistent hypertonicity and fiber shortening in particular muscle groups and is therefore considered to be a secondary impairment. In practice it is often difficult to separate primary and secondary impairments. For example, gastroesophageal reflux, a common problem for many children with cerebral palsy, may be due in part to neurologically based abnormalities in gastrointestinal motility but is clearly influenced by secondary factors such as increased intra-abdominal pressure related to spasticity of the abdominal musculature, constipation related to physical immobility and dietary factors, and abnormalities of position related to the physical characteristics of a particular child. For the pediatrician, awareness of the list of commonly associated problems is the first step toward developing a management strategy for the care of the child with cerebral palsy (Table 111-1).

THE MEDICAL MANAGEMENT OF CEREBRAL PALSY: HABILITATION

The goal for medical management of the child with cerebral palsy is to maximize function and optimize development. In practice this means working to create opportunities for the fullest possible participation in a wide variety of societal settings. The management strategy with this ultimate goal is called *habilitation*. The pediatrician has a pivotal role in the implementation of this strategy. The primary physician who is most familiar with a particular child and his/her family is in the best position to establish goals for medical management that are consonant with the principle of habilitation. Although the many physicians, teachers, and therapists who work with children with cerebral palsy are in an excellent position to define the various impairments and disabilities associated with this condition, families are in the best position to define what "optimizing development," "maximizing function," and "achieving fullest possible participation" actually means for their particular child. The pediatrician is in a position to synthesize the clinical data and the situation-dependent (contextual) data into a coherent picture that forms the basis for medical management and decision-making.

TABLE 111-1
The Medical Management of Cerebral Palsy: Common Medical Problems

PROBLEM/ISSUE	ONSET	FEATURES	THERAPEUTIC APPROACH
Seizures	Neonatal seizures with hypoxic-ischemic encephalopathy; any age for other types	Generalized seizures predominate; partial seizures are common; infantile spasms and Lennox-Gastaut are seen	Individualized; the goal is monotherapy, preferring agents with fewer cognitive side-effects (eg, phenytoin, valproate, and carbamazepine)
Spasticity/dystonia	Develops over first 2 years	Muscle tone abnormalities	Physical therapy is mainstay; a variety of medical and surgical interventions are available (see the Box 111-3)
Contractures	Early childhood, dependent on cerebral palsy type	Permanent shortening/tightness of musculotendinous unit	Lengthening by splinting or serial casting, vigorous physical therapy, surgical lengthening and releases
Hip dislocation	Early childhood, dependent on cerebral palsy type	Subluxation of femoral head out of acetabulum progressing to frank dislocation	Wearing abduction wedge with knee immobilizers to keep femoral head seated in acetabulum at night; soft-tissue releases to prevent subluxation from progressing to dislocation; varus derotational osteotomy and/or complex revision of the acetabulum in complicated dislocations
Scoliosis	All through childhood; worsens with puberty	Curvature of the spine leading to compromise of cardiopulmonary function in severe cases	Early bracing, appropriate seating systems; surgical correction and fixation, preferably after skeletal maturation has been achieved
Other musculoskeletal problems	Any age	Variety of foot deformities; degenerative joint disease	Specific to problem
Poor growth	Typically during infancy, or with changes in diet (eg, bottle feedings to solids) or caregivers	Weight and weight/height < 5th percentile; biochemical evidence of malnutrition (eg, hypoalbuminemia, iron deficiency anemia); poor subcutaneous fat stores, muscle wasting	Behavioral interventions to improve feeding practices; nutritional supplements by mouth; nighttime (temporary) nasogastric tube feedings; permanent gastrostomy or jejunostomy feedings
Gastroesophageal reflux	Infancy/early childhood	Poor growth; irritability; excessive arching; gagging; emesis	Diet modification and positioning; antacids; H_2 blockers (eg, ranitidine, famotidine); prokinetic agents (metaclopromide, cisapride); surgery (fundal plication)

Condition	Age	Features	Management
Constipation	Infancy/early childhood	Infrequent, often hard bowel movements; may complicate feeding/growth problems	Dietary (fiber supplementation); following initial "clean-out," stool softener (eg, docasate sodium, milk of magnesia) coupled with laxative (eg, extract of senna, bisacodyl)
Aspiration pneumonia	Any age	Liquids or solids aspirated as a consequence of poor oral motor function; severe gastroesophageal reflux complicated by aspiration; chemical pneumonitis with infection including anaerobic bacteria	Treatment of underlying cause to prevent aspiration is the key intervention; appropriate supportive therapy (oxygen, antibiotics) as indicated for acute episodes
Developmental delay/sensory impairments	Infancy/early childhood	Delays in a variety of skill areas relative to age-mates; problems with vision, hearing, and somatic sensation	Early developmental, ophthalmologic, and audiologic assessment should be considered mandatory for all children with cerebral palsy. Early intervention services tailored to the profile of cognitive and sensory impairments should be considered in most cases
Strabismus	Infancy/early childhood	Disconjugate gaze may lead to amblyopia ("lazy eye") and permanent preventable loss of vision	Patching; surgery
Dental abnormalities	Any age	Enamel abnormalities may be due to intrauterine abnormalities in development; more often, poor dental hygiene relates to difficulty in on-going care; gingival hyperplasia is seen with the use of phenytoin	Problem specific
Decubitus (pressure) ulcers	Any age	Skin breakdown related to unrelieved pressure, typically over bony prominences, complicated by poor nutrition, absence of adequate subcutaneous fat pads	Pressure relief and adequate nutrition, coupled with good local wound care, are key to healing. Surgical intervention (debridement, surgical closure) is required in selected cases
Spastic bladder	Any age	Recurrent urinary tract infections; urinary frequency related to hypertonicity of the detrusor muscle	Urinalysis and culture; renal ultrasound; urodynamic studies

IV

BIBLIOGRAPHY

Accardo PJ, Capute AJ: *The pediatrician and the developmentally delayed child: A clinical textbook on mental retardation,* Baltimore, 1979, University Park Press.

Freeman JM, Nelson KB: Intrapartum asphyxia and cerebral palsy, *Pediatrics* 82:240–249, 1988.

Hughes I, Newton R: Genetic aspects of cerebral palsy, *Dev Med Child Neurol* 34:80–86, 1992.

Kuban KC, Leviton A: Cerebral palsy, *N Engl J Med* 330(3):118–195, 1994.

Nelson KB, Ellenberg JH: Antecedents of cerebral palsy: Multivariate analysis of risk, *N Engl J Med* 315:81–86, 1986.

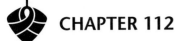

CHAPTER 112

Mental Retardation

Maureen A. Fee

Mental retardation is one of the most common of the major developmental disabilities. Six million Americans of all ages experience mental retardation. One in 10 individuals in this country has a family member with mental retardation. Defined by the American Association on Mental Deficiency, mental retardation refers to substantial limitations in present functioning. It is characterized by significantly subaverage intellectual functioning, existing concurrently with related limitations in two or more of the following applicable adaptive skill areas: communication, self-care, home living, social skills, community use, self-direction, health and safety, functional academics, leisure, and work. Mental retardation manifests before age 18 years. The primary care physician holds an important role in early identification, etiologic evaluation, and coordination of treatment for children with mental retardation. Familiarity with the classification and management issues is essential for fulfilling this role and responsibility.

CLASSIFICATION

The 1992 definition of mental retardation is based on a multidimensional approach intended to broaden the conceptualization of mental retardation, avoid reliance on intelligence quotient (IQ) to assign level of disability (classification), and relate an individual's needs to the level of support required. Hence, the largely IQ-based labels of mild, moderate, severe, and profound will be abandoned in favor of a single diagnostic code for mental retardation with greater emphasis on the individual's needs in various domains (communication, self-help) and the levels of support (intermittent, limited, extensive, pervasive) required to achieve optimal outcome. Thus, the goal is to provide a diagnosis of a "person with mental retardation, who requires limited support in communication, social skills, and self direction" rather than a diagnosis of "mild mental retardation." Because there is an evolution to this method of classification it is prudent to be

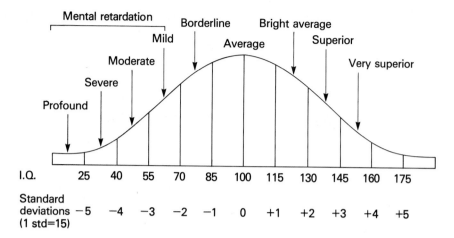

FIG 112-1
Classification of intelligence.

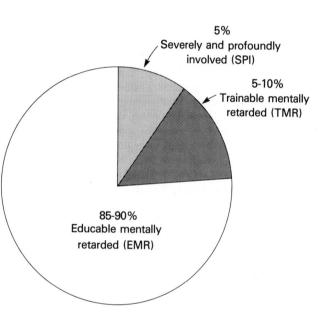

FIG 112-2
Subgrouping of mental retardation, showing that 85% to 90% of individuals are mildly retarded.

aware of the IQ-based classifications that are still in frequent use.

The first step in the classification for mental retardation is determination of an IQ (mental age/chronological age × 100) that is two standard deviations or more below the mean (represented by 100) based on standardized psychological tests (Fig. 112-1). The educational and functional characteristics largely follow the IQ distribution so that individuals with retardation fall into one of four categories: mild, moderate, severe, or profound. Those children with IQ scores in the 70 to 80 range are said to be borderline and are not

labeled mentally retarded. They are considered "slow learners," and are usually academically at the lower end in a regular classroom within the school district. Outside of the educational milieu they show social and vocational independence. The mildly retarded group constitutes the largest subgroup, accounting for 85% to 90% of those individuals labeled mentally retarded (Fig. 112-2). Within the educational sphere they may attend EMR (educable mentally retarded) classrooms where they are able to achieve a fair degree of literacy (reading at the third- to fifth-grade level) in addition to vocational training. More

TABLE 112-1
Functional/Educational Profile of Mental Retardation

IQ	RETARDATION CLASSIFICATION	EDUCATIONAL SETTING	FUNCTIONAL/ADAPTIVE OUTCOME
55–69	Mild	EMR (Learning support)	Identification late preschool, early school years May achieve degree of literacy (read at 3rd–5th grade level) Employed in unskilled or semiskilled capacities May be able to live independently with little supervision
40–54	Moderate	TMR (Life skills)	Identified during preschool years May achieve some basic academic skills Employed in sheltered workshops Independent in self-care and can live in community based home
25–39 <25	Severe Profound	SPI (Multiple handicapped)	Identified in infancy Total dependence, although some very basic self-help skills may be achieved

recently these placements are called learning support classrooms. Such individuals can maintain gainful employment and possibly live independently and marry. Five percent to 10% of those individuals categorized as mentally retarded are in the moderately retarded group and may attend TMR (trainable mentally retarded) classrooms. These classrooms are often now referred to as life skills support classrooms. Here they can learn basic self-help skills that will allow them to live in a community-based home with ample supervision. From a vocational standpoint they are prepared for employment in a sheltered workshop. The remaining 5% fall into the severely and profoundly retarded groups. Their educational needs are very similar and therefore allow them to be grouped together in a SPI (severely and profoundly impaired) classroom or multiple handicapped classroom. Extensive supervision is required, and minimal self-care skills can sometimes be achieved. Limited conversational skills may be seen in the severely retarded, whereas language development in the profoundly impaired is minimal indeed. Table 112-1 illustrates the educational and functional correlates of the various classifications.

PREVALENCE

Overall prevalence is 3%, although prevalence figures vary with age. Because mildly retarded children are often not identified until school-age years, the prevalence of retardation in the preschool years is 0.5%. As the demands increase in the educational setting the prevalence peaks in the age group of 6 to 16 years and may be as high as 10% in some urban settings. When individuals leave the educational environment the more mildly impaired are assimilated into the general population, and the rate in the adult years is approximately 1%. Thus, the prevalence varies with age, based on whether the adaptive behavior is considered deficient. This depends on the setting and consequent expectations rather than on the subaverage intellectual functioning, which is constant. An additional factor in the decreased incidence with age is the increased death rate in the more severely affected. A preponderance of men are affected (55:45), primarily due to the sex-linked disorders (ie, fragile-X syndrome, Menkes syndrome, adrenoleukodystrophy, mucopolysaccharidosis type II).

DIAGNOSIS

Age at diagnosis varies with severity of the disability and with associated clinical findings. Thus, the primary care physician is in a key position for early diagnosis of mental retardation. The diagnosis may be entertained because of a previously known medical diagnosis (eg, chromosomal abnormalities, intrauterine infections, neurocutaneous disorder) or as a result of the patient being in a high-risk category based on past medical history or family history. The more mildly involved youngsters may be devoid of physical stigmata and may only be identified by thorough developmental screening examination in the office. Once a child is suspected of having a developmental lag based on a screening tool such as the Denver Developmental Screening Test (Denver II), a more definitive evaluation (*eg,* Bayley Infant Scale of Mental Development— Revised) may be performed by a developmental psychologist as part of an interdisciplinary developmental assessment.

ETIOLOGY

Once the diagnosis of mental retardation is established, the physician begins the second role, of establishing a cause. The pursuit of a cause is important for identifying the medically treatable causes of mental retardation as well as those that are inheritable. As with any diagnostic problem in medicine, a thorough history is essential, including an in-depth family history as well as prenatal, perinatal, and postnatal history for the affected child. After completion of a thorough history the physician may be able to categorize the mental retardation as being either prenatal, perinatal, or postnatal in onset (Box 112-1). Further delineation of the cause is sought through the physical examination and the growth parameters, especially the serial head circumference measurements. Special attention should be given to any physical stigmata that may prove helpful in establishing a chromosomal or teratogenic cause or a specific syndrome diagnosis. In addition, a thorough ophthalmologic evaluation will aid in the diagnosis of the neurocutaneous syndromes, intrauterine infections, various syndromes, and degenerative disorders manifested by retinal changes.

LABORATORY ASSESSMENT

The laboratory investigation of mental retardation should be based on the history and physical examination and directed toward the identification of the inheritable and treatable causes of mental retardation. It has been shown that routine laboratory tests (*ie,* those that were not indicated by specific history or physical findings) are not usually helpful in eliciting the cause of the child's mental retardation. Also, it is impor-

---

BOX 112-1
Causes of Mental Retardation

Prenatal
  Cranial/cerebral malformations (lissencephaly, holoprosencephaly, congenital hydrocephalus, craniostenosis)
  Chromosomal abnormalities (Down syndrome)
  Intrauterine infections (toxoplasmosis, rubella, cytomegalovirus, herpes, syphilis [TORCH])
  Teratogens (phenytoin, alcohol, irradiation, trimethadione)
  Neurocutaneous disorders (Sturge-Weber syndrome, tuberous sclerosis, neurofibromatosis, linear nevus sebaceous of Jadassohn)
  Placental dysfunction
  Metabolic disorders
    Aminoacidurias (phenylketonuria, homocystinuria, maple syrup urine disease, prolinemia, nonketotic hyperglycinemia, citrullinemia)
    Mucopolysaccharidoses (*eg,* Hunter syndrome, Hurler syndrome)
    Carbohydrate disorders (*eg,* galactosemia)
    Leukodystrophies (*eg,* adrenoleukodystrophy, metachromatic leukodystrophy)
    Purine disorders (Lesch-Nyhan syndrome)
  Hormonal (hypothyroidism, hypoparathyroidism)
Perinatal
  Asphyxia/anoxia
  Infections (sepsis, meningitis)
  Hemorrhage (intraventricular, subarachnoid, fetal-maternal)
  Metabolic (*eg,* hyperbilirubinemia, hypoglycemia)
Postnatal
  CNS trauma
  CNS infections (viral, bacterial)
  CNS toxins (*eg,* lead)
  Anoxic episodes (*eg,* aborted sudden infant death, near drowning)

CNS—central nervous system.

---

tant to realize that 65% to 75% of the retarded population will not have one identifiable biologic or organic cause. The children falling into the mildly retarded range have the lowest yield in terms of an identifiable organic cause. Those in the lower functioning groups will have an increased yield and are more likely to show chromosomal, metabolic, or structural cerebral abnormalities.

Computed tomography (CT) or magnetic resonance imaging may be useful when based on an indication by history or physical examination that is consistent with a progressively enlarging head, a diagnosis of a disorder such as tuberous sclerosis, focal seizures, a focal neurologic examination, or microcephaly in a child. In children with a nonfocal examination and nonspecific mental retardation, the CT scan may be nonspecific and show only cerebral atrophy. A metabolic workup including urine for metabolic screening (amino acids, organic acids, and mucopolysaccharide metabolites) is important in the children functioning below the mildly retarded range; especially in those with poor growth and/or seizure activity. In addition, thyroid screening is often helpful in children with a clinical picture suggestive of hypothyroidism. It is important to consider this diagnosis in children with previously identified causes of mental retardation, such as children with Down syndrome who have an increased incidence of thyroid disease. Chromosome analysis should be performed in children who have three or more congenital abnormalities. Also, this is an important investigation in those children who have a family history consistent with numerous spontaneous abortions. In addition to the routine karyotype analysis with banding, the fragile-X analysis should be performed in boys with an unexplained cause for mental retardation (especially those who display the phenotypic appearance of fragile-X syndrome or have features of pervasive developmental disorder (ie, autism) and girls with mental retardation and a strong family history of retardation in men in the family. Newer techniques such as fluorescent in situ hybridization and analysis of specific DNA sequences detect deletions and rearrangements not identified through standard cytogenetic banding. These techniques will serve to further increase the identifiable causes of mental retardation.

In those children suspected of having a neurodegenerative disorder, a more comprehensive evaluation will need to be undertaken; therefore, referral to a consulting pediatric neurologist is often necessary.

MANAGEMENT

In many ways the diagnosis of mental retardation is a psychological and educational diagnosis. Very few disorders of mental retardation are treatable in the traditional medical model. Although the approach is largely an educational one (whether the education takes place in a fully inclusive setting such as a regular classroom with the appropriate supportive services or in a fulltime special education classroom), the primary care physician plays a vital role in terms of management. The group of children with mental retardation as a whole has more medical complications (seizure disorders, cerebral palsy, feeding disorders, increased incidence of congenital heart disease and chromosomal abnormalities) than the average population. The physician is often in the position of being an advocate for the child and family. In order to do this the primary care physician must have a fund of knowledge and resources that will be beneficial to the handicapped individual. A familiarity with the Individuals with Disabilities Education Act of 1990 (IDEA), ensuring the legal right of education up to the age of 21 years for the handicapped, is essential (see Chapter 121). Being involved with and understanding the educational process is important for assisting parents in obtaining the optimal educational experience for their children. Knowledge of community services such as respite care, the Association for Retarded Citizens, and residential facilities will enable the physician to direct the parents to these resources when needed.

Since IDEA was passed, the primary care physician has had an even more active role in the area of early identification and referral. The law expands services to children 3 to 5 years of age and provides a mechanism of addressing the needs of infants and toddlers (birth through age 3 years) who are experiencing developmental delays or "at risk of having developmental delays if early intervention services are not provided."

Early identification, prior to the school years, will enable the physician to refer to an infant stimulation program with the triple goal of optimizing the infant's development potential, providing parental support, and identifying the child early so that transition into the public school setting is facilitated.

Involvement with the family of a mentally retarded child or adult is an ongoing process. The term chronic sorrow has often been used to describe a feeling within the families of the mentally retarded. Each life milestone for the retarded individual (entry into school, expected time of graduation, sexual maturation, and entry into the work force) may provide further confirmation of the child's deficits. Also, a mentally retarded child places increased stresses on the family structure and on siblings. The primary care physician may be instrumental in exploring these aspects or may need to know resources for referral for the needed support. Thus, the role of the physician only begins with the diagnosis, and continues throughout the child's life. During this extended time, the responsibility is not restricted to the child alone, but must also encompass the family unit as well.

BIBLIOGRAPHY

Chudley AE, Hagerman RJ: Fragile X syndrome, *J Pediatr* 110:821–831, 1987.

Denhoff E: Status of infant stimulation or enrichment programs for children with developmental disabilities, *Pediatrics* 67:32, 1981.

Education of the Handicapped Act Amendments of 1986. Pub L No 99–457, 20 USC §1400, et seq.

Mental retardation: Definition, classification and systems of support, Washington, DC, 1992, American Association on Mental Deficiency.

McLaren J, Brown SE. Review of recent epidemiologic studies of mental retardation: Prevalence, associated disorders and etiology, *Am J Ment Retard* 243–254, 1992.

Miller LG: Toward a greater understanding of the parents of the mentally retarded child, *J Pediatr* 73:699–705, 1968.

President's Committee on Mental Retardation 1987: *Guide for state planning for the prevention of mental retardation and related disabilities,* Rockville, MD, US Department of Health and Human Services, DHHS Publication No 87–21034.

Smith DW: *Recognizable patterns of human malformation,* Philadelphia, 1982, WB Saunders.

Smith DW, Simons FER: Rational diagnostic evaluation of the child with mental deficiency. *Am J Dis Child* 129:1285–1290, 1975.

IV

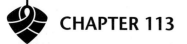

CHAPTER 113

Cleft Lip and Palate

Don LaRossa

In the early weeks of pregnancy, when many women are not certain they are pregnant, the human face and palatal structures are developing. During this time, a cleft of the lip and/or palate will occur in one of 750 to one of 1000 gestations.

During the 3rd to 7th week of pregnancy, the nasofrontal and lateral maxillary processes normally coalesce to form the nose, upper lip, and alveolar structures anterior to the incisive foramen. Failure of normal fusion will result in a cleft of the lip and alveolus (prepalatal structures). The extent of failed fusion determines the severity of the cleft. The cleft may extend completely into the nasal cavity with a gap in the upper arch and a markedly distorted nose (complete cleft). Various degrees of "healing in utero" may occur reducing the severity of the cleft (incomplete cleft). The closure may be almost complete leaving only a minimal notch in the vermilion-cutaneous border of the lip and slight widening and retrodisplacement of the ala nasi on the cleft side. All variations of complete or incomplete clefts may occur unilaterally or bilaterally.

During the 7th to 11th weeks of gestation, the true palate (posterior to the incisive foramen) forms. The head unflexes, mandibular growth occurs, and the tongue moves out from between the two vertically oriented palatal shelves. This allows the two hemipalates to move downward into a horizontal position. They fuse from the incisive foramen posteriorly. Failure of the head to unflex inhibits mandibular growth, prevents the tongue from dropping out from between the palatal shelves, and prevents palatal closure. This is thought to be the etiology for Robin sequence (Pierre Robin sequence), with micrognathia, glossoptosis, and airway obstruction, often associated with cleft palate. In this anomaly, the cleft is often wide and horseshoe-shaped. It is seen commonly in children with Stickler syndrome and velocardiofacial syndrome.

Failure of complete closure of the palate may leave a bifid uvula, an incidental finding seen in approximately 2% of the population. Mucosal fusion without muscular fusion results in a submucosal cleft of the palate seen in approximately one of 10,000 children. A true cleft of the palate occurs when there is a lack of closure or fusion of all layers of the palate and may be associated with a cleft of the lip and prepalatal structures.

Clefts of only the palate are more common in girls, whereas cleft lip is more often seen in boys. A complete, left unilateral cleft of the lip and palate is the most common variant seen. Ethnic variations are noted as well, with Asian children affected more often than white children, who are affected more frequently than black children. Cleft lip can sometimes be seen on uterine ultrasound at 16 weeks gestation, although cleft palate is usually not visualized.

Although heredity can account for a cleft (Table 113-1), most instances are sporadic. Likewise, most clefts are not part of syndromes, although a large number of associated malformations have been described. One of the most commonly seen associated malformations is Stickler syndrome with which the Robin sequence seems to be more prevalent. Velocardiofacial, Van der Woude, Binders, Apert, Crouzon, and Treacher Collins syndromes are commonly seen.

TABLE 113-1
Frequency of Cleft Lip and Palate or Cleft Palate Occurring in Family Members*

AFFECTED RELATIVES	PREDICTED RECURRENCE (%)	
	CLEFT LIP/PALATE	CLEFT PALATE
One sibling	4.4	2.5
One parent	3.2	6.8
One sibling, one parent	15.8	14.9

*From Ross RB, Johnston MC: *Cleft lip and palate,* Baltimore, 1972, Williams & Wilkins. Used by permission.

Drug ingestion has been implicated as causative in mothers taking phenytoin (Dilantin), whereas cortisone can produce clefts in certain strains of laboratory mice. Few commonly used drugs are known to cause the defect. Folic acid deficiency has been implicated, although there is a lack of conclusive evidence in man for this or any other metabolic or vitamin deficiencies causing clefts.

The term *cleft lip and palate* inadequately describes the potential complexity of the deformity. The nose, lip, alveolus, and palate can all be involved. As a consequence, appearance, dentition, dental occlusion, facial growth, speech, and hearing can all be affected. Perhaps more far-reaching are the psychosocial implications for the affected individual.

The birth of an infant with a cleft has a profound effect on the family and presents a challenge to the primary care physician. Because of the complexity of the deformity and the long-term nature of the treatment, a multidisciplinary team approach has been used widely in the United States and worldwide, wherever sophisticated medical care is available. The specialists essential to the team are the plastic surgeon, speech pathologist, orthodontist, pediatrician, and otolaryngologist. In an ideal situation, a psychologist, geneticist, anthropologist, pedodontist, prosthodontist, opthalmologist, and nurse are team members. A team coordinator/educator oversees the team's functioning and its interaction with patients. The evaluation team collaborates to plan treatment strategies, and also serves as a forum for continuing education of the team members by an exchange of knowledge from each specialty area.

GENERAL AND SPECIAL AREAS OF CARE OF THE PATIENT WITH CLEFT LIP OR PALATE

Care in the Newborn Period

The newborn period presents the greatest challenge to the physician, family, and team. Not uncommonly, those who initially provide care for the infant with a cleft are unprepared, despite the relative frequency of clefting. Intervention by someone familiar with the problem should be prompt so as to provide consolation and education to the parents. Outreach by the team nurse, coordinator or parent, of a cleft patient, trained at providing support, is critical at this time. Parents need information about what has happened and where to go for help. Hospital personnel may need advice about feeding and community resources as well.

A general evaluation looking for other anomalies is undertaken. In particular, airway obstruction related to Robin sequence must be assessed. In this anomaly, the dyad of cleft palate size and mandible size interact with each other. The degree of airway obstruction varies directly with jaw size and inversely with cleft size. That is, a wide cleft can help compensate for a small mandible (the tongue size being constant). Hence a child with a small mandible and narrow cleft may quickly get into serious respiratory difficulty, whereas one with a wide cleft may be adequately compensated. Complicating this situation further is the risk of upper airway narrowing or collapse from pharyngeal hypotonia or tracheomalacia. In this case a complete airway assessment and polysomnography are visually indicated.

Feeding Infants with Cleft Lip or Palate

Because clefts of only the lip do not interfere with normal feeding, breastfeeding is often possible. Feeding problems occur in a child with a cleft of the palate who does not suck normally because of his/her inability to create a seal. The nipple on the bottle must be modified to allow milk to flow easily. A preemie nipple should be crosscut with scissors or a Bard Parker® (Becton Dickinson and Company, Lincoln Park, NJ) no. 11 scalpel so that milk drips from the bottle when it is held upside-down. Too much flow will flood the infant's mouth; too little will cause fatigue and malnutri-

tion. The child should be fed in the upright, or football, position and burped frequently, because excess air will be ingested. The infant should sleep in an infant seat or on his/her side. These maneuvers are particularly important in the child with Robin sequence, in which the tongue may fall back into the oropharynx or become lodged above the cleft completely obstructing the airway. Such an infant may have to be fed in an upright position or even tipped forward to get the tongue out of the way to permit feeding. Nasogastric feeding tubes should be used only as a last resort. If one becomes necessary, it is imperative to sham feed the infant with a pacifier during nasogastric feeding lest he/she forgets how to suck.

Children with Robin sequence should be placed on an apnea monitor and have a pulse-oximetry done during feeding to assess the degree of oxygenation. Polysomnography are indicated to fully assess other causes for apnea. If hypoxic episodes occur, the infant may be a candidate for a tongue-lip adhesion procedure or perhaps even a tracheostomy if the obstruction is severe enough. Most children will outgrow their respiratory difficulties (by approximately 3 months of age) as the mandible grows and the infants' neuromuscular function matures.

As a general rule, infants with cleft palate can eat and grow normally. Failure to thrive usually indicates a problem with feeding technique rather than from the mere presence of the cleft. Education and patience can overcome these difficulties. Diet can be advanced normally in these children.

Otologic Problems

Infants with palatal clefts are more prone to develop otitis media. This condition is believed to result from the muscle derangement within the cleft in concert with the drying effects on the eustachian tube orifice exposed to the oral cavity. The tensor palati muscle, which controls the eustachian tube orifice, is more flaccid in the unrepaired cleft interfering with normal opening. Serous otitis media is the rule, creating a milieu for repeated bouts of acute otitis media and reduced hearing. Long-term hearing loss can result from recurrent episodes of acute and chronic otitis media. Virtually all children require myringotomy with tube placement until they have had palate repair. Some have persistent difficulty, and all require close monitoring by the primary care physician, otolaryngologist, and audiologist until their course is clear.

Dental Problems

Dental development is usually delayed in children with cleft palate. Teeth bordering the alveolar cleft may be missing or rotated or may appear within the cleft, depending on the severity of the alveolar cleft. Good dental care is particularly important because many of these children will eventually need fixed bridges or prosthetic teeth to replace those missing from the clefting process. Parents must be cautioned about the milk bottle caries syndrome and directed to good dental care.

Children with clefts of the soft palate do not experience serious orthodontic problems related to the cleft itself. Posterior crossbites may be seen. However, when the cleft involves the alveolus, various degrees of maxillary arch collapse occurs as a consequence of the missing alveolar bone. This collapse results in anterior crossbites and a lack of facial projection or even a concave appearance of the midface. This result can be compounded by surgical scarring, which may inhibit normal facial growth. When children enter the age of mixed dentition (8 to 12 years), the upper dental arches can be orthodontically expanded and the teeth realigned and leveled. Position is then maintained with a prosthetic appliance attached to the teeth (fixed bridge) often with attached prosthetic teeth to replace those that are missing. However, bone grafts from the iliac crest, rib, or cranium can replace the missing alveolar bone. The graft stabilizes the arch, provides for the ingrowth of unstable teeth, and restores the gingival contour. Following this latter approach, missing teeth can be restored via a removable bridge or by bonding them to adjacent teeth (Maryland bridge).

Speech Problems

Children with cleft lip only are not expected to have speech problems related to palatal dysfunction. However, because there is an increased incidence of submucosal clefting of the palate in children with only cleft lip, the stigmata of this problem (bifid uvula, notching of the posterior edge of the hard palate and zona pellucida of the soft palate) should be sought. Most children with submucosal clefting of the palate will not have speech difficulties. However, approximately 20% will exhibit velopharyngeal incompetence producing the typical hypernasal speech associated with poor palatal function. If hypernasal speech becomes evident, surgical repair may be necessary.

Children in whom clefts of the palate have been repaired are evaluated at approximately 2½ years of age by the speech pathologist. The rate of speech development and any evolving problems with velopharyngeal function are particularly noted. Hypernasality and nasal escape are evidence of velopharyngeal incompetence. Lateral static radiographs of the palate obtained with the patient saying the phonemes "M," "D," "S," and "E" will confirm the clinical findings. Where the diagnosis is unclear, videoradiography of the soft palate using the Towne, base, and anterior views with contrast material and nasopharyngoscopy may demonstrate the problems. Mild degrees of velopharyngeal incompetence may be treated with speech therapy. More significant velopharyngeal incompetence may require a pharyngoplasty (posterior pharyngeal flap or sphincter pharyngoplasty) to augment velopharyngeal closure.

Psychosocial Problems

In general, one may anticipate psychosocial problems proportional to the severity of clefting of the lip structures. Interestingly, serious problems are not often seen, perhaps because of the extra attention lavished on these children and their ability to successfully use their mental mechanisms to cope with the difficulties of growing up with a dentofacial deformity or speech impediment. They probably do represent a slightly higher risk group and deserve attention in this sphere. Although the physician or cleft palate team members can manage the psychologic problem, often psychiatric intervention is needed.

The plastic surgeon often oversees the entire treatment of the child, making decisions regarding primary and secondary surgery with input from the team. He/she becomes involved early in the care of the child, meeting with the parents as soon as possible after birth to evaluate the infant and to outline the short- and long-term goals. Education regarding clefting is provided to supplement that given by the outreach person. The first phase of genetic counseling is offered at this time to aid in family planning.

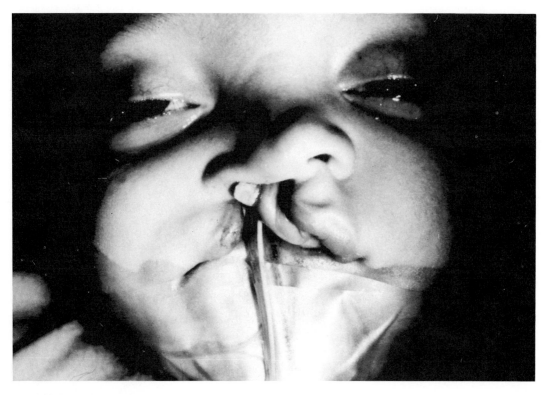

FIG 113-1
A girl, 3 months of age, with complete cleft of the lip and palate at surgery. Note the rudimentary tooth in the cleft adjacent to the nostril rim and the effects on the nose.

IV

Cleft Surgery

In an otherwise healthy infant, surgery is guided by the basic tenets of pediatric surgery, which are 10 weeks of age, 10 lbs of weight, and 10 g of hemoglobin. Hence, lip repairs are usually done at approximately 3 months of age in the uncomplicated cleft. General anesthesia and an overnight hospitalization are usual. Infants can be bottle- or breastfed immediately after surgery without fear of disrupting the repair.

Palatal clefts should be surgically closed by 18 months of age to minimize any deleterious effects on speech. Closure before 12 months of age may improve speech. Even earlier closure (age 3 to 6 months) has not conclusively shown an improvement in speech outcome. The precise timing is dependent on the infant's overall condition and the width of the cleft (Figs. 113-1 and 113-2). Clefts of the soft palate only are usually closed earlier (age 3 to 9 months), whereas closure of complete clefts is delayed (age 6 to 9 months).

Surgery in children with Robin sequence may have to be postponed for as long as 24 months to allow for sufficient mandibular growth and overall increase in the dimensions of the airway. Their palates are rarely closed before 12 months. A longer hospitalization may be needed following cleft palate repair (1 to 3 days) to permit resumption of oral intake. Feeding is done with a cross-cut nipple, as was done preoperatively. Pacifiers are not permitted for 2½ to 3 weeks to prevent pressure on the repair from sucking and to reduce the risk of disruption. The cleft across the alveolus is often left unrepaired to reduce scarring in this area that could impede facial growth. It is closed later, often when bone grafting of the alveolus is done (age 7 to 8 years).

Long-term Care

Following these initial procedures, the child is followed-up by the team on a yearly basis, evaluating growth, speech, dentition, hearing, and

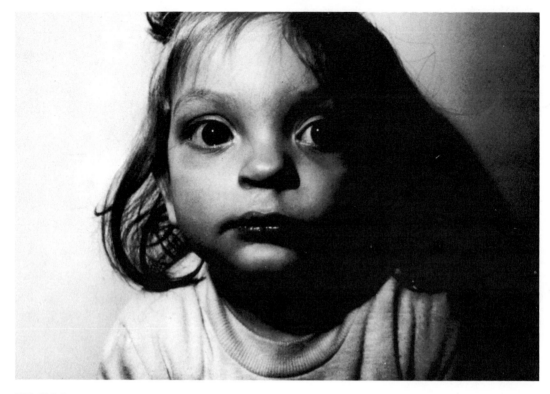

FIG 113-2
The same child in Figure 113-1 at 2 years of age after repair of the lip and palate.

psychosocial development. Revisional operations on the lip, premaxillary bone, and nose to improve speech (posterior pharyngeal flaps or pharyngoplasties) are recommended depending on the team's evaluation and the patient's and family's desires.

As a child enters adolescence, the final phases of treatment are planned. Orthodontics and prosthodontics are completed. When severe derangements of occlusion and the facial skeleton exist, orthognathic surgery may be warranted. This is usually delayed until full facial growth has been achieved (16 years of age for women, 17 to 18 for men). Final revisions are made on the lip and nose, frequently including a rhinoplasty. It is at this time when the second phase of genetic counseling should be offered to the patient. They should be given access to the data they will need to make an informed decision about their risk of having a child with a cleft.

Thus the treatment is complete. The team members have focused on a unique set of anatomic derangements. Appropriate interventions hopefully have been made to equip the young man or woman with the best possible appearance, speech, and confidence to enter the adult community.

BIBLIOGRAPHY

Bennett, et al: Psychotherapy for persons with craniofacial deformities: Can we treat without theory, *Cleft Palate Craniofac J* 30(4):406–410, 1993.

Elmendorfen, et al: Assessment of the patient with cleft lip and palate, *Clin Plast Surg* 20(4): 607–621, 1993.

Fraser FC: The genetics of cleft lip and palate, *Am J Hum Genet* 22:336, 1970.

Kaufman FL: Managing the cleft lip and palate patient, *Pediatr Clin North Am* 38:1127, 1991.

McWilliams BJ, Morris HL, Shelton RL, editors: Cleft Palate Speech, Philadelphia, 1984, BC Decker.

Millard DR: Cleft Craft, vols I, II, III, Boston, 1976, 1977, 1980, Little, Brown & Co.

Ross RB, Johnston MC: Cleft Lip and Palate, Baltimore, 1972, Williams & Wilkins.

CHAPTER 114

Hearing Impairment

Anna-Maria DaCosta
Annie Steinberg

IV

Hearing impairment is often called the "invisible handicap," because it cannot be seen, it is often misunderstood, and its impact is frequently underestimated. Every area of life is affected—familial, social, psychological, economic, and educational. It is important that the pediatrician be aware of the ramifications of hearing impairment and be knowledgeable in its recognition, treatment, and outcome.

DEFINITION AND CLASSIFICATION

Hearing impairment has been defined and classified in several ways (Box 114-1). Audiologists assess hearing impairment by measuring decibel units of loss of the ability to perceive single tones. Functional classification systems that more directly assess the ability to understand the meaning of what is spoken or heard also are used.

Hearing impairment also may be classified according to the time of onset, with prelingual deafness beginning prior to language development (typically before 2 to 3 years of age) and postlingual deafness after language has developed. This method of classification highlights the important relationship between deafness and language acquisition.

The medical community has often classified hearing impairment based on its pathophysiology and etiology. Conductive hearing loss is secondary to middle ear dysfunction. Sensorineural hearing loss is secondary to problems with the cochlea, 8th nerve, and, rarely, the auditory portion of the brain.

In recent years, an alternative view of deafness has emerged, defining it not by its etiology or neurologic symptoms, but rather as a cultural phenomenon with historical, linguistic, social, political, and educational dimensions shared by members of this minority. Membership in the deaf community does not relate just to the degree of hearing loss but rather to an identification with deaf culture and a sharing of language (American Sign Language [ASL]).

PREVALENCE

Estimates of the numbers of people with hearing loss vary, and it is often quite difficult to obtain reliable data on the prevalence among very young

BOX 114-1
Classification of Hearing Impairment

AUDIOLOGIC CLASSIFICATION

	Decibels
Mild	26–40
Moderate	41–65
Severe	66–95
Profound	>96

FUNCTIONAL CLASSIFICATION

Hard of hearing
  Moderate hearing loss
  Requires amplification to understand speech
  Able to attend regular school with supportive services
Partial hearing
  Severe hearing loss
  Requires prolonged auditory and specialized communication training
  Usually benefits from amplification
Deaf
  Profound hearing loss
  Dependence on visual sources for communication
  Amplification of little benefit in understanding verbal communication

BOX 114-2
Risk Factors for Hearing Impairment

Family history of deafness
Congenital infection
Meningitis or encephalitis
Congenital malformations of the head and neck
Prematurity (<1500 g at birth)
Anoxia
Neonatal intensive care admission of >48 hrs

children. In 1991, the Centers for Disease Control and Prevention (CDC) reported that 968,000 youths between 3 and 17 years of age were hearing impaired (1.8% of the population). Of these individuals, 143,000 could not hear and understand normal speech. The National Information Center on Deafness has estimated that between 77,000 and 90,000 hearing impaired children between 3 and 21 years of age are served by special education programs.

DIAGNOSIS

The most important period for language development is generally regarded as the first 3 years of life, and there is consensus regarding the advantage of early identification of hearing impairment and the benefits of timely remediation and treatment. However, the average age at identification of hearing impairment in the United States is close to 3 years, and more than 60% of all deaf children do not enroll in special education classes until 3 to 6 years of age.

Parents are often the first to suspect their child's hearing impairment, but too often they are told that "the child will outgrow the speech delay" or "the child is too young to test." Paren-

tal concern about hearing or speech and language development should always lead to referral for an evaluation of the child's hearing. Other factors that place a child at risk for severe hearing loss have been identified (Box 114-2). However, using these risk factors will identify only approximately 50% of children with significant hearing impairments. Thus, a National Institutes of Health consensus conference has recommended universal hearing screening prior to 3 months of age. They suggest that the screening be performed via two stages: an evoked otoacoustic emissions screen (EOAE) followed by auditory brainstem response (ABR) testing of all those who fail the EOAE. However, there is still debate over the efficacy, cost-effectiveness, and risk-benefit ratio of universal screening. To date, universal screening is not routinely practiced, and resolution of this debate must await further research.

All children who are at risk for hearing impairment should have their hearing tested. Informal tests, such as slamming a door or ringing a bell and observing the child's response, are not useful. A child who startles may still have a significant hearing impairment in a frequency different from the sound produced or may be responding to the vibration or air movement created simultaneously; many children are missed by these inaccurate "screens."

A child of any age can be tested for a hearing loss; however, the appropriate test varies with the child's age and developmental level. For children less than 6 months of age developmentally, two tests are commonly used: the EOAE and the ABR.

The EOAE is a technique for newborn screening. As sound enters the cochlea, the tiny hair cells that transmit the signal to the 8th cranial nerve simultaneously emit an "echo" back through the middle ear, which can be recorded in the external ear. Failure to detect an "echo" indicates the hair cells are not functioning normally. Using this method, it is possible to quickly test a wide range of frequencies objectively.

Another method for testing infant hearing is to record the ABR. Electroencephalogram electrodes are placed on the forehead and behind the ears of the sleeping child. Tones are presented to each ear, following which a burst of neural activity is recorded in the form of waves that represent different parts of the auditory brainstem pathway. Absence of one or more waves suggests an abnormality in this pathway. This screening test is highly sensitive; however, there is a high false-positive rate resulting in overreferral of children with normal hearing.

For children over the age of 6 months developmentally functioning, audiometry is used to assess hearing. Testing through earphones is preferred because sensorineural and conductive losses can be distinguished and information is obtained for each ear individually. However, for children who will not tolerate earphones, audiometric testing can be completed with the use of loudspeakers. Tones presented in audiometry have frequencies ranging from 250 to 4000 Hz and intensities from 0 to 110 dB. Hearing losses from slight to profound can be detected.

ETIOLOGY

Determining the etiology of deafness in children is sometimes difficult, particularly because there is often a lag time between the onset of hearing loss and its diagnosis. A discussion of the etiologies of hearing impairment can best be done by reviewing prenatal, perinatal, and postnatal causes.

Prenatal

Approximately 33% of childhood deafness is hereditary. More than 100 different types of genetic deafness have been identified, with more being discovered each year. In approximately half of these hereditary syndromes, there are other defects as well, which may affect the central nervous, ocular, skin, musculoskeletal, cardiac, or renal systems. The majority of hereditary deafness is autosomal recessive; however, autosomal dominant forms occur in up to 25% of cases, and X-linked forms occur in 1% to 2% of cases.

Some of the more common genetic syndromes associated with deafness include Usher's syndrome, which is associated with retinitis pigmentosa, abnormal gait, and seizures; Waardenberg syndrome, which is associated with heterochromia of the iris, ectopic canthus, and a white forelock; Alport syndrome, which is associated with hematuria, renal failure, and hypertension; and Jervell and Lange-Nielsen syndromes, which are associated with prolonged QT interval and sudden death.

Prenatal environmental factors are also important causes of deafness. There have been reports of teratogenic medications and toxins resulting in deafness. More important, however, is the role of maternal infection including rubella, cytomegalovirus (CMV), toxoplasmosis, and syphilis. Rubella infection, in the first trimester of pregnancy, results in a 50% incidence of deafness in the newborn. In the past, rubella epidemics were a leading cause of acquired deafness; however, since the advent of routine vaccination, this disease has become much less of a threat. Currently, CMV is most prevalent, with sensorineural loss occurring in almost 30% of symptomatic babies and 10% of otherwise asymptomatic babies. Deafness secondary to intrauterine infections frequently co-occurs with neurologic, ocular, and cardiac sequelae.

Perinatal

With the improved survival rates of "ill" newborns, perinatal causes of hearing impairments have been increasing. Anoxia can result in damage to the cochlea. Sepsis and neonatal meningitis, as well as exposure to ototoxic antibiotics and other medications, can increase the risk of hearing impairment. Hyperbilirubinemia, especially at levels associated with the development of kernicterus, can lead to auditory damage. Intracranial hemorrhage also has been associated with hearing loss. Premature infants are at increased risk for all these factors, and 2% to 5% demonstrate significant hearing loss. Additionally, these same risk factors often result in ophthalmologic and neurologic sequelae.

Postnatal

Conductive causes of hearing impairment predominate in the postnatal and early childhood period, with middle ear effusions being the major source.

Sensorineural hearing loss also can develop during this period. The causes include infections such as bacterial meningitis and viral encephalitis, exposure to ototoxic medications, and trauma (both blunt trauma to the cochlea and damage from traumatic noise levels).

ASSOCIATED PROBLEMS

Language Acquisition
Language development is believed to present the central challenge for children who are deaf. For years, the belief has been that educators and parents need to "teach" deaf children language. It has been shown, however, that children who are deaf and who are exposed early to a natural sign language such as ASL, develop sign language on a time table similar to that of spoken language in children who are hearing. Children who are deaf and who are primarily exposed to spoken language alone, however, acquire language much more slowly than do hearing children. Learning to speechread and to speak remains a challenge for many deaf individuals because many spoken words appear identical on the lips, and the correct pronunciation of words that have never been heard must be learned.

Cognitive Development
Intellectual inferiority such as decreased ability to think abstractly has been previously ascribed to individuals who are deaf. However, when testing is conducted in a fully accessible manner a normal range of intelligence can be demonstrated. For reasons that are currently unclear and probably multifactorial, reading remains a source of difficulty for the average deaf student who graduates high school with only a third- to fourth-grade reading level.

Behavior Problems/Psychological Disturbance
Investigators have demonstrated high rates of behavior problems and psychological disturbance in the deaf population (*see* Chapter 131).

Comorbid Conditions
Many of the causes of deafness are frequently associated with other sequelae (*eg,* mental retardation, cerebral palsy, blindness) that may have profound effects on a child's developmental potential and on the educational approach utilized. Of particular importance is the co-occurrence of both visual and hearing impairments that affect the communication strategies and educational approaches used. Vision should be carefully assessed in all individuals presenting with deafness.

INTERVENTIONS

The primary care physician should be aware of the resources, services, and treatment options available to the hearing impaired child and his/her family. Because controversy pervades the field regarding interventions for hearing impairment, it is also important that the physician be able to present information to the family in a nonbiased manner and support the family through the decision-making process.

Audiologic Management
Hearing aids can be used with children of any age and should be fitted as soon as a persistent hearing loss has been identified. Hearing aids amplify sound and transmit this sound to the middle ear. They do not completely correct a hearing loss, but they benefit the majority of children with hearing impairments. Even with optimal amplification, ongoing language intervention is needed.

A relatively new intervention is a cochlear implant. This device is surgically attached to the cochlea to provide direct stimulation of the auditory nerve. It has been approved for individuals over 2 years of age who have profound hearing loss and have not benefitted from amplification. The resultant degree of hearing improvement is variable and currently under investigation.

Educational Management
Public laws mandate early intervention and educational services for all infants and children with hearing impairments. These services include hearing testing, hearing aid fitting, speech and language therapy, and special education. Because 90% of deaf children are born to hearing parents, these programs also provide instruction for parents on the implications of deafness for the family and on possible communication strategies.

Available methods of communication can be described as: oral communication, which emphasizes the development of speech and the use of residual hearing and speechreading; cued speech, which is similar to other oral methods but utilizes hand shapes near the mouth to supplement the information visible on the lips; fingerspelling, in which everything is fingerspelled using a signed manual alphabet; signed exact English, which utilizes signs from ASL as well as other coined signs to encode English grammar and word order into a manual system; and ASL, which is a language of signs that has its own vocabulary, grammar, and idioms. The choice of spoken language–only (oral/aural) versus sign language–only (manual) communication has sparked a more than century-long controversy in the field of deafness. Proponents of the oral/aural approach argue that sign language limits a child's access to the hearing world and lessens the chance that he/she will learn to speak. Supporters of manual communication argue that sign language allows the child easy access to communication and aids in the development of meaningful language. Many educators propose a compromise position, the use of "total communication," in which any and all methods of communication necessary are utilized to allow the child access to language. Communication strategies should be individualized to meet the needs of the child.

Access

A number of devices and strategies have been developed to better allow the deaf individual access to information and to the community.

Telephone devices for the deaf (TDD or TTY) send typewritten messages through telephone lines, permitting conversation in print. If a TDD is not available, a relay service can be used, in which the hearing individual communicates with a special telephone operator who transmits the message to the hearing-impaired person's TDD. All states are mandated to provide relay services.

Closed-caption television decoders enable viewers to read captions on their television screen. Many television shows, movies, and news programs are now captioned.

A number of alerting devices (smoke detector, telephone, doorbell, alarm clock, baby monitor) can substitute a visual or a vibratory signal for an auditory one.

Language barriers frequently restrict an individual's access to appropriate professional services, including, among others, the health care profession. When providing services to people who are hearing impaired it is important that one respect the individual's needs by facing the person when speaking, articulating clearly, and using good lighting. When ASL is the person's preferred mode of communication, the use of interpreters is vital. The Registry of Interpreters for the Deaf, Inc. is a professional organization that maintains a listing of individuals skilled in the use of ASL.

Resources

Various agencies and organizations provide specific services to people who are deaf (Box 114-3). For the family of the newly diagnosed hearing impaired child, exposure to deaf adults can be helpful both in developing a more realistic perspective of deafness and in the decision-making process regarding medical and educational treatment options.

OUTCOME

Deaf Culture

Many people in the deaf community do not view deafness as a disability. Rather, they are a community with their own traditions and a shared

---

BOX 114-3
Resources for Deaf and Hearing Impaired People

Alexander Graham Bell Association for the Deaf
  3417 Volta Place NW, Washington, DC 20007
  Voice/TTY: (202) 337-5220
  Disseminates information on hearing loss.
American Society for Deaf Children
  2848 Arden Way, Suite 210, Sacramento, CA 93825-1373
  Voice/TTY (800) 942-ASDC
  Nonprofit parent-helping-parent organization promoting a positive attitude toward signing and deaf culture.
Captioned Films/Videos
  5000 Park St. N, St. Petersburg, FL 33709
  Voice/TTY: (800) 237-6213
  Free loans of captioned films.
Helen Keller National Center for Deaf-Blind Youths and Adults
  111 Middle Neck Road, Sands Point, NY 11050
  Voice: (516) 944-8900; TTY: (516) 944-8637
  Provides evaluations and vocational training and placement for people who are deaf-blind.
National Information Center on Deafness
  800 Florida Ave. NE, Washington, DC 20002-3695
  Voice: (202) 651-5051; TTY: (202) 651-5052
  Centralized source of up-to-date information on topics dealing with deafness.

IV

language (ASL). These individuals do not wish for a "cure" for their condition. The majority who marry, marry other deaf individuals, and many want to have deaf children. It is through contact with the deaf culture that they gain a sense of acceptance and belonging.

Educational Outcome/Literacy

The Commission on Education of the Deaf reported in 1988 that "The present status of education for persons who are deaf . . . is unsatisfactory." The average deaf child has a third- to fourth-grade reading level at high school graduation. The cause of these difficulties is multifactorial and likely involves many of the factors discussed previously.

There are increasing opportunities for postsecondary education for adolescents and adults who are deaf. Gallaudet University and the National Technical Institute for the Deaf remain the largest programs for college-level education, but community colleges and technical schools now offer programs for the deaf. Some individuals utilize skilled interpreters and/or notetakers to attend other programs, whereas others are enrolled without special support services.

Vocational Outcome and Income

Most career fields are open to the deaf. Choice may depend on degree of hearing loss, communication skills, academic skills, and personal interest. Deaf adults have been employed in many fields, including medicine and other professions. However, according to the CDC, persons with "hearing trouble" are proportionally overrepresented in families with low income. In addition, because of limited interaction with hearing people prior to beginning their careers, many are not well prepared for the interpersonal relationships they encounter in the job market.

SUMMARY

Hearing impairment has profound effects on all aspects of an individual's life. A team including experienced audiologists, otolaryngologists, educators, and primary care physicians is necessary to manage the diagnostic and treatment needs of the hearing impaired child and his/her family.

BIBLIOGRAPHY

Centers for Disease Control and Prevention: *Prevalence and characteristics of persons with hearing trouble: United States, 1990–1991,* Washington, DC, 1994, U.S. Dept. of Health and Human Services.

DiPietro LJ, Knight CH, Sams JS: Health care delivery for deaf patients: The provider's role, *Am Ann Deaf* 126:106–112, 1981.

Dolnick E: Deafness as culture, *The Atlantic Monthly* Sept:37–53, 1993.

Liben LS: *Deaf children: Developmental perspectives,* New York, 1978, Academic Press.

Luterman DM, Ross M: *When your child is deaf: A guide for parents,* Paskton, MD, 1991, York Press.

NIH Consensus Statement: *Early identification of hearing impairment in infants and young children,* Washington, DC, 1993, U.S. Dept. of Health and Human Services.

Schilling LS, DeJesus E: Developmental issues in deaf children, *J Pediatr Health Care* 7(5):161–166, 1993.

Steinberg AG: Deafness, In Vosphitz J, et al: Basic handbook of child and adolescent psychiatry, New York, 1996.

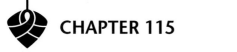

CHAPTER 115

Speech and Language Disorders

Nathan J. Blum
Marleen Ann Baron

Timely detection and appropriate intervention for children with speech and language disorders requires the active involvement of pediatricians and family physicians. Health supervision visits during the toddler and preschool years allow physicians to detect speech and language disorders at the time that they first become evident. In addition, parents often consult their child's physician when they have concerns about their child's speech or language development. Thus, pediatricians and family physicians need to understand the wide range of disorders that can be associated with speech and language problems and when to refer children for further assessment and intervention.

DEFINITIONS

When evaluating a child with a speech or language problem one must determine whether the disorder primarily involves speech, language, or both speech and language. Speech is the motor act of communication, whereas language is knowledge of a symbol system used for interpersonal communication. The symbol system assessed is usually words, but nonverbal symbols (*eg*, waving good-bye, sign language) also should be considered. Language comprehension or receptive language refers to one's ability to understanding the symbol system, whereas expressive language refers to the skills involved in formulating ideas into words or signs.

PREVALENCE

Language disorders affect 5% to 12% of children depending on the criteria used to make the diagnosis. More than half of these children will have primarily expressive language disorders, and the rest will have mixed expressive-receptive disorders. Language disorders are more common in boys than girls.

Speech articulation problems affect 2% to 3% of elementary school–age children and less than 1% of adults. Stuttering of longer than 6 months' duration occurs in 4% of children. By late childhood only 1% of children continue to have stuttering severe enough to interfere with academic or social functioning.

ASSESSMENT

Assessment must involve a thorough history, physical examination, and evaluation of the child's development (*see* Chapter 120). Basic knowledge of speech milestones and receptive and expressive language milestones (Table 115-1) will be helpful in identifying a speech or language delay. The assessment, treatment, and outcome of children with language disorders differs from that of children with speech disorders. Although some children will have both speech and language disorders, this chapter will discuss speech and language disorders separately.

LANGUAGE DISORDERS

Differential Diagnosis
Table 115-2 provides a list of signs that suggest a significant language problem. When one or more of these signs is present a broad differential diagnosis needs to be considered (Box 115-1). The diagnosis of a primary language disorder should be made only after appropriate investigation for these other conditions is completed.

IV

TABLE 115-1
Major Speech and Language Milestones

AGE (MOS)	RECEPTIVE LANGUAGE	EXPRESSIVE LANGUAGE	SPEECH
1–2	Recognizes sounds	Coos	
4–6	Turns to bell	Laughs and squeals	
8–9	Understands name; responds to "no"	"Mama/dada" as sounds; babbles	
10–12	Follows simple command; waves good-bye	"Mama/dada" specific; four words	
14–16	Points to one to two body parts	Six to 12 words	<20% of speech understood by strangers
18–20	Points to pictures/objects; follows two-step commands	Asks for food/drink; 20 to 30 words	50% of speech understood by strangers
22–24	Points to all body parts	Two-word sentences; >50 words	75% of speech understood by strangers
24–30	Understands some prepositions	Uses "me/you," "he/she" correctly; 4- to 8-word sentences	
30–36	Understands concepts: up-down, big-little, loud-soft	Gives use of objects	Almost all speech understood by strangers

TABLE 115-2
Signs of Language Problems Needing Further Evaluation

AGE	
0–6 mos	Child does not respond to sounds or turn toward the speaker who is out of sight.
	Child makes only crying sounds (no cooing or comfort sounds).
1 yr	Child shows only inconsistent responses to sound.
	Child has stopped babbling or does not babble yet.
2 yrs	Child does not understand or attend when spoken to.
	Child does not use any words.
	Vocabulary is minimal (less than eight to 10 words) and is not growing.
	Speech primarily echoes what others say.
2½ yrs	Child is not combining words.
	Child has difficulty following commands or answering simple questions.
3 yrs	Child still echoes.
	Sentences are not used.
	Vocabulary is less than 100 words.
4 yrs	Child has difficulty formulating statements and questions.
	Child has deficient conversational skills and has difficulty learning concepts and/or sequences, such as numbers and the alphabet.
	Language usage is deviant and not used appropriately for social interaction.
5 yrs	Child cannot retain and follow verbal directions.
	Child has difficulty learning sound-symbol relationships.
	Sentence structure is noticeably faulty, and word order in sentences is poor.
	Child cannot describe an event or outing.

Hearing loss must be ruled out by a formal audiologic assessment. Many children with severe hearing loss are not detected until they are 2 to 2½ years of age; lesser degrees of hearing loss that can affect language development are often not detected until children are much older than that. Mild conductive hearing loss caused by chronic serous otitis media may be associated with mild deficits in language (or speech) development but should not be considered a sufficient explanation for more significant deficits.

In 50% of children with mental retardation the parent's initial concern is about the child's language development. Thus, one must also assess milestones that do not involve language function in order to detect more global cogni-

---

BOX 115-1
Differential Diagnosis for Children With Language Delay

Hearing impairment
Mental retardation
Pervasive developmental disorder (autism)
Chronic serous otitis media
Primary language disorders
    Expressive language disorder
    Mixed expressive-receptive language disorder
Acquired language disorder
    Landau-Kleffner (acquired epileptic aphasia)
    Progressive dementia associated with a progressive
        neurologic disorder
Selective mutism
Profound psychosocial deprivation

---

tive deficits. In pervasive developmental disorder (PDD; Chapter 122) the child's social functioning and range of interests will be severely limited.

Children who lose language skills should be referred to a neurologist or developmental pediatrician for assessment. It is not uncommon for children with PDD to lose a few single words between 1 to 2 years of age. However, if a child is losing skills in other areas he/she should be evaluated for a progressive neurologic disorder. Children with Landau-Kleffner syndrome lose language skills because they are having seizure activity in the language areas of the brain. They may or may not have clinical seizures, and they can be difficult to distinguish from children with PDD. A sleep electroencephalogram is needed to make the diagnosis.

Children with selective mutism speak fluently in some situations but refuse to speak in others (*eg*, in school, outside the family). Although some children may not speak in school at the beginning of the year, if there is no improvement in 3 to 4 weeks referral to a psychologist or psychiatrist is indicated.

Severe psychosocial deprivation may cause global delays in development. The history and physical examination usually will identify these children.

Etiology

The primary language disorders (expressive or mixed expressive-receptive) are best viewed as syndromes with multiple etiologies, most of which are not known. Genetics clearly plays a role in these language disorders, but no specific mode of genetic transmission has been identified.

Based on the adult aphasia literature, it was believed that children with primary language disorders have damage to the left hemisphere of the brain. However, brain imaging studies have not consistently identified focal lesions in the left hemisphere. Preliminary research studies using volumetric analysis of brain images on magnetic resonance imaging have reported a larger than normal right perisylvian area in children with language delays. The significance of this finding is not clear.

Treatment

Treatment for children with delays in their language development should be directed by a speech-language pathologist. He/she can help parents or other caregivers learn ways of encouraging and enhancing the child's communication skills. Strategies can be developed to address medical, neurologic, developmental, or behavioral issues that limit the child's ability to acquire or adequately use these skills.

Outcome

The outcome of children with language delay depends on the severity of the delay, the type of language delay (*eg*, expressive vs mixed receptive-expressive), the age of the child, and the child's nonverbal intelligence. Although the majority of children with language delay will demonstrate catch-up in their ability to comprehend and use words, they are at risk for difficulties in language-based academic skills such as reading, spelling, and written expression. They are also at increased risk for behavioral disorders.

Children with a mixed receptive-expressive disorder are at highest risk for later difficulties. As many as 50% to 80% of children aged 4 years with a mixed disorder have been found to require some assistance in early elementary school. Children with isolated expressive language difficulties tend to have a better outcome. Approximately half of these children seem to outgrow their difficulties. The factors associated with a good outcome have not been clearly delineated, although there is some evidence that for toddlers the size of the expressive vocabulary at diagnosis correlates positively with later outcome.

IV

TABLE 115-3
Signs of Speech Problems Needing Further Evaluation

AGE	
2½ yrs	Speech is largely unintelligible to parents.
3 yrs	Parents understand less than half of child's speech.
4 yrs	Speech is largely unintelligible to strangers.
5 yrs	Speech is characterized by many sound substitutions.
	Child has persistent stuttering.
Any age	Stuttering interferes with communication.
	There is noticeable hypernasality or lack of nasal resonance.
	Pitch is not appropriate for the child's age and sex.
	Voice is monotone, extremely loud, largely inaudible, very hoarse, or of poor quality.
	Short lingual frenulum is in question.
	The child is embarrassed or frustrated by communication skills.

SPEECH DISORDERS

Articulation

Speech development is influenced by structural and neuromuscular determinants. Children with abnormal oral structures, such as a cleft palate, a severe malocclusion, or in rare cases an unusually short lingual frenulum (tongue-tie), are likely to have difficulties in acquiring normal speech articulation. Severe malocclusion and a fronting posture of the tongue may result in tongue thrusting and incorrect production of specific sounds. A dental consultation prior to a speech assessment may be necessary to evaluate this complex relationship between occlusion, tongue thrusting, and articulation.

Precise neuromuscular control is necessary to coordinate breathing and the complex oropharyngeal movements that allow normal speech production. A history of early feeding problems may suggest that oral-motor dysfunction is contributing to speech problems. Children with disorders that impair neuromuscular control (eg, cerebral palsy) are at increased risk for speech problems.

Articulation improves with development. Table 115-3 provides some guidelines for when to refer children with articulation problems to a speech-language pathologist. There are developmental norms for sound acquisition. The last sounds to be mastered are "r," "l," "s," and "th." Difficulties with these sounds are not considered a problem in children younger than 5 years of age unless they are combined with other sound errors or are significantly compromising the child's speech clarity.

BOX 115-2
Suggestions for Managing Stuttering

- Provide a positive communication model by speaking in a relaxed, slow manner.
- Allow the child to complete his/her thoughts without interruption or correction of any speech errors.
- Have developmentally appropriate expectations for speech production and fluency.
- Listen to the child without showing concern when the child stutters.
- Do not tell the child to "slow down," "start again," or "take a breath."
- Do not ask the child a lot of questions. Stuttering is more likely to occur in response to questions than during spontaneous speech.
- Professional consultation should be considered if there is no improvement in the child's fluency in 2 to 3 months.

Stuttering

Stuttering occurs frequently in young children and is often a concern of parents. The stuttering may involve syllable, word and/or phrase repetitions, sound prolongations, and excessive hesitations. When stuttering occurs in preschool children and the child does not show signs of reacting to the stuttering (ie, eye blinking or closing, mouth tension, etc.), it is usually a normal disfluency that will be transient. In these cases or if the child is having mild reactions to the disfluency, recommendations provided by the primary care physician may be the only intervention needed (Box 115-2). Preschool children who have a family history of stuttering or other language or communication deficits are at increased risk for persistent stuttering and should be evaluated by a speech-language pathologist.

Children with severe stuttering will have disfluencies in almost every sentence and will show signs of physical struggle during speaking. They may attempt to hide their stuttering or avoid speaking. These children need immediate referral to a speech-language pathologist.

SUMMARY

Pediatricians and family physicians frequently will see children with speech and/or language disorders. Knowledge of normal speech and language milestones and of the wide range of disorders whose primary feature may be a delay in speech or language development should allow early detection and appropriate intervention or referral for these children.

BIBLIOGRAPHY

Bashir AS, Scavuzzo A: Children with language disorders: Natural history and academic success, *J Learn Disabil* 25:53–65, 1992.

Fischel JE, Whitheurst GJ, Caulfield MB, DeBaryshe B: Language growth in children with expressive language delay, *Pediatrics* 82:218–227, 1989.

Guitar B, Conture EG: *The child who stutters: To the pediatrician,* Memphis, TN, 1992, Stuttering Foundation of America.

Montgomery TR: When "not talking" is the chief complaint, *Contemp Pediatr* 11:49–70, 1994.

Owens RE: *Language development: An introduction,* Columbus, OH, 1988, Merrill Publishing.

Plante E: MRI findings in the parents and siblings of specifically language-impaired boys, *Brain Lang* 41:67–80, 1991.

Rescoria L, Schwartz E: Outcome of toddlers with specific expressive language delay, *Appl Psycholinguist* 11:393–407, 1990.

IV

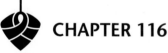

CHAPTER 116

Visual Impairment and Blindness

Annie G. Steinberg
Bernadette Kappen

Because primary care physicians are most often the first professionals to work with families who have a child with a visual impairment, they play a vital role in guiding and supporting the family through the diagnostic process and ongoing care. Vision is a sense that impacts on all areas of early development, including the bonding process and the achievement of motor, social, emotional,

linguistic, and cognitive/academic milestones. After the initial diagnostic phase, the primary care provider can provide referrals to appropriate resources, facilitate the integration of information given by the professionals the family encounters, and provide supportive guidance to the family. In this chapter, the diagnostic process will be discussed as well as the variations of normal development seen in the child with a visual impairment. Some educational considerations are presented, and a list of resources available to families is provided.

CLASSIFICATION AND DEFINITION

There are two categories of children who fall within the classification of visually impaired: children with low vision and children who are blind. Children with low vision are unable to perform visual tasks without the use of special aids such as magnifiers, special lighting, color contrast, or large print. For legal purposes, low vision is described as visual acuity from 20/70 to 20/200 in the better eye after correction. Children with low vision perform visual tasks at reduced speed and precision, even when aided.

The most severe form of visual impairment is blindness, but in most cases blindness is not an all-or-none phenomenon. Children who are totally blind have no useful vision or can only distinguish between dark and light. In the learning process, children who are blind do not have any meaningful visual experiences and must rely primarily or exclusively on other sensory input, such as auditory and tactile input. The legal definition of blindness is corrected visual acuity in the better eye of 20/200 or less, or restriction of the visual field to 20° or less.

PREVALENCE

The incidence of children with low vision is approximately one in 500 births. The incidence of total blindness is four per 10,000 births. In 1977, there were approximately 1.4 million persons in the United States with severe visual impairments. Of these persons, approximately 500,000 were classified as legally blind, and 5.9% were under 18 years of age.

In addition to children with the most severe visual conditions, Prevent Blindness America estimates that more than 12.1 million school-age children, or one in four school-age children, has a vision impairment. Among preschool children, more than 428,000, or one in 20, have a vision problem that can cause permanent vision loss if left untreated. The most common types of eye problems seen in children are myopia (near-

sightedness), strabismus (crossed eyes), and amblyopia (lazy eye).

DIAGNOSIS

Parents often are the first to suspect a visual impairment in their child, often describing visual inconsistencies or lack of response to some visual stimuli. The primary care physician plays an important role in validating parental concerns, recognizing that eyes that appear normal may have significant visual impairment, pursuing necessary evaluation, and avoiding the well-documented tendency to delay referral for diagnostic evaluation.

Practitioners caring for infants commonly will encounter questions regarding fixing (directly examining an object), following (tracking movement of the eye synchronous with the object), alignments/esotropias, periodic movement such as nystagmus, and preferential lateral or eccentric viewing or head tilts. Whenever parental concerns arise, prompt clinical observations of the infant interacting with a parent, rather than with bright objects, should be conducted in the office. This evaluation may be augmented by home videotaping. An alert infant who cannot fix his/her gaze on an object placed in front or to his/her side or who is not attracted to smiling faces should raise concerns by the second month of life. Although transient deviations in eye alignment often resolve during the first few months of life, purposeless wandering eye movements or nystagmus rarely do.

When there are concerns about visual impairment, the age of the child should not delay referral to an opthalmologist. Methods of assessing visual acuity in infants and young children, as well as those with multiple disabilities, are well described. A complete opthalmologic assessment also will include a slitlamp examination of the cornea and lens and measurement of intraocular pressure to rule out glaucoma. This important examination must occur regularly for children with visual impairments, because other ocular conditions may result in secondary glaucoma. In some cases, an electroretinogram, which utilizes a corneal electrode to measure the retinal response to visual stimuli, and visual evoked responses, which measure electrical activity in the visual cortex, may further define the visual impairment. If the ocular examination is

---

BOX 116-1
Causes of Visual Impairment

Retinopathy of prematurity
Congenital cataracts
Congenital infection (rubella, cytomegalovirus, toxo-
    plasmosis, syphilis)
Infection: meningitis, encephalitis
Malformations of visual system (aniridia, coloboma,
    cataracts, glaucoma, optic nerve hypoplasia)
Strabismus
Macular disease: retinitis pigmentosia
Trauma
Cerebral anoxia
Tumors: retinoblastoma
Genetic syndromes (Usher syndrome)

---

normal but the child appears to be functionally blind, a cortical visual impairment may be present. The overt appearance of the eye (*eg*, the iris, retina, presence/density of cataracts, shape/configuration, or presence of a retinoblastoma) or the results of a superficial examination (pupillary reflexes) are not predictive of a child's vision.

Optometrists and teachers can assist the child and the family with determining the functional visual abilities of the child. Even though a child may have extremely low vision, learning its type and how to use the functional vision will assist in optimizing full potential.

Referral of the visually impaired child to an opthalmologist with expertise in low-vision assessment of young children, an optometrist knowledgeable in low-vision techniques for young children, and a teacher or occupational/physical therapist specializing in visual impairment will allow a comprehensive assessment that should facilitate the development of the intervention plan.

ETIOLOGIES

Although visual impairment is a low-incidence disability, the causes the clinician must consider are quite varied (Box 116-1). The epidemiology of causes for visual impairment has varied over time and with the changing patterns of systemic infections (*eg*, rubella) and the increasing survival of premature infants.

Prematurity remains a common cause of visual impairment in infants. Although the role of high levels of oxygen supplementation in retinopathy of prematurity has been recognized, retinopathy of prematurity cannot always be prevented with current treatments of premature infants. Factors other than oxygen supplementation are certainly important but less well understood. In addition, the improved survival of the progressively lower birthweight infants with immature eye development has continued to produce children with severe visual impairment, often accompanied by neurologic damage.

Visual impairment may be associated with almost any form of injury to the brain. In these cases, ultimate visual functioning is difficult to predict because the deficit area lies between the optic nerve and occipital cortex and is dependent on general brain functioning.

Visual impairments may be associated with syndromes such as albinism, retinitis pigmentosa, and Usher syndrome. As with other causes of visual impairment, the visual deficit may be the sole presenting symptom or the condition may have other accompanying disabilities.

In the developing world, vitamin A deficiency, parasitic infections, congenital syphilis or gonorrhea, and malnutrition are but a few of the more common, and preventable, causes of visual impairment affecting as many as 3% to 4% of the population.

CHILD DEVELOPMENT

Adaptation to blindness involves alterations in early communication. Visual regard is so central to human interaction that parents often wonder if their blind child "knows" them. Parents do not intuitively know how to translate their own visual experience of an object into their child's nonvisual way of understanding the world. Thus, blindness can be seen as a communication barrier between caretaker and child that places extraordinary demands on the adaptive capacity of both.

Parents must learn to recognize vocal and tactile responses such as kicking and gurgling so that reciprocal communication can be established early. Verbal interactions also may be altered in children with visual impairment because parents may use more directional and informational language in an effort to provide the child with meaningful and predictive cues about the environment. This interaction may influence early language patterns of the child, but stilted patterns most often resolve with adequate social exposure.

A consensus exists among professionals that some aspects of development are delayed during the early years but can catch up later. The delays are believed to be related to the absence of experience rather than of vision. For example, exploration of the environment with the infant's hands is normally prompted by an enticing visual stimulus; therefore, hand function often is delayed for the child with a visual impairment. Facilitating bimanual exploration is crucial for increasing the experiences of the young child who is visually impaired. However, extra effort aimed at the achievement of some milestones, such as throwing a ball, may be unnecessary and temporarily maladaptive, in that this action reduces opportunities for the tactile exploration of objects.

Several habitual behaviors such as rocking, head-rolling, or gazing at the light were previously referred to as "blindisms." The presence of these behaviors should be carefully evaluated, because they may be stereotypic behaviors less related to the lack of vision than to comorbid conditions. Stereotypic behaviors associated with visual impairment are most often exacerbated by sensory deprivation and improve with stimulating sensory input to the child. Adolescents often describe their awareness of these behaviors and make efforts to discontinue them because of parental or peer reactions.

Body contact and social interaction with family members may be different from that of sighted children. Children who are blind may want to feel parts of the body, hold the arm, sit in the lap, or ask personal questions to fill in the gap resulting from visual impairment. Posture, speech, and facial expression may be different as well. Talking excessively may serve as a means to maintain contact and participation, whereas a "broadcasting" voice may reflect a lack of awareness of the location of others. Parents must educate other family members so that information for the child can be made accessible and so that interpersonal interactions can be facilitated. Peer relationships must be initiated and perpetuated by parents in the early years. If socialization opportunities are unavailable to the child, interpersonal relationships in later years are less likely. Opportunities for normal social interaction and the acquisition of sexual knowledge should not be neglected.

INTERVENTIONS

Intervention begins at the time of diagnosis. Both parents and other family members should be present. Pain, shock, anger, frustration, denial, and grief are among the many responses to the diagnosis, and there is a sudden shift of the family's identity. The practitioner should allow adequate time to respond to questions, such as "Will my baby ever look/smile at me?" A follow-up meeting should be scheduled, and audiotapes or a typed letter may be helpful to the family struggling to integrate overwhelming information.

Support systems for parents and children with visual impairments vary widely but are quite limited in some regions. The primary health care provider should recognize the vital role of both the information and the support provided by their ongoing relationship. They also should recognize the importance of intrafamilial supports, good communication, and a willingness to accept outside help, particularly when the family is stressed by the demands of having a child with special needs.

The stigma of impairment and negative stereotypic misconceptions of individuals who are blind should be explored early after the diagnostic period, so as to afford an opportunity to dispel cultural myths and inaccurate family beliefs. An assessment of how the family feels about and is coping with the visual impairment may reveal less adaptive coping patterns, including minimizing or denying the disability, disavowal of deviance, protectiveness, and an all-consuming commitment to the child. It is important that the health care provider model direct interaction and respect for the child who is blind.

Supporting the family to find the balance between overprotectiveness and independence, and between accommodation to the child's needs and the child's accommodation to the family's lifestyle and interests, will be a lifelong contribution to the well-being of both the child and the family.

Early Intervention Programs

Early intervention programs help families learn to provide the necessary sensorimotor experiences for the child. The families should encourage movement and exploration of the environment. Objects of interest should be made available to the child both by bringing them within reach of the child and by encouraging exploration when developmentally appropriate. A vast array of experiences are necessary to expose the blind child to a variety of environments, objects, animals, and so forth. The need to stimulate creative play cannot be underestimated.

Early intervention programs help parents to understand characteristic behaviors, such as recognizing the blind child's quiet position as attentive waiting. These programs also support the provision of auditory cues that help the infant and child to anticipate what will happen next and facilitate communication. Readiness for braille and the use of electronic and optical aids also can be monitored over time. Children with low vision also must be offered aggressive programs in visual stimulation to optimize visual skills development.

School Programs

For the school-age child, visual impairment can interfere with learning, unless adaptations are made in the materials and devices used as well as in the learning environment. Students must be supported in obtaining and confirming information received through the use of all other senses, rather than through hearing alone. The child is likely to misinterpret auditory cues and will require active engagement with objects and experiences so that spatial concepts, construct formation, and symbolization can emerge.

Legislation mandating an appropriate education in the least restrictive environment has led to the inclusion of many students who are visually impaired in regular classrooms with a specially qualified teacher offering consultation, focused teaching, and the provision of equipment and adaptive materials. This change has led to a highly politicized debate as to what comprises the best educational environment for children with disabilities. This subject should be addressed not as a fixed once-in-a-lifetime decision, but rather as a flexible, needs-based choice addressing specific goals and the environment in which educational and developmental goals can best be achieved. Residential schools or special day programs for children with visual impairments currently serve those students who have multiple disabilities, those who need more constant educational programming, or those from remote areas where there is more limited access to support services for the student. Often residential schools additionally serve as community resource centers.

Adolescence

Adolescence is a critical time for the consolidation of a positive identity as an individual with a visual impairment. The desire to "pass" as sighted and avoid the perceived stigma may be a developmental phase or may signal a disavowal of the external restrictions placed on the adolescent or perceived limitations of the adolescent in the home, school, and community. During adolescence, the individual needs to be offered as many activities as possible. Involvement in community activities and school extracurricular activities should be encouraged. Often the family and school personnel may be fearful of allowing the student to take additional perceived risks. If the risks are not taken, the student is less likely to realize his/her social potential, and the stigma of the visual disability is further perpetuated. During adolescence, the student begins to think about his/her future, and it is essential for appropriate career counseling to be offered, as well as for the student to experience a wide variety of vocational options.

Children and adolescents who have progressive visual impairments require special programs to help them relearn skills in a different way. They also will need counseling to assist them with the psychological aspect of the loss. This is particularly true for those adolescents who have Usher syndrome, which results in deafblindness. Adults who have experienced this type of visual loss as a child share the common feeling that it is critical to let the child or adolescent know what is happening. Trying to protect the child from learning about the potential loss of vision more often results in inappropriate educational/rehabilitative efforts and ineffective preparation for the future. Underlying the difficulty addressing this diagnosis with the child is usually the powerful amalgam of grief, denial, numbing, pain, and the wish to protect the child. The primary care provider can play an important role in facilitating communication among educators, vocational counselors, and parents so that coordinated multidisciplinary planning can occur.

The health care provider may need to make clear recommendations for the implementation of necessary support services in the schools such as alterations of the physical environment, physical or occupational therapy, specialized

IV

equipment, orientation and mobility instruction and support, additional curriculum inclusion (braille, typewriting, etc.), or a special school placement. Resources for professionals and parents are listed at the end of this chapter.

OUTCOMES

Because of the multiplicity of factors involved in the outcome of individuals with visual impairments, accurate predictions of outcome are difficult to make. Children with visual impairments need specialized training to reach their full potential. The curriculum must give special attention to social skills, reading medium (braille or large print), magnification devices, orientation and mobility, and concept development.

Gaps in learning can lead to poor achievement. The ideal program always will focus on the skills the student will need to be successful after high school. In addition to basic curriculum offerings, the child with a visual impairment will need to have training in career and vocational skills. Both educational and rehabilitation agencies have developed transitional services to reduce the high risk of unemployment. Successful programs provide training in social and work skills, on-site job coaching, and a range of work experiences. These programs encourage parental involvement and interagency cooperation. Unfortunately, public attitudes and the stigma of blindness continue to foster the under- and unemployment of blind and visually impaired persons in the vocational setting, and along with practical issues such as transportation, impede community integration. Legislative mandates may help to increase access and pave the way for greater opportunities for the fuller participation in a society of individuals with visual impairments.

RESOURCES

American Foundation for the Blind
15 West 16th Street, New York, NY 10011
(212)620-2000 or (800)232-5463

Blind Children's Center
4120 Marathon Street, PO Box 29159, Los Angeles, CA 90029-0159

Council of Families With Visual Impairment
1155 15th Street, N.W., Suite 720, Washington, DC 20005
(202)393-3666

Glaucoma Foundation
310 East 14th Street, New York, NY 10003
(212)260-1000 or (800)832-EXAM

Helen Keller National Center for Deaf-Blind Youths and Adults
111 Middle Neck Road, Sands Point, New York, NY 11050
(516)944-8900

International Institute for Visually Impaired, 0-7 (Blind Children's Fund)
1975 Rutgers Circle, East Lansing, MI 48823
(517)332-2666

International Society on Metabolic Eye Disease
1125 Park Avenue, New York, NY 10128
(212)427-1246

The Lighthouse, Inc.
800 Second Avenue, New York, NY 10017
(212)808-0077

National Association for Parents of the Visually Impaired (NAPVI)
PO Box 317, Watertown, MA 02272-0317
(800)562-6265

National Eye Research Foundation
910 Skokie Boulevard, Suite 207A, Northbrook, IL 60062
(708)564-0807

National Federation of the Blind
1800 Johnson Street, Baltimore, MD 21230
(410)659-9314

National Information Center for Children and Youth With Disabilities (NICHCY)
PO Box 1492, Washington, DC 20013-1492
(703)893-6061 or (800)999-5599

National Retinitis Pigmentosa Foundation, Inc.
1401 Mt. Royal Avenue, Baltimore, MD 21217
(410)225-9409 or (800)683-5555

Prevent Blindness America
500 East Remington Road, Schaumburg, IL 60173
(800)331-2020

Research to Prevent Blindness
598 Madison Avenue, New York, NY 10022
(212)752-4333 or (800)621-0026

BIBLIOGRAPHY

Barraga NC, Erin JN: *Visual handicaps & learning,* Austin, TX, 1992, Pro-Ed.

Chapman EK, Stone JM: *The visually handicapped child in your classroom,* London, 1988, Cassell Educational Limited.

Fraiberg S: *Insights from the blind,* London, 1977, Souvenir Press.

Friendly DS: Development of vision in infants and young children, *Pediatr Clin North Am* 40:693–703, 1993.

Maloney PL: *Practical guidance for parents of the visually handicapped preschooler,* Springfield, IL, 1981, Charles C. Thomas.

McBroom IW, Tedder NE: Transitional services for youths who are visually impaired, *J Vis Impair Blind* March:69–72, 1993.

Teplin SW: Visual impairment in infants and young children, *Infant Young Child* July:18–51, 1995.

Warren DH, editor: *Blindness and early childhood development,* New York, 1984, American Foundation for the Blind.

Zambone AM: Serving the young child with visual impairments: An overview of disability impact and intervention needs, *Infant Young Child* October:11–21, 1989.

CHAPTER 117

IV

Traumatic Brain Injury

Linda J. Michaud

Traumatic brain injury is one of the major causes of mortality and disability in children and adolescents in the United States. Even for those children who survive the most severe injuries requiring prolonged periods of intensive care and rehabilitation, the primary care physician has a significant role in ongoing health maintenance, recognition of complications of the brain or associated injuries, and coordination of care with outpatient rehabilitation services and special education. Appreciation of the consequences of the different types and severities of traumatic brain injuries, the variability in their sequelae, and the types of interventions available to ameliorate deficits in age-appropriate domains of function should be useful to the primary physician caring for children with traumatic brain injury.

EPIDEMIOLOGY

The incidence of traumatic brain injury resulting in hospitalization is approximately 220 per 100,000 children between birth and 19 years of age per year. The actual numbers of pediatric traumatic brain injuries are much higher because the majority of injuries do not require hospitalization and the majority of the fatalities occur prior to hospital arrival. The most common causes of traumatic brain injury are falls, motor vehicle collisions including both vehicle occupant and nonoccupant (*ie,* bicyclist and pedestrian) injuries, sports and recreation-related injuries, and assaults. The distribution of brain injuries by cause differs with age. Among children between birth and 4 years of age, the majority are due to falls; approximately one fourth of

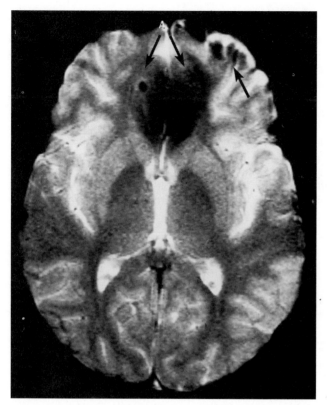

FIG 117-1
Magnetic resonance imaging shows bifrontal contusions *(arrows)* in this 13-year-old pedestrian who was struck by a motor vehicle moving at high speed. Performance on intelligence and academic achievement tests was normal within 6 weeks postinjury; however, short-term memory impairment was severe and warranted special educational support upon the student's return to school.

brain injuries in children younger than 2 years of age are inflicted. In children aged 5 to 9 years, motor vehicle collisions, falls, and sports and recreation-related injuries each account for almost one third of the injuries. Sport and recreation-related activities are the most common cause of brain injury in adolescents from 10 to 14 years of age. Among teenagers aged 15 years and over, the majority of brain injuries are due to motor vehicle collisions. For all age groups, motor vehicle collisions and assaults cause the most severe brain injuries.

The occurrence of traumatic brain injury in boys is twice that for girls. Incidence rates rise slowly in boys after 5 years of age and then dramatically from age 15 years, whereas the rates for girls decline after 3 years of age and then rise modestly after age 12 years. Traumatic brain injuries are more likely to occur during the afternoon and evening, on weekends, and during the spring and summer, when children and adolescents are more likely to be exposed to the previously mentioned causes of injury. Preinjury behavioral characteristics of the child and psy-

chosocial or environmental conditions also predispose some children to traumatic brain injuries.

TYPES OF BRAIN INJURIES

The type of brain injury sustained by a child depends on the nature of the force causing the injury. Primary injuries are caused by impact or inertial forces. Impact forces occur when the head strikes a surface and can result in fractures, focal contusions (Fig. 117-1), and epidural hematomas (Fig. 117-2). Inertial forces occur when the brain undergoes violent motion within the skull and can result in concussions, subdural hematomas (Fig. 117-3), or diffuse axonal injury (Fig. 117-4). Angular acceleration-deceleration and rotational shearing forces, such as those that can occur in motor vehicle collisions, are associated with more severe damage than straight-line forces, such as those occurring in a fall. Greater forces are required to produce progressively deeper lesions, from the cortical surface extend-

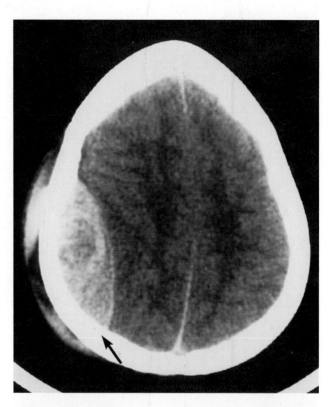

FIG 117-2

Unenhanced axial computed tomography image shows a biconvex area of hyperdensity on the right *(arrow)* producing midline shift to the left in this 8-year-old unhelmeted bicycle rider who fell from her bicycle. The epidural hematoma was promptly evacuated and outcome was without major neurologic sequelae.

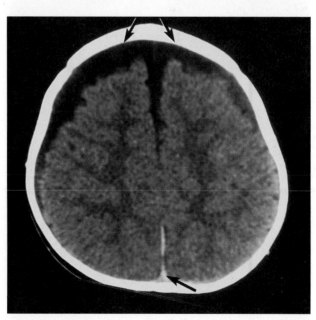

FIG 117-3

Computed tomography imaging reveals evidence of both chronic subdural hematomas *(upper arrows)* and acute interhemispheric blood *(lower arrow)* in this 7-month-old victim of shaking-impact syndrome. Head control remained poor, and the infant was unresponsive to visual and auditory stimuli at discharge from acute hospitalization.

IV

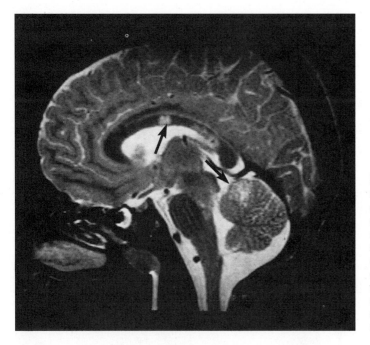

FIG 117-4
Sagittal T2-weighted image reveals diffuse axonal lesions in the corpus callosum *(arrow)* and cerebellum *(arrow)*. This 10-year-old pedestrian was struck by a car, thrown into the air, and landed on his head. Upon discharge from inpatient rehabilitation 6 weeks postinjury, this child was able to ambulate and complete basic self-care with supervision; significant cognitive and linguistic deficits persisted.

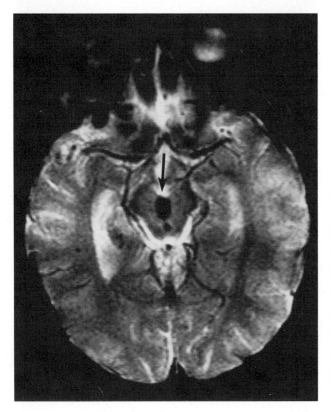

FIG 117-5
This 3-year-old restrained passenger in a motor vehicle collision sustained severe diffuse axonal injury. This magnetic resonance image reveals brain stem hemorrhage *(arrow)* that was associated with bilaterally nonreactive pupils and prolonged coma (44 days). Upon discharge from inpatient rehabilitation 3 months after injury, this child was ambulating with a walker and feeding herself. One pupil remained nonreactive; there was good visual tracking with the other eye and good functional vision. Receptive language recovery was good; the patient remained nonverbal but was communicating expressively with a simple electronic communication board.

ing to the brain stem (Fig. 117-5). Most children with traumatic brain injury have components of injury reflecting both impact and inertial forces. Secondary brain injuries result from increased intracranial pressure, ischemia, hypoxia, hypotension, acidosis, infection, or hydrocephalus. Secondary injury is potentially preventable and is a major focus of therapeutic interventions and current research.

SEVERITY OF BRAIN INJURY

The Glasgow Coma Scale (GCS) is widely used to estimate the severity of traumatic brain injury in both children and adults. The GCS score is based on motor, verbal, and eye opening responses as outlined in Table 1, in Chapter 104. Patients in coma have GCS scores of 8 or less and have severe injury; GCS scores of 9 to 12 reflect moderate injury; and scores of 13 to 15 reflect mild injury. Using these GCS categories, approximately 82% of traumatic brain injuries in children are mild, 14% are moderate to severe, and 5% are fatal.

The GCS score is a more accurate estimate of injury severity if assigned following initial resuscitation. If assigned sooner, short-term factors such as hypotension related to associated injuries, seizures, or intoxication may lead to lower scores and overestimation of the severity of the injury. Although there are limitations of the GCS in pediatric patients, especially with very young preverbal children, it is widely used.

The duration of posttraumatic amnesia is also useful in estimating severity of traumatic brain injury. During this time, which is much longer (3 to 4 times) than the period of unconsciousness, the patient remains amnesic and subsequently will not remember events that occur. The Children's Orientation and Amnesia Test is a measure of duration of posttraumatic amnesia for children and adolescents.

NEUROIMAGING

Neuroimaging is the most useful diagnostic modality following head trauma that results in neurologic signs or severe injury. Computed tomography (CT) is the radiologic method of choice in the acute setting to rapidly identify intracranial hematomas. Cerebral contusions, brain swelling,

and fractures including depressed fractures and most clinically important linear skull fractures also can be detected with CT. Magnetic resonance imaging (MRI) is more sensitive than CT in the detection of diffuse axonal injury and has a role in the subacute stage. Although CT and MRI are helpful in evaluating structural integrity after traumatic brain injury, newer neuroimaging methods may better assess function, such as functional MRI, single photon emission computed tomography, and positron emission tomography. These methods can assess changes in blood flow and metabolism with brain injury. Although not in general clinical use, functional neuroimaging techniques may provide information in the future that will allow increased understanding of the mechanisms of neurologic and functional recovery and evaluation of the effects of therapeutic interventions.

MANAGEMENT

Initial assessment and acute management of head trauma are discussed in Chapter 104. Interventions at the acute stage are directed toward reducing delayed primary or secondary brain damage and preventing secondary complications, including those to other organ systems.

Long-term management varies with type, severity, location, and extent of primary and secondary injury to the brain. Depending on these injury-related factors, neurologic impairment may result in motor, sensory, communication, cognitive, and behavioral dysfunction, as outlined in the Box 117-1. Mild injury most often results in deficits in one or more domains of function that resolve rapidly and spontaneously without intervention. At the other end of the spectrum of injury, severe diffuse neurologic injury usually results in deficits in multiple domains of function that may warrant intensive rehabilitation intervention. Interdisciplinary assessment and rehabilitation using a team approach with physiatrists, physical and occupational therapists, speech and language pathologists, neuropsychologists, special educators, social workers, and rehabilitation nurses may be indicated for those children with severe, multiple deficits. Between the mild injuries with no sequelae and the severe injuries resulting in severe deficits in function are those injuries that result in some disability in one or more areas of

IV

BOX 117-1
**Deficits in Function After Traumatic
Brain Injury**

Motor deficits
  Spasticity
  Incoordination
  Tremor
Sensory deficits
  Visual
  Auditory
  Olfactory
  Gustatory
  Tactile
Communication deficits
  Speech
  Language
    Receptive and/or expressive
    Oral and/or written
Cognitive deficits
  Attention
  Memory
  Information processing
  Speed of performance
  Problem-solving skills
  Abstract information processing
  Organizational skills
  Judgment
Behavioral problems
  Aggression
  Poor anger control
  Hyperactivity
  Impulsivity
  Irritability
  Social withdrawal
  Apathy

---

function but that do not prevent the child from resuming some of his/her previous roles in the family or school. For these children, outpatient rehabilitation services may be warranted. Much of the rehabilitation for children with severe traumatic brain injury is carried out within special educational programs. The Individuals with Disabilities Education Act (IDEA) identified traumatic brain injury as a specific category of disability within special education. Depending on individualized needs, children with traumatic brain injury may receive special educational services in a resource room or self-contained classroom and physical, occupational, and/or speech-language therapies and counseling may be provided as part of the educational program. The primary care physician has a crucial role in the long-term management of the child with traumatic brain injury in identifying new deficits in function that follow injury, referring the child

for appropriate rehabilitation or special education services and coordinating care.

COMPLICATIONS

Complications occurring beyond the acute stage in children with traumatic brain injury include posttraumatic seizures, posttraumatic hydrocephalus, cerebrospinal fluid (CSF) fistulas, "growing" skull fractures, and disorders of endocrine function.

Immediate seizures with onset within minutes of impact are very common and of no long-term consequence. Early seizures occurring within the first week after injury are more common in children than in adults, especially in younger children. Severe brain injury is associated with a higher risk of early posttraumatic seizures, and short-term use of anticonvulsant prophylaxis is indicated to reduce the potential for secondary hypoxic brain injury. Late posttraumatic epilepsy is defined as two or more seizures occurring more than 1 week after brain injury. Even in children with severe injury, the incidence is less than 3%. Because the effectiveness of long-term use of anticonvulsants for prophylaxis has not been demonstrated and the cognitive and behavioral side effects of these medications can be significant in children with brain injury, prophylaxis for late seizures is generally not indicated following closed head trauma.

Posttraumatic hydrocephalus occurs infrequently after pediatric traumatic brain injury. Ventricular enlargement can be associated with either high or normal CSF pressure. Usually, pressures are low and enlarged CSF spaces represent hydrocephalus ex vacuo secondary to cerebral atrophy; shunting is not beneficial in this situation. Occasionally, children will fail to recover function or demonstrate clinical deterioration in association with elevation of CSF pressure; in these cases, clinical improvement typically follows shunting. Subarachnoid hemorrhage is a risk factor for development of posttraumatic hydrocephalus.

CSF fistulas are associated with basilar skull fractures and an increased risk of meningitis. Neurosurgical intervention may be warranted when CSF rhinorrhea or otorrhea persists beyond 1 to 2 weeks after injury. "Growing" skull fractures are an unusual complication of skull fractures that occur in young children, in which the brain or meninges herniate through disrupted dura mater. Prompt recognition and management can prevent further secondary neurologic compromise.

Disruption of the hypothalamic-pituitary area can lead to neuroendocrine dysfunction. Hypothalamic-posterior pituitary disorders include the syndrome of inappropriate antidiuretic hormone secretion and central diabetes insipidus. Although the onset is usually early and these disorders are usually transient, either may occur months after injury and warrant pharmacologic intervention. Dysregulation of thyroid, growth, and adrenocorticotropic hormones, gonadotropins, and prolactin may result from hypothalamic-anterior pituitary injury. Growth and sexual development should be monitored and symptoms and signs of endocrinopathy evaluated, because hormonal replacement may be indicated.

Complications also may occur in other organ systems related to immobilization due to the brain injury and/or to associated injuries. The majority of children with severe brain injuries also have additional injuries to other systems. Respiratory, musculoskeletal, cardiovascular, gastrointestinal, genitourinary, dermatologic, and nutritional problems can complicate the acute and chronic course of children with traumatic brain injury. Detailed discussion of these problems is beyond the scope of this chapter, but are reviewed elsewhere (see References).

PROGNOSIS AND OUTCOME

Mortality after pediatric traumatic brain injury is high in children 2 years of age or less and then steadily decreases to a nadir at 12 years of age before rising again sharply in patients over 15 years of age. The high fatality rates at the two ends of the pediatric age range are associated with mechanisms of injury that result in severe injury, specifically child abuse and motor vehicle collisions.

Outcomes following traumatic brain injury in children who survive range from complete recovery to survival with severe deficits in multiple domains of function. Overall, approximately 20% of injuries result in significant disability, including 10% of those in children with mild injuries and 90% in those with moderate to severe injuries.

Several factors have been associated with outcome following traumatic brain injury in children. Factors associated with survival are not necessarily associated with the severity of the disability in those who do survive. Clinicians should be cautious in prognosticating because none of these factors, either singly or in combination, allows prediction of outcomes of either survival or quality of survival with certainty.

Early clinical status, in the field and emergency room, is highly associated with survival but less predictive of severity of disability in survivors. The severity of the brain injury and associated injuries to other organ systems have been related strongly to both survival and disability. The severity of traumatic brain injury is the major factor associated with severity of disability in survivors. Glasgow Coma Scale scores, especially the motor component, a few days after injury are better predictors of level of disability than those assigned on hospital admission.

The duration of coma and of posttraumatic amnesia are important markers for severity of injury; longer durations are associated with less favorable outcomes. The type of brain injury is also an important predictor of functional outcome. Epidural hematomas that are promptly surgically evacuated are usually associated with good outcomes. In contrast, subdural hematomas, even with rapid neurosurgical intervention, are associated with greater damage to the underlying brain and poorer outcomes. Extensive diffuse axonal injury is associated with persisting functional impairment. Worse outcomes follow focal lesions in addition to diffuse injury as compared with diffuse injury alone. Secondary brain injury such as prolonged increased intracranial pressure reduces the likelihood of a good outcome.

The effect of age at injury on outcome is complex. Several studies have demonstrated worse impairment in cognitive function following severe brain injury in children injured at younger ages. It is likely that there are interactions among the type and severity of injury with mechanism of injury and age. Very young children who are victims of child abuse can suffer severe injuries, including subdural hematomas, and often return to environments with multiple psychosocial stressors. Poor outcome in these children is likely multifactorial and not attributable only to young age at injury.

PREVENTION

Most traumatic brain injury in childhood is preventable. Falls resulting in serious traumatic brain injuries can be prevented by using window bars and gates for stairs, lowering the height of playground equipment to a maximum of 5 feet and modifying playground surfaces to increase energy-absorbing potential, and discouraging the use of baby walkers. The frequency and severity of traumatic brain injuries due to motor vehicle collisions can be reduced through the proper use of car restraints and screening and treatment of alcohol abuse in teenagers. Helmets reduce the risk of brain injury in bicyclists by almost 90% and also should be used for skateboarding, roller blading, and horseback riding. Limiting the availability of firearms, including to children, would reduce brain injuries due to this type of assault. Child abuse has been demonstrated to be less likely to occur in high-risk families in which support and training in parenting skills have been provided. The primary care physician has an important role in prevention through family and community education and through advocacy for appropriate legislation. Until preventive efforts succeed, control of the consequences of the injury on the child and family will remain among the challenges of the physician concerned with the problem of pediatric traumatic brain injury.

BIBLIOGRAPHY

Bijur PE, Haslum M, Golding J: Cognitive and behavioral sequelae of mild head injury in children, *Pediatrics* 86:337–344, 1990.

Duhaime AC, Alario AJ, Lewander WJ, et al: Head injury in very young children: Mechanisms, injury types, and ophthalmologic findings in 100 hospitalized patients younger than 2 years of age, *Pediatrics* 90:179–185, 1992.

Ewing-Cobbs L, Levin HS, Fletcher JM, et al: The Children's Orientation and Amnesia Test: Relationship to severity of acute head injury and to recovery of memory, *Neurosurgery* 27:683–691, 1990.

Jaffe KM, editor: Traumatic brain injury, *Pediatr Ann* 23(1). January, 1994.

Jaffe KM, Fay GC, Polissar NL, et al: Severity of pediatric traumatic brain injury and neurobehavioral recovery at one year—a cohort study, *Arch Phys Med Rehabil* 74:587–595, 1993.

Kraus JF, Rock A, Hemyari P: Brain injuries among infants, children, adolescents, and young adults, *Am J Dis Child* 144:684–691, 1990.

Luerssen TG, Klauber MR, Marshall LF: Outcome from head injury related to patient's age: A longitudinal prospective study of adult and pediatric head injury, *J Neurosurg* 68:409–416, 1988.

Michaud LJ, editor: Pediatric brain injury, *J Head Trauma Rehabil* 10(5) October, 1995.

Michaud LJ, Rivara FP, Grady MS, Reay DT: Predictors of survival and severity of disability after severe brain injury in children, *Neurosurgery* 31:254–264, 1992.

Rosenthal M, Griffith ER, Bond MR, Miller JD, editors: *Rehabilitation of the adult and child with traumatic brain injury,* ed 2, Philadelphia, 1990, FA Davis.

CHAPTER 118

Learning Disabilities

Nathan J. Blum

Achieving success in school is one of the primary tasks of childhood and adolescence. School success is dependent on a wide variety of factors including academic skills, social skills, emotional states and stresses, attentional and motivational factors, and the family and school environments. Although this chapter will focus on children who are having difficulty learning academic skills (ie, children with learning disabilities), it is important to remember that many children who struggle in school have several factors that contribute to their difficulties.

Physicians usually will not make the diagnosis of a learning disability. However, they often are asked by families or school officials to assist in caring for children who are not experiencing success in school. In this role, physicians need to understand current concepts in the diagnosis and remediation of learning disabilities and some of the limitations of the diagnostic process. This understanding will help physicians to recommend and support an appropriate course of action for their patients with school difficulties.

DEFINITION

In 1975 Congress passed the Education for All Handicapped Children Act (Public Law 94-142), which guaranteed "free and appropriate public education" for all handicapped children, including children with learning disabilities. This act, which was reauthorized in 1990 as the Individuals With Disabilities Education Act (IDEA), provides a legal definition of a learning disability as:

". . . a disorder in one or more of the basic psychological processes involved in understanding or in using language, spoken or written, which may manifest itself as an imperfect ability to listen, think, speak, read, write, spell, or to do mathematical calculations. . . The term does not include children who have learning problems that are primarily the result of visual, hearing, or motor handicaps, of mental retardation, of emotional disturbance, or of environmental, cultural, or economic disadvantage." (Office of Education, 1977)

This definition emphasizes that children diagnosed with a learning disability must have a skill deficit that is not primarily explained by a sensory, motor, or generalized cognitive deficit or by emotional or environmental factors. However, the definition is problematic in that the "basic psychological processes" to which it refers are unknown and the level of skill deficit that demonstrates an "imperfect ability" is not specified. Thus, individual states have been left to determine how they will identify children with learning disabilities. More than half of the states have specific operational criteria for the diagnosis of a learning disability, whereas the others employ more general criteria.

When a specific operational definition is used, it involves finding a significant discrepancy (defined variably) between the child's actual achievement and his/her expected achievement. Actual achievement is measured on standardized achievement tests (*see* Assessment), but the mechanism for determining expected achievement can vary greatly. Some states use expected achievement for a child in a specific grade, others base expected achievement on the child's tested level of intelligence, and still others use regression formula, which also are based on intelligence test scores.

All these definitions may limit access to educational assistance for some children who are having difficulty in school. Using grade level to estimate expected achievement makes it difficult for children in the younger grades to qualify.

For instance, a child in first grade may be struggling, but it would be almost impossible for a first-grade child to be two grade levels behind his/her peers. Also, children with superior intelligence who are functioning at grade level, but below the level expected for their intelligence, would not meet the grade level criteria. Although the intelligence-achievement discrepancy formula is generally better accepted for diagnosing learning disabilities, some children with low average intelligence may be 2 years or more behind their classmates in achievement and yet not have a large enough discrepancy between their intelligence and achievement to meet the criteria for a learning disability. In some cases these children may be denied the assistance they need to succeed in school because they are not diagnosed with a learning disability.

PREVALENCE

As is implied in the previous discussion, the criteria for making a diagnosis of a learning disability are not widely agreed upon. The prevalence of learning disabilities will vary with the diagnostic criteria that are used. Most experts estimate that between 3% to 15% of school-age children have a learning disability.

A learning disability in reading, often referred to as *dyslexia,* is the most common learning disability. It is believed to affect approximately 4% of children. Generally, boys are affected somewhat more frequently than girls with a male:female ratio of approximately 1.5:1.

ASSESSMENT

History

Evaluation of children with difficulty in school begins with the history of the problem. The history should include when the problems first began, the parents' and teachers' description of the problems, assessments performed by the school, and the effects of any intervention strategies that have been tried. The physician may offer a unique perspective on the school difficulties because he/she often has knowledge of the child's medical history, developmental history, behavioral history, family history, and family environment, which may not be available to school personnel.

Children with a history of brain injury from trauma, infection, or other causes will be at increased risk of having a learning disability. Chronic medical conditions such as seizures, migraine headaches, asthma, and diabetes can interfere with children's opportunities for learning by affecting multiple factors including attention, energy level, time available for school activities, school attendance, and family functioning. The physician must ensure that these chronic conditions are detected and appropriately managed to minimize their effects on learning.

The history of the child's development and behavior during the toddler and preschool years is often helpful. Children with delays in language development during this period are at increased risk for learning disabilities when they enter school. Children with behavioral characteristics such as hyperactivity, inattention, impulsivity, oppositionality, and anxiety often can be identified in the preschool years. Although these behaviors alone place children at risk for school difficulties, they also occur with increased frequency in children with learning disabilities.

The family history should be investigated for learning disabilities (*see* Etiology), attention deficit/hyperactivity disorder, affective and anxiety disorders, mental retardation, and neurodegenerative disorders. The presence of one of these disorders in the family may help direct further evaluation.

The family environment also will affect school performance. Factors ranging from the degree to which learning is emphasized to stresses such as family illness, conflict, or abuse should be considered.

Physical Examination

There are no physical examination findings that are diagnostic of a learning disability. The examination should focus on dysmorphic or cutaneous findings characteristic of disorders that may be associated with learning disabilities (*eg,* neurofibromatosis, Turner syndrome, etc.). The routine neurologic examination should be normal, although the child with learning disabilities may demonstrate difficulties with fine motor movements, rapid alternating movements, and left-right orientation. Hearing and vision also should be screened.

TABLE 118-1
Intelligence Tests Used in the Assessment of Learning Disabilities

NAME OF TEST	AGE RANGE	DESCRIPTION/SCORING
Wechsler Intelligence Scale for Children—III (WISC-III)	6–16 yrs	Individually administered test of intelligence that provides verbal, performance (nonverbal problem solving), and full-scale (verbal and performance combined) scores. The mean score is 100, and one standard deviation is ± 15 points. Subtest scores often are reported. The mean score of subtests is 10, and one standard deviation is ± 3 points.
Wechsler Preschool and Primary Scale of Intelligence—Revised (WPPSI-R)	36–72 mos	Individually administered test of intelligence that provides verbal, performance, and full-scale scores similar to WISC-III. The mean score is 100, and one standard deviation is ± 16 points.
Stanford-Binet Intelligence Scale—4th Ed	2 yrs to adult	Individually administered test of intelligence. Tasks are grouped by age level. A single IQ score is obtained with a mean of 100, and one standard deviation is ± 16 points. For school-age children test items are heavily weighted toward verbal reasoning skills.

Laboratory Evaluation

There are no routine laboratory or radiologic tests that are helpful in making the diagnosis of a learning disability.

Educational Evaluation

For children who are having difficulty in school an assessment of academic skills is essential to determine if skill deficits are contributing to the school problems. When skill deficits are suspected, a psychoeducational evaluation for learning disabilities should be conducted by a school psychologist. Usually this will involve intelligence quotient (IQ) testing and achievement testing to identify a discrepancy between intelligence and achievement scores as discussed previously.

Information on the most commonly used intelligence tests is summarized in Table 118-1. Achievement tests may be administered to groups of children or individually. Although group tests may be adequate for screening, they should not be used for the diagnosis of learning disabilities, because with group administration one cannot be sure that the child understood the instructions or paid attention to the task. Information on the most commonly used individual achievement tests is summarized in Table 118-2.

ETIOLOGY

Learning disabilities are believed to be of central nervous system origin. Children with a variety of disorders associated with brain injury or dysfunction have been found to have an increased risk for learning disabilities. This group includes children with neurofibromatosis, Tourette syndrome, traumatic brain injury and those who have received craniospinal irradiation. However, children with identifiable brain injuries tend to have the greatest difficulty with visual-perceptual and visual-motor skills, whereas the majority of children with learning disabilities and no identified history of brain injury tend to have the greatest difficulty with language skills.

Children with language-based learning disabilities are believed to have an abnormality in brain development, and this has been studied most extensively in children with reading learning disability. Routine computed tomographic or magnetic resonance brain imaging studies in these children have not found differences between their brains and the brains of control subjects. Research studies using volumetric measurements of specific brain regions often report differences in the corpus callosum, temporal lobes, and planum temporale of children with

IV

TABLE 118-2
Achievement Tests Used in the Assessment of Learning Disabilities

NAME OF TEST	SKILL AREAS ASSESSED	DESCRIPTION/SCORING
Wechsler Individual Achievement Tests (WIAT)	Eight subtests cover reading, writing, mathematics, language comprehension and expression, and spelling. Subtests combined to yield composite scores in reading, mathematics, language, and writing.	Use of reading, mathematics reasoning, and spelling subtests recommended for screening. Provides grade level, percentile, and standard scores.*
Woodcock-Johnson Tests of Achievement—Revised (WJ-R)	Ten subtests cover writing, reading, mathematics, science, social studies, and humanities. Subtests combined to yield cluster scores called the broad reading, broad math, written language, and knowledge scores.	Few easy items so children in kindergarten or first grade can receive high scores without doing many items. Provides grade level, percentile, and standard scores.*
Kauffman Tests of Educational Achievement (K-TEA)	Mathematics application, mathematics computation, reading decoding, reading comprehension, spelling.	Brief and comprehensive forms of test available. Provides standard scores* for each subtest and composite scores for math and reading.
Peabody Individual Achievement Test—Revised (PIAT-R)	Mathematics, reading recognition, reading comprehension, spelling, written expression, general information	Uses multiple-choice format. Provides grade level, percentile, and standard scores.*
Wide Range Achievement Test—Revised (WRAT-R)	Mathematics, single-word reading, spelling	Brief achievement test that assesses a narrow range of skills. Best used as a screening measure. Grade level scores obtained on each subtest.

*Standard scores: mean = 100, standard deviation = ± 15.

reading disability. However, the differences reported are not consistent between studies.

An alternative explanation for reading disability is that reading skills are normally distributed in the population and that children falling below an arbitrary cut-off are diagnosed with reading disability. This explanation would be analogous to the way in which hypertension and obesity are currently diagnosed. There is some epidemiologic data to support this hypothesis for children with reading disability (*see* Shaywitz *et al.* for a further discussion).

Genetic factors do play a role in reading disability. The recurrence rate for reading disability among first-degree relatives of children with dyslexia is 30% to 45%, and the concordance rate is higher among monozygotic than dizygotic twins. These data could be consistent with either of the above hypothesized etiologies for reading disability. Genetic factors could cause abnormal brain development, but it is also known that genetic factors play a role in other human characteristics that are normally distributed in the population (*eg*, height).

TREATMENT

Effective treatments for learning disabilities are primarily educational. They should build on the strengths identified in the psychoeducational testing and provide both remediation and compensation for weaknesses. As an example, a child with a reading disability will require extra instruction in reading (remediation), but he/she also may need instructions or long reading assignments read to him/her and/or extra time to complete these assignments (compensation). If the child has good math skills he/she should be instructed at a level appropriate for the math skills and not be penalized for the reading problems. As children get older there can be increasing emphasis on teaching children strategies for learning new material.

A team approach to treatment is likely to be the most successful. The child's parents, teacher, educational specialist, school psychologist, and physician must work together to develop an individualized educational plan for the child. A speech-language pathologist should be available to help children with language-based learning problems. An occupational therapist may be helpful for children whose motor coordination is interfering with writing or other academic tasks. A mental-health professional should be available to help address emotional, social, and/or family factors that may impact on the child's learning or be a response to the child's learning disability. The child's primary care physician should ensure optimal management of any chronic medical problems and may be involved in providing treatment for attentional problems that often coexist with learning disabilities (*see* Chapter 119).

A number of noneducational treatment approaches to learning disabilities have been suggested. These approaches include the use of large doses of vitamins or trace elements, visual training exercises, tinted lenses, and so forth. These treatments are not recommended because they are often time-consuming and expensive and there is no scientific evidence to support their efficacy (*see* Silver for a review). Also, large doses of some fat-soluble vitamins may be harmful.

OUTCOME

Longitudinal studies indicate that learning disabilities are chronic conditions that tend to persist throughout life. As a group, children with learning disabilities tend to have lower academic achievement and higher school drop-out rates than children without learning disabilities. However, many children with learning disabilities, even those with difficulty in school, are successful once they enter careers that emphasize their strengths. Factors such as the child's overall intelligence, support systems, work ethic, educational interventions, and the severity of the disability may influence outcome. Children with learning disabilities who successfully graduate from high school have a much better chance of being satisfied with their jobs than those who do not graduate.

SUMMARY

Learning disabilities are one of a large number of factors that can contribute to poor school performance. Primary care physicians are in an ideal position to assess medical, developmental, behavioral, and family factors that may be contributing to a child's school difficulties. Knowledge of how learning disabilities are diagnosed and treated should allow these physicians to recommend or support appropriate evaluations and interventions for their patients with learning disabilities.

BIBLIOGRAPHY

Filipek PA: Neurobiologic correlates of developmental dyslexia: How do dyslexics' brains differ from those of normal readers? *J Child Neurol* 10:s63–s69, 1995.

Finlan TG: Do state methods of quantifying a severe discrepancy result in fewer students with learning disabilities? *Learn Disabil Q* 15:129–134, 1992.

Johnson DJ: Educational interventions in learning disabilities: Follow-up studies and future research needs. In Capute AJ, Accardo PJ, Shapiro BK, editors: *Learning disabilities spectrum: ADD, ADHD, & LD,* Baltimore, 1994, York Press.

Office of Education: Assistance to states for education of handicapped children: Procedures for evaluating specific learning disability, *Fed Reg* 42:65–83, 1977.

Pennington BF: Genetics of learning disabilities, *J Child Neurol* 10:s69–s77, 1995.

Shapiro BK, Gallico RP: Learning disabilities, *Pediatr Clin North Am* 40:491–505, 1993.

Shaywitz SE, Fletcher JM, Shaywitz BA: A new conceptual model for dyslexia. In Capute AJ, Accardo PJ, Shapiro BK, editors: *Learning disabilities spectrum: ADD, ADHD, & LD,* Baltimore, 1994, York Press.

Silver LB: Nonstandard therapies of learning disabilities, *Semin Neurol* 11:57–63, 1991.

Wodrich DL, Kush SA: *Children's psychological testing: A guide for nonpsychologists,* Baltimore, 1990, Paul H. Brookes.

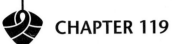

CHAPTER 119

Attention Deficit/Hyperactivity Disorder

Marianne Mercugliano

Hyperactivity and short attention span are childhood symptoms that parents often first discuss with their primary care physician. Many children who manifest these symptoms will ultimately fit the diagnostic criteria for attention deficit/hyperactivity disorder (ADHD). These symptoms, however, are often nonspecific and, therefore, the primary care physician has a critical role in considering other causes for similar behaviors that may require different treatments. This chapter should assist the physician caring for these children and their families in developing strategies for a comprehensive evaluation and coordinated treatment plan.

CLINICAL DESCRIPTION

The core features of ADHD have classically included a short attention span, distractibility, impulsivity, and hyperactivity or restlessness. A parent may present with one or more of these features as chief complaints, but there are often other concerns depending on the age, environment, and nature of the individual child. These concerns may include "immaturity," difficulties with mood lability, motivation or frustration tolerance, peer problems, or academic underachievement. The evaluation of core and associated features is complex because there are no corroborative physical findings or laboratory results, and severity ratings depend on the rater as well as the child. Several of the behaviors commonly associated with ADHD overlap with those behaviors conceptualized within a continuum of temperamental or personality style. ADHD is a diagnosis reserved for those children who meet its diagnostic criteria who are not primarily experiencing another condition, that may result in similar symptoms, and whose symptoms are sufficiently severe to hamper their developmental, social, and/or academic progress. The most pressing reason to strive to understand and treat ADHD is that it causes significant morbidity for a large number of children, their families, and society (prevalence estimates range from 3% to 10%). There is a high incidence of comorbid disruptive behavior, mood, and learning disorders; and symptoms persist to some degree in the majority of adolescents and adults.

EVALUATION

Most clinicians use the diagnostic criteria outlined in the *Diagnostic and Statistical Manual of Mental Disorders–IV* as a starting point in their evaluation. These criteria include six or more of the following symptoms, which have been present for at least 6 months, in at least one of the two major categories (inattention and hyperactivity-impulsivity) plus the four additional requirements listed below.

Symptoms of Inattention
1. Often fails to give close attention to details or makes careless mistakes in schoolwork, work, or other activities
2. Often has difficulty sustaining attention in tasks or play activities
3. Often does not seem to listen when spoken to directly
4. Often does not follow through on instructions and fails to finish schoolwork, chores, or duties in the workplace (not due to oppositional behavior or failure to understand instructions)

5. Often has difficulty organizing tasks and activities
6. Often avoids, dislikes, or is reluctant to engage in tasks that require sustained mental effort (such as schoolwork or homework)
7. Often loses things necessary for tasks or activities (*eg,* toys, school assignments, pencils, books, tools)
8. Is often easily distracted by extraneous stimuli
9. Is often forgetful in daily activities

Symptoms of Hyperactivity/Impulsivity
1. Often fidgets with hands or feet or squirms in seat
2. Often leaves seat in classroom or in other situations in which remaining seated is expected
3. Often runs about or climbs excessively in situations in which it is inappropriate (in adolescents or adults this may be limited to subjective feelings of restlessness)
4. Often has difficulty playing or engaging in leisure activities quietly
5. Is often "on the go" or often acts as if "driven by a motor"
6. Often talks excessively
7. Often blurts out answers before questions have been completed
8. Often has difficulty awaiting turn
9. Often interrupts or intrudes on others (*eg,* butts into conversations or games)

Additional Requirements
1. Some symptoms causing impairment were present before the age of 7 years.
2. Impairment from some symptoms is present in two or more settings.
3. There is clinically significant impairment in social, academic, or occupational functioning.
4. The symptoms are not present exclusively during a diagnosis of pervasive developmental disorder or schizophrenia (or other psychotic disorder) and are not better accounted for by another psychiatric disorder.

The diagnosis of ADHD is then described as either inattentive, hyperactive-impulsive, or combined type. In addition, the diagnosis of "ADHD, not otherwise specified" is available for individuals with prominent symptoms of inattention or hyperactivity-impulsivity who do not meet full criteria for the disorder. It is also important to keep in mind that the symp-

toms must be out of proportion to those expected for the child's *cognitive* age. Thus, ADHD can be diagnosed in the setting of global developmental delay, or mental retardation, but the child's cognitive age must be taken into consideration.

It is common in psychiatric practice to obtain diagnostic information through the use of a standardized diagnostic interview formats. Several questionnaires are available to assist the clinician in gathering diagnostic information in a standardized way and in comparing severity ratings to age- and sex-matched norms. Although these questionnaires tap into the same kinds of symptoms, they also are not specific for DSM-IV criteria. Examples include the Achenbach Child Behavior Checklist and its companion Teacher Report Form, Conners Parent and Teacher Rating Scales, the ADHD Comprehensive Teacher Rating Scales, and the Yale Children's Personal Data Inventory and its companion Yale Teacher's Behavior Rating Scale. It is important that the questionnaires be completed by multiple observers. Issues that may impact on the rater's assessment of the nature and severity of the child's problems also must be considered, particularly when the information from different sources is discrepant.

DIFFERENTIAL DIAGNOSIS

If information provided by both parents and teachers is consistent with ADHD, the primary care physician must then investigate other possible causes for these behaviors. Other conditions may exist instead of, or in addition to, ADHD.

Medical/neurologic conditions include medications (*eg,* anticonvulsants, antihistamines and "mixed" cold preparations, theophylline), visual or hearing impairment, untreated absence or partial complex seizures, lead poisoning, anemia, hyperthyroidism, poor sleep patterns as in obstructive sleep apnea, and neurodegenerative diseases (particularly the leukodystrophies, Wilson disease, and Sanfilippo-type mucopolysaccharidosis). Other neurologic conditions such as mass lesions of the brain and neurocutaneous syndromes may present with cognitive or behavioral symptoms, but usually there are additional signs and symptoms. Syndromes that frequently have ADHD as a component include fetal alcohol

IV

syndrome, fragilex syndrome, Dubowitz syndrome, and Tourette syndrome and neurofibromatosis type 1.

Educational/cognitive conditions refer to undiagnosed learning disabilities, communication disorder, mental retardation, or pervasive developmental disorders (the autistic spectrum disorders) in a child who is therefore educationally misplaced. Behavioral symptoms can arise when a child faces expectations from parents and teachers that are consistently beyond his/her capabilities. Social/environmental conditions include chaotic family environment and physical, sexual, or emotional abuse. Other psychiatric conditions include the other disruptive behavior disorders (conduct and oppositional defiant disorder) and mood and anxiety disorders. In the presence of an active medical or neurologic disorder, pervasive developmental disorder, or extremely dysfunctional social situation, the diagnosis of ADHD is generally suspended.

The primary care physician's objective is to rule out other treatable conditions with a thorough history, general physical examination, and neurologic examination.

The history should include etiologic risk factors in the pre- and perinatal period, health and developmental history, a pedigree focusing on neurodevelopmental and psychiatric conditions, and a thorough review of systems. Referral to a pediatric neurologist is recommended if there are concerns of focal neurologic signs, seizures, or a degenerative course. Routine electroencephalograms and neuroimaging studies are not indicated. A careful assessment of the child's mood, family, and peer functioning is critical. A variety of professionals with training in this type of assessment may perform it including pediatricians, social workers, psychologists, and psychiatrists. The Child Behavior Checklist and Teacher Report Form are helpful in screening for affective and disruptive (internalizing and externalizing) symptoms that may suggest the presence of a different or comorbid disorder. Referral to a child psychiatrist may be helpful if there appears to be significant psychopathology in the child or parent(s).

For educational concerns, a thorough developmental assessment must be performed. For the preschooler, an assessment focusing on cognitive skills (receptive and expressive language and visual-motor problem-solving) by a psychologist or developmental pediatrician is ap-propriate. If language problems are suspected, an evaluation by a speech and language pathologist should be done to assist with diagnosis and treatment planning. For the school-aged child, both cognitive (intelligence quotient) and academic achievement testing by a psychologist and perhaps a special educator are required to distinguish mild global cognitive delay (mild mental retardation) and learning disabilities.

Clearly, the chief complaint of short attention span or hyperactivity requires a complex assessment before ADHD, which is a diagnosis of exclusion, can be made. Further complicating the diagnostic process is the fact that many children with ADHD have learning or psychosocial problems as well. The primary care physician may prefer to be the central coordinator of the evaluation using individual consultants as needed and subsequently providing a synthesis of the results and recommendations for the family. Alternatively, the family may be referred to an interdisciplinary team that specializes in the evaluation of school, behavioral, and developmental problems. Such teams may be found in the child development or child psychiatry divisions of pediatric medical centers or through the school system. The team usually consists of one or more physicians (developmental pediatrician, child psychiatrist, pediatric neurologist), a social worker, and a psychologist with expertise in testing and behavior management. Other consultants such as the special educator, speech and language pathologist, audiologist, geneticist, and occupational therapist are available to the team. The advantage of the team approach is that the evaluators discuss their results together, directly resulting in a better overall understanding of the child and family. Because the evaluations of different professionals may overlap in some areas, the opportunity to have findings corroborated by others as well as the necessity to explain discrepant results may lead to a more in-depth assessment. The need for stepwise intervention and reevaluation may be met more easily by a team because this can be a time and labor-intensive condition to treat. The pediatrician may retain primary responsibility for treatment and follow-up if desired, with guidance from the team, if needed. It should be noted that a comprehensive, multidisciplinary baseline assessment is becoming the standard of care for children with possible ADHD, particularly when medication is being considered.

TREATMENT

Treatment of ADHD consists of educational, behavioral, and, in some cases, pharmacologic intervention. Educational intervention consists of providing the necessary additional help required for the child to master academic skills. It also includes implementing strategies for reducing distractibility in the classroom such as having the child sit at the front of the class near the teacher, providing a carrel for use during independent work, and allowing frequent short breaks or changes in type of activity.

Counseling for the child and family is an important part of treatment and must be presented as such. The main type of counseling used is behavior modification therapy. Parents work with a trained professional (usually, but not always, a psychologist) to learn how to modify the antecedents and consequences of specific behaviors such that positive behaviors are encouraged and negative ones discouraged. This is a labor-intensive undertaking because parents must first learn to become systematic objective observers of the child's behavior, and then must be extremely consistent in applying the techniques they have developed with the psychologist. Parents may become discouraged because changes do not occur as quickly as they would like, but behavior modification has been shown to be effective in improving behavior and academic productivity. Other types of counseling can be helpful in selected cases. The older, insightful child may benefit from individual, cognitively oriented therapy to work on "self-modifying" certain behaviors, as well as self-esteem and social skills. Family therapy can be helpful in resolving specific family issues that may create tension and contribute to increased negative behavior. In addition, family therapy can be helpful in ameliorating the stress experienced by most families raising a child with ADHD. Parents need support because they are often made to think that poor parenting skills are the source of their child's difficulty. When parents do not perceive their child in the same way, or have the same views about discipline, marital discord may result, with the child sensing that he/she is to blame. Finally, the therapist can help a family find ways to ensure that all members' needs are met in a supportive, consistent way, creating the optimal home environment for the child with ADHD.

Methylphenidate (Ritalin), dextroamphetamine (Dexedrine), and magnesium pemoline (Cylert) are the stimulant medications most commonly used to treat ADHD. It has been proposed that children with ADHD have deficient mesocortical dopaminergic transmission, affecting circuits between the frontal lobes and basal ganglia. Other cortical and subcortical circuits are likely to be involved as well. Dextroamphetamine facilitates synthesis and release of norepinephrine and dopamine and inhibits the catabolic enzyme, monoamine oxidase. Methylphenidate primarily blocks dopamine reuptake. Pemoline is an indirect dopamine agonist with fewer sympathomimetic effects.

Stimulants have been shown to improve several aspects of functioning from attention and impulsivity to social and fine motor skills. Improvements in scholastic achievement are controversial and despite substantial improvements in day-to-day functioning, improved long-term outcome has not been clearly documented. This result may be a reflection of the importance of other factors, such as educational intervention, family support, and individual characteristics. Certainly pharmacologic management will accomplish little by itself.

Medication is recommended when educational and behavioral intervention are insufficient. The primary care physician must have a plan for evaluating efficacy and side effects. There is not a single correct way to manage medication for ADHD, but some general principles are important. The family history should be reviewed relative to tics, movement disorders, and neurodegenerative disease. The child's current review of systems should be noted as well as other medications frequently used. Baseline vital signs, including blood pressure, and growth parameters should be obtained. Several parent and teacher rating scales should be completed before medication is started. It is important to speak with the child directly, in age-appropriate terms, about the nature of his/her difficulty and the purpose of medication. In particular, fears of being "bad," "stupid," or "sick" must be addressed. The child should be encouraged to discuss the effects of the medication with parents.

Generally, a dose of 0.3 mg/kg of methylphenidate or 0.15 to 0.25 mg/kg of dextroamphetamine is given before school, and response is monitored by several parent and teacher rating scales.

The dose may be increased weekly until no further benefit is seen or side effects emerge. It is important to assess more than just activity-related items because the optimal dose for improving attention may be smaller than that required for a substantial decrease in physical activity. The lowest dose that results in significant improvement should be used to reduce the risk of side effects. A second dose is often required at lunchtime because the behavioral effects usually last approximately 3 to 4 hours. Older children may benefit from an after-school dose to assist with homework or structured after-school activities. Although some children who receive a dose late in the day will experience insomnia, others who are restless at night may actually sleep better. Many children experience "rebound" as the medication wears off (worsening of baseline symptoms). This effect may be managed by using progressively smaller doses throughout the day, or, for some children, by switching to slow-release capsules. The slow-release, long-acting forms of methylphenidate and dextroamphetamine may allow some children to take medication only once a day, but variable absorption and lack of longer effect can be problems.

Pemoline is given as a single daily dose of 37.5 mg before school and may take up to 3 weeks to take effect. The dose may then be increased by 18.75 mg weekly as needed for optimal effect. Approximately 2.25 mg/kg is usually required. Hypersensitivity reactions involving the liver has occurred, making this a second-line choice and necessitating baseline and periodic liver function tests.

The *Physicians' Desk Reference* (Medical Economics Co., Oradell, NJ) contains an extensive list of reported side effects of stimulants. Those side effects that occur with sufficient regularity to warrant specific anticipatory guidance include insomnia, decreased appetite, dysphoria, irritability, stomachache, headache, weight loss, and small increases in heart rate or blood pressure. Long-term side effects, which are less common but of greater concern, include precipitation of tics and decreased growth. Stimulants may theoretically decrease the seizure threshold so careful attention should be paid to maintaining therapeutic anticonvulsant levels in children who require both types of medication.

A very small proportion of carefully diagnosed children will fail to respond to a stimulant if a range of doses is tried. More often, side effects such as the emergence or exacerbation of tics or anxiety in children with comorbid diagnoses result in the need for consideration of an alternative medication. Antidepressants including the tricyclics (especially imipramine, desipramine, and nortriptyline), the serotonin reuptake inhibitors (especially fluoxetine, sertraline, and clomipramine), and the aminoketone bupropion are possible alternatives, as are the antihypertensives clonidine and, possibly, its newer counterpart, guanfacine.

When properly prescribed and carefully monitored, stimulants appear to be quite safe. There is currently no evidence to suggest that adverse neurobehavioral outcomes are related to medication use in childhood. Appropriate monitoring cannot be overstressed, particularly because most children who benefit from stimulants will need to take them for several years. First, it is imperative that parents have the opportunity to see their child on and off medication during the therapeutic trial so that they may take an active role in assessing its effect. This may be accomplished by having the child take medication on one of the weekend days initially, or by having parents observe their child in a structured activity such as school, sports, or religious instruction with and without medication. Second, several parent and teacher rating scales are required at each dose to obtain the most accurate assessment of effect. Third, during dose adjustment, phone contact every 1 to 2 weeks to discuss side effects is important. Frequent checks of heart rate, blood pressure, and weight are done initially. Once a stable dose is reached, examinations can be done at 3- to 6-month intervals. Fourth, every child deserves an annual trial off medication during the school year so that efficacy can be reassessed.

Parents frequently will raise questions about controversial causes and therapies for ADHD. Immunologic mechanisms and the role of dietary substances are currently under investigation. Large well-controlled studies of additive-free or low-sugar diets have not supported these as causes for the dysfunction. It is certainly possible, however, that selected groups of children have different metabolic characteristics that would be obscured by unselected population studies. If parents elect to try controversial therapies, the primary care physician's responsibility is the same: to help them objectively monitor efficacy and to avoid possible negative consequences.

SUMMARY

ADHD is a common, clinically significant disorder with substantial indirect evidence for an organic basis. Psychosocial and environmental factors are likely to play a significant role in associated symptoms and perhaps outcome. Comorbid diagnoses are common. Treatment may include educational intervention, behavior modification, other types of counseling, and medication. The role of the primary care physician is to rule out other causes of similar symptoms with the aid of consultants as needed, to educate the family about the disorder and available community resources, to provide anticipatory guidance about the particular issues that impact on the child and family at different developmental stages, and to monitor the efficacy and side effects of treatment.

BIBLIOGRAPHY

American Psychiatric Association: *Diagnostic and statistical manual of mental disorders,* ed 4, Washington, DC, 1994, American Psychiatric Association.

Barkley RA: *Hyperactive children: A handbook for diagnosis and treatment,* New York, 1990, Guilford Press.

Weiss G, Hechtman LT: *Hyperactive children grown up: Empirical findings and theoretical considerations,* New York, 1986, Guilford Press.

Culbert TP, Banez GA, Reiff MI: Children who have attentional disorders: Interventions (part 2), *Pediatr Rev* 15(1):5–14, 1994.

Green WH: The treatment of attention-deficit hyperactivity disorder with nonstimulant medications, *Child Adolesc Psychiatr Clin North Am* 4(1):169–195, 1995.

Greenhill LL: Attention-deficit hyperactivity disorder: The stimulants, *Child Adolesc Psychiatr Clin North Am* 4(1):123–168, 1995.

Reiff MI, Banez GA, Culbert TP: Children who have attentional disorders: Diagnosis and evaluation (part 1), *Pediatr Rev* 14(12):455–464, 1993.

Child and Adolescent Psychiatric Clinics of North America, volume 1, number 2, October, 1992. This volume is a series of articles about different aspects of ADHD.

IV

PARENT AND PROFESSIONAL INFORMATIONAL RESOURCES

CHADD (Children and Adults with Attention Deficit Disorders)—The national organization working for education, legislation, and family support for individuals with ADHD.
499 Northwest 70th Avenue, Suite 109, Plantation, FL 33317
(305)587-3700

The ADD Warehouse—A catalogue of sources of information about ADHD for parents, children, and professionals.
300 Northwest 70th Avenue, Suite 102, Plantation, FL 33317
1(800)233-9273

CHAPTER 120

Office Developmental Screening

Susan E. Levy

Routine developmental screening of infants and children by primary care physicians is an effective tool for early identification of developmental disabilities that cause school-related and other problems. The range of developmental disabilities includes motor impairment (*eg*, cerebral palsy), cognitive impairment (*eg*, mental retardation), or communication disorders (*eg*, learning disabilities). During the first 18 months of life, it is easiest to measure motor progress; however, the most common symptom of developmental disability in childhood is delayed development of speech and language, affecting 5% to 10% of all children. Language is the best predictor of future intellectual development and should be the basis of cognitive assessment in the infant and young child.

Early identification of the child with developmental disability allows for referral to appropriate diagnostic and treatment programs. These resources often assist in improving the functional status of the child and family, while providing appropriate educational opportunities and specific intervention services to mitigate the disability.

Office developmental screening should be a three-part process that must include history, physical examination, and developmental screening tests. A thorough medical, family, and developmental history is necessary. A number of medical historical risk factors of the mother's pregnancy and at the time of delivery may alert the primary care physician of increased likelihood of developmental disability (Box 120-1). In addition, a family history of mental retardation, delayed speech, communication disorder, or other developmental disabilities should raise the clinician's index of suspicion for a genetic-based developmental disorder. Several clinical features (neurodevelopmental markers) of the child should alert the primary care physician to the increased risk of developmental disability (Box 120-2). Parental appraisals of the level of developmental functioning and report of current achievements are helpful and have been found to be an effective means of early identification. Parents may be aided in recall of developmental milestones by bringing their child's baby book to the visit. Review of attainment of developmental milestones helps to establish the rate of development and consistency across different developmental streams when compared with norms described by Illingworth and others (Box 120-3).

BOX 120-1
Medical Historical Risk Factors for Developmental Disabilities

Prenatal
  Maternal illness
  Maternal infection
  Maternal malnutrition
  Exposure to toxins
  Exposure to teratogens
  Abnormal fetal movement
  Low birth weight
Perinatal
  Asphyxia
  Abnormal presentation
  Trauma
  Placental dysfunction
Postnatal
  Infection
  Complications of prematurity
  Asphyxia or anoxia
  Seizures
  Presence of congenital defects or syndrome
  Hyperbilirubinemia
  Poor nutrition or feeding difficulties
  Abnormal sleep patterns
  Central nervous system trauma
  Dysmorphic features

BOX 120-2
Neurodevelopmental Markers for
Developmental Disabilities*

Parental concerns about delayed development
Suspected mental retardation
Lack of language development (in absence of
    deafness)
Patient acts as if deaf or blind
Behavioral disturbance
Excessive irritability or lethargy in infancy
Feeding dysfunction or poor sucking
Microcephaly
Dysmorphic physical features
Delay in disappearance of primitive reflexes
Hyperactive or hypoactive fetus
Abnormal fetal presentation
Excessive irritability or lethargy in infancy

---

*These risk factors may be obtained by parental inter-
view or by direct observation and are listed in descending order of importance.

BOX 120-3
Developmental Milestones*

Gross motor
  Chin up (1 mo)
  Head up (wrists) (4 mo)
  Roll (prone to supine) (4 mo)
  Roll (supine to prone) (5 mo)
  Sit alone (8 mo)
  Pull to stand (9 mo)
  Cruise (10 mo)
  Walk alone (13 mo)
  Stairs (mark time; 20 mo)
  Stairs (alternate feet; 30 mo)
  Tricycle (36 mo)
  Two-wheeler (36 mo)

Fine motor/adaptive
  Unfisting (3 mo)
  Reach and grasp (5 mo)
  Transfer (6 mo)
  Handedness (24 mo)
Feeding
  Fingers (10 mo)
  Spoon (15 mo)
  Fork (21 mo)
  Independent feed (36 mo)
Dressing/self-help
  Cooperate (12 mo)
  Pull off socks (15 mo)
  Unbutton (30 mo)
  Button (48 mo)
  Shoe tying (60 mo)

Receptive language
  Social smile (6–8 wk)
  Recognize mother (3 mo)
  Laugh (4 mo)
  Gesture games (9 mo)
  Understand "no" (9 mo)
  One-step command (12 mo)
  Two-step command (24 mo)

Expressive Language
  Coo (3 mo)
  Babble (6 mo)
  Da-da (inappropriate) (8 mo)
  Da/ma (appropriate) (10 mo)
  First word (11 mo)
  Second word (12 mo)
  Two to 6 words (15 mo)
  Two-word phrases (21 mo)
  Two-word sentences (24 mo)
  Three-word sentences (36 mo)
  Echolalia (9–30 mo)
  Four colors (48 mo)

---

*Adapted from Illingworth RS: *The development of the infant and young child: Nor-*
mal and abnormal, New York, 1987, Churchill Livingstone.

Slowed rates of development in cognitive and communication streams may be indicative of mental retardation, whereas a slowed rate in the motor sphere alone may be indicative of cerebral palsy. The rate of developmental progress may be assessed over time, at 3- to 6-month intervals, to determine if the delay is consistent. Significant delays in developmental progress should result in referral for more complete diagnostic assessment.

During the physical examination, particular attention should be directed to identifying abnormalities in growth (especially head circumference), dysmorphic facial or musculoskeletal features, dermal lesions (which may be characteristic of specific neurocutaneous syndromes), and neurologic abnormalities (ie, hypotonia, hypertonia, asymmetric movements, or persistence of primitive reflexes).

A number of standardized developmental screening tests are available for use by the primary care practitioner. They differ in the scope of abilities examined: some assess language development (Peabody Picture Vocabulary Test—Revised [PPVT-R]), others test fine motor and conceptual development (Goodenough Draw-a-Person Test) or examine a broader range of functions (Denver Developmental Screening Test). The amount of time for administration (range 2 to 3 minutes to 45 minutes) and training required for administration also differ. The ideal screening test is quick, simple, inexpensive, reliable, and accurate. No single developmental screening tool meets these requirements. The primary care practitioner should be adept at administering several of the screening tests (eg, a general and language-based tool) in a standardized fashion to facilitate accuracy and promote identification of children at high risk for developmental disability.

DEVELOPMENTAL SCREENING TESTS

Denver II and Revised Prescreening Developmental Questionnaire

The Denver II, a revision and restandardization of the Denver Developmental Screening Test, is administered to children between birth and 6 years of age (Fig. 120-1 A and B). It uses 125 tasks or items to screen a child's performance in four areas of function against that of a standardization sample. The test may be used to screen asymptomatic children for possible problems, to confirm clinical suspicion, or to monitor children at risk (Table 120-1).

The tasks are arranged in four major sectors of function: personal-social, fine motor-adaptive, language, and gross motor. A vertical line is placed at the child's chronologic age, and the tester should administer at least three items to the left and close to the age line as well as all items intersected by the line. As the child passes or fails an item, a "P" or "F" is placed on each task. A "Delay" occurs when a child fails an item that falls to the left of the age line. A "Caution" occurs when a child fails an item for which the age line falls on or between the 75th and 90th percentile (Fig. 120-1 C). The number of delays and/or cautions determines the interpretation of the test result, categorized as normal, suspect, or untestable (Table 120-2).

The Denver II is designed as a single screen or the second stage of a two-stage process. The initial stage is the Revised Prescreening Developmental Questionnaire (PDQ), a parent-answered questionnaire about the child's current developmental status, which takes 10 to 15 minutes to answer. Those children with suspect scores on the Revised-PDQ would then undergo the longer Denver II. Administration of the full Denver II takes 10 to 20 minutes. Children with suspect or untestable results should be rescreened after 1 to 2 weeks. If results are consistent, referral should be made for further diagnosis and possible intervention services.

Many studies have examined the validity of this screening tool. Weaknesses include assessment of language abilities (especially after 3 years of age) and screening in high-risk populations. The new standardization population has a wider representation of minorities and expanded language and personal-social items.

Child Development Inventory

The Child Development Inventory (CDI) (formerly the Minnesota Child Development Inventory) is a parent-completed questionnaire for assessment (and comparison with established norms) of children 15 months to 6 years of age. The CDI booklet includes 270 statements that are grouped according to eight domains and a general development scale: social, self-help, gross

Text continued on p. 882.

TABLE 120-1
Developmental Screening Tests

	AGE	FUNCTION TESTED	RESULTS	COMMENTS	TIME (MIN)	ADMINISTRATION	SOURCE
GENERAL							
Denver II	0–6 years	Sectors of function: personal/social, fine motor-adaptive, language, gross motor	Normal; if suspect or untestable rescreen in 1–2 weeks, refer if persists	Improved standardization	15–20	Parental interview; observation; direct testing	DDM, Inc. P.O. Box 6919 Denver, CO 80206-0919
Revised Prescreening Questionnaire (R-PDQ)	0–6 years	Full range of development; as a 1st stage screening with Denver II as 2nd stage	Suspect or normal	Designed to screen out those children likely to be suspect on Denver II	10–15	Parent-answered if reading comprehension is a problem, questionnaire can be read to parents	DDM, Inc.
Child Development Inventory	15 mo–6 years	Samples 8 domains of devlepment and a General Development Scale	Cutoffs in each domain and General Development tied to 1.3, 1.5, and 2.0 SD below the mean	May be mailed to parents in advance	10–20	Parent-answered questionnaire	Behavior Science Systems, Inc. Box 580274 Minneapolis, MN 55458
Goodenough Draw-A-Person Test							
Pediatric Examination of Educational Readiness (PEER)							
Language							
Peabody Picture Vocabulary Test-Revised (PPVT-R), Forms L & M	26 mo–18 years	Single word	Vocabulary age and standard score	Difficulty generalizing conclusion of overall language and cognitive abilities; cultural bias	10–15	Test administration	American Guidance Service, Publishers Bldg., Circle Pines, MN 55014
Bzoch-League Receptive-Expressive Emergent Language Scale (REEL)	Birth–3 years	Receptive and expressive language	Receptive, expressive and combined language age and language quotients	Primarily parent interview; standardized sample small; revised 1991	10–15	Parental interview; observation	Hawthorne Educational Services, Inc. 800 Gray Oak Dr., Columbia, OH 65201
Clinical Linguistic Auditory Milestone Scale (CLAMS)	0–3 years	Receptive and expressive language and adaptive/fine motor skills	Age of function, Developmental Quotients calculated. If DQ <60 refer; ≤80 twice, refer	Kit not commercially available	5–10	Test administration observation	DMCN 1986; 28:762–771
Early Language Milestone Scale-2 (ELM-2)	0–3 years	Sectors: auditory expressive, auditory receptive, visual	Pass/fail or age equivalent, percentile, or standard score equivalent		1–10	Interview, observation, test administration	PRO-ED 8700 Shoal Creek Boulevard, Austin, TX 78757

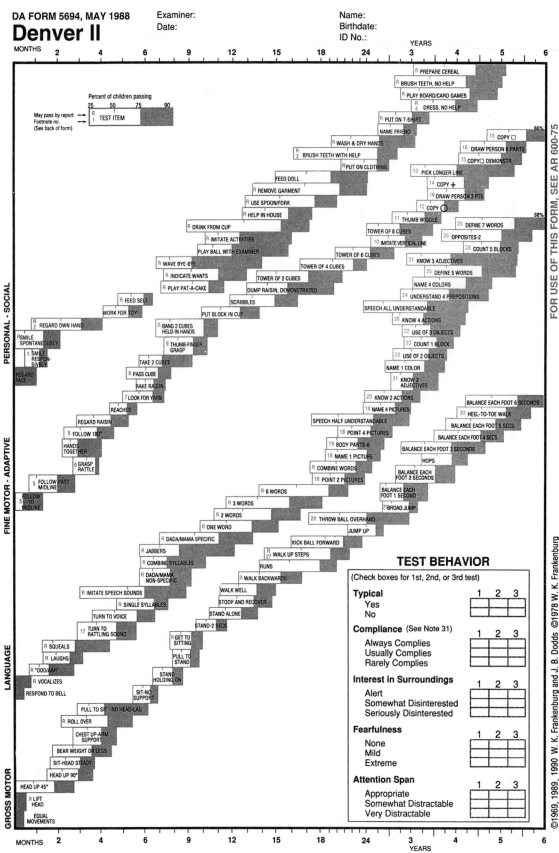

FIG 120-1 For legend see opposite page.

DIRECTIONS FOR ADMINISTRATION

1. Try to get child to smile by smiling, talking or waving. Do not touch him/her.
2. Child must stare at hand several seconds.
3. Parent may help guide toothbrush and put toothpaste on brush.
4. Child does not have to be able to tie shoes or button/zip in the back.
5. Move yarn slowly in an arc from one side to the other, about 8" above child's face.
6. Pass if child grasps rattle when it is touched to the backs or tips of fingers.
7. Pass if child tries to see where yarn went. Yarn should be dropped quickly from sight from tester's hand without arm movement.
8. Child must transfer cube from hand to hand without help of body, mouth, or table.
9. Pass if child picks up raisin with any part of thumb and finger.
10. Line can vary only 30 degrees or less from tester's line. |⁄
11. Make a fist with thumb pointing upward and wiggle only the thumb. Pass if child imitates and does not move any fingers other than the thumb.

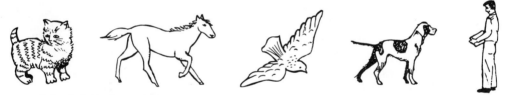

12. Pass any enclosed form. Fail continuous round motions.
13. Which line is longer? (Not bigger.) Turn paper upside down and repeat. (pass 3 of 3 or 5 of 6)
14. Pass any lines crossing near midpoint.
15. Have child copy first. If failed, demonstrate.

When giving items 12, 14, and 15, do not name the forms. Do not demonstrate 12 and 14.

16. When scoring, each pair (2 arms, 2 legs, etc.) counts as one part.
17. Place one cube in cup and shake gently near child's ear, but out of sight. Repeat for other ear.
18. Point to picture and have child name it. (No credit is given for sounds only.)
    If less than 4 pictures are named correctly, have child point to picture as each is named by tester.

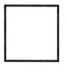

19. Using doll, tell child: Show me the nose, eyes, ears, mouth, hands, feet, tummy, hair. Pass 6 of 8.
20. Using pictures, ask child: Which one flies? . . . says meow? . . . talks? . . . barks? . . . gallops? Pass 2 of 5, 4 of 5.
21. Ask child: What do you do when you are cold? . . . tired? . . . hungry? Pass 2 of 3, 3 of 3.
22. Ask child: What do you do with a cup? What is a chair used for? What is a pencil used for?
    Action words must be included in answers.
23. Pass if child correctly places and says how many blocks are on paper. (1, 5).
24. Tell child: Put block **on** table; **under** table; **in front of** me, **behind** me. Pass 4 of 4.
    (Do not help child by pointing, moving head or eyes.)
25. Ask child: What is a ball? . . . lake? . . . desk? . . . house? . . . banana? . . . curtain? . . . fence? . . . ceiling? Pass if defined in terms of use, shape, what it is made of, or general category (such as banana is fruit, not just yellow). Pass 5 of 8, 7 of 8.
26. Ask child: If a horse is big, a mouse is _____ ? If fire is hot, ice is _____ ? If the sun shines during the day, the moon shines during the _____ ? Pass 2 of 3.
27. Child may use wall or rail only, not person. May not crawl.
28. Child must throw ball overhand 3 feet to within arm's reach of tester.
29. Child must perform standing broad jump over width of test sheet (8 1/2 inches).
30. Tell child to walk forward,   heel within 1 inch of tow. Tester may demonstrate.
    Child must walk 4 consecutive steps.
31. In the second year, half of normal children are non-compliant.

OBSERVATIONS:

FIG 120-1

Denver II (age is given in months). Test 1, Normal; there are no "delays." Because there is only one "caution" (throw ball overhand), the test is normal. Test 2, Normal; there are no "delays" and no "cautions." Failures are to the right of the age line or intersect between the 25th and 75th percentile. This test is normal. Test 3, Suspect; there is one "delay" (hops) and three "cautions" (pick longer line, know three adjectives, balance each foot 3 seconds), which make the test suspect. Test 4, Suspect; there are two "delays" (work for toy, reaches), yielding a suspect test result.

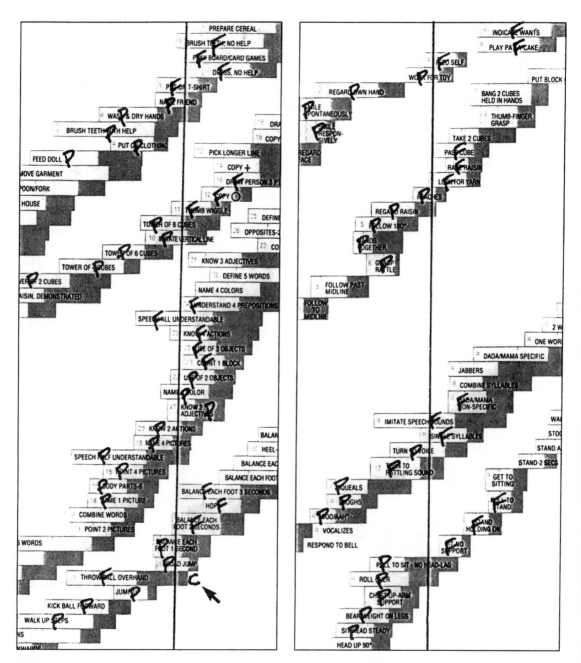

FIG 120-1, cont'd. For legend see p. 879.

motor, fine motor, expressive language, language comprehension, letters, and numbers. Scoring is completed by counting the number of "yes" responses for each of the scales using a single scoring template, plotting the results on the CDI profile, and connecting the points. Children with scores falling below the 30% cut-off (or equivalent to or more than 2 standard deviations below the mean) are in the "Delayed Development Range," and would benefit from referral for further diagnostic services. Studies have shown good sensitivity and specificity for screening.

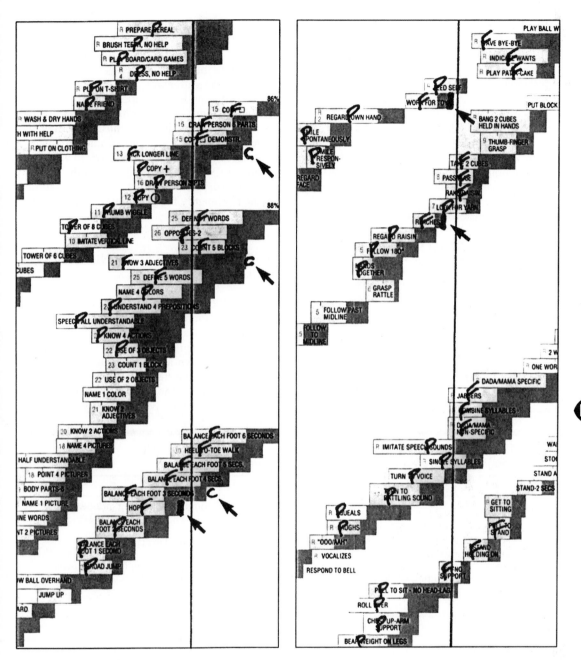

FIG 120-1, cont'd.   For legend see p. 879.

Draw-A-Person Test

The draw-a-person (DAP; Goodenough-Harris drawing test) is a widely used screening test for fine motor and conceptual development. The child aged 3 years and older is asked to draw a person, which can be scored, based on the child's accuracy of observations and conceptual development, approximating a mental age. Points are assigned for each feature of the drawing (Table 120-3). This test does not provide information about the child's language or gross motor development.

The Pediatric Examination of Educational Readiness

The Pediatric Examination of Educational Readiness (PEER) is a standardized observation system designed to predict school performance in the earliest grades and to uncover the need for special services or further evaluations. It includes a physical examination, sensory assessment, and a comprehensive medical and developmental historical review. The multilevel observation of function provides information about the child's developmental attainment, processing efficiency, and neurologic maturation. Simultaneously there is an assessment of the child's behavioral adaptation to the examination, with observations of adaptability, general responsiveness, cooperativeness, and reinforceability. The report provides a profile of strengths and weaknesses, with observations of behavior and attention, resulting in a composite picture of "educational readiness." The neurodevelopmental section of the PEER requires 20 to 30 minutes to complete, with 10 to 15 minutes for the physical and sensory examinations. This examination may be too lengthy for a routine health supervision visit.

LANGUAGE-BASED SCREENING TOOLS

Peabody Picture Vocabulary Test—Revised

The Peabody Picture Vocabulary Test—Revised (PPVT-R) assesses single-word receptive language skills in children 2 to 18 years of age. The child is shown a series of plates with four pictures and given a stimulus word that must be matched with one of the pictures. Scoring results in a single-word receptive vocabulary age and a

TABLE 120-2
Denver II Categories of Scoring

Normal	No delays and a maximum of one "Caution;" conduct routine rescreening at next well-child visit.
Suspect	Two or more "Cautions" and/or one or more "Delays"; rescreen in 1 to 2 weeks to rule out temporary factors such as fatigue, fear, illness.
Untestable	Refusal scores on one or more items completely to the left of the age line or on more than one item intersected by the age line in the 75% to 90% area; rescreen in 1 to 2 weeks.

TABLE 120-3
Goodenough-Harris Draw-a-Person Test Scoring System

ONE POINT ASSIGNED PER FEATURE:	
Head present	Opposition of thumb shown (must include fingers)
Neck present	Hands present
Neck, two dimensions	Arms present
Eyes present	Arms at side or engaged in activity
Eye detail: brows or lashes	Feet: any indication
Nose present	Attachment of arms to legs I (to trunk anywhere)
Nose, two dimensions (not round ball)	Attachment of arms and legs II (at correct point on trunk)
Mouth present	Trunk present
Lips, two dimensions	Trunk in proportion, two dimensions (length greater than breadth)
Both nose and lips in two dimensions	Clothing I (anything)
Both chin and forehead shown	Clothing II (two articles of clothing)
Bridged nose (straight to eyes; narrower than base)	
Hair I (any scribble)	
Hair II (more detail)	
Ears present	
Fingers present	
Correct number of fingers shown	

MENTAL AGE (YR)	POINTS SCORED BY BOYS	POINTS SCORED BY GIRLS
3	4	5
4	7	7
5	11	11
6	13	14
7	16	17
8	18	20

standard score. Some drawbacks of this test are its unrepresentative standardization sample, cultural bias with some pictures, and difficulty with generalizing conclusions as to overall language and cognitive abilities based on single-word receptive vocabulary.

Bzoch-League Receptive-Expressive Emergent Language Scale for Measurement of Language Skills in Infancy

This Receptive-Expressive Emergent Language Scale (REEL) screens the level of receptive and expressive language skills in children aged 1 month to 3 years. It is administered by parental interview, with attempts to confirm questionable items by direct observation of the child. Items of receptive and expressive language skills are grouped in various intervals over 36 months. For example, for the age interval 1 to 2 months, receptive language items include "Frequently gives direct attention to other voices; appears to listen to speaker; often looks at speaker and responds by smiling"; expressive language items include "Has a special cry for hunger; sometimes repeats the same syllable while cooing or babbling; develops vocal signs of pleasure." The items in each interval are scored as plus, minus, or plus-minus. The infant obtains credit for an age interval when he/she scores a plus in at least two of the three items. Results are scored as a receptive, expressive, and combined language age and language quotients may be computed for the highest age interval obtained. Drawbacks of this test include that it is primarily parent interview and the standardization sample is unrepresentative and small.

Clinical Linguistic and Audiotory Milestone Scale

The Clinical Linguistic and Auditory Milestone Scale (CLAMS) is a new tool that assesses language skills in children from birth to 24 months of age, using a series of questions to determine the age of attainment of linguistic and auditory milestones. Both receptive (language comprehension) and expressive (language production) milestones are included. Ages of attainment are recorded to the nearest month and compared with norms described. Ages of attainment of receptive and expressive milestones may then be plotted on a graph demonstrating the normal data (Figs. 120-2, 120-3). Infants whose attainment of milestones is consistently later than the 10th

percentile are at risk of language and cognitive delay.

Early Language Milestone Scale-2

Early Language Milestone (ELM) Scale-2 (Fig. 120-4) assesses language development in children from birth to 3 years of age. It is administered with the ELM Scale-2 scoring form, drinking cup, spoon, crayon, 3-in rubber ball, and 1-in wooden cube, in 1 to 10 minutes. The 43 items of the revised scale are divided into three sections: auditory expressive, auditory receptive, and visual. The ELM Scale-2 may be administered as a screening tool and scored by pass/fail for each section and for the entire scale. This method helps identify the slowest 10% of children with respect to language acquisition. If a subject fails the scale, the examiner has the option to use the point-scoring method, which will result in age equivalents percentile rankings, or standard scores each section plus a global language score.

A vertical line is placed at the child's chronological age. For pass/fail administration all items at or below the chronologic age level are administered. If any item totally to the left of the age bar is failed, the child fails that section and the entire scale. Using the point scoring administration, first a basal level is obtained by passing three consecutive items to the left of the age bar. The ceiling level is obtained by failing three consecutive items to the right of the age bar. Raw scores are calculated by adding 1 point for each item (or part of the item) passed, giving credit for items prior to basal level. Raw scores are then converted using table to age equivalents, percentile values, or standard score equivalents.

REFERRAL

Children suspected of having developmental delay and/or a specific developmental disability should be referred to a team of developmental specialists for further medical and developmental diagnostic assessment. This team may include developmental pediatricians, child neurologists, pediatric geneticists, child psychologists, special education teachers, occupational therapists, physical therapists, and/or speech/language pathologists. Further evaluation should include formal psychological testing with such infant tests as the Bayley Scales of Infant Development, the Gesell Developmental Schedules, or the Catell Infant Intelligence Scale.

IV

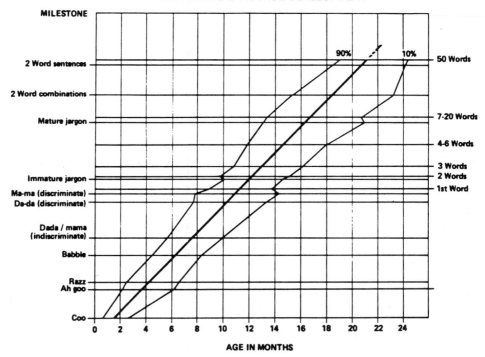

FIG 120-2

Expressive language milestones: 90th and 10th percentiles for normal population. Infants whose attainment of milestones is consistently later than the 10th percentile are at risk for language and cognitive delay. Slope of line through median of each milestone is 1.0 and corresponds to developmental quotient of 100. Milestone attainment can be plotted to depict rate of development as well as plateau or degeneration patterns. (From Capute AJ, Palmer FB, Shapiro BK, et al: *Dev Med Chil Neurol,* 28:762-771, 1986. With permission.)

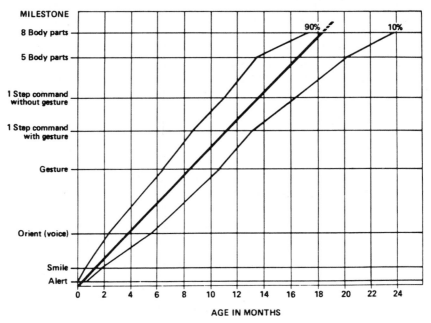

FIG 120-3

Receptive language milestones; 90th and 10th percentiles for normal population (*see* legend for Fig. 120-2). (From Capute AJ, Palmer FB, Shapiro BK, et al: *Dev Med Child Neurol,* 28:762-771, 1986. With permission.)

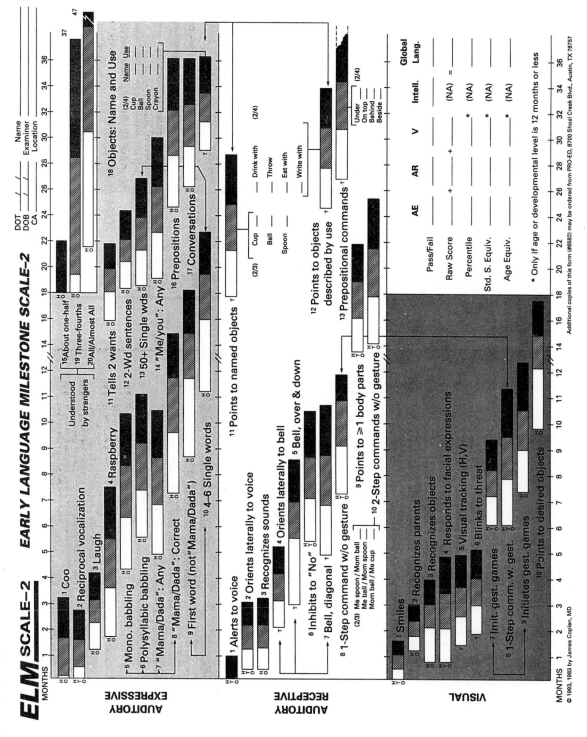

FIG 120-4
Early language milestones-2 (ELM-2) scale sheet.

Continued.

I. General Instructions

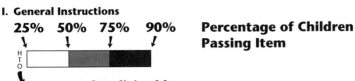

- **Always start with H, where allowed.**
- **Child passes item if passed by any of the allowable means of elicitation for that item.**
- **Basal = 3 consecutive items passed (work down from age line).**
- **Ceiling = 3 consecutive items failed (work up from age line).**

II. Auditory Expressive (AE)
A. Content

AE 1. H: Makes prolonged musical vowel sounds in a sing-song fashion (ooo, aaa, etc.), <u>not</u> just grunts or squeaks.

AE 2. H: Does baby watch speaker's face and appear to listen intently, then vocalize when the speaker is quiet? Can you "have a conversation" with your baby?

AE 4. H: Blows bubbles or gives "Bronx cheer"?

AE 5. H: Makes isolated sounds such as "ba," "da," "ga," "goo," etc.

AE 6. H: Makes repetitive string of sounds: "babababa," or "lalalalala," etc.

AE 7. H: Says "mama" or "dada" but uses them at other times besides just labelling parents.

AE 8. H: Child <u>spontaneously</u>, <u>consistently</u>, and <u>correctly</u> uses "mama" or "dada," <u>just</u> to label the <u>appropriate</u> parent.

AE 9, AE 10, AE 13. H: Child <u>spontaneously</u>, <u>consistently</u>, and <u>correctly</u> uses words. Do not count "mama," "dada," or the names of other family members or pets.

AE 11. H: Uses single words to tell you what he/she wants. "Milk!" "Cookie!" "More!" etc. Pass = 2 or more wants. List specific words.

AE 12. H: Spontaneous, novel 2-word combinations ("Want cookie" "No bed" "See daddy" etc.) <u>Not</u> rotely learned phrases that have been specifically taught to the child or combinations that are really single thoughts (e.g., "hot dog").

AE 14. H: Child uses "me" or "you" but may reverse them ("you want cookie" instead of "me want cookie," etc.)

AE 17. H: "Can child put 2 or 3 sentences together to hold brief conversations?"

AE 18. T: Put out cup, ball, crayon, & spoon. Pick up cup & say "What is this? What do we do with it? (What is it for?)" Child must <u>name</u> the object and give its use. Pass = "drink with," etc., <u>not</u> "milk" or "juice." Ball: Pass = "throw," "play with," etc. Spoon: Pass = "Eat" or "Eat with," etc., <u>not</u> "Food," "Lunch." Crayon: Pass = "Write (with)," "Color (with)," etc. Pass item if child gives <u>name and use</u> for 2 objects.

B. Intelligibility

AE 15, AE 19, AE 20. "How clear is your child's speech? That is, how much of your child's speech can a stranger understand?"

—Less than one-half
—About one-half (AE 15)
—Three-fourths (AE 19)
—All or Almost All (AE 20)

Pick one (H, O)

To score:
If less than one-half: Fail all 3 items in cluster.
If about one-half: Pass AE 15 only.
If three-fourths: Pass AE 19 and AE 15.
If all or almost all: Pass all 3 items in cluster.

III. Auditory Receptive (AR)

AR 1. H, T: Any behavioral change in response to noise (eye blink, startle, change in movements or respiration, etc.).

AR 2. H, T: What does baby do when parent starts talking while out of baby's line of sight? Pass if any shift of head or eyes to voice.

FIG 120-4, cont'd. For legend see p. 885.

AR 3. H: Does baby seem to respond in a specific way to certain sounds (becomes excited at hearing parents' voices, etc.)?

AR 4. T: Sit facing baby, with baby in parent's lap. Extend both arms so that your hands are behind baby's field of vision and at the level of baby's waist. Ring a 2"-diameter bell, first with 1 hand, then the other. Repeat 2 or 3 times if necessary. Pass if baby turns head to the side at least once.

AR 5. T: See note for AR 4. Pass if baby turns head first to the side, then down, to localize bell, at least once. (Automatically passes AR 4.)

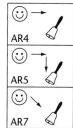

AR 6. H: Does baby understand the command "no" (even though he may not always obey)? T: Test by commanding "(Baby's name), no!" while baby is playing with any test object. Pass if baby temporarily inhibits his actions.

AR 7. T: See note for AR 4. Pass if baby turns directly down on diagonal to localize bell, at least once. (Automatically passes AR 5 and AR 4.)

AR 8. H: Will your baby follow any verbal commands without you indicating by gestures what it is you want him to do ("Stop" "Come here" "Give me" etc.)? T: Wait until baby is playing with any test object, then say "(Baby's name), give it to me." Pass if baby extends object to you, even if baby seems to change his mind and take the object back. May repeat command 1 or 2 times. If failed, repeat the command but this time hold out your hand for the object. If baby responds, then pass item V 8 (1-step command with gesture).

AR 9. H: Does your child point to at least 1 body part on command? T: Have mother command baby "Show me your . . . " or "Where's your . . . " without pointing to the desired part herself.

AR 10. H: "Can child do 2 things in a row if asked? For example 'First go get your shoes, then sit down'?" T: Set out ball, cup, and spoon, and say "(Child's name), give me the spoon, then give the ball to mommy." Use slow, steady voice but do not break command into 2 separate sentences. If no response, then give each half of command separately to see if child understands separate components. If child succeeds on at least half of command, then give each of the following: "(Child's name), give me the ball and give mommy the spoon." May repeat once but do not break into 2 commands. Then "Give mommy the ball, then give the cup to me." Pass if at least two 2-step commands executed correctly. (Note: Child is credited even if the order of execution of a command is reversed.)

AR 11. T: Place a cup, ball, and spoon on the table. Command child "Show me/where is/give me . . . the cup/ball/spoon." (If command is "Give me," be sure to replace each object before asking about the next object.) Pass = 2 items correctly identified.

AR 12. T: Put cup, ball, spoon, and crayon on table and give command "Show me/where is/give me . . . the one we drink with/eat with/draw (color, write) with/throw (play with)." If the command "Give me" is used, be sure to replace each object before asking about the next object. Pass = 2 or more objects correctly identified.

AR 13. T: Put out cup (upside down) and a 1" cube. Command the child "Put the block under the cup." Repeat 1 or 2 times if necessary. If no attempt, or if incorrect response, then demonstrate correct response, saying, "See, now the block is under the cup." Remove the block and hand it to the child. Then give command "Put the block on top of the cup." If child makes no response, then repeat command 1 time but do not demonstrate. Then command "Put the block behind the cup," then "Put the block beside the cup." Pass = 2 or more commands correctly executed (prior to demonstration by examiner, if "under" is scored).

IV. Visual

V 1. H: "Does your baby smile—not just a gas bubble or a burp but a real smile?" T: Have parent attempt to elicit smile by any means.

V 2. H: "Does your baby seem to recognize you, reacting differently to you than to the sight of other people? For example, does your baby smile more quickly for you than for other people?"

V 3. H: "Does your baby seem to recognize any common objects by sight? For example, if bottle or spoon fed, what happens when bottle or spoon is brought into view before it touches baby's lips?" Pass if baby gets visibly excited, or opens mouth in anticipation of feeding.

V 4. H: "Does your baby respond to your facial expressions?" T: Engage baby's gaze and attempt to elicit a smile by smiling and talking to baby. Then scowl at baby. Pass if any change in baby's facial expression.

V 5. T: Horizontal (H): Engage child's gaze with yours at a distance of 18". Move slowly back and forth. Pass if child turns head 60° to left and right from midline. Vertical (V): Move slowly up and down. Pass if child elevates eyes 30° from horizontal. Must pass both H & V to pass item.

V 6. T: Flick your fingers rapidly towards child's face, ending with fingertips 1–2" from face. Do not touch face or eyelashes. Pass if child blinks.

V 7. H: Does child play pat-a-cake, peek-a-boo, etc., in response to parents?

V 8. T: See note for AR 8 (always try AR 8 first; if AR 8 is passed, then automatically give credit for V 8).

V 9. H: Does child spontaneously initiate gesture games?

V 10. H: "Does your child ever point with index finger to something he/she wants? For example, if child is sitting at the dinner table and wants something that is out of reach, how does child let you know what he/she wants?" Pass only index finger pointing not reaching with whole hand.

FIG 120-4, cont'd. For legend see p. 885.

In older children, other tests such as the Stanford-Binet Intelligence Scale, Wechsler Preschool and Primary Scale of Intelligence (WPPSI), Wechsler Intelligence Scale for Children—Revised (WISC-R), and others may be used to determine the level of cognitive or intellectual function.

SUMMARY

Developmental screening in an office setting can be effective when a comprehensive history, physical examination, and selected standardized developmental screening tests are used. A sense of the range of the child's developmental abilities can be determined when tools assessing general and language abilities are used in conjunction.

The primary care physician, therefore, has the first opportunity for early identification of a developmental disability and prevention of secondary complications. Although additional diagnostic and management recommendations may be provided by a consultant team of developmental specialists, the primary care physician maintains the active role as a case manager, and provides ongoing support for the child and family while monitoring medical status and developmental progress in the child.

BIBLIOGRAPHY

American Academy of Pediatrics, Committee on Children with Disabilities: Screening infants and young children for developmental disabilities, *Pediatrics* 93:863–865, 1994.

Casey PH, Swanson M: A pediatric perspective of developmental screening in 1993, *Clin Pediatr* 33:209–212, 1993.

Coplan J, Gleason JR: Quantifying language development using the Early Language Milestone Scale, *Pediatrics* 86:963–971, 1990.

Frankenburg WK: Preventing developmental delays: Is developmental screening sufficient?, *Pediatrics* 93:586–593, 1994.

Frankenburg WK, Dodds J, Archer P, et al: The Denver II: A major revision and restandardization of the Denver Developmental Screening Test, *Pediatrics* 90:477–479, 1992.

Glascoe FP, Dworkin PH: The role of parents in the detection of developmental and behavioral problems, *Pediatrics* 95:829–836, 1995.

Illingworth RS: *The development of the infant and young child: Normal and abnormal,* ed 9, New York, 1987, Churchill Livingstone.

Knobloch H, Pasmanick B: *Gesell and Amatruda's developmental diagnosis,* ed 3, Hagerstown, MD, 1974, Harper & Row.

Levine MD, Carey WB, Crocker AC, et al: *Developmental-behavioral pediatrics,* ed 2, Philadelphia, 1992, WB Saunders.

Levy SE, Hyman SL: Pediatric assessment of the child with developmental delay, *Pediatr Clin North Am* 40:465–477, 1993.

Wachtel RC, Shapiro BK, Palmer FB, et al: CAT/CLAMS: A tool for the pediatric evaluation of infants and young children with developmental delay: Clinical Adaptive Test/Clinical Linguistic and Auditory Milestone Scale, *Clin Pediatr* 33:410–415, 1994.

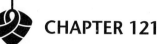

CHAPTER 121

Rights of Children with Developmental Disabilities

Symme W. Trachtenberg

Children with special needs have the right to attain their potential for participation in activities within the family and society at large. Therefore, no matter how severe the disability, children should be provided with the educational programs and services needed to help them reach their greatest potential. The laws, entitlements, and some of the services and resources relevant to helping families of children with special needs are discussed in this chapter.

CIVIL RIGHTS

The Americans with Disabilities Act (ADA) of 1990 (PL 101-336) ensures full civil rights for people of all ages with disabilities. It defines disability as a physical or mental impairment substantially limiting one or more life activity—communication, ambulation, self-care, transportation, employment, socialization, education, training, or housing. The passage of the ADA established the rights of individuals with disabilities to have equal access to employment, transportation, public accommodations, local government services, and telecommunications.

EDUCATIONAL RIGHTS

The Education for All Handicapped Children Act of 1975 (Public Law 94-142) guaranteed free public education for every child with a disability from ages 5 to 21 years. In 1986, amendments to this act (PL 99-457) were passed that mandated preschool programs for children with disabilities from ages 3 to 5 years. It left to the discretion of

each state whether to mandate services for children from birth to 3 years of age. If a state chooses to mandate these services legislatively, they have to include the development of a comprehensive, interdisciplinary, statewide system of early intervention programs for infants and toddlers. Some of these services may not be free to families.

Early intervention programs are available in most states for infants and toddlers who are developmentally delayed. Children diagnosed with a disorder that has a high probability of resulting in developmental delay (eg, fetal alcohol syndrome, sensory impairments, seizure disorder) may be eligible for services. Each child to be served requires an individualized family service plan, which documents the collaborative efforts that will be made to assist the family in enhancing their child's development. The family of each child and at least two professionals participate in the development of the individualized family service plan. Based on the needs of the child and family, other people such as family supports, advocates, and friends may be involved in the process. Services must be provided in natural environments such as home, daycare centers, or preschools.

The Individuals with Disabilities Education Act of 1990 (IDEA; PL 101-476) is a federal statute that reauthorized, retitled, and expanded the Education for All Handicapped Children Act and its amendments. IDEA states that individuals, 3 to 21 years of age, with disabilities are entitled to free and appropriate educational services to meet their unique needs, in the classroom, in the home, or in hospitals. IDEA delineates categories of disabilities under which children can qualify for special education and related services. As of

IV

1995, children who are eligible include those with mental retardation, hearing impairments, visual impairments, deaf-blindness, speech or language impairments, multiple disabilities, serious emotional disturbance, orthopedic impairments, autism, traumatic brain injury, and specific learning disabilities. Other health impairments that limit a child's strength, vitality, or alertness may qualify them for some support services. Such conditions may include chronic or acute health problems such as a heart condition, nephritis, asthma, arthritis, sickle cell anemia, hemophilia, seizure disorder, lead poisoning, leukemia, or diabetes. As the long-term impact of chronic illnesses develop, some children may require special education and related services.

IDEA mandates that every child should be educated in the least restrictive environment, to the maximum extent possible, with nondisabled peers. Through the provision of supplementary supports and aids, parents and school personnel are able to work toward meeting the needs of the child in the school and classroom the child would attend if the child did not have a disability. This is the definition of inclusion.

Local public school districts are responsible for providing unbiased, valid assessments and developing an individualized educational plan. Parents have the right to participate in the evaluation and be a part of the decision-making process in the development of the individualized education plan. The individualized education plan should be reviewed and updated annually or more frequently at the parents' or guardians' request. Assistive technology, behavioral management, vocational and graduation planning, and transition programs, plus adaptive physical education, special transportation, extended school year and health concerns also may be addressed in the individualized education plan.

IDEA requires that parents be trained in all aspects of their child's program. In addition, IDEA requires that school districts provide assistive equipment such as computers and augmentative communication devices for use in school and at home if these devices are needed to meet the educational goals of the child, regardless of the parents' ability to pay for this equipment. Parents have the right to review and receive copies of all educational records kept by the school. Parents have the right to request and receive a due process hearing when there is a disagreement regarding the appropriateness of the identification, evaluation, program, and/or placement of a student with a disability. Mediation is available in some states, and less formal negotiations frequently can avoid the need for a due process hearing.

IDEA is due for reauthorization in 1997. There may be changes in what the law requires as a result.

Another law that has been applied to the school setting is the Rehabilitation Act of 1973, section 504 (PL 93-112). This act is a federal statute that provides additional protection to children who are considered disabled. Under this law developmental disability refers to serious limitations caused by a mental or physical impairment or a combination of both; beginning before the age of 22 years and likely to continue indefinitely; which results in functional limitations in three or more areas of major life activity including self-care, receptive and expressive language, learning, mobility, self-direction, capacity for independent living, and economic self-sufficiency; and reflects the person's need for a combination of special, interdisciplinary, or general care, treatment, or other services over a lifetime or extended time and a need for services to be individually planned and coordinated.

Section 504 states that any program that receives or benefits from federal money is prohibited from discriminating against people who are disabled. It often is used to secure services for those children who do not meet the criteria for special education under IDEA.

Amendments to the Education for All Handicapped Children Act passed in 1983 (PL 98-199) provide educational agencies with incentives to provide transitional services from school to work and other facets of adult living. These services are mandated to begin at 16 years of age or earlier if appropriate.

SERVICES

Federal Funding
In addition to specialized educational settings, various other programs throughout the United States provide services to children with disabilities and their families. Federal funding for such programs is distributed to individual states, which in turn determine how to spend the allo-

cated monies for these services. Each state, city, and county, therefore, offers different programs that may change periodically due to funding allocations. Some states legislate funding to provide services for children and adults with developmental disabilities, whereas other states will only fund services to people with the diagnosis of mental retardation. The services provided in these programs are expected to be family centered and culturally sensitive. Parents are to be valued as the key members of their child's treatment team because of their in-depth knowledge of their child. The child's health care providers should be open to communicating with the child's educational program and the parents in an effort to strengthen family involvement and develop a truly interdisciplinary effort in the best interests of the child. Some parents will need to be encouraged to take a central role in providing advocacy and case management for their child. Other parents may need to be referred to an educational law center, parent training and information center, or protection and advocacy agency to assist them in getting their child's educational needs met.

Evaluations

The family or the physician may request additional diagnostic evaluations. The child then may be referred to hospital-based diagnostic services or clinics for the specific disability. In addition to diagnostic evaluations these programs often serve as a good resource for referral information or treatment. Primary care physicians often play a vital role in providing emotional support and overall guidance for the child and family throughout the diagnostic process.

Interventions

There are programs that provide parents with assistance in finding ways to cope with their child's special needs. They often have supportive counseling for parents and families who may be seen individually, as a family unit, or as part of a professionally run or self-help support group. This supportive experience can mean the difference between a family that is successful and one that is not. Over time, with support and opportunities, parents can learn about their child's disability, their strengths and gifts, and how to help him/her to reach full potential within the family. Some families need additional assistance

with integrating the child with special needs into the family and community.

Families also should be made aware of services that provide concrete help in the day-to-day management of their child. These services fall within two major categories: those that directly contribute to the child's psychosocial growth and the development of important independence skills (eg, special needs and integrated preschool and daycare; Head Start; specialized and integrated day and overnight camps, after-school, recreational, and socialization activities; vocational training, supported employment, transportation) and those that offer relief and assistance to the entire family (eg, respite care, which provides care for the child at home or elsewhere, which could include overnight; homemaker services if the parent is unable to do household activities temporarily). In some cases, the stress created by the intensity of the child's care needs may make it difficult for the parents to cope. Abusive or neglectful behaviors may result. At such times child protective services must be consulted for the child and family.

Children with developmental disabilities tend to remain with their parents longer due to their dependence. Often when children and parents are ready to consider a community living arrangement they are not always available. By beginning transitional services at age 16 or before, a child with a disability has the opportunity to gain the skills needed for community living. These services also teach the skills necessary for competitive or supported employment, leisure activities, and living as independently as possible in the community. The goal is a quality life that provides the opportunity to live, work, and play in the community and to have meaningful personal relationships. Physicians should encourage parents to consider who will care for the child when they are unable to do so. Parents need to be supported in their efforts to investigate the possibilities before they need them. Parents should consider specialized guardianship and estate planning, which is a difficult, but necessary, process.

FINANCIAL ASSISTANCE AND RESOURCES

Supplemental Security Income

Supplemental security income (SSI) is a federal government benefit available to families that have children with disabilities. Social security provides another definition of disability. Social security lists specific medical criteria that include mental or physical impairments that are so severe that they would prevent an adult from working and are going to last for at least 1 year, or impairments that, in the case of a child, would lead to that child's death. This list can be revised yearly by Congress. In 1990, the US Supreme Court ruled in the Zebly Decision to allow children who did not meet the federally regulated medical criteria to receive benefits through Individual Functional Assessments (IFA). Children denied SSI after January 1, 1980, on the basis of their diagnosis and found eligible by an IFA can reapply and may receive retroactive benefits. In addition to SSI cash benefits, these children are eligible for medical assistance as well. As this chapter goes to press, Congress has challenged the Zebly Decision and therefore the eligibility of the children who receive SSI as a result of an IFA.

Early Periodic Screening Diagnosis and Treatment

Early Periodic Screening Diagnosis and Treatment is a free preventive federal health program for children under 21 years of age. The family must be on medical assistance to qualify. This funding covers services that are medically necessary including specialists, equipment, and programs not covered on a state's medical assistance fee schedule, such as home modifications, eye glasses, hearing aids, and braces. This program also would allow for coverage beyond the established limits if a medical necessity for such expanded services exists.

The financial burden of a child with a disability can be enormous. Even with insurance, there may be several uncovered costs, such as medications, house alterations, a wheelchair-accessible van, and so forth. Insurance itself may require the expenditure of significant time and energy in maneuvering through bureaucratic red tape. Some children reach their lifetime cap during the first year of life. Furthermore, if the medical insurance is provided through the parent's place of employment, the ability to change jobs may be limited. The family's choice of housing and location also may be affected by physical barriers or the need to be close to the child's school, doctors, or hospital.

Resource Network

It is important for the primary care physician to develop a list of reliable contacts to establish a resource network in the community. Some organizations with national offices that are helpful to families of children with disabilities are listed at the end of this chapter and in the chapters on hearing and visual impairments. These organizations should be helpful in establishing contact within or nearby the local community. Many have state and local services listed in the local telephone directory. Many county services are listed under the name of the county. Those organizations listed provide free or low-cost educational or social service programs, whereas others are available for information and referral to specialized services within the community. Many national organizations have local support groups and counseling. The social service agencies listed in the telephone book under "Family Services, Children, and Youth" or by religious denomination also can provide counseling and referral information. Parent training and information centers funded under IDEA also are available throughout the country.

SUMMARY

Physicians often are called upon to recommend new services, consult on existing programs, and urge their community to comply with the ADA and become wheelchair accessible. The mandated services outlined barely meet the needs of children with disabilities. Many of these laws must be reauthorized by Congress to continue to fund necessary programs. Currently issues are before Congress and the President regarding the responsibility for programs affecting the lives of people with disabilities. Legislation will surely change what programs will be funded by the federal government. Each state will determine what programs will be funded or cut when they are given the authority over federal grants.

Professionals in health care and educational systems and parents need to be informed about *currently* funded programs and entitlements and the way to access services in their area. A tremendous amount of frequently updated information and parent-to-parent support is available on the Internet (searches can be done using a variety of key words and phrases such as "disability groups," "diagnosis," "government agencies," "children with special health care needs").

Please see the list at the end of this chapter for sources of current information.

BIBLIOGRAPHY

Britton AL: Social integration of adolescents with developmental disabilities, *Int J Adolesc Med Health* 5(2):149–153, 1991.

Davern L, Schnorr R: Public schools welcome students with disabilities as full members, *Child Today* 20(2):21–25, 1991.

Dowrick PW: Key USA statute on the rights of children and youth with disabilities: Selected summaries. Unpublished paper, 1995, Children's Seashore House & University of Pennsylvania.

Hayes A: What the future holds. In Batshaw ML, editor: *Your child has a disability,* Boston, 1991, Little Brown.

Hostler SL: *Family centered care: An approach to implementation,* Charlottesville, VA, 1994, University of Virginia.

Kern L, Delaney BA, Taylor BA: Laws and issues concerning education and related services.
In Kurtz L, Dowrick PW, Levy SE, Batshaw ML, editors: *Children's Seashore House handbook on developmental disabilities: An interdisciplinary sourcebook for professionals,* Gaithersburg, MD, 1996, Aspen Publishers.

Kline DF, Kline AC: *The disabled child and child abuse,* Chicago, 1991, The National Committee for Prevention of Child Abuse Catalog. (To obtain a copy call 800-835-2671.)

Orlin M: The Americans With Disabilities Act: Implications for social services, *Soc Work* 40(2):233–239, 1995.

Reed KL: History of federal legislation for persons with disabilities, *Am J Occup Ther* 46(5): 397–408, 1992.

Romano JL: *Legal rights of the catastrophically ill and injured: A family guide,* Norristown, PA, 1996, Rosenstein & Romano.

NATIONAL SUPPORT GROUPS FOR CHILDREN WITH DISABILITIES

Children and Adults with Attention Deficit Disorder (CH.A.D.D.)
499 Northwest 70th Avenue, Suite 308
Plantation, Florida 33317
305-587-3700

Council for Exceptional Children
1920 Association Drive
Reston, Virginia 22091
703-620-3660

Epilepsy Foundation of America
4351 Garden City Drive
Landover, Maryland 20785
301-459-3700

March of Dimes
1275 Mamaroneck Avenue
White Plains, New York 10605
914-428-7100

Muscular Dystrophy Association
3561 E. Sunrise Drive
Tucson, Arizona 85718
609-529-2000

National Association for Retarded Citizens
PO Box 6109, 2501 Avenue J
Arlington, Texas 76011
800-433-5255

National Easter Seal Society for Crippled Children and Adults
230 W. Monroe Street, Suite 1800
Chicago, Illinois 60606
312-726-6200, TDD: 312-726-4258

Orton Dyslexia Society
724 York Road
Baltimore, Maryland 21204
410-296-0232

Spina Bifida Association of America
4590 McArthur Boulevard NW, Suite 250
Washington, DC 20007-4226
800-621-3141 or 202-944-3285 (local)

United Cerebral Palsy Association
1660 L Street NW, Suite 700
Washington, DC 20036
800-872-5827

Variety Club International (Physical disabilities)
1560 Broadway, Suite 1209
New York, New York 10036
212-704-9872

SOURCES OF CURRENT INFORMATION ABOUT PROGRAMS FOR INDIVIDUALS WITH DISABILITIES

American Association of University Affiliated
  Programs on Developmental Disabilities
8630 Fenton Street, Suite 410
Silver Springs, Maryland 20910
301-588-8252 TDD: 301-588-3319
Can provide contacts for local information.

Educational Resource Information Center
ERIC Clearinghouse on Disabilities and Gifted
  Children
1920 Association Drive
Reston, Virginia 22091
800-328-0272
Can provide contacts for local information.

Federal Information Center Program (FIC)
General Services Administration
18th and F Street NW
Washington, DC 20405
202-501-1937

National Information Center for Children and
  Youth With Disabilities
PO Box 1492
Washington, DC 20013-1492
800-695-0285; 202-884-8200; 703-893-6061 in
  DC TDD: 703-893-8614

National Organization on Disability
910 16th Street, NW #20006
Washington, DC 20006
202-293-5960

Title I Programs for Students With Special Needs
Elementary and Secondary Education Act
United States Department of Education
Compensatory Education Program
600 Independence Avenue, SW
Washington, DC 20202-6132
202-260-0826

A special thank-you goes to Ruth Landsman, a
parent of a young man who has exceeded
everyone's expectations, the Director of Parents' Exchange, and a parent advocate, who
reviewed and added to this work and always
keeps me current.

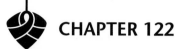

CHAPTER 122

Autism and Other Pervasive Developmental Disorders

Joyce Elizabeth Mauk

Autism is one of several disorders under the general heading of pervasive developmental disorders (PDD). This group of disorders is characterized by abnormalities in communication, socialization and activities, and interests. Children with PDD frequently present to the primary care physician with delayed language development and/or social unresponsiveness to parents. The physician has an important role in diagnosis and referral for treatment of these children.

CLASSIFICATION

Pervasive developmental disorder is a general term that describes the heterogeneous group of disorders in Table 122-1. These disorders have the following characteristics in common: abnormalities in communication, abnormalities in social relatedness, and stereotyped patterns of behavior and a restricted repertoire of activities and interests. Some differentiating features are outlined in Table 122-1. In the past, terms such as *childhood psychosis, autism, PDD,* and *atypical development* were used to describe children with this triad of abnormalities. The following classification system is based on the current diagnostic schema outlined in Diagnostic and Statistical Manual of Mental Disorders (DSM-IV).

AUTISTIC DISORDER

Autism is the most severe expression of the PDDs. Communication is markedly impaired in affected children who may be completely nonverbal.

When spoken language does develop, it commonly is idiosyncratic and echolalic. These patients typically do not use language in order to communicate, but as a method of self-stimulation. Receptive language is also impaired, and sometimes the children appear to be deaf. Nonverbal aspects of communication, such as eye contact and body posture, are also severely abnormal. Social relatedness is impaired, and the child may be oblivious to others. Children with autism exhibit a variety of unusual behaviors such as stereotypies, excessive desire for sameness, and lack of representational or pretend play. Self-injurious behavior, hyperactivity, and tantrums may complicate educational attempts. Children diagnosed with an autistic disorder frequently also have mental retardation, although this is not an invariant finding.

RETT SYNDROME

Rett syndrome is a degenerative neurologic disorder, so far described only in female patients, that may present with autistic features. Its other essential features include a normal perinatal period, acquired microcephaly, and loss of purposeful hand use. The hands become engaged in constant, stereotypic writhing or wringing midline movements. The disorder typically is associated with severe to profound mental retardation and development of spasticity and seizures. Its early presentation may be indistinguishable from autistic disorder, but its characteristic features become more apparent over time.

IV

TABLE 122-1
Types of Pervasive Developmental Disorders

	MENTAL RETARDATION	REGRESSION	MOTOR PROBLEMS
Autistic disorder	+	−	−
Rett disorder	+	+	+
Childhood disintegrative disorder	+	+	+/−
Asperger disorder	−	−	Clumsiness
Pervasive developmental disorder–not otherwise specified	Variable	Variable	−

CHILDHOOD DISINTEGRATIVE DISORDER

Childhood disintegrative disorder describes individuals with a loss of multiple areas of functioning after approximately 2 years of normal development. The typical areas of disintegration include language, social, or adaptive skills; excretory control; and play and motor skills. It is particularly important to rule out metabolic and neurodegenerative diseases in any child with a history of loss of developmental milestones. The diagnosis of childhood disintegrative disorder is only a description of behavior and a diagnosis of exclusion following workup for known degenerative diseases. It should be emphasized that some individuals with autism may manifest subtle signs of developmental regression such as losing the use of a few inconsistent words. These losses usually are poorly defined and do not include hard signs of neurologic regression such as loss of excretory or motor control as in childhood disintegrative disorder.

ASPERGER DISORDER

Asperger disorder describes individuals with no delays in global cognitive and language development, but with other autistic-like features. For example, spoken language may be unusually pedantic and formal, and the nonverbal aspects of communication such as eye contact and body position may be abnormal. Affected individuals exhibit unusual activities such as flicking light switches and intense interests in trivia such as maps and train schedules. Delayed motor milestones and clumsiness are also characteristic. Their social ineptitude prevents them from developing friendships and other relationships. It is believed that some individuals who are diagnosed

as schizoid personality disorder may fit the diagnostic criterion for Asperger disorder as well.

PERVASIVE DEVELOPMENTAL DISORDER–NOT OTHERWISE SPECIFIED

Pervasive developmental disorder–not otherwise specified (PDD-NOS) is a term reserved for those individuals with abnormal social and communication skills and stereotyped behaviors that are of relatively brief duration, develop later in life, or are of insufficient severity to warrant another PDD diagnosis. It is not uncommon for a child who ultimately is diagnosed with a language-based learning disability to appear "autistic-like" at 2 or 3 years of age, but later to exhibit few or no autistic features. PDD-NOS would be an appropriate diagnostic label for such a child.

PREVALENCE

Autism occurs in approximately four to five per 10,000 live births. Rett syndrome and childhood disintegrative disorder are more rare, both in the range of less than one per 10,000. The milder forms of PDD, including Asperger and PDD-NOS are somewhat more common and may occur in approximately ten per 10,000 live births. Except for Rett syndrome, which has been described only in girls, the male:female ratio for all PDDs is 4 to 5:1.

DIAGNOSIS

Children with PDD usually present for evaluation between 2 and 4 years of age. Those children with the most severe deficits in cognitive, social, or language function are the first to come to medical attention. The most frequent presenting problems are delays in talking and, in many cases, the impression of deafness. Parents rarely suspect the diagnosis of autism. A careful history and examination should help guide the diagnostic and referral process.

Children with severe to profound hearing impairment may appear to be autistic because of their inconsistent responses to verbal and social interaction. All children with developmental delays and a suspicion of an autistic-like disorder should have an assessment by an audiologist. Although family and social problems are not believed to cause autism, severely neglected or depressed children can appear autistic; therefore, evaluation of the social condition and caregivers is important.

Unrecognized seizure disorders also can complicate the diagnostic picture. Metabolic or degenerative disorders often are characterized by a history of a loss of skills, episodes of dehydration, coma, or growth difficulties. Symptoms suggestive of seizures or metabolic disorders should be sought historically and evaluated by laboratory study if the history is suggestive.

In the majority of cases the diagnosis of a PDD is based on the triad of deficits in communication, social deficits, and an impaired repertoire of activities and interests. Very few of these youngsters will have a metabolic or degenerative disorder. Individuals suspected of having a PDD should be evaluated by a psychologist, developmental pediatrician, and speech pathologist. Standardized tests of intelligence quotient (IQ) should be administered, as well as questionnaires and observational scales regarding autistic behaviors. In general, children with PDD show relatively higher nonverbal skills and depressed language and play skills. The experienced examiner will note abnormalities in interactions with the environment and with other people. These abnormalities may include abnormal sensitivity to sound and unusual environmental exploration such as sniffing or licking.

ETIOLOGY AND EVALUATION

Autistic disorder, Asperger disorder, and PDD-NOS can be thought of as one disorder with variations of severity. There are several known causes of mental retardation that also are associated with autistic-like disorders including phenylketonuria, tuberous sclerosis, and Cornelia de Lange syndrome. The fragile X syndrome may be associated with autism but probably is more closely related to mental retardation. The precise cause of autistic disorder, Asperger disorder, and PDD-NOS is unknown, but this group may share a common etiology. Some cases show an increased incidence of problems during pregnancy and early infancy (eg, asphyxia), which may or not be causal.

Multiple studies have identified an increased familial incidence of all autistic disorders. Psychiatric disorders and affective and cognitive disabilities also are more common in family members. Because PDD is not just one specific disorder, but a heterogeneous group, the inherited causes of PDD may be similarly varied. The recurrence risk for PDD in subsequent pregnancies after the birth of a proband is approximately 8.6%.

Rett syndrome is likely to be genetic and unrelated to the other PDDs. It appears to be an X-linked disease that is lethal in boys. The latter conclusion is suggested by the observation that no male patients have been identified with the disorder.

The laboratory evaluation of suspect cases is limited. If a thorough physical examination and history are not concerning for neurocutaneous stigmata, neurologic degeneration, or specific syndromes, most laboratory studies are not helpful. A thorough metabolic screening test will rule out a large number of biochemical disorders. Macro- or microcephaly should prompt central nervous system imaging studies. All children suspected of having autism should have a hearing evaluation, including brain stem–evoked potentials if behavioral audiometry is not successful. If the history is suggestive of seizures, an electroencephalogram (EEG) may be indicated. Rett syndrome has a characteristic EEG pattern, and up to 25% of children with an autistic disorder also may have epilepsy.

In contrast to most children in the autistic group, those who meet the criteria for childhood disintegrative disorder should have an extensive evaluation for degenerative disorders.

Researchers have identified some structural and biochemical characteristics of autistic children. Several studies have identified underdevelopment of two cerebellar vermal lobules. In addition, abnormalities in the neurotransmitters serotonin and the endogenous endorphins have been identified. These reports implicate a biologic basis for these disorders, but, to date, these features cannot be considered diagnostic.

ASSOCIATED PROBLEMS

Two thirds of individuals with PDD have mental retardation. In 60% of patients with PDD, the IQ is less than 50, and in 20%, it ranges between 50 and 70. Of those individuals with a normal IQ (greater than 70), the majority have unusual profiles on formal testing. They show evidence of a learning disability, uneven development, or scatter of abilities. Typically nonverbal or performance skills are higher than language skills. This result is true of profoundly affected patients as well as those who are more mildly involved such as those with Asperger syndrome.

Approximately 25% of individuals with PDD will develop seizures, commonly not until adolescence. These seizures generally are easily treated with antiepileptic drugs.

Severe behavioral disorders are strongly associated with autism, including severe disruptive behaviors such as aggression and hyperactivity as well as self-injurious behaviors. Affected individuals often have stereotypies such as rocking and other repetitive, purposeless movements. Withdrawal, excessive irritability, a desire for sameness, and emotional lability may present major social problems. The incidence of disabling psychiatric conditions, including psychosis and depression, is increased in individuals with autism. Unusual attachments to inanimate objects, such as a piece of string or a Tupperware lid, are frequent. Play skills are very poorly developed, and pretend play is usually completely lacking. The severe behavioral manifestations of the syndrome often are the most handicapping aspect of these complex disorders.

Unusual responses to sensory input are not uncommon, such as insensitivity to pain or heat or overreaction to environmental noises. Food selectivity, food refusal, or resistance to food textures may lead to compromised nutrition or constipation. Sleep disturbances also are associated with the PDDs.

TREATMENT

Autistic spectrum disorders can be some of the most frustrating and devastating problems for families and professionals to manage and understand. Fortunately, increased recognition of these disorders has led not only to improvements in treatment but to stimulated research and investigation. Unfortunately, the eagerness to find a treatment or cure often leads to rapid acceptance and promotion of therapeutic techniques before they have had adequate trials.

It appears that early enrollment in a specialized program with an intensive language focus improves the patient's outcome. In many centers parents also are trained as treatment providers. Several curricula have been developed, most notably TEACCH (Treatment and Education of Autistic and related Communication handicapped CHildren), which has been replicated in schools across the country. Much enthusiasm currently surrounds an intense individualized program based on the work of Dr. Ivar Lovaas. A few patients who were educated using his intense discreet trial learning methods have showed unusual successes. This pilot work now is being replicated at a number of centers. All curricula for young children with PDD need to include intensive teaching of social and language skills and to develop opportunities to generalize and practice these skills. The level of academic achievement attained by the large group of individuals diagnosed with PDD is very variable. Current educational law entitles individuals access to education in the least restrictive environment. Some interaction with typically developing peers is optimum.

Behavioral interventions designed to decrease maladaptive behaviors and increase adaptive behaviors are often a part of treatment.

Despite the intense interest in structural and biochemical brain abnormalities in autism, a specific medication or therapeutic technique has not been identified as curative. Pharmacologic management is secondary to educational and behavioral interventions. Medications should be used to target specific symptoms such as withdrawal, overactivity, or irritability, which may interfere with a child's global functioning. Haloperidol, Naltrexone, and others have been shown to alleviate some symptoms. Prescribing psychotropic medications in this population requires careful evaluation of treatment goals and side effects. Medication should be prescribed by a professional with extensive experience with this population.

OUTCOME

Prognosis is closely linked to verbal ability and intelligence. In general, predictions of adult intellectual functioning should be deferred until age 5 or 6 years. Earlier predictions tend to be inaccurate, and the more prominent autistic symptomatology often resolves over time. Independent functioning is more difficult to predict because it is related to social ability and behavioral issues as well. It is somewhat reassuring, however, that evidence exists to show that individuals with PDD will continue to acquire new adaptive skills throughout their lives. A small percentage of higher-functioning individuals will be self-supporting, but the majority of adults (70%) with some form of PDD will require supervised living arrangements.

BIBLIOGRAPHY

American Psychiatric Associates: *Diagnostic and statistical manual of mental disorders,* ed 4, Washington, DC, 1994.

Courchesne E, Yeung-Courchesne R, Press GA, et al: Hypoplasia of cerebellar vermal lobules VI and VII on autism, *N Engl J Med* 318:21, 1349–1359, 1988.

Folstein SE, Piven J: Etiology of autism: Genetic influences in an update on autism: A developmental disorder, *Pediatrics* 87(suppl):767, 1991.

Mauk JE: Autism and pervasive developmental disorders, *Pediatr Clin North Am* 40(3):567–578, 1993.

Schreibman L: Autism, *Developmental clinical psychology and psychiatry,* vol 15. CA, 1988, Sage Publications.

Volkmar FR, Klin A, Siegel B, et al: Field trial for autistic disorder in DSM-IV, *Am J Psychiatry* 151:9, 1994.

IV

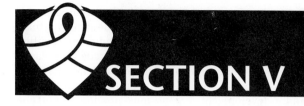

SECTION V

Behavioral Problems

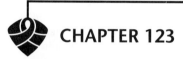

CHAPTER 123

Child and Family Psychosocial Assessment

John Sargent

Primary care physicians are frequently the first to be consulted concerning problems of child behavior and development. These physicians also may observe that some families need assistance in coping with acute and chronic illness, school problems, and transitions in family life. Because of their special role in the lives of the families, they are in an excellent position to provide assistance to parents concerning psychosocial problems of their children, which are estimated to be the reason for 10% to 20% of primary care visits.

To diagnose and manage the child's problems, primary physicians will need a model for assessment of the child's emotional and behavioral capacity. They also should be able to analyze family functioning to define these difficulties accurately and arrange for treatment.

The family, like other living systems, is organized as a hierarchy that allows for the accomplishment of several tasks:

1. Development and maintenance of integrity of family
2. Ongoing development and function of all members
3. Expression of affection, authority, and affiliation
4. Negotiation of changes and responses to stress
5. Conflict resolution, problem solving, decision making
6. Behavior control-socialization coupled with encouragement for individual action and expression

Any individual is simultaneously an independent entity, a member of the family, and a member of smaller groupings within the family. The family encourages the development of all members toward the goal of being successful as a person and in a social setting. The family is a major area for the expression of affection and affiliation as well as for displeasure and anger for children and adults. Responses to change and stress are developed within the family, problems are solved, and conflict and disagreement are negotiated so that the family maintains its integrity at the same time as it fosters individual development and achievement. The family also establishes mechanisms for behavior control that allow for both socialization and individual expression of all family members. Successful participation in all of these family endeavors promotes the emotional and behavioral development of children.

Each of the family members and subgroups (eg, spouses, parental figures, siblings, and individuals) has special tasks and responsibilities within the family. The members of the subgroupings must be able to work together, but there needs to be enough separation among them so that each can pursue individual tasks and gain competence to achieve its goals. As two adults form a family, they develop methods of interaction that encourage the expression of mutual satisfaction, psychological needs, and confirmation of accepted behaviors. Conflicts and disagreements are negotiated. Spouses help each other succeed and support each other when stress occurs. The experience and growth that occur both within and outside the family must be incorporated into the development of the spouse relationship. At the same time, the spouses must be able to be separate enough from the children and from their own parents to maintain their relationship and resolve their disagreements. The spouse relationship also can provide the children with examples of both affection and support, as well as the resolution of conflict, which can become part of the children's values and expectations and model for successful development of intimate relationships. Components of spouse behavior are summarized below:

1. Support and encouragement
2. Intimacy, affection, sex
3. Potential for procreation
4. Creation of a new culture with continuity with families of origin
5. Resolution of disagreements, collaboration

Divorce and remarriage, single parenthood, and alternate family forms have made achieving these goals more difficult for some adults in families; however, parents must still pursue these tasks.

In our society, the child's caretakers have the major responsibility for promoting growth and development. Parents must provide support and nurturance to the child to establish an emotional bond. When such attachment is present, the child will desire parental approval and usually will respond to parental authority. The parents need to provide enough socialization to set limits on the child's behavior and to be able to define the child's world in such a way that the child feels safe and protected. The parents should promote their child's efforts in age-appropriate tasks. These tasks will include consistent school performance, school attendance, relating to peers, and assuming increasing autonomy within the family as development proceeds. Parents also will need to instill within the child a sense of competence and mastery at each developmental level, so that the child successfully integrates new knowledge and new experiences and develops an ever-increasing sense of self-worth and self-esteem. Finally, parents or parental figures will need to assist their child in coping with unexpected failures, disappointments, and losses. Parental figures will need to negotiate and decide on a course of action with respect to their children in situations in which there is no clear and obvious right answer. As the parents negotiate these issues and achieve a course of action, they can increasingly gain a sense of competence and confidence in their own ability as parents and transmit these positive feelings to their children. If there are difficulties in the spouse relationship so that conflicts are not negotiated effectively, parents may find it increasingly difficult to resolve disagreements concerning their children and the children will receive inconsistent direction.

Through *parent-child interaction,* children experience support appropriate to their developmental level and learn to expect that authority and limits can be rational and predictable. Considerations in parent-child interaction include:

1. Congruence between parental behavior and child's needs and skills is important.
2. Varying parental responses and styles of parent-child interaction are required at different stages of development (eg, infancy, pre-

school, school age, adolescence, young adulthood).

3. Major components of parental behavior are:
   Support and nurturance
   Structure, limits, definition of the world
   Affiliation (appreciation of the child for his/her own sake, based on accurate understanding of the child's skills).

If the parents appreciate and recognize the child's abilities and competencies, the child can learn self-esteem, which will then assist him/her in the development of further skills. The child's own development serves, in turn, to increase the parents' sense of their own adequacy. As the child grows and develops, parent-child interaction must change. Parents must provide the older child more opportunities to make independent decisions and solve problems while also requiring the child to take increasing responsibility for his/her actions. The parents' own actions move from control and rule-setting to supervision, monitoring, and availability.

Sibling relationships within the family allow each child to learn and experience competition and cooperation among peers, learn specific abilities to negotiate conflict, establish autonomy, and achieve recognition for development among siblings, which can then assist the child in similar situations outside the family. It is important for the family to encourage siblings' opportunities to interact directly with one another, both to cooperate and to resolve disagreements or conflicts.

CHILD AND FAMILY ASSESSMENT

Through history taking, observation of family interaction, and assessment of the manner in which the family relates to the physician, it is possible to assess the family's patterns of interaction, their skills, capacities, assets, and difficulties as the family members relate to the presenting problem. Methods used in family evaluation are:

1. Observing interaction, monitoring
   Leadership
   Predominant features of relationships: closeness vs distance
   Flexibility of relationships
   Verbal-nonverbal congruence of communication

Involvement of all family members
Task orientation

2. Response to stress or change
   Degree of disruption
   Support generated
   Commitment to cooperation
   Problem-solving behaviors
   Appreciation of new information

3. Ability to utilize extrafamilial resources effectively

The physician will want to note what takes place in his/her office as well as what is described by the family. The physician should appreciate not only how the family relates to the problem in question, but also how the family functions on a day-to-day basis in relationship to the tasks outlined above. As the physician recognizes particular skills and assets of a given family and identifies and works with them, these skills will enable the family to be more confident and competent in dealing with their child and the presenting problem. To assess families, the physician will need to have an organized framework to guide the evaluation process. Parameters for family evaluation are:

1. Relationships
2. Leadership
3. Boundaries
4. Negotiation and conflict resolution
5. Communication and expression of emotion
6. Problem solving
7. Relationship with physician

ELEMENTS OF EVALUATION

Relationships

Relationships between family members should be flexible so that each member can work together for support and growth and can maintain distance when limits and discipline are important. Parental figures should be able to establish relationships with the children appropriate to the situation and the children's needs. The physician should be concerned when either excessive closeness or excessive distance characterizes the relationship between parent and child. An overly close affiliation between parent and child may interfere with the parent's ability to establish important rules. The parent may hold back, either because of inability to get angry at the child or fear of upsetting the child by taking a firm stand. Such relationships may be revealed when the child and overinvolved parent are sitting close to each other, the parent answers for the child or describes how the child feels rather than encouraging the child to speak for himself/herself, or when the parent uses the pronoun "we" to describe difficulties pertaining to the child. Very often in problematic families, one parent establishes and maintains an overly close relationship with the child in question, whereas the other parent is overly distant. Parents often argue with one another about appropriate responses to the child and frequently each responds independently, counterbalancing the other and confusing the child.

Excessively distant relationships may occur in disorganized families in which the parents are so involved with their own problems that the needs of the child are neglected. In such families, the child is given more autonomy than is age-appropriate and rules are either nonexistent or enforced inconsistently. Such families may be unable to focus on the child's problem, and the parents may be primarily concerned about the effect of the child's problem on their lives and less concerned about the child's distress. The child also may be blamed or made a scapegoat by the parents as the source of all parental difficulties. Excessively distant or underinvolved parents may appear apathetic and unresponsive to the child's distress, leaving the child to either increasingly withdraw, persist in disturbed behavior, or try to mask his/her sadness.

Leadership

All families require leadership to set direction, accomplish tasks, solve problems, and satisfy the needs of the children as determined by the children's developmental status and skills. Parents are expected to set rules, enforce behavior, and respond with support, encouragement, and reinforcement for positive outcomes. Within the family, rules should be agreed on by the parental figures to minimize undermining and subversion. The physician needs to learn from each family who the leadership group is and to be sure that members of that group recognize their participation and agree on who takes part in making decisions. In general, in a nuclear family, parents take on that role, with grandparents and relatives having secondary or subordinate roles. In some families, however, grandparents maintain a leadership position, especially in single-parent families. In families with problems, there exists confusion and disagreement about the identity of the family leaders and a lack of collaboration between parental figures. The primary care physician will need to note this, especially as it relates to problem behavior or emotional responses on the part of the children. The children may be allowed to voice complaints with the understanding that the parents are the final arbiters of decisions.

Boundaries

The physician should note whether family subgroupings exist and function independently. In observing the family interactions, the physician should try to decide if parents and children can act independently and as a family unit depending on the situation. The physician should pay attention to whether the spouses can protect and develop their relationship without excessive interference by the children or extended family. The physician also will want to note whether the siblings can cooperate and work together to support one another, and whether the parents can make decisions and implement them without significant intrusion from outside the family. It should be noted whether the boundary around the family allows for family participation in the extrafamilial world, at the same time as it identifies the family as a separate entity reinforcing a sense of belonging and participation. An exclusive, overly close parent-child relationship in a family in which discipline is inadequate and marital strife apparent is indicative of an ineffective boundary between the parents and the children. Such overinvolvement with the child may occur in a family with a special child, such as one with a physical handicap or chronic physical illness. Parents in such families may be overprotective of the child, while assuming functions for the child and speaking for him/her. The child also may avoid speaking for himself/herself out of a limited sense of self-esteem, assertiveness, and autonomy. In such situations, the child's development of independence and maturity is often significantly delayed.

Negotiation and Conflict Resolution

All families have disagreements among their members. In some families, conflicts are acknowledged and confronted directly, whereas in others potential conflict is consistently avoided. Some families disagree openly but are unable to reach a constructive resolution of the problem at hand. The physician should assess the capacity of the family for conflict resolution because unresolved disagreements typically lead to chronic hostility, undermining, and ineffective parenting. Families that tolerate and resolve disagreement are usually more open in their discussion of family problems and more able to use external resources and the guidance of the physician in addressing behavioral and developmental difficulties. As history is given, the physician can observe discussion and the resolution of disagreements as they occur spontaneously or as negotiation is directed through his/her intervention. If conflict is apparent but denied, family tension may increase as problems of the children are discussed. Families that are unable to resolve conflict directly usually have significant marital problems that are denied but cause one parent to become overinvolved with one of the children. The child may become caught in the marital struggle of the parents and more involved in the family, further reinforcing behavior difficulties and emotional immaturity. This difficulty can persist following divorce and should be investigated when evaluating a behavior problem in a child with divorced parents.

Communication and Expression of Emotion

The primary care physician, while assessing the family, will note whether communication is clear and whether nonverbal and verbal communication between family members is consistent and congruent. He/she will pay attention to whether family members listen to and respond to one another or act as though they haven't heard the other's statement. Confusion of verbal and nonverbal messages is especially common in the face of emotional or behavioral problems of the children or in response to significant psychosomatic symptoms.

The physician also will note whether emotional upset on the part of any family member is recognized and supported by other family members. He/she also should observe whether emotional expression interferes with important family functions, so that rules are not enforced for family members who are perceived as being particularly upset or stressed. The child's emotional upset then affects family members in a way that disrupts the family's ability to respond to his/her difficulties and to support his/her development of improved self-esteem and increased self-reliance.

Capacity for Problem Solving

Families vary in their ability to assess situations, gather information, decide among possible alternatives, and implement strategies to resolve problems. Components of effective problem-solving are:

1. Gaining knowledge: background understanding
2. Information gathering, in specific situations
3. Information processing: assessing specific situations
4. Decision making: choosing among alternative strategies
5. Implementation: carrying out strategies
6. Assessing results and modifying strategies

Within a family, these steps are shared, negotiated, and carried out collaboratively. Some families readily address themselves to the difficulties and are effective in marshaling their resources to resolve them. Through effective problem solving, these families gain increased confidence and competence and are more adequately prepared to resolve future difficulties. Other families, because of tenuous or difficult family relationships and an inability to resolve disagreements, fail to gather information effectively and fail to implement strategies to resolve problems. These families are likely to attempt the same solutions over and over again and to perceive other remedies as inaccessible or impossible. Their repertoire of behaviors becomes extremely limited and their responses to problems are stereotyped, rigid, and ineffective.

To resolve problems successfully, disagreeing parents must find a way to put aside their differences in the interest of the child and family. They must develop a mutually acceptable plan for responding to their child's difficulties, and, therefore, soften rigid and polarized positions. Through his/her assessment of the family, the physician will want to pay particular attention to the ways in which parents end up in mutually opposing positions, and, therefore, are unable to address themselves to problem situations.

Relationship With the Physician

The physician should assess the family's ability to relate to him/her and respond to the interventions. If the family approaches the physician in an open, interested, and friendly fashion, the physician should feel more comfortable in responding to the problem and expecting parental collaboration and cooperation. The physician also should expect to experience a different, but effective, relationship with each family member as he/she meets with the family. Families in which members are guarded or inaccessible are more likely to have serious difficulties. The physician also should expect that the observed family behavior will be indicative of the family's responsiveness to other extrafamilial resources, which may need to be utilized in order to solve the presenting problem. Teachers, therapists, and social agencies may either be welcomed by a family or resisted.

These characteristics of family functioning are interdependent and mutually reinforcing, so that a family with several positive characteristics is likely to have others. These competencies lead to further success in a circular fashion. Taken together, the presence of the qualities listed above describes a family that is flexible and capable of change over time as well as a family that will be able to resolve difficulties with appropriate input from the physician.

ASSESSMENT OF THE CHILD'S BEHAVIORAL CAPACITIES

Evaluation of the child's emotional and behavioral status will take place at the same time as the physician is evaluating the family. Parameters of child assessment are:

1. Physical functioning: neurologic, sensory
2. Integration ability: visual-motor, auditory-motor
3. Communication ability: understanding and expression
4. Mood and emotional tone
5. Affect: variety, expression, appropriateness, and regulation
6. Relationships: capacity for attachment, friendship, and intimacy
7. Competence and mastery, problem-solving ability
8. Self-esteem
9. Content and style of thought
10. Temperament: behavioral style
11. Impulse control
12. Appropriateness based on developmental

stage and intrinsic capacities (eg, intelligence, physical integrity, well-being)

The physician should have a framework for appreciating the child's abilities in relationship to the age and developmental level. The physician should observe the child's *behavioral style,* ability to approach new stimuli, and curiosity. The doctor should note whether the behavior is goal-directed and modulated, rapid and diffuse, or slow and withdrawn. The physician should note the child's ability to control his/her behavior in response to the demands of the examining room situation and in response to the requests of the physician and parents. In estimating the child's degree of *impulse control,* the doctor can differentiate times when children have difficulties responding to consistent directions from situations in which the child is generally responsive but the directives are inconsistent and inappropriately given. The physician should notice the child's ability to speak directly and coherently and the overall content and manner of the child's *thinking.* Such elements as spontaneity, coherence, and articulation of speech are important, as well as the overall coherence and goal-directedness of the child's thinking and verbal communication. The physician may want to ask for the child's wishes, fantasies, and views of the future as a reflection of the child's self-esteem and self-concept. The doctor should also evaluate the overall *mood* or emotional tone of the child during his/her assessment as well as the child's ability to express and experience a variety of *affects.* The affect should reflect the content of the issue under discussion, and the child should be able to respond to and mirror the physician's affect as he/she interacts with the child.

The physician should observe the child's ability to *relate* to him/her during the assessment process. If the child is unusually withdrawn or shy, or unusually responsive and open, these cues will indicate potential difficulties to the physician. The degree of eye contact and spontaneous speech, the degree of trust the child demonstrates in the physician, and the extent to which the child desires the physician's approval and warmth should be noted. The final component of the assessment of the child for the physician is a clear appreciation of the child's strengths in relationship to any particular difficulties that may be present. This component is especially important in situations in which the child's difficulty is associated with developmental delay, physical handicap, or chronic illness. It will be through these strengths that the physician will enable the family to encourage the child in the development of appropriate self-esteem, competence, and mastery and in the achievement of maximum psychosocial adaptation.

SYNTHESIS AND SUMMARY

The assessment of both family and child will take place for the physician throughout history taking, observations of family interaction, physical examination, and review and assessment of the visit. This assessment will lead the physician to a recognition of the family's strengths and capacities and their accomplishments with respect to child-rearing. It also will help the physician determine the areas of difficulty or weakness within the family corresponding to the problems the family has identified. The physician should be able to feel comfortable with the assessment and to expect that the impressions of the child

and of the family make sense. A successful family in which child rearing has proceeded without significant difficulties may be having specific problems at a point of developmental stress at which previously mastered parenting skills are no longer effective. A family in which the child demonstrates significant behavior problems may have marked unresolved conflicts between the parents, with significant overinvolvement on the part of one parent with the child so that the rules and directives of parenting are ineffective. In a family in which a psychosomatic symptom is present, there may be significant parental concern for either the meaning of the symptom or for the vulnerability of the child in question. As the physician recognizes increasingly the consistency between family assessment and child assessment, he/she will be able to intervene effectively with the family to promote their successful achievement of the tasks of child rearing and also to be able to utilize external resources or refer a family for additional assistance when the presenting problem and family difficulties require such intervention.

BIBLIOGRAPHY

Carter B, McGoldrick M, editors: *The changing family life cycle,* ed 2, New York, 1988, Gardner Press.

Falicov C, editor: *Family transitions: Continuity and change over the life cycle,* New York, 1988, Guilford Press.

Greenspan SI: *The clinical interview of the child,* New York, 1981, McGraw-Hill.

Hodas GR, Sargent J: Psychiatric emergencies. In Fleisher G, Ludwig S, editors: *Textbook of pediatric emergency medicine,* ed 2, Baltimore, 1988, Williams & Wilkins.

Minuchin S: *Families and family therapy,* Cambridge, MA, 1974, Harvard University Press.

Minuchin S, Minuchin PL: The child in context: A systems approach to growth and treatment. In Talbot NB, editor: *Raising children in modern America,* Boston, 1976, Little Brown & Co.

Sargent J: The family: A pediatric assessment, *J Pediatr* 102:973-976, 1983.

Simons J: *Psychiatric examination of children,* ed 2, Philadelphia, 1974, Lea & Febiger.

Walsh F, editor: *Normal family process,* New York, 1982, Guilford Press.

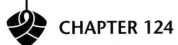

CHAPTER 124

Family Treatment of Childhood Behavior Problems

John Sargent

Family therapy has attracted the attention of many practitioners because it deals not only with the individual who presents with a problem but also with the family who lives with the patient. This chapter describes some of the principles of family therapy and strategies used by family therapists in treating children and their families.

The primary care physician's role in working with children with behavioral problems is to make an accurate diagnosis of the child's problem and of the family's functioning and to intervene in family operations directly or to refer the family for family-oriented psychotherapy. It is important for the physician to recognize that when dealing with a child's emotional or behavioral problem, the family also must be considered. In order for the interventions to have the most beneficial effect, the assessment of the family should be complete and should reflect an appreciation of the role of the family in relationship to the child's symptom. The physician, then, will require a model of how family interaction influences the child's problem.

Family therapy is a method to change family interactions so that their functioning is effective in relationship to the child's development, adaptation, and socialization. The goal of family therapy is to assist the family to solve its own problems, to manage and direct the development of the children, and to appreciate the unique needs, skills, and abilities of each child. To effectively intervene in family interaction, the physician should have in mind a model of effective family organization and functioning and an appreciation of the influence of the family in the development and maintenance of their children's symptomatic behavior. This is not to suggest that all behavior problems are a result of faulty family interaction. Some, such as attention-deficit disorder, psychosis, and mood disorders may reflect an underlying physiologic difference on the part of the affected child. The physician has a responsibility to help the family adapt to and cope with each of their children's individual capabilities and needs, allowing maximal psychosocial functioning and adaptation on the part of each child.

Family therapy is based on the concept that symptomatic behavior in a family member arises within a family context and is an attempt to adapt to that situation.

VIEWPOINT OF FAMILY THERAPY

1. Symptomatic behavior arises within the family and is adaptive to the family.
2. Symptoms are maintained by family interaction and play a role in maintaining the stability of the family.
3. The symptom affects the entire family; the entire family affects the symptom.
4. Symptoms tend to arise in families at points of change or transition.
5. Interactions of families with symptoms are constricted. More skills and possibilities exist within the family than are utilized currently.
6. Most families can successfully respond to symptoms, foster their children's development, and accomplish other family goals.

Families with a symptomatic member are dysfunctional, that is, not capable of effectively meeting the needs for all members at the time of problem expression. The symptom is not limited to the member with a problem, but embedded in patterns of family interaction and continued by those family transactions. The problem also maintains family stability in a circular fashion. The entire family affects the symptomatic member, whose behavior, in turn, affects the entire family. Symptoms tend to arise within families at times of change or stress, especially at transitions in the family life cycle. At these times, previously adaptive patterns of family interaction are no longer satisfactory for family members. New responses are not available or are perceived as threatening because interactions among family members are inappropriately rigid. Because limited aspects of any individual's capacities are utilized by the family, family problem solving is deficient and the symptom remains or may worsen.

The basic assumption of family therapy is that families with symptoms possess unused capabilities and unapplied strengths. Encouraging those interactions that utilize family strengths more effectively can enable the family to resolve the symptoms or adapt to underlying differences in their children. These new interactions can be integrated into the family responses, ultimately altering the family system and achieving more effective family functioning.

Dysfunctional families have inadequate leadership that occurs when there is disagreement or conflict between the parents or between a single parent and another important caretaker. Unresolved disagreement between parenting figures leads to inconsistent direction and may result in undermining decisions. As long as the caretakers have problems with their own interaction, the symptoms in the children will persist. Each parent encourages the child to side with him/her in the persistent disagreements, therefore encouraging further participation of the child in family matters, leaving the child less available to peer group and less able to develop self-control and effective self-esteem.

Problems occur when there is a blurring of the boundary between parent and child. A secret coalition of one parent and the child may develop, with the two of them acting against the other parent. These alliances may shift, with the child alternatively aligned with each parent. The physician should recognize that the child is an active participant but may not have the insight nor autonomy necessary to refuse to take sides with one parent. The child may not recognize the parents' vulnerability or may not be aware that they are rewarded with increased attention for participation in the parents' disagreement. The child's problem diminishes the stress of unresolved parental conflict and distracts the family, as a whole, from other unaddressed and important stresses. Communication among family members is likely to be confused and incomplete, with nonverbal and verbal communications contradicting each other. Within the family, there is also likely to be a chronic state of tension and stress. As each family member plays a role in the perpetuation of the child's problem, it becomes evident that the difficulty is actually a problem of the family rather than just the child.

Relationships among family members become excessively rigid and stereotyped and attempts to resolve the problem by one parent or by the child individually become part of the cycle that maintains or worsens the problem. At that point, advice that does not alter the rules of family organization and habitual family interaction also further maintains the problem. Interventions that directly change family organization and the actions that maintain the problem are required so that the parents, together, can collaborate to assist the child to grow, appropriate to his/her developmental stage and age. Treatment will require change on the part of all family members. The parents will need to work together more effectively, the child will need to be supported when in trouble and yet limited when out of control, and the siblings will need to be able to cooperate more effectively. As the parents collaborate to resolve the difficulty or appreciate the special needs of their child, they then can be encouraged to resolve their marital difficulties at the same time as the child is encouraged to learn skills and develop maturity. Indications for family therapy are listed below.

INDICATIONS FOR FAMILY THERAPY

1. Poor compliance with medical treatment
2. Poor control of chronic illness and repeated hospitalizations
3. Less than expected physical function despite adequate medical treatment, or psychosomatic symptoms
4. Social withdrawal, depression, emotional immaturity in a child
5. Poor school performance with adequate learning skills

6. Aggressive, reckless, out-of-control behavior
7. Family strife in raising children
8. Family concern about child's ability to mature into adolescence or adulthood
9. Psychosis, suicidal behavior
10. Nonorganic failure to thrive, parent-child attachment disorders
11. Substance abuse
12. Child abuse or neglect with appropriate legal supervision

Several distinct models of family-oriented treatment for childhood behavior problems have been developed. Each model responds to the symptomatic behavior of children by assisting the family to resolve the child's symptoms and proceed with family life successfully. One clearly articulated model of family treatment has been developed and described by Salvador Minuchin. Derived from a consistent model of effective family functioning, it has been utilized in response to a variety of emotional and behavioral problems of children. Outcome studies have shown Minuchin's structural family therapy to be effective for serious psychosocial and psychophysiologic disorders in children including psychosomatic disorders and adolescent drug abuse and habituation. It is particularly relevant for physicians caring for children because of its focus on change and development throughout family life and its normative expectations of parental and child behavior, especially in response to problems or stress. The treating person assists the family in responding to crises and transitions and then expects the family to reestablish control over its behavior and functioning as soon as the problem is resolved. The treating person remains available to the family for assistance in future crises. This therapist, then, has a role with the family analogous to that of primary care physician for illnesses. Primary care physicians can learn the techniques of family therapy and can, with interest, training, and experience, treat a variety of uncomplicated behavioral, emotional, and psychosomatic problems of children. The following discussion reflects this and identifies the physician as a treating person. The approach to treatment and the techniques of treatment will be similar if the primary care physician chooses to refer the family and patient to a family-oriented therapist.

STRUCTURAL FAMILY THERAPY

1. Therapy is aimed at changing family relationships and family behavior in the present.
2. Therapy highlights family strengths and assists the family in developing confidence and ability to manage the child's care and development.
3. Therapy is geared toward action.
4. A clear understanding of the child's physical and intellectual capacities must be developed and agreed on by the parents.
5. Therapy uses family concern about the disabled or ill child to change family relationships.
6. The parents must work together.
7. The parents can then enhance treatment and require maturity of the child.
8. As the child's symptoms become manageable for the family, the focus of therapy can shift to other issues troubling the family: the marriage, difficulties of the siblings, and so forth.

The primary goal of structural family therapy is to alter inappropriate patterns of family interaction by reestablishing and restructuring family relationships. The physician, then, can create and support more effective family activity, at the same time as the parents encourage and support the child's development and maturity. Treatment supports effective functioning of all family members and requires that the family actively solve problems in the presence of the physician. Changes in family relationships induce changes in behavior of all members—first the child and subsequently the parents—and these changes can be reinforced, first by the physician and ultimately by family members in their lives at home.

Initial Evaluation

The initial treatment stage is one in which the physician completes an assessment of the child's physiologic, emotional, and behavioral functioning and integrates that assessment into his/her appreciation of the family system's operation. The physician can note whether the parents collaborate effectively, whether both parents appreciate the child's difficulties in the same way, which pattern of family interaction interferes with successful approaches to the presenting problems, and which areas of family difficulty are reflected in the parents' inability to deal effectively with the child's behavior problem. The first step in successful treatment is for the physician to work with the family developing a relationship with each family member and appreciating each individual point of view without blaming anyone. The physician also learns and respects the culture, idiosyncrasies, and style of the family, and notices and highlights strengths and competencies of each family member in the family as a whole. The physician also should maintain an attitude of impartiality, which will convey the belief that each family member is presenting only that individual's perspective of the family reality.

During the evaluation phase, the physician will identify predominant family relationships and preferred patterns of interaction, noting who talks to whom, what the tone of the conversation is, what the predominant features of the relationships between both parents and the identified patient are, and how family members address the problem. A hypothesis is developed about the family structure and the difficulties in family organization that are impeding resolution of the symptoms. During this assessment, the physician may note significant overprotectiveness on the part of one parent; marked rigidity that leaves one parent overly close to the child with the problem, whereas the other parent is excessively distant and critical; and significant difficulty in negotiation and conflict resolution between the parents. The physician also should develop an appreciation of the role of the child's symptoms in the family. Are there stresses on family members that the symptoms are masking or diverting attention from? Does the symptom play a role in maintaining contact between the child and a distant or undervalued parent? Is there a particular reason why the parents are having difficulties with this child with this set of problems?

It is important for the physician to remember at this time that it is not the child's particular temperament or behavioral style that is important in any family, but rather the fit between that child's style and the family's expectations and abilities to respond effectively to that child. As the physician gathers history concerning the presenting problem, attention should be paid to methods that each family member has used to try to resolve the problem and what other family members have done when a particular member was attempting to apply his/her preferred solution. Does the father provide support and encouragement to the child as the child misbehaves for the mother, or does the father rather support and encourage the mother's disciplinary efforts? Is the mother overly close or protective of the child, whereas the father is harsh and disciplinary? When the child becomes symptomatic, does the mother or father become anxious, confused, and therefore unable to respond? The physician, gaining experience in observing family interactions, will note the same patterns occurring over and over again in any particular family and will observe the ways in which parents interfere with each other's efforts, leaving the child unsupported and without consistent direction. As history is obtained concerning recent family circumstances, the physician also may note other unresolved difficulties that the family has and incompetencies that the family has recognized, but is not able to address. Examples of this may be recent death, concern about the child's overall well-being, economic stress, or interference of extended kin.

Intervention in Family Operation

The physician's first goal in working with the family is to establish a spirit of teamwork and collaboration with the parents, with the expectation that all three adults will gain the same appreciation of the child's needs and work together to come up with effective solutions to the child's problems. At this point, the physician should be clear about the definition of the child's problems and gradually and directly help the parents to share this assessment. Often, however, a direct statement of the child's capabilities and problems by the physician may only lead to increased family resistance and denial of the child's problems. It is important for the physician to develop ways of asking parents to note and recognize the child's behavior in response to parental directives. As the parents become increasingly adept at observing and identifying their child's skills, and negotiating between themselves a consistent appreciation of the child, they will then be able to develop ways of acting to limit problematic behaviors and support effective behaviors of the child. This may include the parents' noticing that the child has difficulty following inconsistent directions, therefore becoming able to address more consistent rules and expectations to the child. It also may include the parents' reinforcing impulse control, expecting performance of homework, or expecting continued functioning despite moderate interfering functional physical symptoms. As the parents monitor their child's behavior and negotiate actively between themselves a response that they can both carry through and feel comfortable with, they will increasingly become competent at limiting the child's behavior and supporting the child's need for nurturance and attention.

The physician generally will ignore ineffective family operations, encourage a task-orientation on the part of the parents, and demonstrate optimism and support of the family's success. At the same time as he/she encourages the parents to be more competent and successful with the child, the physician will want to support the child's self-esteem and encourage the child to achieve appropriate developmental and behavioral goals. The physician will need to encourage the family to express sadness and disagreement and provide support and congratulations when interventions are successful. The physician should monitor the family's success in dealing with the child and intermittently encourage the parents to collaborate more effectively with each other on other issues of their lives, especially with regard to particular family stresses. Specific techniques for treatment for the child, including relaxation training so that the child can deal effectively with painful or fearful experiences, drug treatment (eg, using stimulants for attention-deficit disorder), and consistent responses to problematic behaviors through the use of behavior modification techniques may be useful and integrated into the therapy. As treatment progresses, the physician may want to meet independently with the parents to identify with them any particular stresses in their marriage that will need to be addressed either by the physician or through referral to a therapist. The physician also may want to meet independently with the child, especially for older children and adolescents, to be sure that the child's self-esteem is improving and interest in the world of peers is increasing. The techniques of family therapy are summarized below:

1. The therapist should be aware of the child's physical condition and intellectual capacity.

2. The therapist develops and conveys respect for family problems and possibilities.
3. The therapist collaborates with medical and educational specialists working with the child and family.
4. Family members resolve problems and interact during therapy.
5. The therapist maintains focus of the session on issues of his/her choice.
6. The therapist highlights the responsibility of the family to solve problems.
7. The therapist builds disagreements among family members during the sessions so that motivation is developed to resolve conflict and develop plans that all are committed to following.
8. The therapist regulates participation in the sessions, allowing for the creation of new family relationships and the most effective methods of family operation.
9. The therapist monitors family performance supporting new relationships and skills.
10. The therapist can shift to sessions for marital therapy with the parents and individual sessions for the child as indicated.

These interventions are directed at changing boundaries within the family, the family's beliefs about their relationships and their child's abilities, and the realities of family relationships. Family members become increasingly flexible and able to respond to the child's problem and other stresses. As increasing capacity and competency on the part of the family as a whole is noted, the physician can decrease the involvement and return to a primary care approach, remaining available to the family to provide assistance in future stressful or crisis situations. For many behavior problems and emotional problems, the physician can carry through the interventions described here independently. The parents can achieve an experience of success that reinforces their effectiveness in raising the children. In some situations, such as those described in this section, the child's problems may be significant. In other situations, unresolved marital difficulties and severe communication problems among family members also may be noted. In these situations, it is necessary to refer these families for psychotherapy.

The physician, attuned to family problems as a basis for many of the complaints of children, will develop skills for detection and early intervention. For more details, consult the works by Minuchin listed in the bibliography.

BIBLIOGRAPHY

Allmond B, Buckman W, Goffman H: *The family is the patient,* St Louis, 1979, CV Mosby.

Coherty W, Baird M: *Family therapy and family medicine,* New York, 1983, Guilford Press.

Crouch M, Roberts I, editors: *The family in medical practice,* New York, 1987, Springer-Verlag.

Haley J: Toward a theory of pathological systems. In Watzlawick J, Weakland J, editors: *The interactional view,* New York, 1977, WW Norton.

Heneo S, Grose N, editors: *Principles of family systems in family medicine,* New York, 1985, Bruner-Mazel.

Hodas GR, Sargent J: Psychiatric emergencies. In Fleisher G, Ludwig S, editors: *Textbook of pediatric emergency medicine,* ed 2, Baltimore, 1988, Williams & Wilkins.

Hoffman L: *Foundation of family therapy,* New York, 1981, Basic Book.

Langsley DG, Kaplan DM: *Treatment of families in crisis,* New York, 1968, Grune & Stratton.

Minuchin S: *Families and family therapy,* Cambridge, MA, 1974, Harvard University Press.

Minuchin S, Fishman HC: *Family therapy techniques,* Cambridge, MA, 1981, Harvard University Press.

Mirkin M, Koman S, editors: *Handbook of adolescents and family therapy,* New York, 1985, Gardner Press.

Pittman F: *Turning points: Treating families in transition and crisis,* New York, 1987, Norton.

Sargent J: Family therapy: A view for pediatricians, *J Pediatr* 102:977–981, 1983.

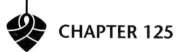

CHAPTER 125

Effective Use of Psychiatric Consultation

Henry G. Berger

In a psychiatric consultation a psychiatrist and primary care physician work together in evaluating a child's emotional climate and well being, formulating a treatment plan, or facilitating the execution of the plan. Effective use of psychiatric consultation requires the physician to 1) have a good working relationship with the consultant, 2) learn to recognize and respond to emotional "red flags" in his/her patients and families, 3) recognize what issues are beyond his/her own expertise and time limitations, and 4) know how to enable the child and family to overcome their fears and reluctance in obtaining necessary help. Part of the job of a consulting psychiatrist is to help the practitioner to fulfill these requirements. This chapter describes each of these in detail.

WORKING RELATIONSHIP BETWEEN CONSULTANT AND PHYSICIAN

The primary tools of a psychiatric consultant are the ability to establish rapport and sensitivity to the feelings of others, as well as the more specialized diagnostic and therapeutic skills. The physician who cannot feel comfortable in discussing problems with the psychiatrist and develop confidence in the consultant's abilities may well ask how the troubled patients might feel with the same individual. The lack of an open, cooperative working relationship may force the physician to avoid utilizing the consultant until there is a "serious problem." Finally, the practitioner may inadvertently give away a feeling of discomfort or distrust to the child or family, thus affecting their relationship with the psychiatrist. The primary care physician also should consider his/her own attitudes toward emotional issues and psychotherapy in general. On the other hand, the psychiatrist should be interested and comfortable with medical issues, while acknowledging a lack of expertise in these areas. One of the most destructive obstacles to resolving a child's and family's emotional difficulties is a conflict between the practitioner and psychiatrist. Even the most positive teamwork is often tested and stressed by the disruptive nature of certain emotional difficulties. Thus, it is particularly important to select the right psychiatric consultant and to maintain a sound working relationship.

"RED FLAGS"

The primary care physician should be alert to signs and signals that suggest a need for further exploration and perhaps immediate or eventual therapeutic intervention. Although a more detailed description of the diagnostic categories and criteria can be found in the *Diagnostic and Statistical Manual of Mental Disorders* (third edition, revised) prepared by the American Psychiatric Association, a physician will want to be alert at least to signals suggesting underlying disorders or difficulties. Such warning signs range from the severe and more obvious one, suggesting psychiatric disorders, to the more common emotional problems and family dysfunction. The problems suggesting underlying disorders and certain associated diagnostic or

etiologic categories are listed in Table 125-1. These categories are not meant to be all-inclusive, nor are the symptoms or signs pathognomonic.

Various studies of pediatric inpatient, outpatient, and physically disabled populations show a high incidence of undiagnosed psychopathology. This suggests at least the need to be alert to complaints and receptive to a family's requests for help and to be willing to take the time, when necessary, to explore these complaints adequately to develop a treatment plan. Stressful episodes and conditions that should alert the physician to the need for further exploration to determine the impact on the child and the possible need for intervention are listed below. This list is certainly not complete but is meant as a demonstration of the need for a broader perspective in considering the child's emotional environment as well as his/her individual symptoms and behavior.

1. Loss of family member through death or divorce
2. Depressed or psychotic parent or guardian
3. Chronically or severely ill child, parent, or sibling
4. Chronic parental conflict or other type of severe family dysfunction
5. Child with learning disability or attention-deficit disorder
6. Physical or sexual abuse of child or other family member

FORMULATING A SOLUTION TO THE PROBLEM

Once a decision is made that a particular behavior or situation requires further evaluation, a practitioner must decide whether to proceed alone or to call in a consultant. In either case, time needs to be set aside for a meeting for all family members to discuss the particular situation or complaint. Although this sometimes can be done immediately, often it requires a return visit for all family members scheduled at a time that is convenient for both the practitioner and the family and child. The purpose of such a meeting is to gather necessary information, both by hearing from all family members as well as by observing their relationships together. During this meeting a treatment program also can be

TABLE 125-1
Underlying Disorders and Diagnostic Categories

PROFILE	DIAGNOSTIC CONSIDERATION
Preschool	
Numerous developmental and behavioral delays in language, social, and motor skills	Mental retardation
Severely withdrawn; noncommunicative; emotionally unresponsive	Childhood autism; pervasive developmental disorder
Significantly anxious or depressed; delayed development; evidence of repeated physical injury; aggressive behavior	Child abuse or neglect
Chronic sleep or eating difficulties; oppositional behavior	Inconsistent or irregular parenting; lack of nurturance
Mild complaints in apparently well-developed child, with age-appropriate behavior	Overwhelmed, emotionally unsupported, anxious parent
School Age	
Poor school performance; aggressive behavior; tantrum; overactivity	Attention-deficit disorder; learning disability
Chronic somatic complaints, with frequent school absence	School avoidance, with family dysfunction
Severe moodiness; social isolation; poor school performance	Childhood affective disorders
Poorly controlled childhhood asthma or diabetes, or other "psychosomatic illness"	Stress; family dysfunction
Frequent behavior problems; stealing; fighting; oppositional behavior	Family dysfunction
Adolescence	
Severe personality changes; withdrawn or bizarre behavior; agitated behavior becoming worse; confused behavior	Schizophrenia
Severe weight loss; frequent compulsive vomiting; frequent laxative use	Anorexia nervosa, bulimia
Self-destructive behavior; continual moodiness; school failure; sleep difficulties	Affective disorder
School failure; delinquent behavior; drug abuse; promiscuity	Attention-deficit disorder; learning disability; borderline personality disorder
Poorly controlled chronic illness; asthma, diabetes, colitis	Family dysfunction
School failure, labile mood, personality change	Drug and alcohol abuse

developed with the cooperation and consent of the family. This therapy can mean immediate suggestions and intervention on the part of the practitioner to alleviate problems that are more simple or the involvement at the next stage of the psychiatric consultant for further assessment and possible intervention. The meeting avoids the risk of the practitioner reassuring a family about a particular complaint without adequate data or prematurely dismissing a complaint as something the parents "might want to see a psychiatrist about." Furthermore, such a meeting increases the chances of enlisting the cooperation of all family members in pursuing a particular decision or treatment plan. In a family meeting, the physician can obtain a history while simul-

taneously observing family members' reactions to one another. The physician should encourage a family discussion of the problem so that interactions can be observed better. Such family sessions also are useful to discuss relevant medical findings, school reports, or testing data. If a problem-solving approach is maintained in a supportive and accepting atmosphere, most families will readily accept appropriate advice. Methodical data gathering through conjoint family meetings helps the physician to avoid becoming involved in an overly complex, explosive, or time-consuming situation.

Most primary care physicians will find they have neither the training nor the time to deal with problems such as a severely dysfunctional family, significantly depressed child or adult, or the variety of problems created by some of the more serious issues mentioned previously. Thus, one possible outcome of the evaluation meeting is a decision to consult a psychiatrist for further evaluation and possible treatment. To carry out this decision, it is often necessary for the practitioner to help the family overcome their resistance and anxieties concerning psychiatric involvement.

Often the primary care physician is involved in short-term counseling and in prescribing psychotropic medication. It is estimated that more than 50% of emotionally ill patients are being seen by the primary care physician. In such situations, it may be particularly important for the primary care physician to maintain an ongoing relationship with a consulting psychiatrist.

FACILITATING A DIRECT MEETING BETWEEN FAMILY AND PSYCHIATRIC CONSULTANT

The value of considering the psychiatric consultation as a joint process involving the practitioner, family, and consultant makes it possible to view the psychiatrist as participating as an advisor prior to his/her beginning therapy with the family. In this role, the psychiatrist may help the practitioner identify the problem, gather information, and evaluate the information prior to meeting the family. Such a process naturally means that the practitioner must have a comfortable, ongoing, working relationship with the consultant and that the consultant be available (at least by phone) as needed. Often the practitioner's comfort with the psychiatric consultant will be apparent to the family and enable them to be comfortable in meeting with him/her. Even under these conditions, however, the most sensitive and supportive physicians may meet enormous resistance to involving a psychiatrist. At this point, the family may attempt to minimize a potentially serious problem to convince the practitioner that they can handle it themselves with a little help, stating it is really just "the teacher's problem" or "the child will grow out of it." Helping the family and child overcome this resistance can be extremely beneficial, both to obtain the necessary assistance and to help them solve problems realistically and cooperatively.

There are a few general approaches and techniques that are useful in overcoming such resistance. First, it is helpful to try to determine its cause. Is the family trying to protect the child? Does someone feel they are to blame for the problem and wish to avoid being criticized? Has there been a previous bad experience with a psychiatrist? Is the involvement of a psychiatrist viewed as an admission of failure? These and other difficulties may be at the root of such resistance and may be clues to more underlying family dysfunction. Sometimes the first visit can be set up as a consultation and a "test," just as a referral to a radiologist is a consultation to find out if anything is wrong and if further treatment is necessary. Whatever the underlying issue may be, the physician will want to maintain a clear stance concerning his/her opinion about obtaining psychiatric help, whereas, on the other hand, recognizing the legitimate fears of family members. The physician's strongest ally in overcoming such fears is an ongoing positive relationship with the patient and family. In certain instances, friendly understanding but firm encouragement is not enough. In acute crises, one may look for extended family members, friends, church, or school personnel as allies—both in efforts in supporting a disorganized, fragmented family and in assisting further encouragement in obtaining psychiatric help. In other instances, further private consultation between the psychiatrist and physician can be useful and possibly a decision may be reached and agreed to by the family to have a meeting with the psychiatrist in the family physician's office as a form of further evaluation.

SYSTEMS OF CARE AND MENTAL HEALTH CONSULTATION

It is important to consider the system of health care delivery as part of the environment that may affect the process of mental health consultation. Although the underlying principles remain the same, their application must take into account the effects of the system of health care delivery. Issues such as continuity of care, physician-patient relationship, physician-consultant relationship, and availability of consultation may all be influenced for better or worse as traditional fee-for-service medical care is replaced by the newest systems of delivery and managed care. Although the validity of many of our own biases will surely be tested in the future, accumulated evidence and experience suggest the following:

1. Early intervention is important in avoiding more serious and, therefore, more costly behavioral dysfunction.

2. A positive, continuous doctor-patient relationship is important in obtaining treatment compliance for both medical and behavioral intervention.

3. The availability of mental health experts as a resource to the treating physician and the family is both necessary and cost-effective. Ideally a framework for ongoing discussion and consultation between the physician and the mental health provider should strengthen the skills of the primary care physician with consequent improved patient care and cost-effectiveness.

How such programs are implemented in the newer health care systems is a challenge to all those involved as patient advocates and health care providers.

SUMMARY

As in working with any other consultant, the primary care physician's relationship with the psychiatric consultant requires a mutual respect and rapport. A general broad focus on the part of the primary care physician is needed to recognize a wide array of problems, including psychosocial dysfunction and to respond to and adequately assess these problems. Naturally, the physician must be able to recognize personal limitations and be able to ask for help when indicated. The psychiatric consultation, however, requires special consideration because of the unique discomfort that families and individuals have in dealing with and working through psychosocial problems and in requesting the help of a psychiatric consultant.

BIBLIOGRAPHY

Beardslee WR, Benporad J, Keller MB, et al: Children of parents with major affective disorders, a review, *Am J Psychiatry* 140:825–832, 1983.

Bennett LA, Wolin SJ, Reiss D: Cognitive, behavioral and emotional problems among school-age children of alcoholic parents, *Am J Psychiatry* 145:185–190, 1988.

Borus JF: Psychiatry and the primary care physician. In Kaplan H, Sadock B, editors: *Comprehensive textbook of psychiatry,* vol 4, Baltimore, 1985, Williams & Wilkins.

Breslau N: Psychiatric disorders in children with physical disabilities, *J Am Acad Child Psychiatry* 24:87–94, 1985.

Campo JV, Fritch SL: Somatization in children and adolescents, *J Am Acad Child Adolesc Psychiatry* 33(9):1223–1235, 1994.

Christophersen ER: Incorporating behavioral pediatrics into primary care, *Pediatr Clin North Am* 29:261–296, 1982.

Fritz GK, Mattison RE, Nurcombe B, Spirito A: *Child and adolescent mental health consultation in hospitals, schools and courts,* Washington, DC, 1993, American Psychiatric Press.

Hauts CB, Turbett JA, Arnold E, Krase E: Cost of medical/surgical delays: Prevented by psychiatric treatment, *J Am Acad Child Psychiatry* 24:227–230, 1985.

Last CG, Hersen M, Kayden A, et al: Psychiatric illness in mothers of anxious children, *Am J Psychiatry* 144:1580–1583, 1987.

Livingston R, Taylor JL, Crawford SL: A study of somatic complaints and psychiatric diagnosis in children, *J Am Acad Child Adolesc Psychiatry* 27:185–187, 1988.

Orleans CT, George LK, Haupt JL, et al: How primary care physicians treat psychiatric disorders. A national survey of family practitioners, *Am J Psychiatry* 142:52–57, 1985.

CHAPTER 126

Depression

Gordon R. Hodas

Depression during childhood and adolescence is a serious and potentially life-threatening condition that implies imbalance at three distinct levels: individual, interpersonal, and biochemical. At the individual level, childhood and adolescent depression implies a significant disturbance in mood, most commonly persistent sadness, self-deprecation, and suicidal ideation. There are myriad presentations, varying from a full-blown depressive syndrome with physiologic concomitants to a less complete but often equally serious adjustment reaction with serious alterations of mood toward sadness and hopelessness. At the interpersonal level, childhood and adolescent depression signifies a breakdown in the process of care-taking and support on the part of the adults, and an interference in the capacity of child and family to acknowledge and talk about the problem. The biochemical level becomes especially relevant in severe cases of childhood and adolescent depression in which disturbances in mood and self-concept are accompanied by physiologic and other associated impairments in functioning. In such instances there is often a family history of depression. Medication decisions are beyond the scope of the office-based physician and should be deferred until the child has been referred for psychotherapy and fully assessed.

Although some children and adolescents have been depressed for a prolonged period, depression usually implies a recognizable change from an earlier, more adaptive mode of functioning. The office-based physician should recognize that depression in childhood and adolescence may present directly, in the form of overt sadness, or indirectly, in the form of persistent somatic complaints, frequent office visits, and school avoidance patterns. Similarly, depression may be readily acknowledged by some children and

adolescents and their parents and strongly denied by others. Because parents may not be able to recognize depression in a child at times, the office-based physician can serve a crucial role in identifying the depression and making a referral when indicated.

PRESENTATION

For a previously well-functioning child, irritability, as manifested by strained personal relationships, and decreased concentration, as manifested by a deterioration in school performance, may be early signs of depression and may be recognized by the parents and/or the child. Depression in childhood and adolescence may include any of the following presentations:

1. Sad, hopeless mood
2. Suicide attempts
3. Recurrent "accidents"
4. Impaired relationships
5. Impaired academic performance
6. Recurrent somatic complaints
7. School avoidance
8. Alcohol and drug abuse
9. Exacerbation of a medical condition
10. Conduct disorders
11. Eating disorders

The findings may occur singly or in combinations. The child or adolescent may describe directly his/her sad, hopeless feeling, or the mood state may be so evident that the physician recognizes it readily and the patient confirms it. When the patient shows a capacity to acknowledge his/her depression and discuss it with the physician, there is a more favorable prognosis, even if the symptoms are severe. Any overt suicide attempt should be regarded as serious, because all suicidal behavior represents a genuine statement of distress and self-destructive urges. Repeated accidents are a frequent manifestation of depression and may take the form of unconscious recklessness or risk-taking, or deliberate life-endangering acts. It would appear that many accidents, especially motor vehicle collisions, are really unacknowledged suicide attempts.

The depressed child may have impaired relationships and academic performance, at times accompanied by recurrent somatic complaints and school avoidance. The somatic complaints (such as headaches, abdominal pain, nausea, and dizziness) typically have no organic basis despite repeated evaluation. Deterioration of academic performance may occur in both high-achieving children and in children with ongoing attention or learning problems.

Some children, unable to face the painful affect of depression directly, mask the depression through other behaviors, including drug and alcohol abuse and conduct disorders. Depression also should be suspected with an unexplained exacerbation of a medical condition and with eating disorders such as anorexia nervosa and bulimia.

RECOGNITION

The cardinal features that assist the office-based physician in recognizing overt or underlying depression are presented in the following lists. The diagnosis of depression is best made by seeing the child with the parent(s) and also by talking with the child or adolescent alone and observing the patient for signs of depression, while noting the relationship that unfolds. In most instances, a gently sympathetic approach on the part of the physician will make the sad affect more apparent and will enable the child to begin to discuss some of the sources of distress. The three major criteria for recognizing depression are dysphoric mood (a pervasive sense of distress and ill-being), self-deprecatory ideation, and associated impairments of functioning.

The major feature of the *dysphoric mood* of depression is a persistent sense of sadness; features of this mood are:

1. Sad affect
2. Irritability
3. Anxiety
4. Lability
5. Crying
6. Exhaustion

The other characteristics listed may occur singly or in combination. Lability refers to persistent moodiness and the tendency to be verbally abusive. The sense of exhaustion may be overwhelming and may be experienced both emotionally and physically.

Self-deprecatory ideation frequently manifests itself in terms of self-doubt and indecisiveness. The subjective expressions of self-deprecation are:

1. Self-doubt
2. Low self-esteem
3. Sense of worthlessness
4. Indecisiveness
5. Sense of guilt
6. Sense of powerlessness and helplessness
7. Sense of hopelessness
8. Suicidal ideation

Suicidal wishes are likely to occur when the child sees himself/herself as powerless, helpless, and hopeless.

In general, *associated impairments of functioning* occur in more severe depressions and may have physical, academic, interpersonal, and behavioral manifestations. These impairments of functioning are:

1. Physical alterations
   Sleep pattern
   Eating pattern
   Energy pattern
   Somatic preoccupations
   Exacerbated medical condition
2. Academic
   School absence
   Visits to school nurse
   Drop in grades
3. Interpersonal
   Withdrawal from peers and family
   Increased isolation
   Increased conflict at home
4. Behavioral
   Suicide attempts
   Acting out
   Eating disorders

Physical alterations may involve changes in three physiologic patterns: sleep (excessive sleep or insomnia), eating (poor appetite and weight loss), and energy (psychomotor retardation, fatigue, and inability to concentrate). Exacerbation of both psychosomatic and chronic medical illnesses also may occur. Academic impairments may involve lower grades, poor work habits, school absence (often unreported), and visits to the school nurse.

A careful drug history is helpful in making the diagnosis. In general, exogenous substances tend to produce symptoms that mimic acute schizophrenia rather than acute depression. Amphetamine, cocaine, and hallucinogen withdrawal may produce some depression, but usually this effect is superficial and is often accompanied by severe agitation. Depression can be distinguished from schizophrenia because the depressed patient, however withdrawn and preoccupied, speaks in a goal-directed manner and may exhibit some warmth. Hallucinations and delusions are uncommon in adolescent depression and, when present, relate to themes of worthlessness.

Recognition and diagnosis of depression are the office-based physician's primary tasks. It is not always easy to distinguish between significant adolescent depression and the moodiness and lability that often accompanies this developmental period. However, in view of the increasing acceptability of self-destructive behavior among adolescents, both through individual acts and suicide pacts, it is especially prudent for the office-based physician to remain alert to the possibility of depression and to take a cautious approach. Screening for signs of depression should be done with every child and adolescent and should include questions about drug and alcohol use, school performance and attendance, family relationships, future plans, suicidal thoughts, and direct self-destructive behavior.

When discussion elicits concern on the part of the physician about a sad or suicidal child or adolescent, the physician should talk further to that patient, seeking to learn sources of stress, attempts at coping, and available sources of support. The physician should ask about the child's relationship with parents, the extent to which the child has shared his/her concerns with the parents, and how the child would expect the parents to react if they were aware of his/her crisis. Additional questions about suicide should focus on the immediate possibility of suicide on the part of the child or adolescent and

on the child's ability to make a firm nonsuicide agreement, first to the physician and later to the parents. With actively suicidal patients, immediate psychiatric referral, either to the pediatric emergency room or to an immediately available private psychiatrist, should be made. The physician should make certain that both parents are present or should have them come in immediately so that the parents can deal with the crisis together.

REFERRAL

The referral process may be more difficult with a depressed but not actively suicidal patient who needs psychiatric referral, because rationalization and denial may set in. The urgency created by an acutely suicidal or psychotic patient is absent in these cases. In addition, the referral recommendation is typically made by the physician only to the mother; as a result, the father may feel excluded and not support referral. To promote a successful psychiatric referral by avoiding some of these pitfalls, it is recommended that the office-based physician regularly take the following steps:

1. The physician, after talking with the child alone, should arrange for a family conference at which both parents (or other responsible adults) and the child are present. When the physician's relationship has been primarily with the mother rather than with both parents, the physician can offer, when relevant, to personally call the other important caretaker to request participation at the family conference.

2. The physician should help the child determine what he/she wants to share with the family at the conference. The physician should also review with the child what the physician plans to discuss at the family meeting, so that the child feels supported and his/her confidentiality is respected.

3. At the family conference, the physician needs to understand the primary concerns of the parents. If the parents identify the child's depression as a concern, the physician can recommend psychiatric referral on that basis. If the parents are not concerned about depression but identify specific changes in the child's functioning (eg, deterioration of school

performance, personal relationships, or participation in team sports), the physician can link these behavioral changes to the child's depression and offer psychiatric referral as a way to help the child resume his/her normal level of competence. If the parents are unreceptive to psychiatric referral and the child is not in crisis, the physician can propose a second meeting at a designated future time to review the child's progress. When making a referral the physician gives the family the name of a specific psychiatrist to call, whenever possible, and encourages the family to make immediate contact. The physician also assures the family that he/she will actively communicate with the psychiatrist and will remain available to the child and family.

BIBLIOGRAPHY

Brent DA: Depression and suicide in children and adolescents, *Pediatr Rev* 14(10):380–388, 1993.

Carter BD, Edwards JF, Kronenberger WG, et al: Case control study of chronic fatigue in pediatric patients, *Pediatrics* 95(2):179–186, 1995.

Ferro T, Carlson GA, Grayson P, Klein DN: Depressive disorders: Distinctions in children, *J Am Acad Child Adolesc Psychiatry* 33(5): 664–670, 1994.

Lewinsohn PM, Clarke GN: Major depression in community adolescents: Age at onset, episode duration, and time to recurrence, *J Am Acad Child Adolesc Psychiatry* 33(6):809–818, 1994.

Myers K, Troutman B: Developmental aspects of child and adolescent depression, *Curr Opin Pediatr* 5(4):419–424, 1993.

Pedersen W: Parental relations, mental health, and delinquency in adolescents, *Adolescence* 29(116):975–990, 1994.

Summerville MB, Kaslow NJ: Psychopathology, family functioning, and cognitive style in urban adolescents with suicide attempts, *J Abnorm Child Psychol* 22(2):221–235, 1994.

CHAPTER 127

Suicide Attempt

Gordon R. Hodas

The acutely suicidal patient, together with the acutely psychotic patient, represent the two most serious psychiatric emergencies that the office-based physician faces. Broadly defined, suicidal behavior involves thoughts or actions that may lead to self-inflicted serious injury or death. Suicidal ideation involves the wish or plan to die, not yet acted upon, whereas a suicidal attempt implies that actual behavior to take one's life has occurred. It is important for the office-based physician to regard all suicide attempts as serious and reject the notion of "suicidal gesture" for apparently less serious attempts, because many of these children may remain strongly suicidal and try again.

A suicide attempt by a child or adolescent signifies a cry for help as well as a breakdown in the system of mutual supports in the family that guides and protects a child while also promoting his/her autonomy. Therefore, the physician must select the treatment that addresses the needs of child and family and not just child alone. Most suicidal children are depressed, and all share a pervasive sense of hopelessness and helplessness. Alternate solutions are viewed as absent or unrealistic, and suicide is seen as the only solution for the child's and family's problems. In addition to depression, suicide attempts occur in the context of major losses (eg, serious illness or death in the family), major family conflict or instability (eg, separation, divorce, and physical or emotional abuse), and psychosis. Beyond the specific identified precipitants, childhood and adolescent suicide attempts are usually the culmination of preexisting problems of several years' duration.

Although incidence figures for both suicide attempts and successful suicides have climbed rapidly over the past 30 years, there has been some stabilization of incidence during the 1980s and 1990s. This trend is significant but should not be falsely reassuring. In contemporary American society, too often suicidal behavior is seen as an acceptable response to personal crisis and distress. At times suicide is even viewed as heroic. One consequence of these changing social values is adolescent suicide pacts, in which groups of adolescents try to kill themselves either by prior agreement or through a process of negative modeling. Such events have been common during the past decade and have created tragedies in many communities.

In addition to the recent trends described, it has been recognized for some time that suicide attempts and completed suicides often are underreported and are at times classified as accidents to avoid shame for the child and family. For children under 10 years of age, suicide is not even classified as a cause of death in registries. Available data indicate that suicide attempts occur in children as young as 5 years of age. For persons between 15 and 24 years of age, suicide is now the second leading cause of death. Furthermore, many accidents, especially motor vehicle collisions, are believed to be masked suicides.

Suicidal thinking is not uncommon in childhood and adolescence and can present in many psychiatric conditions. For example, 72% of children ages 6 to 12 years who were sequentially admitted to a psychiatric inpatient unit were found to have suicidal ideation or attempts. Suicidal thinking is even more common in depressed children. In one study, more than 80% of outpatient depressed children reported suicidal ideation during some point in their depression.

A suicide attempt by a boy is two times more likely to be fatal than one by a girl; on the other hand, girls attempt suicide at least three times more often than boys. Overall, approximately 80% of suicide attempts are by ingestion. More lethal methods (such as jumping, shooting, or attempted hanging) are more common with boys and often express greater suicidal intent. It would be incorrect to assume that other methods do not often reflect a genuine wish to die.

Because the majority of children and adolescents who have engaged in suicidal behavior have not been identified or treated by mental health professionals, the office-based physician can play an important screening role.

The office-based physician should suspect a possible suicide attempt with "accidental" ingestions, vehicular collisions, and other suspicious accidents. The index of suspicion is higher if the child appears sad, has made a previous suicide attempt, or comes from an unstable family environment. When younger children present with an accident or injury, the possibility of inadequate parental supervision or child abuse must be considered.

Immature conceptions of death by preadolescent children complicate the assessment of suicide attempts in that age group. Although variability exists, an appreciation of the irreversibility of death usually does not occur until the age of 9 years; even then the child may believe that, in his/her case, death will not be irreversible and will be pleasant. It is not until adolescence that the adult concept of an irreversible death is firmly in place.

OFFICE EVALUATION

Common characteristics associated with suicide attempts in children aged 6 to 12 years are:

1. Depression
2. Hopelessness
3. Low self-esteem
4. Worthlessness
5. Positive family history
6. Positive wish to die
7. Death seen as temporary

These characteristics distinguish high-risk suicidal children from other emotionally disturbed, but nonsuicidal children. The first four features, all related to significant depression, are juxtaposed with a wish to die without fully appreciating the irreversibility of death. A family history of suicide attempts increases the risk.

The sequence of events commonly associated with adolescent suicide attempts is summarized below, following the work of Joseph Teicher.

1. Continuing family instability
2. Withdrawal from parents and communication breakdown
3. Acute precipitating event, with loss of self-esteem

Typically, there is a history of family instability of many years' duration, characterized by residential and environmental changes and unexpected losses through divorce, illness, and suicide. With the onset of adolescence, a period of mutual alienation between parents and adolescent may occur, characterized by withdrawal, misunderstandings, and communication breakdown. This further loss of support, coming at a time of developmental transition, lowers the adolescent's self-esteem, rendering him/her vulnerable to an acute disappointment (eg, peer rejection, broken romance, poor grades), which may precipitate a suicide attempt.

High-risk suicide situations for children and adolescents are summarized below.

1. Attempted suicide
2. Threatened or planned suicide
3. Desire for death
4. "Accidental" ingestion or other questionable accident
5. Severe depression
6. Significant interpersonal withdrawal
7. Sadness and recurrent somatic complaints
8. Violence
9. Psychosis

As can be seen, many different clinical situations may be associated with a high risk for suicide.

The office-based physician should be alert to these possibilities so that further assessment and treatment can be pursued when indicated.

MANAGEMENT

With an immediate suicide attempt, the goal is to get the child and family to the pediatric emergency room as soon as possible so that proper medical treatment can be provided and further evaluation pursued. With a child who admits to serious suicidal intent without an overt attempt, either emergency room evaluation or direct psychiatric referral is indicated. When a child or adolescent admits to a recent suicide attempt that no longer requires medical evaluation or treatment, psychiatric referral is appropriate unless continuing suicidal intent necessitates emergency room evaluation and possible hospitalization.

As a general guide, the following four principles of assessment and management are offered:

1. *Routinely screen for suicide ideation.* The screening for suicidal ideation, especially with adolescents, should not be neglected even when a patient does not appear depressed or under obvious stress. The physician should raise the question of suicide in a matter-of-fact manner. (Physician: "How often do you feel down?" "When you get really down, do you sometimes wish you were dead or think of killing yourself?") With higher-risk children, questioning about suicide should be more extensive. (Physician: "When you're really sad like this, do you sometimes wish you were dead?" "Have you been feeling that way lately?" "Have you tried to kill yourself?")
2. *Consider all suspicious accidents to be possible suicide attempts.* In this way, the office-based physician may detect a seriously depressed child and prevent a completed suicide.
3. *Regard all suicide attempts as serious.* Some suicide attempts may have only limited medical consequences but that does not mean they are not serious (the child who takes 10 diazepam [Valium] tablets and survives may be just as suicidal as the child who takes 10 digitalis pills and dies). It is suicidal intent that matters. It is important for the physician

to ask not only about the immediate precipitant to the suicide attempt but also about long-standing sources of concern to the child.

4. *Determine the level of suicidal intent—the actual wish to die—with all suicide attempts.* This includes the child's direct statements about dying and is also reflected in the child's overall mental status and in the nature of the actual suicide attempt.

The systematic assessment of a suicidal child or adolescent involves an appreciation of the child's current medical status and his/her wish to die and context of support. Critical information is gained through assessment of medical lethality, suicidal intent, and strengths of the child, the family, and social context.

Medical lethality refers to the severity of the medical consequences of a suicide attempt.

Assessing Medical Lethality

1. Need for emergency room treatment
2. Vital signs
3. Loss of consciousness
4. Evidence of drug/alcohol intoxication (*eg*, pupils, smell on breath)
5. Need for emesis, lavage, and catharsis
6. Acute medical complications: cardiac complications, respiratory arrest, convulsions
7. Indications for medical hospitalization
8. Indications for intensive care treatment
9. Residual abnormalities

The physician assesses such factors as the necessity for emergency room treatment, alteration of vital signs, loss of consciousness, signs of drug or alcohol intoxication, and development of acute complications such as cardiac complications, or respiratory arrest and seizures. The physician also should evaluate the requirement of medical or intensive care hospitalization and possible residual effects of the attempt.

Suicidal intent is inferred by the physician following a suicide attempt based on the circumstances of the attempt, the patient's self-report of the seriousness of his/her intent at the time of the attempt, and an assessment of the child's mental status.

Assessing Suicidal Intent—Wish to Die

- Circumstances of suicide attempt (from child and family)
   Use of violent means (hanging, shooting, jumping, deliberate car accident)
   All available pills ingested

   Use of multiple pills and alcohol
   Hidden suicide note
   Child found unexpectedly
   Previous suicide attempts
- Child's self-report
   Premeditation of attempt
   Irreversible concept of death
   Nature of precipitating stresses
   Anticipation of death
   Desire for death, then and now
   Attempt to conceal suicide attempt
- Child's mental status
   Orientation and possible psychosis
   Unwillingness to relate to or cooperate with physician
   Unwillingness to accept family support
   Negative orientation toward future
   Continuing suicidal impulses

It is important to determine how serious the suicide intent was and the extent of continuing suicide risk. It is strongly recommended that the physician rely not only on the data regarding circumstances and self-report, but also on his/her overall impression of the child as revealed in the physician-patient relationship. A child who relates warmly to the physician and expresses remorse is usually a better risk than one who verbalizes the risk to die or continues to deny the attempt.

Finally, the physician should evaluate the *strengths of child, family, and social context.*

Assessing Strengths and Supports

- Strengths and assets of child
   Ability to relate to physician
   Ability to utilize parents
   Ability to acknowledge problem
   Positive orientation toward future
- Strengths and assets of family
   Commitment to child
   Ability to unite during current crisis
   Ability to unite during past crises
   Problem-solving abilities
   Capacity to supervise child
   Ability to utilize external supports
- Nature of external supports
   Family physician, pediatrician, psychiatrist
   Extended family
   Neighbors, other significant adults
   Religious community

Because a suicide attempt represents a fundamental crisis in child development and parenting, it is essential that the physician seek out all possible strengths and supports. As listed above, these include strengths of the family and child and the strengths offered by external supports. It is only by appreciating these strengths that a safe and realistic plan can be undertaken.

Every suicide attempt, regardless of its apparent seriousness, requires psychiatric consultation for that patient, and some patients will require psychiatric hospitalization. The nature of the psychiatric involvement will depend on the circumstances of the suicide attempt. The alert child can be interviewed alone and with the parents in the emergency room, whereas the obtunded child may need to be seen the next morning on the medical floor on which he/she is hospitalized. When psychiatric hospitalization is deemed necessary, it should be effected as soon as the child has been cleared medically. Psychiatric hospitalization becomes substantially easier when the office-based physician prepares the child and parents for the possibility and then supports the decision once made. On occasion, the emergency psychiatrist may need to initiate an involuntary commitment for psychiatric hospitalization.

The primary physician should arrange for immediate psychiatric referral for those patients who do not require psychiatric hospitalization. This is best achieved by addressing both parents, either alone or in the presence of the child. The physician should contact the family shortly after this to be sure that his/her recommendations for psychiatric care were followed. In like manner, when the physician learns about a suicide attempt made weeks or months earlier, it is imperative that he/she not be lured into the denial pattern that the patient may be demonstrating. *All suicide attempts, regardless of when they are detected, should receive psychiatric consultation and referral.* Hospitalization is indicated under the following circumstances: 1) the physician has had difficulty in gaining the cooperation of the child and family, 2) the child has made a serious suicide attempt and continues to have strong suicidal intent, 3) the child has made a repeated suicide attempt, 4) the child is psychotic, 5) the family appears unable to provide necessary supervision and support to the child, and 6) there is rapid denial by child and family of the significance of a serious suicide attempt.

After psychiatric referral, the office-based physician maintains a health-oriented primary care relationship with child and family. The physician and treating psychiatrist should communicate regularly so that each is aware of and can support the other's efforts. The physician should appreciate that, with appropriate individual and family psychotherapy, suicidal children and adolescents with their families are often able to reverse the self-destructive cycle and move constructively ahead into the future.

BIBLIOGRAPHY

Adams DM, Overholser JC, Lehnert KL: Perceived family functioning and adolescent suicidal behavior, *J Am Acad Child Adolesc Psychiatry* 33(4):498–507, 1994.

Brent DA: Depression and suicide in children and adolescents, *Pediatr Rev* 14(10):380–388, 1993.

Duncan J: The immediate management of suicide attempts in children and adolescents: Psychological aspects, *J Fam Pract* 4:77–80, 1977.

Garfinkel BD, Golombek H: Suicide and depression in childhood and adolescence, *Can Med Assoc J* 110:1278–1281, 1974.

Hofman A: Adolescents in distress: Suicide and out of control behavior, *Med Clin North Am* 59(6):1429–1437, 1975.

Teicher J: Children and adolescents who attempt suicide, *Pediatr Clin North Am* 17:687–697, 1970.

CHAPTER 128

Drug and Alcohol Abuse

John Sargent

In recent years, it has been estimated that between 80% and 90% of adolescents in the United States have used a drug for nonmedical purposes. The use of these substances to alter mood, perception, and behavior has become an integral part of coming of age in our society. Many young people experiment with drugs and do not repeat the experience. Others use the drugs intermittently, or regularly, in a controlled fashion and suffer few adverse consequences. For some, however, early experimentation may progress to a pattern of abuse that becomes compulsive and repetitive and may become associated with physical and psychosocial deterioration. In addition to psychological difficulties that can arise as a result of the effects of the drug use, these substances interfere with other developmentally important behaviors and experiences during adolescence. Furthermore, irresponsible drug and alcohol use can lead to death or disability due to accidents that occur under the influence of these substances.

It is important for the primary care physician to be familiar with different categories of adolescent drug use. The majority of adolescent drug use is *experimental* and carried out for its effects on mood or behavior. Experimental drug use is controlled and limited to specific situations and the adolescent ingests enough of the drug to alter his/her mood, but rarely enough to cause acute intoxication or overdose. *Intoxication* refers to significant use of a given drug on a particular occasion that will lead to a dramatic alteration in mood, behavior, and physical status that interferes with judgment, inhibition, and control of behavior and places the drug user at significant risk, especially if engaging in dangerous activities. *Overdose* refers to the excessive use of a drug that interferes with bodily functions and can lead to significant physiologic impairment or death. *Habituation* describes a pattern of repetitive drug use that is compulsive and engaged in regardless

of external circumstances. *Addiction* implies physical dependency on a drug with physiologic symptoms resulting from abrupt cessation of its use. Addiction occurs only with substances that induce *tolerance,* a decreased effect from repeated administration of the same dose of a specific drug. Habituation and addiction describe patterns of drug use over time, whereas intoxication and overdose refer to a response to a drug ingestion on one particular occasion.

As the physician deals with adolescent substance use, it is always important for him/her to bear in mind the age and developmental stage of each adolescent and the expectations and mores of that adolescent's family and culture. The primary care physician will find that drug or alcohol use may be a problem for particular teenagers or their families at different stages of use. Some families may find infrequent use of drugs to be problematic, even though it is intermittent and controlled by the adolescent, whereas other families may not be significantly concerned even though the adolescent's use of a drug has become repetitive and may be interfering with that adolescent's overall functioning.

Drug and alcohol use among adolescents is culturally influenced and can be supported by the teenager's peer group. An adolescent's use of a particular substance may reflect both use in the adolescent's family as well as the activities of that adolescent's peers. Studies of adolescents who use drugs repeatedly indicate that these youths, who harbor a more critical attitude toward conventional society, often place a higher value on independence and autonomy and lower values on academic achievement. The use of drugs also may be reinforced by a perceived lack of confidence and competency, lack of attention and support within the family, and a lack of overall adaptation to the academic environment.

Drug use is an age-graded behavior. It can be

seen by adolescents as a developmental milestone and, therefore, is identified as a marker of enhanced maturity. There is often a hierarchy of drug use. Cigarettes and alcohol often are tried first, marijuana subsequently. A smaller proportion of adolescents may try other drugs of abuse, including opiates, hallucinogens, cocaine, or amphetamines. Drug use is a learned behavior. The adolescent experiences a sense of belonging and participation within the peer group through the use of drugs or alcohol, and often drugs are used as recreation. The adolescent then associates stress reduction and social pleasure with drug use, and this association continues through repetitive use. The adolescent also may gain a feeling of independence through drug use. The adolescent's view of himself/herself begins to include substance use as well as the lack of other enjoyments without drug use. As the adolescent increasingly withdraws from other experiences and fails to continue to participate in other aspects of teenage behavior, developmental lags can occur that further reinforce repetitive drug or alcohol use. Substance abuse, then, can lead to a stance of pseudoindependence and pseudoconfidence for the adolescent who believes that he/she is in control of his/her behavior. However, the adolescent does not take responsibility for problems resulting from the drug use. At the same time, family, school, and other social systems often react in a helpless fashion, leaving the adolescent increasingly isolated and his/her drug use out of control.

Drug use during adulthood most closely resembles the amount and frequency of drug use in an individual's family, rather than drug use among adolescent peers. Excessive drug use is commonly a time-limited behavior, with a decrease in use often occurring after approximately 10 years. There is evidence that individuals are more likely to have difficulty with substance abuse if they begin to use drugs or alcohol prior to age 15, as opposed to beginning use in later years. The physician should identify patterns of substance use in parents and adult relatives as he/she works with adolescents who have difficulties with drug use. Drug use is more worrisome when associated with other problem behaviors such as truancy, marked aggressiveness, communication problems within the family, runaway behavior, or sexual promiscuity. Drug and alcohol use is also a greater concern when the substance use interferes with school or work performance or with participation in other peer group activities

that might lead to a sense of increased competency and social effectiveness. Both alcohol and marijuana are depressants, and although their use may be relaxing, it can also lead to a worsening of pre-existing depression in an adolescent. Because adolescents with mood or adjustment disorders more commonly have chronic drug use, it is important for the physician to pay attention to the potential for suicide, either through the adolescent's deliberate or inadvertent overdosage or through self-destructive behavior such as driving a car under the influence of an exogenous substance.

An adolescent who is confused about goals for his/her life may use drugs and alcohol more excessively. Drug use is likely to become a more significant problem when poverty or educational deficiencies are also present. This is also the case when the adolescent experiences education and other peer group activities as ritualized, uninvolving, and unsatisfying. Adolescents may use drugs in a repetitive fashion when they are experiencing significant emotional distress. In these situations, the drug or alcohol use may actually be an attempt to relieve the pain of a psychiatric disorder through self-medication. It is also important for the primary care physician to remember that adolescents may have accurate information about the effects of drugs on their mood or behavior at the same time as they are misinformed about the effects of drugs on their judgment or physiology. Adolescents often do not recognize these effects on their judgment, leading them when intoxicated, to engage in highly risky behavior, especially unprotected sexual activity or violence. It is not unusual for teenagers, when under the influence of alcohol or drugs, to engage in date rape or unwanted sex, for which they later feel extremely guilty or ashamed. In general, the teenager's use of drugs is goal-directed, although the adolescent's lack of judgment or control in specific circumstances may affect the amount consumed.

TYPES OF DRUGS

Table 128-1 reviews commonly abused substances and describes toxic signs, treatment of intoxication, signs of overdose, and treatment of acute overdoses. References are provided in the bibliography for further information concerning the treatment of severe overdosages with these substances. Alcohol, the most commonly used

TABLE 128-1
Common Drug Poisonings, Signs of Toxic Effects, and Treatment*

DRUG	MILD TOXIC SIGNS	SPECIMEN FOR DIAGNOSIS	TREATMENT	SEVERE OVERDOSE SIGNS	TREATMENT
Opiates					
Heroin Morphine Demerol Methadone	"Nodding" drowsiness, small pupils, urinary retention, slow and shallow breathing; skin scars and subcutaneous abscesses; duration 4–6 hr; with methadone, duration to 24 hr	Blood, urine	Naloxone (Narcan) 0.01 mg/kg intravenously	Coma; pinpoint pupils, slow irregular respiration or apnea, hypotension, hypothermia, pulmonary edema	Naloxone
Depressants					
Alcohol	Confusion, rousable drowsiness, delirium, ataxia, nystagmus, dysarthria, analgesia to stimuli	Blood, urine, breath	Alcohol excitement: diazepam or chlorpromazine	Stupor to coma; pupils reactive, usually constricted; oculovestibular response absent; motor tonus initially briefly hyperactive then flaccid; respiration and blood pressure depressed; hypothermia; with glutethimide, pupils moderately dilated, can be fixed; with meprobamate, withdrawal seizures common; with methaqualone, coma, occasional convulsions, tachycardia, cardiac failure, bleeding tendency	Intubate, ventilate, gavage; drainage position; antimicrobials; keep mean blood pressure above 90 mm Hg and urine output 300 mL/hr; avoid analeptics; hemodialyze for severe phenobarbital poisoning
Barbiturates		Blood			
Glutethimide (Doriden)		Blood	None needed for acute toxicity; withdraw drug under supervision if patient is chronic user		
Meprobamate (Equanil)		Blood			
Methaqualone (Quaalude, Sopor, Mandrax)	Hallucinations, agitation, motor hyperactivity, myoclonus, tonic spasms	Blood, urine			
Chlordiazepoxide (Librium)	Usually taken with another sedative if poisoning is attempted	Blood			As above; diuresis of little help
Diazepam (Valium)		Urine			

*From Wyngaarden JB, SMith LH, editors: *Cecil textbook of medicine,* 17th ed, Philadelphia, 1985, WB Saunders. Used by permission.

substance of abuse consumed by adolescents, is used most often in social situations. Within the past 10 years initiation into alcohol use has occurred at increasingly younger ages, frequently in junior high school. The psychoactive effects of alcohol are similar to those of other depressants and tranquilizers. The degree of intoxication depends on the amount of alcohol consumed and correlates roughly with blood alcohol levels. Mild intoxication may lead to reduction in anxiety, and individuals who are mildly intoxicated may feel that they perform more readily in social situations. Alcohol use becomes a significant problem as the user becomes increasingly depen-

TABLE 128-1
Common Drug Poisonings, Signs of Toxic Effects, and Treatment—cont'd

DRUG	MILD TOXIC SIGNS	SPECIMEN FOR DIAGNOSIS	TREATMENT	SEVERE OVERDOSE SIGNS	TREATMENT
Stimulants					
Amphetamines Methylpheni- date	Hyperactive, ag- gressive, some- times paranoid, repetitive be- havior; dilated pupils, tremor, hyperactive re- flexes; hyper- thermia, tachy- cardia, arrhyth- mia; acute tor- sion dystonia	Blood, urine	Reassurance if mild Diazepam or chlorproma- zine if severe	Agitated, assaul- tive and para- noid excite- ment; occa- sionally convul- sions; hypother- mia; circulatory collapse	Chlorpromazine
Cocaine	Similar but less prominent than above; less par- anoid, often eu- phoric	Blood	Reassurance Diazepam or chlorproma- zine	Twitching, irregu- lar breathing, tachycardia	Sedation
Psychedelics LSD Mescaline Psilocybin STP Phencyclidine	Confused, disori- ented, percep- tual distortions, distractable, withdrawn or eruptive, lead- ing to accidents or violence; wide-eyed, di- lated pupils; restless, hyper- reflexic; less of- ten, hyperten- sion or tachy- cardia		Reassurance; "talk down;" do not leave alone Diazepam	Panic	Reassure; diaz- epam satisfac- tory; avoid phe- nothiazines Symptomatic supportive; Acidify urine with ammonium chloride
Atropine- scopolamine (Sominex)	Agitated or con- fused, visual hallucinations, dilated pupils, flushed and dry skin		Reassure	Toxic disoriented delirium, visual hallucination; later, amnesia, fever, dilated fixed pupils, hot flushed dry skin, urinary re- tention	Reassure; sedate lightly; 1) avoid phenothiazines; 2) do not leave alone
Antidepressants Imipramine (Tofranil) Amitriptyline (Elavil)	Restlessness, drowsiness, tachycardia, ataxia, sweating	Blood		Agitation, vomit- ing, hyperpy- rexia, sweating, muscle dysto- nia, convul- sions, tachy- cardia or ar- rhythmia	Symptomatic; gastric lavage
MAO inhibitors Tranylcypro- mine (Parnate) Phenelzine (Nardil) Pargyline (Eutonyl)	Hypertensive cri- ses, agitation, drowsiness, ataxia	Blood	Withdrawal	Hypotension; headache; chest pain; agitation; co- ma, seizures, and shock	Symptomatic; gastric lavage
Phenothiazines	Acute dystonia, somnolence, hypotension	Blood	Benadryl 0.50; withdrawal	Coma; convul- sions (rare); arrhythmias; hypotension	Symptomatic; gastric lavage

dent on the alcohol for its effect in reducing anxiety and increasing ease of performance in social situations. Problem drinking also may develop as a reaction to a stressful situation, especially within the adolescent's family or peer group. Alcohol consumption then becomes increasingly frequent and may begin to occur when the adolescent is alone as he/she prepares for worrisome or potentially stressful situations. The acute intoxicating effects of alcohol are important causes of disability and death among young people. These acute effects may include overdosage, suicide, violent behavior, or accidents. Any physician working with adolescents will need to strongly reinforce the fact that adolescents should never drive when drinking (or after). Alcoholism is rare among adolescents, but chronic alcohol use can lead to significant worsening in school performance and social adjustment.

Marijuana is the second most commonly used substance by adolescents. Half of those teenagers who use alcohol also use marijuana. It affects perception, behavior, and emotional state. It may lead to an increased sense of well-being or euphoria, accompanied by feelings of relaxation or sleepiness. Differential effects of marijuana may be seen due to differences in amount ingested of its active substance tetrahydrocannabinol (THC). With increasing ingestion, marijuana may significantly interfere with information processing, attention, and perception, as well as performance of simple motor tasks and reaction time. Thinking may become confused and disorganized, and altered time perception is a frequently noticed effect. Excessive doses of marijuana can induce hallucinations and depersonalization, although most smokers can adjust the dosage to avoid severely unpleasant effects. It is important for adolescents to appreciate that marijuana use may significantly interfere with performance of motor tasks, especially driving a car.

Adolescents currently use other drugs much less frequently and often in an experimental fashion. Less than 0.5% of all adolescents use any other drug in a repetitive fashion. Phencyclidine (PCP) is a commonly used hallucinogen that may lead to bizarre behavior, an inability to integrate sensory input, changes in body image, and marked disorganization of thinking. PCP is generally used to increase sensitivity to external stimuli and to elevate mood, but it may induce hallucinations and a frightening disorientation

that may persist for up to 2 to 3 days. The use of LSD and other psychedelic drugs also alters perceptions and leads to hallucinations, alteration of subjective time, and marked lability of mood. The use of LSD appears to be increasing again among adolescents, especially younger teenagers and teens with significant emotional difficulties, which increases the risk of dangerous or frightening experiences while under the influence of the drug. Acute and chronic use of PCP warrants complete medical evaluation, and the patient may require hospitalization when acutely intoxicated for monitoring, protection, and support, while the symptoms of disorientation and panic persist.

Stimulants such as amphetamines and cocaine are used to heighten the sense of accomplishment, induce a feeling of well-being, and reduce fatigue. Amphetamines and cocaine also may lead to a feeling of euphoria, excitement, and a perception of enhanced clarity of thinking. Their use may be extremely reinforcing, leading to chronic repetitive use. Acute overdosage may lead to extreme anxiety, assaultiveness, hallucinations, and psychotic effects. Chronic overdosage with both cocaine and amphetamines can lead to visual hallucinations and paranoid delusions; chronic use of cocaine can lead to increased craving of the drug, with heightened irritability and depression and discomfort when the user is not able to obtain the substance. Massive overdose of cocaine also can lead to cardiac arrest and sudden death.

Recently there has been a significant increase in the use of cocaine. Most worrisome has been the popularity of smoking the crystalline form of cocaine, crack. This has become readily available and inexpensive and has been used regularly by disaffected adolescents involved in alcohol and drug abuse. Crack is especially dangerous because of its powerful addictive quality. Physicians who learn that an adolescent is using crack regularly will want to discuss the danger of that substance frankly with the adolescent and refer the young person for inpatient drug rehabilitation treatment.

Sedatives are less frequently used by adolescents and are generally used in association with other drugs. They induce a feeling of peace and tranquility and a reduction in anxiety and inhibition. It is possible, but unusual, to find adolescents physically dependent on sedatives. The use of opioids, including heroin, has become more common among adolescents within the past 20 years. However, their use continues to depend on availability and patterns of substance abuse among a particular teenager's peer group. Heroin use continues to be more common in poor environments where adolescents have limited alternative opportunities for expression and accomplishment. Users of opioids often develop a pattern of addiction and physical dependence. Physical problems seen in drug addicts including phlebitis, endocarditis, and malnutrition are common complications of chronic heroin use that the physician must be prepared to identify and treat in individuals with a history of opioid ingestion. The risk of exposure to HIV, through the use of unsterilized needles among intravenous drug users, also must be considered.

During routine outpatient care, the primary care physician should question adolescents about drug use. The adolescent's pattern of drug use and associated psychosocial adjustment should be ascertained. It is rare that an adolescent will visit the physician specifically for difficulties with drugs or alcohol, although visits for somatic symptoms or anxiety or psychologic concerns may mask worries about substance abuse. In obtaining the history, the physician should identify which drugs are used, how much is ingested at any particular time, and how frequently and under what circumstances the drug is used. It is also extremely important for the physician to determine from the adolescent the reason why he/she is using a particular substance and to appreciate the adolescent's knowledge about the effects and dangers of the drugs used. As has been stated previously, tension, boredom, anxiety, a feeling of inadequacy, curiosity, or an attempt to alter perceptions or activity level may lead an adolescent to experiment with drugs or use them regularly. The physician may learn more about an adolescent's drug use by interviewing the teenager alone. The physician also should determine what the parents know about the teenager's drug use and their response to it. The physician also should note the parents' appreciation of the difficulties the adolescent is experiencing that may be reinforcing drug use and their attempts to help the teenager decrease these stresses.

The primary care physician also should obtain a profile of the adolescent's functioning in school and peer-group activities; identify the adolescent's interests, overall accomplishments, sense of competency, and self-esteem; and understand the adolescent's relationship within his/her family. In addition to obtaining a history concerning drug or alcohol use, the physician should learn the teenager's impressions of his/her drug use and ability to control the drug use and to vary his/her sources of recreation. The physician also should learn if the adolescent experiences any difficulties in association with his/her drug use, including social isolation because of the drug use. Use of drugs and alcohol in adolescence becomes drug abuse when it is an ineffective way of coping with developmental or environmental stresses or when the drug use itself leads to further difficulties in overall psychosocial functioning. The physician will also want to obtain information from parents concerning their impressions of the adolescent's psychologic well-being and social functioning. A complete examination is often helpful in identifying any physical effects of drug use and especially in identifying physical difficulties associated with repetitive use of substances such as amphetamines or sedatives.

At the close of his/her evaluation, the physician will have developed an impression of 1) the seriousness of the drug use itself and its potential acute and chronic ill effects, 2) the adolescent's psychosocial level of adaptation, and 3) the opinions of the adolescent's family concerning both drug use and emotional and behavioral difficulties associated with it. As a result of this evaluation, the pediatrician can determine whether an adolescent's use of drugs is experimental and controlled or if it is repetitive or habitual and indicative of severe adjustment problems.

MANAGEMENT

For the group of adolescents for whom drug use is experimental and for whom there are no significant associated difficulties in functioning, the physician should involve the family to support the adolescent's accomplishments, to encourage alternative recreational experiences, and to provide adequate supervision for the adolescent. The physician should discuss drug use during health maintenance visits and will especially want to ensure that adolescents and their families have accurate information concerning alcohol, drugs, and smoking. The physician should point out the addictive qualities of nicotine, alcohol, cocaine, and crack and help adolescents recognize the danger of street drugs and PCP.

Adequate supervision will include helping the parents set rules about drug use. These rules should be aimed at preventing irresponsible drug use and drug or alcohol use in unsupervised situations or among younger adolescents. The physician also should strongly encourage communication and emotional support within the family. Consideration of the adolescent's age, the type of substance, and the circumstances of substance use are important in these decisions. The physician should avoid power struggles with adolescents and help parents recognize that they are capable of limiting their teenager's behavior and ensuring his/her safety. It is probable that adolescents under the legal drinking age may experiment with alcohol use, and parents need to strongly reinforce and support good judgment concerning this. The parents need to feel that they can limit drinking or drug use in an uncontrolled fashion and can prevent driving when under the influence of either alcohol or marijuana. The physician's goal should be to help the family and the teenager to make responsible choices about drug and alcohol use. The physician will then help the family to ensure that the adolescent continues to develop in other areas of his/her life, learns varied methods of obtaining pleasure and enjoyment, and learns to be able to identify and discuss stresses and anxieties that he/she is experiencing and to react to difficult circumstances without habitually using exogenous substances.

Adolescents with patterns of frequent or habitual drug use will require referral for mental health treatment, ideally treatment involving the entire family. Patterns of frequent drug use in association with other evidence of poor adaptation and family difficulties require outpatient psychotherapy for the entire family. Adolescents with habitual drug use, significant underlying psychopathology, and serious family problems may need inpatient care followed by regular outpatient individual and family therapy and regular urine monitoring for drug use. Patients with physical dependency on a drug will need hospitalization to supervise withdrawal from the drug. The physician and psychiatric consultant also will identify specific adolescents and families with serious drug-related problems who require the special expertise of an inpatient drug-treatment program for adolescents.

ANTICIPATORY GUIDANCE

The physician can counsel families with adolescents concerning drug and alcohol use as part of anticipatory guidance in adolescent primary care. The physician should ensure that both teenagers and their families have adequate information concerning the potentially dangerous effects of alcohol and psychoactive drugs and prepare them as a family to make decisions concerning appropriate recreational use of drugs. A family will do better by discussing these issues openly. In areas where there are not organized programs for education, the physician will need to work with school personnel and the school system to heighten parents' sense of responsibility and surveillance concerning the use of these substances at parties. Schools often have programs to deal with substance abuse that can be reinforced by the pediatrician. The physician can support strong community efforts to limit teenage substance use and driving under the influence of either alcohol or marijuana. Physicians also can help school personnel to identify adolescents with particular adjustment difficulties and associated substance abuse and then assist in referral for appropriate mental health treatment.

BIBLIOGRAPHY

Adger H Jr: Problems of alcohol and other drug use and abuse in adolescents, *J Adolesc Health* 12(8):606–613, 1991.

Johnson RL: Drug abuse, *Red Rev* 16(5):197–199, 1995.

Swadi H: Drug abuse in children and adolescents: Update, *Arch Dis Child* 67(10):1245–1246, 1992.

CHAPTER 129

Eating Disorders

John Sargent

Anorexia nervosa and bulimia, prototypes of biopsychosocial disorders, represent diagnostic and therapeutic challenges for the primary care physician who must complete physical, psychologic, and familial assessments and direct the interventions necessary to have the patient recover and change the pattern of adapting to stress. Because the management of these serious and potentially fatal disorders is beyond the area of primary care, the doctor must recognize early signs and symptoms and be able to refer the patient for appropriate therapy. This chapter also will explain the dynamics of families of these patients and several therapeutic plans.

ANOREXIA NERVOSA

Anorexia nervosa is the diagnosis applied to individuals, mostly women, who demonstrate a relentless pursuit of thinness and an absolute refusal to maintain minimum body weight. Weight loss is achieved through reduction in dietary caloric intake, especially foods containing carbohydrates and fats. For some patients, weight loss also is achieved through the use of diet pills, vomiting, laxatives, or diuretics. Because of a marked disturbance in body image, the patient experiences himself/herself as fat even when underweight, and feels strongly that he/she needs to diet to lose more weight. The term *anorexia* is, in fact, a misnomer because there is no loss of appetite, only the absolute control of appetite by the patient. In anorexia there is no known physical or psychiatric disorder to account for the weight loss. However, anorexia nervosa can occur in association with chronic underlying physical and psychiatric illness. The identification and treatment of anorexia nervosa should occur when a patient is under a minimum healthy weight for age, sex, and height; continues to diet; and strongly believes that he/she needs to lose more weight. The diagnosis of anorexia is a positive diagnosis that is reached through obtaining a history of relentless, intractable dieting and weight loss and an absolute refusal to begin to eat more to maintain normal weight. Ninety-five percent of cases of anorexia are in women. The onset of the disorder occurs more often in adolescence, and currently one in 200 adolescent girls develops the symptoms of anorexia. There is no identified specific organic etiology for anorexia nervosa. Anorexia can and often does become chronic, with the symptoms extending over years. Mortality associated with anorexia has been estimated to be 5% to 10%.

Clinical Features

The primary physical features of anorexia nervosa occur as a result of starvation. Patients with anorexia have significant disturbances in endocrine function associated with starvation-induced hypothalamic disturbances that usually resolve with weight gain. Patients generally have low body temperature, low pulse rate, and low blood pressure. They may have significant gastrointestinal complaints, including abdominal pain, and may experience bloating when eating small amounts of food. At significantly low weight, patients have muscle wasting, weakness, and slow movements. They may have marked thinning of their hair as well as the development of fine lanugo hair over their body. Although thyroid hormone levels are generally within normal limits, patients usually complain of being cold when others are warm; often the patients are amenorrheic. At moderate amounts of weight loss, there are generally no other significant physical disturbances and results of most laboratory studies are within normal limits. Patients may have a slight amount of leukopenia, with white blood cell counts in the range of 4000/mm³, and hemoglobin level may be increased, usually on the basis of chronic dehydration and reduction in level of total body fluids. Death generally occurs because of cardiovascular collapse only after more than a 40% weight loss. Patients often think slowly and in a rigid fashion. They may identify problems in concentrating. With severe weight loss, an organic psychosis can occur. Patients who use laxatives or vomit regularly also can have alterations in electrolyte levels, with vomiting resulting in hypokalemic alkalosis and laxative abuse leading to dehydration.

Resumption of normal dietary intake and cessation of vomiting generally lead to physical recovery. Upon refeeding, some patients, after prolonged periods of malnutrition, may have gastrointestinal complaints, malabsorption, and diarrhea. This generally occurs only in patients whose dietary intake has been under 500 calories/day. Dramatic increases in caloric intake from 500 calories/day to 3500 to 5000 calories/day over a short period of time have resulted in the development of cardiac failure, which was reversed when caloric intake was reduced. Moderate caloric intake of 2500 to 3000 calories/day after slowly increasing caloric intake by 200 calories/day has been tolerated well by patients recovering from anorexia.

Psychologic and Behavioral Features

Patients with anorexia nervosa demonstrate characteristic psychologic and behavioral disturbances. They deny other problems and state that they feel fine, have no physical complaints, and only need to lose a few more pounds. They report a pervasive sense of helplessness and ineffectiveness and, when asked, generally have little respect for their previous accomplishments. An individual with anorexia also may be markedly nonassertive. He/she is generally perfectionistic and may describe himself/herself as feeling out of control. His/her weight loss gives him/her a sense of mastery and control. He/she generally does not disagree overtly and yet maintains a stance of intractability through resistance. The patient usually is brought to the physician's attention by someone else (most often his/her parents) rather than coming voluntarily. The patient may be very attentive to his/her parents' feelings and highly concerned for the well-being of his/her family.

Patients with anorexia nervosa may have bizarre or unusual eating habits; they may eat in a compulsive fashion and often refuse to eat with others, eating only in private. They also may compulsively exercise, usually performing it in a ritualized fashion and not for fun, but rather for its continued effect on caloric consumption, inducing weight loss. Most patients continue to attend school, studying excessively for hours at a time. The patient is usually socially isolated and withdrawn from peers and group activities. Individuals with anorexia also may become highly emotional and upset when frustrated. The symptoms of anorexia may develop after a significant psychosocial stress such as loss of a boyfriend or divorce or death of a parent or may develop following an increased awareness of one's body or disappointment with one's accomplishments or attractiveness. Individuals who develop anorexia have been unhappy and dissatisfied with themselves for some time prior to the onset of dieting and weight loss. Dieting and weight loss lead to a worsening of the psychologic state and increased social withdrawal, which further reinforce focus on weight and dieting behavior.

Differential Diagnosis

The differential diagnosis for anorexia nervosa includes other causes of weight loss and appetite restriction. It is rare, however, for significant organic illnesses to mimic the psychologic and behavioral features of anorexia as well as its purposeful and relentless course. Chronic gastrointestinal disease including Crohn disease or ulcerative colitis can present with reduction in food intake and abdominal pain and frequently diarrhea, gastrointestinal bleeding, and evidence of malabsorption. Patients with cancer may have significant weight loss and reduction in appetite. However, these patients do not diet and lose weight on purpose. Central nervous system tumors and Addison disease have also, at times, been confused with anorexia. However, in the appropriate age range, history and physical examination appear to clearly differentiate anorexia from chronic organic illness.

The Family and Anorexia

Minuchin and colleagues investigated the interaction of families with an anorectic member at the time the symptoms were present. Five predominant characteristics of family interaction were present in these families and detrimental to overall family functioning: enmeshment, overprotectiveness, rigidity, lack of conflict resolution, and involvement of the sick child in unresolved parental conflict.

Enmeshment refers to a tight web of family relationships in which family members are highly sensitive to one another. They often infer moods and needs of others and submerge individual interests for the good of the whole. Overt criticism is rare. Enmeshment characterizes appropriate relationships between spouses or parents and adolescents or young adults. *Overprotectiveness* describes a relationship in which autonomy is sacrificed and highly nurturant interactions predominate. Family members feel a strong sense of vulnerability. The anorectic patient is often as highly protective of his/her parents and siblings as they are of him/her. Within these families, the interactions of enmeshment, protectiveness, and conflict avoidance are rigidly preferred. Even at times of stress or necessary developmental change, one observes the family to utilize, repeatedly and ineffectively, a narrow range of behaviors. In dealing with the anorectic child, the family responds as they would to a much younger child. Families with anorectic members have marked difficulty allowing for and encouraging the resolution of disagreement. As these disagreements remain, a chronic state of tension and stress develops. These characteristics are mutually reinforcing creating a family organization that is fragile and unable to respond effectively to the symptoms of anorexia. The final common feature of these families is *involvement of the symptomatic child in unresolved parental conflict.* The patient helps maintain family integrity by joining the side of one parent in a stable coalition against the other parent, by providing a focus for common concern and action through his/her symptoms, or by being caught between the parents in a loyalty conflict. Because of the *rigidly* preferred family patterns of interaction, the parents may be more concerned with the rightness of their own actions rather than their effectiveness. They may try (one parent by pleading, the other parent by demanding) to help the patient to eat, but then when each fails, each parent recoils and leaves the anorectic patient alone and without support. Because the family members do not resolve conflict well, they do not compromise and work together.

If the family is highly overinvolved with the patient, he/she need not perceive his/her own sensations. Others may recognize them first or deny their presence. The child must also be vigilant to perceive and respond to the signs of distress from others. In a context in which everyone is vulnerable and protection is necessary, interpersonal trust does not develop. When conflict and distress are denied or not resolved, the child does not develop a sense of competence and an appropriate use of problem-solving skills.

It is important to remember that the family does not cause their child's anorexia. The cause is unknown, and it is essential for the pediatrician to not blame the family for the occurrence of the disorder.

BULIMIA

Bulimia is a syndrome in which patients eat excessively and then follow these periods of overeating with episodes of purging through vomiting, laxative abuse, or diuretic use. We reserve the term *bulimia* for patients who are of at least normal weight at the time of diagnosis. Most bulimic patients weigh between normal and 10% to 15% above normal. Approximately one third of anorectic patients develop episodic binging and purging as they regain and maintain normal weight. Other patients who are bulimic may never have been significantly underweight. The frequency of binges generally varies from patient to patient and may vary also in any individual patient. Some patients can go days or weeks without binging or purging; other patients may pursue this activity daily or several times daily. The exact incidence of bulimia is unknown, although recent studies of eating habits of women college students indicate that some 10% to 20% of high school and college students engage in this behavior. Bulimia also occurs much more frequently in women (80% to 90% of cases). Foods consumed during binging are frequently high in carbohydrates. These periods of binging occur in addition to normal eating at regular mealtimes. However, some patients report episodes of excessive dieting or fasting, fluctuating with binges that then result in purging. Bulimic patients also may have a history of drug or alcohol abuse.

Physical Features

The physical difficulties associated with bulimia in patients with normal weight are caused by repetitive purging. Patients who induce vomiting may have calluses on the backs of their hands; they also may have parotid swelling. They may experience epigastric distress associated with chronic esophagitis or may have episodes of mild to moderate gastrointestinal bleeding occurring as a result of excessive repetitive vomiting. All patients with significant repetitive vomiting have some degree of tooth enamel erosion as a result of chronic irritation by gastric acid. Cardiac arrhythmias may result from hypokalemic alkalosis associated with significant chronic vomiting. Patients who use laxatives excessively may become dehydrated.

Psychologic Features

Bulimic patients are aware of their problem and are distressed by their symptoms. They report that the bulimic symptoms are habitual and outside of their control. Usually acting in secrecy, the patients are generally quite ashamed of their symptoms and reluctant to admit to them. Many patients describe that the binges are planned; others will describe periods of overeating that occur almost involuntarily. They also describe a point in eating at which they are sure that they have eaten too much and, therefore, will purge after finishing eating. This decision then leaves them free to continue to eat as much as they would like with the knowledge that they will be able to get rid of the food after completing the binge. Usual caloric intake in a binge often exceeds 2500 calories. Patients describe a battle with themselves to gain control over the symptoms and prevent future binges. They continually fail to master the problem that leads to worsening of the symptoms. Increase in frequency of binging can lead to lessening of their self-esteem and increased social isolation. Many bulimic patients, however, report successful performance in work, school, or social activities. Patients describe binges occurring during periods of loneliness, boredom, anxiety, or anger so that the eating and purging can be used to dissipate disturbing emotions. The loss of food relieves the anxiety but also leads to increased self-criticism and increased frequency of the binging. The entire experience of overeating and purging also is physically and psychologically consuming and exhausting. Patients then experience a period of quiet and relaxation, distracting them from stresses in their environment. The cycle then repeats itself.

Differential Diagnosis

As with anorexia, the diagnosis of bulimia is made through confirmation of symptoms by history and elimination of organic causes for the vomiting by physical examination. Causes of repetitive vomiting, such as Addison disease, need to be considered; however, the self-induced nature of the purging and excessive calorie intakes in episodes of binge eating are not present in other organic diseases.

The Family with a Bulimic Member

Enmeshment, rigidity, and poor conflict resolution are frequent in families with patients with bulimia. Patients maintain a stance of independence and act as if they are responsible for themselves, yet they are often sad, lonely, and unsupported. Although the patient frequently will state that the symptoms are secret, family members are aware and concerned about the eating disorder. The family fluctuates between attempting to stop the symptoms through injunctions or cajoling and retreating when ineffective. The family then becomes angry, blames the patient, and abandons him/her. This stance persists for awhile, and then the cycle occurs again. The fluctuation between overinvolvement and abandonment is characteristic of families with bulimic members. It happens concerning the symptoms of bulimia and in other areas of family life. Within these families, conflict is apparent. However, it is still not resolved. The parents may not have gotten along for many years. This fixed arrangement of argument, retreat, and reconciliation is stabilized by concern for the symptomatic child with bulimia. There also may be other overt and recognized difficulties with impulse control in families with bulimic members. One or both parents may have difficulty with their temper, often leading to explosive behavior in the house. There may be a history of substance abuse within the family, especially alcohol abuse, and concern that one or both parents may become depressed and incapacitated. There also may be a history of incest in the family, reflecting the lack of personal boundaries and poor impulse control.

OFFICE EVALUATION

The physician's evaluation of an eating disorder should include a determination of the patient's physical status, an assessment of the patient's psychosocial difficulties and developmental level, and an assessment of the family. The physician's efforts with respect to the physical symptoms and medical difficulties related to the eating disorder must be coordinated with efforts to deal with psychosocial and familial difficulties that occur simultaneously. The treatment approach must be one in which the body and mind of the patient are dealt with in concert and the patient is treated in relationship to the family. The goals of the medical evaluation of a patient with an eating disorder are 1) identification of underlying disease processes present at the time of the referral and ascertainment that no physiologic process explains the weight loss, 2) clarification of the patient's physiologic condition and the nature of any metabolic difficulties resulting from the patient's symptoms that require immediate remediation, and 3) effective preparation of the patient and family for resolution of the physical, psychosocial, and familial difficulties associated with the eating disorder.

The physician's evaluation can be performed on an outpatient basis. The presence of all parental figures is essential and underscores the need of parents and all family members to be involved in the treatment. The physician obtains history concerning the development of the symptoms, methods utilized to achieve weight reduction if this has occurred, current dietary practices, and information concerning the use of self-induced vomiting or exogenous substances. The physician also should obtain history concerning other physical symptoms including weakness, faintness, muscle cramping, loss of concentration, periods of dehydration, and difficulties with fluid retention. For women, menstrual history should be accurately established and any further medical difficulties should be noted. In particular, the physician will want to pay attention to the presence of symptoms that are not generally associated with either anorexia or bulimia, such as frequent diarrhea or bloody stools indicative of possible inflammatory bowel disease, neurologic signs or symptoms associated with central nervous system tumors, or evidence of an endocrine disorder. The patient's report that he/she is actively pursuing dieting or purging after eating is a positive indication of the presence of an eating disorder.

After obtaining each parent's perception of the problem, the symptoms should be discussed with the patient in the parents' presence. The physician should inform the patient that the frequency and severity of eating-related symptoms cannot be kept secret because of the seriousness of the symptoms and because all family members will be involved in the treatment of the eating disorder. The physician will also want to ask the patient directly concerning his/her weight goal and his/her feelings about his/her body shape. The physician should also learn from each parent how they have tried to resolve the eating-related symptoms.

The physician also can obtain information concerning the patient's psychosocial adaptation, the family medical history, recent changes in the home, and other current family stresses. The physician should ask the patient about emotional difficulties and suicidal ideation or behavior. The patient's level of functioning should be determined, including such factors as school or work attendance and performance, peer relationships, social activity, career interests, level of self-esteem, and sense of competency. As the patient is questioned, the physician should attempt to help the parents to remain silent and to listen. Overinvolvement within the family is demonstrated when one or both parents interrupts frequently, corrects the patient, or offers alternative explanations. The physician also will want to develop an initial assessment of the family system by noting whether the parents act together and respect each other during their meeting with him/her. The physician's evaluation of the family will include an assessment of family leadership and the commitment of the family as a whole to effective problem resolution.

The physician also will need to carry out a thorough physical examination and appropriate laboratory studies to be certain of the medical diagnosis and the patient's physical condition. It is our strong impression that the diagnosis of the eating disorder is a positive diagnosis achieved through recognition of symptoms and history of anorexia or bulimia. Usually a complete blood cell count, a sedimentation rate, urinalysis, and chemical profile studies are adequate tests. In patients with significant weight loss, who may have an arrhythmia, an electrocardiogram is performed. If there is concern about the patient's neurologic condition, computed tomography of the brain may be ordered. Patients who describe significant gastrointestinal (GI) tract symptoms that would not be expected in either bulimia or anorexia should have GI radiographs, including an upper GI study and barium enema. If there is sufficient concern about the patient's endocrine status beyond that expected on the basis of the weight loss, thyroid studies and cortisol studies can be performed. However, in uncomplicated cases of anorexia nervosa or bulimia, these values are usually normal. The female patient's estrogen levels in anorexia will be low, purely on the basis of starvation-induced hypothalamic dysfunction.

Most patients with mild to moderate symptoms have normal physical examination and laboratory studies. On physical examination, in underweight patients, the pulse rate and blood pressure may be significantly lower. A pulse rate of 120 beats per minute and a blood pressure of 110 to 120 over 85 to 90 mm Hg may be indicative of significant dehydration in a patient who is severely underweight and whose usual pulse rate is 50 beats per minute and usual blood pressure is 80 to 90 over 50. Worrisome findings of laboratory studies in patients with eating disorders include leukopenia, indicating potential immune compromise; hypoglycemia; and elevation in values of hemoglobin, hematocrit, and blood urea nitrogen, indicative of dehydration. The patient's electrolyte levels deserve special attention. Hypokalemic alkalosis may be seen in patients with repetitive vomiting. A disturbing sign, the absence of ketones in the urine of a patient who is acutely starving may indicate the total utilization of muscle stores for energy. Abnormalities in liver enzyme levels usually occur after significantly chronic and severe malnutrition. Any unusual findings of laboratory studies or unexplained physical signs on examination require further evaluation.

MANAGEMENT

The initial assessment includes the patient's diagnosis, physical condition, medical status, developmental level, and the family's organizational and functional status. The presence of acute medical complications (such as dehydration, electrolyte abnormalities, or impending cardiovascular collapse indicated by postural hypotension) necessitates immediate medical hospitalization and appropriate physical treatment. Psychiatric hospitalization is recommended for patients with eating disorders when the patient's weight is dangerously low and when the symptoms are sufficiently out of control to seriously compromise the patient's functioning in other areas of his/her life. Suicidal ideation or behavior or psychotic behavior requires hospitalization of the patient. An inpatient psychiatric program can be used to demonstrate the severity of the symptoms to the family and to augment outpatient treatment that previously has been ineffective. Medical or psychiatric hospitalization is required in 15% to 20% of patients with anorexia nervosa or bulimia, either to deal with acute complications or crises in treatment.

All patients with anorexia or bulimia and their families will require outpatient treatment that addresses both the physical and psychosocial problems of the patient and the problems in organization and interaction within the family. Treatment is a collaborative effort among family, patient, physician, and therapist. The physician will need to remain available to monitor the patient's physical condition, to reinforce the goals of treatment for the patient including goal weight and expected rate of weight gain, and to provide dietary information as necessary. Patients who purge either through vomiting or laxative abuse will require regular medical evaluation in order to be certain that the patient's physical condition is stable, to reinforce improvement, and to be certain that the patient remains safe for treatment on an outpatient basis.

Early referral and effective treatment can lead to resolution of eating disorders. The physician can follow patients with small amounts of weight loss, but the follow-up period should be brief. In situations that fail to improve with the physician's intervention or in situations for which the physician believes psychotherapeutic attention is required following his/her initial assessment, patients should be referred to a therapist who is experienced in treating eating disorders, capable of working successfully with adolescents and their families, and willing to collaborate with the physician concerning the medical aspects of treatment. The therapist also should be able to use the physician's information and his/her determinations of the patient's condition to foster improvement of the family and the patient. The physician should inform the therapist of his/her impressions, his/her availability to monitor the patient physically and his/her desire to collaborate in treatment. The physician's referral for psychotherapy should be made in a positive fashion, orienting the family and patient toward resolution of the eating disorder symptoms. Frequently, families with members with eating disorders will either deny the severity of the symptoms or deny the presence of psychologic difficulties. It is important for the physician to help the family appreciate that psychotherapy is necessary.

The physician should arrange a follow-up meeting with the family after making a referral for psychotherapy to discuss the family's initial impressions of psychotherapy and to ensure that the family has begun therapy. The physician can reiterate his/her expectation that the family continue treatment as well as encourage them to resolve any questions concerning their initial impressions of treatment with the therapist. Throughout the course of treatment, it is important that the physician and therapist communicate regularly and work actively to resolve any areas of disagreement, either concerning the impressions of the patient or family, therapeutic approach, or goals of treatment.

PHYSICIAN'S ROLE IN THE PREVENTION OF EATING DISORDERS

The physician can take an active role in the prevention and early identification of eating disorders. Media reports and advertisements suggest that anyone can be thin while eating whatever he/she would like. Especially for women, one's physical appearance is viewed as a sign of one's worth as a person. The family physician can work with families to support the development of a more moderate approach to physical appearance and dieting behavior as he/she provides primary care. The physician also should be particularly attuned to difficulties in the development of effective control and effective autonomy throughout adolescence and young adulthood. A complete dietary history, including questions concerning dietary behavior and the existence of binging and purging, should be part of the physician's routine evaluation of adolescent health. The physician should monitor the adolescent's sense of self-esteem, autonomy, and personal control. Finally, the physician will need to be attentive to the ability of the family to respond effectively to the adolescent's need for supervision and direction, and for autonomy and privacy. While working with families, the physician may note that there are some in which parents have significant difficulty in encouraging the young person's individuation and sense of personal responsibility. In some of these families, the symptoms of an eating disorder may occur and be reinforced through family behavior. Early diagnosis of the eating disorder and institution of effective treatment is essential.

The physician also can work with school nursing personnel to identify instances in which dieting and eating-related behavior have caused problems. Early identification of these situations can then lead to treatment and their effective resolution. The physician also can encourage early identification and treatment of eating disorders and the individual's satisfaction with his/her own physiology and acceptance of the limitations of his/her own body through working with schools and within the community. This will include advocating a more thoughtful and patient and a less impulsive and moralistic approach to food and diet. If the physician also encourages alternative means of expression, appropriate and adequate family relationships, and an increased acceptability of varieties of body shape, the incidence and the severity of eating disorders can be reduced, whereas symptoms can be treated in an effective and humane manner.

BIBLIOGRAPHY

Boskind-White M, White WC: *Bulimarexia: The binge/purge cycle,* New York, 1983, Norton.
Bruch H: *Eating disorders,* New York, 1973, Basic Books.

Bruch H: *The golden cage,* Cambridge, MA, 1978, Harvard University Press.
Collins M, Hodas GR, Liebman R: Interdisciplinary model for the inpatient treatment of an-

orexia nervosa, *J Adolesc Health Care* 4:3–8, 1983.

Crow SJ, Mitchell JE: Rational therapy of eating disorders: A review, *Drugs* 48(3):372–379, 1994.

Edwards KI: Obesity, anorexia, and bulimia, *Med Clin North Am* 77(4):899–909, 1993.

Garfinkel P, Garner D: *Anorexia nervosa: A multidimensional perspective,* New York, 1982, Brunner/Mazel.

Garner D, Garfinkel P, editors: *Handbook of psychotherapy for anorexia nervosa and bulimia,* New York, 1984, Guilford Press.

Halmi KA, Falk JR, Schwartz E: Binge-eating and vomiting: A survey of a college population, *Psychol Med* 11:697–706, 1981.

Harkaway J, editor: *Eating disorders: The family*

therapy collection, vol 20, Rockville, MD, 1987, Aspen Publications.

Hirschmann J, Zaphiropoulos L: *Are you hungry?* New York, 1985, Random House.

Johnson C, Connors M: *The etiology and treatment of bulimia nervosa: A biopsychosocial perspective,* New York, 1987, Basic Books.

Minuchin S, Rosman BL, Baker L: *Psychosomatic families: Anorexia nervosa in context,* Cambridge, MA, 1978, Harvard University Press.

Sargent J, Liebman R, Silver M: Family therapy for anorexia nervosa. In Garner DM, Garfinkel PE, editors: *The treatment of anorexia nervosa and bulimia,* New York, 1984, Guilford Press.

Sargent J, Liebman R: The outpatient treatment of anorexia nervosa, *Psychiatr Clin North Am* 7:235–245, 1984.

CHAPTER 130

School Refusal

Gordon R. Hodas

School refusal, also known as school phobia and school avoidance, has been called "the great imitator" because the patient frequently presents with other symptoms, often recurrent somatic complaints such as headache or abdominal pain. Although school refusal may on occasion be the presenting concern, usually this diagnosis is made by the office-based physician's considering this possible diagnosis and pursuing it in the history.

School refusal implies a separation problem between child and parents, usually the mother, and a block in the development of competence and autonomy on the part of the child. School refusal is distinguished from truancy because school refusal occurs with the knowledge and accommodation of the parents, whereas truancy usually occurs in the absence of parental awareness. Even when the medical evaluation is normal children who still refuse to attend school may be seen by parents as too sick and too upset to return to class.

Incidence figures for school refusal are not available, but the condition is not uncommon and is probably underdiagnosed. School absence may be long and continuous, sporadic over time, or interspersed with regular attendance the majority of each week. The primary care physician should appreciate the frequent association between chronic somatic complaints, depression, and school refusal.

Overprotected children with somatic symptoms are at highest risk for school refusal and may include previously vulnerable but now healthy children, special children, and children from families at risk for divorce and from families in which parents have physical symptoms and possible disability. Children with chronic medical illnesses more typically strive actively to remain in school.

OFFICE EVALUATION AND DIAGNOSIS

The triad of findings that leads to the diagnosis of school refusal includes: 1) poor school attendance, 2) vague physical symptoms, and 3) normal physical and laboratory findings. These findings often occur in association with depression and anxiety.

School attendance patterns vary from continuous to intermittent. Sporadic school absence occurs most commonly in the fall after the school year begins, and following holidays and weekends. The child may function quite well without physical complaints and anxiety when school is not in session, but symptoms develop when classes resume. This pattern may have occurred over several academic years. On the other hand, when a child has missed several consecutive weeks of school or more, this situation represents a major crisis and must be responded to immediately and decisively by the physician. The child with good grades who misses 1 or 2 days of school each week can more easily escape detection; it is here that the careful history of the office-based physician is rewarded.

The vague physical complaints and symptoms that, despite a normal medical evaluation, may accompany the school refusal pattern are as follows:

1. General
   Insomnia
   Excessive sleeping
   Fatigue
   "Fever"
2. Skin
   Pallor
3. Ear, nose, and throat
   Recurrent sore throat
   Constant "sinus trouble"
4. Respiratory
   Hyperventilation
   Coughing tics
5. Cardiovascular
   Chest pain
   Palpitations
6. Gastrointestinal
   Abdominal pain
   Anorexia
   Nausea
   Vomiting
   Diarrhea
7. Renal
   None
8. Genital
   Dysmenorrhea
9. Skeletal
   Bone pain
   Joint pain
   Back pain
10. Neuromuscular
    Headaches
    Dizziness
    Syncope
    "Weakness"

Although the most common symptom is abdominal pain, there may be multiple complaints. Anorexia in the absence of weight loss may occur, as may diarrhea. Nausea may be present, with or without associated vomiting. Vomiting often follows stressful events. The serious complaint of vomiting should not mislead the physician into an overly extensive workup that unwittingly reinforces disability. Similar considerations apply to skeletal complaints that may occur—bone pain, joint pain, and back pain. Other possible symptoms that may mask the school refusal syndrome include chest pain, dysmenorrhea, muscle weakness, coughing, tics, and recurrent sore throats.

Certain family characteristics of the child with school refusal have been identified. Berger described four important elements: 1) An overprotective attitude toward the patient. The child is excused from family responsibilities, and his/her wishes are quickly granted. 2) A belief in the physical or emotional vulnerability of the mother. This belief may be fostered by the mother herself, who may express fear of emotional breakdown and complain of various physical symptoms. 3) An isolated and devalued father, frequently seen as uninterested and unreliable, perhaps even as violent. There may be accompanying marital tension. 4) Occurrence of a major change in family composition (such as the departure from home of an older sibling), which has focused new attention on the younger child.

The major responsibility of the office-based physician is the detection of school refusal. Hints in history taking include the following: 1) The child has had multiple somatic complaints or recurrent complaints involving one somatic symptom, in the absence of significant medical findings. 2) A substantial amount of missed school has occurred. 3) Child and parents may be evasive about how much school has been missed and under what circumstances. 4) The parents may agree to the child's remaining home out of frustration, to avoid further conflict, after the child cries out in distress, refuses to leave home, and the parents argue fruitlessly with the child and with each other. 5) The child may function well at home after the morning crisis has passed and may do well on the weekends also. 6) The child may have a history of limited peer relationships and of previous episodes of school refusal. 7) Some major family event—illness, depression, or a family member leaving home—often preceded the school refusal by several weeks or months.

MANAGEMENT

The office-based physician can manage many cases of uncomplicated childhood school refusal himself/herself. The physical examination should be done in the presence of the parent(s) in a thorough manner, with the physician emphasizing the absence of physical findings. Appropriate, but not excessive laboratory work should be performed, and medication should not be prescribed. *No letters condoning further school absence should be written.*

Once the physician has established the absence of organic disease, he/she should set up a family conference with both parents present and the child outside the office. At the family conference, the physician should ask the parents to describe their child's temperamental style, ways of coping, and responses to stress. While acknowledging the child's subjective physical pain and probable anxiety, the physician should reassure the parents that the child has no serious illness and needs to learn to attend school despite his/her symptoms. Building on the child's strengths, the physician and parents then develop a specific strategy to help the child understand the need for an immediate return to school. When the child joins the meeting, the physician and parents review the findings and discuss together the plan for the child's improved functioning and return to school. The legitimacy of the child's symptom and his/her anxiety, when present, is made clear, as well as the readiness of parents and physician to support the child. The child is invited to cooperate so that the entire family can work together and is informed, when necessary, that the parents will persist even if he/she fails to cooperate.

This approach is effective with many cases of childhood school refusal. When it fails (*eg,* the parents are unable to make an agreement or to carry it out successfully), psychiatric referral is indicated. Psychiatric referral is also indicated in the following situations: long-standing continuous school refusal, recurrent episodes, severe anxiety or depression, psychosis, and most cases occurring in adolescence.

When the office-based physician manages school refusal himself/herself, it is important that he/she contact the school nurse to reassure him/her of the child's state of health, describe his/her proposed approach to the school refusal, and obtain the nurse's support. The physician should encourage the family to maintain close telephone contact with him/her over the next several days until he/she sees the child and family again, ideally after the first day of successful return to school. When psychiatric referral is made, the physician should underline the urgency of this process and make sure that the family follows through. The family-oriented treatment of this problem addresses both the child's return to school and underlying stresses. The physician frequently needs to support the treatment actively; with the most difficult cases, the physician and psychiatrist may need to meet with the family jointly to clarify issues and underline the need for treatment. Following completion of treatment, the office-based physician should continue to encourage the child during the primary care visits, while remaining alert to the possibility of recurrence.

BIBLIOGRAPHY

Berger H: Somatic pain and school avoidance, *Clin Pediatr* 13:819–826, 1974.

Nader PR, Bullock D, Caldwell B: School phobia, *Pediatr Clin North Am* 22:605–716, 1975.

Schmitt B: School phobia: The great imitator: A pediatrician's viewpoint, *Pediatrics* 48:433–442, 1971.

CHAPTER 131

Behavioral and Emotional Adjustment in Children Who Are Deaf or Hearing Impaired

Annie G. Steinberg
Anna-Maria DaCosta

In Chapter 114, the importance of the early recognition of hearing impairment and rapid implementation of audiologic, educational, and communication-based interventions was examined. Although sensory impairment does not itself result in mental health problems, hearing loss can have a profound effect on family and peer communication, interactions in the community, identity formation, and self-esteem. Additionally, the diagnosis and treatment of emotional and behavioral disorders in children who are deaf or hearing impaired may be delayed by clinicians who ascribe the problem to the hearing loss rather than pursue usual assessments and treatment options. The clinician evaluating the clinical symptoms of a child who is deaf must integrate information from a number of sources and consider the many factors (including but not limited to biologic, social, educational, and linguistic) that impact on the life of the child and family. Additionally, deafness can serve as a model for other sensory disabilities of communi-

cation disorders that also present what appears to be insurmountable cultural or linguistic barriers and affect many aspects of the clinician's usual diagnostic and therapeutic practice. This chapter will examine common behavioral and emotional symptoms of the child who is deaf or hearing impaired and will guide the clinician in their evaluation and treatment.

CLASSIFICATION AND DIAGNOSIS

The same mental health problems exist in children who are deaf or hearing impaired as in children without hearing impairments. However, behavioral and/or emotional problems are compounded by the presence of this sensory disability; symptoms such as depression, anxiety, and paranoia are exacerbated by fewer expressive outlets. Reduced receptive language also leads to fewer opportunities for learning about emotional states due to linguistic and information gaps, *eg,* regarding self-soothing and the management of emotional experiences in general. To complicate matters further, co-morbid conditions such as neurologic dysfunction, learning disabilities, mental retardation, and other handicapping conditions obscure the diagnostic picture in approximately 30% of hearing-impaired children.

In assessing the child who is deaf, it is necessary to examine the dynamic interplay of the etiologic factors and avoid the "deficit assumption" (the assumption that the child who is deaf will have a number of problems and difficulty achieving his/her potential based solely on deafness). Rather, the emphasis should be on the question, "How does this impairment interface with the developmental process and/or the environment and what have been the adaptive responses?"

Limitations of Current Descriptive Classifications

Prior reports have attempted to characterize the personalities and problem behaviors of children who are deaf; however, for the most part, these studies were descriptive, based on nonvalidated measures for this population and may have reflected the lack of linguistic and cultural awareness of the examiner. An example of this can be seen in the examination of attentional and hyperactivity symptoms. A number of the problem behaviors reported in children who are deaf are similar to those seen in children with attention-deficit hyperactivity disorder (ADHD), including impulsivity and increased activity level. Indeed, children who are deaf are likely to have a higher risk of these symptoms given that some etiologies of deafness also can result in ADHD. However, few guidelines exist on which to base a decision regarding the presence of ADHD in this population. Several of the criteria used to make the diagnosis refer to speaking, listening, or language comprehension that may not be available to the child who is deaf, and normative data for standardized measures of ADHD do not currently exist for this population. Additionally, increased psychomotor activity can be viewed as an appropriate expressive outlet for the child with few other means for self-expression. Diagnoses such as ADHD or impulse control disorder must be differentiated from the motoric expression of a mood or affect such as frustration in a child who has had few opportunities to develop the language and cognitive skills necessary for impulse control.

The complexity of diagnosing symptoms in a child who is deaf also can be seen when the child presents with bizarre behaviors such as talking or signing to him/herself, conversing with imaginary friends beyond the usual phase of development, altered social/emotional reciprocity, gaze aversion, and social awkwardness. All of these presenting complaints can be manifestations of an undersocialized and sensorially deprived child who is deaf, a severe developmental disorder, or a major psychiatric disturbance. Children who are deaf or hearing impaired have the full spectrum of behavioral and emotional problems including depressive, anxiety, habit, posttraumatic, conduct, personality, and developmental disorders.

ETIOLOGY

A wide variety of emotional and behavioral symptoms are neuropsychiatric manifestations of some of the etiologies of deafness. Hereditary syndromes such as Usher syndrome have known associations with major psychiatric disorders, although these usually accompany the progression of the disease. Maternal intrauterine infections are associated with a number of central nervous system manifestations. Prematurity often is accompanied by intraventricular hemorrhages or anoxia, and meningitis, encephalitis, or other infectious or traumatic etiologies all can result in neurologic damage and neuropsychiatric symptoms. Communication problems may be the primary cause of emotional and behavioral symptoms etiology in many circumstances. This unique etiologic factor will be addressed here.

Although clinicians often ascribe most behavioral problems in children who are deaf to the hearing impairment, deafness per se is not usually accompanied by such symptoms. However, language is a central theme in the life of a child with a hearing impairment, and no emotional or behavioral symptoms can be understood without considering the degree to which family members enjoy a meaningful shared language. Whereas hearing children acquire language through environmental exposure and without special efforts, children with hearing impairments (born to parents who are hearing) must be helped to gain exposure to language through the use of manual or sign language, amplified auditory stimuli, and/or oral training in speechreading and speech. Regardless of the child's speech and lipreading aptitude, oral training is slow and difficult for the preschool-aged child. Therefore, a deaf child's usable language skills in the preschool years are typically less than optimal. Despite parental and familial efforts to communicate, communicative frustration and linguistic and social isolation constitute a significant psychosocial stressor in the early years of the child's life. A relationship between emotional and behavioral disturbances and the inability of children to communicate with their family members in a shared language can be demonstrated; this may be more a function of the quality of family dialogue and communication than the specific communication method or language utilized.

EMOTIONAL AND BEHAVIORAL MANIFESTATIONS

The primary care provider often will encounter the following clinical situations (which are not mutually exclusive):

1. The child with minimal language or minimal shared language in the family and behavioral symptoms due to confusion, frustration, sensory isolation, or loneliness
2. The child with a co-morbid condition, either overt, such as a dual sensory impairment or cerebral palsy, or previously undiagnosed, such as a learning disability or a coordination disorder, which makes the acquisition of speech or sign language more difficult
3. The child with a significant mental health problem that has eluded diagnosis or intervention due to the lack of accessible pediatric care

Deafness can impact on the life of the child and family throughout the life cycle.

Infancy and Toddlerhood

Much emotion is communicated nonverbally in the first year of life. The early ability to communicate love and to engender a sense of trust nonverbally helps a child to develop a sense of self and awareness of others, regardless of hearing status. There are differences, however, for the deaf child. Usually, a parent immerses his/her infant in speech that becomes integral in the development of the parent-child relationship. Language, usually in the speech medium, serves as a link to the parent. In later months, objects and words are connected, and words, rhymes, and songs all evoke parent connections and are used for soothing, pleasure, and supporting the achievement of developmental milestones. This result can occur only if the language is accessible to the child. The hearing mother of a deaf infant may not intuitively know how to transcend sensory modalities and provide comparable sensory stimulation in a visual form or how and when to give the child's nonverbal communication a verbal form, particularly about emotions and the inner experiences of the child.

The initial diagnostic period often is characterized by a lack of professional support during the immediate evaluative phase, followed by a period of overwhelming and conflicting information. Guilt and reactive depression compound the frustration regarding the inability to communicate fully as language becomes increasingly more important. Parents report the disorienting recommendations to "raise your child in a different culture, in a language other than your own . . ." and often yearn for the time when their child "belonged to them." News of the deafness often serves as a catalyst for underlying marital or familial discord. Immediate financial expenditures for hearing aids and medical appointments, as well as time lost from work, all stress the family system. Family elders often bear family and cultural myths regarding deafness, which may further the negative perception of deafness and lower expectations for the child. Maternal depression and anxiety, perceived lack of social supports, and reported stressful life events have all been correlated with the deaf child's degree of behavioral problems, although the causal relationship is unclear.

A deaf child's toddler years bring frustration, which is greatly magnified as compared with the experience of the hearing toddler. Often the child has little to no understanding of what the parent is asking, or of why, for instance, the child's chin is suddenly jerked toward the mother (to establish eye contact). Safety concerns often necessitate that the parent intervene in a physical manner with the child who cannot hear either the prohibition or its explanation. Parents also often have different expectations for their deaf child's behavior than for their hearing children and impose fewer consequences and more restrictive limitations (based on perceived risk). The process of separation and individuation often is affected by these interactions.

Childhood

Parents may express bewilderment as to how to establish reasonable behavioral expectations for a child without verbal explanations. Delayed toilet training, feeding problems, as well as the imposition of stringent safety measures, are common complaints of parents of children who are deaf. Seeking a shared modality of communication, parents may insist on the child's production of spoken words, which in turn may paradoxically lead to an oppositional resistance to later speech and language therapy. Initiative may be affected, because purposeful behavior, expression of intent, and the resultant reinforcement and encouragement require a communicative channel.

In the absence of verbal language or an alternative to it, children are left with motoric responses to their affective expression until a shared language is established. If a deaf child does not learn or use a language during his/her early years, not only are language skills inadequate, but the opportunity for communication and exploration with family and peers is sorely missed. Inadequate communication between parents and children often leads to impulsive, motoric responses to vent frustration, disappointment, and anger by both parent and child.

Even children with unilateral or mild hearing loss are required to observe visual cues with a vigilance uncharacteristic of young children and may appear to have poor frustration tolerance or attentional problems when actually fatigued. This effect may be exacerbated by increased degrees of hearing loss, particularly in the absence of a visually accessible or manual language.

Cognitive and social lags of the deaf child are most often related to experiential deficiencies. The deaf child usually lacks available role models, information, and opportunities for mutual communication with peers, parents, and teachers.

The educational setting can exacerbate rather than ameliorate problem behaviors. In recent years, there has been a trend away from residential and toward day-school programs and mainstreaming. Although this direction has offered many children excellent educational programs as well as the opportunity to live with their families, in many regions, school districts are unable to provide a challenging program and the child is placed in a "generic" special needs classroom. Additionally, in the absence of significant exposure to individuals who are deaf, individual teachers' and peers' negative predictions and beliefs about deafness will have a profound impact on the child's educational environment.

Adolescence

Puberty brings great challenges for the adolescent who must develop a sense of identity and self-acceptance. Rapid physical growth and sexual development often occur without the benefit of adequate information regarding the normal maturation process, instinctual urges and appropriate outlets, opportunities to discuss values, the meaning of consent and consensual activities, or the prevention of sexually transmitted diseases. Ensuing confusion and isolation may lead to a preoccupation with normal developmental changes.

During adolescence, an identity and self-concept that integrate deafness must be consolidated. In the absence of adult deaf role models, manifestations of this struggle may include "practicing" or pretending to be hearing, by refusing to use hearing aids, request clarifications, lipread, or sign. The deaf adolescent's separation-individuation may involve increased deaf peer activities with communication exclusively in American Sign Language, often excluding the nonsigning parents. Such behavior can be used by the adolescent to test limits and challenge parental authority and competence. The use of alcohol or drugs often serves as a means of social integration with hearing peers; many teens are initiated into the drug world by hearing siblings, family members, or peers with whom there was little previous interaction.

Separation-individuation issues often are intensified by familial struggles regarding driving, dating, college departure, or leaving home. Transition to adulthood is further challenged by difficulties in obtaining babysitting or part- or full-time employment. Unfortunately, despite the opportunity to extend educational programming to age 21 years, many deaf students leave high school with no work experience, unrealistic career goals, and few vocational training options.

INTERVENTIONS

Parents often are overwhelmed with information and with the biases of professionals, and tension often is related to disagreements regarding communication approach. It is critical that the primary care provider avoid the "communication debate" and help parents to view their current choices without further polarization. In particular, the use of sign language does not interfere with speech acquisition and can augment oral training, whereas involvement with an auditory-verbal program or cochlear implantation need not eliminate the use of sign language. Children benefit from all modes of access to language, and parents should be helped to recognize that their treatment options are neither mutually exclusive nor irreversible. By addressing myths such as, "if my child signs, he'll never learn to talk," or "if you don't use sign language, then you haven't fully accepted your child's deafness," the intense pressure to choose may be reduced. Parents also benefit from exposure to successful role models who are deaf and involvement in local and national parent-led support groups.

The goals for a successful intervention include family adaptation to and acceptance of the child's special communication needs and a positive language-accessible home and school environment. Parents in a postdiagnostic state of disequilibrium need support because they suddenly lack the usual language resources to communicate with their own child and need to have confidence and joy restored to their parenting role.

Primary care providers need to have an awareness of the unique communication needs of hearing-impaired children and their families. An understanding of the various forms of communication, as well as the special technologies that can be used when providing services, is important. Resources such as professionals with expertise in deafness, parent support/advocacy groups, community resource centers, and interpreter referral agencies can help the clinician to evaluate and refer the child. In general, providing mental health services to deaf children and adolescents requires specialized knowledge and communicative skills.

The primary care provider must have the usual opportunities to evaluate the child and the presenting problem. The usual diagnostic interview, physical examination, and observation of the parent-child interaction must be conducted with careful consideration to ensuring direct communication with the child rather than relying on the parent as interpreter. A barrier to an effective evaluation is present when the "interpreter" is a family member, who often is embroiled in the conflict precipitating the evaluation. With support from interpreter referral agencies and subspecialized professionals, clinicians can modify their practice and accommodate themselves so as to be accessible to the child who is deaf or hearing impaired. Even observation of parent-child communication is difficult if parental translations are simply assumed to be accurate. If the parent and child do not have mutual comprehension (eg, if the child's speech is unintelligible to the parent and no sign language or gestural communication is used), this is likely to be a significant component of the problem. Understanding both sides of the dialogue allows the clinician to evaluate the degree to which the parent and child work to communicate until comprehension is achieved, regardless of the communication method or the reliance on gesture, lipreading, writing, pronounced articulation, or repetition, as well as the patience, warmth, acceptance, and pride accompanying these mutual efforts.

In addition to the interview with the child and family, consultation with the child's teachers can help the primary care provider to understand the degree to which the educational environment is knowledgeable of, accessible to, and challenging for the child. Questions about the seating arrangements, degree of itinerant support, tutor and notetaking services, reliance on the child's lipreading skills vs. interpreter provision, home-school communication, support for appropriate peer interaction, opportunities for leadership roles, and so forth can help the primary care provider assess the manner in which the educational program is impacting on the social and emotional life of the child.

Family therapy with a therapist knowledgeable about the impact of deafness on the life of the child and family can help to address a variety of issues, including unresolved grief related to the diagnosis of deafness, familial communication problems and perceptions (eg, "oh, she understands when she wants to understand"), parental expectations and overprotectiveness, negative attributions to the behaviors, and information derived from diagnostic assessment such as genetic testing results or an abnormal electroencephalogram or magnetic resonance imaging. Family therapy can play an important role in resolving intrafamilial conflicts, exploring choices regarding educational and vocational placement, and facilitating the achievement of independent living skills.

Individual psychotherapy, including art, drama, play, and/or movement therapy, can be helpful to the hearing-impaired child or adolescent with emotional or behavioral problems. Behavioral interventions in families with limited communication can help the child to anticipate what will happen next, clarify consequences for behaviors, and offer parents direction and a simple communication channel. Pictorial or photographic representations of the day or week can be extremely helpful if the child is prelingual.

Psychopharmacologic interventions only should be used with a clear diagnosis, treatment goals, and identified outcome measures. If clinical symptoms are inconsistent with the pattern expected in hearing children (eg, hyperactive at home but fine in high-demand and minimally structured school situations), medications are unlikely to benefit the child and may further confound the picture.

School-based treatment allows for the development of an intervention that may be implemented consistently across environments. Many parents of children who are deaf utilize school staff when problems arise in the home, so the involvement of the primary care providers may uncover inconsistencies in the expectations or responses of family and school staff and strengthen the school-family collaboration. Children and adolescents who are deaf are extremely responsive to group interventions with peers and/or group leaders who are also deaf. School settings are often the ideal milieu for group therapy addressing general interpersonal problem-solving and socialization skills or special problems related to victimization, parental addiction to drugs, and so forth. Integrated deaf-hearing peer group interactions, such as organized sports and expressive arts, and role models of successful deaf-hearing interactions should be a component of a mainstreamed educational program.

Buddy and mentor programs can be vital in enhancing self-esteem and growth. After-school and evening therapeutic recreation and an extended school year can be included in the child's individualized educational plan and can make an enormous difference in the life of the child and family. If the emotional disturbance is severe, day treatment, partial hospitalization, and respite care may be necessary. This is an area in which most regions are deficient, because few programs are communication accessible for a deaf patient. When a child or adolescent who is deaf has the need for intensive psychiatric services, parents most often must choose between inaccessible but local services and accessible but out-of-state services with far less potential for family involvement.

OUTCOMES

The child who is deaf can reach his/her optimal potential when core cultural and linguistic identity issues, familial expectations, and negative stereotypes of deafness have been examined. Positive self-esteem can reduce depressive vulnerability, and access to a rich educational program can reduce information gaps and improve vocational outcome. Even with these factors addressed, some children and adolescents who are deaf will have emotional or behavioral problems that necessitate prompt diagnostic evaluations and treatment. These services should be provided by or in collaboration with professionals knowledgeable about the impact of deafness on child development and the life of the family.

Primary care providers should avail themselves of the expertise of organizations and professionals experienced in providing general and mental health services to children and adolescents who are deaf or hearing-impaired. Although demanding, work with this population is a unique challenge that is both compelling and highly rewarding.

BIBLIOGRAPHY

Densham J: *Deafness, children and the family: A guide to professional practice,* Brookfield, VT, 1995, Ashgate Publishing.

Gregory S, Bishop J, Sheldon L: *Deaf young people and their families,* Cambridge, 1995, Cambridge University Press.

Jenkins I, Chess S: Psychiatric evaluation of perceptually impaired children: Hearing and visual impairments. In Lewis M, editor: *Child and adolescent psychiatry: A comprehensive textbook,* Baltimore, 1991, Williams & Wilkins.

Liben LS: *Deaf children: Developmental perspectives,* New York, 1978, Academic Press.

Marshack M: *Psychological development of deaf children,* New York, 1993, Oxford University Press.

Meadow-Orlans KP: Socialization of deaf children and youth. In Higgins PC, Nash JE, editors: *Understanding deafness socially,* Springfield, IL, 1996, Charles C. Thomas.

Meadows KP: Studies of behavioral problems of deaf children. In Stein LK, Mindel ED, editors: *Deafness and mental health,* New York, 1981, Grune & Stratton.

Meadow KP, Trybus RJ: Behavioral and emotional problems of deaf children: An overview. In Branford LJ, Hardy WG, editors: *Hearing and hearing impairment,* New York, 1979, Grune & Stratton.

Mindel ED, Vernon M: *They grow in silence—The deaf child and his family,* Silver Spring, 1971, National Association of the Deaf.

Padden C, Humphries T: *Deaf in America,* Cambridge, 1988, Harvard University Press.

Schlesinger H, Meadow K: *Sound and sign—Deafness and mental health,* Berkeley, 1972, University of California Press.

CHAPTER 132

Behavioral, Psychologic, and Psychiatric Sequelae of Physical and Sexual Abuse

Laurie Robbins Appelbaum

Physical and sexual child abuse significantly affect multiple dimensions of a child's emotional and behavioral life. These traumatic experiences frequently shape outward behavior, cognition, self-concept, and relationships and often are associated with psychiatric disorders. However, there is no one syndrome of disturbances exhibited by all abused children. The sequelae displayed by any one child is quite individual and reflects the characteristics of that child, the characteristics of the abusive experience or experiences, the specific experiences relating to disclosure of the abuse, and the events, reactions, and interactions of people and systems following the disclosure.

In addition to the abuse itself, the child often experiences multiple stressors, which may include family disruption, threats, family blame, pressure to retract the disclosure, family stress associated with protective services investigations, court appearances, educational disruption, loss of privacy because many people (teachers, doctors, lawyers, social workers, therapists) know of the abuse, housing moves, foster placement, shelter stays, and medical examinations and treatment. Those factors that protect children are not well understood, but family support (believing, nonblaming, taking steps to keep the child safe from further abuse) appears to diminish negative sequelae.

BEHAVIORAL PROBLEMS

Caregivers are most likely to seek help for the outward behavioral manifestations of traumatic experiences. Abused children often display acting-out behaviors, which are most likely to disturb adults. Aggression is common, whatever the abusive experience may have been. Abused children often have tremendous rage, which may be beyond any optimally expectable developmental coping capacities. Moreover, these children have reason to utilize suboptimal or deviant coping strategies. They have learned a coping model of aggression by their direct experience or by witnessing aggression. Some children, particularly boys, may cope with their fears and humiliation by identifying with the aggressor (which is a form of "if you can't beat them, join them"). Neuropsychiatric impairment, whether preexisting or secondary to abusive head trauma, can further limit the repertoire of coping mechanisms for anger.

Other common acting-out behaviors include inappropriate sexual behavior and sexual provocativeness. Some children display an inappropriate physical closeness, not understanding the normal physical distances people keep and how those distances vary with strangers vs. family. Sexualized behavior makes adults uncomfortable and may result in adults keeping a distance, both physical and emotional, from the child. Parents of other children may not allow their children to play with the child. These adult reactions, which may be understandable, convey to the child a sense of diminished worth and limit the appropriate avenues to get emotional needs met. The child's sexualized behavior also increases the risk for further victimization and may cause others to disbelieve reports of further victimization. Lying is another common behavior that can damage relationships and further decrease the likelihood that the child will be believed if she/he is again abused.

Children who do not "act out" may display other behavioral changes. Some may exhibit social isolation or withdrawal from normal activities. School performance may deteriorate. Less subtle manifestations of distress include suicide attempts and even substance abuse.

PSYCHOLOGIC ISSUES

Because child abuse is psychologic trauma, the sequelae always include psychologic issues. Abused children frequently have difficulties around their sense of self. They often feel damaged and have a poor or distorted body image. They feel guilty because they believe that they are responsible for the abuse or for the consequences of the disclosure. They also feel shame; adolescents sometimes focus on a sense of difference from peers. They may feel that their sexual identity is defined by the abuse rather than by their own feelings and preferences. For example, a victim of homosexual abuse may believe that the abusive experience means that he/she must be homosexual. Having experienced profound powerlessness, abused children may see themselves as insignificant. Those who have been deliberately unprotected by their family may feel unloved and unworthy.

Abused children commonly have problematic psychologic constructs of relationships. Trust is a major issue for many abused children, who are slow to drop their guard. Because relationships in families of abuse often involve secrecy, manipulation, lying, exploitation, and selfish disregard for others, abused children may perpetuate these relationship patterns with others. Because abused children also often have poor social skills, their peer relationships often are quite problematic.

Abused children most commonly experience a very high level of anger and grief. They have difficulty in regulating affect and may distort reality. They tend to see the world as dangerous. They also have a higher incidence of cognitive difficulties. The sequelae of abuse often create powerful issues of grief and loss for a child. Many children have powerful ambivalent feelings toward their abuser and may miss absent parents or siblings if the family is disrupted. There may be moves, changes of caregivers or schools, diminished economic resources, and changes of friends.

The entire family may be experiencing anger, guilt, grief, loss, and the effects of the disruption. In particular, social service agency involvement and criminal justice system processes can be extremely stressful.

PSYCHIATRIC DISORDERS

Another way of viewing the sequelae of abuse is from the framework of psychiatric diagnosis. This framework provides a rational approach to choosing treatment modalities. Although not all abused children's difficulties fit the diagnostic criteria for a specific psychiatric disorder, some psychiatric disorders are prevalent in abused children. Particularly common are posttraumatic stress disorder, dissociative disorders, depressive disorders, anxiety disorders, disruptive behavior disorders, and adjustment disorders. These disorders may not be recognized by caregivers, who may only be aware of the most behaviorally prominent manifestations.

The diagnosis of posttraumatic stress disorder involves 1) a traumatic event or events; 2) reexperiencing the event, which may involve repetitive play of some aspect of the trauma, nightmares, recall, or distress on exposure to cues that recall the event; 3) avoidance of stimuli associated with the trauma and a general numbness; and 4) persistent symptoms of increased arousal, which may include sleep problems, irritability, angry outbursts, hypervigilance, difficulty concentrating, and an exaggerated startle response. Posttraumatic stress disorder may be acute, chronic, or delayed in onset. Some abused children may display only partial symptoms of the disorder, and may thus meet the criteria for either atypical anxiety disorder or for an adjustment disorder.

Children who have been abused are at risk for dissociative disorders. In particular, they may experience dissociative states, which are characterized by a trancelike disturbance of consciousness, in which the child is able to ignore the reality of his/her immediate experience. Some children who are severely and chronically abused may dissociate into different identities to cope with the abuse and develop multiple personality disorder. The existence of multiple personality disorder in childhood, however, is controversial. The diagnosis requires careful discrimination from the developmentally appropriate expression of imagination (especially imaginary friends).

TREATMENT

Disclosure of abuse is a crisis point for the child and family. The first goal in office management is to prevent further harm to the child. Beyond filing a report for suspected abuse, the physician can minimize harm from the sequelae of abuse. Physical examination can cause retraumatization if not conducted sensitively. Whenever possible, the child should be accompanied by a supportive, familiar adult during the examination, be given opportunities to make choices, and have procedures explained in advance. Fears and refusals need to be dealt with gently; if medically safe, some parts of the examination or procedures may have to be deferred if a child is too frightened or resistant. When an abused child is particularly afraid of one gender, medical personnel may need to be of the opposite gender.

Particular attention needs to be paid to protecting the privacy of the child and family—abuse can be stigmatizing. Abuse is also a prime subject for gossip, even for medical, educational, child welfare, and legal professionals. Information that a particular child has been abused should be conveyed only to those who need to know in order to work with or for the child (and only in accord with the legal and ethical constraints on confidentiality).

The office-based physician also can provide an important source of support to the child and family in dealing with the many significant stressors that appear after abuse is disclosed. A supportive attitude and specific advocacy for the child's needs can significantly help the child with the many interviews (with child welfare workers, police, and prosecutors) and with the ordeals of courtroom appearances. The physician can be alert to signs that family disruption is disturbing the child and can counsel the family and child to minimize the impact on the child.

Every abused child should be referred to a qualified mental health professional who is experienced in the evaluation and treatment of abused children. The child should have an evaluation to identify his/her needs and to screen for specific psychiatric disorders, especially suicide risk. Children who display significant difficulties should be referred to a child and adolescent psychiatrist.

The outcome of the evaluation should be a treatment plan tailored to the child's individual needs. Most children will need some form of expressive therapy to specifically deal with the abuse; the choice of individual, group, and/or family therapy should be based on the issues to be addressed and not on the preferences of the therapist. Parents usually need involvement in their child's treatment so as to parent the child sensitively and effectively. When the parents have been abusive or neglectful, they may need intensive parenting training as well. Serious problematic behaviors require behavioral therapy. Specific psychiatric disorders require specific treatment. Children who are suicidal or whose behavior is dangerous may require psychiatric hospitalization.

Disclosure of abuse may be associated with transient school difficulties. The physician may need to counsel patience in light of the trauma. If the child has missed classroom time because of the abuse or treatment, support or tutoring may be sufficient to allow the child to catch up on academics.

Other family members may need support as well. Adults who love a child may experience extreme rage, guilt, anxiety, and depression over the child's abuse. Their distress is usually even greater if they themselves were abused in childhood. Family members who exhibit extreme distress or signs of decompensation should be gently referred for their own treatment. Some parents may be more concerned about their own needs than those of the child. They should be reminded to respond to the child's needs. Family members should be encouraged to utilize whatever healthy supports are available, such as family, friends, and clergy.

Many sequelae of child abuse are long term. Recovery is slow; new difficulties may surface as the child faces new developmental issues or tasks or as painful issues surface in treatment. Legal proceedings may drag on for years, with repeated court dates and testimony. Children need to be prepared and supported for the rigors of testifying. The role of the primary care physician continues to be crucial in providing support, advocacy, and sensitive medical care. Many abused children have long-term difficulty with physical examinations and gender of medical personnel; somatization, fears about disease, and fears about bodily abnormality are common and require realistic reassurance. The physician also needs to be alert for signs of further abuse. However, the abused child's fragile self-esteem can be damaged if the child perceives the physician as overemphasizing the abuse without displaying enough emphasis on emotional growth and other strengths.

Chronic school difficulties may require a change in educational placement if there are underlying learning difficulties or if behavioral or psychologic problems interfere with learning.

The best prognosis is for children who are kept safe from further abuse, whose families respond sensitively and appropriately to the child's needs, and who experience minimal losses or other stressors.

CHAPTER 133

Psychosis

Gordon R. Hodas

Psychosis is a state of severe impairment in functioning characterized by a loss of contact with reality, poor interpersonal relationships, and disturbances in thinking. Behavior may be aggressive, withdrawn, or both. Younger children express psychosis as a global withdrawal from relationships and reality in a way that may affect nearly all phases of development. Adolescents with acute onset of schizophrenia or manic episodes show a clinical picture similar to that of adults with these conditions. Psychoses of childhood and adolescence can be divided into two categories: organic and psychiatrically based psychosis. The distinction between these two is based on the presence of some identifiable physical source for organic psychosis, such as a medical or traumatic condition or an exogenous substance, whereas no such identifiable source can be ascertained for psychiatrically based psychosis.

Psychiatrically based psychosis of childhood and adolescence is divided into four major categories: 1) infantile autism (onset prior to the age of 30 months), 2) pervasive developmental disorders (onset between 30 months and 12 years), 3) schizophrenic episodes (onset in adolescence), and 4) manic-depressive illness (onset in adolescence).

ORGANIC PSYCHOSIS

Although the majority of psychoses are psychiatrically based, the primary care physician must be alert to the possibility of organic psychosis and consider possible sources. This possibility is especially pertinent given the increasing use of nonprescription drugs by adolescents. The four major sources of an organic psychosis are medical conditions, trauma, prescribed medications, and drug intoxications.

Causes of Organic Psychosis
Medical conditions
- Central nervous system lesions
    Tumor
    Brain abscess
    Cerebral hemorrhage
    Meningitis or encephalitis
    Temporal lobe epilepsy
- Cerebral hypoxia
    Pulmonary insufficiency
    Severe anemia
    Cardiac failure
    Carbon monoxide poisoning
- Metabolic and endocrine disorders
    Electrolyte imbalance
    Hypoglycemia
    Hypocalcemia
    Thyroid disease (hyperthyroidism and hypothyroidism)
    Adrenal disease (hyperadrenocorticism and hypoadrenocorticism)
    Uremia
    Hepatic failure
    Diabetes mellitus
    Porphyria
- Rheumatic diseases
    Systemic lupus erythematosus
    Polyarteritis nodosa
- Infections
    Malaria
    Typhoid fever
    Subacute bacterial endocarditis
- Miscellaneous conditions
    Wilson disease
    Reye syndrome
Trauma
- Acute
- Chronic
Prescribed medication(s)
- Side effect

- Toxicity
- Discontinuation

Drug intoxications (toxic psychosis)
- Accidental ingestion
- Proprietary medications
- Drug experimentation or abuse
- Alcohol abuse
- Suicide attempt

Most of the medical conditions will have been previously diagnosed, but some (eg, cerebral lupus erythematosus and Reye syndrome) may present as acute psychosis. Chronic trauma can be more easily overlooked and requires a careful history and neurologic evaluation. Prescribed medications may cause psychosis, either as a side effect when the medication is given in high doses or as an untoward effect when it is being tapered off and discontinued.

Drug or alcohol experimentation is the most common cause of organic psychosis in adolescence. The following exogenous substances may induce a toxic psychosis either singly or in combination: alcohol, barbiturates, antipsychotics (eg, phenothiazines), amphetamines, cocaine, crack, hallucinogens (eg, LSD, peyote, mescaline), marijuana, phencyclidine (PCP), methaqualone (Quaalude), anticholinergic compounds, heavy metals, corticosteroids, reserpine, opiates (eg, heroin, methadone). The physician should always consider the possibility of a suicide attempt when an adolescent presents with an organic psychosis.

ACUTE ADOLESCENT SCHIZOPHRENIA

Schizophrenia, despite substantial research efforts remains a mystery. Although a genetic predisposition exists, it is not entirely clear what factors produce this state of emotional disorganization and why it occurs when it does. The prognostic range is extremely wide, from individuals who experience a single psychotic break and recover completely, to persons who remain symptomatic and require either institutional or supervised living arrangements.

Schizophrenia occurs in 1% of the population. Schizophrenia, equally distributed between men and women, is more common in nonwhite populations and in lower socioeconomic groups. There is a significantly greater likelihood for schizophrenia in an individual whose parent(s) or sibling has the disorder. Although the peak age for patients to have hospital admission for schizophrenia is 25 to 34 years, acute schizophrenic episodes occur commonly in middle to late adolescence and young adulthood, prior to the age of 25 years, and can begin as early as 12 years of age.

Many individuals with an acute schizophrenic episode are found to have led isolated lives prior to the psychosis. Other individuals may have achieved higher levels of functioning and may have a better prognosis. In general, positive outcomes are proven when the patient and his/her family are informed about schizophrenia, participate actively in treatment, and work to create a stable, predictable living environment.

MANIC-DEPRESSIVE ILLNESS

Manic-depressive illness usually occurs prior to the age of 30 years, and there is increasing recognition that the disorder can occur in late childhood and in adolescence. Manic-depressive illness may present in different ways: 1) as an acute manic state, with or without prior history of mania and depression; 2) as an acutely depressed state, in a patient with one or more manic attacks in the past; 3) as rapid alternation between mania and depression.

An acute manic episode may emerge suddenly in adolescence, but often there are early clues. A family history of depression or manic-depressive illness often can be obtained. The patient may have had previously untreated depressive episodes or have been regarded as "moody." The patient may identify past and present mood swings with irritability and an accompanying loss of personal control.

INFANTILE AUTISM AND PERVASIVE DEVELOPMENTAL DISORDER OF CHILDHOOD

Together, infantile autism and pervasive developmental disorder of childhood account for most cases of psychosis in children from birth to 12 years of age. Both disorders, which are three times more common in boys than girls, are extremely rare, with approximately two cases per

TABLE 133-1
Differentiating Features of Organic Psychiatrically Based Psychosis

ASSESSMENT FEATURE	ORGANIC	PSYCHIATRIC
History		
Nature of onset	Acute	Insidious
History before illness	Prior illness or drug use	Prior psychiatric history (self or family)
Physical evaluation		
Level of consciousness	May be impaired	Normal
Vital signs	May be impaired	Usually normal
Pathologic autonomic signs	May be present	Normal
Laboratory studies, including urine screening	May be abnormal	Normal
Mental status evaluation		
Orientation	May be impaired	Intact
Recent memory	May be impaired	Intact
Intellectual functioning	May be impaired	Intact
Nature of hallucinations	Not auditory (eg, visual, tactile)	Auditory
Response to support and medication	Often dramatic	Often limited

10,000 children. The major distinguishing feature is age at onset, with infantile autism by definition occurring prior to 30 months of age. Tasks of the primary care physician for these children are to diagnose the condition, refer the child and family for appropriate service, and work collaboratively with this treatment network.

Infantile Autism
The cardinal feature of autistic children is a generalized lack of responsiveness to people, together with a failure to develop normal attachment behavior. The manner of presentation can be quite variable, and the diagnosis is usually made after the child is 12 months of age. Often the mother can describe sensing a "differentness" or "strangeness" about the child going back to the first several months. The child often is described as having been aloof. Developmental milestones may be erratic or delayed. Only 30% of autistic children have an intelligence quotient above 70. Some of these children have an underlying medical condition such as maternal rubella syndrome or previous encephalitis or meningitis, but the etiology for the vast majority of autistic children is unknown. The autistic child uses toys inappropriately and in a bizarre manner. Stereotyped behaviors (such as rocking, twirling, or whirling) may occur. The single most important prognostic sign is the development or absence of language by the age of 5 years.

Pervasive Developmental Disorder
Children with a pervasive developmental disorder have had apparently normal development during the first 2½ years of life. Typically, the child acquires language. Developmental milestones are often variable and mental retardation, when present, is less severe than with infantile autism. The key deficiency again is in social relationships and attachment. Pervasive development disorder accounts for most cases of psychosis in children under the age of 12 years.

OFFICE EVALUATION

Table 133-1 indicates some of the differentiating features of organic and psychiatrically based psychosis. *History* often reveals an acute onset for an organic psychosis, as compared with a more gradual, insidious onset for psychiatrically based psychosis. With the latter, a history of prior psychotic episodes or a family history of psychosis may be obtained. With an organic psychosis, the panicked patient sometimes admits to an ingestion of drugs or a history of drug use is obtained from family or friends. History of the circumstances of the ingestion, including the possibility of a suicide attempt, should be obtained. On *physical examination,* alteration of vital signs may occur with organic psychosis, or there may be other findings of an underlying medical or traumatic disorder. *Mental status evaluation* points toward an organic psychosis if there is impairment in orientation, recent memory, and other cognitive functioning. In organic psychosis, *hallucinations* tend to be visual and also may be tactile, olfactory, and gustatory; in contrast, psychiatrically based psychosis is most frequently accompanied by auditory hallucinations. Finally, the immediate response to *support, reassurance,* and small doses of *medication* are frequently more dramatic with organic psychosis than with psychiatrically based psychosis.

A patient experiencing an *acute schizophrenic episode* appears strange, preoccupied, and private. Affect is flat, and the patient has little interest in relating to the physician. Speech appears disconnected, lacking goal-directedness and clear transitions. There may be inappropriate smiling and/or giggling or other inappropriate comments. The patient typically finds it excruciatingly difficult to make decisions, such as that of agreeing to psychiatric treatment.

The following are the most commonly found signs and symptoms of acute schizophrenic episodes: auditory hallucinations, flatness of affect, thoughts spoken aloud, and delusions of external control. Auditory hallucinations typically involve voices of persons talking negatively about the patient in the third person. At times, the voices also may direct the patient toward suicidal or homicidal acts. The patient may feel that others can read his/her mind or can either add to or take away the patient's ideas at will. The patient also has delusions of external control that involve the belief that the patient's mind, thoughts, behavior, spirit, and/or body are being externally controlled by some outside force or person. An acutely psychotic individual also may be depressed and may have suicidal and homicidal ideations.

An acute schizophrenic episode can be differentiated from an organic psychosis on the basis of history, which usually reveals chronic deterioration in functioning and the gradual emergence of psychotic symptoms. A positive family history of schizophrenia may be helpful. Findings of physical examination of the acutely schizophrenic patient are usually negative, except for that of possible tachycardia associated with anxiety.

The *manic patient* presents with an expansive, often grandiose, and elevated mood. The patient reports feeling extremely good and readily describes his/her exploits, which may include great achievements and plans, lack of sleep, and buying sprees. The patient speaks rapidly with pressured speech and may show a "flight of ideas," rapidly shifting from one topic to the next without completing earlier thoughts. The patient also may become irritable and emotionally labile if someone disagrees with him/her. Extremely aggressive and combative behavior may be displayed. The patient overestimates himself/herself and has little or no awareness of his/her distortion of reality. If the patient also is experiencing a significant depression, emotional lability will be even greater. Overall, the range of sudden emotional responses may include any of the following: euphoria, anxiety, irritability, combativeness, panic, and depression. There also may be a history of previous episodes of mania or depression.

The office-based physician can make the diagnosis of *infantile autism* on the basis of the history, the mother's concerns, and the findings of regular visits during the first 2½ years of life. Children with a *pervasive developmental disorder* also may be identified through history and clinical presentation. The patient may demonstrate extreme anxiety, difficulty in separation, hypersensitivity to sensory stimuli, irregular physiologic patterns, and extreme mood lability. Posturing and self-mutilation may occur. Speech may be abnormal, and affect may be inappropriate. Typically, these children appear to have a "strange" quality noted by the physician.

In encountering an acutely psychotic adolescent, the office-based physician should recognize that the patient as well as the family are often extremely anxious. The patient's mood may be extremely labile, because the world is seen as dangerous, threatening, and unpredictable. Whether agitated or withdrawn, the patient may pose a suicidal and/or violent risk, and violence can be directed at the physician and emergency room staff as well as the family and outside world.

MANAGEMENT

The management of psychosis in the acute phase includes the following goals:

1. Differentiating Organic Psychosis From the Psychiatrically Based Psychosis.—This distinction is made on the basis of history (individual, family, illness, and drug histories), mental status, physical examination, and laboratory studies, including toxicology screen. When in doubt, the patient should be observed for a longer period of time. This differentiation of organic from psychiatrically based psychosis will influence all subsequent management decisions.

2. Determining Possible Suicidal Danger or Other Risk of Self-Harm.—All acutely psychotic patients may represent an immediate suicide risk due to impaired judgment and possible depression. In addition, the patient may harm himself/herself unintentionally. It is essential to ascertain from the patient, friends, and family whether any deliberate or accidental life-endangering events have taken place. The patient should be asked directly about suicidal thoughts. This assessment will influence significantly the decision of whether or not to hospitalize the patient.

3. Determining the Nature of Family Resources.—To address the emergency created by the acutely psychotic patient, the office-based physician should call in all important family members. The nature of the family response and the degree to which the family can collaborate with the physician in developing a treatment plan for the patient guide the physician in deciding on treatment and disposition.

4. Determining the Need for Medical Hospitalization.—Medical hospitalization may be necessary in cases of organic psychosis due to newly diagnosed or exacerbated chronic illness or toxic psychosis to manage medical complications. With an intoxication, the patient and family often deny the significance of the acute episode after it resolves. Therefore, it is essential that the psychiatrist see the patient and family as soon as he/she is able to speak coherently. If medical hospitalization is employed, the patient should be placed on a floor that is experienced in the acute management of psychotic and possibly suicidal patients. A psychiatrist should be available on an emergency basis.

5. Determining the Need for Psychiatric Hospitalization.—Under ideal circumstances, the acute schizophrenic or manic patient is managed on an outpatient basis, with intensive psychiatric intervention beginning at the time of diagnosis. Outpatient treatment for acute psychiatrically based psychosis is indicated under the following circumstances: *a)* the patient is not suicidal, homicidal, or at significant risk of acci-

dental self-harm; *b)* the patient recognizes his/her own impairment and is cooperative; *c)* the family is organized and appears capable of supervising the patient; *d)* a therapist is available at the time of the crisis to work immediately with patient and family; *e)* the patient responds to antipsychotic medication in the emergency room.

Psychiatric hospitalization, on the other hand, is required in the following cases: *a)* the patient is suicidal, violent, or incapable of supervised self-care; *b)* the family is absent or unable to assume responsibility for the patient; and *c)* no therapist is available to assume immediate control of the case.

6. Using Psychotropic Medication, When Indicated.—Antipsychotic medication may be utilized in the acute management of both organic and psychiatrically based psychosis. Many toxic psychoses resolve with support and reassurance, involvement of the family, isolation from other patients, the passage of time, and physical restraint, if needed. When these measures fail, and especially when the ingested drug is known, low doses of an antipsychotic agent may be quite helpful. When severe psychiatrically based psychosis requires psychiatric hospitalization or when no therapist is available to take responsibility for the case, it is recommended that the patient *not* be given antipsychotic medication on an emergency basis, because the partial response to this medication may result in the patient's being turned away by the psychiatric hospital. In such circumstances, the intramuscular or intravenous use of diphenhydramine (Benadryl), 20 to 50 mg, and physical restraints, when necessary, are preferable. Other minor tranquilizers such as diazepam (Valium), oxazepam (Serax), and alprazolam (Xanax) also may be utilized.

Common antipsychotic medications, relative potency, and usual dosage ranges are listed in Table 133-2. It is recommended that the office-based physician select several drugs and gain familiarity with their usage in emergency situations. The physician also should be familiar with common side effects of antipsychotic medications and inform patients and parents of these. Lethargy, dizziness, and hypotension may occur with those drugs given in high doses (chlorpromazine, thioridazine), and vital signs should be monitored. Extrapyramidal side-effects are common with low-dosage drugs (haloperidol, trifluoperazine, fluphenazine); these side effects

TABLE 133-2
Common Antipsychotic Medications

GENERIC NAME (BRAND NAME)	ESTIMATED EQUIVALENT DOSAGE (MG)	TOTAL DAILY DOSAGE (MG)
Phenothiazines		
Chlorpromazine (Thorazine)	100	5–1000
Thioridazine (Mellaril)	100	50–800
Trifluoperazine (Stelazine)	5	5–30
Fluphenazine (Prolixin)	2	1–20
Butyrophenones		
Haloperidol (Haldol)	2	2–40

include acute dystonia (abnormal muscle contractions); akathisia (abnormal motor restlessness); pseudo-Parkinsonism (rigidity, slowness, stooped posture, drooling, inexpressive facies). Tardive dyskinesia (often irreversible, with long-term use) may occur with either high- or low-dose antipsychotic medication.

Acute dystonic reactions are common in the adolescent and young adult age group and can be treated prophylactically with benztropine, 1 to 4 mg/day orally. Emergency treatment of dystonia involves the intramuscular or intravenous use of diphenhydramine, 25 to 50 mg. For manic-depressive illness, lithium is the mainstay of treatment but requires 1 week or more to achieve maximum beneficial effect. The administration of lithium should be the responsibility of the treating psychiatrist.

FOLLOW-UP

Once the acute psychotic episode has resolved, whether organic or psychiatric, the office-based physician can broaden his/her own relationship with the adolescent, encourage personal competence, and help the family deal with important issues, such as parental limit setting and appropriate levels of closeness, as well as independence, autonomy, and eventual separation. If the patient requires continuing medication, the physician supports this. If specialized education is required or treatment programs are needed, the physician becomes familiar with these programs and serves as an advocate for the patient, ensuring that appropriate services are being provided and that communication between institutions also occurs.

BIBLIOGRAPHY

Campbell M, et al: Treatment of autistic disorder, *J Am Acad Child Adolesc Psychiatry* 35(2): 134–143, 1996.

Fields JH, Grochowski S, Lindenmayer JP, et al: Assessing positive and negative symptoms in children and adolescents, *Am J Psychiatry* 151(2):249–253, 1994.

Livingston R, Bracha HS: Psychotic symptoms and suicidal behavior in hospitalized children, *Am J Psychiatry* 149(11):1585–1586, 1992.

Weller EB, Weller RA, Fristad MA: Bipolar disorder in children: misdiagnosis, underdiagnosis, and future, *J Am Acad Child Adolesc Psychiatry* 34(6):709–714, 1995.

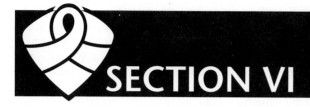

SECTION VI

Talking With Parents and Patients

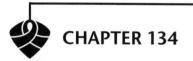

CHAPTER 134

Innocent Murmur

Sidney Friedman

Approximately 90% of children referred to a cardiologist for evaluation are referred because of the presence of a cardiac murmur. The two common types of heart disease in childhood, congenital and rheumatic heart disease, usually present with a cardiac murmur. Skill in cardiac auscultation is important in pediatrics, because approximately 40% of normal children between the ages of 2 and 12 years have so-called functional or innocent murmurs. Thus, physicians are beset with the problem of determining in every second or third patient examined whether a murmur is a significant one, indicating the presence of heart disease, or an innocent one, indicating the absence of heart disease.

A label of functional or innocent murmur has the following implications: 1) no pathologic changes are present in the heart or great vessels, 2) the cardiac murmur does not affect the future health or prognosis of the patient, 3) no further

diagnostic investigation or long-term follow-up systematic observation is necessary, 4) no prophylaxis against bacterial endocarditis is necessary, 5) no antistreptococcal prophylaxis is needed to prevent a recurrence of rheumatic fever.

There is abundant evidence in the literature and from the personal experience of pediatric cardiologists that functional or innocent murmurs can be identified accurately by simple auscultation. A recent study by Newberger and associates supported the concept that a qualified pediatric cardiologist can identify accurately the categories of "no heart disease" or "definite heart disease" without the use of simple or complex diagnostic testing. The close correlation of the separate clinical examinations of Friedman and Wells in a survey of approximately 5000 schoolchildren in Philadelphia also supports this concept. There is ample evidence that innocent

959

murmurs are truly benign with regard to future cardiac health. A 20-year follow-up study by Marienfeld and associates, published in 1962, demonstrated that the incidence of real heart disease in a group of adults identified as having an innocent murmur 20 years earlier was the same as in a group of controlled patients without a cardiac murmur in childhood.

In a survey of more than 20,000 schoolchildren, Bergman and Stamm pointed out the high incidence of the false diagnosis of heart disease resulting from the misinterpretation of innocent murmurs and suggested the term *cardiac nondisease*. The inaccuracy in diagnosis often resulted in unnecessary restriction and anxiety about heart disease in children and parents. The authors pointed out the frequency of confusion in the layperson's understanding of heart disease in children—specifically, fear of heart attacks from overexertion, a concept derived from the symptoms of adult degenerative heart disease. They concluded that the amount of disability from cardiac nondisease was greater than that due to actual heart disease in children. Failure of adequate communication between physicians and parents and the false diagnosis of heart disease resulting from the misinterpretation of innocent murmurs were the main sources of the cardiac nondisease.

Because many children are examined in routine school physical examinations or in presports or precamp examinations by physicians other than their family physician, and because many children are followed in group practices in which examinations are carried out by a number of different doctors, it is wise to mention the presence of a cardiac murmur to parents and to enter this information into the written records.

The skill and subjective confidence of physicians in deciding whether a cardiac murmur is innocent or significant vary widely. Nevertheless, an effective policy of management of children with cardiac murmurs can be established. If the presence of the murmur is reported to the family, the primary care physician must first decide whether he/she is certain or uncertain about the identification of the cardiac murmur. If the murmur is an innocent one, then the physician can proceed with the verbal type of communication outlined below. The physician may decide to observe the cardiac murmur on several occasions and come to a final conclusion at a later date. This scheme should be carried out

without involving the parents in one's own indecision. If the diagnosis is uncertain, or if the parents are aware of the presence of the murmur, the physician must take further steps promptly to clarify the situation by appropriate consultation and study. It is unwise and unfair to permit parents with an unsettled question about the presence or absence of heart disease in their offspring to suffer this indecision for any significant length of time. When logistically possible, the use of such basic studies as an electrocardiogram (ECG) or chest radiograph is expected as a further confirmation and should be ordered to enhance the attitude of certainty. However, these studies are not a substitute for a skillful physical examination.

The following dialogue is an example of an appropriate approach to the discussion of the diagnosis of innocent murmurs with parents.

I can hear a heart murmur in my examination of John, but I do not think it is of any importance. It falls in the category of heart murmurs that are called functional *or* innocent. *Are you familiar with these terms? (The answer is usually "no.")*

There are a large number of children who have heart murmurs that we know from experience are not related to heart disease or a heart defect. These murmurs are called functional or innocent murmurs, because they have no relationship to any defect of the structure of the heart but rather are related to the function or working of the heart. These murmurs are due to a vibration of the heart muscle itself rather than to the turbulence of blood flow related to a defect such as a hole between two of the chambers or an abnormality of one of the valves in the heart.

There is a considerable and lengthy experience in following patients with functional or innocent murmurs. It has been shown by long-term follow-up studies that patients with functional or innocent murmurs do not have any higher incidence of heart disease than patients without such murmurs, even after they are observed for 20 or 30 years. Therefore, you can be certain that this murmur will not turn into something else in the future. It is not the beginning of some other condition that will be a problem later on.

I think it would be a good idea to do a routine survey of your child's heart to gain even more reassurance that the murmur is of no importance. I think that we should do an ECG and a chest radiograph in order to get further information indicating that the heart is normal. If results of these studies are normal, then I do not think there is any need to pursue this matter further. If results of these studies are normal, which I expect they will be, the accuracy of the diagnosis is extremely high, approaching 100% in the presence of a murmur of this character.

At this point, it is appropriate to answer any questions that arise and to send the family off to have the studies done. This provides parents with some time to think over what has been said and to identify any questions they want answered. When they return, I look at the radiograph and ECG. If results of these are normal, then I have a further conversation with the parents along the following lines:

Both of the tests, the radiograph and the ECG, are entirely normal so everything seems to fit together, the physical examination and the studies. There are a few things I want to be sure you understand about functional or innocent murmurs. First and foremost, there is nothing anatomically wrong with your child's heart. He can be on the football team. This murmur does not mean that he has any structural defect or disease of his heart. The second point I want to make is this: Although it is true that approximately 90% of these murmurs disappear when the child is around 10 or 14 years of age, not 100% of them disappear. However, it makes no difference whether the murmur disappears or does not disappear, as far as the future cardiac health of your child is concerned. For this reason, it is not necessary to have any follow-up examinations in children with functional or innocent murmurs. It is important to identify the murmur, but there is no need to continue to examine this child until the murmur is no longer audible. That will not contribute anything to the future health care of your child. The identification of the murmur is what we are doing today, and it is clear that the murmur is a functional or innocent one.

The third point I want to make is that you may, indeed, heart about this murmur again. These functional or innocent murmurs are variable

in how loud they sound on different occasions. They are made to sound louder by any condition that increases the work of the heart. Thus, if a child has a fever or is anemic, or perhaps is apprehensive about something, these functional or innocent murmurs will sound very loud to the listener. Sometimes, when the murmurs are quite loud, they are interpreted by the person who is examining the child to be more important and significant than they really are. In this way, you may hear about the presence of a loud murmur again, particularly at a time when the heart is working hard. The clinical setting in which this sequence may occur is a school physical examination, or during a family trip when the child develops an illness with fever. A physician who does not know the child from previous examinations may mention to you, under these circumstances, that a loud heart murmur is present, and advise further evaluation. You must remember not to push the panic button under these circumstances, because the murmur will almost certainly be the same murmur present today, but will have been accentuated by fever or apprehension.

The goal of this presentation is to transmit a sense of certainty to both parents and child about the absence of heart disease. Contributing to this are 1) firmness of expression by the physician. This is largely an expression of the confidence he/she has in his/her own cardiac auscultation skills. Expressions such as "he can be on the football team" offer more reassurance to parents than the expression, "no restrictions are necessary" or "don't worry about it". 2) The lack of need for follow-up is a strong point of reassurance for parents and should be stressed and the rationale repeated. 3) Some form of diagnostic testing should be employed to support the clinical diagnosis. This may not be essential on a statistical analysis for an experienced pediatric cardiologist, but testing provides a great deal of additional psychological support for parents and referring physicians.

Above all, be definite!

BIBLIOGRAPHY

Bergman AB, Stamm SJ: The morbidity of cardiac nondisease in school children, *N Engl J Med* 276:1008–1013, 1967.

Friedman S, Robie WA, Harris TN: Occurrence of innocent adventitious cardiac sounds in childhood, *Pediatrics* 3:782–789, 1949.

Friedman S, Wells CR: Experience in secondary screening of cardiac suspects of school age, *J Pediatr* 49:410–416, 1956.

Marienfeld CJ, Telles N, Silvera J, et al: A 20-year follow-up study of "innocent" murmurs, *Pediatrics* 30:42–48, 1962.

Newberger JW, Rosenthal A, Williams RG, et al: Noninvasive tests in the initial evaluation of heart murmurs in children, *N Engl J Med* 308:61–64, 1983.

SUGGESTED READING

Friedman S: The innocent (functional) cardiac murmurs of childhood, *Clin Pediatr* 4:77–81, 1965.

Friedman S: Some thoughts about functional or innocent murmurs, *Clin Pediatr* 12:678–679, 1973.

Caceres CA, Perry LW, editors: *The Innocent Murmur—A Problem in Clinical Practice,* Boston, 1967, Little, Brown & Co.

CHAPTER 135

Mental Retardation

Thomas A. Curry

During the course of monitoring a child's development, the primary care physician will be able to detect children who fail to progress through established normal ranges of development. Using a developmental screening test such as the Denver Developmental Screening Test, the physician can identify children in need of more extensive evaluation. The team involved in the evaluation includes developmental pediatricians, geneticists, neurologists, and psychologists. This panel of health professionals permits a refined approach to the multitude of problems. Unfortunately, the diversity of styles and methods of individual team members often can be a source of uncertainty to the family. Either as the coordinator of the evaluation or as the translator of the recommendations from the diagnostic team, the primary care physician is frequently the one who must tell the parents that their child is retarded.

Discussion with the parents of a mentally retarded child requires sensitivity and forethought. The pressure of time can severely impair the physician's ability to appropriately explain a diagnosis, interpret an evaluation, and react to parental concerns. Prior to a parent conference, the physician must prepare for the meeting. A few seconds to review documents immediately prior to talking with the parents is insufficient and frequently can lead to a most unsatisfactory outcome. The physician should understand the details of the evaluation that has taken place, the nature of the testing that was performed, and the specific results of the testing.

A short list of goals to be accomplished during the meeting is helpful in focusing the discussion and developing a general format for the meeting.

THE CONFERENCE

Although working parents frequently find it difficult to arrange a time that both may be present, efforts should be made to avoid delivering the news to one person. The absent parent will frequently demand explanations and ask questions that the parent who was present finds difficult or impossible to answer. It is helpful to determine in advance of the conference if the parents wish other members of the extended family to attend the meeting. This conference may require several sessions. The amount of time spent at the meeting is dependent on the ability of the parent to comprehend and absorb all the facts and attitudes that are presented.

Structuring the parent conference is important. A typical outline is presented below.

Structure of Parent Conference

- **The diagnosis**
    Interpretation of diagnosis
    Review of tests
- **Emphasis on normal features**
  Planning
    Effect on child
    Effect on family
- **Closing**
    Need for second opinion
    Definite follow-up

Giving the results of the evaluation at the beginning of the conference rather than at the end permits the parents to react to the diagnosis throughout the interview. For some, the shock of the diagnosis may cease any further meaningful dialogue. Because many parents have some idea that their child is retarded, the risk of stating the diagnosis early is limited. The diagnosis can be expressed in a variety of terms, such as below-normal intelligence or below-average potential. It is important, however, for the parents to hear the term *retardation* from the physician. If retardation is not mentioned, parents may leave the meeting feeling their child is just slow or delayed but not retarded. Occasionally, a physician will spend considerable time enumerating in great detail the results of testing prior to giving a final diagnosis. This technique only heightens the parents' tension and anxiety as they wait for the conclusion.

After presenting the diagnosis, the physician can interpret the diagnosis for the family. This discussion should include review of the tests performed. The physician's demonstration of a working knowledge of the tests employed will understandably enhance the parents' acceptance of the diagnosis. Clarification of the results of psychologic testing or other evaluations from the subspecialists should be done prior to the meeting so that the physician's poor understanding of the tests does not give the parents an excuse to doubt the diagnosis.

During the conference, the parents need to hear positive statements about their child. A special effort should be made to emphasize those aspects of the child's evaluations that are normal. If appropriate, this is the time to state that the child will walk or speak but at a slower rate than peers. Although parents may focus on the areas of delay, the positive features such as ability to attend school or participation in sports should be mentioned.

Even though the diagnosis is mentioned at the outset of the conference, the problem needs to be put in the perspective of the child and the family. Parents will want to know the effect this diagnosis will have on their child. What are the recommendations for the short term as to the special educational placement, schooling, and therapy? The child should be given an opportunity to use all of his/her capabilities. Overprotection is not helpful for the child; optimal training is. Specific opportunities for schooling should be reviewed. Federal and state mandates regarding educational services and their availability in the community should be addressed. Achieving full potential, however limited, is the goal that must be reinforced several times in the discussion.

The physician should attempt to deal with the potential effect of the diagnosis on the family. Usually the parents worry about the possibility of this occurring in another child. They may try affixing blame on themselves or others for this problem. This concern about genetic implications should have been anticipated in the evaluation. If appropriate, metabolic screening or genetic evaluation is helpful in detecting an inherited disorder. Parents want to know if they are responsible for their child's retardation. Mothers have questions about events in their

VI

pregnancies that may have caused the problem. The parents may need help in explaining the diagnosis to their other children. This explanation should be brief and appropriate to the level of understanding of the child. Obviously, sensitivity is needed in dealing with this issue. The family also may appreciate help in how to explain the diagnosis with its difficult implications to nonfamily members.

Finally, a complete parent conference deals with the parents' need to doubt the diagnosis. The parents can be told that it is normal to have doubts about the diagnosis, and they may need to have a second opinion. The mention of another opinion should be followed by a list of facilities or personnel who can provide this service rather than allowing the parents to seek out persons who provide advice that either is unhelpful or delays acceptance or training. A file of American Academy of Pediatrics Committee Reports can be offered to the family to help them understand problems of vitamin therapy or exercise in treating retardation. Not all families will require another opinion, reflecting either their own personality and experience or the adequacy of the evaluation and conference. Rather than interpret the need for a second opinion as a threat to intelligence or skill, the physician should be a facilitator to make this second opinion a learning experience and an ability for the family to build confidence in their physician. During the conference it is appropriate to pause and permit periods of silence to aid the family in adjusting to the information and to allow an opportunity to formulate questions on sensitive topics.

At the conclusion of the conference, a specific follow-up appointment should be made. This second meeting serves to continue the dialogue about the problem as well as to indicate to the parents that they are not being abandoned by their physician who will be part of their support system.

PROBLEMS AND PITFALLS

Some parents have anticipated the diagnosis of mental retardation. By comparing their child with peers or siblings, they are aware that development is delayed. Others may be upset and alarmed. Their response is similar to the grief response popularized by Kubler-Ross—denial, rage, depression, acceptance, and adjustment. Some parents may have to symbolically bury

their expectations for an ideal child before they can begin to deal with their child. On occasion, the initial reaction of the parents to the specific diagnosis or the specific test results is so overwhelming that the remainder of the material anticipated for the conference must be postponed. The physician needs to be willing to reschedule a conference under these circumstances. To plow through the remaining agenda with parents who are unable to focus or participate in the conference is inappropriate.

More commonly, the parents demonstrate resistance to the diagnosis. The physician should appreciate at least some degree of denial. It is understandable that the parents hope that the information is inaccurate or incorrect. Expressing an understanding that the family may wish that these facts were not true permits alignment with the family at a crucial time. The physician needs to remain firm, however, in the presentation of the conclusion.

Infrequently, anger is directed toward the person conducting the parent conference. Hostility by the physician does not aid the parents in the acceptance of the news. Quietly pointing out their anger and asking them to explain their feelings are of greater value.

During the discussion highly technical aspects should be avoided. Parents cannot always appreciate the intricate detail of testing or of laboratory evaluations. It is important to explain the test results with a language that is appropriate for the parent. Pausing frequently and asking if they wish an explanation repeated or restated is helpful.

Making very specific long-term predictions of outcome is inappropriate. Repeatedly, parents relate anecdotes of physicians who told parents that their child would never respond to treatment, only to prove the physician wrong. Physicians' expectations of eventual outcome have been shown at times to be too pessimistic compared with those of other health professionals. The long-term outcome needs to be addressed, but an attempt at the initial conference with the parents to make specific predictions is hazardous.

SUMMARY

Mental retardation often is suspected by the primary care physician, who will also be the individual responsible for presenting the diagnosis to the family. To be effective, the physician must have familiarity with the tests, present the diagnosis in a firm but gentle manner, and then be prepared to support the family as they accept the diagnosis and make plans for the future.

BIBLIOGRAPHY

Kaminer RK, Cohen HJ: How do you say, "Your child is retarded"? *Contemp Pediatr* 5:36–49, 1988.

Korsch BM: What do patients and parents want to know? What do they need to know? *Pediatrics* 74:917–919, 1984.

Myers BA: The informing interview: Enabling parents to "hear" and cope with bad news, *Am J Dis Child* 137:572, 1983.

Nursey AD, Rohde JR, Farmer RD: Ways of telling new parents about their child and his or her mental handicap: A comparison of doctors' and parents' views, *J Ment Defic Res* 35:48–57, 1991.

Olson J, Edwards M, Hunter JA: The physician's role in delivering sensitive information to families with handicapped infants, *Clin Pediatr* 26:231–234, 1987.

Wolraich ML, Superstein GN, O'Keefe P: Pediatricians' perceptions of mentally retarded individuals, *Pediatrics* 80:643–649, 1987.

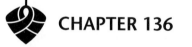

CHAPTER 136

Down Syndrome

Deborah L. Eunpu
Elaine H. Zackai

Down syndrome, the most common cause of mental retardation, occurs in approximately one in 600 live births. Because of the high incidence, most pediatricians will be confronted at some time with the necessity of informing parents that their child has this condition. How the physician informs the parents about the diagnosis can be a critical determinant of how well the parents accept this unexpected event and adjust to its implications.

CONFIRMING THE DIAGNOSIS

As soon as the diagnosis is suspected, the physician should arrange the confirming chromosome analysis so that parents can be told the diagnosis at the earliest time. Results of the study usually can be obtained 72 hours after culture initiation if prior arrangements are made with the referral laboratory. When asked their preference, the vast majority of parents of children with Down syndrome express a desire to be informed of the diagnosis as soon as possible. Many parents are aware that a problem exists before the physician has mentioned the suspicion, and a delay in providing the diagnostic information can result in parents being informed inappropriately by another source. Early informing also will allow the parents to consider all options for the care of the child with Down syndrome. Delaying the disclosure also can reduce the parents' trust of the primary care physician.

When an infant has associated problems requiring immediate medical attention (eg, a congenital heart defect or duodenal atresia), it is equally important that the parents be apprised of the diagnosis of Down syndrome as soon as possible. This will help them to view the infant's problem(s) in the context of the overall diagnosis and not to focus on isolated aspects of the child's condition.

Although most often the mother is first informed alone, most parents prefer to be told together. Telling both parents together allows them to support each other and permits each one to obtain answers to his/her questions. Other parent preferences include being told in a private setting and if possible having the baby present during the discussion. Parents have found it beneficial if there is another professional present who can be available to them for questions and discussion after the initial informing session. The physician must also consider the specific family constellation in deciding how to proceed with informing the parents.

INFORMATION FOR PARENTS

The information relayed to the parents should include an explanation of the chromosomal basis of the diagnosis, the risk of recurrence, the availability of prenatal diagnosis in a future pregnancy, a description of the associated physical features and medical problems, and a discussion of the developmental expectations for children with Down syndrome. The discussion should be in language and terms that the parents can understand. Telling parents their child will be mentally retarded can have very different meanings to different parents. Some associate retardation with violent behavior; others have a concept that retardation implies no development. Thus,

it is most important to use descriptive examples to provide a frame of reference that parents can comprehend meaningfully. Parents need to know that although acquisition of milestones is expected to be delayed, the child with Down syndrome is expected to sit, walk, talk, and be able to manage self-care tasks such as dressing, going to the toilet, and feeding. The physician must also describe the expected limits. Because individuals with Down syndrome continue to learn by rote rather than by progressing to higher cognitive levels of integrative learning, they will not be able to attain full independence as adults. Again, the physician should give specific, concrete examples that are more helpful than simply giving an expected intelligence quotient level (mean, 50 to 60) or telling parents the child will probably function in the trainable range of retardation. Overall, one should present a balanced view of the significance of the diagnosis of Down syndrome. Expected limitations, potential medical problems, and positive characteristics all merit discussion.

Every parent deserves to know the possible alternatives for caring for their child with Down syndrome. Although most parents will want to raise the infant in their family, it is important that parents at least know that foster care (temporary or leading to adoption) can be arranged. Residential placement may not be an option in the newborn period, because many residential facilities will not accept infants for admission. In addition, it is agreed that children with Down syndrome do best in a one-to-one care setting. Temporary foster care can serve as a valuable alternative if the parents are ambivalent about their plans for the child. Foster care leading to adoption is a very feasible option if the parents decide not to rear their child with Down syndrome. Because infants with Down syndrome are regarded as being very adoptable, local social service agencies usually can provide ready access to adoption agencies and resources. In presenting such information, the physician should encourage the parents to consider these possible options and help them see that the choice they make should be determined by what best suits their specific family situation. Parents should not be told which choice to select nor should they be urged to make permanent decisions without adequate consideration.

Parents who will raise their child with Down syndrome in their home should be apprised of locally available infant stimulation programs, the local Association for Retarded Citizens, parent support groups, and other supportive services (financial, social, and psychological).

Follow-up discussions frequently will be required to cover all information. Many parents, on hearing the diagnosis, cannot absorb additional information. These couples will require time to adjust to the shock of the unexpected news and to grieve for the lost normal child that they anticipated. One must tailor the length and content of the discussion to the parents' needs and abilities.

Even if the parents are ready to hear all of the information, follow-up is still important. New questions will arise and parents will need clarification of information that was heard only partially or incorrectly. One study of parental adjustment found that parents typically experience a second wave of grief that is initiated by delayed acquisition of a social smile and poorer eye contact than expected for the infant's age. At later times, follow-up visits also can prove beneficial by providing parents an opportunity to discuss their child's progress and their own adjustment, questions, or concern. At times of transition (eg, first school placement and completion of formal education), intervention in the form of anticipatory guidance can be particularly helpful to parents. In fact, such follow-up is desired by most parents.

Parents who have other children often ask how to tell the older siblings and whether the child with Down syndrome will have an adverse effect on them. One should urge parents to answer the other children's questions at their level of understanding because older siblings usually detect the parents' sadness and preoccupation and are, therefore, aware that a problem exists. Although siblings may show some sadness at learning of the problem and experience some initial awkwardness in talking about the problem, siblings (and their friends) are typically understanding of the child's limitations, will include him/her in activities, and usually assume a protective role toward the child.

Throughout all dealings with parents who are trying to understand the significance of the diagnosis of Down syndrome in their child, the primary care physician should use sensitivity in the disclosure and maintain a stance of openness and acceptance. Such an approach will assist the parents in exploring their fears, hopes, and feelings to allow the healthiest adjustment to their experience.

BIBLIOGRAPHY

Carr J: Effect on the family of a child with Down syndrome, *Physiotherapy* 62(1):20–24, 1976.

Cunningham CC, Morgan PA, McGucken RB: Down's syndrome: Is dissatisfaction with disclosure of diagnosis inevitable? *Dev Med Child Neurol* 26:33–39, 1984.

Davis H: *Counseling parents of children with chronic illness or disability.* Leicester, 1993, BPS Books.

Gath A: Parental reactions to loss and disappointment: The diagnosis of Down's syndrome, *Dev Med Child Neurol* 27:392–400, 1985.

Hockey A: Evaluation of adoption of the intellectually handicapped: A retrospective analysis of 137 cases, *J Ment Defic Res* 24:187–202, 1980.

Pueschel S, Murphy A: Assessment of counseling practices at the birth of a child with Down syndrome, *Am J Ment Defic* 81:325–330, 1976.

Pueschel SM: Changes of counseling practice at the birth of a child with Down syndrome, *Appl Res Ment Retard* 6:99–108, 1985.

Pueschel SM, Pueschel JK: *Biomedical concerns in persons with Down syndrome,* Baltimore, 1992, Paul H. Brookes Publishing.

Pueschel SM, Tingey C, Rynders JE, et al, editors: *New perspectives on Down syndrome,* Baltimore, 1987, Paul H. Brookes Publishing.

Smith R, editor: *Children with mental retardation: A parents' guide,* Rockville, MD, 1993, Woodbine House.

Solnit AJ, Stark MH: Mourning and the birth of a defective child, *Psychoanal Study Child* 16: 523–537, 1961.

VI .

CHAPTER 137

Potentially Fatal Disease

R. Beverly Raney, Jr.

Discussing death is one of the most difficult tasks for the primary care team. This chapter offers an approach to help communicate the serious nature of the child's disease to the parents. There are three stages in the course of a life-threatening illness at which the possibility of death must be faced. The first occurs at the time of diagnosis of a potentially lethal disease. The second stage takes place at the time of relapse, after some period of active treatment, or when the disease fails to respond to initial therapy. The third stage is that period during which further medical intervention, with the goal of cure, is no longer feasible. At that time palliative measures may be used, but eventual death has become a certainty and life expectancy is limited to days or weeks.

DIAGNOSIS

How should the primary care physician describe to the parents the diagnosis and management of a possibly lethal disorder? The physician should outline the symptoms and signs of the child's illness and then discuss the diagnosis, attempting to keep the conversation simple and limited to practical issues such as the need for hospitalization, the types of treatment available, and the expected outcome of therapy. Ideally, both parents should be present in a quiet, private room, separate from the child so they can feel free to react emotionally and to ask questions without frightening the child. The parents are told calmly and sympathetically that the child has a life-threatening and potentially fatal disease. In many cases, treatment can alleviate the symptoms, perhaps permanently. The probability of control of the disease should be stressed, as should curability if that is possible.

The diagnosis of acute lymphoblastic leukemia is used here as an example. Once the diagnosis is confirmed by examination of the bone marrow, we inform the parents by saying, "Your child has acute leukemia. That is why the child is pale and feels tired and sometimes has fever. The bone marrow is producing the wrong kind of blood cells. We can nearly always eradicate leukemia for a period of time by giving the child several drugs. If the disease goes away and does not reappear within 3 years, your child may eventually be cured."

Parents also need to know at this point whether hospitalization is advisable. We believe that the shock of the diagnosis of cancer, for example, is such that outpatient management is psychologically very difficult for the parents and may be inadvisable for the child. Also, the parents need time to learn about the disease and to become familiar with medical terms and procedures. The parents also should be told whether imminent death is likely. In addition, they need to know whether the child can lead a virtually normal life, both during and after the period of treatment. The time required for this discussion should ideally not exceed 30 minutes, because parents are generally incapable of absorbing and retaining overly detailed information when under stress. The physician should close by emphasizing that he/she will be available to talk with them again and will answer their ongoing questions as much as possible. It may be helpful at this point to schedule a regular time to talk with one or both parents each day. We then say, "If you think of a question when we are not around, write it down and we can discuss it at our next meeting." It is important to warn them that neighbors and friends will give opinions and anecdotes about similar cases. These stories, which may confuse the parents, should be brought to the conference for discussion.

After the methods of management have been instituted, further instruction of the parents can take place. The parents may need assistance or encouragement in informing their child with words and explanations that are not frightening. The child needs to know that he/she has a serious disease that requires treatment. The child should be reassured that the medicine will help make him/her well again. We inform the parents and the child about the benefits and side effects of treatment, citing primarily the major and most noticeable types of toxic effects. For example, we say, "Your child with acute lymphoblastic leukemia will need injections, blood cell counts, bone marrow tests, and occasionally spinal taps to eliminate the leukemia cells and determine when they have disappeared. The drugs will probably cause increased appetite (glucocorticosteroids) and hair loss (vincristine); sometimes vomiting or constipation occurs. We can help minimize the stomach and bowel problems with other medicines, but your child may want to wear a hat at school or when outside the home."

Other caregivers such as nurses, social workers, and psychiatrists specially trained to work with families of seriously ill children are part of the management team and provide additional counseling and information. Educational material should be distributed and discussed. As parents see their child's health becoming restored, they become more capable of asking cogent questions about the disease, the treatment, their child's outlook for survival, and the quality of life. We emphasize that the attainment of remission is the first and most important goal, because children who cannot be rendered free of detectable disease are not likely to survive. Often parents' anxieties begin to dissipate after remission is documented. The parents need to be encouraged to treat the child as normally as possible during the period of remission, because cure is possible and perhaps likely.

RELAPSE

Relapse, or recurrence of the disease, is as difficult and frustrating for the patient, parents, and physician as is the diagnosis. In fact, the period of relapse is often perceived as worse, because it is known that relapse nearly always signifies death from the disease. Thus there is actually less hope for long-term survival after recrudescence

of the illness than there was before. Nonetheless, it is realistic and honest to emphasize that some children do recover after relapse. To provide the child another opportunity to overcome the disorder, further therapy should be undertaken, even if the likelihood of a successful outcome is low. At this stage parents need to understand the various options for further management and the problems that may arise as the therapeutic choices become more limited. Both parents should be present for support and to minimize misunderstanding. During this and subsequent interviews the primary physician can reevaluate the emotional state of the parents and determine how well they are able to cope with distressing events. The parents may need help explaining to the patient that the previous treatment is no longer working and that new medicine and possibly other measures are needed to regain control of the disease. The primary physician also can begin to prepare for the likelihood that the child will die in a relatively finite period of time. As an example, the physician may say, "The tests show that the medicines are no longer effective, because the malignant cells have returned. That is bad, because we give our best drugs at the beginning, and the disease has clearly become resistant to them. Still, there are some different medicines that have helped other children in this situation, and we would like to use them to try once more to eradicate the disease. Although permanent cure is now much less likely, it is not necessarily impossible."

IMPENDING DEATH

Once it becomes clear that active medical management can no longer control the disease, the physician is faced with having to tell the parents that death is a certainty. At this time the physician must be compassionate but honest. As an example, the physician may say, "We have now tried all the reasonable forms of treatment and yet the disease continues to come back. We really have nothing left to fight the disease, except some new experimental drugs that may well make your child even sicker. We can try one of them, if you want, but you know as well as we do that miracles don't usually happen when you need one."

The dying child often will have some psychologic distress, such as fear of separation from the parents or fear of intractable pain. The child also will experience increasing loss of control and of stamina. The child's difficulties are intensified if a vital organ such as the liver, lungs, or brain is involved, adding physical distress to the emotional trauma. During this period the physician should strive to alleviate symptoms whenever possible, being liberal about the use of narcotics for pain control and sedatives to help the patient sleep at night. The physician should encourage the family and patient to live for each day. The physician also should avoid the temptation to appear definite about the duration of a child's survival. We believe that it is preferable to give parents some guide, such as the statement that the child probably has several weeks to a few months to live, rather than a finite time. If the child is of school age, home tutoring and visits by friends and classmates should be arranged. Often a trip to a favorite vacation spot or to a child's playground or amusement park can help the family realize a worthwhile goal that the patient would enjoy and that the survivors will later recall with pleasure. The physician also can help by suggesting that the parents should not become completely antidisciplinarian; goals still need to be set and accomplished within the limits of the child's diminishing capabilities. The more normal each day can be, the better. Referral to a hospice association for support during this phase can be very helpful.

There is always discussion about how much to tell the child who is about to die. This area is complex and varies with each person's particular situation. We believe that most children already know when they are dying, but they generally avoid seeking a point-blank confirmation, because all hope is thereby removed. However, honesty and trust must be maintained. It is not usual in our experience for a child to ask either the physician or a parent, "Am I going to die?" If the child does ask, one may begin by responding, "Do you feel that bad? Does the thought of dying scare you? Let's talk about that now." Then the child can express feelings openly. If he/she asks "Am I dying now?", one may answer, "Yes, it is possible, and some children do die from the disease you have. But we will do everything we can to prevent it, and we will be here with you, even if things become worse."

The primary physician also should advise the parents that the sick child's siblings may, like the parents, have considerable feelings of stress, including depression and guilt. The parents need help to understand that the surviving children must not be shunted aside as the sick child is dying. The siblings also need to comprehend the gravity of the illness and know that their brother or sister may die within a short time. We suggest that the parents gather the whole family and outline the fact that the affected child's condition is not improving, that he/she may need more sleep and be less capable than formerly. The parents can say, "It is not anyone's fault, but your brother (sister) is really not getting better just now, and we all need to think about just how we can help. Maybe there is something we can all do together as a family, soon, in case he (she) becomes sicker as time goes by."

Ideally, in advance of the child's death the parents should discuss with the physician how to begin to make funeral arrangements. This area is difficult and sometimes painful to address, but the actual shock of a child's demise intensifies the parents' distress and renders them less capable of making decisions afterward. At this point the physician may say, "I wonder if you have any questions about what is going on. Sometimes families request an autopsy to learn more about their child's disorder and possibly to help the physicians learn more to benefit other children later. Would you like me to explain what is involved?"

The primary physician can and should strive to be available when the patient dies. That physician who has known the child through many years is the medical person best qualified to be with the family at or just after the moment of death, to pronounce the patient dead, and to assist the family by providing a limited amount of sedatives if requested. In this way the grieving parents will not be forced to take the child's body to an emergency room for pronouncement of death. The physician should help the parents tell the siblings that the child has stopped breathing and is no longer alive on earth. The clergy, especially if previously involved, should be notified right away.

Even after the child has died, the physician can help the parents by recalling with them the good times of the child's life, by being thankful that the struggle is over for that child, and by emphasizing that everything reasonable was done before death supervened. Any lingering questions should be answered, and contact by letter, telephone, or personal visit should be maintained with the family after the child has died. Even after the death, families may need reassurance from the physician that a new treatment described in the newspaper would not have saved the child's life and that everyone involved did everything possible to prolong the child's period of useful life.

BIBLIOGRAPHY

Adams-Greenly M: Psychological staging of pediatric cancer patients and their families, *Cancer* 58:449–453, 1986.

Conatser C: Preparing the family for their responsibilities during treatment, *Cancer* 58:508–511, 1986.

Coody D: High expectations: Nurses who work with children who might die, *Nurs Clin North Am* 20:131–142, 1985.

Koocher GP: Psychosocial issues during the acute treatment of pediatric cancer, *Cancer* 58:468–472, 1986.

Newton RW, Bergin B, Knowles D: Parents interviewed after their child's death, *Arch Dis Child* 61:711–715, 1986.

Pollock GH: Childhood sibling loss: A family tragedy, *Pediatr Ann* 15:851–855, 1986.

Siegel BS: Helping children cope with death, *Am Fam Physician* 31:175–180, 1985.

Speece MW, Brent SB: Children's understanding of death: A review of three components of a death concept, *Child Dev* 55:1671–1686, 1984.

Spinetta JJ, Deasy-Spinetta P: The patient's socialization in the community and school during therapy, *Cancer* 58:512–515, 1986.

SUGGESTED READING

Eden OB, Black I, MacKinlay GA, Emery AEH: Communication with parents of children with cancer, *Palliat Med* 8:105–114, 1994.

Koocher GP, Berman SJ: Life threatening and terminal illness in childhood. In Levine MD, Carey WB, Crocker AC, et al, editors: *Developmental-behavioral pediatrics,* Philadelphia, 1983, WB Saunders.

Redd WH: Advances in psychosocial oncology in pediatrics, *Cancer* 74(suppl 4):1496–1502, 1994.

Spinetta JJ, Deasy-Spinetta P: *Living with childhood cancer,* St Louis, 1981, CV Mosby.

VI

CHAPTER 138

Chronic Illness

Balu H. Athreya

The primary care physician is in an ideal position to help children with chronic illness and their families because he/she knows the family background and the strengths and weaknesses of the family members and establishes lasting relationships with them. The major differences between the management of patients with acute illness and of those with chronic illness are that there is often hope of "cure" in acute illness, whereas the main theme in chronic illness is "care," and in acute illness, the physician is in full control of the management, whereas in chronic illness, the physician is only one member of a multidisciplinary team. This shift from "cure" to "care" and the need to share decision-making powers may be difficult for some physicians. Some physicians may be concerned that they do not have the time or resources to handle the psychosocial problems of the child with chronic illness. Caring for these children requires time, and time is what busy physicians lack. Also, there is no financial reward for the enormous amount of time needed to coordinate the care and to talk with the families of these children. These issues have assumed greater importance in the context of major changes occurring in the delivery of medical care.

Considering the magnitude and importance of the problem and the unique position the family physician occupies, it makes good sense for family physicians to be the team leaders in giving coordinated long-term care to children with chronic illness and handicapping conditions. Indeed, in the managed care setting, they will be expected to play this role.

TALKING WITH PARENTS

In managing serious and chronic disease, information must be gathered before advice is given. Therefore, it is important to determine what the family wants to know and hear about before presenting to the family an elaborate discussion on the etiology, pathogenesis, and treatment of the disease in question. Effective, sympathetic, and sensitive listening is the first step.

SETTING

It is important to have a proper setting in terms of time, place, and emotional climate in order to have worthwhile discussions with these families. Busy offices with multiple interruptions from telephone calls and office staff or bustling hospital corridors are not good settings. Ideally, the physician should be prepared to set aside a period of approximately 45 to 60 minutes for discussion.

For the initial discussion, it is essential that both parents be present. An emotionally relaxed atmosphere is essential as well. The parents should realize by the physician's posture, the way he/she prompts them, and the way he/she answers their questions that he/she is interested in their problems and that he/she is listening.

COLLECTING INFORMATION

The educational and intellectual level of the parents, their socioeconomic conditions, anxiety levels, support systems, and coping abilities should be determined before the physician can answer their questions. The physician has to look for clues by observing and listening carefully.

One has to know the strengths and weaknesses of these families. Strengths may be apparent or potential. Similarly, weaknesses may be real or hidden. It is important to build on the strengths. The strength may be a schoolteacher who is especially interested in this child or a social worker in an agency who knows the family well and speaks their language. It is also essential not to stress their weaknesses and vulnerabilities.

In my personal observation, families of children with chronic illness who cope well and lead a reasonably "normal" life have the following characteristics:

1. Parents who have a good marital relationship before the onset of the chronic illness
2. Parents who mutually agree on issues after some reasonable discussion
3. An extended family support system
4. Religious faith
5. Faith in their physician

These personal observations were confirmed by Schulman in his study of families of children with leukemia. For families with "weakness" in these areas, early counseling may be helpful.

The usual concerns and questions of the family are:

1. What is the diagnosis? How sure are you about the diagnosis?
2. What is the cause? Could we have prevented it? Is it my fault?
3. What can you do about it? How can I help?
4. Why me? Why us?
5. What are the tests? Why are they done? At what cost?
6. What is the future likely to be?
7. Will it go away?
8. Can he/she get married and have children?
9. What are the vocational possibilities and problems?

PROVIDING ANSWERS

It is not necessary to answer all the questions at one meeting. It may be better to give only as much information as the family can handle at one time. The first task is to answer questions that are of major concern. Both the physician and the family have to learn that answers to some questions come only with time.

It is easy, given the mystique of being a physician, to come up with definite answers for all questions. The physician, having been trained to be certain and to know everything, finds it difficult to say "I don't know," but the physician should be bold enough and secure enough to say "I don't know" if that is a truthful statement.

Most parents will accept and appreciate honesty. But for certain technical questions, an appropriate answer may be, "I don't know, but I will find out." If the physician says this, he/she should make sure he/she finds the answer as soon as possible.

Simple words should be used to describe the diagnosis. If there are doubts about the diagnosis, or if there is a possibility that the diagnosis will have to be added to or changed, this should be indicated at the initial conference. A good booklet with a diagram of the organ involved (or a clay or plastic model of that organ) may help the families understand the explanation better. The physician can suggest that the family return with their questions during the next visit.

There are a number of patient education booklets that are available. Physicians may be able to obtain more information from social service agencies, national clearing houses (see bibliography), or the local chapter of the foundation dealing with the disease in question (eg, Arthritis Foundation).

In addition, the physician also may wish to refer the families to a parent support group or to a parent of a patient with a similar problem. This may help some families realize that there are other children with similar problems and lessens the feelings of having been singled out for bad luck. Parents also are more likely to ask other parents, rather than the physician, about their personal concerns. Parents who have similar problems can be extremely supportive. However, some families may feel negative to such controls. If the physician is not aware of any such parent support group, information such as this can be obtained from a nearby academic medical facility.

The explanation the physician gives on the disease may have to be repeated many times before the message is fully understood. Soon after the diagnosis is made, parents are often in a state of shock, grief, and denial and are not prepared to hear all the physician may have to say. They may not comprehend and may deny much of what the physician has told them. It is necessary for the physician to be patient, not to defend himself/herself, but to repeat his/her explanations often.

Another idea, used by many physicians, is to audiotape the discussion with the family's permission and give the tape to them. They can listen to this at their leisure. This tape also will

VI

provide other family members and other caretakers with the same information.

When parents inquire about the cause of the disease, they are not asking just for medical explanations. They also want to know if they did something wrong—by omission or by commission. This feeling of "guilt," a universal phenomenon, should be addressed with sensitivity and honesty.

Questions such as "Why did it happen to me?" or "Why did it happen to my child?" are personal, philosophic questions. Some parents tend to dwell indefinitely on these questions and are immobilized because of their preoccupation with this unanswerable question. This occurs less commonly in people with deep religious faith. In fact, some families turn to religion after a chronic illness is diagnosed in a child. Some families with deep problems regarding this question tend to become depressed and socially isolated and may require special help.

Another major area of concern for the children and their families is the use of laboratory tests. Most families want to know what tests are being done, when they are being done, and at what cost. They also wish to know why some tests are repeated and whether they have to be repeated so often. Special efforts must be made to explain the tests being ordered, and how these tests will help in the management of the child's disease. Risks and benefits should be explained, whenever necessary, depending on the physician's relationship with the family and the invasiveness of the procedure. Some children and adults need sufficient notice to enable them to get prepared. Others want to be told just prior to the test. Truthfulness is necessary, but not at the expense of frightening the children and their families.

Questions on prognosis are difficult to answer, particularly for a disease with indefinite course, such as juvenile rheumatoid arthritis and systemic lupus erythematosus. It is hard to live with uncertainty. Families cope better when they know what to expect. But, unfortunately, the physician cannot be definite in giving a prognosis for certain diseases. Therefore, it becomes a fine balancing act for the physician to be truthful and realistic, without being too optimistic or pessimistic.

Physicians need to understand themselves and their strengths and weaknesses before answering questions on prognosis. Some cannot give bad news and tend to soften the news that may then be interpreted as good news by families. Others tend to be overly pessimistic, even with mild disease. Both these extremes are to be avoided.

It is possible to convey bad news without shocking the parents to numbness, and it is unnecessary to constantly crush their hopes. Families need hope to sustain them. As long as parents are planning for and dealing with the current situation appropriately, do not be concerned if they periodically express their hopes that the disease will miraculously go away. It does not matter what they say. It is what they do that the physician should observe. If what they do suggests that they are coping well, leave things alone, encourage them, "cruise along." If what they do suggests poor coping, get involved quickly.

When parents inquire about prognosis, they have three other hidden concerns: 1) The first concern is related to the genetic nature of the disease and whether it can occur in a sibling or future offspring. 2) The second question relates to the chances of the affected child being able to grow up, marry, and have children. They are asking whether the affected child may pass the disease on to his/her offspring. 3) The third concern centers around physical activity and independence. The parents want to know if their child can go through the educational program and be able to earn a living.

When discussing treatment, simple explanations should be given. Written instructions should be helpful. Also, instructions should not be unrealistic or strain the family's resources. Compliance decreases as the treatment plan becomes more and more complicated.

The family should know that they are the principal members of the treatment team. Each family has its own special problems and special solutions. It is important to listen to them, and allow enough room in the plans for them to manage their problems in their own way. Plans should be made to suit the needs of each family, and support structures should be built to make sure the plan is carried out. For example, it is unwise to give an elaborate morning care plan to the mother of a child with myelomeningocele if she also has other school-aged children. Contacts with the school principal, local social service agency, or child guidance clinic may have to be arranged to help these families. At times, it is better for the physician not to be too specific with his/her recommendations. Most chronic diseases have an unpredictable course, unique in each child, that requires flexibility in planning on the part of the parent and the physician.

SUMMARY

Taking care of patients with chronic illness is a difficult task. Yet it is an area that brings into focus all the components of the "Art of Medicine." It helps the physician grow and mature.

Ambroise Paré said that "we seek to cure sometimes, relieve often, and comfort always." That is the essence of taking care of patients with chronic illness. Primary care should become more interesting and rewarding by including a few children with chronic illness.

BIBLIOGRAPHY

Batshaw ML, Perret YM: *Children with handicaps. A medical primer,* ed 3. Baltimore, 1992, Paul H. Brooks Publishing.

Brewer EJ, McPherson M, Magrab PR, Hutchins VL: Family-centered, community-based coordinated care for children with special health care needs, *Pediatrics* 83:1055–1060, 1989.

Community checklist for care of children with special needs, Publication of Association for the Care of Children's Health, Washington, DC, 1987.

Grant WW: What parents of a chronically ill or dysfunctioning child want to know, but may be afraid to ask, *Clin Pediatr* 17:915–917, 1978.

Green M: Coming of age in general pediatrics, *Pediatrics* 72:275–282, 1983.

Hobbs N, Perrin JM, Ireys HT: *Chronically ill children and their families,* San Francisco, 1985, Jossey Bass Publishers.

Liptak GS, Ravell GM: Community physician's role in case management of children with chronic illnesses, *Pediatrics* 84:465–471, 1989.

Martin EW: Pediatricians' role in the care of disabled children, *Pediatr Rev* 6:275–282, 1985.

McCollum AT: *The chronically ill child: A guide for parents and professionals,* ed 2, New Haven, 1981, Yale University Press.

National Resources from National Information Center for Children and Youth with Disabilities. PO Box 1492, Washington, DC 20013–1492.

Newacheck PW, Taylor WR: Childhood chronic illness: Prevalence, severity and impact, *Am J Public Health* 82:364–370, 1992.

Pless IB, Power C, Peckham CS: Long-term psychosocial sequelae of chronic physical disorders in childhood, *Pediatrics* 91:1131–1136, 1993.

Stein RK, Bauman LJ, Westbrook LE, et al: Framework for identifying children who have chronic conditions: The case for a new definition, *J Pediatrics* 122:342–347, 1993.

VI

CHAPTER 139

Child Abuse and Neglect

Toni Seidl

When working with the diagnosis of child abuse, good communication is crucial. We are, for the most part, dealing with psychologically fragile adults whose children have been, and will continue to be, dependent on them at least until the mandatory agencies or the courts intervene. Physicians and nurses find it difficult to accept the very concept that these children need and want the parents who have caused them pain. In child abuse cases there are in effect two patients: the adult(s) and the child. Thus the practitioner needs to promote parental involvement within the bounds of safety for the child and to facilitate healing of both parent and child. To accomplish this task, a bond of trust has to be created between the practitioner and the parents. This relationship need not compromise the care of the child or prevent practitioners from contacting those systems they are mandated to report to. Practitioners must be familiar with the presentations and dynamics of child abuse or neglect, skillful at obtaining factual histories, and capable of treating and providing care in a neutral and nonthreatening setting.

Child abuse is an unacceptable but common phenomenon as well as an all too often predictable event when the parent is childlike, frustrated, isolated, emotionally impoverished, poor, unemployed, and has minimal parenting skills. In addition the practitioner should not view the reporting process as necessarily resulting in a loss of rapport with the family or the automatic creation of an adversarial situation but as a legal duty essential to the treatment process. An understanding of ourselves and of the child's parents is the only way the practitioner can position himself/herself to communicate effectively and therapeutically with the child and family.

Alternatively the caregiver could suspect child abuse and consider intervention as someone else's responsibility. Although this distancing does provide the practitioner with a temporary absence of conflict, it does not affect change in the family nor provide safety for the abused child and his/her siblings, or facilitate a working relationship between the practitioner and the family. The subject of violence toward children and the more insidious but equally devastating neglect have historically been avoided by our culture and the helping professions. The language and appropriate style required to cope with this problem are alien to most professionals.

A pivotal constraint to productive communication is the common and deeply held myth that those individuals who abuse and neglect their children have essentially different goals for their children than other caregivers do. This is inaccurate; even abusive and neglectful parents want their children to thrive and become productive human beings. It must be emphasized that the creation of an understanding between parties will require that practitioner to search beyond surface presentations such as detachment and defensiveness. Another myth is that child abusers are alcoholic, psychotic, or both. This perception can serve to hamper communication profoundly unless dispelled. In fact, psychosis occurs in less than 5% of abusers, and the prevalence of alcoholism is similar in abusive and nonabusive parents.

Providers need to take responsibility for learning how to interpret parental hostility and resistance as potent symptoms of fear and inadequacy. They also should acknowledge that, given the same set of variables, they might very well be capable of abusing or neglecting a child. Individuals who act out assaultively with children are likely to be passive to a fault when dealing with authority figures whom they perceive to be powerful and in control. Fear of retribution is another common anxiety that impedes physicians functioning as parent counselors. However, when a reality-based relationship develops between the parents and health workers, retribution is unlikely.

THE CONFERENCE

In talking to parents in the hospital or in the office, the physician must be "in charge" in every sense of the word. Arrange the conference site so that it is private, quiet, and free from interruptions. An unhurried appearance on the part of the practitioner and single-minded purpose is essential to reinforce the seriousness of the conference. Positioning of the conference participants is especially important when the subject for discussion is child abuse. Threatened individuals need us to firmly establish that we are comfortable and that we are in control of ourselves and of them. To do this, we must convey a sense of calm, a sense of direction, and a sense of eagerness for involvement with the parents.

The following points reflect a helpful style of managing the conference. Sit close and lean forward to demonstrate attentiveness to the parents as individuals. Do not be intimidated by their predictable passivity, hostility, or hyperactivity. The articulation of the role of reporter of suspected child abuse and caregiver rather than apportioner of blame or investigator needs to be threaded throughout the contacts with the family. By maintaining a child-focused stance, parental anxiety and anger can be successfully avoided.

It is preferable to begin the parent conference with a positive or approving comment such as, "I am glad that you brought Lilly to the hospital today; it was the right thing to do. She is a very pretty infant." After such an opening, the parents' conversation, body language, and posture usually will become less defensive and more open in response to our approval, which they will translate as a degree of acceptance.

The next step is the sharing of the medical facts without establishing etiologic conclusions. This needs to be done clearly and concretely, with explanations of medical terminology and concepts in a nonpatronizing manner. Individuals who abuse and neglect their children constantly struggle with feelings of incompetence.

Try to avoid the possibility of this negative attitude, which creates a fertile atmosphere for the escalation of hostility and other aberrant behaviors. The following is the type of dialogue often used: "We are glad that Lilly is breathing by herself now, but we are still worried about the blood under the covering of her brain." These same parents will need generous amounts of reassurance and a sense of a plan. "We are doing more tests to find out just how serious the injury is so that we can treat your daughter in the best way possible." By doing this, the practitioner's expertise is established and the stage is set with the deliberate use of the word "injury" for the discussion of nonaccidental trauma or child abuse. Then, to demonstrate again a nonrejecting atmosphere and to validate the parent-child relationship, a comment such as: "We will let you see your daughter as soon as we can, because we know how much she needs you." This avoids the abusive and neglectful parents' compulsion to prove to us that they love their child when, of course, the issue for us is not one of love but of behaving in a caring and protective manner.

Next obtain a history of the events leading up to the presentation of symptoms. This is an extraordinarily important step, both diagnostically and in terms of separating accidental from nonaccidental injury or neglect and to become prepared psychologically and factually. To proceed in relative comfort and with credibility, one needs to be secure in the suspicion of abuse or neglect. Only when the information is gathered personally and meshed with the physical findings can the suspicion be presented to the parents in a clear and unwavering manner. After the parents have presented their version of the events they can be gently confronted with the reality that their presentation of the history does not fit their child's physical findings. "Mr. and Mrs. Jones, what you are telling me is puzzling in that we see hundreds of children each year who fall off beds and they do not have the type and severity of injury Lilly has. Is there anything else you can think of that might have injured her?" Here reality is supportively threaded into the conversation while giving the parents an opportunity to acknowledge the abuse. If the answer is no, move on to further explain the configuration and mechanism of injury in as concrete a way as possible. This should be supplemented with radiographs, a computed tomography scan, any

VI

other aids available, and an explanation of the syndrome of child abuse.

It is productive to preface this portion of the discussion with the comment, "I have something to tell you that is going to be upsetting for you to hear and difficult for me to say." By doing this, we are reinforcing a partnership in treatment. An effective follow-up comment can be "We see children every day who are abused and neglected by parents and caretakers, and because of my training, knowledge, and judgment, I believe Lilly's injury is the result of child abuse." By doing this, we are carefully avoiding the establishment of blame while reemphasizing our expertise and being straightforward with concern. The use of the powerful words "child abuse" also serves to decrease the potential for denial and misinterpretation later.

Requirements to report child abuse, as stated in the specific civil and criminal statutes of the particular community, plus information regarding the process and implications of reporting and protective services investigation must be explained to the parents. Most practitioners feel compelled to do this in a rather formal style, realizing that families are not necessarily able to internalize all that is said. This serves not only to cause the family to appreciate how firmly the suspicion of child abuse or neglect is held but also to appreciate the commitment to reporting child abuse. Middle- and upper-class educated families who may very well try to derail the reporting process can be effectively managed with this approach. "When I have a suspicion of child abuse, the law clearly states that I must report it to children's protective services for investigation, and that is what I have done." In addition, messages of caring and mutuality need to be transmitted. "This does not mean that I will be less involved with you or that your daughter's care will be compromised. The staff and I are here to help you and Lilly." Assurances of confidentiality within the parameters of legal mandates need to be reiterated. Parents also deserve information regarding the implications and process of the protective services and criminal investigations.

With all of this said, the physician must keep in mind that child abuse is not necessarily an isolated form of family violence. Therefore, an adequate medical and psychosocial evaluation should include exploration for the coexistence of domestic violence. Violence toward children can be the event that flags a relationship between parents as an abusive one. Spousal abuse can be the antecedent to, or a contributing factor in, the child abuse, or the child may have been caught in the crossfire between parents, rather than the intended recipient of the assault. Once identified, intervention with domestic violence requires a set of skills and interventions beyond most pediatric practitioners and pediatric sites. The best the line practitioner can expect to accomplish, without immediate or on-site access to a specialized service or team, is calm acknowledgment of the problem, support, and the encouragement to seek out referral to the appropriate service providers. In the absence of life-threatening circumstances criminal justice system reporting for adult victims of family violence remains voluntary in most jurisdictions.

All of this is best accomplished with a multidisciplinary approach, because the needs of abusive or neglectful families are overwhelming and complex, requiring varied expertise and monumental energy. This, coupled with the requisite involvement with the criminal and civil systems, is more than any individual or discipline can master and manage alone.

The medical and psychosocial management of child abuse or neglect offers an extraordinary challenge to us as practitioners, not only in terms of rescuing children but in terms of restoring a significant group of adults to their functional role as parents.

BIBLIOGRAPHY

AMA News: Family violence and the physician. Jan:3–39, 1992.

Council on Scientific Violence: American Medical Association: Violence Against Women:

Relevance for medical practitioners, *JAMA* 267(23):3184–3189, 1992.

Finkelhor D, Gelles RJ, Hotaling GT, et al: *The dark side of families: Current family violence research,* Beverly Hills, CA, 1983, Sage Publications.

Goldberg G: Breaking the communication barrier: The initial interview with an abusing parent, *Child Welfare* 54:4, 1985.

Hartman C, Reynolds D: Resistant clients: Confrontations, interpretation, and alliance, *Social Casework,* April 1987.

CHAPTER 140

Explaining Epilepsy

Robert Ryan Clancy

Epilepsy, a common chronic neurologic disorder, affects millions of persons worldwide. After the physician has concluded that the diagnosis of epilepsy is warranted, the patient and family usually have many questions and concerns regarding the nature and significance of this condition. The physician should anticipate these healthy questions and be prepared to respond in a clear and timely manner. The purpose of this chapter is to review common questions raised by individuals with epilepsy and their families and to illustrate one approach to answering these questions. The physician's response constitutes a vehicle to patient self-education and participation in the comprehensive management of the disorder.

What is "epilepsy"?

The term *epilepsy* refers to an individual's tendency to experience repeated seizures. Each seizure is the individual attack of altered brain function that arises from temporary abnormal electrical patterns in the brain. Some individuals with epilepsy may have only two seizures in their lifetime; others have more frequent attacks.

Is there a difference between "epilepsy," "seizure disorder," and "convulsions"?

The terms *epilepsy* and *seizure disorder* are synonymous. Because of the stigma attached to the term *epilepsy* by some members of society, there has been an increased emphasis on the diagnostic label *seizure disorder* rather than *epilepsy;* however, they are the same condition. Medically speaking, the term *convulsion* is not strictly identical to epilepsy or seizure disorder, even though the diagnosis convulsive disorder is encountered occasionally. For example, after some individuals faint they may display a brief *nonepileptic* convulsion. The convulsion appears as jerks or twitches of the muscles of the face or limbs, due to the brief period of low blood pressure during the fainting episode. However, convulsion does not indicate excessive brain electrical activity from a tendency for recurrent seizures. On the other hand, seizures in some people with epilepsy are properly described as convulsive if they display forceful, repeated contractions or movements of the musculature.

Who gets epilepsy?

Anyone can have epilepsy. It is estimated that approximately 1% of the population is prone to recurrent seizures and thus warrants the diagnosis. When all types of seizures are collectively considered (including febrile seizures, single seizures, and epilepsy), the incidence of affected individuals increases to 10%. Seizures can arise at any age, from newborn infants to the elderly.

Epilepsy occurs with equal frequency in all parts of the world and in all races.

What happens to the brain during each individual seizure?

Let's start with a more familiar experience. Most individuals have had an opportunity to undergo electrocardiography. You may recall that electrodes were attached to your arms, legs, and chest. The electrical signals that control the heart are detected and monitored with each heartbeat. The brain also runs on electrical impulses. Normal electrical signals are very orderly and tightly controlled by the brain. During an individual epileptic seizure, excessive amounts of electricity temporarily take over the normal function of part or all of the brain. This results in the seizure and the temporary interruption of normal brain function.

How many kinds of seizures are there?

Because the brain is a complicated and specialized organ, it has many ways to express seizures. Historically, epileptic seizures were broadly characterized as big seizures (grand mal epilepsy) and little seizures (petit mal epilepsy). Today we recognize numerous types of epileptic seizures. It is for this reason that you must provide your physician with a careful description of the seizures. It is on the basis of this careful description of the components of the attack that the physician can best diagnose the specific type of seizure.

Most individuals with epilepsy experience only one or a few different types of seizures. Slight differences in the duration or intensity of a typical seizure do not warrant the diagnosis of a new type of seizure. Rather, this is reserved for seizures that are distinctively different in their quality.

What causes the tendency for seizures?

Anything that is potentially harmful to the brain may be a cause for seizures. A serious head injury, encephalitis, meningitis, chemical imbalances, drugs, stroke, or even a brain tumor can disrupt the normal functioning of the brain and give rise to the excessive electrical activity that is the basis for the individual seizure. It is for this reason that the doctor conducts a careful history and physical examination of the patient with newly diagnosed seizures. In some cases, additional blood testing, a computed tomography scan of the brain, or magnetic resonance imaging may be suggested. Still, in many individuals, no specific cause for the recurring seizures is discov-

ered. The cause of the seizures may then be described as idiopathic. This reflects our incomplete knowledge of the cause(s) of seizures in many individuals. Sometimes the seizures arise from genetic (inherited) influences, but in most cases medical science has simply failed to uncover the fundamental cause of the seizures.

Is epilepsy contagious?

Absolutely not! There is no way you can catch epilepsy by observing a seizure or associating with an affected individual. However, inheritance may play an important role in some cases of epilepsy. In others, inheritance seems to play little or no role. According to some medical authorities the risk for seizures occurring in close relatives of those with epilepsy varies from 2% to 50% depending on the specific type of seizures. When one parent has epilepsy, the risk of epilepsy in their children is approximately 6%; if both parents have epilepsy, the risk of epilepsy in their children increases to approximately 10%.

What is the difference between epilepsy, cerebral palsy, and mental retardation?

These three conditions are entirely different. Epilepsy refers only to the tendency for recurring seizures. Cerebral palsy represents a physical handicap in which the individual has faulty muscle control due to a central nervous system disorder. This may result in abnormal walking, impaired use of the hands, or speech difficulties. Mental retardation reflects an impairment of intellectual skills (subnormal intelligence), visible as slow mental development and a reduced ability to learn. It is true that some individuals with multifaceted neurologic problems can have *combinations* of these three separate problems. For example, some individuals with cerebral palsy also may be mentally retarded and experience recurring seizures (epilepsy).

Who is qualified to treat epilepsy?

Any knowledgeable general practitioner, family physician, internist, pediatrician, general neurologist, or epileptologist may successfully diagnose and treat seizure disorders. In addition to individual practitioners who care for patients with epilepsy, there are a variety of comprehensive epilepsy clinics available throughout the United States and Canada. The Epilepsy Foundation of America (EFA) can provide the names and locations of physicians who are especially knowledgeable in the diagnosis and treatment of seizure disorders.

What is the purpose of treating epilepsy?

The physician usually recommends medication to prevent the individual seizures of the epilepsy. Such medications are called *antiepileptic drugs* or *anticonvulsants*. The physician selects the drug most likely to be effective from a wide choice of available medications. The purpose of medication is to help protect the patient from future seizures. Drug treatment does not necessarily erase or remove the underlying tendency for the seizures but rather provides protection against the individual attacks. Because most individuals cannot predict when a seizure will occur, it is necessary to faithfully consume antiepileptic drugs on a daily basis to prevent recurrence. This is a difficult chore for most individuals, because few are accustomed to taking medications on a regular basis. However, the price of poor compliance is high: seizures may recur during play, school, driving, or work.

How successful is treatment with antiepileptic drugs?

Approximately 80% of individuals with epilepsy are successfully treated with medications. They enjoy a total or substantial reduction of their seizures. As long as they faithfully use their medications as prescribed, they can reasonably expect good seizure control. Unfortunately, approximately 20% of people do not adequately respond to the medications currently available. For some of these patients, neurosurgery may be necessary.

Can one stop worrying about seizures once started on medications?

No. The faithful consumption of medication is not a 100% guarantee against the possibility of future seizures. It would be more reasonable to consider the medication as a safety net rather than as total ironclad protection. One should always be aware of the possibility of an unexpected seizure arising even if previously well controlled. For this reason, individuals with seizures should maintain constant vigilance for their personal health and safety.

How long will antiepileptic drugs be continued?

For many types of epilepsy, medications can be withdrawn 2 to 5 years after total seizure control. This is especially true for some of the so-called benign epilepsy syndromes of childhood. Those are considered benign because the majority of affected people are entirely healthy aside from the seizures and eventually outgrow their tendency for seizures. For a few types of seizures, the outlook is less optimistic and withdrawal of treatment may result in a relapse of the seizures. Consequently, although the goal of withdrawing medications several years after establishing total seizure control is desirable, it is not attainable in all individuals.

When the time does come to discontinue medication, the reduction is always conducted gradually. In this clinical setting, anticonvulsants are never abruptly withdrawn. Precipitous discontinuation of antiepileptic drugs can cause serious consequences including the appearance of repeated or prolonged seizures.

Do antiepileptic drugs have side effects?

The person who consumes medication must remain alert to the possibility of side effects: just as individuals are different so may be their reaction to medications. Each antiepileptic medication has its own individual spectrum of side effects. The physician should discuss the possible side effects of each drug you may be consuming. This serves to inform you of possible adverse effects and help minimize their occurrence.

Don't be overly concerned about the initial side effects of antiepileptic drugs. It takes a little while for most people to adjust to their temporary initial reactions. Some medications have more lasting side effects than others. Ask your doctor about choosing the anticonvulsant that is least likely to interfere with your lifestyle.

In general, there are two broad types of side effects: physical and mental. Examples of physical side effects include swollen gums, increased hair growth, weight gain or loss, facial cosmetic changes, or alterations of internal organs such as the liver. Examples of mental side effects include sleepiness, irritability, poor attention or concentration, or slurred speech.

What side effects should be reported to the doctor?

Drowsiness or trouble concentrating are common after starting some antiepileptic drugs and need not be reported unless severe or persistent. Swollen glands, rash, hives, or ulcers in the mucous membranes may indicate an allergic reaction and should be reported. Unusual nosebleeding, easy bruisability, or blood in the urine or stool should be promptly reported.

Can one become addicted to antiepileptic medications?

Usually not. Most antiepileptic medications are not physically addicting. For example, there is no physical dependency created from the long-term consumption of phenytoin, carbamazepine, or valproate. Physical dependency can result from the long-term consumption of benzodiazepam drugs (including diazepam, Valium; clorazepate dipotassium, Tranxene; and clonazepam, Klonopin) and barbiturates (including phenobarbital; mephobarbital, Mebaral; and primidone, Mysoline). When the time comes to taper these medications, they are slowly withdrawn over an extended period to minimize any possible physical signs of withdrawal. Because phenobarbital normally leaves the body very slowly, it automatically provides its own slow method of tapering.

Psychologic addiction to anticonvulsants can occur in some individuals who enjoy the comforting thought of safety from seizures symbolized by the drug. They understandably react adversely when advised to discontinue their medications. Individuals can become psychologically dependent on medications even though there is no physical addiction. This depends as much on their personality as on the nature of the drug.

Do antiepileptic drugs cause mental retardation?

Antiepileptic drugs do not lower the intelligence quotient (IQ) or cause mental retardation. However, they do affect the workings of the nervous system as they achieve their desired effects (seizure control) and in the process introduce unwanted neurologic side effects. These side effects can be expressed as disturbances of behavior, mood, sleeping, attention span, or concentration. For some individuals, these side effects may be trivial; for others, they materially impair the speed and accuracy of some mental processes. In that circumstance, it is sometimes necessary to reduce the dose or switch to a different antiepileptic drug.

Can antiepileptic drugs be taken with other medications?

In general, yes. Most medications can be safely administered with antiepileptic drugs without any untoward side effects. However, there are some important drug interactions that your physician knows about. It is wisest to check with your doctor or pharmacist before taking drugs together. For example, some women who consume antiepileptic medications are at risk for failure of oral birth control pills. Because some seizure medications increase the rate of drug elimination by the liver, birth control pills may be metabolized too rapidly. This may result in conception or breakthrough bleeding. Even vitamins can be removed from the body too quickly while consuming seizure medications. Therefore, many doctors recommend taking a daily multivitamin supplement.

What is the purpose of the blood test recommended by the doctor?

The dosage of individual antiepileptic drugs usually is given on a per-pound basis; lighter individuals receive smaller doses than heavier individuals. The completeness of absorption from the intestinal tract and the rate of drug breakdown in the body also differ between individuals. In the final analysis, what is most important is how much medication appears in the bloodstream available for delivery to the tissues of the brain. Adequate seizure control often depends on maintaining a specific concentration of medication in the bloodstream. Your doctor may request that a drug level be obtained to measure the exact concentration of medication in your body. This allows more rational dose manipulation to achieve optimal seizure control. A low blood level may indicate a marginal protection against seizures. A high blood level may indicate impending signs of overmedication.

For some medications it is also advised that periodic blood tests be obtained to monitor the health of some internal body organs such as the liver, kidneys, pancreas, or the blood-forming organs. Your doctor will use these tests to evaluate how your body reacts to the drugs.

What about generic antiepileptic drugs?

Many physicians prefer that their patients do not consume some generic anticonvulsants. Generic phenobarbital is the rule rather than the exception. However, manufacturers' formulations of phenytoin (Dilantin), carbamazepine (Tegretol), and valproate (Depakene, Depakote) may differ sufficiently to cause a change in blood levels that could result in the reappearance of seizures (if the levels fall too low) or intoxication (if the levels rise too high).

For some families, the expense of purchasing antiepileptic medications is a major burden. Do not be afraid to shop around to find the least expensive supplier of medication. If possible, buy in bulk rather than in small 1-month amounts, which are generally more expensive. The EFA offers a mail-order pharmacy that may be less expensive than your local retailers.

What can I do to help the doctor manage the seizure disorder?

The patient and family are the eyes and ears of the doctor. It is rare for the physician to personally witness the patient's seizures. Therefore it is most helpful for a clear description of all the events before, during, and after the seizure to provide the physician with accurate information to make the most precise diagnosis. Many physicians recommend that their patients maintain a seizure calendar or log. This provides a written record of the time, duration, description, and circumstances of the seizures.

The patient with epilepsy and the family must become informed partners with the doctor for successful health care. It is recommended that they be as knowledgeable as possible about seizures, take the time to read about the condition, and keep the doctor informed of the patient's status.

Patients should also be familiar with the name(s) and dose(s) of prescribed medication and with expected common drug side effects. Pill organizers can be purchased at the pharmacy to help you keep the medication schedules straight.

How can I help reduce the risk of seizures?

By maintaining a seizure calendar, it is occasionally possible to identify factors in the environment that trigger the attacks. By keeping an accurate seizure calendar, you and the physician may identify and avoid such precipitating factors. The second major job of the individual is to be totally compliant with prescribed medications. This is easier said than done, but the medication cannot help while safely stored in the medicine cabinet! Any physical illness such as the flu or fever can lower the resistance to seizures and possibly precipitate an attack. Similarly, extreme sleep deprivation or the immoderate consumption of alcohol and some illicit drugs can substantially increase the risk of seizures. Unnatural degrees of emotional distress may precipitate seizures. However, the normal healthy stresses that are encountered in everyday life do not aggravate seizures. It is not recommended to keep the patients perpetually calm. All patients with epilepsy should shoulder their fair share of life's excitement, challenges,

stresses, and disappointments. Indeed, it seems that some people are more prone to seizures while they are idle. In general, the advice "keep busy" is healthy.

Are seizures painful?

Seizures are almost never painful. In fact, most persons have no recollection of the event at all.

What do you do at the scene of a seizure?

When most people first witness a seizure, their immediate reaction is: "He/she is dying." This is not true. The seizure will pass, and the individual will be safe and sound in only a few minutes, so keep calm. There is nothing you can do to stop the seizure sooner; it will run its course. Most seizures last only a few minutes. Remove glasses or dentures if possible, and place something soft under the person's head so they do not bump it on the ground. Do not attempt to restrain the movements. Tight clothing may be loosened. Some people will have erratic breathing during the seizure, but this is a natural part of the attack. Roll the person on his/her side so he/she does not choke on vomit or his/her saliva. Do not attempt to insert anything into the mouth. Although some can bite their tongue, you cannot stop this. It is a myth that individuals can swallow their tongue during a seizure. In the rarest of circumstances, individuals may not resume breathing after a seizure, and so cardiopulmonary resuscitation (CPR) should be started. Some families make it a point to learn CPR through qualified instructors at the American Red Cross.

It also is recommended that persons with epilepsy possess a "medical alert" bracelet, neck chain, or wallet card that describes their condition and provides relevant phone numbers.*

What happens after a seizure?

After a grand mal seizure, most individuals will awaken but seem confused or groggy and may fall asleep soon afterward. Headache, muscle soreness, or bloody saliva (if the tongue was bitten) may be noted. The person's color improves quickly even if he/she was pale, gray, or bluish (cyanotic) during the seizure. A deep state of relaxation immediately follows the attack,

VI

---

*Medical alert items are available from: Medic Alert Foundation International, Box 1009, Turlock, CA 95381 (1-800-ID-Alert); Emergency Information, American Medical Association, 535 N. Dearborn St., Chicago, IL 60610; National Identification Co, Inc, 3955 Oneida Street, Denver, CO 80207.

984   TALKING WITH PARENTS AND PATIENTS

during which the person remains still and offers no resistance to movement. Even the muscle sphincters of the bladder and rectum can relax and lead to incontinence of urine and stool.

Some people bounce back immediately after a seizure, others require more time to recuperate. If consciousness is not regained promptly, medical attention should be sought. Do not offer the individual anything to eat or drink until he/she is awake and able to swallow safely.

Are seizures harmful to the brain?

Although they are dramatic and may be frightening to the onlooker, individual seizures do not produce brain damage or result in a lower IQ.

Do you automatically take the child to a hospital after a seizure?

It is not obligatory to take a child to the doctor or hospital after each and every seizure. It would be best to clarify with your doctor when to go. If any injury occurred during the seizure (such as a laceration from falling), the patient obviously should be examined. Similarly, if the episode is unusually long, different from previous seizures, or recovery incomplete after the attack is over, the individual should be evaluated by a physician.

Can seizures occur during sleep?

Yes. Nocturnal epilepsy refers to some individuals' tendency to have seizures during sleep. Indeed, some people have their attacks only while asleep. Unfortunately, this sometimes means that seizures are unrecognized or poorly described. Parents find this unsettling because many desire to be with their child during the seizure. There is no perfect solution to this dilemma. An inexpensive auditory home intercom (usually intended to monitor a baby's crying) can allow the parents to hear the child's activities in their own room during the night.

What are "status seizures"?

Although the vast majority of seizures occur as brief individual attacks, long uninterrupted seizures may rarely occur and are potentially harmful. Prolonged seizures lasting hours can result in brain damage or death. This can be avoided by prompt medical attention. If a single seizure lasts 15 minutes or more, many physicians recommend that the family bring the patient for medical evaluation. It would be best to have a specific plan of action prepared in advance in the case of such an emergency.

In what circumstance could a seizure be harmful?

As already discussed, individual seizures themselves are not harmful to the brain. However, harm can occur if the seizure occurs in a circumstance that would produce an injury. For example, a person who has a seizure while swimming could drown unless there was immediate help from a partner or supervising adult. Bicycling amidst traffic could produce harm if the child lost control and swerved into the path of a vehicle. A seizure at great heights (*eg*, rock climbing) could produce a serious fall. Similarly, seizures while operating heavy machinery or driving could result in personal injury.

What restrictions or limitations apply to the child with epilepsy?

All parents and guardians should exercise a healthy degree of authority and discipline over their children, including those with epilepsy. Most physicians recommend that they receive no special treatment or sheltering lest they stigmatize themselves as incapable or different. They should not be removed from challenges, excused from their transgressions, or spared the normal disappointments that constitute formative experiences of childhood.

Driving restrictions are enforced for most individuals, but all states permit driving once complete seizure control has been established for 6 months to 2 years. Unfortunately, some employers do restrict individuals with epilepsy from filling some types of jobs.

What about school?

It is generally recommended that school personnel be informed of the presence of a seizure disorder. The teacher can be a valuable asset because he/she has ample opportunity to directly observe the child for seizures and potential drug side effects. The teacher will be best prepared to help the student during a seizure with foreknowledge of what to expect and instructions about what to do. The teacher also can be encouraged to read and learn more about seizure disorder.

It is known that learning disabilities and attention deficit disorders are overrepresented in epileptic school-aged children. If the teacher observes these in your child, be prepared to deal realistically with the problems because specific treatment may be available that may materially improve school performance.

What about employment?

Children with epilepsy should plan their education with realistic career goals. For example, children with uncontrolled seizures will not be issued licenses to drive commercial vehicles or pilot airplanes. Naturally, they should be advised against pursuing such careers. Vocational counselors in school may be helpful in determining the individual's strengths, weaknesses, and aptitude for a host of appropriate careers.

Are there any limitations on participation in sports?

There is generally no restriction in participation in athletics, including contact sports such as football. However, participation in any athletic competition inherently conveys some risk, and the individual contemplating such athletics should be physically well and capable of participation. Ideally, this includes good seizure control.

What about planning for a family?

It is strongly suggested that women who desire to raise a family should confer with their doctor long before conceiving. Some medications may be harmful to the developing fetus and should be withdrawn before conception. Dietary supplementation of folic acid is commonly advised. Seizure control can deteriorate during pregnancy so the physician may wish to follow-up the patient or monitor drug levels more frequently until delivery.

Is it difficult to obtain life insurance with epilepsy?

Life insurance is obtainable through many companies. Some companies have overpriced their premiums to discourage people with epilepsy from seeking a policy. However, other companies offer reasonably priced insurance. A listing is available through the EFA.

What other sources of services are available to me?

Individuals seeking specific services may direct inquiries to their Public Health Department or Public Health Nurse. Most states also provide vocational rehabilitation and disability counsels. The State Department of Social Services or Mental Health Services also may provide assistance in some circumstances.

Where can I find more information about epilepsy?

A series of well-written and informative brochures is available on request from the EFA.* Several books about epilepsy are also available for patients and families.

---

*The Epilepsy Foundation of America, 4351 Garden City Drive, Landover, MD 20785 (301-459-3700).

BIBLIOGRAPHY

Chee C, Clancy R: Children with epilepsy. In Fithian J, editor: *Understanding the child with chronic illness at school,* Phoenix, 1984, Oryx Press.

Commission on Classification and Terminology of the International League Against Epilepsy: Proposal for classification of epilepsies and epileptic syndromes, *Epilepsia* 26:268–278, 1985.

Devinsky O: *A guide to understanding and living with epilepsy,* FA Davis, 1994, Philadelphia.

Freeman JM, Vining EP, Pillas D: *Seizures and epilepsy in childhood: A guide for parents,* Baltimore, 1990, The Johns Hopkins University Press.

Jan JE, Ziegler RG, Erba G: *Does your child have epilepsy?* Baltimore, 1983, University Park Press.

Jennings T, Bird TO: Genetic influences in the epilepsies, *Am J Dis Child* 135:450–455, 1981.

Lin JT-Y, Ziegler DK, Lai C-W, et al: Convulsive syncope in blood donors, *Ann Neurol* 11:525–528, 1982.

Newmark ME, Penry JK: *Genetic aspects of the epilepsies: A review,* New York, 1981, Raven Press.

Reisner H, editor: *Children with epilepsy: A parents guide.* Kensington, MD, 1988, Woodbine House.

VI

CHAPTER 141

Congenital Anomalies

Richard Polin

Few events are more emotionally devastating for new parents than to be told their newborn child is not properly formed. Most frequently, either the pediatrician or family practitioner is the physician with whom parents speak first and, therefore, these individuals must have an organized approach to such meetings. The purpose of this chapter is to provide practical guidelines for speaking with families about children with congenital anomalies or malformations.

Before meeting the parents of a child with a congenital anomaly, it is vitally important to perform a careful physical examination. Parents need and seek an accurate diagnosis and detailed description of abnormalities—not a general impression that their child is not properly formed. Nothing is more frustrating for families than to have multiple meetings with their physician, each meeting describing an additional problem. Frequently, small cleft palates are overlooked, and so it is important to examine this area carefully. The overall pattern of both major and minor malformations must be considered. Even minor malformations can be significant when found in association with other anomalies. In general, a child with a single defect should not be considered to have a specific syndrome. When two or more malformations are present, however, the risk of detecting a major malformation rises to 90%. Attention should be directed to describing and categorizing the anomalies and, if possible, determining which of the defects occurred earliest in morphogenesis. This information can help determine the timing of the embryonic insult. Funduscopic examination by an experienced ophthalmologist may be especially informative, because many eye abnormalities are unique and suggest a specific diagnosis. Laboratory tests (eg, cytogenetic studies, radiographs) should be obtained to evaluate abnormalities in specific organ systems rather than used as a "fishing expedition" that can be both costly to parents and not very fruitful.

The first meeting with the parents following the child's birth is often the most important in the counseling process. Whenever possible, both parents should be present at all conferences. Because of cultural teachings, however, some husbands will attempt to exclude their wives from meeting any physician and insist that all communications occur through them. The husbands assume this attitude because they fundamentally believe their wives are not capable of accepting unpleasant news. Contrary to these beliefs, women often accept the truth better than their husbands and frequently are more communicative. Other family members (eg, grandparents) can be included in these meetings; however, they should be passive participants, allowing the parents of the child to formulate their own questions and reach their own conclusions. Parents need to know that they alone will best be able to support each other emotionally.

The initial meeting with the parents of a child with congenital anomalies generally follows a common format whether the child has a single abnormality or multiple-malformation syndrome. The purpose of this meeting is three-fold: 1) to state and describe the problem, 2) to obtain pertinent historical information, and 3) to answer parental questions.

EXPLAINING THE PROBLEM

A description of the anomalies should be given in the simplest possible terms. It is inadvisable to give parents a list of all possible diagnoses and the outcome for each disorder. Too much information given to families is likely to overwhelm and confuse them. An exception to this rule exists when the physician is talking with the parents of a child with a suspected chromosome abnormality. In retrospect, most of these families wished to know the diagnosis as soon as it was suspected by a physician. It is appropriate in these situations to inform parents that the overall pattern of malformations suggests a chromosome disorder and to briefly describe the significance of such an abnormality. The parents should be encouraged not to focus on any one single anomaly but should be told that the presence of many abnormal features indicates the chromosome problem.

The prognosis for single or multiple malformations should be realistically communicated. When a single malformation such as cleft lip is present, the correctable nature of this defect should be emphasized. Discussions with parents concerning nonlethal malformations ideally should take place with the infant in the room. The physician should demonstrate that their child is normal, with the exception of a single anomaly. The discussion concerning the child with multiple congenital anomalies should be approached in a similar fashion. Even when the prognosis for survival or normalcy is poor, parents should be encouraged to interact with and touch their child.

Some parents may find themselves unable to make an emotional commitment to a child with congenital anomalies. This refusal to bond to these children may be an attempt by these families to protect themselves from further emotional suffering. Occasionally, families will try to abandon a child with only a cosmetic problem. In these situations the stimulus for continuing parental involvement should come from other family members, physicians, nurses, and social service personnel. No attempt should be made to discuss withdrawal of life support systems at the first meeting. Parents must first understand the seriousness and extent of the anomalies before they are able to reach a decision concerning ongoing intensive care.

HISTORY

A second goal of the parent conference should be to obtain historical information that will help make a diagnosis. The age, sex, and past and present health of parents, siblings, and other closely related family members should be determined. The ethnic background of the infant's family and the geographic area from which they originated also may be important. Specifically, a history of maternal diabetes, polyhydramnios, or epilepsy should be sought. A detailed description of drug exposure and viral illness during the pregnancy should be obtained; however, it is important to emphasize to both parents that neither maternal drug use nor an upper respiratory tract infection in the first trimester of pregnancy is likely to be related to congenital malformations in the infant.

ANSWERING QUESTIONS

The four most common parental questions are: 1) What caused the malformations? 2) Will my child be mentally retarded? 3) Will my child survive? 4) Have we done something that caused the malformations? Although a detailed discussion of the causes of malformations might be left for a genetic counselor when there is one available, there are certain fundamental concepts that can be transmitted by the family physician. The simplest response to the first question regarding cause is that until a specific diagnosis is determined, there can be no definite answer. Parents can be told that there are four general etiologic categories for malformations: mendelian disorders (eg, achondroplasia), multifactorial disorders (eg, cleft lip), environmental disorders (eg, thalidomide-induced phocomelia), and chromosome disorders (eg, Down syndrome); however, it must be emphasized that their child's anomaly is most probably unrelated to something the parents did or neglected to do at the time of conception or during the pregnancy.

The question of handicap also should be dealt with in general terms. If the malformation is a single structural anomaly such as club foot, the remedial nature of this malformation should be stressed, as well as what is normal with the rest of the body. The prognosis for multiple malformation syndromes will vary with etiology. Trisomy chromosome disorders are uniformly associated with moderate to severe mental retardation. Other malformation syndromes (such as the VATER association: vertebral, anal anomaly, tracheoesophageal, radial upper limb, hypoplasia, and renal defects) have a normal mental outlook despite the severity of malformations.

VI

Most parents assume their children will survive, regardless of the extent of their anomalies. Survival ultimately will depend on the severity of cardiac and central nervous system malformations. If the infant requires assisted ventilation, the parents should be told the life support will continue until they have had sufficient time to evaluate the appropriateness of continued care. The question of discontinuation of ventilation should be raised by the physician once it is clear that the neurologic outlook for the infant is extremely poor or if the child has malformations that are incompatible with an existence outside the hospital and are not correctable. The life-support issue is generally broached by the practitioner once the family has been given a definitive statement regarding prognosis. At that meeting, the parents should be told they will be permitted as much time as needed to reach a decision; however, the date of future meetings with the family should not be left open-ended, and a new time should be set. Many families find the involvement of a clergyman welcome support at this stage. When discontinuing support is considered, the hospital ethics committee also will help define the issues and offer an opinion.

If the decision is made to remove an infant from the ventilator, some families request that they be allowed to hold their infant while the lines and tubes are removed. *All families should be encouraged to hold their infants.* This may be their only opportunity to truly function like a parent with their son or daughter. The child should be wrapped in a blanket and given to the family in a quiet area where they can be left alone to grieve. After the child has died, it is important to have the family schedule a return visit to the office for postdeath counseling and discussion of autopsy findings.

The majority of infants with malformations can be cared for in smaller hospitals without immediate referral to a tertiary center. Chromosome studies as well as standard radiologic procedures and biochemical tests can be obtained in most community hospitals. It is advisable, however, to consult a geneticist before discharging the infant from the hospital, so that the family can meet the individual who will provide the majority of counseling. Infants with life-threatening anomalies involving the central nervous system, heart, or lungs should be cared for in a hospital with an intensive care nursery and surgical subspecialists. The pediatric geneticist should be consulted as quickly as possible in such cases to facilitate the diagnostic process.

SUMMARY

The initial meeting with the family should be considered the first step in the process of genetic counseling and emotional support. Further meetings should be attended by a geneticist, but not at the exclusion of the generalist. The tenor set by these initial meetings will determine parental attitude and ability to cope with their child.

BIBLIOGRAPHY

Aase JM: *Diagnostic dysmorphosis,* New York, 1990, Plenum Medical Book Co.

Bergoffen J, Zackai FH: The infant with multiple anomalies. In Polin RA, Yoder MC, Burg FD, editors: *Workbook in practical neonatology,* Philadelphia, 1993, WB Saunders.

Jones KL: *Smith's recognizable patterns of human malformation,* ed 4, Philadelphia, 1987, WB Saunders.

Miller LG: Towards a greater understanding of the parents of the mentally retarded child, *J Pediatr* 73:699, 1968.

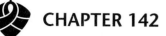

CHAPTER 142

Communicating With the Adolescent Patient

Kenneth R. Ginsburg

SETTING THE STAGE FOR OPTIMAL COMMUNICATION

To be able to impact on the lives of adolescents, the primary care physician needs to discuss intimate topics. The typical adolescent expects to get a check-up, shots, and their forms completed—not to be asked to disclose personal information. If the provider does not "set the stage" for a deeper level of communication, the history elicited is likely to be far from the truth, and the patient is unlikely to be receptive to anticipatory guidance. To optimize communication, the provider should use the beginning of the visit to address all of the teenager's concerns regarding the purpose of the interview and its boundaries. Teenagers will not disclose personal information without having a sense of the following issues: 1) Why is the provider asking personal questions? 2) What will he/she do with the answers; will he/she judge me or share my secrets? 3) Is it worth sharing private information; can this person do anything to help me? After addressing all of these issues, the final parameters that need to be explained are the limits of confidentiality. If these are not addressed before obtaining the history, the provider risks losing the patient's trust if he/she needs to intervene. Strict confidentiality must be the norm in the adolescent-provider relationship. However, situations under which confidentiality can never be offered include the history of abuse and the disclosure of suicidal or homicidal plans. Ideally, the parent(s) can be included in this initial relationship-defining conversation. If they are present, they are more likely to understand that although the provider must honor confidentiality, he/she does so to encourage the patient to communicate openly. The parents also will be reassured that there are boundaries to confidentiality in life-threatening situations and that in all situations the provider will be an advocate of appropriate parental involvement.

"Setting the stage" can begin with a discussion regarding the importance of the adolescent in taking more responsibility for his/her own health. If the provider desires, the teenager can be told that he/she can begin calling the office independently with any concerns regarding his/her body, mind, or emotions and that the teenager may seek any kind of advice that will keep him/her healthy. Next, the patient should be informed that the provider is committed to preventing problems instead of just waiting for them to happen. Then the teenager should be given an opportunity to surmise what topics he/she would discuss with other teenagers if they themselves were professionals committed to preventing the kind of problems that most harm teenagers. In my experience, younger teens initially respond "nutrition," whereas older teens tend to respond "HIV, violence, and drugs." Whatever his/her response, the provider gains insights into the teenager's primary concerns and receives tacit permission to discuss these subjects.

THE PSYCHOSOCIAL ASSESSMENT

Once the stage is set for optimal communication, the history can be obtained. Because of the personal nature of the psychosocial interview, the teenager must be interviewed privately. However, chief complaints, past medical history, and family history can be elicited with the parent present. It may encourage the parent to allow for private time if the primary care physician emphasizes the importance of parental participation in the beginning of the visit and remembers to elicit parental concerns before they leave the room.

Once in a private setting, the provider should first ask the youth if there were any major concerns he/she did not feel comfortable stating in the parents' presence and then should proceed to screen the youth for high-risk behaviors. There are a few overriding rules about the screen. First, the interview should proceed from general, less intimate topics to those more personal. Next, questions within these topics initially should be impersonal (eg, "Are many of the teens in your school doing drugs?"). Finally, all questions must be asked without judgment, and the provider must take care not to express shock or dismay to the responses. There is time later for the provider to offer guidance to the patient. A quick reaction may disrupt disclosure of the full history.

It is important to take a comprehensive psychosocial history. SHADSSS (school, home, activities, depression, substance use, sexuality, safety) is a mnemonic intended to remind interviewers to be comprehensive and to progress from the least to the most personal items. Following are suggested approaches to each area of interest. However, screens must be tailored for each patient and community.

School

School is the proxy measure for well-being. Worrisome responses here are predictive that problems will be revealed later in the screen.
"How is school going?"; "Are you doing as well as you think you can?"; "What is your favorite subject in school?"

The beginning of the screen is also an opportune time to ask, "What would you like to do when you get older?" The response to this question is very revealing. Adolescents with no plans for the future may not believe they have one and consequently may be at greater risk for many of the behavioral morbidities.

Home

Although all teenagers have tensions in their relationship with their parents, it is critical to determine for whom the relationship is reaching crisis proportions. If caught early, families can be guided into the use of more appropriate levels of communication and discipline.

"How are things at home?"; "Do you get along well with your parents/siblings?"; "Do you feel that people at home understand you?"; "If you have a problem, who can you go to?"

Activities

Peer relationships and activities are of exceptional importance to the teenager. Knowing what a patient's friends are doing offers a strong clue into what type of pressures the patient is likely to encounter and what type of behaviors they are at greatest risk of exhibiting.
"What kind of things do you do outside of school?"; "Who is your best friend?"; "What is he/she like?"; "What kind of things do you do together?"; "What does he/she plan for the future?"; "Do you have many other friends, what are they like?"; "Sometimes I worry about teenagers being influenced by their friends—do you think your friends are a good or bad influence on you?"

Depression

Suicide is the third leading cause of death in teenagers. Not all adolescents who commit suicide are depressed; some are impulsive. Even those youth who are depressed often do not exhibit classic vegetative signs. Therefore, teenagers must be asked questions about depression and suicide directly.
"How is life going for you?"; "Would you describe yourself as a happy or a sad person?"; "Who can you talk to if you have a problem?"; "Have you ever thought of hurting yourself?"

If any of the responses are positive the teenager deserves a comprehensive screen. This screen should include a past history of a suicide attempt by the patient or a person close to the patient, existence of a plan to commit suicide, and access to the means to carry out the plan. If the patient has suicidal intention or strong ideation, he/she must be referred to mental health services immediately. As stated in the provider's introduction to the patient, suicidal intention is never treated with confidentiality. Although the interview is focused on mental health, the provider can explore self-esteem and body image:
"You are at the age when your body is going through a lot of changes, do you feel like you understand these changes?"; "How do you feel about the way your body is developing? . . . about how you look?"

Substance Use

Mind-altering substances contribute sharply to the mortality related to accidents and the morbidities of school failure and depression. In addition, they become an independent risk factor for the transmission of sexually transmitted diseases. Concern over the use of cigarettes and alcohol should not be minimized because these substances can lead to long-term addictions with dire health consequences.

"Are many teens in your area smoking cigarettes/ drinking alcohol/using drugs?"; "Are any of your friends doing the same?"; "Have you ever used . . . ?"; "How often . . . ?"; "Do you think you have a problem with . . . ? If not, convince me!"

Sexuality

It is important for the provider to approach the subject of sexuality with no preconceptions. The provider should not transmit the assumption that the patient has or has not engaged in sexual activity. Special care should be taken not to communicate the assumption that the patient is heterosexual.

"Have you begun dating?"; "Are you currently seeing someone?"; "What is the person like?"; "Have you begun to become sexual with that person, by this I mean hugging, kissing, or even touching in private places?"; "What do you think makes a person ready for intercourse?"; "Have many of your friends become sexually active?"; "Have you had intercourse with this or any other person?"; "How many sexual partners have you had?"; "Are you aware of the negative consequences of sexual intercourse (disease, pregnancy, and emotional pain)?"; "Have any of the consequences ever happened to you?"; "Are you doing anything to make sure that none of these consequences will happen to you?"

Safety

Interpersonal violence is a primary concern for many adolescents. Determining who is likely to be a victim or perpetrator of violence can save lives. It is imperative for the provider to learn whether the patient carries a weapon. Many youth operate under the belief that a weapon will protect them without even considering that it puts them at much greater risk of death.

"Do you feel safe at school?"; "Are there a lot of fights at your school?"; "Do people bring weapons to school?"; "Do you get in fights?"; "What
makes you mad enough to fight?"; "Are you able to walk away from fights, how do you do that?"; "What do you usually do when you are really mad or frustrated?"; "Have you ever been severely injured in a fight?"; "Do you think a knife or gun would make you safer . . . do you carry one?"

If the provider is treating teenagers for a violence-related injury it is of critical importance to explore whether he or she has plans to get even. Finally, the provider should take this opportunity to explore for a history of physical or sexual abuse.

"Do you feel safe at home?"; "Is there anyone who hurts you or touches you when you don't want to be touched?"

THE BRIEF PSYCHOSOCIAL SCREEN

Although the comprehensive psychosocial screen should be an integral part of every well adolescent visit, its length precludes it from being realistically incorporated into every encounter. Teenagers are known to present to medical care with a hidden agenda. They may state a vague complaint such as fatigue, chest pain, abdominal pain, or headache, whereas, in reality, they are reaching for help. They may be testing to see if the provider is savvy enough to uncover their distress and get them appropriate help. With this in mind, I use a three-part screen that can be quickly incorporated into *any* visit. The provider first should ask, "How is school going?" Because school is a proxy measure for general well-being, life's stressors are likely to adversely affect school performance. Common concerning responses include: "I had a bad quarter," "Not as well as it used to be," or "I'm not going very much." These responses represent a challenge from the teenager to see if the adult will further explore the causative factors. However, the teenager whose life is stressful, but for whom school is a successful respite, may be missed by this question. Therefore, to be sure all youth are screened, the provider should also ask, "Are you happy?" or "How is life going for you?" No matter what the response is, the provider should follow quickly with "When you are not happy how do you handle it, who do you talk to?" The teenager who is unhappy and has no one to talk to is at risk. This teenager deserves a comprehensive screen, with special attention to

VI

depression and suicidal intent, no matter what the presenting complaint is.

BEHAVIORAL CHANGE

The ultimate goal of the provider is to support the teenaged patient in the acquisition of safe behaviors and avoidance of risky behaviors. The psychosocial screen offers a glimpse into those behavioral areas that pose the greatest risk to the patient. Through a combination of discussion and role playing, the provider can offer information to the patient and help him/her to develop the skills needed to resist pressures and retain control over his/her own behaviors.

Before the provider offers anticipatory guidance, he/she must be familiar with the cognitive level of the patient. Adolescents are in transition between the concrete thinking of childhood and the abstract thinking of adulthood. A child thinks concretely: he/she sees things as they are, without regard to future consequences. The world and the people in it are viewed as "good" or "bad." Concrete thinkers do not have the capability to look beyond an individual's actions to determine his/her underlying motivations. In contrast, abstract thinking empowers the adult to see the shades of gray, to consider future consequences, and to evaluate the underlying motivations of others. Thus, abstract thinking serves to be highly protective. Understanding the degree to which each adolescent is able to absorb abstract ideas is a critical first step in communicating with him/her. If a patient is unable to contemplate the future, warnings about how current actions may have long-term consequences are useless. For example, although cigarettes cause cancer and heart disease, the young adolescent cares more that they make you smell and cough when you're running and cost a lot of money.

In adolescence a child undergoes a transition from concrete perceptions to the more protective styles of adulthood. Children progress along this transition zone both because of neurologic maturation and through life experiences. With each new experience and its consequences, the adolescent takes a small step toward more abstract thinking. This is no different today than it ever has been, but the consequences of error may be much more severe. Fights still bloody noses, but they also may provoke a shooting. Sex still brings the risk of pregnancy, but it also may bring HIV. To the extent that it is possible, the provider can guide the teenager verbally through "life experiences" allowing him/her to make "mistakes" in the safety of a medical setting rather than in the peril of the real world. I call this the "cognitive aha" experience. The hope is that the realizations made in the safe setting may hold a portion of the effectiveness of those mistakes made in the dangerous world. The key to this style of guidance is in the breaking down of abstract concepts into multiple concrete steps. The teenager is guided through each step until he/she comes to an abstract realization.

One style of producing the "cognitive aha" is the "decision tree." This method is used for discussions when teenagers seem to have no grasp of future consequences. The provider discusses the teenager's fantasies and draws a map toward the future. At each junction, the provider inquires whether the fantasy is realistic and suggests other possible outcomes. The teenager who wants to have a baby is an ideal candidate for this technique. Many teenage girls believe that a baby will give them the love they seek and that the father will stay loving and involved. The provider can draw a timeline and describe challenges along the way. The teenager should be asked at each juncture what it is really like for her friends at that point (ie, how many fathers stay with the mothers). Another good candidate for this technique is the teenager about to engage in a retributive violent act. He/she wants the immediate emotional release but is unaware of the peril. I have used this opportunity to walk the patients through alternative outcomes. Using both a diagram and slow-motion role playing, I demonstrate the potential outcomes of his/her death, maiming, as well as life in jail. I take him/her through the length of his/her jail time, including the sadness inflicted on his/her family, the loss of his/her education, and the prevention of his/her parenthood. Finally, we discuss the teenager's old age when he/she is alone and poor because of the family and education he/she has forsaken. Ultimately, the one day when the teenager will feel bad for not getting even seems minimal when compared with a life outcome that is more to his/her liking.

The "cognitive aha" also can be used, via diagrams and role playing, to demonstrate numerous other concepts, including the epidemiologic transmission of disease and the danger of carrying a weapon for protection. Teenagers often base their decision on whether or not to use condoms on how much they trust their partner. They lack the understanding that HIV is invisible and that sexual contact with one clean partner belies the number of people from whom one can catch diseases. A diagrammatic representation reveals that the teenager exposes himself/herself to his/her partner's partners, and so on. As the teenager looks at the expanding numbers, I ask whether he/she "trusts" all of these people. In the case of the teenager who is considering carrying a weapon, reverse role playing in which the patient plays a weapon-carrying foe and the provider plays the teenager can be used. First, the provider should teach that the best option is to keep walking or avoid the conflict entirely. Then, the provider should swing at the patient (do everything in slow motion so as never to produce an immediate emotional response). The provider should ask the teenager how a person with the gun would respond. The answer is that he/she probably would swing back, although he/she may pull out his/her gun and threaten. Now, the provider should create the same conflict, reach toward his/her belt, as if for a gun, and ask the teenager how he/she would respond. The answer becomes clear to the teenager, if he/she reaches for a gun, or even has the reputation of being a gun carrier, he/she is more likely to get shot in a conflict situation.

Bringing patients to new abstract realizations can only fulfill part of the goal of achieving changes in behavior. Adolescents also have to be offered skills. Several complex behavioral change theories have been posited to guide programs and practitioners in optimizing the potential for change. In the simplest of terms, the process of change involves five steps. 1) An individual must recognize that there is a problem with his/her behavior. 2) The individual must decide that a behavioral change is desired. 3) The individual must implement the new behavior using the appropriate skills. 4) The individual evaluates the benefits versus the costs of the new behavior. 5) The individual determines whether to adapt the new behavior as permanent. The classic medical communicative style, in which providers offer facts alone, cannot therefore effect behavioral change for an adolescent. Although information can take an individual through the first two steps, it offers none of the skills needed to implement change. Thus, offering information alone produces smarter, motivated, but frustrated, patients.

Teenagers often have the desire to advocate for health behaviors but are thwarted by their peers or sexual partners. There are three refusal techniques that health professionals can easily teach to patients through discussion or role playing. If the provider creates a scenario using unrealistic language, he/she will hear the teenager say, "it's not like that." These words signal the end of effective communication. Therefore, if role playing is used, the provider should offer only short, universally accepted phrases.

The first refusal skill is the ability to say "NO!" effectively. Teenagers, in sexual or drug situations, believe that saying "yes" labels them as an unsavory character. As a consequence, they have created a language in which the word "no" stated meekly means that they want to be pushed further. Consequently, the word "no" often invites further pressure. Providers can teach patients how to let people know they mean "NO!" by not giggling or smiling while saying it and repeating it as often as it takes to get the point across.

The second refusal skill is the ability to reverse pressure. Young teenagers need first to be informed that lines such as "I love you" and "everybody is doing it" are, indeed, lines. The provider should inquire with teenagers what lines their peers use to pressure them into engaging in unwanted behaviors. Then, through role playing, the provider can strategize with them how to reverse those pressure lines.

The final refusal skill is the ability to replace risky activities and behaviors with safer ones. The provider should learn what his/her patient does with friends. For example, if the patient either plays basketball or does drugs, he/she should be taught to always carry a basketball. This allows the patient to keep his/her friends—a critical point for adolescents—while avoiding negative behaviors. As obvious as this skill seems to adults, it is new to younger teenagers. Another refusal skill is to have the teenager create a code with his/her parents. If the parent receives a phone call during which the teenager uses the code, it signals the parent to demand that the teenager return home immediately. Teenagers find it very difficult to leave their friends but have no problem blaming their parents for ruining all of their fun. Thus, the teenager retains control over his/her actions without worrying about loss of esteem in the eyes of his/her friends.

VI

Health providers cannot independently change the lives of our adolescent patients. However, if we make ourselves consistently available to them as trustworthy adults, we can position ourselves to make a difference. If we are familiar with the community resources available to teenagers in crisis, then our role as assessors can be invaluable. For those adolescents not in crisis, we can serve as adults who offer gentle, respectful guidance and who teach effective strategies to maintain healthy behaviors. A first step is in the commitment to communicate effectively with them.

SUGGESTED READINGS

Clark LR, Ginsburg KR: How to talk to your teenaged patients, *Contemp Adolesc Gynecol* 1: in press, 1995.

Dryfoos JG: *Adolescents at risk: Prevalence and prevention,* New York, 1990, Oxford University Press.

Ginsburg KR, Slap GB, Cnaan A, et al: Adolescents' perceptions of factors affecting their decisions to seek health care, *JAMA* 273:1913–1918, 1995.

Hodgman CH, Jack MS: Interviewing. In Mc-Anarney ER, Kreipe RE, Orr DP, Comerci GD, editors: *Textbook of adolescent medicine,* Philadelphia, 1992, WB Saunders.

Irwin CE: Why adolescent medicine? *J Adolesc Health Care* 7: 2S–12S, 1986.

Millstein SG, Peterson AC, Nightingale EO, editors: *Adolescent health promotion,* New York, 1992, Oxford University Press.

Slap GB, Vorter DF, Khalid N, et al: Adolescent suicide attempters: Do physicians recognize them? *J Adolesc Health* 13:286–292, 1992.

APPENDIX

Formulas and Diets

Beth Leonberg McCoy

Formula and diet intolerances are common occurrences among infants and young children; however, they are rarely of a serious nature. Making changes in diet should be done thoughtfully, because transient intolerance may resolve quickly without intervention. Permanent changes in diet may result in significant cost to the family as well as stigma to the child whose diet is "special." The following information is provided to help guide formula or diet choices when a change is clearly indicated.

The material contained in this appendix is intended for use by the practitioner in instructing parents on formula selection and basic diet modifications. Compliance to dietary changes is highly dependent on counseling on how to incorporate changes in ways that are consistent with individual and family preferences, lifestyle, and available resources. Consultation with a registered dietitian (RD) is recommended to assist the patient and family in making the necessary adjustments while preventing secondary nutrient deficiencies. Qualified RDs may be found through hospitals or local public health departments or by calling the American Dietetic Association's referral network at 1-800-366-1655.

INFANT FORMULAS

The American Academy of Pediatrics recommends breast milk as the feeding of choice for all healthy term infants. When mothers are unable to or choose not to breastfeed, formula feeding is an appropriate alternative. Infant formulas are designed to provide nutrients in quantities mimicking those of breast milk, allowing for differences in absorption and bioavailability of nutrients.

Standard infant formula is made from modified cow's milk and is well tolerated by almost all infants. It is important to note that cow's milk protein allergy has been estimated to occur in 0.3% to 7% of American children and that congenital lactose intolerance in infants occurs very rarely. The remaining majority of infants tolerate cow's milk–based formulas well. For those infants who do not, a soy-based formula can be used, however, as many as 50% of infants allergic to cow's milk protein are similarly allergic to soy protein. Soy formulas provide comparable nutrients as cow's milk-based formulas and result in similar growth patterns.

Premature infants have unique nutrient requirements due to underdeveloped physiologic and metabolic systems; premature infant formulas have been developed to compensate for these differences and to promote growth patterns resembling those in utero. Major modifications include decreased lactose content, increased protein content (whey-predominant), significantly increased concentrations of calcium and phosphorous, and increased concentrations of sodium, potassium, and chloride.

Standard infant formulas are designed for use through the first year of life at which time the infant may be switched to whole cow's milk. For the child with milk protein allergy or lactose intolerance, soy-based toddler formulas may be used. The significantly greater cost of toddler formulas when compared with whole or 2% milk makes their routine use difficult to justify.

Transient formula intolerance due to viral illness is generally unresponsive to formula changes. Feeding through a gastrointestinal viral illness, using standard infant formula, has been associated with less weight loss and comparable time for resolution of symptoms. If a formula change is indicated, it should not be viewed as a permanent change and an attempt to return to a

TABLE A-1
Infant Formulas

Formula Type	Indications	Unique Properties	Available Products
Milk-based	Breast milk substitute for term infants	• +/− iron • Ready to feed, powder or liquid concentrate • 20 kcals/oz • Variable whey: casein	Enfamil Gerber Good Start Similac SMA
Soy-based	Breast milk substitute for infants with cow's milk protein allergy or lactose intolerance	• Lactose-free • Some also corn- or sucrose-free • 20 kcals/oz • May contain added fiber • Iron fortified	Gerber Soy Isomil Isomil DF Isomil SF Nursoy Prosobee
Premature	Breast milk substitute for infants <38 wks gestational age	• Low lactose • Fat modified to contain medium-chain triglycerides • Higher calcium and phosphorous • 22 or 24 kcals/oz • Iron fortified • Nutrient dense	Enfamil Premature Neocare Similac Special Care SMA "Preemie"
Older Infant	Transitional formulas for infants >6 mos	• 20 kcals/oz • Iron fortified	Follow-up Formula Next Step Next Step Soy
Hypoallergenic	Milk or soy protein allergy	• Hydrolyzed protein • Sucrose- and lactose-free	Nutramigen
Elemental	Indicated for malabsorption	• Lactose-free • Contain either hydrolyzed protein or free amino acids	Alimentum Neocate Pregestimil
Amino Acid–Modified	Inborn errors of metabolism	• Low or devoid of specific amino acids that cannot be metabolized	Protein Free Diet Powder 80056 Pro Phree Multiple other specific products
Fat-Modified	Defects in digestion, absorption, or transport of fat	• Contain increased % of kcal as medium-chain triglycerides	Alimentum Portagen Pregestimil
Carbohydrate-Modified	Simple sugar intolerance	• 3232A and RCF require addition of complex carbohydrate to be complete	3232A Lactofree RCF
Low Electrolyte	Renal or cardiac disease, or other conditions requiring low renal solute load	• Decreased sodium content	Similac PM 60/40 SMA

standard formula should be made when the illness resolves.

Table A-1 illustrates the types of infant formulas currently available, their indications and unique properties, and commercially available products of these types. Formula manufacturers are developing new formulas rapidly, continually expanding the range of choices. It is important to note that newly introduced formulas are generally more expensive and targeted at small patient populations.

SUPPLEMENTING ORAL DIETS

Inadequate intake may be a significant contributor to poor growth in infants and children with primary failure to thrive or chronic disease. After establishing, via careful diet history, the need for caloric supplementation, there are a number of options for increasing the calorie density of the diet. In choosing an approach to adding calories to the diet, consideration must be given to the child's age, food preferences, the

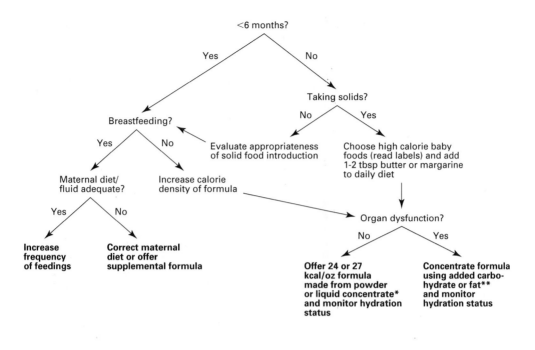

* See formula concentration instructions in Table A-2.
** See available additives in Table A-3.

FIG A-1
Supplementing oral diets of infants less than 1 year of age.

family's dietary habits, and the family's resources.

The algorithm presented in Figure A-1 illustrates decision making that may be used to select appropriate means of increasing the calorie density of oral diets for infants. Tables A-2 and A-3 provide information on preparing and concentrating infant formulas and additives that may be used with infant or pediatric formulas or foods. Figure A-2 illustrates decision making for supplementing oral diets of children over 1 year of age.

TUBE FEEDING

Infants and children who are unable to meet their daily nutrient requirements orally but have all or some normal gastrointestinal function may be enterally supplemented by tube. Bolus or nocturnal continuous enteral feedings may be used to provide supplemental nutrition, allowing the child to take orally what he/she is able and

TABLE A-2
Formula Preparation

Concentration	Amount of Powder or Liquid Concentrate	Water (oz)
20 kcal/oz (0.67 kcal/mL)	1 cup powdered formula	29
	4 scoops powdered formula	8
	13 oz liquid concentrate	13
24 kcal/oz (0.8 kcal/mL)	1 cup powdered formula	24
	5 scoops powdered formula	8
	13 oz liquid concentrate	9
27 kcal/oz	1 cup powdered formula	21
	5.5 scoops powdered formula	8
	13 oz liquid concentrate	6
1 scoop = 1 tablespoon		

TABLE A-3
Formula and Oral Diet Additives

Substrate	Example	Source	Provides	Standard Dose	Advantages	Disadvantages
Carbohydrate	Honey	Glucose, fructose	4 kcal/mL		Inexpensive	Cannot give to children < 2 years of age
	Karo, light Moducal*	Corn syrup Maltodextrin	4 kcal/mL 19 kcal/tbsp		Inexpensive Less osmotically active than glucose polymers	May be too sweet Increases osmolality
	Polycose†	Glucose polymers	23 kcal/tbsp 2 kcal/mL		Less sweet	Increases osmolality
	Rice cereal	Complex starch	4 kcal/tsp		Minimal osmotic activity; beneficial to patients with reflux	May clog feeding tubes
	Sucrose Sumacal‡	Cane sugar Maltodextrin	52 kcal/tbsp 19 kcal/tbsp		Inexpensive Tasteless; less osmotically active than glucose polymers	May be too sweet Increases osmolality
Fat	Corn oil	Long-chain triglycerides	8.6 kcal/mL	0.5 mL/oz	Does not increase osmolality; calorically dense	Not liquid miscible; may adhere to tubing
	Margarine/butter	Long-chain triglycerides	102 kcal/tbsp		Does not increase osmolality; calorically dense	Not liquid miscible; may adhere to tubing
	MCT Oil*	Medium-chain triglycerides	7.7 kcal/mL	Infants: 1 mL 4×/day; increase as tolerated. Children: 1 tbsp 3–4×/day	Does not require bile salts for absorption; absorbed directly into portal circulation bypassing lymphatics	Will not meet requirement for essential fatty acids; cannot be mixed into formula; strong odor
	Microlipid‡	Long-chain triglycerides	4.5 kcal/mL	0.5–1 mL/oz	Does not increase osmolality; liquid miscible	Less calorically dense

Protein	Casec*	Calcium caseinates	4 g/tbsp	Also a significant source of calcium	Must be mixed with water before adding to formula or other liquids
	Elementra§	Whey protein, hydrolyzed	4.5 g/tbsp	More elemental for patients with malabsorption	
	Powdered skim milk	Cow's milk protein	2.7 g/tbsp	Inexpensive	Contraindicated for patients with cow's milk allergy or lactose intolerance
	Promix¶	Whey protein	3.75 g/tbsp		
	Promod†	Whey protein	3 g/tbsp		
	Propac‡	Whey protein	4 g/tbsp		
	Propac Plus‡	Whey protein	3.3 g/tbsp	Contains electrolytes and some minerals	Trace amounts of lactose
	ProViMin†	Casein	2.1 g/tbsp	Contains vitamins and minerals	Additional iron may be necessary
Carbohydrate and fat	Duocal**		64 kcal/tbsp	Calorie dense; water soluble	

*Mead Johnson & Company, Evansville, IN
†Ross Products Division, Abbott Laboratories, Columbus, OH
‡Sherwood Medical, St. Louis, MO
§Clintec Nutrition Company, Deerfield, IL
¶Corpak Inc, Wheeling, IL
**Scientific Hospital Supplies, Inc, Gaithersburg, MD

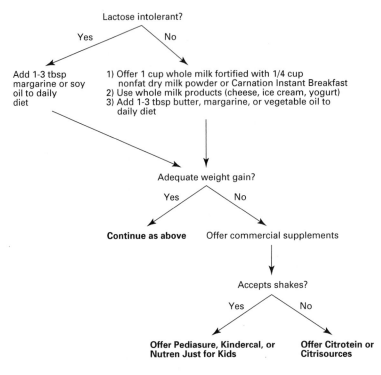

Lactose intolerant?

Yes / No

Add 1-3 tbsp margarine or soy oil to daily diet

1) Offer 1 cup whole milk fortified with 1/4 cup nonfat dry milk powder or Carnation Instant Breakfast
2) Use whole milk products (cheese, ice cream, yogurt)
3) Add 1-3 tbsp butter, margarine, or vegetable oil to daily diet

Adequate weight gain?

Yes / No

Continue as above   Offer commercial supplements

Accepts shakes?

Yes / No

Offer Pediasure, Kindercal, or Nutren Just for Kids   **Offer Citrotein or Citrisources**

FIG A-2
Supplementing oral diets of children greater than 1 year of age.

proceed with normal activities during the day. Although initiation of enteral feedings may require a short hospital stay for tube placement, teaching, and assessment of tolerance, these processes are increasingly being conducted as outpatient procedures with qualified nursing and RD follow-up in the home.

A thorough discussion of enteral feeding of children is beyond the scope of this appendix; however, two algorithms are presented that may assist in the decision to use enteral nutrition support, the route of tube feeding indicated, and the selection of product to be used. Figure A-3 provides a "decision tree" for choosing the route of nutrition support. Figure A-4 presents commonly used enteral products for children over 1 year of age and their indications for use. For infants who are being tube fed, the infant formulas presented in Table A-1 may be used.

LACTOSE-RESTRICTED DIETS

Lactose-restricted diets are indicated for individuals with lactose intolerance resulting from congenital, primary, or secondary lactase deficiency. Intolerance varies significantly in degree. Whereas children with congenital lactase deficiency have very low or absent enzyme activity, those with primary deficiency acquired after 3 to 5 years of age often have adequate enzyme activity to tolerate moderate amounts of lactose-containing foods. Secondary lactase deficiency is transient in nature and usually improves with resolution of gastrointestinal disease; however, recovery of enzyme activity may be incomplete.

Dietary restriction of lactose-containing foods and drugs results in resolution of symptoms. Because most children are able to tolerate small amounts of lactose-containing products, reintro-

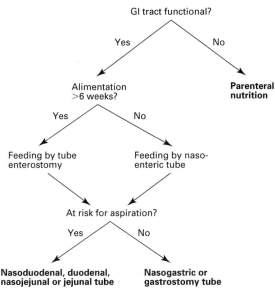

GI tract functional?

Yes / No

Alimentation >6 weeks?

Parenteral nutrition

Yes / No

Feeding by tube enterostomy

Feeding by naso-enteric tube

At risk for aspiration?

Yes / No

Nasoduodenal, duodenal, nasojejunal or jejunal tube

Nasogastric or gastrostomy tube

FIG A-3
Decision tree for provision of enteral feeds.

duction of these products should be tried until symptoms develop. Careful reading of labels on food packages is essential for those children with severe intolerance. Low-lactose commercial food products, including milk, cheese, and ice cream, are available and may be used as tolerated. Over-the-counter lactase enzyme replacements are available in a variety of forms including chewable tablets taken with meals or liquid drops added to fluid milk. For infants who are lactose intolerant, lactose-free infant formulas include Lactofree and soy-based formulas. Fortified soy milks available in health food stores or formulas such as Next Step Soy may be used as milk replacements for older children.

The lactose-restricted diet may be low in calcium, phosphorous, vitamin D, and riboflavin. Vitamin D deficiency is rarely a problem for American children; however, calcium supplementation in the form of calcium glucontate, calcium citrate, or calcium lactate may be indicated. Calcium-fortified foods such as orange juice and bread also may be used to meet daily calcium requirements.

Table A-4 provides a listing of allowed and restricted foods for the child who requires a lactose-restricted diet.

SODIUM-RESTRICTED DIETS (2000 TO 4000 mg)

Restrictions in the sodium content of the diet may be indicated for children and adolescents on adrenocorticoid therapy, with hypertension, or with renal, liver, or cardiac disease if edema or hypertension is present. Although dietary sodium may be restricted over a range of intakes from 250 mg/day to 3000 to 4000 mg/day, the most commonly prescribed diets are the moderately restricted 2000 mg/day and the no-added-salt diet of 3000 to 4000 mg/day. For both of these diets, salt is not permitted in the preparation of food or at the table. Label reading is essential to avoid foods with added salt; information about sodium-containing ingredients that should be avoided in 2000 mg/day and stricter sodium restrictions is provided in Table A-5. Commercially available salt substitutes generally contain salts of other minerals whose restriction also may be indicated. Spices and spice blends that do not

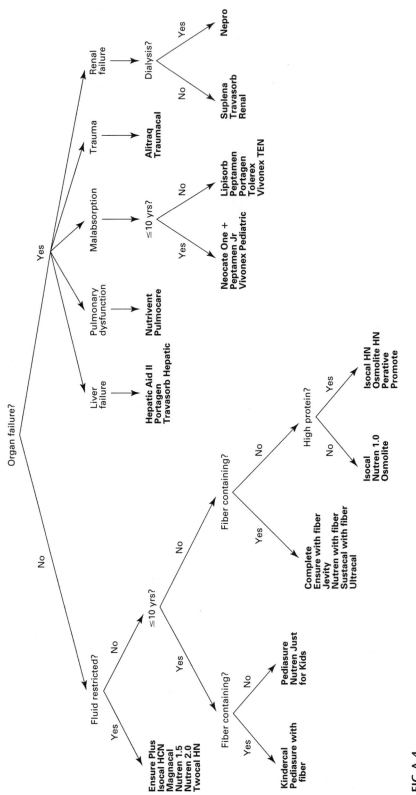

FIG A-4

Selecting an enteral formula for children greater than 1 year of age.

TABLE A-4
Lactose Restricted Diet

Food Groups	Foods Allowed	Foods Restricted
Milk	Soy milk products, yogurt, and buttermilk in small amounts if tolerated	All other milk and milk drinks, cocoa, cocoa malt, Ovaltine
Vegetable	All except those "Restricted"	Any canned or frozen vegetables prepared with milk or milk solids or seasoned with butter, margarine (if not tolerated), cream or cheese sauces
Bread/starch	• Water breads, hard rolls, French bread, biscuits, muffins, waffles and pancakes not made with milk or milk solids • Dry and cooked cereals, cereals that do not contain milk solids (read labels) • Rice, all pastas, potatoes prepared without milk or milk solids	Bread made with milk or milk solids, crackers made with butter or margarine (if not tolerated), French toast made with milk Cereals containing milk, milk solids or lactose (eg, cream of rice, Special K, Fortified Oat Flakes, Cocoa Krispies); commercial french fries, creamed or instant potatoes
Fruit	All fruits and juices unless listed as "Restricted"	Orange Julius or other fruit-based "milk shakes"
Meat	All except those listed as "Restricted"	Cold cuts or frankfurters containing milk solids, creamed or breaded meats, fish, poultry or sausage; cheese, if not tolerated
Fat (in moderation)	Milk-free margarine, gravies, mayonnaise, if tolerated, butter or margarine made with milk solids	Oil if not tolerated; butter or margarine made with milk solids; sauces made with milk
Beverage (in moderation)	Coffee, tea, carbonated drinks, instant coffee, and cereal beverages (read labels)	Instant coffee or cereal beverages containing milk solids
Dessert (in moderation)	Gelatin, angel food cake, homemade cake made with vegetable oils and no milk solids; water and fruit ices	Cake mixes or other baked product mixes containing milk solids; any product made with milk or milk solids
Seasoning (in moderation)	Pure seasonings and spices	Monosodium glutamate or artificial sweeteners with any lactose added
Soup (in moderation)	Meat- and vegetable-base soups	Cream soups and all soups made with milk
Sweets (in moderation)	Sugar, jams, jellies, and candies made without milk or milk solids; corn syrup, honey	All sweets made with milk; products such as chocolate, peppermints, and butterscotch, caramel
Miscellaneous	Popcorn, nut butters	Chewing gum, milk gravies, ascorbic acid tablets (in moderation), certain vitamin and mineral preparations—check with your druggist
Lactose-free commercial products	It is wise to check the label for all ingredients when purchasing any processed foods, because ingredients may change from time to time. Avoid products that include milk, milk products, or lactose as an ingredient.	
Lactose-free formulas and supplements	This is a list of only a few of the most commonly used foods. Some come in various flavors. • Milk substitutes: Edensoy, Rice Dream, Allmond Amasame, "Nut" Milk, West Soy Milk • Infant soy formulas: Isomil, Prosobee, Nursoy • Lactose-free infant formula: Lactofree • Lactose-free supplements: Pediasure, Sustacal, Peptamen, Tolerex, Ensure, Isocal, Osmolite, Resource, Ensure Plus, Nutren	

From *Pediatric diet manual,* Marriott Health Care Services, 1995. Reprinted with permission.

contain sodium may be recommended to patients as alternatives to table salt for flavoring foods in cooking and at the table.

The average American diet contains approximately 6000 mg of sodium per day, relying heavily on processed, prepared, and fast foods. Adolescents who consume many of their meals away from home and who may prepare their own meals at home are heavy consumers of these types of foods that have especially

TABLE A-5
Ingredients Containing Sodium

Products containing these ingredients should be avoided if:
1) Any of these ingredients is among the first three ingredients on the label
2) Three or more of these ingredients are present

Sodium (Na)
Salt (NaCl)
Brine (salt and water)
Monosodium glutamate (MSG)
Sodium nitrate
Sodium bicarbonate (baking soda)
Baking powder
Sodium propinate
Sodium benzoate
Sodium caseinate
Sodium phophate
Disodium inosinate
Meat stock
Milk or dry milk solids

TABLE A-6
Sodium Content of Fast Foods

Fast Food	Sodium (mg)
Biscuit sandwich	
With egg and ham	1310
With egg and sausage	1130
Croissant	
With bacon, egg, and cheese	790
With egg, cheese, and ham	1390
English muffin with egg, cheese, and Canadian bacon	730
French toast sticks	490
Pancakes with butter and syrup, 3	1103
Hash browns, ½ cup	290
Hamburger, ¼ lb	690
Cheeseburger, ¼ lb	1160
Roast beef sandwich, 5 oz	792
Chicken nuggets, six pieces	530
Chicken, breaded and fried	
Light meat, two pieces	975
Dark meat, two pieces	756
Chicken fillet sandwich	750
Broiled chicken sandwich	600
Fish fillet, batter-dipped and fried, 3 ounce piece	484
Fish sandwich with tartar sauce	615
Burrito with meat and beans, 1 small	668
Enchilada with beef and cheese, 1 large	1320
Nachos, 4 oz, with cheese	816
With cheese, beans, and beef	1800
Taco, 1 small	802
Taco salad	1060
Grilled chicken salad	690
Pizza, ¼ of 12" pizza with cheese, meat and vegetables	630
Submarine sandwich with coldcuts	1650
Hot dog with chili, 1	480
Chili con carne, 1 cup	1008
Baked potato, 1	
With cheese sauce and bacon	1280
With cheese sauce and broccoli	440
Coleslaw, ½ cup	260
Potato salad, ⅓ cup	312
French fries	
Regular	150
Large	290
Supersize	350
Hush puppies, 1	965
Onion rings	810

high sodium contents. Table A-6 provides the approximate sodium content of popular fast foods.

A diet restricted to 2000 mg of sodium should not result in significant nutrient deficiencies; however, if milk products are not consumed in recommended amounts, calcium supplementation may be indicated. Table A-7 provides a listing of allowed and restricted foods for the child who requires a 2000-mg sodium diet. Table A-8 provides a similar listing for the child who requires a no-added-salt (3000 to 4000 mg/ day) diet.

FAT-CONTROLLED DIETS

Diets restricted in fat are indicated for children with elevated serum triglycerides or cholesterol or for those needing to control weight gain.

The American Academy of Pediatrics has recommended selected screening of children over 2 years of age whose family history indicates a risk of developing coronary vascular disease (CVD). The primary therapy for all individuals with elevated risk of CVD is adherence to the "prudent" diet, which involves restricting fat to less than 30% of total calories, saturated fat to less than 10% of total calories, and cholesterol to less than 300 mg/day. Although individual response varies, diet therapy alone has proven to be effective in decreasing serum cholesterol. If the prudent, or step 1, diet fails to meet minimal treatment goals within 3 months, the step 2 diet may be implemented. This diet further restricts saturated fat to less than 7% of total calories and cholesterol to less than 200

Text continued on p. 1010.

TABLE A-7
2000-mg Sodium Diet (Sodium-Restricted)

Food Groups	Foods Allowed	Foods Restricted
Milk 120 mg Na/ 8 oz (2 cups daily)	Whole, 2%, skim, evaporated (½ cup), powdered (3 tbsp), reconstituted milk; yogurt, cocoa powder	Buttermilk, instant cocoa mix, other commercial instant milk beverages, malted milk
Vegetable Group A 9 mg Na/½ cup (as desired)	Fresh or low-sodium canned vegetables, frozen vegetables not in group B, salt-free canned vegetable juices	Sauerkraut or other vegetables prepared in brine, regular mixed vegetable juices, regular tomato juice
Group B 100 mg Na/½ cup (1 serving daily)	Frozen lima beans, peas, frozen peas and carrots, beet greens, swiss chard	Regular canned vegetables and those with salt added during cooking, frozen vegetables in sauce
Group C 230 mg Na/½ cup (1 serving daily)	Regular canned vegetables and those with salt added during cooking	More than one serving daily
Bread/starch Group A 120 mg Na/serving (5 servings daily)	Regular bread (1 slice), dry cereal (¾ cup), Melba toast (4), Graham crackers (3), bagel, English muffin, frankfurter bun, hamburger roll (½), yeast donut, seasoned macaroni, noodles, rice, spaghetti, potatoes, lentils, parsnips, split peas (½ cup)	Breads, crackers, and rolls with salted tops, corn chips, potato chips, pretzels, instant cooked cereals, salted popcorn; stuffing mixes, rice mixes, prepared dinners (eg, spaghetti, macaroni and cheese)
Group B Low-sodium 5 mg Na/serving (as desired)	Low-sodium bread (1 slice), unsalted regular cooked cereal (½ cup), Puffed Rice, Puffed Wheat, Shredded Wheat (1 cup), salt-free popcorn (1 cup), salt-free potato chips, salt-free pretzels, salt-free crackers (6 sq), matzo (6" sq), low sodium biscuits (4), flours—all purpose (2½ tbsp), unsalted macaroni, noodles, rice, spaghetti, potatoes, dried lentils, parsnips, split peas (½ cup)	All others, commercial mixes
Fruit 2 mg Na/serving (as desired)	Any fresh, frozen, or canned fruit or fruit juice, avocado	All crystallized and glazed fruit, maraschino cherries, fruit dried with sodium sulfite, olives
Meat Group A 69 mg Na/oz 6 oz daily	Fresh or frozen meat, poultry, or fish seasoned as in recipe; shellfish cooked with no added salt	Regular canned or smoked meat, poultry, or fish; bacon, luncheon meats, ham, chipped or corned beef, frankfurters, salt pork, sausage, meats koshered by salting
Group B 25 mg Na/oz Used in moderation	Unsalted cottage cheese (¼ cup), low-sodium peanut butter (2 tbsp), fresh meat, fish, poultry, low-sodium canned meat, fish, poultry, low-sodium cheese	Regular cheese, regular peanut butter
Eggs 60 mg Na (1 daily)	Fresh or whole egg substitutes	Frozen with salt, pickled
Fat 50 mg Na/serving (5 servings daily)	Butter or margarine (1 tbsp), cream, half & half, mayonnaise. The following may be used in moderation: butter or margarine, cooking oil or fat, salt-free nuts, low-sodium salad dressings, oil or fat, unsalted	Bacon, bacon fat, salt pork, salted nuts, party spreads and dips, regular salad dressings (2 tsp)
Beverage Negligible amount of Na (as desired)	Coffee, tea, coffee substitutes, soft drinks	Limited use of carbonated beverages to that amount equal to 50 mg Na
Dessert Group A Negligible amount of Na (as desired)	Low-sodium pudding and gelatin fruit ices	All others

Continued

TABLE A-7
2000-mg Sodium Diet (Sodium-Restricted)—cont'd

Food Groups	Foods Allowed	Foods Restricted
Group B 50 mg Na/serving (2 servings)	Cookies, plain (1), ice cream, sherbet, flavored gelatin (½ cup); pound cake (1 slice); vanilla wafers (5)	All others
Group C 150 mg Na/serving (not more than 1 serving daily)	Angel food cake, plain cake with frosting; custard and pudding (½ cup)	Pies, pastries, any desserts containing salted nuts
Soup 40 mg Na/1 cup	Homemade cream or meat broth soups made without salt or low-sodium canned soups. If cream soup is served, count sodium value of milk used in recipe. Use only vegetables listed in Group A	Regular canned soup, stews, or bouillon cubes, liquid or powder
Miscellaneous Neglible amount of Na (as desired)	Jelly, jam, unflavored gelatin, lemon, lime, vinegar, cream or tartar, yeast, chocolate, cocoa, low-sodium candy, nonsalt herbs and spices, low-sodium catsup, low-sodium mustard	Catsup, chili sauce, cooking wine, celery salt, garlic salt, onion salt, pickle relish, prepared mustard, soy sauce, meat sauces, meat tenderizers, monosodium glutamate, barbecue sauce, Worcestershire sauce, Dutch processed cocoa

From *Pediatric diet manual,* Marriott Health Care Services, 1995. Reprinted with permission.

TABLE A-8
3000- to 4000-mg Sodium Diet (No Added Salt)

Food Groups	Foods Allowed	Foods Restricted
Milk	All	None
Vegetable	All except those restricted; low-sodium tomato juice and low-sodium mixed vegetable juice	Regular tomato juice, mixed vegetable juice, pickles, sauerkraut, and others prepared in brine
Bread/starch	All except those restricted	Bread, crackers, and rolls with salted tops; salted potato chips, corn chips, or any other salted chips, salted pretzels, salted popcorn
Fruit	All except those restricted	Olives
Meat, poultry, fish, eggs, and cheese	All meats and poultry except those restricted Bacon, limit to two strips (70 mg) Any fish except those restricted Cottage cheese, cream cheese, natural cheeses such as cheddar or Swiss All regular peanut butter	Cured and smoked: luncheon meats, ham, chipped or corned beef, frankfurters, salt pork, sausage; meats koshered by salting; sardines, salty or smoked fish, anchovies, caviar, salted herring; processed cheese or cheese spreads; Roquefort, Camembert, or Gorgonzola cheese
Eggs	All	None
Fat	All	None
Beverage	All	None
Dessert	Any except those containing restricted items	Salted nuts
Soup	Homemade cream or meat broth soups, made with allowed ingredients, low-sodium canned soups	Regular canned soups, stews, or bouillon cubes, liquid or powder
Miscellaneous	All except those made with salt	Salt, catsup, chili sauce, cooking wine, celery salt, garlic salt, relishes, barbecue sauces, meat sauces, meat tenderizers, soy sauce, Worcestershire sauce

From *Pediatric diet manual,* Marriott Health Care Services, 1995. Reprinted with permission.

TABLE A-9
Fat-Controlled Diets

Meat, poultry, fish, and shellfish	Age	Recommended oz/day	
		Step 1	Step 2
	2–3	2	2
	4–6	5	5
	7–18	6	6
	Step 2 diet allows only the leanest cuts of meat, fish, and poultry.		

Choose	Decrease

Lean cuts of meat with fat trimmed such as:
  Beef—round, sirloin, chuck, loin
  Lam—leg, arm, loin, rib
  Pork—tenderloin, leg, shoulder (arm or picnic)
  Veal—all trimmed cuts except ground
Poultry without skin
Fish and shellfish
Luncheon meat such as turkey ham, turkey, lean ham, lean roast beef, or chicken hot dogs
	Fatty cuts of meat such as:
	  Beef—regular ground, short ribs, corned beef brisket
	  Pork—spareribs, blade roll
	  Bacon, sausage
	  Organ meats such as liver, kidney, sweetbread, brain
	Poultry with skin, fried chicken
	Fried fish and shellfish
	Regular luncheon meat such as bologna, salami, sausage, and beef or pork hot dogs

Eggs	Age	Recommended Servings/wk	
		Step 1	Step 2
	2–6	3	2
	7–18	3	1

Choose	Decrease
Eggs whites (two whites equal one whole egg in recipes) Cholesterol-free egg substitutes	Eggs yolks beyond suggested number of servings per week (includes egg used in cooking)

Breads, cereals, pasta, rice, dry peas and beans	Age	Recommended servings/day	
		Step 1	Step 2
	2–3	5	5
	4–6	6	6
	7–10	7	7
	11–14		
	Boys	9	9
	Girls	8	8
	15–18		
	Boys	12	12
	Girls	8	8

Choose	Decrease
Bread (1 slice)—whole grain bread; hamburger and hot dog bun (½); corn tortilla (1) Cereal (1 cup ready-to-eat, ⅓ cup bran or ½ cup cooked)—oat, wheat, corn, multigrain Pasta (½ cup cooked) such as plain noodles, spaghetti, macaroni Rice (½ cup cooked) Low-fat crackers—animal crackers (8); Graham (3); saltine-type (6); low-fat snack chips (15); thin pretzels (7); low-fat popcorn (3½ cups)	Bread in which eggs are a major ingredient; croissants, flour tortilla, taco shell, taco chips Granola-type cereals Egg noodles and pasta containing egg yolk Pasta and rice prepared with cream, butter, or cheese sauces High-fat crackers such as cheese crackers, butter crackers, those made with saturated fats; potato and corn chips; popcorn made with oil or butter sauce

Continued

TABLE A-9
Fat-Controlled Diets—cont'd

Choose	Decrease
Homemade baked goods using unsaturated oil, skim or 1% milk, and egg substitutes—quick bread (1 slice); 2-in biscuit (1); cornbread muffin (1); bran muffin (1); 4-in pancake (1); 9-in diameter waffle (¼)	Commercial baked pastries, muffins, biscuits, dough-nuts, sweet rolls, Danish pastry using saturated fats
Dry peas and beans (½ cup cooked), such as split peas, black-eyed peas, chick peas, kidney beans, navy beans, lentils, soybeans, soybean curd (tofu)	Dry peas and beans prepared with butter, cheese, or cream sauce

		Recommended servings/day	
Dairy products	Age	Step 1	Step 2
	2–6	3	3
	7–18	4	4
	Step 2 diet allows only milk and yogurt with 1% milk fat or less and cheeses with not more than 2 g of fat per oz.		

Choose	Decrease
Milk (1 cup)—skim milk, 1% milk (fluid, powdered, evaporated); buttermilk	Whole milk (fluid, evaporated, condensed); 2% low-fat milk; imitation milk
Yogurt (1 cup)—nonfat or low-fat yogurt; yogurt beverages	Whole-milk yogurt; custard-style yogurt; whole milk yogurt beverages
Cottage cheese (½ cup)—low-fat, nonfat, or dry curd (0 to 2% fat)	Cottage cheese (4% fat)
Cheese (1 oz)—low-fat cheeses labeled no more than 6 g of fat per oz on step 1 (no more than 2 g of fat per oz on step 2	High-fat cheese such as American, bleu, brie, cheddar, colby, edam, monterey jack, parmesan, Swiss, Neufchatel
Frozen dairy dessert (½ cup)—ice milk, frozen yogurt (low-fat and nonfat)	Cream cheese, ice cream
Nonfat creamers, nonfat whipped toppings, and non-fat sour cream substitutes	Cream, half & half, whipping cream, nondairy creamer, whipped topping, sour cream

		Recommended servings/day	
Vegetables	Age	Step 1	Step 2
	2–10	3	3
	11–18		
	Boys	4	4
	Girls	3	3

Choose	Decrease
Vegetables (½ cup)—fresh, frozen, or canned	Vegetables prepared with butter, cheese, or cream sauce

		Recommended servings/day	
Fruits	Age	Step 1	Step 2
	2–3	2	2
	4–6	3	3
	7–10	3	4
	11–14	3	3
	15–18		
	Boys	5	5
	Girls	3	3

Choose	Decrease
Fruit (½ cup or medium-size piece)—fresh, frozen, canned, or dried	Fried fruit or fruit served with butter or cream sauce
Fruit juice (½ cup)—fresh, frozen, or canned	

Continued

TABLE A-9
Fat-Controlled Diets—cont'd

Sweets and snacks		Recommended serving/day	
	Age	Step 1	Step 2
	2–3	1	1
	4–10	2	2
	11–18		
	Boys	4	4
	Girls	3	3

Choose	Decrease
Beverages (6 fluid oz)—fruit-flavored drinks; lemonade, fruit punch	
Sweets (1½ tbsp)—sugar, syrup, honey, jam, preserves; candy (¾ oz) made primary with sugar (candy corn, gum drops, hard candy); fruit-flavored gelatin (½ cup)	Candy made with chocolate, butter, cream, coconut oil, palm oil, palm kernel oil
Low-fat frozen desserts (⅓ cup)—sherbet, sorbet, fruit ice, popsicles, low-fat frozen yogurt	Ice cream and frozen treats made with cream and whole milk
Cookies (2), cake (1 slice), pie (1 slice), pudding (½ cup)—all prepared with egg whites, egg substitute, skim milk, or 1% milk, and unsaturated oil or margarine; gingersnaps (2); fig bar cookies (1); angel food cake	Commercial baked high-fat cookies, cakes, cream pies, doughnuts

Fats and oils		Recommended servings/day	
	Age	Step 1	Step 2
	2–3	4	5
	4–6	5	6
	7–10	5	7
	11–14		
	Boys	7	9
	Girls	5	8
	15–18		
	Boys	10	12
	Girls	5	8

Step 2 diet allows tub margarines and oils very low in saturated fats. In order to keep total calories from fat at approximately 30%, while reducing saturated fats, step 2 diet allows more servings of unsaturated fats.

Choose	Decrease
Unsaturated oils (1 tsp)—corn, olive, peanut, rapeseed (canola oil), safflower, sesame, soybean	Coconut oil, palm kernel oil, palm oil
Margarine (1 tsp)—made from unsaturated oils listed above; light or diet margarine (2 tsp)	Butter, lard, bacon fat, shortening
Salad dressings (tbsp)—dressings made with unsaturated oils listed above; low-fat or oil-free dressings (serving size depends on amount of oil)	Dressing made with egg yolk, cheese, sour cream, whole milk
Seeds and nuts (1 tbsp)—peanut butter, other nut butters	Coconut
Cocoa powder (as desired), olives (5 small), avocado (⅛ of whole)	Chocolate

From *Pediatric diet manual,* Marriott Health Care Services, 1995. Reprinted with permission.

TABLE A-10
Recommended Serving Sizes for Children 1 to 18 Years of Age

	Milk and Milk Products	Meat	Breads and Cereals	Fruits	Vegetables
Servings per day	3–4	2–3	4–6	2–4	3–5
Ages 1–3 yrs	½–¾ cup milk (skim milk not recommended before 2 years of age)	1.5–2 oz meat, fish, or poultry	½–1 slice bread; ¼–⅓ cup rice or pasta; ¼–⅓ cup cooked cereal; ⅓–½ cup dry cereal	¼ cup juice or canned fruit; 3–4 slices fresh fruit without skins	⅛–¼ cup cooked vegetables
Ages 4–6 yrs	¾ cup milk	2 oz meat, fish, or poultry	1 slice bread; ½ cup rice or pasta; ½ cup cooked cereal; ⅓–½ cup dry cereal	½ cup juice or canned fruit; 1 small piece fresh fruit	¼ cup cooked vegetables; ½ cup raw vegetables
Ages 7–10 yrs	¾ cup milk	2 oz meat, fish, or poultry	1 slice bread; ½ cup rice or pasta; ½ cup cooked cereal; ¾ cup dry cereal	½ cup juice or canned fruit; 1 small piece fresh fruit	½ cup cooked vegetables; 1 cup raw vegetables
Ages 11–18 yrs	1 cup milk	2–2½ oz meat, fish, or poultry	1 slice bread; ½ cup rice or pasta; ½ cup cooked cereal; 1 cup dry cereal	½ cup juice or canned fruit; 1 average piece fresh fruit	½ cup cooked vegetables; 1 cup raw vegetables
		Meat equivalent (1 oz) = 1 egg; 1 oz cheese; ¼ cup cottage cheese; ½ cup dried peas or beans; 1 tbsp peanut butter	Include whole grains to increase fiber	Include a good source of vitamin A and C daily	Include a good source of vitamin A and C daily

mg/day; the recommendation for total fat in the diet is unchanged. Table A-9 provides a listing of foods to choose and decrease in the diet to achieve the step 1 and step 2 diets for the child with documented risk of CVD.

The National Cholesterol Education Program has recommended the prudent diet for all healthy children and adolescents over the age of 2 years. Although overzealous application of low-fat diets may lead to inadequate calorie intake resulting in poor weight gain and growth, the prudent diet is not intended to be a low-calorie diet and should not result in any significant nutrient deficiencies.

Dietary intake studies show the typical Ameri-can diet is approximately 38% fat. Concurrently, studies show the incidence of obesity in children to be 25% to 27% and in adolescents to be 15% to 21%, reflecting an increase of 40% to 55% over the past 20 years. The use of very low–calorie diets in children is still controversial and gener-ally not recommended except in carefully super-vised settings. Instead, the first line of approach in weight control for children is the achievement of weight maintenance, allowing the child to "grow into" his/her weight without compromis-ing linear growth. The prudent diet, using age-appropriate portions, may be used to provide the overweight child with an appropriate diet to slow the rate of weight gain. Table A-10 provides

TABLE A-11
Milk Protein–Free Diet

MILK PROTEIN–FREE DIET

This food allergy list is intended to be used as a general guideline and is not all-inclusive. Read food labels for any ingredients that may be contraindicated.

AVOID THE FOLLOWING FOODS AND FOOD ADDITIVES:

Artificial butter flavor
Butter, butter fat, buttermilk
Casinates (ammonium, calcium, magnesium, potassium, sodium)
Cheese
Cottage cheese
Cream cheese
Cream soup/chowder
Cream
Curds
Custard
Foods with the following description: ice cream, au gratin, escalloped, creamed
Half & half
Hot cocoa
Hydrolysates (casein, milk protein, protein, whey, whey protein)
Junket
Lactalbumin, lactalbumin phosphate
Lactoglobulin
Lactose
Milk (condensed, derivative, dry, evaporated, low-fat, malted, nonfat, powdered, protein, skim, solids, whole)
Meats (containing milk solids mixes—weiners)
Mixes
Nougat
Pudding
Rennet casein
Sauces (check for milk)
Sherbet (check for milk)
Simplesse
Sour milk solids
Sour cream, sour cream solids
Whey (delactosed, demineralized, protein concentrate)
Yogurt
Zweiback
Common infant formulas containing milk protein include: Enfamil, Lactofree, Next Step (manufactured by Mead Johnson); Gerber Baby Formula (manufactured by Gerber); Follow-up Formula, Good Start* (manufactured by Carnation); Similac, Similac PM 60/40 (manufactured by Ross); SMA (manufactured by Wyeth).

Continued

TABLE A-11
Milk Protein–Free Diet–cont'd

ADDITIVES THAT MAY INDICATE THE PRESENCE OF MILK PROTEIN:

Brown sugar flavoring
Caramel flavoring
Chocolate
High-protein flour
Margarine
Natural flavoring

NOTE: A "D" on a product label next to a "K" or circled "U" may indicate the presence of milk protein.
Casein hydrolysates found in hypoallergenic infant formulas are allowed, *ie,* Nutramigen (Mead Johnson), Alimentum (Ross).
*Carnation Good Start contains hydrolyzed whey and may be less allergenic than other milk-based infant formulas.
From *Pediatric diet manual,* Marriott Health Care Services, 1995. Reprinted with permission.

information on appropriate portion sizes for children based on age.

Because obesity is a multifactorial disease that includes multiple psychosocial factors, the most effective treatment approaches are similarly multifactorial. Diet is only one component of an effective weight-management program, which also includes exercise and behavior modification.

FOOD ALLERGY DIETS

Diets eliminating one or more types of foods are indicated for children who experience adverse gastrointestinal, respiratory, skin, or cardiovascular reactions following their consumption. Common allergens for infants include cow's milk protein, soy protein, fish, egg, and wheat. Most infants outgrow cow's milk allergy by 3 to 4 years of age. Common allergens for older children include peanuts, tree nuts, chocolate, shellfish, citrus, and other grains such as corn and oats.

Food allergies and intolerances present a significant challenge to providing a balanced, nutritious diet to children. Because these diets necessarily eliminate certain foods and food types, nutrient deficiencies may result, and careful planning is required to ensure adequate intake. Supplementation, especially of calcium for children with milk protein allergy, may be indicated.

Tables A-11 through A-16 provide lists of foods and food additives to be avoided for children with food allergies based on their specific needs. Because food manufacturers change ingredients frequently based on availability, price, and consumer preference for certain ingredients, parents must be taught to carefully read all food labels. Table A-17 lists additional resources for parents and professionals seeking information on managing food allergies and manufacturers who can provide information on ingredients used in their food products.

TABLE A-12
Soy Protein–Free Diet

SOY PROTEIN–FREE DIET

This food allergy list is intended to be used as a general guideline and is not all-inclusive. Read food labels for any ingredients that may be contraindicated.

AVOID THE FOLLOWING FOODS AND FOOD ADDITIVES:

Hydrolyzed Veg protein (HVP)
Miso
Shoyu sauce
Soy (flour, grits, milk, nuts, sprouts)
Soybean (curd, granules)
Soy protein (concentrate, isolate)
Soy sauce
Tamari
Tempeh
Teriyaki sauce
Textured vegetable protein (TVP)
Tofu
Common infant formulas containing soy protein include: Gerber Soy Formula (manufactured by Gerber); Isomil (manufactured by Ross); Nursoy (manufactured by Wyeth); Prosobee (manufactured by Mead Johnson); I-Soyalac and Soyalac (manufactured by Mt. Vernon Foods, Inc.); Next-Step Soy (manufactured by Mead Johnson).

ADDITIVES THAT MAY INDICATE THE PRESENCE OF SOY PROTEIN:

Flavorings	Vegetable starch
Hydrolyzed plant protein	Vegetable gum
Hydrolyzed soy protein	Vegetable broth
Natural flavoring	

NOTE: Soybean oil and soy lecithin are fats and are generally safe for most soy-allergic children to eat.
From *Pediatric diet manual,* Marriott Health Care Services, 1995. Reprinted with permission.

TABLE A-13
Wheat-Free Diet

WHEAT-FREE DIET

This food allergy list is intended to be used as a general guideline and is not all-inclusive. Read food labels for any ingredients that may be contraindicated.

AVOID THE FOLLOWING FOODS AND FOOD ADDITIVES:

Bagels
Batter/breaded foods
Biscuits
Bread
Bread crumbs
Bran
Cake and cake mix
Cereal extract
Cookies and cookie mix
Cornbread
Crackers
Cracked wheat
Cracked meal
Cream of wheat
Enriched flour
Farina
Gluten
Graham crackers
Graham flour
Gravy
High-gluten flour
High-protein flour
Muffins and muffin mix
Pasta (noodles)
Pie crust
Pizza crust
Vital gluten
Waffles
Wheat bran
Wheat germ
Wheat gluten
Wheat starch
Whole wheat flour

ADDITIVES THAT MAY INDICATE THE PRESENCE OF WHEAT PROTEIN:

Gelatinized starch
Hydrolyzed vegetable protein (HVP)
Modified food starch
Modified starch
Natural flavoring
Soy sauce
Starch
Textured vegetable protein
Vegetable gum
Vegetable starch

From *Pediatric diet manual,* Marriott Health Care Services, 1995. Reprinted with permission.

TABLE A-14
Egg-Free Diet

Egg-free diet

This food allergy list is intended to be used as a general guideline and is not all-inclusive. Read food labels for any ingredients that may be contraindicated.

Avoid the following foods and food additives:

Angel cake
Albumin
Challah (a Jewish bread)
Cookies
Crepes
Custard
Eggs (dried, hard boiled, powdered, solids, white)
Egg substitutes
Egg bagels
Egg noodles
Egg rolls
Eggnog
French toast
French vanilla (flavored)
Globulin
Hollandaise sauce
Ice cream
Low-cholesterol eggs (eg, Egg Beaters)
Lysozyme
Mayonnaise
Meringue
Omelettes
Ovalbumin
Ovomucin
Ovomucoid
Ovovitellin
Popovers
Simplesse (fat substitute)
Souffle
Tartar sauce

Additives that MAY indicate the presence of egg:

(Question or avoid foods whose ingredients are uncertain.)
Cakes
Casseroles
Chinese, Thai, and other ethnic dishes (including soups cleared with egg)
Cooked puddings, custards
Cocomalt
Corn bread
Cream candies
Cream pie
Foods breaded or coated (eg, fried or baked fish, meat, poultry, vegetables)
Fried rice
Malted drinks
Meatloaf
Muffins

Continued

TABLE A-14
Egg-Free Diet–cont'd

Additives that MAY indicate the presence of egg:

Pancakes
Pastries
Potato salad
Pudding
Quick breads
Sherbet
Waffles

From *Pediatric diet manual,* Marriott Health Care Services, 1995. Reprinted with permission.

TABLE A-15
Tree Nut–Free Diet

Tree nut–free diet

This food allergy list is intended to be used as a general guideline and is not all-inclusive. Read food labels for any ingredients that may be contraindicated.

Avoid the following foods and food additives:

Almond extract
Almond paste
Almonds
Brazil nuts
Cashews
Chestnuts
Filberts
Gianduja (a creamy mixture of chocolate and chopped toasted nuts found in premium or imported chocolate)
Hazel nuts
Hickory nuts
Macadamia nuts
Marzipan
Nougat
Nu-Nuts artificial nuts (flavored peanuts)
Nut butters
Nut oil
Nut paste
Nuts
Pecans
Pine nuts
Pinyon nuts
Pistachios
Walnuts
Wintergreen extract

NOTE: Imitation or artificial flavorings or extracts may be used if not made with additives listed above.

From *Pediatric diet manual,* Marriott Health Care Services, 1995. Reprinted with permission.

TABLE A-16
Peanut Protein–Free Diet

PEANUT PROTEIN–FREE DIET
This food allergy list is intended to be used as a general guideline and is not all-inclusive. Read food labels for any ingredients that may be contraindicated.

AVOID THE FOLLOWING FOODS AND FOOD ADDITIVES:
Cold pressed peanut oil Ground nuts Mixed nuts Nu-Nuts artificial nuts, (flavored peanuts) Peanuts Peanut butter Peanut flour

ADDITIVES THAT MAY INDICATE THE PRESENCE OF PEANUT PROTEIN:
(Question or avoid foods whose ingredients are uncertain.) African, Chinese, Thai, and other ethnic dishes Baked goods (pastries, cookies, etc.) Candy Chili Chocolate (candy, candy bars) Egg rolls Hydrolyzed plant protein Hydrolyzed vegetable protein Ice cream (homemade) and ice cream toppings containing nuts Marzipan Nougat

NOTE: Peanut oil is a fat and generally considered safe for most peanut-allergic children to eat (avoid cold pressed peanut oil).

From *Pediatric diet manual,* Marriott Health Care Services, 1995. Reprinted with permission.

TABLE A-17
Additional Resources for Food Allergies

For general information:
American Dietetic Association
National Center for Nutrition and Dietetics
216 West Jackson Boulevard
Chicago, Illinois 60606-6995
1-800-977-1600, ext. 4854

The Food Allergy Network
4744 Holly Avenue
Fairfax, Virginia 22030-5647
1-800-929-4040

US Department of Agriculture
Human Nutrition Information Service
6505 Belcrest Road
Hyattsville, Maryland 20782
1-301-436-5724

For production information:
Gerber Products
Consumer Relations
445 State Street
Fremont, Michigan 49413
1-800-4-GERBER

Hershey Foods Corporation
Consumer Relations
100 Crystal A Drive
Hershey, Pennsylvania 17033-0815
1-800-468-1714

Kraft General Foods Consumer Center
250 North Street
White Plains, New York 10625
1-800-431-1003

Kellogs
Consumer Affairs Division
PO Box CAMB
Battle Creek, Michigan 49016-3447
1-800-962-1413

Nabisco Foods Group
Consumer Information Services
PO Box 1911
East Hanover, New Jersey 07936-1911
1-800-932-7800

Nestle Food Company
Consumer Affairs
800 North Brand Boulevard
Glendale, California 91203
1-800-637-8537

The Pillsbury Company
Consumer Relations
Box 550
Minneapolis, Minnesota 55440-0550
1-800-767-4466

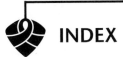

INDEX

Note that page numbers in italic indicate figures; those followed by "t" indicate tables.

A

ABCD evaluation, 766
Abdomen
  acute. *See* Abdominal pain, acute
  palpation of, 402
  protuberant, 190, 265
  surgical, 188, 189
Abdominal distention, 191, 213, 398, 402
Abdominal epilepsy, 192
Abdominal examination, 186
Abdominal gas, 43, 44, 61
Abdominal mass(es), 40, 177-181, 400, 428-430
Abdominal migraine, 192
Abdominal pain
  acute, 181-189, *184, 188,* 429, 685
  in adolescents, 102
  chronic, 190-194, 455
  colicky, 182, 183, 185
  in cystic fibrosis, 751
  with diarrhea, 228
  in newborn, 43, 61
  NSAIDs and, 761
  rectal exam in, 186, 191, 193
  recurrent, 190
  in sickle cell disease, 624
  with vomiting, 398-402
Abdominal peristalsis, 399, 402
Abdominal trauma, 182
  child abuse and, 178, 182, 186, 187, 482
Abdominal tumors, 178, 609, 610t
Abdominal ultrasound, 74, *179*-181, 194
Abdominal wall lesions, 428-430
ABO incompatibility, 293, 593
Abrasions, 772, 773, 752
Abscess(es). *See also* Cyst(s)
  appendiceal, 183
  Bartholin gland, 682
  brain, 271
  breast, 428
  dental, 271, 273
  felon, 801, *802*
  in liver, 302
  lymph node, 799
  paronychia, *803*
  perianal, 430, 799-800
  peritonsillar, 726
  pulmonary, 280, 661
  secondary, 800
Abscess cavity, packing of, 799, 801
Abscess drainage, 797-803, *798, 802, 803*
  contraindications to, 799
Absence seizures, 702
Abstract thinkers, 992
Abuse. *See also* Alcohol abuse; Child abuse; Drug abuse; Sexual abuse
  physical. *See* Physical abuse
  spousal, 978
Academic performance, maturation and, 114
Acanthosis nigricans, 538
Accident(s), prevention of, 151-157, 156t
Accidental death, 135
Accidental hypothermia, 795
Accidental pregnancy, 121, 121t
Acetaminophen, 421, 449, 452t-454, 759
Acetylcholinesterase, amniotic, 810

Acetylcysteine, in cystic fibrosis, 748, 751
Acetylsalicylic acid, side effects of, 761t
Achenbach Child Behavior Checklist, 869, 870
Achievement tests, 865, 866t
Achilles tendonitis, 791
Acholic stools, 295, 306
Achondroplasia, 321
Acid burn of eye, 773
Acidosis, 795, 560
Acne, 518, 519t
Acoustic neuroma, 243
Acquired immunodeficiency syndrome. *See* AIDS
Acrodynia, 314
ACTH stimulation test, 537, 539
Acute abdomen. *See* Abdominal pain, acute
Acute chest syndrome, 624
Acyclovir, 420, 448, 511, 615, 644, 690, 982
Addison disease, 537
Adenoidectomy, 726
Adenomas, 117, 118, 197, 198, 302
Adenosine, 391
Adenovirus(es), enteric, 228
Adenovirus infection, 217, 687
  in mesenteric lymphadenitis, 183
Adipocyte proliferation, 143
Adipose tissue, development of, 142-143
Adjusted age, 71, 80
Adnexal mass, 185, 186, 685
Adolescence, phases of, 112-113
Adolescent(s)
  behavioral change in, 992-994
  blind, 853
  blood pressure of, 106
  breast exam of, *107*
  "cognitive aha" experience of, 992
  communicating with, 989-994
  concrete vs. abstract thinking by, 992
  confidentiality and, 989
  in crisis, 990, 994
  depression in, 990, 992
  developmental tasks of, 6t, 7, 112-114
  dieting of, 148, 150
  effect of divorce on, 168
  family and social history of, 105, 990, 991
  fantasies of, 992
  growth and development of, 104, 106
  gynecomastia in, 203
  HIV infection in, 629-637, 989
  home issues of, 990
  hypersomnia in, 96, 99
  immunizations for, 102, *103,* 104
  interview of, 101, 102, 989-994
  laboratory tests for, 108-111
  legal issues and, 101, 989
  menstrual history of, 105
  mental health of, 990, 992
  myelomeningocele in, 820
  nutritional history of, 104
  obese, 143, 147, 148, 150
  peer pressures and, 990-993
  pelvic exam of, 108
  physical exam of, 105-110, *106-110*
  pregnancy in, 136, 992
  psychosocial concerns of, 112-114
  psychosocial screening of, 989-992
  refusal skills of, 993

Adolescent(s)—*cont'd*
  relationship to parents, 989, 990, 993
  risk behaviors in, 990, 992
  routine examination of, 101-111
  safety of, 990
  school issues of, 990
  scoliosis screening of, 106, *109, 110*
  sexual abuse of, 991
  sexual history of, 104, 120, 991
  substance abuse by, 104, 991
  suicidal ideation in, 990, 992
  violence and, 991-993
Adoption, in Down syndrome, 966
Adrenal crisis, 537
Adrenal failure, 536
Adrenal hyperfunction, and anovulation, 117
Adrenal hyperplasia, 538, 541
Adrenal insufficiency, 536-538, 400
Adrenarche, 116, 539
Adrenocorticotropic hormone stimulation test, 537, 539
Adult respiratory distress syndrome, 661
Adverse drug reactions, 741-742
Aerosol therapy, 748
Agammaglobulinemia, 678, 679
Age
  cognitive, 869
  corrected, 71, 80
  gestational, 38
Agenda, 14, 15t, 27
Aggressive conduct disorder, 90
Aggressiveness, in toddler, 89
AIDS. *See* HIV infection
AIDS indicator illness, 633
Airbags, 155
Airway, artificial, 284
Airway collapse, 218
Airway inflammation, 733
Airway obstruction, 217, 726
  in cleft deformity, 834, 835
  in cystic fibrosis, 747, *748,* 749
  and enuresis, 254
  by foreign body, 217, 726
  sleep-associated, 99
Alagille syndrome, 293
Alanine aminotransferase (ALT), 305, 306
Alarms, enuresis, 254-257
Albuterol, 734, 734t
Alcohol abuse, 104, 265, 136, 926-932
Alcohol bath, 421
Alcohol use, by teens, 991
Aldosteronism, 538
Alkali burn of eye, 773
Alkali denaturation test, 347
Alkylating agents, 616
Allergens, 731, 736, 1011-1012
Allergic bronchopulmonary aspergillosis, 735, 749
Allergic conjunctivitis, 361, 364, 731, 736-737
Allergic contact dermatitis, 515
Allergic disorders, 731, 736-742. *See also* specific types
Allergic hives, 512-513
Allergic pneumonitis, 761
Allergic reactions, and edema, 250, 252
Allergic rhinitis/conjunctivitis, 731, 736-737
Allergic "shiners," 731, 736
Allergy(ies)
  and abdominal pain, 190